Lecture Notes in Computer Science 9351

More information about this series at http://www.springer.com/series/7412

Nassir Navab · Joachim Hornegger
William M. Wells · Alejandro F. Frangi (Eds.)

Medical Image Computing and Computer-Assisted Intervention – MICCAI 2015

18th International Conference
Munich, Germany, October 5–9, 2015
Proceedings, Part III

Springer

Editors
Nassir Navab
Technische Universität München
Garching
Germany

William M. Wells
Brigham and Women's Hospital
Harvard Medical School
Boston
USA

Joachim Hornegger
Friedrich-Alexander-Universität
Erlangen-Nürnberg
Erlangen
Germany

Alejandro F. Frangi
University of Sheffield
Sheffield
UK

ISSN 0302-9743 ISSN 1611-3349 (electronic)
Lecture Notes in Computer Science
ISBN 978-3-319-24573-7 ISBN 978-3-319-24574-4 (eBook)
DOI 10.1007/978-3-319-24574-4

Library of Congress Control Number: 2015949456

LNCS Sublibrary: SL 6 – Image Processing, Computer Vision, Pattern Recognition, and Graphics

Springer Cham Heidelberg New York Dordrecht London

Printed on acid-free paper

Springer International Publishing AG Switzerland is part of Springer Science+Business Media
(www.springer.com)

Preface

In 2015, the 18th International Conference on Medical Image Computing and Computer-Assisted Intervention (MICCAI 2015) was held in Munich, Germany. It was organized by the Technical University Munich (TUM) and the Friedrich Alexander University Erlangen-Nuremberg (FAU). The meeting took place in the Philharmonic Hall "Gasteig" during October 6-8, one week after the world-famous Oktoberfest. Satellite events associated with MICCAI 2015 took place on October 5 and October 9 in the Holiday Inn Hotel Munich City Centre and Klinikum rechts der Isar. MICCAI 2015 and its satellite events attracted word-leading scientists, engineers, and clinicians, who presented high-standard papers, aiming at uniting the fields of medical image processing, medical image formation, and medical robotics.

This year the triple anonymous review process was organized in several phases. In total, 810 valid submissions were received. The review process was handled by one primary and two secondary Program Committee members for each paper. It was initiated by the primary Program Committee member, who assigned a minimum of three expert reviewers. Based on these initial reviews, 79 papers were directly accepted and 248 papers were rejected. The remaining papers went to the rebuttal phase, in which the authors had the chance to respond to the concerns raised by reviewers. The reviews and associated rebuttals were subsequently discussed in the next phase among the reviewers leading to the acceptance of another 85 papers and the rejection of 118 papers. Subsequently, secondary Program Committee members issued a recommendation for each paper by weighing both the reviewers' recommendations and the authors' rebuttals. This resulted in "accept" for 67 papers and in "reject" for 120 papers. The remaining 92 papers were discussed at a Program Committee meeting in Garching, Germany, in May 2015, where 36 out of 75 Program Committee members were present. During two days, the 92 papers were examined by experts in the respective fields resulting in another 32 papers being accepted. In total 263 papers of the 810 submitted papers were accepted which corresponds to an acceptance rate of 32.5%.

The frequency of primary and secondary keywords is almost identical in the submitted, the rejected, and the accepted paper pools. The top five keywords of all submissions were machine learning (8.3%), segmentation (7.1%), MRI (6.6%), and CAD (4.9%).

The correlation between the initial keyword counts by category and the accepted papers was 0.98. The correlation with the keyword distribution of the rejected papers was 0.99. The distributions of the intermediate accept and reject phases was also above 0.9 in all cases, i.e., there was a strong relationship between the submitted paper categories and the finally accepted categories. The keyword frequency was essentially not influenced by the review decisions. As a conclusion, we believe the review process was fair and the distribution of topics reflects no favor of any particular topic of the conference.

This year we offered all authors the opportunity of presenting their work in a five-minute talk. These talks were organized in 11 parallel sessions setting the stage for further scientific discussions during the poster sessions of the main single-track conference. Since we consider all of the accepted papers as excellent, the selection of long oral presentations representing different fields in a single track was extremely challenging. Therefore, we decided to organize the papers in these proceedings in a different way than in the conference program. In contrast to the conference program, the proceedings do not differentiate between poster and oral presentations. The proceedings are only organized by conference topics. Only for the sake of the conference program did we decide on oral and poster presentations. In order to help us in the selection process, we asked the authors to submit five-minute short presentations. Based on the five-minute presentations and the recommendations of the reviewers and Program Committee members, we selected 36 papers for oral presentation. We hope these papers to be to some extent representative of the community covering the entire MICCAI spectrum. The difference in raw review score between the poster and oral presentations was not statistically significant ($p > 0.1$). In addition to the oral presentation selection process, all oral presenters were asked to submit their presentations two months prior to the conference for review by the Program Committee who checked the presentations thoroughly and made suggestions for improvement.

Another feature in the conference program is the industry panel that features leading members of the medical software and device companies who gave their opinions and presented their future research directions and their strategies for translating scientific observations and results of the MICCAI community into medical products.

We thank Aslı Okur, who did an excellent job in the preparation of the conference. She took part in every detail of the organization for more than one year. We would also like to thank Andreas Maier, who supported Joachim Hornegger in his editorial tasks following his election as president of the Friedrich Alexander University Erlangen-Nuremberg (FAU) in early 2015. Furthermore, we thank the local Organizing Committee for arranging the wonderful venue and the MICCAI Student Board for organizing the additional student events ranging from a tour to the BMW factory to trips to the world-famous castles of Neuschwanstein and Linderhof. The workshop, challenge, and tutorial chairs did an excellent job in enriching this year's program. In addition, we thank the MICCAI society for provision of support and insightful comments as well as the Program Committee for their support during the review process. Last but not least, we thank our sponsors for the financial support that made the conference possible.

We look forward to seeing you in Istanbul, Turkey in 2016!

October 2015

Nassir Navab
Joachim Hornegger
William M. Wells
Alejandro F. Frangi

Organization

General Chair

Nassir Navab	Technische Universität München, Germany

General Co-chair

Joachim Hornegger	Friedrich-Alexander-Universität Erlangen-Nürnberg, Germany

Program Chairs

Nassir Navab	Technische Universität München, Germany
Joachim Hornegger	Friedrich-Alexander-Universität Erlangen-Nürnberg, Germany
William M. Wells	Harvard Medical School, USA
Alejandro F. Frangi	University of Sheffield, Sheffield, UK

Local Organization Chairs

Ralf Stauder	Technische Universität München, Germany
Aslı Okur	Technische Universität München, Germany
Philipp Matthies	Technische Universität München, Germany
Tobias Zobel	Friedrich-Alexander-Universität Erlangen-Nürnberg, Germany

Publication Chair

Andreas Maier	Friedrich-Alexander-Universität Erlangen-Nürnberg, Germany

Sponsorship and Publicity Chairs

Stefanie Demirci	Technische Universität München, Germany
Su-Lin Lee	Imperial College London, UK

Workshop Chairs

Purang Abolmaesumi	University of British Columbia, Canada
Wolfgang Wein	ImFusion, Germany
Bertrand Thirion	Inria, France
Nicolas Padoy	Université de Strasbourg, France

Challenge Chairs

Björn Menze	Technische Universität München, Germany
Lena Maier-Hein	German Cancer Research Center, Germany
Bram van Ginneken	Radboud University, The Netherlands
Valeria De Luca	ETH Zurich, Switzerland

Tutorial Chairs

Tom Vercauteren	University College London, UK
Tobias Heimann	Siemens Corporate Technology, USA
Sonia Pujol	Harvard Medical School, USA
Carlos Alberola	University of Valladolid, Spain

MICCAI Society Board of Directors

Stephen Aylward	Kitware, Inc., NY, USA
Simon Duchesne	Université Laval, Quebéc, Canada
Gabor Fichtinger (Secretary)	Queen's University, Kingston, ON, Canada
Alejandro F. Frangi	University of Sheffield, Sheffield, UK
Polina Golland	MIT, Cambridge, MA, USA
Pierre Jannin	INSERM/INRIA, Rennes, France
Leo Joskowicz	The Hebrew University of Jerusalem
Wiro Niessen (Executive Director)	Erasmus MC - University Medical Centre, Rotterdam, The Netherlands
Nassir Navab	Technische Universität, München, Germany
Alison Noble (President)	University of Oxford, Oxford, UK
Sebastien Ourselin (Treasurer)	University College, London, UK
Xavier Pennec	INRIA, Sophia Antipolis, France
Josien Pluim	Eindhoven University of Technology, The Netherlands
Dinggang Shen	UNC, Chapel Hill, NC, USA
Li Shen	Indiana University, IN, USA

MICCAI Society Consultants to the Board

Alan Colchester	University of Kent, Canterbury, UK
Terry Peters	University of Western Ontario, London, ON, Canada
Richard Robb	Mayo Clinic College of Medicine, MN, USA

MICCAI Society Staff

Society Secretariat	Janette Wallace, Canada
Recording Secretary	Jackie Williams, Canada
Fellows Nomination Coordinator	Terry Peters, Canada

Program Committee

Acar, Burak
Barbu, Adrian
Ben Ayed, Ismail
Castellani, Umberto
Cattin, Philippe C.
Chung, Albert C.S.
Cootes, Tim
de Bruijne, Marleen
Delingette, Hervé
Fahrig, Rebecca
Falcão, Alexandre
Fichtinger, Gabor
Gerig, Guido
Gholipour, Ali
Glocker, Ben
Greenspan, Hayit
Hager, Gregory D.
Hamarneh, Ghassan
Handels, Heinz
Harders, Matthias
Heinrich, Mattias Paul
Huang, Junzhou
Ionasec, Razvan
Isgum, Ivana
Jannin, Pierre
Joshi, Sarang
Joskowicz, Leo
Kamen, Ali
Kobashi, Syoji
Langs, Georg
Li, Shuo
Linguraru, Marius George
Liu, Huafeng
Lu, Le
Madabhushi, Anant
Maier-Hein, Lena
Martel, Anne
Masamune, Ken
Moradi, Mehdi
Nielsen, Mads
Nielsen, Poul
Niethammer, Marc
Ourselin, Sebastien
Padoy, Nicolas
Papademetris, Xenios
Paragios, Nikos
Pernus, Franjo
Pohl, Kilian
Preim, Bernhard
Prince, Jerry
Radeva, Petia
Rohde, Gustavo
Sabuncu, Mert Rory
Sakuma, Ichiro

Salcudean, Tim
Salvado, Olivier
Sato, Yoshinobu
Schnabel, Julia A.
Shen, Li
Stoyanov, Danail
Studholme, Colin
Syeda-Mahmood, Tanveer
Taylor, Zeike
Unal, Gozde
Van Leemput, Koen
Wassermann, Demian
Weese, Jürgen
Wein, Wolfgang
Wu, Xiaodong
Yang, Guang Zhong
Yap, Pew-Thian
Yin, Zhaozheng
Yuan, Jing
Zheng, Guoyan
Zheng, Yefeng

Additional Reviewers

Abolmaesumi, Purang
Achterberg, Hakim
Acosta-Tamayo, Oscar
Aerts, Hugo
Afacan, Onur
Afsari, Bijan
Aganj, Iman
Ahad, Md. Atiqur Rahman
Ahmidi, Narges
Aichert, André
Akbari, Hamed
Akhondi-Asl, Alireza
Aksoy, Murat
Alam, Saadia
Alberola-López, Carlos
Aljabar, Paul
Allan, Maximilian
Allassonnieres, Stephanie
Antani, Sameer
Antony, Bhavna
Arbel, Tal
Auvray, Vincent
Awate, Suyash
Azzabou, Noura
Bagci, Ulas
Bai, Wenjia
Baka, Nora
Balocco, Simone
Bao, Siqi
Barmpoutis, Angelos
Bartoli, Adrien
Batmanghelich, Kayhan
Baust, Maximilian
Baxter, John
Bazin, Pierre-Louis
Berger, Marie-Odile
Bernal, Jorge
Bernard, Olivier
Bernardis, Elena
Bhatia, Kanwal
Bieth, Marie
Bilgic, Berkin
Birkfellner, Wolfgang
Blaschko, Matthew
Bloch, Isabelle
Boctor, Emad
Bogunovic, Hrvoje
Bouarfa, Loubna
Bouix, Sylvain
Bourgeat, Pierrick
Brady, Michael
Brost, Alexander
Buerger, Christian
Burgert, Oliver
Burschka, Darius
Caan, Matthan
Cahill, Nathan
Cai, Weidong
Carass, Aaron
Cardenes, Ruben

Cardoso, Manuel Jorge
Carmichael, Owen
Caruyer, Emmanuel
Cathier, Pascal
Cerrolaza, Juan
Cetin, Mustafa
Cetingul, Hasan Ertan
Chakravarty, M. Mallar
Chamberland, Maxime
Chapman, Brian E.
Chatelain, Pierre
Chen, Geng
Chen, Shuhang
Chen, Ting
Cheng, Jian
Cheng, Jun
Cheplygina, Veronika
Chicherova, Natalia
Chowdhury, Ananda
Christensen, Gary
Chui, Chee Kong
Cinar Akakin, Hatice
Cinquin, Philippe
Ciompi, Francesco
Clarkson, Matthew
Clarysse, Patrick
Cobzas, Dana
Colliot, Olivier
Commowick, Olivier
Compas, Colin
Corso, Jason
Criminisi, Antonio
Crum, William
Cuingnet, Remi
Daducci, Alessandro
Daga, Pankaj
Dalca, Adrian
Darkner, Sune
Davatzikos, Christos
Dawant, Benoit
Dehghan, Ehsan
Deligianni, Fani
Demirci, Stefanie
Depeursinge, Adrien
Dequidt, Jeremie
Descoteaux, Maxime
Deslauriers-Gauthier, Samuel
DiBella, Edward
Dijkstra, Jouke
Ding, Kai
Ding, Xiaowei
Dojat, Michel
Dong, Xiao
Dowling, Jason
Dowson, Nicholas
Du, Jia
Duchateau, Nicolas
Duchesne, Simon
Duncan, James S.
Dzyubachyk, Oleh
Eavani, Harini
Ebrahimi, Mehran
Ehrhardt, Jan
Eklund, Anders
El-Baz, Ayman
El-Zehiry, Noha
Ellis, Randy
Elson, Daniel
Erdt, Marius
Ernst, Floris
Eslami, Abouzar
Fallavollita, Pascal
Fang, Ruogu
Fenster, Aaron
Feragen, Aasa
Fick, Rutger
Figl, Michael
Fischer, Peter
Fishbaugh, James
Fletcher, P. Thomas
Florack, Luc
Fonov, Vladimir
Forestier, Germain
Fradkin, Maxim
Franz, Alfred
Freiman, Moti
Freysinger, Wolfgang
Fripp, Jurgen
Frisch, Benjamin
Fritscher, Karl

Fundana, Ketut
Gamarnik, Viktor
Gao, Fei
Gao, Mingchen
Gao, Yaozong
Gao, Yue
Gaonkar, Bilwaj
Garvin, Mona
Gaser, Christian
Gass, Tobias
Gatta, Carlo
Georgescu, Bogdan
Gerber, Samuel
Ghesu, Florin-Cristian
Giannarou, Stamatia
Gibaud, Bernard
Gibson, Eli
Gilles, Benjamin
Ginsburg, Shoshana
Girard, Gabriel
Giusti, Alessandro
Goh, Alvina
Goksel, Orcun
Goldberger, Jacob
Golland, Polina
Gooya, Ali
Grady, Leo
Gray, Katherine
Grbic, Sasa
Grisan, Enrico
Grova, Christophe
Gubern-Mérida, Albert
Guevara, Pamela
Guler, Riza Alp
Guo, Peifang B.
Gur, Yaniv
Gutman, Boris
Gómez, Pedro
Hacihaliloglu, Ilker
Haidegger, Tamas
Hajnal, Joseph
Hamamci, Andac
Hammers, Alexander
Han, Dongfeng
Hargreaves, Brian
Hastreiter, Peter
Hatt, Chuck
Hawkes, David
Hayasaka, Satoru
Haynor, David
He, Huiguang
He, Tiancheng
Heckel, Frank
Heckemann, Rolf
Heimann, Tobias
Heng, Pheng Ann
Hennersperger, Christoph
Holden, Matthew
Hong, Byung-Woo
Honnorat, Nicolas
Hoogendoorn, Corné
Hossain, Belayat
Hossain, Shahera
Howe, Robert
Hu, Yipeng
Huang, Heng
Huang, Xiaojie
Huang, Xiaolei
Hutter, Jana
Ibragimov, Bulat
Iglesias, Juan Eugenio
Igual, Laura
Iordachita, Iulian
Irving, Benjamin
Jackowski, Marcel
Jacob, Mathews
Jain, Ameet
Janoos, Firdaus
Janowczyk, Andrew
Jerman, Tim
Ji, Shuiwang
Ji, Songbai
Jiang, Hao
Jiang, Wenchao
Jiang, Xi
Jiao, Fangxiang
Jin, Yan
Jolly, Marie-Pierre
Jomier, Julien
Joshi, Anand

Joshi, Shantanu
Jung, Claudio
K.B., Jayanthi
Kabus, Sven
Kadoury, Samuel
Kahl, Fredrik
Kainmueller, Dagmar
Kainz, Bernhard
Kakadiaris, Ioannis
Kandemir, Melih
Kapoor, Ankur
Kapur, Tina
Katouzian, Amin
Kelm, Michael
Kerrien, Erwan
Kersten-Oertel, Marta
Khan, Ali
Khurd, Parmeshwar
Kiaii, Bob
Kikinis, Ron
Kim, Boklye
Kim, Edward
Kim, Minjeong
Kim, Sungmin
King, Andrew
Klein, Stefan
Klinder, Tobias
Kluckner, Stefan
Kobayahsi, Etsuko
Konukoglu, Ender
Kumar, Puneet
Kunz, Manuela
Köhler, Thomas
Ladikos, Alexander
Landman, Bennett
Lang, Andrew
Lapeer, Rudy
Larrabide, Ignacio
Lasser, Tobias
Lauze, Francois
Lay, Nathan
Le Reste, Pierre-Jean
Lee, Han Sang
Lee, Kangjoo
Lee, Su-Lin
Lefkimmiatis, Stamatis
Lefèvre, Julien
Lekadir, Karim
Lelieveldt, Boudewijn
Lenglet, Christophe
Lepore, Natasha
Lesage, David
Li, Gang
Li, Jiang
Li, Quanzheng
Li, Xiang
Li, Yang
Li, Yeqing
Liang, Liang
Liao, Hongen
Lin, Henry
Lindeman, Robert
Lindner, Claudia
Linte, Cristian
Litjens, Geert
Liu, Feng
Liu, Jiamin
Liu, Jian Fei
Liu, Jundong
Liu, Mingxia
Liu, Sidong
Liu, Tianming
Liu, Ting
Liu, Yinxiao
Lombaert, Herve
Lorenz, Cristian
Lorenzi, Marco
Lou, Xinghua
Lu, Yao
Luo, Xiongbiao
Lv, Jinglei
Lüthi, Marcel
Maass, Nicole
Madooei, Ali
Mahapatra, Dwarikanath
Maier, Andreas
Maier-Hein (né Fritzsche), Klaus Hermann
Majumdar, Angshul
Malandain, Gregoire

Mansi, Tommaso
Mansoor, Awais
Mao, Hongda
Mao, Yunxiang
Marchesseau, Stephanie
Margeta, Jan
Marini Silva, Rafael
Mariottini, Gian Luca
Marsden, Alison
Marsland, Stephen
Martin-Fernandez, Marcos
Martí, Robert
Masutani, Yoshitaka
Mateus, Diana
McClelland, Jamie
McIntosh, Chris
Medrano-Gracia, Pau
Meier, Raphael
Mendizabal-Ruiz, E. Gerardo
Menegaz, Gloria
Menze, Bjoern
Meyer, Chuck
Miga, Michael
Mihalef, Viorel
Miller, James
Miller, Karol
Misaki, Masaya
Modat, Marc
Moghari, Mehdi
Mohamed, Ashraf
Mohareri, Omid
Moore, John
Morales, Hernán G.
Moreno, Rodrigo
Mori, Kensaku
Morimoto, Masakazu
Murphy, Keelin
Müller, Henning
Nabavi, Arya
Nakajima, Yoshikazu
Nakamura, Ryoichi
Napel, Sandy
Nappi, Janne
Nasiriavanaki, Mohammadreza
Nenning, Karl-Heinz
Neumann, Dominik
Neumuth, Thomas
Ng, Bernard
Nguyen Van, Hien
Nicolau, stephane
Ning, Lipeng
Noble, Alison
Noble, Jack
Noblet, Vincent
O'Donnell, Lauren
O'Donnell, Thomas
Oda, Masahiro
Oeltze-Jafra, Steffen
Oh, Junghwan
Oktay, Ayse Betul
Okur, Aslı
Oliver, Arnau
Olivetti, Emanuele
Onofrey, John
Onogi, Shinya
Orihuela-Espina, Felipe
Otake, Yoshito
Ou, Yangming
Ozarslan, Evren
Pace, Danielle
Papa, Joao
Parsopoulos, Konstantinos
Paul, Perrine
Paulsen, Rasmus
Peng, Tingying
Pennec, Xavier
Peruzzo, Denis
Peter, Loic
Peterlik, Igor
Petersen, Jens
Petitjean, Caroline
Peyrat, Jean-Marc
Pham, Dzung
Piella, Gemma
Pitiot, Alain
Pizzolato, Marco
Plenge, Esben
Pluim, Josien
Poline, Jean-Baptiste
Prasad, Gautam

Prastawa, Marcel
Pratt, Philip
Preiswerk, Frank
Preusser, Tobias
Prevost, Raphael
Prieto, Claudia
Punithakumar, Kumaradevan
Putzer, David
Qian, Xiaoning
Qiu, Wu
Quellec, Gwenole
Rafii-Tari, Hedyeh
Rajchl, Martin
Rajpoot, Nasir
Raniga, Parnesh
Rapaka, Saikiran
Rathi, Yogesh
Rathke, Fabian
Rauber, Paulo
Reinertsen, Ingerid
Reinhardt, Joseph
Reiter, Austin
Rekik, Islem
Reyes, Mauricio
Richa, Rogério
Rieke, Nicola
Riess, Christian
Riklin Raviv, Tammy
Risser, Laurent
Rit, Simon
Rivaz, Hassan
Robinson, Emma
Roche, Alexis
Rohling, Robert
Rohr, Karl
Ropinski, Timo
Roth, Holger
Rousseau, François
Rousson, Mikael
Roy, Snehashis
Rueckert, Daniel
Rueda Olarte, Andrea
Ruijters, Daniel
Samaras, Dimitris
Sarry, Laurent
Sato, Joao
Schaap, Michiel
Scheinost, Dustin
Scherrer, Benoit
Schirmer, Markus D.
Schmidt, Frank
Schmidt-Richberg, Alexander
Schneider, Caitlin
Schneider, Matthias
Schultz, Thomas
Schumann, Steffen
Schwartz, Ernst
Sechopoulos, Ioannis
Seiler, Christof
Seitel, Alexander
Sermesant, Maxime
Seshamani, Sharmishtaa
Shahzad, Rahil
Shamir, Reuben R.
Sharma, Puneet
Shen, Xilin
Shi, Feng
Shi, Kuangyu
Shi, Wenzhe
Shi, Yinghuan
Shi, Yonggang
Shin, Hoo-Chang
Simpson, Amber
Singh, Vikas
Sinkus, Ralph
Slabaugh, Greg
Smeets, Dirk
Sona, Diego
Song, Yang
Sotiras, Aristeidis
Speidel, Michael
Speidel, Stefanie
Špiclin, Žiga
Staib, Lawrence
Stamm, Aymeric
Staring, Marius
Stauder, Ralf
Stayman, J. Webster
Steinman, David
Stewart, James

Styles, Iain
Styner, Martin
Su, Hang
Suinesiaputra, Avan
Suk, Heung-Il
Summers, Ronald
Sun, Shanhui
Szekely, Gabor
Sznitman, Raphael
Takeda, Takahiro
Talbot, Hugues
Tam, Roger
Tamura, Manabu
Tang, Lisa
Tao, Lingling
Tasdizen, Tolga
Taylor, Russell
Thirion, Bertrand
Thung, Kim-Han
Tiwari, Pallavi
Toews, Matthew
Toh, Kim-Chuan
Tokuda, Junichi
Tong, Yubing
Tornai, Gábor János
Tosun, Duygu
Totz, Johannes
Tournier, J-Donald
Toussaint, Nicolas
Traub, Joerg
Troccaz, Jocelyne
Tustison, Nicholas
Twinanda, Andru Putra
Twining, Carole
Ukwatta, Eranga
Umadevi Venkataraju, Kannan
Unay, Devrim
Urschler, Martin
Uzunbas, Mustafa
Vaillant, Régis
Vallin Spina, Thiago
Vallotton, Pascal
Van assen, Hans
Van Ginneken, Bram
Van Tulder, Gijs
Van Walsum, Theo
Vandini, Alessandro
Vannier, Michael
Varoquaux, Gael
Vegas-Sánchez-Ferrero, Gonzalo
Venkataraman, Archana
Vercauteren, Tom
Veta, Mtiko
Vignon-Clementel, Irene
Villard, Pierre-Frederic
Visentini-Scarzanella, Marco
Viswanath, Satish
Vitanovski, Dime
Voigt, Ingmar
Von Berg, Jens
Voros, Sandrine
Vrtovec, Tomaz
Wachinger, Christian
Waechter-Stehle, Irina
Wahle, Andreas
Wang, Ancong
Wang, Chaohui
Wang, Haibo
Wang, Hongzhi
Wang, Junchen
Wang, Li
Wang, Liansheng
Wang, Lichao
Wang, Linwei
Wang, Qian
Wang, Qiu
Wang, Song
Wang, Yalin
Wang, Yuanquan
Wee, Chong-Yaw
Wei, Liu
Wels, Michael
Werner, Rene
Wesarg, Stefan
Westin, Carl-Fredrik
Whitaker, Ross
Whitney, Jon
Wiles, Andrew
Wörz, Stefan
Wu, Guorong

Wu, Haiyong
Wu, Yu-Chien
Xie, Yuchen
Xing, Fuyong
Xu, Yanwu
Xu, Ziyue
Xue, Zhong
Yagi, Naomi
Yamazaki, Takaharu
Yan, Pingkun
Yang, Lin
Yang, Ying
Yao, Jianhua
Yaqub, Mohammad
Ye, Dong Hye
Yeo, B.T. Thomas
Ynnermann, Anders
Young, Alistair
Yushkevich, Paul
Zacharaki, Evangelia
Zacur, Ernesto
Zelmann, Rina
Zeng, Wei
Zhan, Liang
Zhan, Yiqiang
Zhang, Daoqiang
Zhang, Hui
Zhang, Ling
Zhang, Miaomiao
Zhang, Pei
Zhang, Shaoting
Zhang, Tianhao
Zhang, Tuo
Zhang, Yong
Zhao, Bo
Zhao, Wei
Zhijun, Zhang
Zhou, jinghao
Zhou, Luping
Zhou, S. Kevin
Zhou, Yan
Zhu, Dajiang
Zhu, Hongtu
Zhu, Yuemin
Zhuang, ling
Zhuang, Xiahai
Zuluaga, Maria A.

Contents – Part III

Quantitative Image Analysis I: Segmentation and Measurement

Quantitative Image Analysis II: Microscopy, Fluorescence and Histological Imagery

Quantitative Image Analysis I: Segmentation and Measurement

Deep Convolutional Encoder Networks for Multiple Sclerosis Lesion Segmentation

Tom Brosch[1,4], Youngjin Yoo[1,4], Lisa Y.W. Tang[4], David K.B. Li[2,4], Anthony Traboulsee[3,4], and Roger Tam[2,4]

[1] Department of Electrical and Computer Engineering, UBC
[2] Department of Radiology, UBC
[3] Division of Neurology, UBC
[4] MS/MRI Research Group, University of British Columbia, Vancouver, Canada

Abstract. We propose a novel segmentation approach based on deep convolutional encoder networks and apply it to the segmentation of multiple sclerosis (MS) lesions in magnetic resonance images. Our model is a neural network that has both convolutional and deconvolutional layers, and combines feature extraction and segmentation prediction in a single model. The joint training of the feature extraction and prediction layers allows the model to automatically learn features that are optimized for accuracy for any given combination of image types. In contrast to existing automatic feature learning approaches, which are typically patch-based, our model learns features from entire images, which eliminates patch selection and redundant calculations at the overlap of neighboring patches and thereby speeds up the training. Our network also uses a novel objective function that works well for segmenting underrepresented classes, such as MS lesions. We have evaluated our method on the publicly available labeled cases from the MS lesion segmentation challenge 2008 data set, showing that our method performs comparably to the state-of-the-art. In addition, we have evaluated our method on the images of 500 subjects from an MS clinical trial and varied the number of training samples from 5 to 250 to show that the segmentation performance can be greatly improved by having a representative data set.

Keywords: Segmentation, multiple sclerosis lesions, MRI, machine learning, unbalanced classification, deep learning, convolutional neural nets.

1 Introduction

Multiple sclerosis (MS) is an inflammatory and demyelinating disease of the central nervous system, and is characterized by the formation of lesions, primarily visible in the white matter on conventional magnetic resonance images (MRIs). Imaging biomarkers based on the delineation of lesions, such as lesion load and lesion count, have established their importance for assessing disease progression and treatment effect. However, lesions vary greatly in size, shape, intensity

N. Navab et al. (Eds.): MICCAI 2015, Part III, LNCS 9351, pp. 3–11, 2015.
DOI: 10.1007/978-3-319-24574-4_1

and location, which makes their automatic and accurate segmentation challenging. Many automatic methods have been proposed for the segmentation of MS lesions over the last two decades, which can be classified into unsupervised and supervised methods. Unsupervised methods do not require a labeled data set for training. Instead, lesions are identified as an outlier class using, e.g., clustering methods [1] or dictionary learning and sparse coding to model healthy tissue [2]. Current supervised approaches typically start with a large set of features, either predefined by the user [3] or gathered in a feature extraction step, which is followed by a separate training step with labeled data to determine which set of features are the most important for segmentation in the particular domain. For example, Yoo et al. [4] proposed performing unsupervised learning of domain-specific features from image patches from unlabelled data using deep learning. The most closely related methodology to our currently proposed one comes from the domain of cell membrane segmentation, in which Cireşan et al. [5] proposed to classify the centers of image patches directly using a convolutional neural network [6] without a dedicated feature extraction step. Instead, features are learned indirectly within the lower layers of the neural network during training, while the higher layers can be regarded as performing the classification. In contrast to unsupervised feature learning, this approach allows the learning of features that are specifically tuned to the segmentation task. Although deep network-based feature learning methods have shown great potential for image segmentation, the time required to train complex patch-based methods can make the approach infeasible when the size and number of patches are large.

We propose a new method for segmenting MS lesions that processes entire MRI volumes through a neural network with a novel objective function to automatically learn features tuned for lesion segmentation. Similar to fully convolutional networks [7], our network processes entire volumes instead of patches, which removes the need to select representative patches, eliminates redundant calculations where patches overlap, and therefore scales up more efficiently with image resolution. This speeds up training and allows our model to take advantage of large data sets. Our neural network is composed of three layers: an input layer composed of the image voxels of different modalities, a convolutional layer [6] that extracts features from the input layer at each voxel location, and a deconvolutional layer [8] that uses the extracted features to predict a lesion mask and thereby classify each voxel of the image in a single operation. The entire network is trained at the same time, which enables feature learning to be driven by segmentation performance. The proposed network is similar in architecture to a convolutional auto-encoder [9], which produces a lower dimensional encoding of the input images and uses the decoder output to measure the reconstruction error needed for training, while our network uses the decoder to predict lesion masks of the input images. Due to the structural similarity to convolutional auto-encoders, we call our model a convolutional encoder network (CEN). Traditionally, neural networks are trained by back-propagating the sum of squared differences of the predicted and expected outputs. However, if one class is greatly underrepresented, as is the case for lesions, which typically comprise less than

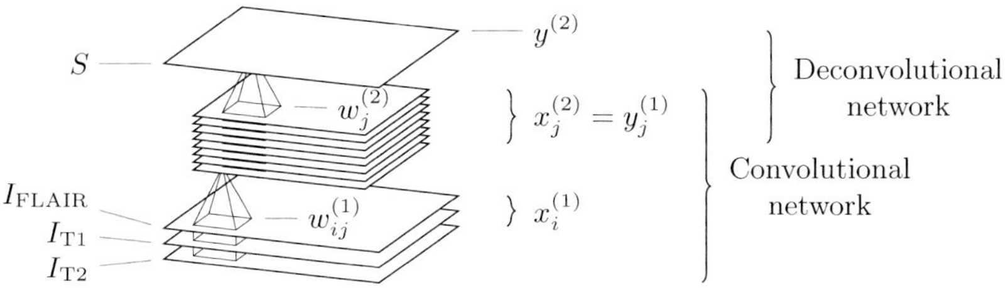

Fig. 1. Convolutional encoder network used to produce a lesion segmentation, S, from multi-modal images, $I = (I_{\mathrm{FLAIR}}, I_{\mathrm{T1}}, I_{\mathrm{T2}})$. The first two layers form a convolutional neural network with trainable filter kernels $w_{ij}^{(1)}$, and the last two layers form a deconvolutional neural network with trainable filter kernels $w_j^{(2)}$.

1 % of the image voxels, the algorithm would learn to ignore the minority class completely. To overcome this problem, we propose a new objective function based on a weighted combination of sensitivity and specificity, designed to deal with unbalanced classes and formulated to allow stable gradient computations.

2 Methods

In this paper, the task of segmenting MS lesions is defined as finding a function s that maps multi-modal images I, e.g., $I = (I_{\mathrm{FLAIR}}, I_{\mathrm{T1}}, I_{\mathrm{T2}})$, to corresponding lesion masks S. Given a set of training images I_n, $n \in \mathbb{N}$, and corresponding segmentations S_n, we model finding an appropriate function for segmenting MS lesions as an optimization problem of the following form

$$\hat{s} = \arg\min_{s \in \mathcal{S}} \sum_n E(S_n, s(I_n)) \tag{1}$$

where $\mathcal{S}$ is the set of possible segmentation functions, and E is an error measure that calculates the dissimilarity between ground truth segmentations and predicted segmentations.

The set of possible segmentation functions is modeled by the convolutional encoder network illustrated in Fig. 1. Our network consists of three layers: an input layer, a convolutional layer, and a deconvolutional layer. The input layer is composed of the image voxels $x_i^{(1)}(\boldsymbol{p})$, $i \in [1, C], C \in \mathbb{N}$, where i indexes the modality, C is the number of modalities, and $\boldsymbol{p} \in \mathbb{R}^3$ are the coordinates of a particular voxel. The convolutional layer automatically learns features from the input images. It is a deterministic function of the following form

$$y_j^{(1)} = \max\left(0, \sum_{i=1}^{C} \tilde{w}_{ij}^{(1)} * x_i^{(1)} + b_j^{(1)}\right) \tag{2}$$

where $y_j^{(1)}, j \in [1, F], F \in \mathbb{N}$, denotes the feature map corresponding to the trainable convolution filter $w_{ij}^{(1)}$, F is the number of filters, b_j is a trainable bias term, $*$ denotes valid convolution, and $\tilde{w}$ denotes a flipped version of w. The deconvolutional layer uses the extracted features to calculate a probabilistic lesion mask as follows

$$y^{(2)} = \operatorname{sigm}\left(\sum_{j=1}^{F} w_j^{(2)} \circledast x_j^{(2)} + b^{(2)}\right) \tag{3}$$

where $x_j^{(2)} = y_j^{(1)}$, $w_j^{(2)}$ and $b^{(2)}$ are trainable parameters, $\circledast$ denotes full convolution, and $\operatorname{sigm}(z)$ denotes the sigmoid function defined as $\operatorname{sigm}(z) = (1 + \exp(-z))^{-1}, z \in \mathbb{R}$. To obtain a binary lesion mask from the probabilistic output of our model, we chose a fixed threshold such that the mean Dice similarity coefficient is maximized on the training set.

The parameters of the model can be efficiently learned by minimizing the error E on the training set using stochastic gradient descent [6]. Typically, neural networks are trained by minimizing the sum of squared differences (SSD)

$$E = \frac{1}{2}\sum_{\boldsymbol{p}} \left(S(\boldsymbol{p}) - y^{(2)}(\boldsymbol{p})\right)^2. \tag{4}$$

The partial derivatives of the error with respect to the model parameters can be calculated using the delta rule and are given by

$$\frac{\partial E}{\partial w_j^{(2)}} = \delta^{(2)} * \tilde{x}_j^{(2)}, \qquad \frac{\partial E}{\partial b^{(2)}} = \frac{1}{N^3}\sum_{\boldsymbol{p}} \delta^{(2)}(\boldsymbol{p}) \tag{5}$$

with

$$\delta^{(2)} = \left(y^{(2)} - S\right) y^{(2)} \left(1 - y^{(2)}\right) \tag{6}$$

where N^3 is the number of voxels of a single input channel. The derivatives of the error with respect to the first layer parameters can be calculated by applying the chain rule of partial derivatives and is given by

$$\frac{\partial E}{\partial w_{ij}^{(1)}} = x_i^{(1)} * \tilde{\delta}_j^{(1)}, \qquad \frac{\partial E}{\partial b_j^{(1)}} = \frac{1}{M^3}\sum_{\boldsymbol{q}} \delta_j^{(1)}(\boldsymbol{q}) \tag{7}$$

with

$$\delta_j^{(1)} = \left(w_j^{(2)} \circledast \delta^{(2)}\right) \mathbb{I}\left(y_j^{(1)} > 0\right) \tag{8}$$

where M^3 is the number of voxels of a feature map, $\boldsymbol{q} \in \mathbb{R}^3$, and $\mathbb{I}(z)$ denotes the indicator function defined as 1 if the predicate z is true and 0 otherwise.

The sum of squared differences is a good measure of classification accuracy, if the two classes are fairly balanced. However, if one class contains vastly more samples, as is the case for lesion segmentation, the error measure is dominated by the majority class and consequently, the neural network would learn to completely ignore the minority class. To overcome this problem, we use a combination of sensitivity and specificity, which can be used together to measure classification performance even for vastly unbalanced problems. More precisely, the final error measure is a weighted sum of the mean squared difference of the lesion voxels (sensitivity) and non-lesion voxels (specificity), reformulated to be error terms:

$$E = r\frac{\sum_{\boldsymbol{p}} \left(S(\boldsymbol{p}) - y^{(2)}(\boldsymbol{p})\right)^2 S(\boldsymbol{p})}{\sum_{\boldsymbol{p}} S(\boldsymbol{p})} + (1-r)\frac{\sum_{\boldsymbol{p}} \left(S(\boldsymbol{p}) - y^{(2)}(\boldsymbol{p})\right)^2 \left(1 - S(\boldsymbol{p})\right)}{\sum_{\boldsymbol{p}} \left(1 - S(\boldsymbol{p})\right)} \quad (9)$$

We formulate the sensitivity and specificity errors as squared errors in order to yield smooth gradients, which makes the optimization more robust. The sensitivity ratio r can be used to assign different weights to the two terms. Due to the large number of non-lesion voxels, weighting the specificity error higher is important, but the algorithm is stable with respect to changes in r, which largely affects the threshold used to binarize the probabilistic output. In all our experiments, a sensitivity ratio between 0.10 and 0.01 yields very similar results.

To train our model, we must compute the derivatives of the modified objective function with respect to the model parameters. Equations (5), (7), and (8) are a consequence of the chain rule and independent of the chosen similarity measure. The update for $\delta^{(2)}$ can be derived analogously to the SSD case, and is given by

$$\delta^{(2)} = \left(\alpha S + \beta(1 - S)\right)\left(y^{(2)} - S\right)y^{(2)}\left(1 - y^{(2)}\right) \quad (10)$$

where $\alpha = 2r(\sum_{\boldsymbol{p}} S(\boldsymbol{p}))^{-1}$ and $\beta = 2(1 - r)(\sum_{\boldsymbol{p}}(1 - S(\boldsymbol{p})))^{-1}$.

3 Experiments and Results

To allow for a direct comparison with state-of-the-art lesion segmentation methods, we evaluated our method on the FLAIR, T1-, and T2-weighted MRIs of the 20 publicly available labeled cases from the MS lesion segmentation challenge 2008 [10], which we downsampled from the original isotropic voxel size of $0.5\,\text{mm}^3$ to an isotropic voxel size of $1.0\,\text{mm}^3$. In addition, we evaluated our method on an in-house data set from an MS clinical trial of 500 subjects split equally into training and test sets. The images were acquired from 45 different scanning sites. For each subject, the data set contains T2- and PD-weighted MRIs with a voxel size of $0.937\,\text{mm} \times 0.937\,\text{mm} \times 3.000\,\text{mm}$. The main preprocessing steps included rigid intra-subject registration, brain extraction, intensity normalization, and background cropping.

We used a CEN with 32 filters and filter sizes of $9 \times 9 \times 9$ and $9 \times 9 \times 5$ voxels for the challenge and in-house data sets, respectively. Training on a single GeForce GTX 780 graphics card took between 6 and 32 hours per model depending on the training set size. However, once the network is trained, segmentation of trimodal 3D volumes with a resolution of, e.g., $159 \times 201 \times 155$ voxels can be performed in less than one second. As a rough[1] comparison, Cireşan et al. [5] reported that their patch-based method required 10 to 30 minutes to segment a single 2D image with a resolution of 512×512 voxels using four graphics cards, which demonstrates the large speed-ups gained by processing entire volumes.

[1] Cireşan et al. used a more complex network that is composed of 11 layers. However, their network was trained on much smaller images, which roughly compensates for the increased complexity.

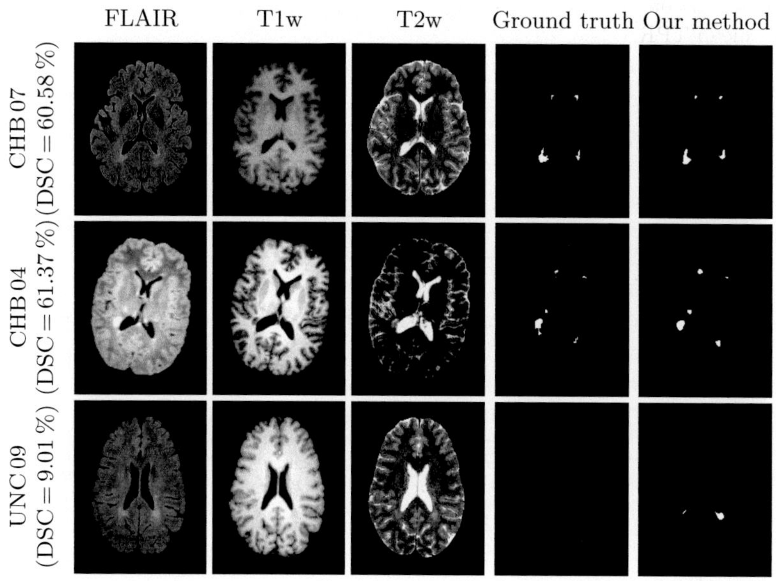

Fig. 2. Example segmentations of our method for three different subjects from the challenge data set. Our method performed well and consistently despite the large contrast differences seen between the first two rows. In the third row, our method also segmented lesions that have similar contrast, but these regions had not been identified as lesions by the manual rater, which highlights the difficulty in distinguishing focal lesions from diffuse damage, even for experts.

We evaluated our method on the challenge data set using 5-fold cross-validation and calculated the true positive rate (TPR), positive predictive value (PPV), and Dice similarity coefficient (DSC) between the predicted segmentations and the resampled ground truth. Figure 2 shows a comparison of three subjects from the challenge data set. The first two rows show the FLAIR, T1w, T2w, ground truth segmentations, and predicted segmentations of two subjects with a DSC of 60.58 % and 61.37 %. Despite the large contrast differences between the two subjects, our method performed well and consistently, which indicates that our model was able to learn features that are robust to a large range of intensity variations. The last row shows a subject with a DSC of 9.01 %, one of the lowest DSC scores from the data set. Our method segmented lesions that have similar contrast to the other two subjects, but these regions were not classified as lesions by the manual rater. This highlights the difficulty of manual lesion segmentation, as the difference between diffuse white matter pathology and focal lesions is often indistinct. A quantitative comparison of our method with other state-of-the-art methods is summarized in Table 1. Our method outperforms the winning method (Souplet et al. [1]) of the MS lesion segmentation challenge 2008 and the currently best unsupervised method reported on that data set (Weiss et al. [2]) in terms of mean TPR and PPV. Our method performs comparably to a

Table 1. Comparison of our method with state-of-the-art lesion segmentation methods in terms of mean TPR, PPV, and DSC. Our method performs comparably to the best methods reported on the MS lesion segmentation challenge data set.

Method	TPR	PPV	DSC
Souplet et al. [1]	20.65	30.00	—
Weiss et al. [2]	33.00	36.85	29.05
Geremia et al. [3]	39.85	40.35	—
Our method	39.71	41.38	35.52

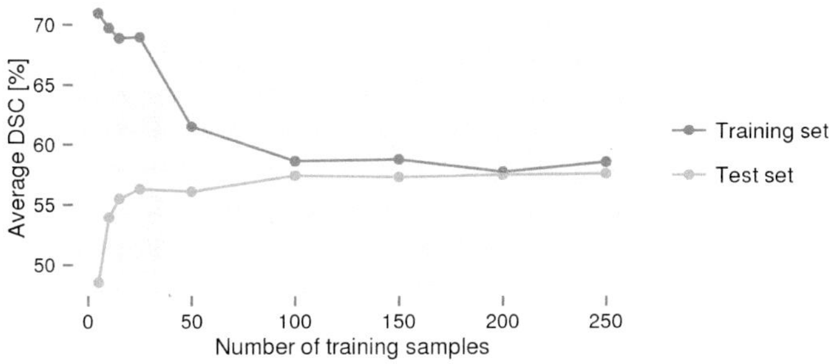

Fig. 3. Comparison of DSC scores calculated on the training and test sets for varying numbers of training samples. At around 100 samples, the model becomes stable in terms of test performance and the small difference between training and test DSCs, indicating that overfitting of the training data no longer occurs.

current method (Geremia et al. [3]) that uses a carefully designed set of features specifically designed for lesion segmentation, despite our method having learned its features solely from a relatively small training set.

To evaluate the impact of the training set size on the segmentation performance, we trained our model on our in-house data set with a varying number of training samples and calculated the mean DSC on the training and test sets as illustrated in Fig. 3. For small training sets, there is a large difference between the DSCs on the training and test sets, which indicates that the training set is too small to learn a representative set of features. At around 100 samples, the model becomes stable in terms of test performance and the small difference between training and test DSCs, indicating that overfitting of the training data is no longer occurring. With 100 training subjects, our method achieves a mean DSC on the test set of 57.38 %, which shows that the segmentation accuracy can be greatly improved compared to the results on the challenge data set, when a representative training set is available.

4 Conclusions

We have introduced a new method for the automatic segmentation of MS lesions based on convolutional encoder networks. The joint training of the feature extraction and prediction layers with a novel objective function allows for the automatic learning of features that are tuned for a given combination of image types and a segmentation task with very unbalanced classes. We have evaluated our method on two data sets showing that approximately 100 images are required to train the model without overfitting but even when only a relatively small training set is available, the method still performs comparably to the state-of-the-art algorithms. For future work, we plan to increase the depth of the network, which would allow the learning of a set of hierarchical features. This could further improve segmentation accuracy, but may require larger training sets. We would also like to investigate the use of different objective functions for training based on other measures of segmentation performance.

Acknowledgements. This work was supported by NSERC and the Milan and Maureen Ilich Foundation.

References

1. Souplet, J.C., Lebrun, C., Ayache, N., Malandain, G.: An automatic segmentation of T2-FLAIR multiple sclerosis lesions. In: MIDAS Journal - MICCAI 2008 Workshop (2008)
2. Weiss, N., Rueckert, D., Rao, A.: Multiple sclerosis lesion segmentation using dictionary learning and sparse coding. In: Mori, K., Sakuma, I., Sato, Y., Barillot, C., Navab, N. (eds.) MICCAI 2013, Part I. LNCS, vol. 8149, pp. 735–742. Springer, Heidelberg (2013)
3. Geremia, E., Menze, B.H., Clatz, O., Konukoglu, E., Criminisi, A., Ayache, N.: Spatial decision forests for MS lesion segmentation in multi-channel MR images. In: Jiang, T., Navab, N., Pluim, J.P.W., Viergever, M.A. (eds.) MICCAI 2010, Part I. LNCS, vol. 6361, pp. 111–118. Springer, Heidelberg (2010)
4. Yoo, Y., Brosch, T., Traboulsee, A., Li, D.K.B., Tam, R.: Deep learning of image features from unlabeled data for multiple sclerosis lesion segmentation. In: Wu, G., Zhang, D., Zhou, L. (eds.) MLMI 2014. LNCS, vol. 8679, pp. 117–124. Springer, Heidelberg (2014)
5. Ciresan, D., Giusti, A., Schmidhuber, J.: Deep neural networks segment neuronal membranes in electron microscopy images. In: Advances in Neural Information Processing Systems, pp. 1–9 (2012)
6. LeCun, Y., Bottou, L., Bengio, Y., Haffner, P.: Gradient-based learning applied to document recognition. Proceedings of the IEEE 86(11), 2278–2324 (1998)
7. Kang, K., Wang, X.: Fully convolutional neural networks for crowd segmentation. arXiv preprint arXiv:1411.4464 (2014)

8. Zeiler, M.D., Taylor, G.W., Fergus, R.: Adaptive deconvolutional networks for mid and high level feature learning. In: 2011 IEEE International Conference on Computer Vision (ICCV), pp. 2018–2025. IEEE (2011)
9. Masci, J., Meier, U., Cireşan, D., Schmidhuber, J.: Stacked convolutional auto-encoders for hierarchical feature extraction. In: Honkela, T. (ed.) ICANN 2011, Part I. LNCS, vol. 6791, pp. 52–59. Springer, Heidelberg (2011)
10. Styner, M., Lee, J., Chin, B., Chin, M., Commowick, O., Tran, H., Markovic-Plese, S., Jewells, V., Warfield, S.: 3D segmentation in the clinic: A grand challenge II: MS lesion segmentation. In: MIDAS Journal - MICCAI 2008 Workshop, pp. 1–6 (2008)

Unsupervised Myocardial Segmentation for Cardiac MRI

Anirban Mukhopadhyay[1], Ilkay Oksuz[1], Marco Bevilacqua[1], Rohan Dharmakumar[2], and Sotirios A. Tsaftaris[1,3]

[1] IMT Institute for Advanced Studies Lucca, Italy
[2] Biomedical Imaging Research Institute, Cedars-Sinai Medical, Los Angeles, USA
[3] Department of Electrical Engineering and Computer Science, Northwestern University, Evanston, USA

Abstract. Though unsupervised segmentation was a de-facto standard for cardiac MRI segmentation early on, recently cardiac MRI segmentation literature has favored fully supervised techniques such as Dictionary Learning and Atlas-based techniques. But, the benefits of unsupervised techniques e.g., no need for large amount of training data and better potential of handling variability in anatomy and image contrast, is more evident with emerging cardiac MR modalities. For example, CP-BOLD is a new MRI technique that has been shown to detect ischemia without any contrast at stress but also at rest conditions. Although CP-BOLD looks similar to standard CINE, changes in myocardial intensity patterns and shape across cardiac phases, due to the heart's motion, BOLD effect and artifacts affect the underlying mechanisms of fully supervised segmentation techniques resulting in a significant drop in segmentation accuracy. In this paper, we present a fully unsupervised technique for segmenting myocardium from the background in both standard CINE MR and CP-BOLD MR. We combine appearance with motion information (obtained via Optical Flow) in a dictionary learning framework to sparsely represent important features in a low dimensional space and separate myocardium from background accordingly. Our fully automated method learns background-only models and one class classifier provides myocardial segmentation. The advantages of the proposed technique are demonstrated on a dataset containing CP-BOLD MR and standard CINE MR image sequences acquired in baseline and ischemic condition across 10 canine subjects, where our method outperforms state-of-the-art supervised segmentation techniques in CP-BOLD MR and performs at-par for standard CINE MR.

Keywords: Unsupervised Segmentation, Dictionary Learning, BOLD, CINE, MRI.

1 Introduction

Cardiovascular Disease (CVD) is the leading cause of mortality worldwide, and the modern analysis of cardiac function using imaging techniques (specifically

N. Navab et al. (Eds.): MICCAI 2015, Part III, LNCS 9351, pp. 12–20, 2015.
DOI: 10.1007/978-3-319-24574-4_2

Cardiac CINE MR) is an effective way of diagnosing CVD. An emerging cine-like cardiac modality is Cardiac Phase-resolved Blood Oxygen-Level-Dependent (CP-BOLD) MR, a truly noninvasive method that identifies the ischemic myocardium by examining changes in myocardial signal intensity patterns as a function of cardiac phase [19].

Fully supervised myocardial segmentation (i.e., separating myocardium from the rest of the anatomy) developed for standard CINE MR, however, underperform in the case of CP-BOLD MR due to the spatio-temporal intensity variations of the myocardial BOLD effect [14,19]. Thus, in addition to violating shape invariance (as with standard CINE MR), the principal assumption of appearance invariance (consistent intensity [12]) is violated in CP-BOLD MR as well. As a result, no automated CP-BOLD MR myocardial segmentation algorithms exist, and semi-automated methods based on tracking are currently employed [18]. We hypothesize that this is due to the lack of exploiting the unsupervised techniques in a sparse representation setting, which can be an effective tool for developing features that are invariant to temporal and inter-subject variabilities, yet unique and descriptive. In addition, we also argue that the temporal consistency assumption for myocardial segmentation of standard CINE MR is a special case of the more generalized spatio-temporal variability observed in CP-BOLD MR. Consequently, developing generalized features for CP-BOLD MR should also address the problems of myocardial segmentation of standard CINE MR.

In this paper, rather than relying on low-level features often used for representing the myocardium when developing segmentation methods for standard CINE MR, which are inconsistent for CP-BOLD MR, a fully unsupervised motion and sparse representation-based feature selection technique has been developed to accommodate the myocardial BOLD effect. The only assumption is that the myocardium moves differently than its surrounding background anatomy. This strategy is also motivated by the findings of [9] where sparse representation using dictionaries are shown to be invariant under intensity changes. In addition, the sparse representation is capable of retaining semantic information of the myocardium [21]. This essentially enables myocardial segmentation in cardiac MR image sequences (i.e. CINE stack) without any form of manual intervention e.g., landmark selection, ROI selection, spatio-temporal alignment to name a few. The unsupervised motion and sparse-representation strategy is designed to facilitate this key observation. Each frame is coarsely segmented (over-segmented) based on the optical flow vectors, inspired by [10]. The appearance and motion of the coarsely-segmented background is sparsely represented in a patch-based discriminative dictionary learning technique. A one-class Support Vector Machine (SVM) [15] is employed on the learnt sparse representation of all the pixels in the image sequence to classify myocardium from the background.

The main contributions of the paper are twofold. First of all, we revisit fully unsupervised myocardial segmentation technique employing no manual intervention and minimal myocardial motion-pattern assumption for solving general myocardium segmentation problem in standard and emerging cardiac MR imaging modalities. Secondly, we have employed a joint motion and sparse representation based technique, where the motion not only generates a rough estimate of the myocardium, but also guides the sparse representation stage to a smooth solution based on the motion of the myocardium.

The remainder of the paper is organized as follows: Section 2 discusses the related work, Section 3 presents the proposed method with results are described in Section 4. Finally, Section 5 offers discussion and conclusion.

2 Related Work

The automated myocardial segmentation for standard CINE MR is a well studied problem [12]. Most of these algorithms can be broadly classified into two categories based on whether the methodology is unsupervised or supervised one.

Unsupervised segmentation techniques with no or weak priors were employed early-on for myocardial segmentation of cardiac MR, almost all of which require minimal or advanced manual intervention [12]. Among the very few unsupervised techniques which are fully automated, most similar ones to our proposed method are those considering motion as a way to propagate an initial segmentation result to the whole cardiac cycle [5], [6] and [11]. Only Lynch et. al. [8] considered motion as an intrinsic entity in a temporal deformation model with level-sets for fully automatic unsupervised segmentation.

However, supervised segmentation techniques have received more attention in recent years and in particular, Atlas-based supervised segmentation techniques have achieved significant success [12]. The myocardial segmentation masks available from other subject(s) are generally propagated to unseen data in Atlas-based techniques [2] using non-rigid registration algorithms like diffeomorphic demons (dDemons) [20], FFD-MI [3], probabilistic label fusion or SVM [2]. Segmentation-only class of supervised techniques, on the other hand, mainly focuses on feature-based representation of the myocardium. Texture information is generally considered as an effective feature representation of the myocardium for standard CINE MR images [22]. Patch-based static discriminative dictionary learning technique (SJTAD) [16] and Multi-scale Appearance Dictionary Learning technique [4] have achieved high accuracy and are considered as state-of-the-art mechanisms for supervised myocardial segmentation. The hindsights of all the supervised methods are the requirements of lots of data for training and a robust feature matching framework, which is especially critical for emerging cardiac modalities such as CP-BOLD MR. In this paper, we follow a segmentation approach where the major feature includes using motion information and discriminative dictionary learning based sparse representation in a fully unsupervised fashion.

3 Method

Our proposed Unsupervised Motion and Sparsity based Segmentation (UMSS) method (as shown in Figure 1) for segmenting 2D Cardiac MR (both standard CINE and CP-BOLD) image sequences is described here in details.

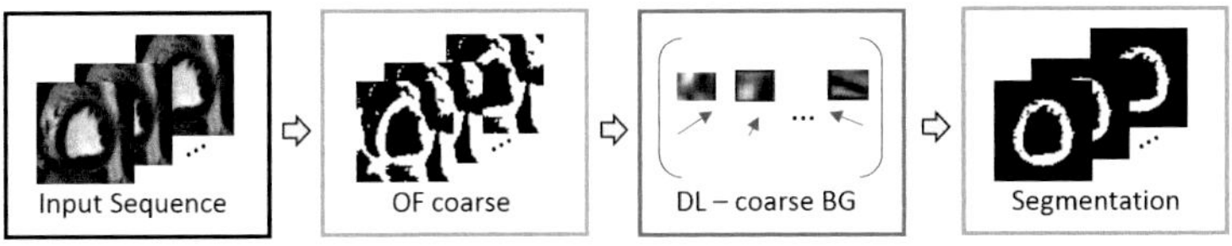

Fig. 1. Description of the proposed method. (see text for details)

Optical Flow Based Coarse Segmentation: Our first step is to compute optical flows between two subsequent frames (I_t, I_{t+d}) of the given image sequence using [7]. The motion boundary of the optical flow can be measured simply by calculating the gradient. We have computed the coarse segmentation by applying a threshold T_c on the gradient vectors as shown in Algorithm 1.

Dictionary Learning of Background: Given a sequence of images $\{I_t\}_{t=1}^{T}$ and corresponding coarse segmentation labels obtained from Optical Flow motion boundary as described earlier, we can obtain a matrix, $\{Y = [Y^{cB}Y^{cF}]\}$, where the matrix Y^{cB} and Y^{cF} contains the coarse background and Foreground information respectively. Information is collected from image and motion patches: squared patches centered around each pixel of the image and its corresponding motion matrix. More precisely, the p-th column of the matrix Y^{cB} is obtained by concatenating the normalized patch vector of pixel intensities and motion vectors taken around the p-th pixel in the coarse background. The Dictionary Learning part of our method takes as input this matrix Y^{cB}, to learn a dictionary D^{cB} and a sparse feature matrix X^{cB}. Dictionaries and sparse features are trained via the K-SVD algorithm [1]. We use the "Gram matrix" $(G^{cB} = (Y^{cB})^T Y^{cB})$ to promote diversity in the initialization step. The idea is to have a subset of patches as much diverse as possible to train dictionaries and sparse features. To ensure a proper discriminative initialization, patches that correspond to high values in the Gram matrix are discarded from the training before performing K-SVD. We sort the training patches w.r.t. the sum of their related coefficients in the Gram Matrix, and we prune them by choosing a certain percentage.

One-Class SVM for Segmentation: The goal of the segmentation problem is to assign to each pixel of the image sequence a label, i.e. establish if the pixel is included in the background or the myocardium. To perform this classification, we use the coarse Background dictionary $\{D^{cB}\}$ previously learnt with Discriminative Dictionary Learning technique for sparse representation of the appearance and motion features. We compute the sparse feature matrix $X = [X^{cB}X^{cF}]$ for all the pixels of the image sequence with OMP [17]. The classification is performed by constructing the classifier from only the sparse-features of coarse Background class X^{cB} (the p-th column of the matrix X^{cB}, x_p^{cB}, is considered as the discriminative feature vector for the particular pixel p) using a one-class SVM framework [15]. Supposing for each pixel p of coarse Background class, there is a high dimensional feature space F, then each sample is represented in F by $\Phi(x_{p\in cB})$ and the objective function is formulated as follows:

Algorithm 1. Unsupervised Motion and Sparsity based Segmentation (UMSS)

Input: Image sequence from single subject

Output: Predicted Myocardium masks across the sequence

1: Calculate Optical Flow $\vec{f}_p$ at each pixel p between pairs of frames (I_t, I_{t+d})

2: Measure motion boundary from gradient of Optical Flow $B_p = 1 - exp(-\lambda \left\| \nabla \vec{f}_p \right\|)$ where λ is the parameter controlling steepness, $B_p \in [0, 1]$.

3: Compute Coarse segmentation $C_p \in {}^{cB, if\, B_p < T_c}_{cF, if\, B_p \geq T_c}$

4: Collect all $C_p \in cB$ and Calculate $Y_p^{cB} = [I_{p\pm\Delta}; \vec{f}_{p\pm\Delta}]$

5: Discard atoms with high values in intra-class Gram matrix G^{cB}

6: Learn dictionary and sparse feature matrix with the K-SVD algorithm

$$\underset{D^{cB}, X^{cB}}{\text{minimize}} \|Y^{cB} - D^{cB} X^{cB}\|_2^2 \quad \text{s. t.} \quad \|x_{p\in cB}\|_0 \leq L$$

7: Train one-class SVM on X^{cB} using Equation 1

8: Test on all sparse features $X \in x_{p\in(cF \cup cB)}$ for final classification

$$\underset{W\in F, \eta\in\mathbb{R}^l, b\in\mathbb{R}}{\text{minimize}} \frac{1}{2} W^T W + \frac{1}{\nu l} \sum\nolimits_{p\in cB} \eta - b \quad \text{s. t.} \quad W \cdot \Phi(x_{p\in cB}) \geq b - \eta, \eta \geq 0 \quad (1)$$

Here, W is the normal vector that represents the support, b is the threshold of function f, $\eta_{p\in cB}$ is the slack variable and ν is the parameter that represents the fraction of sample that should be accepted as the other class. During testing, sparse features for all the pixels of the image sequence, stored in matrix $\hat{X}$ are fed to the classifier learnt on the coarse Background features, to classify the myocardial region as the other class. In addition, a Hough transformation-based post processing step is employed by fitting parametric circles to enforce the shape constraint of the myocardium. Note that the later step is a rudimentary way of ensuring shape-based constraints. Treating it in a more sophisticated way, using probabilistic models (e.g. Graph-cut with coarse Background as a sink) or level-set, can potentially improve the performance.

4 Results

This section offers a qualitative analysis and quantitative comparison of our proposed UMSS method w.r.t. state-of-the-art methods, to demonstrate its effectiveness for myocardial segmentation. Note that our method outperforms all supervised methods from current literature in both baseline and ischemia cases of CP-BOLD MR, whereas yields state-of-the-art results for both baseline and ischemia cases of standard CINE MR.

Data Preparation and Parameter Settings: 2D short-axis images of the whole cardiac cycle were acquired at baseline and severe ischemia (inflicted as stenosis of the left-anterior descending coronary artery (LAD)) on a 1.5T Espree (Siemens Healthcare) in the same 10 canines along the mid ventricle using both standard CINE and a flow and motion compensated CP-BOLD acquisition within few minutes of each other [19].

As for the parameters of UMSS, in this paper we have empirically chosen a d of 5 and a threshold T_c of 0.4 for coarse segmentation based on Optical Flow, 9×9 as the patch size, λ of 0.5, ν of 0.2 and a pruning of 10% for Gram Filtering. Each sparse feature has been represented by 5 non-zero elements whereas a dictionary of 10 atoms is chosen for coarse Background representation. We computed the myocardium segmentation across the whole stack of image sequences for each subject and tested the parameter sensitivity within a reasonable range, but the detailed performance chart is omitted for brevity.

Quantitative Comparison: As segmentation quality metric, the Dice coefficient, which measures the overlap between ground truth segmentation masks and those obtained by the algorithm(s), is employed. For our implementation of *Atlas-based segmentation methods*, the registration algorithms dDemons [20] and FFD-MI [3] are used to propagate the segmentation mask of end-diastole image from all other subjects to the end-diastole image of the test subject, followed by a majority voting to obtain the final myocardial segmentation. For *supervised classifier-based methods*, namely Appearance Classification using Random Forest (ACRF) and Texture-Appearance Classification using Random Forest (TACRF) random forests are used as classifiers to get segmentation labels from different features. To provide more context, we compare our approach with *dictionary-based methods*, SJTAD and RDDL. SJTAD is an implementation of the method in [16], whereas the discriminative dictionary learning of [13] is used for RDDL. Finally to showcase the strengths of our design choice of sparse representation using discriminative dictionary learning, we have considered two additional variants of UMSS, without Dictionary Learning (UMSS No DL) and without concatenating optical flow features with intensity for Dictionary Learning (UMSS No Motion). All quantitative analysis for supervised methods are performed using strict leave-one-subject-out cross validation.

As Table 1 shows, overall, for standard CINE, most algorithms perform adequately and the presence of ischemia slightly reduces performance. However, when BOLD contrast is present, other approaches fail to accommodate changes in appearance due to contrast, but UMSS obtains consistent performance. Specifically, Atlas-based methods are shown to perform well in standard CINE but poorly in CP-BOLD. ACRF and TACRF, instead, show very low performance in both cases. Among dictionary-based methods, SJTAD performs well in standard CINE MR, but under-performs in CP-BOLD MR. When comparing with its variants, UMSS shows that both Dictionary Learning and motion information are extremely beneficial.

Qualitative Analysis: The quality of myocardial segmentation by UMSS for both baseline and ischemia cases across standard CINE and CP-BOLD MR is shown in Figure 2. Note that UMSS results in very smooth endo- and epicardium contours which closely follow ground truth contours generated by the experts and can be attributed to the successful representation of myocardial motion.

Table 1. Dice coefficient (mean (std)) for segmentation accuracy in %.

Methods	Baseline		Ischemia	
	Standard CINE	CP-BOLD	Standard CINE	CP-BOLD
Atlas-based methods				
dDemons [20]	60(8)	55(8)	56(6)	49(7)
FFD-MI [3]	60(3)	54(8)	54(8)	45(6)
Supervised classifier-based methods				
ACRF	57(3)	25(2)	52(3)	21(2)
TACRF	65(2)	29(3)	59(1)	24(2)
Dictionary-based methods				
SJTAD [16]	71(2)	32(3)	66(3)	23(4)
RDDL [13]	42(15)	50(20)	48(13)	61(12)
Proposed Unsupervised method				
UMSS No DL	25(9)	26(12)	19(5)	18(7)
UMSS No Motion	49(15)	42(19)	51(14)	53(12)
UMSS	62(20)	71(10)	65(14)	66(11)

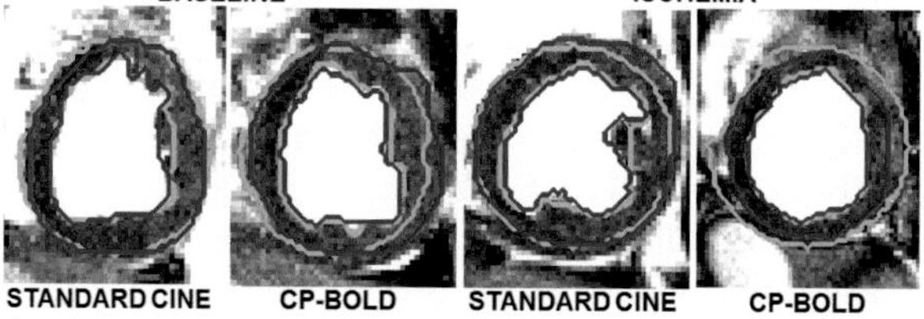

Fig. 2. Segmentation result (green) of UMSS for both CP-BOLD MR and standard CINE MR at baseline and ischemic condition superimposed with corresponding Manual Segmentation (red) contours delineated by experts.

5 Discussions and Conclusion

This study motivates us to rethink the standard assumptions regarding the segmentation of the myocardium in MR image sequences, especially to accommodate emerging cardiac MR imaging modalities. In particular, deviating from fully supervised techniques (the performance of which heavily depends on the amount of training data) towards unsupervised ones can benefit in multitude of ways: from operating on no training data, better handling of variability in image contrast to no manual intervention. In addition, this work has shown that unsupervised methods can still deliver state-of-the-art performance even for standard CINE MR. The proposed algorithm does not exploit the spatio-temporal information across cardiac phases and doing so by introducing graph-based formulation should increase performance in future extensions. UMSS can be an effective tool in challenging datasets where inter-acquisition variability prohibits the effectiveness of supervised segmentation strategies. Finally, such post-processing tools are expected to be instrumental in advancing the utility of emerging cardiac MR imaging techniques, e.g., CP-BOLD MR, towards clinical translation.

Acknowledgement. This work is supported by NIH 2R01HL091989-05.

References

1. Aharon, M., et al.: K-SVD: An Algorithm for Designing Overcomplete Dictionaries for Sparse Representation. TSP 54(11), 4311–4322 (2006)
2. Bai, W., et al.: Multi-atlas segmentation with augmented features for cardiac MR images. MIA, 98–109 (2015)
3. Glocker, B., et al.: Dense image registration through MRFs and efficient linear programming. MIA 12(6), 731–741 (2008)
4. Huang, X., et al.: Contour tracking in echocardiographic sequences via sparse representation and dictionary learning. MIA 18, 253–271 (2014)
5. Jolly, M.-P., Xue, H., Grady, L., Guehring, J.: Combining registration and minimum surfaces for the segmentation of the left ventricle in cardiac cine MR images. In: Yang, G.-Z., Hawkes, D., Rueckert, D., Noble, A., Taylor, C. (eds.) MICCAI 2009, Part II. LNCS, vol. 5762, pp. 910–918. Springer, Heidelberg (2009)
6. Lin, X., Cowan, B.R., Young, A.A.: Automated detection of left ventricle in 4D MR images: Experience from a large study. In: Larsen, R., Nielsen, M., Sporring, J. (eds.) MICCAI 2006. LNCS, vol. 4190, pp. 728–735. Springer, Heidelberg (2006)
7. Liu, C.: Beyond Pixels: Exploring New Representations and Applications for Motion Analysis. Doctoral Thesis MIT (2009)
8. Lynch, M., et al.: Segmentation of the left ventricle of the heart in 3D+t MRI data using an optimised non-rigid temporal model. TMI 27(2), 195–203 (2008)
9. Mukhopadhyay, A., Oksuz, I., Bevilacqua, M., Dharmakumar, R., Tsaftaris, S.A.: Data-driven feature learning for myocardial segmentation of CP-BOLD MRI. In: van Assen, H., Bovendeerd, P., Delhaas, T. (eds.) FIMH 2015. LNCS, vol. 9126, pp. 189–197. Springer, Heidelberg (2015)
10. Papazoglou, A., et al.: Fast object segmentation in unconstrained video. In: ICCV (2013)
11. Pednekar, A., et al.: Automated left ventricular segmentation in cardiac MRI. TBME 53(7), 1425–1428 (2006)
12. Petitjean, C., et al.: A review of segmentation methods in short axis cardiac MR images. MIA 15(2), 169–184 (2011)
13. Ramirez, I., et al.: Classification and clustering via dictionary learning with structured incoherence and shared features. In: CVPR, pp. 3501–3508 (2010)
14. Rusu, C., et al.: Synthetic generation of myocardial blood-oxygen-level-dependent MRI time series via structural sparse decomposition modeling. TMI, 1422–1433 (2014)
15. Scholkopf, B., et al.: Estimating the support of a high-dimensional distribution. Neural Computation 13(7), 1443–1471 (2001)
16. Tong, T., et al.: Segmentation of MR images via discriminative dictionary learning and sparse coding: Application to hippocampus labeling. NeuroImage, 11–23 (2013)
17. Tropp, J., et al.: Signal recovery from random measurements via orthogonal matching pursuit. T. Inf. Theo. 53(12), 4655–4666 (2007)
18. Tsaftaris, S.A., et al.: A dynamic programming solution to tracking and elastically matching left ventricular walls in cardiac CINE MRI. In: ICIP, pp. 2980–2983 (2008)

19. Tsaftaris, S.A., et al.: Detecting Myocardial Ischemia at Rest With Cardiac Phase-Resolved Blood Oxygen Level-Dependent Cardiovascular Magnetic Resonance. Circ. Card. Imag. 6(2), 311–319 (2013)
20. Vercauteren, T., Pennec, X., Perchant, A., Ayache, N.: Non-parametric diffeomorphic image registration with the demons algorithm. In: Ayache, N., Ourselin, S., Maeder, A. (eds.) MICCAI 2007, Part II. LNCS, vol. 4792, pp. 319–326. Springer, Heidelberg (2007)
21. Wright, J., et al.: Sparse representation for computer vision and pattern recognition. Proc. IEEE 98(6), 1031–1044 (2010)
22. Zhen, X., Wang, Z., Islam, A., Bhaduri, M., Chan, I., Li, S.: Direct estimation of cardiac Bi-ventricular volumes with regression forests. In: Golland, P., Hata, N., Barillot, C., Hornegger, J., Howe, R. (eds.) MICCAI 2014, Part II. LNCS, vol. 8674, pp. 586–593. Springer, Heidelberg (2014)

Multimodal Cortical Parcellation Based on Anatomical and Functional Brain Connectivity

Chendi Wang, Burak Yoldemir, and Rafeef Abugharbieh

BiSICL, University of British Columbia, Vancouver, Canada
chendiw@ece.ubc.ca

Abstract. Reliable cortical parcellation is a crucial step in human brain network analysis since incorrect definition of nodes may invalidate the inferences drawn from the network. Cortical parcellation is typically cast as an unsupervised clustering problem on functional magnetic resonance imaging (fMRI) data, which is particularly challenging given the pronounced noise in fMRI acquisitions. This challenge manifests itself in rather inconsistent parcellation maps generated by different methods. To address the need for robust methodologies to parcellate the brain, we propose a multimodal cortical parcellation framework based on fused diffusion MRI (dMRI) and fMRI data analysis. We argue that incorporating anatomical connectivity information into parcellation is beneficial in suppressing spurious correlations commonly observed in fMRI analyses. Our approach adaptively determines the weighting of anatomical and functional connectivity information in a data-driven manner, and incorporates a neighborhood-informed affnity matrix that was recently shown to provide robustness against noise. To validate, we compare parcellations obtained via normalized cuts on unimodal vs. multimodal data from the Human Connectome Project. Results demonstrate that our proposed method better delineates spatially contiguous parcels with higher test-retest reliability and improves inter-subject consistency.

Keywords: Anatomical connectivity, brain network analysis, clustering, functional connectivity, multimodal cortical parcellation.

1 Introduction

Brain cortical parcellation refers to subdividing the cerebral cortex into regions that exhibit internal homogeneity in certain properties [1]. Connectivity-based parcellation (CBP) is a promising method for brain cortical parcellation, where voxels in the brain are divided into a coarser collection of functionally or anatomically homogeneous brain regions by clustering voxels with similar connectivity profiles [2]. Among CBP techniques, functional connectivity (FC) based parcellation is the predominant approach, where voxels are grouped according to the statistical dependencies between their functional magnetic resonance imaging (fMRI) time courses [1]. However, even with advanced clustering methods, reliable brain parcellation remains challenging due to the notoriously low signal-to-noise ratio (SNR) of fMRI data. Given the close relationship between anatomical

N. Navab et al. (Eds.): MICCAI 2015, Part III, LNCS 9351, pp. 21–28, 2015.
DOI: 10.1007/978-3-319-24574-4_3

connectivity (AC) and FC in the brain [3], we argue that simultaneous analysis of AC and FC information for CBP is beneficial. Despite its promising potential, multimodal CBP remains a relatively unexplored direction. To the best of our knowledge, the only existing approach to multimodal CBP uses the overlap among probabilistic parcellation maps derived from different modalities to generate a consensus map [4,5]. A major disadvantage of this approach is its late fusion, i.e the unimodal parcellation is performed in isolation on each modality then combined in a subsequent fusion step rather than jointly analyzing multimodal data in a truly unified framework.

In this paper, we propose a multimodal CBP method where AC and FC, inferred through diffusion MRI (dMRI) and fMRI, are combined. To prevent bias towards any particular task, we use resting state fMRI (RS-fMRI) data, which captures the intrinsic functional brain connectivity. Our rationale in combining AC and FC is that FC estimates tend to contain many false positive correlations due to structured noise arising from confounds such as head movements and cardiac pulsations, whereas AC estimates tend to contain false negatives mainly due to the crossing fiber problem during tractography. Combining both data should thus help alleviate the problems linked to individual modalities. To fuse AC and FC, we use a data-driven adaptive weighting scheme that is based on the reliability of local FC information. To encode AC and FC information, we use a neighborhood-information-embedded multiple density (NMD) affinity matrix which has been recently shown to facilitate adaptive adjustment of voxel affinity values and provide robustness against noise [6].

To evaluate our proposed approach, we use the real data obtained from the Human Connectome Project (HCP) [7]. We apply our approach on normalized cuts (Ncuts) [8] and Ward clustering which are two of the most popular clustering methods for parcellation [1]. We demonstrate the benefits of incorporating AC information by comparing unimodal FC-based vs. multimodal parcellation. We show that our multimodal method achieves higher test-retest reliability and increases inter-subject consistency compared to unimodal parcellation. Further, we qualitatively illustrate that subject-specific parcellation maps better resemble the group parcellation maps when the multimodal approach is used.

2 Materials

In this work, we used the publicly available multimodal HCP Q2 dataset [7]. Along with other imaging modalities, this dataset comprises dMRI and RS-fMRI scans of 38 subjects with no history of neurological disease (17 males and 21 females, ages ranging from 22 to 35).

2.1 RS-fMRI Data

The RS-fMRI data comprised two sessions, each having a 30 minute acquisition with a TR of 0.72 s and an isotropic voxel size of 2 mm. Preprocessing already applied to the data by HCP [9] included gradient distortion correction, motion correction, spatial normalization to MNI space, and intensity normalization. Additionally, we regressed out motion artifacts, mean white matter and cerebrospinal fluid signals, and principal components of high variance voxels. Next, we applied a bandpass filter with cutoff frequencies of 0.01 and 0.1 Hz to minimize the effects of low frequency drift and high frequency noise. The data were finally demeaned and normalized by the standard deviation.

2.2 dMRI Data

The dMRI data had an isotropic voxel size of 1.25 mm, three shells (b=1000, 2000 and 3000 s/mm^2) and 288 gradient directions with six b=0 images. The data, which have already been corrected for EPI distortion, eddy current, gradient nonlinearity and motion artifacts by HCP [9], were downsampled to 2 mm isotropic resolution to reduce the computational cost.

3 Methods

Our approach starts by estimating the AC and FC from dMRI and fMRI data, respectively, in Section 3.1. Subsequently, we construct our multimodal connectivity model by fusing anatomical and functional connectivity information into a single connectivity metric in Section 3.2. We provide an overview of how we encode our connectivity metric into a neighborhood-informed affinity matrix in Section 3.3, on which parcellation is finally performed using clustering method.

3.1 Estimating Brain Connectivity

AC Estimation: We perform whole-brain deterministic global tractography on dMRI data using MITK [10] to reconstruct all fiber tracts in the brain simultaneously, which alleviates error propagation along tracts. Given the tracts, we define an AC fingerprint for each voxel [11] as the number of tracts connecting that voxel to each target region. Target regions can be taken as every other voxel, or parcels from an initial parcellation map. Since the human brain has a sparse AC structure, we opt to use the 116 regions in the Automated Anatomical Labeling (AAL) atlas as target regions instead of using individual voxels. This reduces the number of unknowns to be estimated, i.e. elements of AC fingerprints, from more than 100,000 to 116 per voxel, resulting in more robust AC estimates in addition to reducing computational complexity. Finally, our AC estimate is defined as the cross-correlation between the computed AC fingerprints of voxels of interest. Depending on the application, voxels of interest can be defined as the voxels in the whole brain or specific regions.

FC Estimation: Let $\mathbf{Z}$ be a $t \times N$ matrix of preprocessed fMRI time courses, where t is the number of time points and N is the number of voxels of interest. We estimate the FC matrix using Pearson's correlation: $\mathbf{FC} = \mathbf{Z}^T\mathbf{Z}/(t-1)$. Although the interpretation of negative correlations is currently an open research problem, there is a lack of anatomical evidence for negative correlations unlike positive correlations [12]. We thus set negative values in the FC matrix to zero.

3.2 Adaptively Weighted Multimodal Connectivity Model

To reduce false positive correlations in FC estimates and false negatives in AC estimates, we propose a multimodal CBP model that we later demonstrate to outperform the unimodal approach.

Multimodal Connectivity Model: To generate our multimodal connectivity matrix **MC**, we deploy the following linearly weighted model:

$$\mathbf{MC}_{ij} = \rho_{ij}\mathbf{FC}_{ij} + (1 - \rho_{ij})\mathbf{AC}_{ij}, \tag{1}$$

where $\mathbf{AC}_{ij}$ and $\mathbf{FC}_{ij}$ are estimates of AC and FC between voxels i and j, and ρ_{ij} is the relative weighting term.

Normalization: It is important to note that naive combination of AC and FC values may not be suitable since their distributions are largely divergent. FC distribution has a mean value of 0.2564 as empirically estimated from a group of 38 healthy subjects, while AC distribution has a mean value of 0.7295. The difference in their distribution makes a single value in two distributions represent different measures of connectivity, leading to misleading combined correlation value. To compensate for this, we map the AC values to match the FC distribution using histogram matching as follows. Let $a_1 \leq a_2, \ldots, \leq a_M$ be the raw AC data, and $f_1 \leq f_2, \ldots, \leq f_M$ be the FC values, where M is the number of voxel pairs. We compute the histograms of AC and FC, followed by their cumulative distribution functions $F_a(x) = P(X \leq x), x \in [a_1, a_M]$ and $F_f(y) = P(Y \leq y), y \in [f_1, f_M]$. $P(X \leq x)$ is the probability that the random variable X takes on a value less than or equal to x. Next, we replace each AC value a_i with the FC value f_j which satisfies $F_a(a_i) = F_f(f_j)$. This normalization enables unbiased multimodal AC and FC data fusion, where each AC value after normalization is used in the multimodal connectivity model in (1).

Adaptive Weighting: To set the relative weighting term ρ_{ij} in (1) in a data-driven manner, we construct a measure of local reliability in fMRI observations. The idea is to weigh down the effect of FC in voxels where fMRI observations are deemed to be unreliable. We estimate a reliability metric γ_i for a given voxel i as the cross-correlation of its local FC fingerprints estimated from the first and second halves (indicated as **FC1** and **FC2**) of its time points. The local FC fingerprint of voxel i refers to the FC profiles within its neighborhood δ_i, i.e. $\{\mathbf{FC}_{ik}\}$, $\forall k, k \in \delta_i$. Presumably, the local FC fingerprint of a voxel should be similar in two different time windows in the absence of an explicit task and noise. The reliability values γ_i will be low for voxels where noise in fMRI time courses is more pronounced, and more weight will be assigned to AC. This metric can be mathematically expressed as:

$$\gamma_i = \frac{n_{\delta_i} \sum\limits_{k \in \delta_i} \mathbf{FC1}_{ik}\mathbf{FC2}_{ik} - \sum\limits_{k \in \delta_i} \mathbf{FC1}_{ik} \sum\limits_{k \in \delta_i} \mathbf{FC2}_{ik}}{\sqrt{n_{\delta_i} \sum\limits_{k \in \delta_i} \mathbf{FC1}_{ik}^2 - (\sum\limits_{k \in \delta_i} \mathbf{FC1}_{ik})^2} \sqrt{n_{\delta_i} \sum\limits_{k \in \delta_i} \mathbf{FC2}_{ik}^2 - (\sum\limits_{k \in \delta_i} \mathbf{FC2}_{ik})^2}} \tag{2}$$

where n_{δ_i} is the number of neighbors of voxel i. We set δ_i to be the 26 nearest neighborhood of voxel i. We use the information from the immediate neighbors of a given voxel, as it has been shown that larger neighborhoods might make the analysis more prone to acquisition and registration artifacts [3]. The reliability of a functional connection, ρ_{ij}, is implicitly bounded by the voxel $v, v \in \{i, j\}$, having relatively lower reliability. As such, we define ρ_{ij} as the minimum reliability of voxels i and j as shown in (3).

$$\rho_{ij} = min(\gamma_i, \gamma_j) \tag{3}$$

3.3 Affinity Matrix Estimation

Traditionally, correlations or distances are mapped using a Gaussian kernel to produce an affinity matrix for clustering. However, this entails an inherent assumption of fixed density distribution of affinity values, which rarely holds true in practice. We thus adopt the NMD affinity matrix [6], which embeds local neighborhood information into the affinity matrix and adaptively tunes the density distribution of affinity values. The NMD affinity matrix is defined as:

$$\mathbf{A}_{ij}^{\mathbf{MC}} = \exp(-\frac{K_i K_j d_{ij}^2}{\overline{d_i}\,\overline{d_j}}), \tag{4}$$

where d_{ij} is the distance between voxels i and j defined as $1 - \mathbf{MC}_{ij}$, $\overline{d_i}$ is the average distance between voxel i and the one fourth of its nearest neighbors [6], and K_i is a measure of the spread of $\{d_i\}$, the set of distance values from voxel i to all of its neighbors as we proposed in [6]. This formulation effectively modifies the $\mathbf{A}_{ij}$ values based on putative cluster memberships of voxels i and j. Specifically, it scales the affinity value down when i and j are likely to be in different clusters since the spread of $\{d_i\}$ and $\{d_j\}$ would presumably be large, resulting in a large $K_i K_j$. The opposite holds true when voxels i and j are likely to be in the same cluster. $\mathbf{A}_{ij}^{\mathbf{FC}}$ values for unimodal parcellation can be generated by defining d_{ij} in (4) as $1 - \mathbf{FC}_{ij}$.

In our experiments, we use $\mathbf{A}_{ij}^{\mathbf{FC}}$ and $\mathbf{A}_{ij}^{\mathbf{MC}}$ as the inputs to clustering methods for unimodal and multimodal parcellation, respectively. We highlight that the estimation of multimodal connectivity model and affinity matrices are independent of the clustering method chosen and they can be used in conjunction with any clustering algorithm that takes an affinity matrix as its input. Similar results have been observed using Ward clustering, however we only show the results obtained using Ncuts due to the space limitations.

4 Results and Discussion

In this work, we focused on parcellating the inferior parietal lobule (IPL) and the visual cortex (VC), both known to possess functional and anatomical heterogeneity [13,14]. The voxels of interest are thus taken to be the voxels within the IPL and VC from the left hemisphere in the AAL atlas. In the HCP dataset, dMRI data are in the native diffusion space of each subject whereas fMRI data are in the standard MNI space. To fuse AC and FC in a common space, we warped the fractional anisotropy image of each subject to the MNI space using affine registration. The resulting transformation was then used to map the AC matrices of each individual subject to the MNI space using nearest neighbor interpolation.

Cortical parcellation maps are challenging to validate due to the lack of ground truth. However, assuming there truly is a functional parcellation, it should presumably remain stable for each subject and consistent across subjects. Thus, we base our quantitative validation on intra-subject stability and inter-subject consistency of the resulting brain parcels, which we measure using Dice similarity coefficient after relabeling parcels using the Hungarian algorithm [15]. Further, we qualitatively evaluate our method by visually comparing the group parcellation map with those estimated from individual subjects. Our rationale here is that the group map is expected to be more reliable since it is generated by pooling data across subjects, effectively increasing the SNR. It can thus be used as pseudo ground truth to compare individual parcellation maps against. As common in literatures [13,14], we divided the IPL into six and the VC into nine subregions in our experiments.

4.1 Quantitative Results

Intra-Subject Test-Retest Reliability: To evaluate the intra-subject test-retest reliability of our proposed approach, we calculated the subject-specific parcellation maps from the two RS-fMRI sessions of each subject separately. We then compared the resulting two parcellation maps for each subject and averaged the results across subjects. In the IPL, our proposed multimodal CBP method improved the test-retest reliability from 0.92 ± 0.09 to 0.94 ± 0.08 compared to unimodal parcellation. In the VC, our method increased the average Dice coefficient from 0.88 ± 0.08 to 0.90 ± 0.08. The difference between the two techniques are statistically significant for both regions at $p < 0.05$ based on the Wilcoxon signed rank test, which was also used in inter-subject validation.

Inter-Subject Consistency: We adopted the leave-one-out cross-validation approach to assess inter-subject consistency. Taking one subject at a time, we compared the group parcellation map obtained using the remaining subjects with the subject-specific parcellation map. For generating group parcellation maps, we first concatenated the voxel time courses temporally across scans and S=38 subjects. Group FC matrices were then computed using the pooled time courses, and group AC matrices were generated by averaging AC matrices from S-1 subjects prior to applying Ncuts. In the IPL, using multimodal parcellation instead of unimodal improved the Dice coefficient from 0.85 ± 0.1 to 0.89 ± 0.1. In the VC, Dice coefficient improved from 0.85 ± 0.1 to 0.88 ± 0.09. For both regions, the difference is statistically significant at $p < 0.05$.

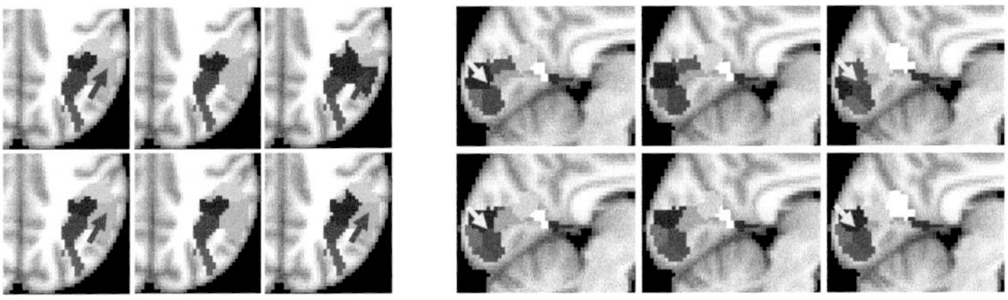

Fig. 1. Qualitative results for the IPL (left) and the VC (right) using the HCP data. For each region, top row shows the results of FC-based parcellation, and bottom row shows the results of the proposed multimodal parcellation. 1st column: Group maps, 2nd and 3rd columns: The subject-specific maps with the highest and lowest Dice coefficient with the group maps. The significant differences are highlighted with arrows.

4.2 Qualitative Results

To qualitatively evaluate the reliability of our proposed method, we generated a group parcellation map using the group affinity matrix of all subjects, and compared it with subject-specific parcellation maps. For brevity, we only present subjects showing the highest and lowest similarity with the group map indicated by Dice coefficient in Fig. 1. The group maps obtained using FC-based unimodal parcellation and the proposed multimodal CBP did not exhibit major differences indicating that using unimodal parcellation suffices when there is enough data. However, the subject-specific map having the lowest Dice coefficient (top right) shows major differences compared to the group map (top left) when the unimodal method is used. It can be observed that there are differences in the number of parcels and the parcel boundaries on the slices shown. In contrast, more reliable results can be obtained using our proposed multimodal method. Taken collectively, our results indicate that incorporating AC information into parcellation can increase the robustness of the analysis, resulting in more reproducible parcels both among different scans of the same subject and across different subjects.

5 Conclusions

We proposed a multimodal approach to cortical parcellation based on joint analysis of anatomical and functional brain connectivity. Our method determines the weighting between AC and FC in a data-driven manner, by adaptively assigning higher weight to AC at voxels where FC is deemed less reliable. On real data from 38 healthy subjects, we quantitatively demonstrated the potential of our method compared to FC-based unimodal parcellation in terms of test-retest reliability and inter-subject consistency. Qualitatively, we showed that subject-specific parcellations better resemble the group maps using our multimodal CBP model. We thus argue that multimodal parcellation may enable more reliable identification of brain regions leading to potentially more accurate higher-level brain network analyses. Our future work will focus on the metric learning for the fusion method, and the application of our method to whole-brain parcellation.

References

1. Thirion, B., Varoquaux, G., Dohmatob, E., Poline, J.-B.: Which fmri clustering gives good brain parcellations? Frontiers in Neuroscience 8 (2014)
2. de Reus, M.A., Van den Heuvel, M.P.: The parcellation-based connectome: limitations and extensions. Neuroimage 80, 397–404 (2013)
3. Honey, C., Sporns, O., Cammoun, L., Gigandet, X., Thiran, J.P., Meuli, R., Hagmann, P.: Predicting human resting-state functional connectivity from structural connectivity. Proceedings of the National Academy of Sciences 106(6), 2035–2040 (2009)
4. Wang, J., Yang, Y., Fan, L., Xu, J., Li, C., Liu, Y., Fox, P.T., Eickhoff, S.B., Yu, C., Jiang, T.: Convergent functional architecture of the superior parietal lobule unraveled with multimodal neuroimaging approaches. Human Brain Mapping 36(1), 238–257 (2015)
5. Zhang, D., Snyder, A.Z., Shimony, J.S., Fox, M.D., Raichle, M.E.: Noninvasive functional and structural connectivity mapping of the human thalamocortical system. Cerebral Cortex 20(5), 1187–1194 (2010)
6. Wang, C., Yoldemir, B., Abugharbieh, R.: Improved functional cortical parcellation using a neighborhood-information-embedded affinity matrix. In: IEEE International Symposium on Biomedical Imaging, pp. 1340–1343. IEEE Press (2015)
7. Van Essen, D.C., Smith, S.M., Barch, D.M., Behrens, T.E., Yacoub, E., Ugurbil, K., Consortium, W.M.H., et al.: The wu-minn human connectome project: an overview. Neuroimage 80, 62–79 (2013)
8. Craddock, R.C., James, G.A., Holtzheimer, P.E., Hu, X.P., Mayberg, H.S.: A whole brain fmri atlas generated via spatially constrained spectral clustering. Human Brain Mapping 33(8), 1914–1928 (2012)
9. Glasser, M.F., Sotiropoulos, S.N., Wilson, J.A., Coalson, T.S., Fischl, B., Andersson, J.L., Xu, J., Jbabdi, S., Webster, M., Polimeni, J.R., et al.: The minimal preprocessing pipelines for the human connectome project. Neuroimage 80, 105–124 (2013)
10. Neher, P.F., Stieltjes, B., Reisert, M., Reicht, I., Meinzer, H.P., Fritzsche, K.H.: Mitk global tractography. In: SPIE Medical Imaging, International Society for Optics and Photonics, pp. 83144D–83144D (2012)
11. Johansen-Berg, H., Behrens, T., Robson, M., Drobnjak, I., Rushworth, M., Brady, J., Smith, S., Higham, D., Matthews, P.: Changes in connectivity profiles define functionally distinct regions in human medial frontal cortex. Proceedings of the National Academy of Sciences of the United States of America 101(36), 13335–13340 (2004)
12. Skudlarski, P., Jagannathan, K., Calhoun, V.D., Hampson, M., Skudlarska, B.A., Pearlson, G.: Measuring brain connectivity: diffusion tensor imaging validates resting state temporal correlations. Neuroimage 43(3), 554–561 (2008)
13. Wang, J., Fan, L., Zhang, Y., Liu, Y., Jiang, D., Zhang, Y., Yu, C., Jiang, T.: Tractography-based parcellation of the human left inferior parietal lobule. Neuroimage 63(2), 641–652 (2012)
14. Montaser-Kouhsari, L., Landy, M.S., Heeger, D.J., Larsson, J.: Orientation-selective adaptation to illusory contours in human visual cortex. The Journal of Neuroscience 27(9), 2186–2195 (2007)
15. Munkres, J.: Algorithms for the assignment and transportation problems. Journal of the Society for Industrial & Applied Mathematics 5(1), 32–38 (1957)

Slic-Seg: Slice-by-Slice Segmentation Propagation of the Placenta in Fetal MRI Using One-Plane Scribbles and Online Learning

Guotai Wang[1], Maria A. Zuluaga[1], Rosalind Pratt[1,2], Michael Aertsen[3], Anna L. David[2], Jan Deprest[4], Tom Vercauteren[1], and Sebastien Ourselin[1]

[1]Translational Imaging Group, CMIC, University College London, UK
[2]Institute for Women's Health, University College London, UK
[3]Department of Radiology, University Hospitals KU Leuven, Belgium
[4]Department of Obstetrics, University Hospitals KU Leuven, Belgium

Abstract. Segmentation of the placenta from fetal MRI is critical for planning of fetal surgical procedures. Unfortunately, it is made difficult by poor image quality due to sparse acquisition, inter-slice motion, and the widely varying position and orientation of the placenta between pregnant women. We propose a minimally interactive online learning-based method named Slic-Seg to obtain accurate placenta segmentations from MRI. An online random forest is first trained on data coming from scribbles provided by the user in one single selected start slice. This then forms the basis for a slice-by-slice framework that segments subsequent slices before incorporating them into the training set on the fly. The proposed method was compared with its offline counterpart that is with no retraining, and with two other widely used interactive methods. Experiments show that our method 1) has a high performance in the start slice even in cases where sparse scribbles provided by the user lead to poor results with the competitive approaches, 2) has a robust segmentation in subsequent slices, and 3) results in less variability between users.

1 Introduction

The placenta plays a critical role in the health of the fetus during pregnancy. Abnormalities in the placental vasculature such as occur in twin-to-twin transfusion syndrome (TTTS) [4], can result in unequal blood distribution and a poor outcome or death for one or both twins. Placenta accreta, which is caused by an abnormally adherent placenta invading the myometrium, increases the risk of heavy bleeding during delivery. Minimally-invasive fetoscopic surgery provides an effective treatment for such placental abnormalities, and surgical planning is critical to reduce treatment-related morbidity and mortality.

With advantages such as large field of view, lack of ionizing radiation and good soft tissue contrast, Magnetic Resonance Imaging (MRI) is widely used for general surgical planning, but high-quality MRI for a fetus is difficult to achieve, since the free movement of the fetus in the uterus can cause severe motion artifacts [7]. The Single Shot Fast Spin Echo (SSFSE) allows the motion

N. Navab et al. (Eds.): MICCAI 2015, Part III, LNCS 9351, pp. 29–37, 2015.
DOI: 10.1007/978-3-319-24574-4_4

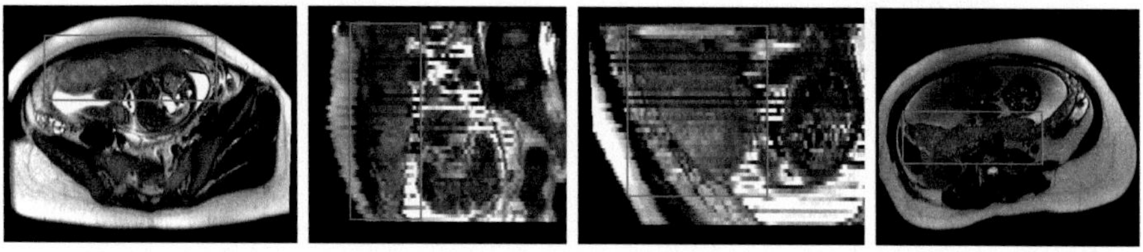

(a) axial view (b) saggital view (c) coronal view (d) axial view

Fig. 1. Examples of fetal MRI. (a), (b) and (c) are from one patient while (d) is from another. Note the motion artifacts and different appearance in odd and even slices in (b) and (c). The position of the placenta is anterior in (a), but posterior in (d).

artifacts to be nearly absent in each slice, but inter-slice motions still corrupt the volumetric data. The slices are acquired in an interleaved spatial order, which leads to different appearance between odd and even slices as shown in Fig. 1. In addition, fetal MRI is usually sparsely acquired with a large inter-slice spacing for a good contrast-to-noise ratio. Although some novel reconstruction techniques [5] can get super-resolution volume data of fetal brain from sparsely acquired slices, they have yet to demonstrate their utility for placental imaging and require a dedicated non-standard acquisition protocol. These factors bring several challenges to the segmentation of the placenta from clinical MR data.

The low-quality volumetric data with high-quality slices motivates employing 2D segmentation methods with a slice-by-slice strategy. Automatic methods rarely work well with medical images due to ambiguous appearance cues. Prior-knowledge brought from different patients in the form of shape/appearance models or propagated atlases [6] may help make the segmentation more robust, but the position and orientation of the placenta within the uterus varies greatly between pregnancies (see Fig. 1(a) and Fig. 1(d)), making it hard to model such statistical prior-knowledge. In contrast, interactive segmentation has been widely used in practice, where scribbles given by user provide useful information for accurate segmentation. A convenient interactive method should make full use of scribbles to get accurate segmentation with only a few number of user interactions. Traditional methods such as snakes or generalized gradient vector flow (GGVF) [10] use only the spatial information of an initial contour provided by the user, others such as Graph Cuts [2] and Geodesic Framework [1,3] take advantage of low level features to estimate the probability that a pixel belongs to the foreground or background.

In this paper, we propose a learning-based semi-automatic approach named Slic-Seg for segmentation of the placenta in fetal MRI. It is different from traditional interactive segmentation methods in the following ways: 1) It aims to make full use of user inputs to improve the accuracy and reduce number of user interactions. 2) Online Random Forest (RF) is employed for effective learning based on mid-level features, allowing the training set to be expanded on the fly. As a result, the method can achieve a high performance with a minimal number of user inputs.

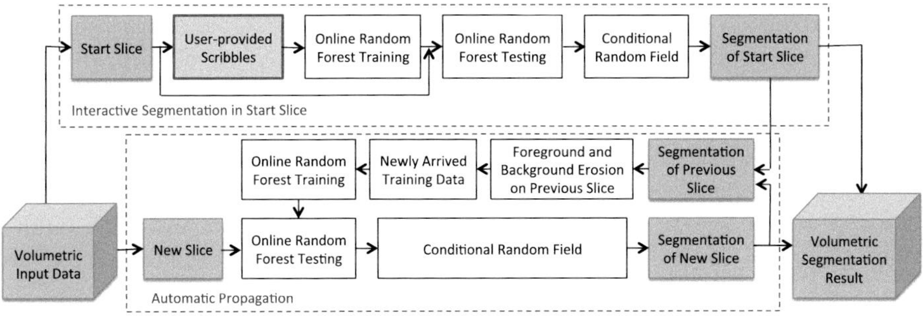

Fig. 2. The workflow of our Slic-Seg framework. User interaction is only required in the start slice. Other slices are segmented sequentially and automatically.

2 Methods

The workflow of our proposed Slic-Seg is shown in Fig. 2. A user selects a start slice and draws a few scribbles in that slice to indicate foreground and background. Online RF efficiently learns from these inputs and predicts the probability that an unlabeled pixel belongs to foreground or background. That probability is incorporated into a Conditional Random Field (CRF) to get the segmentation result based on which new training data is automatically obtained and added to the training set of RF predictor on the fly. To get the segmentation result from a volumetric placenta data, other slices are segmented sequentially and automatically without more user interactions.

Preprocess and Feature Extraction. Odd and even slices are rigidly aligned together to correct the motion artifacts, and histogram matching is implemented to address the different contrast between slices. For each pixel, features are extracted from a 9×9 pixel region of interest (ROI) centered on it. In each ROI, we extract gray level features including mean and standard deviation of intensity, texture features acquired by gray level co-occurrence matrix (GLCM) and wavelet coefficient features based on Haar wavelet.

Online Random Forests Training. A Random Forest [9] is a collection of binary decision trees composed of split nodes and leaf nodes. The training set of each tree is randomly resampled from the entire labeled training set (label 1 for the placenta and label 0 for background). At a split node, a binary test is executed to minimize the uncertainty of the class label in the subsets based on Information Gain. The test functions are of the form $f(\mathbf{x}) > \theta$, where $\mathbf{x}$ is the feature vector of one sample, $f(\cdot)$ is a linear function, and θ is a threshold. At a leaf node, labels of all the training samples that have been propagated to that node are averaged, and the average label is interpreted as the posterior probability of a sample belonging to the placenta, given that the sample has fallen into that leaf node.

The training data in our application is obtained in one of two ways according on segmentation stage. For the start slice, training data comes from the scribbles provided by the user. During the propagation, after one slice is segmented, skeletonization of the placenta was implemented by morphological operators, and the background is eroded by a kernel with a certain radius (e.g., 10 pixels). New training data is obtained from the morphological operation results in that slice and added to existing training set of RF on the fly. To deal with online training, we use the online bagging [8] method to model the sequential arrival of training data as a Poisson distribution Pois(λ) where λ is set to a constant number. Each tree is updated on each new training sample k times in a row where k is a random number generated by Pois(λ).

Online Random Forests Testing. During the testing, each pixel sample $\mathbf{x}$ is propagated through all trees. For the nth tree, a posterior probability $p_n(\mathbf{x})$ is obtained from the leaf that the test sample falls into. The final posterior is achieved as the average across all the N trees.

$$p(\mathbf{x}) = \frac{1}{N} \sum_{n=1}^{N} p_n(\mathbf{x}) \tag{1}$$

Inference Using Conditional Random Field. In the prediction of RF, the posterior probability for each pixel is obtained independently and it is sensitive to noise. To reduce the effect of noise and obtain the final label set for all the pixels in a slice, a CRF is used for a global spatial regularization. The label set of a slice is determined by minimizing the following energy function:

$$E(\mathbf{c}) = -\alpha \sum_{i} \Psi(\mathbf{c}_i|\mathbf{x}_i, I) - \sum_{i,j} \Phi(\mathbf{c}_i, \mathbf{c}_j|I) \tag{2}$$

where the unary potential $\Psi(\mathbf{c}_i|\mathbf{x}_i, I)$ is computed as $\log p(\mathbf{c}_i|\mathbf{x}_i, I)$ for assigning a class label $\mathbf{c}_i$ to the ith pixel in a slice I, and p comes from the output of RF. The pairwise potential $\Phi(\mathbf{c}_i, \mathbf{c}_j|I)$ is defined as a contrast sensitive Potts model $\phi(\mathbf{c}_i, \mathbf{c}_j, \mathbf{g}_{ij})$ [2] where $\mathbf{g}_{ij}$ measures the difference in intensity between the neighboring pixels and can be computed very efficiently. α is a coefficient to adjust the weight between unary potential and pairwise potential. The energy minimization is solved by a max flow algorithm [2]. A CRF is used in every slice of the volumetric image, and after the propagation, we stack the segmentation of all slices to construct the final volumetric segmentation result.

3 Experiments and Results

Experiment Data and Setting. MRI scanning of 6 fetuses in the second trimester were collected. For each fetus we had two volumetric data in different views that were used independently: 1), axial view with slice dimension

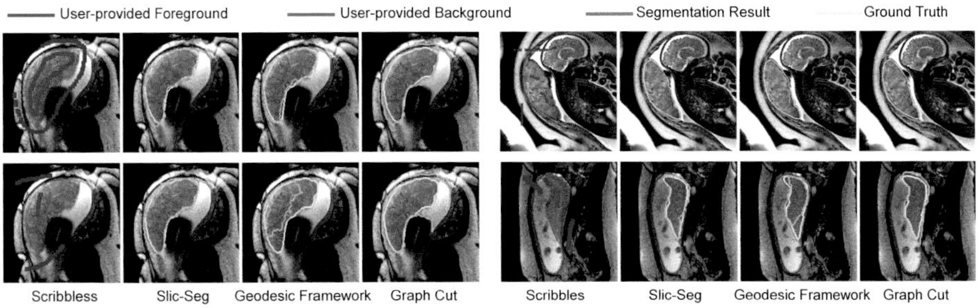

Fig. 3. Visual comparison of segmentation in the start slice by different methods. Upper left: user inputs are extensive, all methods result in a good segmentation. Lower left: user inputs are reduced in the same slice, only Slic-Seg perserves the accuracy. Right: two more examples show Slic-Seg has a better performance than Geodesic Framework and Graph Cut with only a few user inputs.

512×448, voxel spacing 0.7422 mm×0.7422 mm, slice thickness 3mm. 2) sagittal view with slice dimension 256×256, voxel spacing 1.484mm×1.484mm, slice thickness 4mm. A start slice in the middle region of the placenta was selected from each volumetric image, and 8 users provided scribbles in the start slice. A manual ground truth for each slice was produced by an experienced radiologist. The algorithm was implemented in C++ with a MATLAB interface. Parameter setting was: $\lambda=1$, $N=20$, $\alpha=4.8$. We found the segmentation was not sensitive to α in the range of 2 to 15 (see supplementary). The depth of trees was 10.

Results and Evaluation. We compared Slic-Seg with two widely used interactive segmentation methods: Geodesic Framework[1] of Bai and Sapiro [1] and Graph Cut [2]. Fig. 3 shows four examples of interactive segmentation in the start slice. In each subfigure, the same scribbles were used by different segmentation methods. On the left side of Fig. 3, the same slice was used with different scribbles. In the upper left case, scribbles provided by the user almost roughly indicate the boundary of the placenta, and all of the three methods obtain good segmentation results. In the lower left case, scribbles are reduced to a very small annotation set, Geodesic Framework and Graph Cut fail to preserve their performance, but Slic-Seg can still get a rather accurate segmentation. Two more cases on the right of Fig. 3 also show Slic-Seg can successfully segment the placenta using only a few number of scribbles.

In the propagation, the above three methods used the same morphological operations as mentioned previously to automatically generate foreground and background seeds for a new slice. In addition, we compared Slic-Seg with its offline counterpart where only user inputs in the start slice were used for training of an offline RF. Fig. 4 shows an example of propagation by different methods with the same user inputs in the start slice. S_i represents the ith slice following the start slice. In Fig. 4, though a good segmentation is obtained in the start

[1] Implementation from: `http://www.robots.ox.ac.uk/$\sim$vgg/software/iseg/`

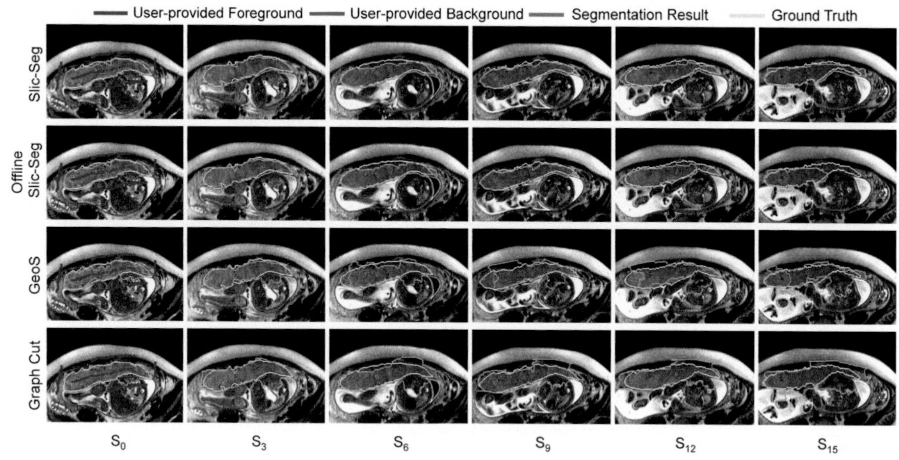

Fig. 4. Propagation of different methods with the same start slice and scribbles. S_i represents the ith slice following the start slice. User provided scribbles in S_0 are extensive and all methods have a good segmentation in that slice. However, during the propagation, only Slic-Seg keeps a high performance. (More slices are shown in the supplementary video).

slice due to an extensive set of scribbles, the error of Geodesic Framework and Graph Cut become increasingly large during the propagation. In a slice that is close to the start slice (e.g. $i \leq 9$), offline Slic-Seg can obtain a segmentation comparable to that of Slic-Seg. When a new slice (e.g. $i \geq 12$) is further away from the start slice, offline Slic-Seg fails to track the placenta with high accuracy. In contrast, online Slic-Seg has a stable performance during the propagation.

Quantitative evaluation was achieved by calculating the Dice coefficient and symmetric surface distance (SSD) between segmentation results and the ground truth. Fig. 5 shows the Dice coefficient and SSD for each slice in one volumetric image (the same image as used in Fig. 4). For each slice, we use error bars to show the first quartile, median and the third quartile of the Dice coefficient and SSD. Fig. 5 shows that Slic-Seg has a better performance in the start slice and during the propagation than offline Slic-Seg, Geodesic Framework and Graph Cut. The less dispersion of Slic-Seg indicates its less variability between users. Fig. 6 shows the evaluation results on data from all the patients. We present Dice and SSD in both the start slice and the whole image volume.

Discussion. The experiments show that Slic-Seg using RF, CRF and segmentation propagation has better performances in the start slice and during propagation than Geodesic Framework and Graph Cut. This is due to the fact that the last two methods use low level appearance features to model placenta and background, which may not be accurate enough in fetal MRI images with poor quality. In contrast, the RF in our method uses mid-level features of multiple aspects including intensity, texture and wavelet coefficients, which may provide

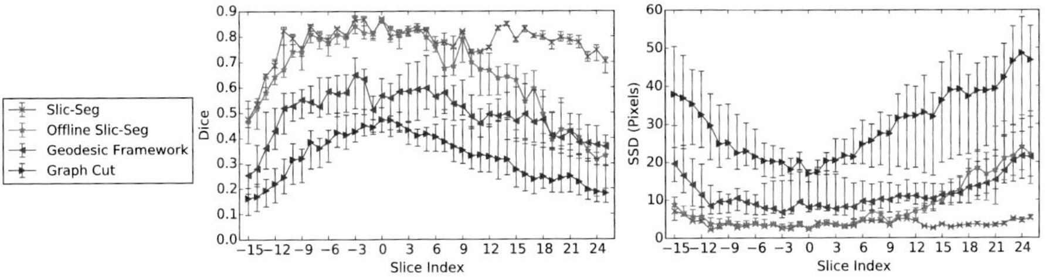

Fig. 5. Evaluation on one image volume in terms of Dice (left) and SSD (right) in each slice (evaluation on other image volumes can be found in the supplementary). Each error bar shows the median, first quartile and third quartile across all the 8 users, each of which segmented the image twice with different scribbles. Note that Slic-Seg has a high accuracy in the start slice and during the propagation, with low variability among different users.

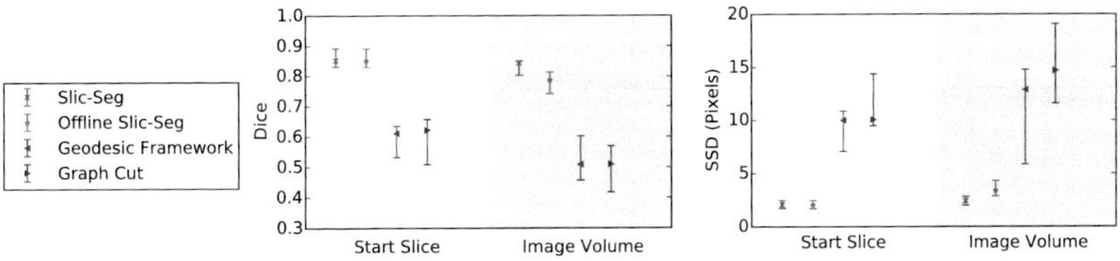

Fig. 6. Evaluation on data from all the 6 patients (each having 2 orthogonal datasets) in terms of Dice (left) and SSD (right) in the start slice and the whole image volume. Each of 8 users segmented these images twice with different scribbles. Note Slic-Seg and offline Slic-Seg get the same result in the start slice. Slic-Seg has a high performance with less variability in both the start slice and the whole image volume. The p value between Slic-Seg and offline Slice-Seg on the image volumes is 0.0043 for Dice, and 0.0149 for SSD.

a better description of the differences between the placenta and background. Because the appearance of the placenta in a remote slice could be different from that in the start slice, the offline RF that only uses user-provided scribbles for training may give a poor prediction after propagating along several slices. The online RF that accepts sequentially obtained training data addresses this problem and is adaptive to the appearance change, which leads to a more robust segmentation during the propagation. The short error bars of Slic-Seg in Fig. 5 and Fig. 6 indicate that the performance of this method has a low variability among different users. Though our method requires user interactions only in the start slice, it could allow user corrections with some additional scribbles when the segmentation propagates to terminal slices. Since it needs fewer user interactions and allows the training data to be expanded efficiently, the segmentation can be conveniently improved with little additional user efforts.

4 Conclusion

We present an interactive, learning-based method for the segmentation of the placenta in fetal MRI. Online RF is used to efficiently learn from mid-level features describing placenta and background, and it is combined with CRF for labelling. The slice-by-slice segmentation only requires user inputs in a start slice, and other slices are segmented sequentially and automatically to get a volumetric segmentation. Experiments show that the proposed method achieves high accuracy with minimal user interactions and less variability than traditional methods. It has a potential to provide an accurate segmentation of the placenta for fetal surgical planning. In the future, we intend to combine sparse volumetric data in different views for a 3D segmentation.

Acknowledgements. This work was supported through an Innovative Engineering for Health award by the Wellcome Trust [WT101957]; Engineering and Physical Sciences Research Council (EPSRC) [NS/A000027/1], the EPSRC (EP/H046410/1, EP/ J020990/1, EP/K005278), the National Institute for Health Research University College London Hospitals Biomedical Research Centre (NIHR BRC UCLH/UCL High Impact Initiative), a UCL Overseas Research Scholarship and a UCL Graduate Research Scholarship.

References

1. Bai, X., Sapiro, G.: A Geodesic Framework for Fast Interactive Image and Video Segmentation and Matting. IJCV 82(2), 113–132 (2008)
2. Boykov, Y., Jolly, M.P.: Interactive graph cuts for optimal boundary & region segmentation of objects in N-D images. In: ICCV 2001, vol. 1, pp. 105–112, July 2001
3. Criminisi, A., Sharp, T., Blake, A.: GeoS: Geodesic image segmentation. In: Forsyth, D., Torr, P., Zisserman, A. (eds.) ECCV 2008, Part I. LNCS, vol. 5302, pp. 99–112. Springer, Heidelberg (2008)
4. Deprest, J.A., Flake, A.W., Gratacos, E., Ville, Y., Hecher, K., Nicolaides, K., Johnson, M.P., Luks, F.I., Adzick, N.S., Harrison, M.R.: The Making of Fetal Surgery. Prenatal Diagnosis 30(7), 653–667 (2010)
5. Gholipour, A., Estroff, J.A., Warfield, S.K., Member, S.: Robust Super-Resolution Volume Reconstruction From Slice Acquisitions: Application to Fetal Brain MRI. IEEE TMI 29(10), 1739–1758 (2010)
6. Habas, P.A., Kim, K., Corbett-Detig, J.M., Rousseau, F., Glenn, O.A., Barkovich, A.J., Studholme, C.: A Spatiotemporal Atlas of MR Intensity, Tissue Probability and Shape of the Fetal Brain with Application to Segmentation. NeuroImage 53, 460–470 (2010)
7. Kainz, B., Malamateniou, C., Murgasova, M., Keraudren, K., Rutherford, M., Hajnal, J.V., Rueckert, D.: Motion corrected 3D reconstruction of the fetal thorax from prenatal MRI. In: Golland, P., Hata, N., Barillot, C., Hornegger, J., Howe, R. (eds.) MICCAI 2014, Part II. LNCS, vol. 8674, pp. 284–291. Springer, Heidelberg (2014)

8. Saffari, A., Leistner, C., Santner, J., Godec, M., Bischof, H.: On-line random forests. In: ICCV Workshops 2009 (2009)
9. Schroff, F., Criminisi, A., Zisserman, A.: Object class segmentation using random forests. In: BMVC 2008, pp. 54.1–54.10 (2008)
10. Xu, C., Prince, J.L.: Snakes, Shapes, and Gradient Vector Flow. IEEE TIP 7(3), 359–369 (1998)

GPSSI: Gaussian Process for Sampling Segmentations of Images

Matthieu Lê[1], Jan Unkelbach[2], Nicholas Ayache[1], and Hervé Delingette[1]

[1] Asclepios Project, INRIA Sophia Antipolis, France
[2] Department of Radiation Oncology, Massachusetts General Hospital and Harvard Medical School, Boston, MA, USA

Abstract. Medical image segmentation is often a prerequisite for clinical applications. As an ill-posed problem, it leads to uncertain estimations of the region of interest which may have a significant impact on downstream applications, such as therapy planning. To quantify the uncertainty related to image segmentations, a classical approach is to measure the effect of using various plausible segmentations. In this paper, a method for producing such image segmentation samples from a single expert segmentation is introduced. A probability distribution of image segmentation boundaries is defined as a Gaussian process, which leads to segmentations that are spatially coherent and consistent with the presence of salient borders in the image. The proposed approach outperforms previous generative segmentation approaches, and segmentation samples can be generated efficiently. The sample variability is governed by a parameter which is correlated with a simple DICE score. We show how this approach can have multiple useful applications in the field of uncertainty quantification, and an illustration is provided in radiotherapy planning.

1 Introduction

Medical image analysis, and in particular medical image segmentation, is a key technology for many medical applications, ranging from computer aided diagnosis to therapy planning and guidance. Medical image segmentation is probably the task most often required in those applications. Due to its ill-posed nature, the quantification of segmentation accuracy and uncertainty is crucial to assess the overall performance of other applications. For instance, in radiotherapy planning it is important to estimate the impact of uncertainty in the delineation of the gross tumor volume and the organs at risk on the dose delivered to the patient.

A straightforward way to assess this impact is to perform *Image Segmentation Sampling* (ISS), which consists of gathering several plausible segmentations of the same structure, and estimate the variability of the output variables due to the variability of the segmentations. For computer generated segmentations, ISS could simply be obtained by varying the parameters or initial values of the algorithm producing the segmentations. However, in many cases, parameters of the algorithms cannot be modified, and segmentations are partially edited by a user. For manual or semi-manual segmentations, it is possible to estimate the

N. Navab et al. (Eds.): MICCAI 2015, Part III, LNCS 9351, pp. 38–46, 2015.
DOI: 10.1007/978-3-319-24574-4_5

inter-expert variability on a few cases but it usually cannot be applied on large databases due to the amount of resources required.

This is why it is important to automate the generation of "plausible segmentations" that are "similar to" a given segmentation of a region of interest (ROI). This is the objective of this paper which, to the best of our knowledge, has not been tackled before. It is naturally connected to several prior work in the field of medical image segmentation. For instance, [1] have proposed segmentation approaches based on Markov Chain Monte Carlo where parameter sampling leads to an estimation of the posterior probability of obtaining a segmentation given an image. However in those approaches, the algorithm defines the likelihood and prior functions and then estimate the most probable (or the expected) segmentation whereas in ISS the objective is to sample directly from the posterior distribution, knowing only its mean or mode. Therefore they are not readily suitable to the task of ISS.

Other related approaches [2,3,4] are aiming at producing a consensus segmentation given several expert segmentations, or several atlas segmentations. They define probabilities of having a given segmentation based on a reference one, and their generative nature makes them suitable for ISS. Typical examples are the STAPLE algorithm [2], the log-odds maps [3] and their refinement [4]. However, as shown in section 2, the segmentations generated from a single expert segmentation lack plausibility, and the spatial regularity of the contours cannot be finely controlled.

In this paper, a novel framework is introduced to sample segmentations automatically leading to plausible delineations. More precisely, the proposed approach incorporates knowledge about image saliency of the ROI such that the sampled contours variability may be greater at poorly contrasted regions. Furthermore the proposed approach is mathematically well grounded, and enforces the spatial smoothness of the contours as it relies on Gaussian processes defined on implicit contours. Finally, segmentation sampling can be performed efficiently even on large medical images thanks to an original algorithm based on discrete Fourier transform. Variability in the samples is easily controlled by a single scalar, and an application to radiotherapy dose planning is described.

2 Existing Generative Models of Segmentations

This section reviews relevant generative models of segmentations proposed in the literature. Results are illustrated on a synthetic image (Fig. 1) for which the structure border is surrounded by regions of low and high contrast.

The probabilistic atlases [3] derived from log-odds of signed distance functions assume that voxels are independently distributed with a Bernouilli probability density function of parameter b whose value depends on the distance to the structure border. The STAPLE algorithm [2] is a region formulation for producing consensus segmentations. Given a binary segmentation T and expert sensitivity p and specificity q, the algorithm is associated with a generative model for which a segmentation D can be sampled knowing T as a Markov Random Field with

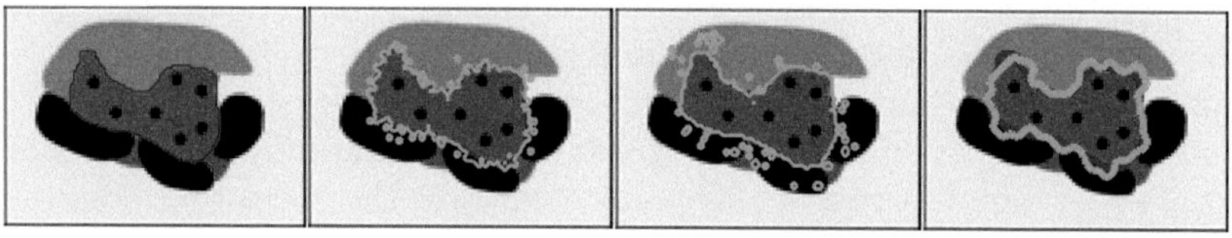

Fig. 1. From left to right: synthetic image with region of interest outlined in red; segmentation sampling based on log-odds; segmentation sampling based on STAPLE without ICM steps ($p = 68\%$ and $q = 66\%$); ISS based on STAPLE with ICM steps ($p = 68\%$ and $q = 66\%$). The ground truth is outlined in red, the samples are outlined in orange.

the likelihood term $P(D_i = 1) = pP(T_i = 1) + (1 - q)P(T_i = 0)$ and a prior accounting for local spatial coherence. Segmentations are generated by sampling independently the Bernoulli distribution at each voxel followed by a number of Iterated Conditional Modes (ICM) relaxation steps. Various ISS results are obtained in Fig. 1 for the log-odds and STAPLE generative models with specified parameters.

In all cases, the produced segmentations are not realistic for 2 reasons. First of all, the variability of the segmentation does not account for the intensity in the image such that borders with strong gradients are equally variable as borders with weak gradient. This is counter intuitive as the basic hypothesis of image segmentation is that changes of intensity are correlated with changes of labels. Second, borders of the segmented structures are unrealistic mainly due to their lack of geometric regularity (high frequency wobbling in Fig. 1 (Right)). While anatomical or pathological structure borders are not necessarily smooth (e.g. highly diffuse tumors), the generated samples show irregular generated contours in the presence of regular visible contours in the image which is not plausible.

3 GPSSI

3.1 Definition

We propose a generative model of image segmentation that overcomes the two limitations of previous approaches. First of all, spatial consistency of the sampled segmentations is reached by describing a probabilistic segmentation with a Gaussian process with a squared exponential covariance, which allows to easily control the spatial coherence of the segmentation. Second, sampled segmentations do take into account the image intensity by replacing the signed distance functions with signed geodesic distance. The geodesic distance makes voxels far away from the mean segmentation if they are separated from it by high gradient intensity regions. Therefore a random perturbation on the mean segmentation is unlikely to reach those voxels with high contrast, and more likely to affect voxels with low geodesic distance, i.e. voxels neighboring the mean segmentation with similar intensity values.

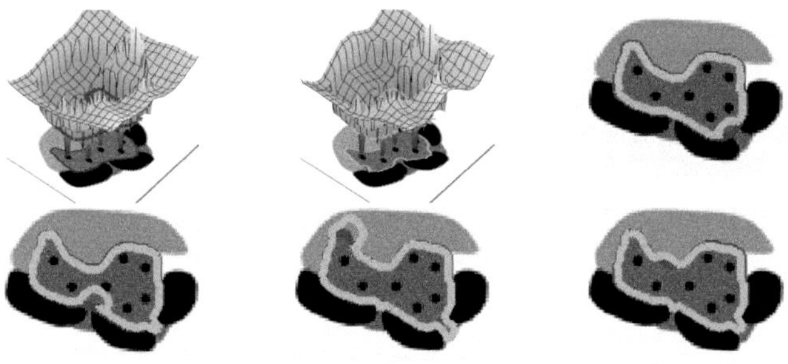

Fig. 2. (Top Left) Mean of the GP μ; (Top Middle) Sample of the level function $\varphi(\mathbf{x})$ drawn from $\mathcal{GP}(\mu, \Sigma)$; (Others) GPSSI samples. The ground truth is outlined in red, the GPSSI samples are outlined in orange.

A novel probabilistic framework of image segmentation is introduced by defining a level set function via a Gaussian process (GP). The mean of the GP is given by a signed geodesic distance, and its covariance is defined with a squared exponential driven by the Euclidean distance between voxels. Gaussian process implicit surfaces have been introduced previously by Williams *et al.* [5] as a generalization of thin plate splines and used recently [6] for surface reconstruction. However, our approach combining geodesic and Euclidean distance functions for the mean and covariance is original and specifically suited to represent probabilistic image segmentations.

Geodesic Distance Map. Signed geodesic distance map are computed as $\mathcal{G}(\mathbf{x}) = \min_{\Gamma \in \mathcal{P}_{\mathrm{seg},x}} \int_0^1 \sqrt{||\mathbf{\Gamma}'(s)||^2 + \gamma^2(\nabla\mathcal{I}(\mathbf{\Gamma}(s)) \cdot (\mathbf{\Gamma}'(s)/||\mathbf{\Gamma}'(\mathbf{s}))||)^2} ds$, where $\mathcal{I}$ is the input image, $\mathcal{P}_{\mathrm{seg},x}$ is the set of all paths between the voxel x and the segmentation $\mathcal{C}$, and Γ one such path, parametrized by $s \in [0,\ 1]$. The parameter γ sets the trade-off between Euclidean distance ($\gamma = 0$) and gradient information. Its implementation is based on a fast grid sweeping method as proposed in [7] where the gradient is computed with a Gaussian kernel convolution controlled by parameter h. Geodesic distance is set negative inside the segmentation and positive outside.

GPSSI. Gaussian processes (GP) are a generalization of multivariate Gaussian distributions, and provide a framework to define smooth probability distributions over functions. GP are widely used in machine learning for solving inference problems [8] over spatially correlated datasets. In this paper, it is the generative nature of GP that is of interest since they naturally produce spatially smooth samples in a straightforward manner. This is a key advantage over previous approaches such as Markov Random Fields which enforce the connectivity between labels rather than the geometric regularity of the boundary of a ROI.

In GPSSI, a segmentation is defined via a level function $\varphi(\mathbf{x})$, $\mathbf{x} \in \Omega$ such that its zero level set corresponds to the boundary of the ROI. Smoothness in the level function $\varphi(\mathbf{x})$ translates into the smoothness of the boundary $\mathcal{B}_\varphi = \{\mathbf{x}|\varphi(\mathbf{x}) = 0\}$. A GP is fully defined by its mean and covariance functions: its mean value is set to the signed geodesic distance $\mu(\mathbf{x}) = \mathcal{G}(\mathbf{x})$ while its covariance is chosen as the squared exponential function, $\Sigma(\mathbf{x}, \mathbf{y}) = w_0 \exp(-\|\mathbf{x} - \mathbf{y}\|^2 / w_1^2)$. This choice of covariance enforces the smoothness of the segmentation, with parameter w_1 characterizing the typical correlation length between two voxels while w_0 controls the amount of variability of the level function.

3.2 Efficient Sampling

Sampling of a GP is simply performed through the factorization of the covariance matrix at sample points. More precisely, let $\Omega_M = \{\mathbf{x}_i\}$, $i = 1 \ldots M$ be the set of M discrete points $\mathbf{x}_i$ where the level function $\varphi(\mathbf{x})$ is defined. Typically Ω_M may be the set of all voxel centers in the image. The covariance matrix $\Sigma_{ij}^{MM} = w_0 \exp(-\|\mathbf{x}_i - \mathbf{x}_j\|^2 / w_1^2)$ at sampled points is of size $M \times M$. To sample from a GP $\mathcal{GP}(\mu, \Sigma)$, a factorization of the covariance matrix $\Sigma^{MM} = LL^\top$ is required, such that given normally distributed variables $z \sim \mathcal{N}(0, 1)$, GPSSI are simply computed as the zero crossing of $\mu + L(w_0, w_1)z \sim \mathcal{GP}(\mu, \Sigma)$.

A classical issue with GP sampling is that the factorization of Σ^{MM} becomes ill-conditioned and computationally expensive for large values of M. Since in practice $M \approx 10^7$, a regular matrix factorization would not be feasible. To make the problem tractable, we take advantage of the regular grid structure of the image and make the additional assumption that periodic boundary conditions on the image apply. In this case, Σ^{MM} is a Block Circulant with Circulant Blocks (BCCB) matrix such that each row of Σ^{MM} is a periodic shift of the first row of Σ^{MM}, $C \in \mathrm{R}^M$. C can be seen as an image of M voxels, whose voxel value is the evaluation of the square exponential covariance for every shift present in the image. Theoretical results on the BCCB matrix spectral decomposition allow for a straightforward computation of $\Sigma^{MM} = \mathrm{F}^{-1}\mathrm{diag}(\mathrm{F}C)\mathrm{F}$, where F is the $M \times M$ discrete Fourier transform matrix. Hence, the eigenvalues of Σ^{MM} are the discrete Fourier transform of C. As such, if $z_1, z_2 \sim \mathcal{N}(0, \mathbb{I})$ i.i.d, then the real and imaginary part of $\mathrm{F}\sqrt{\mathrm{diag}(\mathrm{F}C)}(z_1 + iz_2)$ are two independent samples from the GP [9]. This can be efficiently computed using the Fast Fourier Transform without storing F.

4 Results

4.1 Parameter Setting

In the proposed approach, segmentation sampling depends on the scale h of the gradient operator, the parameter γ of the geodesic map, and the parameters ω_0 and ω_1 of the covariance function. The parameter h depends on the level of noise in the image (typically chosen as 1 voxel size) whereas γ controls the importance of the geodesic term. In our experiments, we set $\gamma = 100/\mathbb{E}(\mathcal{I})$, where $\mathbb{E}(\mathcal{I})$ is the mean of the image. Parameter w_1 controls the smoothness scale of the structure, and is chosen as the radius of the equivalent sphere given the volume V of the ROI: $w_1 = (\frac{3}{4\pi}V)^{\frac{1}{3}}$. Finally ω_0 controls the variability around the mean shape:

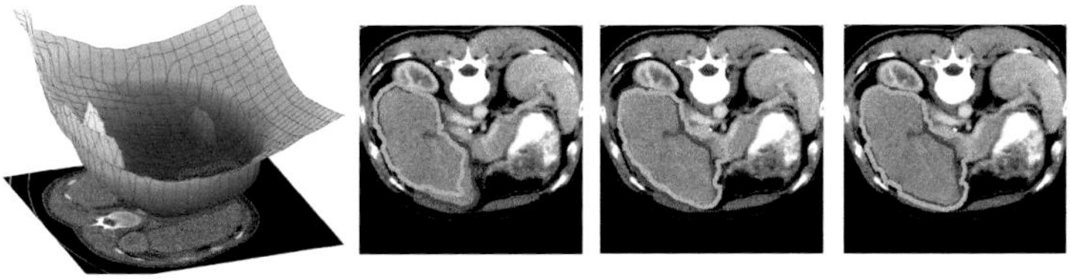

Fig. 3. From left to right, mean μ of the GP and three samples from $\mathcal{GP}(\mu, \Sigma)$. The clinician segmentation is outlined in red, the GPSSI samples are outlined in orange.

the greater ω_0, the greater the variability. Such variability may be practically quantified for instance in terms of mean DICE index between any pair of expert segmentations. In such case, it is easy to find ω_0 corresponding to a given DICE score (see Fig. 4). This approach offers an intuitive way to semi-automatically set the parameter ω_0. Instead of DICE score, one could also use quantiles of histograms of symmetric distances between contours.

4.2 Segmentation Sampling

Samples of the 2D synthetic segmentation case can be seen on Fig. 2 with $\omega_0 = 38$ corresponding to an inter sample DICE of 90%. Samples are coherent with the visible image boundary since most samples do not include highly contrasted (black) regions of the image but instead invade low contrast regions of the image.

Sampling of liver segmentation in CT image is shown in Fig. 3 with $\omega_0 = 4$ corresponding to an inter sample DICE index of 88%. The generation of each sample takes less than 1s on a PC laptop despite the size of the image ($256 \times 256 \times 104$). Samples tend to leak on structures with similar intensity as the liver parenchyma.

Segmentation sampling was also performed on a 3D T1 post contrast MRI (T1Gd MRI) where the proliferative part (active rim) of a grade IV glioma was segmented by an expert (Fig. 4 left). The strong correlation between the covariance parameter ω_0 and the inter-sample DICE coefficient was computed after generating 40 samples for each value of ω_0 (Fig. 4 right). Thus the user may easily choose ω_0 as a function of the desired DICE index.

Note that the likelihood of samples generated from $\mathcal{GP}(\mu, \Sigma)$ is not very informative as it is computed over the whole image and not just the generated contour.

5 Tumor Delineation Uncertainty in Radiotherapy

The proposed method is applied to the uncertainty quantification of radiotherapy planning. The standard of care for grade IV gliomas (Fig. 4) is the delivery of 60 Gray (Gy) to the Clinical Target Volume (CTV) which is defined as a 2-3cm extension of the Gross Tumor Volume (GTV) visible on a T1Gd MRI [10]. For the patient shown in Fig. 4, 40 segmentations of the GTV are sampled from a

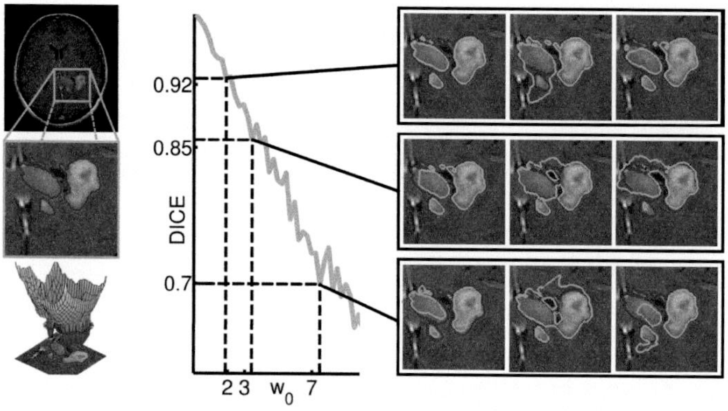

Fig. 4. (Left) Segmentation of brain tumor active rim from T1 MR image with Gadolinium contrast agent; (Right) Relationship between the parameter ω_0 and the inter-sample DICE score. The clinician segmentation is outlined in red, the GPSSI samples are outlined in orange. When ω_0 increases, the inter-sample DICE score decreases.

given segmentation with parameter ω_0 set to achieve a mean DICE coefficient of 85% between the sampled segmentations (Fig. 4). For each sample, a CTV is generated by considering a 2cm isotropic extension taking into account the natural barriers of the tumor progression (ventricles and falx cerebri).

Fig. 5 shows the mean target dose and its standard deviation derived from the 40 sampled CTVs. Several strategies could be applied to take into account the uncertainty in the GTV delineation. Generally, radiotherapy planning has to find a compromise between delivering radiation to the tumor, and avoiding dose to radiosensitive tissues. Visualization of dose uncertainty may guide the physician in this process. For example, the radiation dose could be reduced in regions of high uncertainty if this allows for dose reductions in radiosensitive organs, and thereby reduces the risk of side effects substantially. Technically, the standard deviation of the target dose could be used in the optimization of the radiation beams to weight differently voxels at the border of the CTV where the dose target is less certain. Moreover, it is important to visualize areas that represent

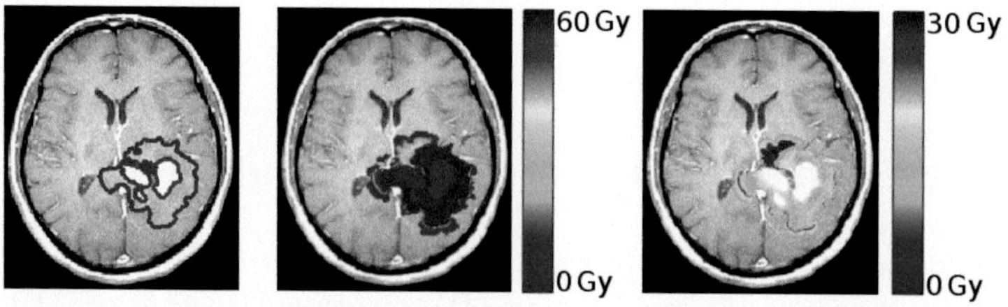

Fig. 5. (Left) Original GTV in red and CTV in blue overlaid on the T1Gd MRI; (Middle) Mean target dose from 40 samples ($\omega_1 = 19, \omega_0 = 4$); (Right) Standard deviation of the target dose.

tumor with near certainty and should be treated to the prescribed dose. In the long term, tumor segmentation samples could be used for radiotherapy planning based on models of tumor control probability (TCP).

6 Conclusion

In this paper, an original image segmentation sampling framework has been proposed to generate plausible segmentations close to a given one. The approach leads to spatially smooth contours that take into account the presence of salient features of the ROI in the image. Samples are efficiently generated, with a variability around a reference segmentation easily controlled by a single scalar.

Future work will further explore the incorporation of uncertainty in the radiotherapy dose planning. The proposed method could have several additional applications for instance to produce consensus segmentations from several expert ones. It could also be used to assess the confidence of the performance of segmentation algorithms in the context of segmentation challenges, by providing several likely segmentations around the ground truth segmentations.

Acknowledgments. Part of this work was funded by the European Research Council through the ERC Advanced Grant MedYMA 2011-291080.

References

1. Fan, A.C., Fisher III, J.W., Wells III, W.M., Levitt, J.J., Willsky, A.S.: MCMC curve sampling for image segmentation. In: Ayache, N., Ourselin, S., Maeder, A. (eds.) MICCAI 2007, Part II. LNCS, vol. 4792, pp. 477–485. Springer, Heidelberg (2007)
2. Warfield, S.K., Zou, K.H., Wells, W.M.: Simultaneous truth and performance level estimation (STAPLE): an algorithm for the validation of image segmentation. IEEE Transactions on Medical Imaging 23(7), 903–921 (2004)
3. Pohl, K.M., Fisher, J., Bouix, S., Shenton, M., McCarley, R.W., Grimson, W.E.L., Kikinis, R., Wells, W.M.: Using the logarithm of odds to define a vector space on probabilistic atlases. Medical Image Analysis 11(5), 465–477 (2007)
4. Sabuncu, M.R., Yeo, B.T., Van Leemput, K., Fischl, B., Golland, P.: A generative model for image segmentation based on label fusion. IEEE Transactions on Medical Imaging 29(10), 1714–1729 (2010)
5. Williams, O., Fitzgibbon, A.: Gaussian process implicit surfaces. In: Gaussian Proc. in Practice (2007)
6. Gerardo-Castro, M.P., Peynot, T., Ramos, F.: Laser-radar data fusion with gaussian process implicit surfaces. In: Corke, P., Mejias, L., Roberts, J. (eds.) The 9th Int. Conf. on Field and Service Robotics, Brisbane, Australia (2013)
7. Criminisi, A., Sharp, T., Blake, A.: GeoS: Geodesic image segmentation. In: Forsyth, D., Torr, P., Zisserman, A. (eds.) ECCV 2008, Part I. LNCS, vol. 5302, pp. 99–112. Springer, Heidelberg (2008)

8. Rasmussen, C.E.: Gaussian processes for machine learning (2006)
9. Kozintsev, B.: Computations with Gaussian random fields (1999)
10. Mason, W., Del Maestro, R., Eisenstat, D., Forsyth, P., Fulton, D., Laperrière, N., Macdonald, D., Perry, J., Thiessen, B., Committee, C.G.R., et al.: Canadian recommendations for the treatment of glioblastoma multiforme. Current Oncology 14(3), 110 (2007)

Multi-Level Parcellation of the Cerebral Cortex Using Resting-State fMRI

Salim Arslan and Daniel Rueckert

Biomedical Image Analysis Group, Department of Computing,
Imperial College London, London, UK

Abstract. Cortical parcellation is one of the core steps for identifying the functional architecture of the human brain. Despite the increasing number of attempts at developing parcellation algorithms using resting-state fMRI, there still remain challenges to be overcome, such as generating reproducible parcellations at both single-subject and group levels, while sub-dividing the cortex into functionally homogeneous parcels. To address these challenges, we propose a three-layer parcellation framework which deploys a different clustering strategy at each layer. Initially, the cortical vertices are clustered into a relatively large number of supervertices, which constitutes a high-level abstraction of the rs-fMRI data. These supervertices are combined into a tree of hierarchical clusters to generate individual subject parcellations, which are, in turn, used to compute a groupwise parcellation in order to represent the whole population. Using data collected as part of the Human Connectome Project from 100 healthy subjects, we show that our algorithm segregates the cortex into distinctive parcels at different resolutions with high reproducibility and functional homogeneity at both single-subject and group levels, therefore can be reliably used for network analysis.

1 Introduction

Parcellation of the cerebral cortex constitutes one of the core steps to reveal the functional organization of the brain. It is usually followed by network analyses devised to generate graphical models of the connections between the parcellated regions. Such analyses have the potential to uncover the neural mechanisms behind the human behavior and to help understand neurological disorders [8]. It is of great importance to obtain reliable parcellations, since errors at this stage propagate into the subsequent analysis and consequently affect the final results. Among others, there are two notable attributes that define "reliability" in the context of a cortical parcellation: 1) parcellated sub-regions should be functionally consistent and comprise similar vertices, since network nodes are typically represented by a single entity (such as the average time series of the constituent vertices) and 2) both individual subject and groupwise parcellations should be reproducible to some extent, that is, multiple parcellations obtained from different datasets of the same subject as well as groupwise parcellations computed from the subsets of the same population should exhibit functional and structural similarity.

N. Navab et al. (Eds.): MICCAI 2015, Part III, LNCS 9351, pp. 47–54, 2015.
DOI: 10.1007/978-3-319-24574-4_6

With this motivation, we propose a whole-cortex parcellation framework based on resting-state functional magnetic resonance imaging (rs-fMRI). The brain is still functional in the absence of external stimuli, thus rs-fMRI time series can be utilized to parcellate the cortical surface into functionally homogeneous sub-regions. The majority of the literature on the rs-fMRI driven parcellation techniques consists of methods (i) that aim to discover the cortical networks (e.g. default mode network) [10,5] and (ii) that propose to subdivide the entire cortical surface in order to produce a baseline for connectome analysis [3,2,7]. Hierarchical clustering, independent component analysis (ICA), region growing, spectral graph theory, and k-means are some of the many statistical models proposed to compute cortical parcellations as reviewed in [6]. Although promising solutions exist among them, there still remain challenges to be overcome, especially in order to obtain reliable parcellations that fulfill the aforementioned requirements at both single-subject and group levels.

We address these challenges with a three-layer parcellation framework in which each layer makes use of a clustering technique targeting a specific problem. First, we pre-parcellate the cortical vertices into highly consistent, relatively large number of homogeneous supervertices with a hybrid distance function based on rs-fMRI correlations and geodesic distance. This stage does not only reduce the dimensionality of the data and decrease the computational cost, but also improves the SNR. Second, we build hierarchical trees on top of the supervertices to obtain individual parcellations reflecting the functional organization of the cortex without losing the spatial integrity within the parcels. Third, we compute a graphical model of the parcel stability across the individual parcellations and cluster this graph in order to generate a groupwise representation of the subjects in the population. Our framework is capable of parcelleting the cortical surface into varying number of sub-regions (50 to 500 per hemisphere), thus allowing the analysis at multiple scales.

The most closely related work to our approach is a single-subject parcellation method composed of region growing and hierarchical clustering [2]. The major differences to our proposed work are twofold. First, we introduce a new pre-parcellation technique based on supervertices instead of relying on regions derived from stable seeds. Second, our method is capable of generating parcellations at the group level, thus can be used for population network analysis as opposed to [2]. We also compare our approach to another state-of-the-art cortical parcellation method based on spectral clustering with normalized cuts [3] and demonstrate that the proposed framework is more effective than the other approaches at both single-subject and group levels, achieving high reproducibility while preserving the functional consistency within the parcellated sub-regions.

2 Methodology

2.1 Data Acquisition and Preprocessing

We evaluate our algorithm using data from the Human Connectome Project (HCP). We conducted our experiments on the rs-fMRI datasets, containing scans from 100 different subjects (54 female, 46 male adults, age 22-35). The data for each subject was acquired in two sessions, divided into four runs of approximately 15 minutes each. Data was preprocessed and denoised by the HCP structural and functional minimal preprocessing pipelines [4]. The outcome of the pipeline is a standard set of cortical time series which were registered across subjects to establish correspondences. This was achieved by mapping the gray matter voxels to the native cortical surface and registering them onto the 32k standard triangulated mesh at a 2 mm spatial resolution. Finally, each time series was temporally normalized to zero-mean and unit-variance. We concatenated the time series of 15-minute scans acquired in the same sessions, obtaining two 30-minute rs-fMRI datasets for each of the 100 subjects and used them to evaluate our approach.

2.2 Initial Parcellation via Supervertex Clustering

We start the parcellation process by clustering the cortical vertices into a set of functionally uniform sub-regions. This stage does not only enforce spatial continuity within clusters, but is also beneficial for delineating more reproducible parcellations. To this end, we propose a k-means clustering algorithm inspired by SLIC superpixels [1]. Differently from the classical k-means, we limit the search space for each cluster to reduce the number of distance calculations and we define a hybrid distance function[1] which is capable of grouping highly correlated vertices, yet ensuring spatial continuity within clusters.

The cortical surface is represented as a smooth, triangulated mesh with no topological defects. Initially, k seeds are selected as the singleton clusters by uniformly sub-sampling the mesh. The algorithm iteratively associates each vertex with a cluster by computing their similarity using an Euclidean function in the form of $\sqrt{(d_c/N_c)^2 + (d_g/N_g)^2}$, where d_c and d_g correspond to the functional and spatial distance measures, respectively. Functional similarity between two vertices is measured by the Pearson's distance transformation of their corresponding time series. This transformation ensures the distance between highly correlated vertices being close to zero, thus increases their likelihood of being assigned to the same cluster. Spatial proximity is measured by the geodesic distance along the cortical surface, which is approximated as the length of the shortest path between the nodes in the mesh graph. N_c and N_g refer to the normalization factors, which are set to their corresponding maximal values in a cluster[2]. The algorithm converges when none of the clusters change between two consecutive iterations. Clustering decreases the dimensionality of the dataset to the number of supervertices, thus reduces the computational cost of the subsequent stages. Each supervertex is now represented by the average time series of the constituent vertices, minimizing the effects of noisy signals throughout the dataset.

[1] Please note that our distance function is not a metric, since it does not necessarily satisfy the triangle inequality.

[2] We straightforwardly set N_c to 2, since the Pearson's distance values fall within the range $[0, 2]$. Similarly, N_g is set to the predefined local search limit, since the maximum distance within a cluster cannot exceed it.

2.3 Single-Level Parcellation via Hierarchical Clustering

The supervertices over-parcellate the cortical surface, therefore a second stage should be deployed in order to obtain a reasonable number of parcels without losing the ability to represent the functional organization of the cortex and having non-uniform functional patterns within sub-regions. Towards this end, we join supervertices into non-overlapping parcels using agglomerative hierarchical clustering. This approach builds a hierarchy of clusters using a bottom-up strategy in which pairs of clusters are merged if their similarity is the maximal among the other pairing clusters. We only join adjacent clusters into a higher level in order to ensure the spatial continuity throughout the parcellation process. The algorithm is driven by Ward's linkage rule and the similarity between pairing clusters is computed by Pearson's distance. The algorithm iteratively constructs a dendrogram, in which the leaves represent the supervertices and the root represents an entire hemisphere. Cutting this tree at different levels of depth produces parcellations with the desired precision. We investigate the effect of different granularities on the parcel reproducibility and functional consistency in the following section.

2.4 Groupwise Parcellation via Spectral Clustering

Connectome analyses usually require a reliable groupwise representation for identifying common functional patterns across groups of healthy or disordered subjects and compare how the connectivity changes, for example, through aging. To this end, we deploy a final clustering stage in order to identify the group parcellations. We compute a graphical model of the parcel stability across the whole population [9], in which an edge between two vertices is weighted by the number of times they appear in the same parcel across all individual parcellations. Notably, the spatial integrity of the parcels is automatically guaranteed, since only vertices sharing the same cluster membership can have a correspondence between each other. The graph is subdivided by spectral clustering with normalized cuts [3] into pre-defined number of sub-regions, thus similar to individual parcellations, allowing analysis of the connectome at different levels of detail.

3 Results

We assess the parcellation performance in two ways: (a) reproducibility and (b) functional consistency. Reproducibility is measured with a two-pass Dice score-based method suggested in [2]. In the first pass, overlapping sub-regions are matched and given the same label based on their Dice scores. Functional inconsistency due to low SNR usually results in a higher number of parcels than desired. To eliminate its effect on the performance, a second-pass is applied to the parcellations and over-segmented sub-regions are merged. A group of parcels is considered as over-segmented if at least half of it overlaps with a single parcel in the other parcellation. After locating and merging over-segmented parcels, the average Dice score is used to assess the accuracy of the resulting parcellations. Functional consistency of a parcellation is assessed with respect to homogeneity and silhouette width [3]. Homogeneity is computed as the average pairwise correlations within each parcel after applying Fisher's z-transformation. Silhouette width combines homogeneity with inter-parcel separation[3], in order to assess the effectiveness of the parcellation algorithm in terms of generating functionally consistent sub-regions[4]. Algorithms were run on the left and right hemispheres separately and performance measurements were computed at different scales, starting from 500 parcels per hemisphere and in decrements of 50. Subsequently, results for the left and right hemispheres were averaged for the final plots.

We present single-subject reproducibility and functional consistency results obtained by our approach (3-LAYER), region growing (RG-HC), and normalized cuts (NCUT) in Fig. 1. Each subject has two rs-fMRI datasets, therefore reproducibility can be computed by matching parcellations derived from them separately. Functional homogeneity of the first parcellation was computed using the second rs-fMRI dataset, and vice versa, to avoid bias that may have emerged during the computation of the parcellations. Both 3-LAYER and RG-HC were run with $\sim$2000 initial clusters, each cluster having $\sim$30 cortical vertices on average. Results indicate that RG-HC and 3-LAYER perform similarly in terms of computing functionally segregated parcels; the former having slightly better performance at the lower resolutions, whereas the latter is able to generate single-subject parcellations with higher homogeneity, having 1-5% better scores. This is primarily due to the fact that we represent the cortical surface by functionally uniform supervertices and incorporate a flexible spatial constraint into our distance function, enabling any vertex to be assigned to a cluster if they exhibit high correlation and are spatially close (but not necessarily neighbors) as opposed to the region growing, which is based on stable seed points and a more strict definition of spatial proximity. However, region growing shows moderately better performance in terms of reproducibility when the same seed set (RG-HC2) is used at both parcellations, but this has no impact on the functional homogeneity. Although NCUT generates highly reproducible parcellations at low resolutions, it produces the least homogeneous sub-regions and shows a poor performance in silhouette width. Its high reproducibility can be attributed to the bias emerging from the structure of the cortical meshes that were used to drive the algorithm, which tends to generate evenly shaped parcels at the expense of losing functional segregation ability as also discussed in [2] and [3].

Functional consistency of the parcellations was also qualitatively measured by inspecting the connectivity profiles of the parcellated sub-regions thoroughly. We identified that sharp transitions across functional patterns are more significantly aligned with our parcellation boundaries compared to the other algorithms.

[3] Inter-parcel separation is computed as the average of the correlations between the vertices constituting a parcel and the remaining vertices across the cortex.

[4] Silhouette width is defined as $\frac{(H-S)}{max\{H,S\}}$, where H is the within-parcel homogeneity and S is the inter-parcel separation for a given parcel. Obtaining silhouette widths of close to 1 indicates a highly reliable and functionally consistent parcellation.

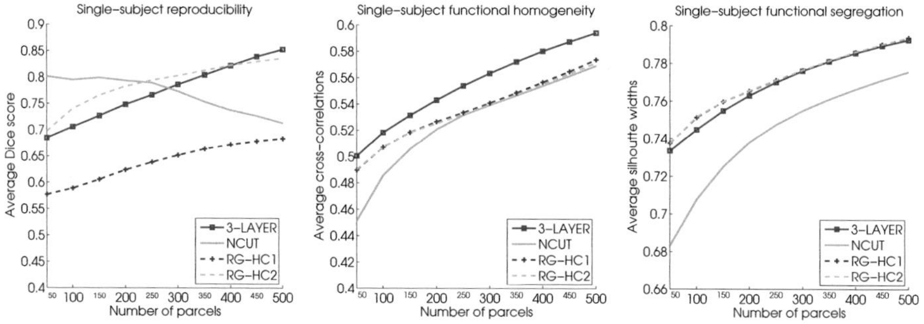

Fig. 1. Single-subject reproducibility (*left*), functional homogeneity (*middle*), and functional segregation (*right*) results obtained by our approach (3-LAYER), region growing with different (RG-HC1) and same seeds (RG-HC2), and normalized cuts (NCUT). See the text for the experimental setup.

Further examinations on the parcellations revealed that our boundaries matched well with the borders in cytoarchitectonic cortical areas, especially within the somato-sensory and vision cortex, showing agreement with the findings in [2].

The group level parcellations were assessed by dividing the subjects into two equally sized subgroups by random permutation and then computing a group parcellation for each subset. Reproducibility was measured by matching two group parcellations using the same Dice score method. Functional consistency of the groupwise parcellations was computed by measuring the parcel homogeneity and silhouette width based on each individual subject's rs-fMRI time series and then averaging them within the subgroups. All measurements were repeated for 10 times, each time forming subgroups with different subjects. Performance scores computed in each repetition were then averaged and plotted in Fig. 2. Groupwise parcellations were computed by using the stability graphs obtained from each method's single-level parcellations. In addition, we also computed a groupwise parcellation by averaging the rs-fMRI datasets of all subjects (after applying Fisher's z-transformation) and parcellating this average dataset by spectral clustering (MEAN) [3]. In general, the group-level results exhibit a similar tendency with those of the individual subjects. MEAN and NCUT show higher reproducibility at low resolutions, however 3-LAYER outperforms them for increasing number of parcels, obtaining upto 15% better scores. It generates the most functionally consistent parcellations at almost all resolutions achieving up to 4% higher homogeneity and 3% better functional segregation than the other approaches, except for 50-150 parcels, where RG-HC performs slightly better. These results may indicate that our parcellations can effectively reflect common functional characteristics within the population, being minimally affected by the functional and structural variability across different subjects.

Finally, for visual review, we present the parcellations of an arbitrary subject and the groupwise parcellations of the population obtained by the proposed algorithm in Fig. 3. We also provide the Dice scores computed between the single-level parcellations and their respective group representations in order to show

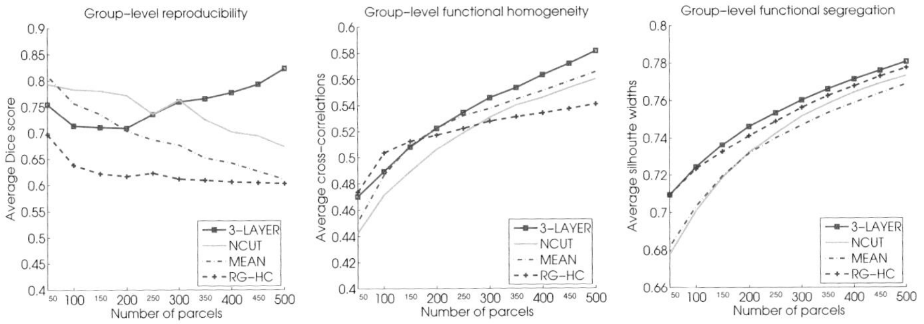

Fig. 2. Group-level reproducibility (*left*), functional homogeneity (*middle*) and functional segregation (*right*) results obtained by our approach (3-LAYER), region growing (RG-HC), normalized cuts (NCUT) and averaging rs-fMRI datasets (MEAN). See the text for the experimental setup.

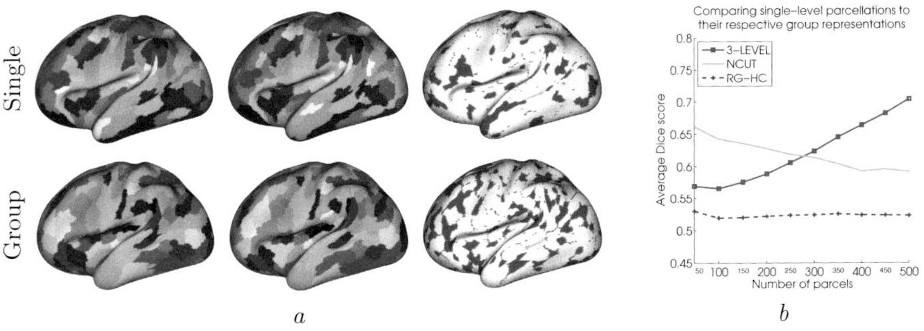

Fig. 3. (*a*) Parcellations obtained by the proposed method (3-LAYER) for 200 parcels. Single-level and groupwise parcellations in the first two columns were derived from different rs-fMRI datasets of the same subject and from different subgroups of the population, respectively. The third column shows the differences between the first and second parcellations in each row. (*b*) Average Dice scores computed between the single-level parcellations and their respective group representations.

the robustness of the proposed method in terms of coping with the functional variability within the population, especially at high resolutions.

4 Conclusions

We presented a new three-layer clustering approach to parcellate the cerebral cortex using resting-state fMRI. Our experiments at the single-subject and group levels demonstrated that the proposed algorithm can produce reliable parcellations, with higher reproduciblity and functional consistency compared to state-of-the-art approaches, therefore can be reliably and effectively used for network analysis. The three-layer method is in general more successful in grouping correlated vertices together, thus fulfills a critical requirement of connectome studies.

Having these promising results using solely rs-fMRI, we are now working on a multi-modal approach to improve the precision of the parcellation borders by incorporating task-fMRI into the parcellation framework. Another challenge in the parcellation problem is finding an optimal number of parcels. Our initial experiments showed that, the functional transitions in the connectivity profiles can be utilized to drive an objective function at the hierarchical clustering stage, thus can be used for this purpose.

Acknowledgments. Data were provided by the Human Connectome Project, WU-Minn Consortium (Principal Investigators: David Van Essen and Kamil Ugurbil; 1U54MH091657). The research leading to these results received funding from the European Research Council under the European Unions Seventh Framework Programme (FP/2007-2013) / ERC Grant Agreement no. 319456.

References

1. Achanta, R., Shaji, A., Smith, K., Lucchi, A., Fua, P., Susstrunk, S.: SLIC superpixels compared to state-of-the-art superpixel methods. IEEE T. Pattern Anal. 34(11), 2274–2282 (2012)
2. Blumensath, T., Jbabdi, S., Glasser, M.F., Van Essen, D.C., Ugurbil, K., Behrens, T.E., Smith, S.M.: Spatially constrained hierarchical parcellation of the brain with resting-state fMRI. NeuroImage 76, 313–324 (2013)
3. Craddock, R.C., James, G., Holtzheimer, P.E., Hu, X.P., Mayberg, H.S.: A whole brain fMRI atlas generated via spatially constrained spectral clustering. Hum. Brain Mapp. 33(8), 1914–1928 (2012)
4. Glasser, M.F., Sotiropoulos, S.N., Wilson, J.A., Coalson, T.S., Fischl, B., Andersson, J.L., Xu, J., Jbabdi, S., Webster, M., Polimeni, J.R., Van Essen, D.C., Jenkinson, M.: The minimal preprocessing pipelines for the Human Connectome Project. NeuroImage 80, 105–124 (2013)
5. Power, J.D., Cohen, A.L., Nelson, S.M., Wig, G.S., Barnes, K.A., Church, J.A., Vogel, A.C., Laumann, T.O., Miezin, F.M., Schlaggar, B.L., Petersen, S.E.: Functional network organization of the human brain. Neuron 72(4), 665–678 (2011)
6. de Reus, M.A., van den Heuvel, M.P.: The parcellation-based connectome: Limitations and extensions. NeuroImage 80, 397–404 (2013)
7. Shen, X., Tokoglu, F., Papademetris, X., Constable, R.T.: Groupwise whole-brain parcellation from resting-state fMRI data for network node identification. NeuroImage 82, 403–415 (2013)
8. Sporns, O., Tononi, G., Ktter, R.: The Human Connectome: A structural description of the human brain. PLoS Comput. Biol. 1(4), e42 (2005)
9. van den Heuvel, M., Mandl, R., Hulshoff Pol, H.: Normalized cut group clustering of resting-state fMRI data. PLoS One 3(4), e2001 (2008)
10. Yeo, B.T., Krienen, F.M., Sepulcre, J., Sabuncu, M.R., Lashkari, D., Hollinshead, M., Roffman, J.L., Smoller, J.W., Zollei, L., Polimeni, J.R., Fischl, B., Liu, H., Buckner, R.L.: The organization of the human cerebral cortex estimated by intrinsic functional connectivity. J. Neurophysiol. 106(3), 1125–1165 (2011)

Interactive Multi-organ Segmentation Based on Multiple Template Deformation

Romane Gauriau[1,2], David Lesage[1], Mélanie Chiaradia[3], Baptiste Morel[4], and Isabelle Bloch[2]

[1] Philips Research MediSys, Paris, France
[2] Institut Mines-Telecom, Telecom ParisTech, CNRS LTCI, Paris, France
[3] H. Mondor Hospital APHP, Medical Imaging Department, Créteil, France
[4] A. Trousseau Hospital APHP, Radiology Department, Paris, France

Abstract. We present a new method for the segmentation of multiple organs (2D or 3D) which enables user inputs for smart contour editing. By extending the work of [1] with user-provided hard constraints that can be optimized globally or locally, we propose an efficient and user-friendly solution that ensures consistent feedback to the user interactions. We demonstrate the potential of our approach through a user study with 10 medical imaging experts, aiming at the correction of 4 organ segmentations in 10 CT volumes. We provide quantitative and qualitative analysis of the users' feedback.

1 Medical Motivation and Overview

Despite constant improvements of fully automatic segmentation approaches, perfect accuracy remains unreachable in many image processing scenarios, especially when inter- and intra-patient variabilities are important. In a clinical context, the possibility of incorporating user corrections is particularly valuable. From a user point of view, the interactions should be: (i) simple, easy to perform, (ii) fast (ideally with real-time feedback), (iii) intuitive (well-behaved algorithm feedback). Designing efficient and user-friendly algorithms meeting these criteria is particularly difficult.

Many works on interactive segmentation can be found in the literature. For instance, the live wire technique [2] is a highly interactive approach, close to fully manual 2D delineation. This approach can be extended to 3D and performed in real-time [3], but it remains very time-consuming for the end user. Various methods aim at optimizing globally an energy taking into account image information and user-provided initializations (e.g. through strokes). This problem is often tackled within discrete optimization frameworks [4,5,6,7,8]. The different formulations found in the literature propose different properties in terms of robustness, speed and sensitivity to initialization. Image partitioning from user inputs can also be formulated as a continuous variational problem [9] and include more global and contextual information. Globally optimizing an energy that changes with each new user input can have counter-intuitive effects, as the algorithm *forgets* previous results while not putting particular emphasis on the

N. Navab et al. (Eds.): MICCAI 2015, Part III, LNCS 9351, pp. 55–62, 2015.
DOI: 10.1007/978-3-319-24574-4_7

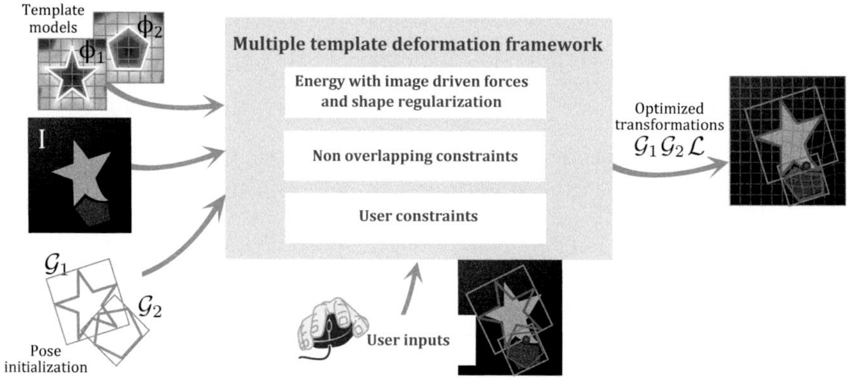

Fig. 1. Illustration of the framework principle on a toy example with two objects.

latest inputs. The non-convexity of some segmentation formulations can be exploited to derive sequential approaches [10,11]. After each user interaction, the contour evolves towards a local minimum of the new energy, starting from its previous location. With these methods, the impact of new inputs remains global. Resulting contours may change at locations distant from the latest inputs. Few methods were proposed for more local corrections [12,13] but they generally do not guarantee shape consistency. Finally, very few works are dedicated to the simultaneous segmentation of multiple objects [14], even less so in 3D [15].

In this work, we propose a framework for multi-organ interactive segmentation with: (i) simple interactions (point-wise mouse clicks), (ii) fast and *on the fly* user interactions, (iii) intuitive results (good tradeoff between user input and image information). We rely on the multiple template deformation framework of [1] for its efficiency and robustness, with shape priors and non-overlapping constraints. We extend it with user inputs expressed as hard optimization constraints (Sec.2). As an important refinement, we show how to handle user interactions in a spatially local fashion. Our approach is evaluated through a user study with 10 medical imaging experts, aiming at the correction of 4 organ segmentations in 10 CT volumes (Sec.3). The qualitative and quantitative feedback highlights the user-friendliness of our framework, which, we believe, is a decisive criterion towards its suitability to clinical workflows.

2 Methodology

This work is based on the multiple template deformation framework of [1]. We extend it with user constraints and propose a fast numerical optimization making possible real-time user interactions. The approach is illustrated in Fig.1.

2.1 Multiple Implicit Template Deformation with User Constraints

We denote an image $I : \Omega \rightarrow \mathbb{R}$ where $\Omega \in \mathbb{R}^d$ is the image domain ($d = 3$ in this work). For each object indexed by $n \in [\![1, N]\!]$ we associate an implicit shape template $\phi_n : \Omega_n \rightarrow \mathbb{R}$ where Ω_n are the template referentials (ϕ_n is positive inside and negative outside the contour). In general the implicit shape template is a distance function whose zero level corresponds to the contour. For each object we define the transformations $\psi_n : \Omega \rightarrow \Omega_n$ that map back the image domain to the template domains. Each of these transformations is advantageously decomposed as $\psi_n = \mathcal{G}_n \circ \mathcal{L}$, where $\mathcal{G}_n : \Omega \rightarrow \Omega_n$ corresponds to the pose of object n (e.g. a similarity transformation) and $\mathcal{L} : \Omega \rightarrow \Omega$ corresponds to the local deformation common to the set of templates in the domain Ω.

The approach aims at finding the transformations $\mathcal{G}_n$ and $\mathcal{L}$ that best fit the template onto the image while following image-driven forces (specific to each object and defined by $f_n : \Omega \rightarrow \mathbb{R}$) and not deviating too much from the original shape. To prevent the objects from overlapping, specific penalizations are added on template pairs intersections (Eq.2) after pose transformation $\mathcal{G}_n$ [1]. The corresponding energy equation is given below (Eq.1), where H is the Heaviside function, λ is a constant balancing the shape prior and U is a reproducing kernel Hilbert space defined by a Gaussian kernel. We use the same forces f_n as in [1] integrating both region intensities and edge information.

$$\min_{\mathcal{G}_1,..\mathcal{G}_N,\mathcal{L}} \left\{ E(\mathcal{G}_1, .., \mathcal{G}_N, \mathcal{L}) = \sum_{n=1}^{N} \left(\int_\Omega H(\phi_n \circ \mathcal{G}_n \circ \mathcal{L}(x)).f_n(x)dx \right) + \frac{\lambda}{2} \|\mathcal{L} - Id\|_U^2 \right\} \tag{1}$$

subject to

$$\forall (i,j) \in [\![1, N]\!]^2, i < j,\ C_{i,j} = \int_\Omega H(\phi_i \circ \mathcal{G}_i(x)) H(\phi_j \circ \mathcal{G}_j(x))dx = 0, \tag{2}$$

$$\forall n \in [\![1, N]\!], \forall q_n \in [\![1, K_n]\!],\ \gamma_{q_n}\, \phi_n \circ \mathcal{G}_n \circ \mathcal{L}(x_{q_n}) \geq 0,\ \gamma_{q_n} \in \{-1, 1\} \tag{3}$$

We integrate user inputs into this framework as point-wise hard constraints similarly to [16]. These correspond to very simple interactions (mouse clicks). To modify the contour of object n, the user can add a point x_{q_n} *outside* (denoted as $\gamma_{q_n} = 1$) or *inside* ($\gamma_{q_n} = -1$) the object. Adding a point outside (respectively inside) the object indicates that the template should be deformed to include (respectively exclude) the point. These constraints can be expressed with regards to the sign of the deformed implicit template ϕ_n, as formulated in Eq. 3. For instance, for an outside point ($\gamma_{q_n} = 1$), the implicit template is constrained to become positive, i.e. to include point x_{q_n}: $\gamma_{q_n} \phi_n \circ \mathcal{G}_n \circ \mathcal{L}(\mathbf{x}_{q_n}) \geq 0$.

2.2 Numerical Optimization

To optimize the constrained problem of Eq. 1-3 we do not use the penalty method as in [1], as it may suffer from instability due to ill-conditioning. Instead, we use the augmented Lagrangian scheme presented in [17] to turn the problem into a series of unconstrained minimizations:

$$\min_{\mathcal{G}_1,...,\mathcal{G}_N,\mathcal{L}} \left\{ \hat{E}_k = E + \sum_{\substack{1\leq i\leq N \\ i<j\leq N}} h(C(\mathcal{G}_i,\mathcal{G}_j),\alpha^k_{i,j},\mu_k) + \sum_{\substack{1\leq n\leq N \\ 1\leq q_n\leq K_n}} h(\gamma_{q_n}\phi_n\circ\mathcal{G}_n\circ\mathcal{L}(x_{q_n}),\alpha'_{q_n},\mu'_k) \right\} \tag{4}$$

where we denote $E = E(\mathcal{G}_1,...,\mathcal{G}_N,\mathcal{L})$ and $\hat{E}_k = \hat{E}_k(\mathcal{G}_1,...,\mathcal{G}_N,\mathcal{L})$, $\alpha^k_{i,j}$ and α'_{q_n} are the Lagrange multipliers, μ_k and μ'_k are the penalty parameters of the constraints, and h is the function defined by:

$$h(c,\alpha;\mu) = \begin{cases} -\alpha c + \frac{\mu}{2}c^2 & \text{if } c - \frac{\alpha}{\mu} \geq 0, \\ -\frac{\alpha^2}{2\mu} & \text{otherwise.} \end{cases} \tag{5}$$

The unconstrained energy of Eq.4 can then be optimized following a gradient descent. At each optimization step k, the Lagrange multipliers are fixed, the energy is optimized and new Lagrange multipliers estimates can be obtained for the optimization step $k+1$. As in [1], the parameters of the transformations $\mathcal{G}_n$ and $\mathcal{L}$ are updated jointly and iteratively.

Efficient Implementation. Note that the gradients of the energy can be efficiently computed as: (i) integrals over the volume can be turned into integrals over surfaces, (ii) many terms are only needed near the zero level of the implicit functions, (iii) a collision detection step can be added to prevent the systematic computation of the non-overlapping constraints, (iv) if a constraint gets verified then it is not optimized. For instance the automatic segmentation of 6 organs in a typical abdominal CT takes about 30 seconds to converge in the absence of user corrections (including localization). New user inputs add relatively localized constraints taking minimal effort to satisfy, in general within a few seconds.

Convergence. The optimization procedure ensures the convergence towards a local minimum of the (non-convex) energy, which is not guaranteed to be the global minimum. In our applicative scope, this turns into an advantage. In complex medical imaging tasks, the global minimum rarely corresponds to the exact desired result. Intuitively, user constraints will quickly drive the segmentation to the desired local minimum. Note also that contradictory constraints can be easily detected and mitigated in practice.

2.3 Enhancing the Framework for Local Contours Editing

When correcting the contours of pre-segmented objects, a user may expect the impact of his inputs to remain spatially local. A proper algorithm behavior would take into account the user inputs while relying on the image information in a ROI around the user input location. In such a case we suppose that the objects are already correctly positioned in the image and that only local deformations occur. Hence we propose a new formulation of the energy E of Eq.1:

$$E(\mathcal{L}) = \sum_{n=1}^{N} \left\{ \int_{\Omega} \left(K_\sigma * \sum_{q_n=1}^{K_n} \delta_{q_n}(x) \right) H(\phi_n\circ\mathcal{L}(x)).f_n(x)dx \right\} + \frac{\lambda}{2}\|\mathcal{L} - Id\|^2_U \tag{6}$$

where K_σ is a Gaussian kernel with fixed width (in practice 2-3cm) and $\delta_{q_n} = \delta(x - x_{q_n})$ (δ is the Dirac distribution). With this new energy, the image-driven forces act in the neighborhood of the user inputs only. Note that the shape contours remain consistent.

The numerical optimization with this new energy equation is similar to the one presented in Sec.2.2, except that the pose transformations are not optimized and the non-overlapping constraint term is reduced to the empty set.

2.4 Flexibility of the Framework

The method proposed is very flexible and can be adapted to different usages. Any type of image-driven forces can be implemented. The algorithm can work in automatic mode (given an initialization of the models, e.g. with regression localization as in [1]) or with user inputs. The user constraints can be added while the algorithm is running, which allows for live interactions[1].

3 A Study for the Evaluation of the User Interactions

The idea behind our experiments is to *reproduce* a clinical context where the clinicians could use automatic segmentation results (given from the original framework [1], possibly run off-line) and correct them with our method with local corrections (energy of Eq.6) if needed.

Material. Our database is composed of 156 3D CT images coming from 130 patients with diverse medical conditions and from different clinical sites (which implies different fields of view, resolution etc.). Slice and inter-slice resolutions range from 0.5 to 1 mm and from 0.5 to 3 mm, respectively. The organs of interest have been manually segmented on all the database. The database has been split randomly into 50 and 106 volumes for training (localization part) and testing, respectively. Our method was implemented in C++.

A Simple Interface. The interface is made as simple as possible. There is one button to activate the corrections and one button to remove the last correction. Once the correction button is pressed, the algorithm runs continuously and the user can add point constraints in any orthogonal view and at any moment without waiting. The right mouse button is used to select the organ to correct and the left one is used to add a point constraint in the volume. A left click oustide the selected object will attract the contour (*inside* constraint) while a left click inside the object will move away the contour (*outside* constraint).

Protocol. To ensure clinical-like conditions we propose to use our framework without user constraints to segment 4 abdominal organs (liver, kidneys and spleen) on our database of 106 CT volumes. The volumes are sorted with regards

[1] Demonstration video: `http://perso.telecom-paristech.fr/~gauriau/`

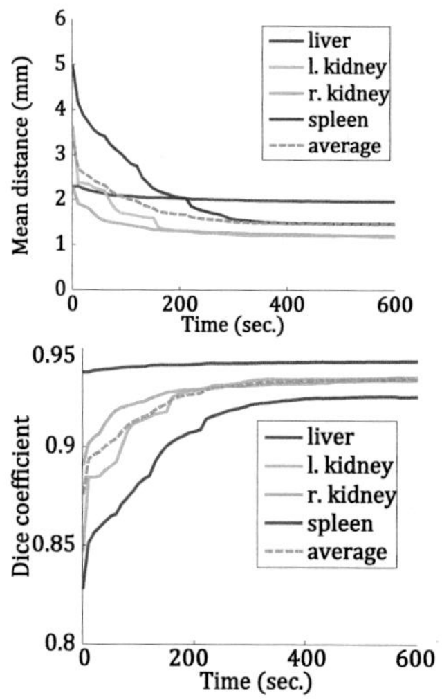

Fig. 2. Average mean distance and dice results per image in function of the correction time.

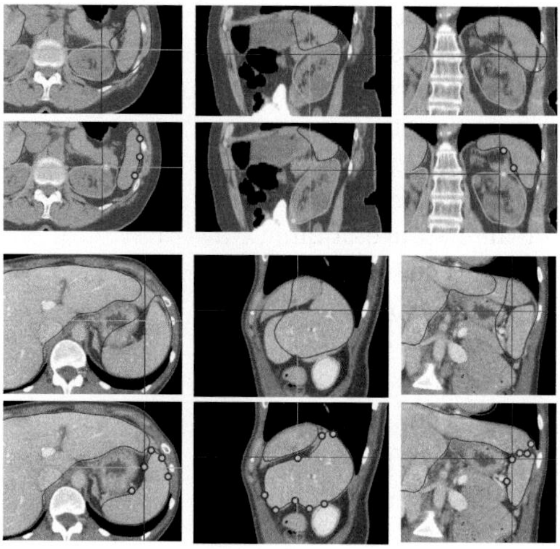

Fig. 3. Examples of results in two different volumes, after automatic segmentation (1st and 3rd lines) and after user constraints (2nd and 4th lines) in the three orthogonal views.

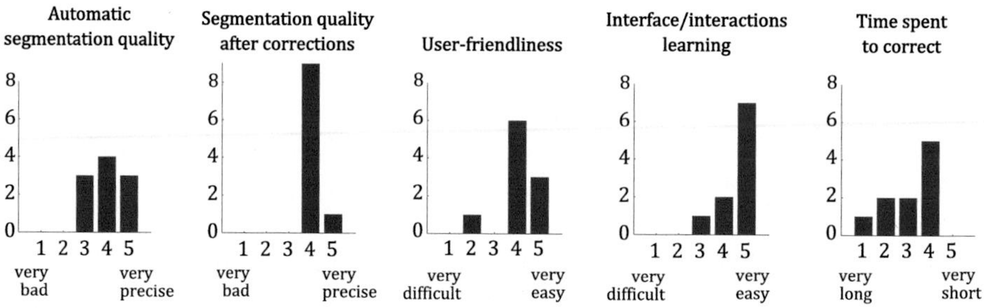

Fig. 4. Feedback form results from the 10 experts.

to their Dice coefficient to the ground truth and we select 10 volumes uniformly spread on this basis. We have then a sample of CT volumes representing the variability of the automatic segmentation results that we could find in a clinical context with an automatic method. Then 10 experts of the medical imaging domain (among them two radiologists) were asked to correct the results of the automatic segmentation in these volumes. Note that they were not asked for extreme precision. None of them knew the interface and the algorithm before using it. They only had few minutes to understand the tool before starting the experiments. Note that the experiments were performed on different computers with various configurations. During the experiments, each click was recorded and intermediate segmentation results were saved. At the end of the experiments, each user was asked to fill a form and give their feedback.

Results of the User Study. On average the users spent 345 seconds per volume (median: 228s). Figure 2 gives, for each organ, the average mean distance and dice coefficient according to the ground truth in function of the correction time. Note that the accuracy converges rather rapidly. After about 300 seconds an average distance of 1.5mm is reached. Considering that there are 4 organs to look at and correct, this remains reasonable in terms of time. The liver reaches a mean distance of 2mm explained mainly by the user variability and tolerance (e.g. sometimes the user includes or not part of the aorta and the inferior vena cava). Figure 3 shows examples of results before and after corrections. We observe that small corrections as well as important deformations can be handled by the algorithm. Finally, Fig. 4 shows the results of the feedback survey. The users seem satisfied with the final segmentation results. They confirm that the tool is very easy to learn. They suggest that some effort should be spent on the reactivity of our prototype, which is expected to be much improved with further code optimization. They also highlighted one limit of this approach: as large deformations are penalized (with the regularization term), large errors are more difficult to correct.

4 Conclusion

In this article we presented a fast and robust multi-organ segmentation method integrating user inputs in an intuitive manner. While benefiting from the original template deformation framework of [1], the efficient numerical optimization scheme with augmented Lagrangian results in a fast and stable algorithm allowing live user interactions. We also proposed a new formulation of the energy to take into account user inputs in a spatially local fashion. This extended framework can be used to build a complete and coherent tool chain: organs can be automatically segmented off-line (in about 30 sec.) and the clinicians can correct these results if needed. Thanks to our study with 10 users, we showed that this tool is easy to learn and results in fast, coherent and accurate corrections. Our experiments gave us precious insight for possible improvements. First, our local correction scheme could be made more adaptive, e.g. by adapting the width of the kernel K_σ to the distance between the user input and the object contour. Second, we are working on improving the performance of our software through code optimization and parallelization, as reactivity is a crucial aspect of such clinical tools. Finally, we saw that our approach may have difficulties with large errors, requiring large deformations to be corrected. We are currently exploring refinements better suited to such use cases.

Acknowledgments. This work is supported in part by an ANRT grant (008512012). We are very thankful to Vincent Auvray, Maxim Fradkin, Hélène Langet, Thierry Lefèvre, Paolo Piro and Jean-Michel Rouet for their participation in the study.

References

1. Gauriau, R., Ardon, R., Lesage, D., Bloch, I.: Multiple template deformation. application to abdominal organ segmentation. In: ISBI, pp. 359–362 (2015)
2. Mortensen, E., Morse, B., Barrett, W., Udupa, J.: Adaptive boundary detection using live-wire two-dimensional dynamic programming. In: IEEE Computers in Cardiology, pp. 635–638 (1992)
3. Falcao, A.X., Udupa, J.K., Miyazawa, F.K.: An ultra-fast user-steered image segmentation paradigm: live wire on the fly. IEEE TMI 19(1), 55–62 (2000)
4. Boykov, Y., Jolly, M.-P.: Interactive organ segmentation using graph cuts. In: Delp, S.L., DiGoia, A.M., Jaramaz, B. (eds.) MICCAI 2000. LNCS, vol. 1935, pp. 276–286. Springer, Heidelberg (2000)
5. Grady, L.: Random walks for image segmentation. IEEE PAMI 28(11), 1768–1783 (2006)
6. Bai, X., Sapiro, G.: A geodesic framework for fast interactive image and video segmentation and matting. In: IEEE ICCV, pp. 1–8 (2007)
7. Criminisi, A., Sharp, T., Blake, A.: GeoS: Geodesic image segmentation. In: Forsyth, D., Torr, P., Zisserman, A. (eds.) ECCV 2008, Part I. LNCS, vol. 5302, pp. 99–112. Springer, Heidelberg (2008)
8. Zhang, J., Zheng, J., Cai, J.: A diffusion approach to seeded image segmentation. In: IEEE CVPR, pp. 2125–2132 (2010)
9. Zhao, Y., Zhu, S.C., Luo, S.: Co3 for ultra-fast and accurate interactive segmentation. In: International Conference on Multimedia, pp. 93–102. ACM (2010)
10. Cremers, D., Fluck, O., Rousson, M., Aharon, S.: A probabilistic level set formulation for interactive organ segmentation. In: SPIE, vol. 6512 (2007)
11. Mory, B., Ardon, R., Yezzi, A.J., Thiran, J.: Non-euclidean image-adaptive radial basis functions for 3D interactive segmentation. In: IEEE International Conference on Computer Vision, pp. 787–794 (2009)
12. Grady, L., Funka-Lea, G.: An energy minimization approach to the data driven editing of presegmented images/volumes. In: Larsen, R., Nielsen, M., Sporring, J. (eds.) MICCAI 2006. LNCS, vol. 4191, pp. 888–895. Springer, Heidelberg (2006)
13. Harrison, A.P., Birkbeck, N., Sofka, M.: IntellEditS: Intelligent learning-based editor of segmentations. In: Mori, K., Sakuma, I., Sato, Y., Barillot, C., Navab, N. (eds.) MICCAI 2013, Part III. LNCS, vol. 8151, pp. 235–242. Springer, Heidelberg (2013)
14. Boykov, Y.Y., Jolly, M.P.: Interactive graph cuts for optimal boundary & region segmentation of objects in N-D images. In: IEEE ICCV, vol. 1, pp. 105–112 (2001)
15. Fleureau, J., Garreau, M., Boulmier, D., Leclercq, C., Hernandez, A.: 3D multi-object segmentation of cardiac MSCT imaging by using a multi-agent approach. In: IEEE Annual International Conference, pp. 6003–6006. EMBS (2009)
16. Mory, B., Somphone, O., Prevost, R., Ardon, R.: Real-time 3D image segmentation by user-constrained template deformation. In: Ayache, N., Delingette, H., Golland, P., Mori, K. (eds.) MICCAI 2012, Part I. LNCS, vol. 7510, pp. 561–568. Springer, Heidelberg (2012)
17. Nocedal, J., Wright, S.J.: Numerical optimization. Springer, New York (2006)

Segmentation of Infant Hippocampus Using Common Feature Representations Learned for Multimodal Longitudinal Data

Yanrong Guo[1], Guorong Wu[1], Pew-Thian Yap[1], Valerie Jewells[2], Weili Lin[1], and Dinggang Shen[1,*]

[1] Department of Radiology and BRIC, University of North Carolina at Chapel Hill, NC, USA
[2] Department of Radiology, University of North Carolina at Chapel Hill, NC, USA
dgshen@med.unc.edu

Abstract. Aberrant development of the human brain during the first year after birth is known to cause critical implications in later stages of life. In particular, neuropsychiatric disorders, such as attention deficit hyperactivity disorder (ADHD), have been linked with abnormal early development of the hippocampus. Despite its known importance, studying the hippocampus in infant subjects is very challenging due to the significantly smaller brain size, dynamically varying image contrast, and large across-subject variation. In this paper, we present a novel method for effective hippocampus segmentation by using a multi-atlas approach that integrates the complementary multimodal information from longitudinal T1 and T2 MR images. In particular, considering the highly heterogeneous nature of the longitudinal data, we propose to learn their common feature representations by using hierarchical multi-set kernel canonical correlation analysis (CCA). Specifically, we will learn (1) *within-time-point common features* by projecting different modality features of each time point to its own modality-free common space, and (2) *across-time-point common features* by mapping all time-point-specific common features to a global common space for all time points. These final features are then employed in patch matching across different modalities and time points for hippocampus segmentation, via label propagation and fusion. Experimental results demonstrate the improved performance of our method over the state-of-the-art methods.

1 Introduction

Effective automated segmentation of the hippocampus is highly desirable, as neuroscientists are actively seeking hippocampal imaging biomarkers for early detection of neurodevelopment disorders, such as autism and attention deficit hyperactivity disorder (ADHD) [1, 2]. Due to rapid maturation and myelination of brain tissues in the first year of life [3], the contrast between gray and white matter on T1 and T2 images undergo drastic changes, which poses great challenges to hippocampus segmentation.

Multi-atlas approaches with patch-based label fusion have demonstrated effective performance for medical image segmentation [4-8]. This is mainly due to their ability

* Corresponding author.

N. Navab et al. (Eds.): MICCAI 2015, Part III, LNCS 9351, pp. 63–71, 2015.
DOI: 10.1007/978-3-319-24574-4_8

to account for inter-subject anatomical variation during segmentation. However, infant brain segmentation introduces new challenges that need extra consideration before multi-atlas segmentation can be applied. *First*, using either T1 or T2 images alone is insufficient to provide an effective tissue contrast for segmentation throughout the first year. As shown in Fig. 1, the T1 image has very poor tissue contrast between white matter (WM) and gray matter (GM) in the first three months (such as the 2-week image shown in the left panel), as WM and GM become distinguishable only after the first year (such as the 12-month image shown in the right panel). However, the T2 image has better WM/GM contrast than the T1 image in the first few months. *Second*, some time periods (around the 6-month age as shown in the middle panel of Fig. 1) are more challenging to decipher because of very similar WM and GM intensity ranges (as shown by green and blue curves in Fig. 1) as partial myelination occurs.

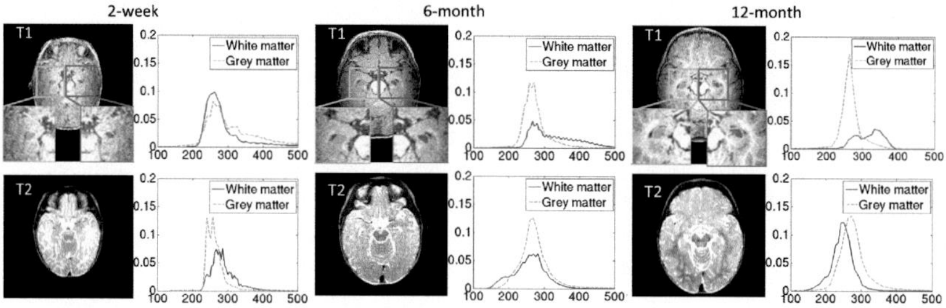

Fig. 1. Typical T1 (top) and T2 (bottom) brain MR images acquired from an infant at the 2 weeks, 6 months and 12 months, with the zoom-in views of local regions of hippocampi (green and red areas) shown at the bottom of T1 images. The WM and GM intensity distributions of T1 and T2 images on these local regions are also given to the right of each image.

Since the infant brain undergoes drastic changes in the first year of life, across-time-point feature learning is significant to help normalize cross-distribution differences and to borrow information between subjects at different time points for effective segmentation. Therefore, we propose to combine information from multiple modalities (T1 and T2) and different time points together via a patch matching mechanism to improve the label propagation in tissue segmentation. Specifically, to overcome the issue of significant tissue contrast change across different time points, we propose a hierarchical approach to learn a common feature representation. First, we learn the common features for the T1 and T2 images at each time point by using the classic kernel CCA [9, 10] to estimate the highly nonlinear feature mapping between the two modalities. Then, we further map all these within-time-point common features to a global *common* space to all different time points by applying the multi-set kernel CCA [11, 12]. Finally, we utilize the learned common features for guiding patch matching and propagating atlas labels to the target image (at each time point) for hippocampus segmentation, via a sparse patch-based labeling [13]. Qualitative and quantitative experimental results of our method on multimodal infant MR images acquired from 2-week-old to 6-month-old infants confirm more accurate hippocampus segmentation.

2 Method

2.1 Hierarchical Learning of Common Feature Representations

Suppose our training set consists of the longitudinal data including S subjects, each with T time points and two modalities (1: T1; 2: T2), denoted as $\boldsymbol{A} = \left\{(I_{s,t}^{(1)}, I_{s,t}^{(2)}) | s = 1, \dots, S, t = 1, \dots, T\right\}$. $I_{s,t}$ denotes the intensity image for subject s at time point t. We first register each training image $I_{s,t}^{(m)}$ $(m = \{1,2\})$ to a template image by deformable registration [14][1], thus producing a registered image $\tilde{I}_{s,t}^{(m)}$. We then gather the images into $2 \times T$ groups, one for each modality m and time point t, consisting of S registered images $\tilde{\boldsymbol{I}}_t^{(m)} = \left\{\tilde{I}_{s,t}^{(m)} | s = 1, \dots, S\right\}$, as shown in the left panel of **Fig. 2**. The patches from Q randomly sampled locations $V = \left\{v_q | q = 1, \dots, Q\right\}$ in the template domain are similarly organized into $2 \times T$ image patch groups $\boldsymbol{P} = \left\{\boldsymbol{P}_t^{(m)} | t = 1, .., T; m = 1,2\right\}$, where $\boldsymbol{P}_t^{(m)} = \left[\boldsymbol{p}_{1,t}^{(m)}(v_1), \dots, \boldsymbol{p}_{s,t}^{(m)}(v_q), \dots, \boldsymbol{p}_{S,t}^{(m)}(v_Q)\right]$ is a matrix for each patch group with $N = Q \times S$ columns of patches sampled from $\tilde{\boldsymbol{I}}_{\cdot,t}^{(m)}$. Each patch $\boldsymbol{p}_{s,t}^{(m)}(v_q)$ is rearranged as a column vector in $\boldsymbol{P}_t^{(m)}$. For simplicity, we omit the location v and denote the i-th column of $\boldsymbol{P}_t^{(m)}$ as $\boldsymbol{P}_t^{(m)}(i), i = 1, \dots, N$. In the following, we describe the hierarchical feature learning in two steps as illustrated in Fig. 2.

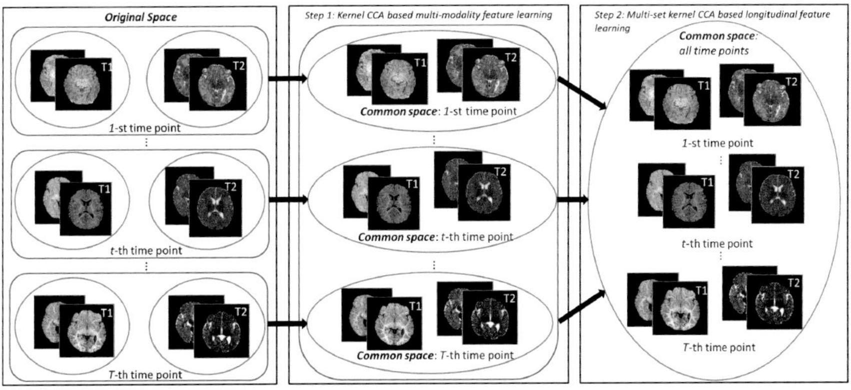

Fig. 2. Schematic diagram of the proposed hierarchical feature learning method.

[1] For the training images, we used our in-house joint registration-segmentation tool to accurately segment the intensity image into WM, GM, and cerebrospinal fluid (CSF). Therefore, the impact of the dynamic change in image contrast is minimized for the deformable registration. The diffeomorphic Demons is set with the smoothing sigma for updating field as 2.0 and the number of iterations as 15, 10, and 5 in low-, mid-, and high-resolution, respectively.

Step 1: Learning Within-Time-Point Common Features. Learning a common feature representation for all patch groups $\boldsymbol{P}$ simultaneously is challenging, since features vary significantly across groups. To overcome this problem, we first determine the common feature representation across modalities by employing the kernel CCA to learn the non-linear mappings of $\boldsymbol{P}_t^{(1)}$ and $\boldsymbol{P}_t^{(2)}$ for each time point t.

Specifically, we apply the Gaussian kernel $\phi(\cdot,\cdot)$ to measure similarity of any pair of image patches in $\boldsymbol{P}_t^{(1)}$ and obtain a $N \times N$ kernel matrix $\boldsymbol{K}_t^{(1)} = [\phi(\boldsymbol{P}_t^{(1)}(i), \boldsymbol{P}_t^{(1)}(j))]_{N\times N}$ $(i,j = 1,\ldots,N)$. Similarly, we can obtain a $N \times N$ kernel matrix $\boldsymbol{K}_t^{(2)}$ for group $\boldsymbol{P}_t^{(2)}$. Then, kernel CCA aims to find two sets of linear transforms $\left\{\boldsymbol{W}_t^{(m)} = \left[\boldsymbol{w}_t^{(m)}(1),\ldots,\boldsymbol{w}_t^{(m)}(r),\ldots,\boldsymbol{w}_t^{(m)}(R)\right]_{N\times R} | m = 1,2\right\}$ for $\boldsymbol{P}_t^{(1)}$ and $\boldsymbol{P}_t^{(2)}$, respectively, such that the correlation between mapped features $(\boldsymbol{w}_t^{(1)}(r))^T\boldsymbol{K}_t^{(1)}$ and mapped features $(\boldsymbol{w}_t^{(2)}(r))^T\boldsymbol{K}_t^{(2)}$ is maximized in the common space:

$$\mathrm{argmax}_{\boldsymbol{w}_t^{(1)}(r),\boldsymbol{w}_t^{(2)}(r)} \frac{\left(\boldsymbol{w}_t^{(1)}(r)\right)^T \boldsymbol{K}_t^{(1)}\left(\left(\boldsymbol{w}_t^{(2)}(r)\right)^T \boldsymbol{K}_t^{(2)}\right)^T}{\left[\left(\boldsymbol{w}_t^{(1)}(r)\right)^T \boldsymbol{K}_t^{(1)}\left(\left(\boldsymbol{w}_t^{(1)}(r)\right)^T \boldsymbol{K}_t^{(1)}\right)^T\right]\left[\left(\boldsymbol{w}_t^{(2)}(r)\right)^T \boldsymbol{K}_t^{(2)}\left(\left(\boldsymbol{w}_t^{(2)}(r)\right)^T \boldsymbol{K}_t^{(2)}\right)^T\right]} \tag{1}$$

where $R = \min\left(rank\left(\boldsymbol{K}_t^{(1)}\right), rank\left(\boldsymbol{K}_t^{(2)}\right)\right)$. The denominator of Eq. (1) requires that the distribution of the mapped features should be as compact as possible within each group. Partial Gram-Schmidt orthogonalization method [9] can be sequentially used to find the optimal $\boldsymbol{w}_t^{(1)}(r)$ and $\boldsymbol{w}_t^{(2)}(r)$ in Eq. (1), where the rth pair of $\boldsymbol{w}_t^{(1)}(r)$ and $\boldsymbol{w}_t^{(2)}(r)$ are orthogonal to all previous pairs and also maximize Eq. (1). By transforming $\boldsymbol{P}_t^{(1)}$ and $\boldsymbol{P}_t^{(2)}$ with $\boldsymbol{W}_t^{(1)}$ and $\boldsymbol{W}_t^{(2)}$, respectively, we obtain a common-space feature representation at time point t as $\widehat{\boldsymbol{F}}_t^{(1)} = \left(\boldsymbol{W}_t^{(1)}\right)^T \boldsymbol{K}_t^{(1)}$ and $\widehat{\boldsymbol{F}}_t^{(2)} = \left(\boldsymbol{W}_t^{(2)}\right)^T \boldsymbol{K}_t^{(2)}$.

Step 2: Learning Across-Time-Point Common Features. After concatenating the features obtained in Step 1 as $\widehat{\boldsymbol{F}}_t = \left[\left[\widehat{\boldsymbol{F}}_t^{(1)}\right]^T, \left[\widehat{\boldsymbol{F}}_t^{(2)}\right]^T\right]^T_{2R\times N}$, the $N \times N$ kernel matrix $\widehat{\boldsymbol{K}}_t$ can be computed for each $\widehat{\boldsymbol{F}}_t$. We then estimate the feature transformations $\boldsymbol{Z}_t = [\boldsymbol{z}_t(1), \ldots \boldsymbol{z}_t(g), \ldots, \boldsymbol{z}_t(G)]_{N\times G}$ for each $\widehat{\boldsymbol{F}}_t$, which maximize the correlations of all the transformed features in a global common space with $G = \min_t rank(\widehat{\boldsymbol{K}}_t)$. This can be solved using the multi-set kernel CCA [11, 12], which maximizes the correlations of multiple transformed features between each pair of time points t and t':

$$\begin{gathered}\mathrm{argmax}_{\boldsymbol{z}_t(g)|_{t=1}^T} \sum_{t=1}^{T}\sum_{t'=1,t'\neq t}^{T}\left[\left(\boldsymbol{z}_t(g)\right)^T \widehat{\boldsymbol{K}}_t\left(\left(\boldsymbol{z}_{t'}(g)\right)^T \widehat{\boldsymbol{K}}_{t'}\right)^T\right] \\ s.t., \forall t, \left(\boldsymbol{z}_t(g)\right)^T \widehat{\boldsymbol{K}}_t\left(\left(\boldsymbol{z}_t(g)\right)^T \widehat{\boldsymbol{K}}_t\right)^T = 1\end{gathered} \tag{2}$$

By transforming $\widehat{\boldsymbol{F}}_t$ with $\boldsymbol{Z}_t$, we can obtain a common-space feature representation across different time points as $\widehat{\boldsymbol{D}}_t = (\boldsymbol{Z}_t)^T\widehat{\boldsymbol{K}}_t$.

2.2 Patch-Based Label Fusion for Hippocampus Segmentation

Hierarchical Feature Representation. Before adopting the segmentation algorithm, each original intensity patch from both target images and atlas images is mapped into an across-time-point common space by our proposed hierarchical feature learning method in Section 2.1. Specifically, for segmenting a target subject $\left\{I_{0,t}^{(m)}, m = 1,2\right\}$ at time point t, where we use "0" for representing the current target *subject*, we first align its T1 image with T2 image and then linearly register H atlas subjects $\left\{\left(I_{h,t}^{(m)}, L_{h,t}\right), m = 1,2; t = 1, \ldots, T; h = 1, \ldots, H\right\}$ to them. Here, $L_{h,t}$ indicates the respective hippocampus mask. Instead of simply using the original T1 and T2 intensity patches $\left\{\boldsymbol{p}_{h,t}^{(m)}(v), m = 1,2\right\}$ as the features at location v in the target image ($h = 0$) or atlas images ($h = 1, \ldots, H$), we apply the following steps to map all these original image patches to the across-time-point common space: (1) obtain the within-time-point features by $\hat{\boldsymbol{f}}_{h,t}^{(m)}(v) = \left(\boldsymbol{W}_t^{(m)}\right)^T \phi\left(\boldsymbol{p}_{h,t}^{(m)}(v), \boldsymbol{P}_t^{(m)}\right), m = 1,2$, where Gaussian kernel $\phi(\cdot,\cdot)$ measures the similarity between $\boldsymbol{p}_{h,t}^{(m)}(v)$ and all patches in $\boldsymbol{P}_t^{(m)}$ (defined in Section 2.1); (2) concatenate $\hat{\boldsymbol{f}}_{h,t}^{(1)}(v)$ and $\hat{\boldsymbol{f}}_{h,t}^{(2)}(v)$ to form a within-time-point feature $\hat{\boldsymbol{f}}_{h,t}(v)$; and (3) obtain the feature in the across-time-point common space by $\hat{\boldsymbol{d}}_{h,t}(v) = (\boldsymbol{Z}_t)^T \phi\left(\hat{\boldsymbol{f}}_{h,t}(v), \hat{\boldsymbol{F}}_t\right)$, where $\hat{\boldsymbol{d}}_{h,t}(v)$ is the final learned feature vector for target image ($h = 0$) or atlas images ($h = 1, \ldots, H$) at location v.

Patch-Based Label Fusion. To determine the label $l_{0,t}(u)$ at each target image point u, we collect a set of candidate multi-modality patches along with their corresponding bels $\left\{\left(\boldsymbol{p}_{h,t}^{(m)}(v), l_{h,t}(v)\right), m = 1,2; t = 1, \ldots, T; h = 1, \ldots, H; v \in \Omega(u)\right\}$ in a certain search neighborhood $\Omega(u)$ from H aligned atlases. After mapping all candidate atlas image patches for obtaining the common feature representations $\left\{\hat{\boldsymbol{d}}_{h,t}(v), t = 1, \ldots, T; h = 1, \ldots, H; v \in \Omega(u)\right\}$ across H atlas subjects at different time t, we can construct a dictionary matrix $\boldsymbol{\mathcal{D}}(u)$ by arranging $\left\{\hat{\boldsymbol{d}}_{h,t}(v)\right\}$ column by column. Since each atlas patch bears the anatomical label ("1" for hippocampus and "-1" for non-hippocampus), we can also construct a label vector $\boldsymbol{l}(u)$ from the labels of candidate atlas patches $\left\{l_{h,t}(v), t = 1, \ldots, T; h = 1, \ldots, H; v \in \Omega(u)\right\}$ by following the same order of $\boldsymbol{\mathcal{D}}(u)$, where each element $l_{h,t}(v)$ is the atlas label at $v \in \Omega(u)$. Then, the label fusion can be formulated as a sparse representation problem as:

$$\operatorname{argmin}_{\boldsymbol{\xi}(u)} \left\{\left\|\hat{\boldsymbol{d}}_{0,t}(u) - \boldsymbol{\mathcal{D}}(u)\boldsymbol{\xi}(u)\right\|_2^2 + \lambda\|\boldsymbol{\xi}(u)\|_1\right\}, \tag{3}$$

where λ controls the strength of sparsity constraint. $\boldsymbol{\xi}$ is the weighting vector where each element is associated with one atlas patch in the dictionary and a larger value in $\boldsymbol{\xi}$ indicates the high similarity between the target image patch and the associated atlas patch. SLEP [15] is used to solve the above sparse representation problem. Finally, the label at the target image point u can be determined by $l_{0,t}(u) = sign(\boldsymbol{\xi}^T(u)\boldsymbol{l}(u))$.

3 Experimental Results

We evaluate the proposed method on infant MR brain images of twenty subjects, where each subject has both T1 and T2 MR images acquired at 2 weeks, 3 months, and 6 months of age. Standard image pre-processing steps, including resampling, skull stripping, bias-field correction and histogram matching, are applied to each MR images. We fix the patch size to $9 \times 9 \times 9$ and the weight λ in Eq. (3) to 0.002. FLIRT in the FSL software package [16] with 12 DOF and correlation as the similarity metric is used to linearly align all atlas images to the target image. The twenty subjects are divided into two groups for training and testing, respectively.

Discriminative Power of Learned Common Features. Fig. 3 compares the sample distribution represented by the four different features: T1 intensities, T2 intensities, within-time-point features given by kernel CCA features, and across-time-point features by multi-set kernel CCA features. Based on the projected feature distribution (reduced to three dimensions for visualization) shown in Fig. 3, kernel CCA and multi-set kernel CCA can better separate hippocampus from non-hippocampus samples.

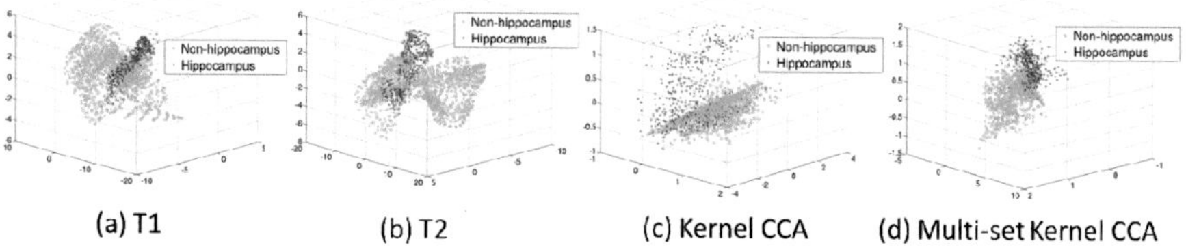

Fig. 3. Distributions of voxel samples with four types of features, respectively. Red crosses and green circles denote hippocampus and non-hippocampus voxel samples, respectively.

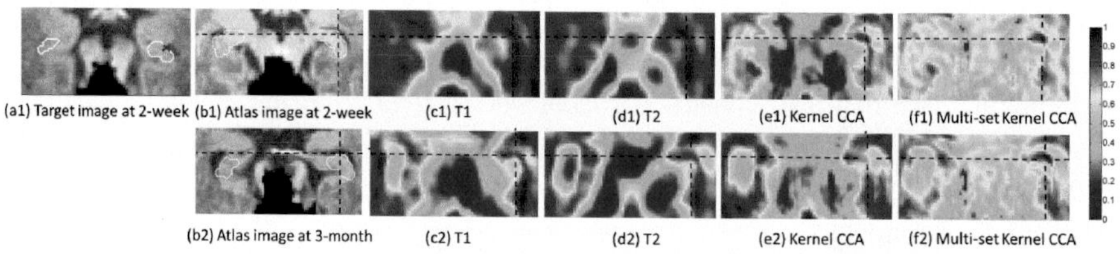

Fig. 4. Comparison of similarity maps for four different feature representations between a key point (red cross) in the target image (a1) and all points in the two atlas images (b1 & b2). (b1) An atlas from the same time point as (a1); (b2) An atlas from a different time point as (a1).

In Fig. 4, we further show the similarity maps resulting from different feature matching between a key point (red cross) on the boundary of the hippocampus (white contours) in the target image (a1) and all points in each of the two atlas images (b1 & b2), respectively. Four feature representation methods: T1 (c1 & c2), T2 (d1 & d2), kernel CCA (e1 & e2), and multi-set kernel CCA (f1 & f2) are compared. For the first row, the target and atlas images are from the same time point. The results demonstrate the effectiveness of the within-time-point common features. For the second row, the target and atlas images are from different time points. The results demonstrate the effectiveness of the across-time-point common features.

Quantitative Evaluation on Hippocampus Segmentation. The mean and standard deviation of the Dice ratios and the average symmetric surface distance (ASSD) of the segmentation results based on the four feature representations are listed in Table 1. The best results are marked in bold. Our feature learning method based on multi-set kernel CCA achieves significant improvement over all other methods in terms of overall Dice ratio (paired t-test, $p<0.014$) and ASSD (paired t-test, $p<0.049$). It is worth noting that, although segmenting the 6-month images seems to be the most challenging among all time points, all comparison methods achieve their longitudinally highest segmentation accuracy at 6 months. This is partially due to the large increase of hippocampus volume during early brain development (i.e., average around 20% growth rate of hippocampus volume from 2-week-old to 6-month-old infants), making large hippocampus volumes in the 6-month-olds relatively easy to segment. Besides, the Dice ratios for combined T1 and T2 are 59.3%, 67.2%, and 70.2%, respectively, for 2-week, 3-month, and 6-month images, which are 5.9%, 3.1%, and 2.4% lower than our proposed method. To test consistency in hippocampal volume measured by different raters, an overall inter-rater reliability ICC (intra-class correlation coefficient) between segmentation techniques for each rater is calculated for hippocampal volumes. The inter-rater ICC is 79.4% for the manual segmentations. Fig. 5 further shows some typical results of surface distances between automatic segmentations and manual segmentations by the four feature representation methods. Our proposed hierarchical feature learning achieves the best performance.

Table 1. Mean and standard deviation of Dice ratio (Dice, in %) and average symmetric surface distance (ASSD, in mm) for the segmenations obtained by four feature representation methods.

	Age	T1	T2	Kernel CCA	Multi-set kernel CCA
	2-Week	60.3±14.5	50.7±13.8	63.1±12.1	**65.2±10.1**
Dice	3-Month	66.7±11.9	59.5± 8.8	69.2± 4.9	**70.3± 5.3**
(%)	6-Month	69.6±10.1	66.9± 8.3	71.5± 7.9	**72.6± 7.0**
	Average	65.5±12.5	59.0±12.4	67.9± 9.3	**69.3± 8.2**
	2-Week	0.96±0.49	1.20±0.39	0.89±0.37	**0.88±0.33**
ASSD	3-Month	0.79±0.33	0.97±0.21	0.78±0.14	**0.76±0.17**
(mm)	6-Month	0.79±0.31	0.84±0.24	0.75±0.25	**0.72±0.22**
	Average	0.85±0.38	1.00±0.32	0.81±0.27	**0.79±0.25**

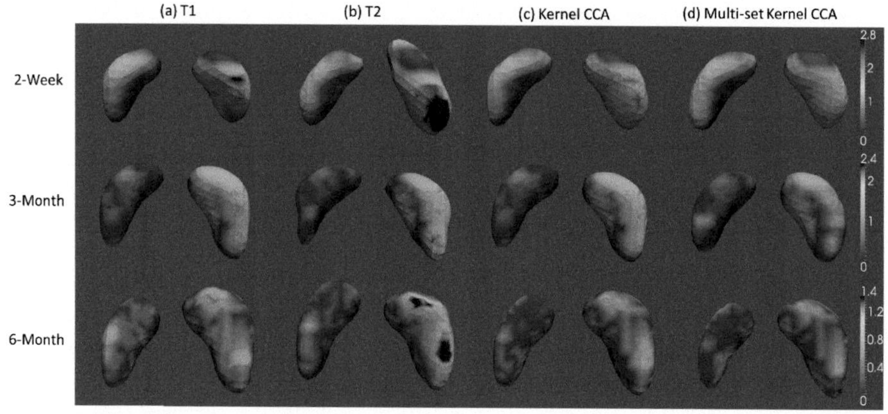

Fig. 5. Visualization of surface distance (in mm) for hippocampus segmentation results.

4 Conclusion

In this paper, we proposed a multi-atlas patch-based label propagation and fusion method for the hippocampus segmentation of infant brain MR images acquired from the first year of life. To deal with dynamic change in tissue contrast, we proposed a hierarchical feature learning approach to obtain common feature representations for multi-modal and longitudinal imaging data. These features resulted in better patch matching, which allowed for better hippocampus segmentation accuracy. In the future, we will evaluate the proposed method using more time points from infant data.

References

1. Bartsch, T.: The Clinical Neurobiology of the Hippocampus: An integrative view, vol. 151. OUP, Oxford (2012)
2. Li, J., Jin, Y., Shi, Y., Dinov, I.D., Wang, D.J., Toga, A.W., Thompson, P.M.: Voxelwise spectral diffusional connectivity and Its applications to alzheimer's disease and intelligence prediction. In: Mori, K., Sakuma, I., Sato, Y., Barillot, C., Navab, N. (eds.) MICCAI 2013, Part I. LNCS, vol. 8149, pp. 655–662. Springer, Heidelberg (2013)
3. Cohen, D.J.: Developmental Psychopathology, 2nd edn. Developmental Neuroscience, vol. 2. Wiley (2006)
4. Coupé, P., et al.: Patch-based Segmentation using Expert Priors: Application to Hippocampus and Ventricle Segmentation. NeuroImage 54, 940–954 (2011)
5. Rousseau, F., et al.: A Supervised Patch-Based Approach for Human Brain Labeling. IEEE Trans. Medical Imaging 30, 1852–1862 (2011)
6. Tong, T., et al.: Segmentation of MR Images via Discriminative Dictionary Learning and Sparse Coding: Application to Hippocampus Labeling. NeuroImage 76, 11–23 (2013)
7. Wang, H., et al.: Multi-Atlas Segmentation with Joint Label Fusion. IEEE Trans. Pattern Anal. Mach. Intell. 35, 611–623 (2013)
8. Wu, G., et al.: A Generative Probability Model of Joint Label Fusion for Multi-Atlas Based Brain Segmentation. Medical Image Analysis 18, 881–890 (2014)

9. Hardoon, D.R., et al.: Canonical Correlation Analysis: An Overview with Application to Learning Methods. Neural Computation 16, 2639–2664 (2004)
10. Arora, R., Livescu, K.: Kernel CCA for Multi-view Acoustic Feature Learning using Articulatory Measurements. In: Proceedings of the MLSLP (2012)
11. Lee, G., et al.: Supervised Multi-View Canonical Correlation Analysis (sMVCCA): Integrating Histologic and Proteomic Features for Predicting Recurrent Prostate Cancer. IEEE Transactions on Medical Imaging 34, 284–297 (2015)
12. Munoz-Mari, J., et al.: Multiset Kernel CCA for Multitemporal Image Classification. In: MultiTemp 2013, pp. 1–4 (2013)
13. Liao, S., et al.: Sparse Patch-Based Label Propagation for Accurate Prostate Localization in CT Images. IEEE Transactions on Medical Imaging 32, 419–434 (2013)
14. Vercauteren, T., et al.: Diffeomorphic Demons: Efficient Non-parametric Image Registration. NeuroImage 45, 61–72 (2009)
15. Liu, J., et al.: SLEP: Sparse Learning with Efficient Projections. Arizona State University (2009), `http://www.public.asu.edu/~jye02/Software/SLEP`
16. Jenkinson, M., et al.: Improved Optimization for the Robust and Accurate Linear Registration and Motion Correction of Brain Images. NeuroImage 17, 825–841 (2002)

Measuring Cortical Neurite-Dispersion and Perfusion in Preterm-Born Adolescents Using Multi-modal MRI

Andrew Melbourne[1], Zach Eaton-Rosen[1], David Owen[1], Jorge Cardoso[1], Joanne Beckmann[2], David Atkinson[3], Neil Marlow[2], and Sebastien Ourselin[1]

[1] Centre for Medical Image Computing, University College London, UK
[2] Academic Neonatology, EGA UCL Institute for Women's Health, London, UK
[3] Medical Physics, University College Hospital, London, UK

Abstract. As a consequence of a global increase in rates of extremely preterm birth, predicting the long term impact of preterm birth has become an important focus of research. Cohorts of extremely preterm born subjects studied in the 1990s are now beginning to reach adulthood and the long term structural alterations of disrupted neurodevelopment in gestation can now be investigated, for instance with magnetic resonance (MR) imaging. Disruption to normal development as a result of preterm birth is likely to result in both cerebrovascular and microstructural differences compared to term-born controls. Of note, arterial spin labelled MRI provides a marker of cerebral blood flow, whilst multi-compartment diffusion models provide information on the cerebral microstructure, including that of the cortex. We apply these techniques to a cohort of 19 year-old adolescents consisting of both extremely-preterm and term-born individuals and investigate the structural and functional correlations of these MR modalities. Work of this type, revealing the long-term structural and functional differences in preterm cohorts, can help better inform on the likely outcomes of contemporary extremely preterm newborns and provides an insight into the lifelong effects of preterm birth.

1 Introduction

Very preterm birth (birth at less than 32 weeks completed gestational age) occurs at a time of rapid neurological development supported by changes in blood flow and distribution. Preterm birth leads to an increased risk of adverse neurodevelopmental outcome [1] and this is believed to be related to delay or disruption to normal developmental and subsequent longterm deficits. Investigation of the long term impacts of prematurity in early adulthood allows us to infer the impact of early injury on later functional development. The effect of preterm birth on the cardiovascular system has recently been investigated [2] where raised blood pressure and increased cardiac wall thickness were observed. These effects are thought to be related to the long term impact of the early switch from a placental circulation to a driven pulmonary circulation, although this is likely to be complicated by intrauterine infection, hypoxia and poor postnatal organ

N. Navab et al. (Eds.): MICCAI 2015, Part III, LNCS 9351, pp. 72–79, 2015.
DOI: 10.1007/978-3-319-24574-4_9

growth. The consequential impact of preterm birth on the cerebrovascular system is an open area of research and combined measurement of both flow and cortical architecture are likely to be important in establishing both the impact of prematurity on function and also providing early evidence of cerebrovascular disease in adulthood.

Arterial Spin Labelled (ASL) MRI has achieved some success in recent years, linked to the increased availability of 3T MRI, as an endogenous tracer technique for measuring blood flow and perfusion [3]. The technique has found many applications and here we apply the technique to investigating the long term influence of preterm birth and relate this to cortical microstructure as assessed by diffusion weighted MRI (DWI). Measurement of changes to cerebral blood flow (CBF) allows investigation of the functional properties of the tissue. Accurate measurement of alterations in brain perfusion as a result of preterm birth may have substantial benefit for predicting lifelong risk of vascular disorders and thus preventative steps can be taken at an early age. Combined with multi-compartment diffusion imaging, the joint role of ASL and microstructure can be investigated and in this work we make this possible by combining two such modalities.

Substantial changes in architecture and appearance occur in the cortex during the last 10 weeks of gestation. The appearance of intra-cortical arborisation and new cortico-cortical connections can be observed using diffusion weighted MRI (DWI). Recent biophysically motivated models of grey and white matter diffusion characteristics can be used to observe these changes *in vivo* [4]. These structural changes occur in tandem with changes to the microvascular environment and preterm birth results in much of this development taking place in altered developmental conditions. A combination of focal brain tissue injury and developmental disturbances is thought to be responsible for many of the functional deficits seen at later ages [5] and would be reflected in structural and function changes measured using a range of MR modalities.

There is some support for the theory that oxygen delivery is limited by the propensity of oxygen to diffuse through extra-vascular tissue and that this explains some of the relationships observed using arterial spin labelled and blood-oxygenation level dependent MRI [6,7]. The cortical microenvironment observed by the diffusion of water in DWI is also the environment that provides a barrier to oxygen diffusion and thus it is plausible that a relationship would be observed. Specifically, this would imply that the local structure and local tissue composition relate to blood delivery to the cortex and specifically that increased cortical orientation dispersion (and thus a more complex local tissue arrangement) would correlate with increased local cerebral, and thus cortical, blood flow.

In this work, we use a novel modified diffusion model-fit that makes use of T2-weighted images to separate contributions from tissue and free isotropic volume fractions and use this to investigate the relationship of these parameters with the measured CBF from ASL. This is the first time that correlations of this type have been shown in this extremely-preterm born adolescent cohort.

2 Methods

Data. Data was collected from 43 preterms (born at less than 26 weeks completed gestation) and 21 term-born adolescents at 19 years of age. On a Philips 3T Achieva we acquired Pseudo-Continuous ASL (PCASL) for 30 control-label pairs with PLD=1800ms+41ms/slice, label duration (τ)=1650ms (3x3x5mm). Acquisition was carried out using 2D EPI in the same geometry as the DWI ensuring similar levels of distortion. Diffusion weighted data was acquired across four b-values at $b = \{0, 300, 700, 2000\} s.mm^{-2}$ with $n = \{4, 8, 16, 32\}$ directions respectively at TE=70ms (2.5x2.5x3.0mm). T2 weighted data was acquired in the same space as the diffusion imaging with five echo times at TE={40,50,85,100,150}ms. In addition we acquired a 3D T1-weighted volume at 1mm isotropic resolution for obtaining a segmentation and region labels [8].

Arterial Spin Labelled MRI. PCASL data can be used to estimate a cerebral blood flow map (CBF) using the following relationship [3]:

$$\mathrm{CBF} = \frac{6000\lambda}{2\alpha} \frac{e^{\mathrm{PLD}/\mathrm{T1}_{\mathrm{blood}}}}{\mathrm{T1}_{\mathrm{blood}}(1 - e^{-\tau/\mathrm{T1}_{\mathrm{blood}}})} \frac{(S_C - S_L)}{S_{PD}} [\mathrm{ml}/100g/\mathrm{min}] \quad (1)$$

where λ is the plasma/tissue partition coefficient (0.9ml/g), PLD the post-labelling delay after the end of the bolus, $\mathrm{T1}_{blood}$ the blood T1 value ($1650ms$), α the labelling efficiency (0.85) and τ the labelling pulse duration.

Multi-compartment Diffusion Weighted Imaging. We fit a multi- compartment signal model to the multi-shell data using non-linear least squares [9]. We fit the model simultaneously to the diffusion weighted and T2 data, treating the T2 data as unweighted diffusion data with variable echo time. We provide a modification of the method of [9] to explicitly incorporate a two-compartment T2 distribution allowing correction of volume fractions in regions of mixed T2, such as voxels containing both GM and CSF which are of interest for this work.

$$S(b, \mathbf{x}) = S_0 \left[v_{iso} e^{-bd_{iso}} e^{-\mathrm{TE}/\mathrm{T2}_{iso}} + (v_{in} A_{in} + v_{ex} A_{ex}) e^{-\mathrm{TE}/\mathrm{T2}_{tis}} \right] \quad (2)$$

The signal model attributes the grey matter signal measured by DWI to three compartments; an intra-neurite space, with volume fraction v_{in} and signal modelled by $A_{in}(\gamma, \mathbf{x}, \theta, \phi, d_{||})$, and an extra-neurite space, with volume fraction v_{ex} with signal modelled by $A_{ex}(v_{in}, \gamma, \mathbf{x}, \theta, \phi, d_{||})$ and a free-isotropic space with volume fraction, v_{iso} modelled as a function of isotropic diffusivity d_{iso} [10]. The two angular parameters θ and ϕ define the principal diffusion direction whilst $d_{||}$ and d_{iso} describe parallel (to the principal direction) and isotropic diffusivities respectively. Given the experimental b-value, b, and gradient direction, $\mathbf{x}$, the signal from the intra and extra-neurite spaces is coupled by a specific distribution, $f(\mathbf{n}, \gamma)$, which is assumed to represent axonal dispersion; formally a Watson distribution of oblateness γ, varying between 0, for highly oriented axons, up to

1 when there is no preferred structural orientation [9]. This distribution couples the intra and extra neurite spaces. The multi-compartment diffusion fitting routine above can be enhanced by the inclusion of T2 relaxometry data. In this case we give the algorithm additional information, ostensibly to give a higher precision estimate of the v_{iso} volume fraction. Analysis is simplified by only varying the TE of the b0 images, in which case the equation simplifies in the absence of diffusion-weighting to become a two-component T2 relaxometry fit and, using literature values at 3T, we fix the two T2 values to $T2_{tis} = 100ms$ and $T2_{iso} = 300ms$.

3 Results

3.1 Comparison of DWI with and without Additional T2 Imaging

Figure 1 shows examples of model-fitting with and without T2 weighted images on two preterm-born subjects. Figure 1, panel A illustrates differences seen in posterior white matter regions, with lower fitted isotropic volume fraction, whilst panel B illustrates less noisy fitting in regions of pure CSF, albeit in an extreme case. The inclusion of T2-weighted images helps suppress high white matter v_{iso} values and reduces noisy parameter values in regions of CSF. We use this to motivate the use of the joint model fitting technique.

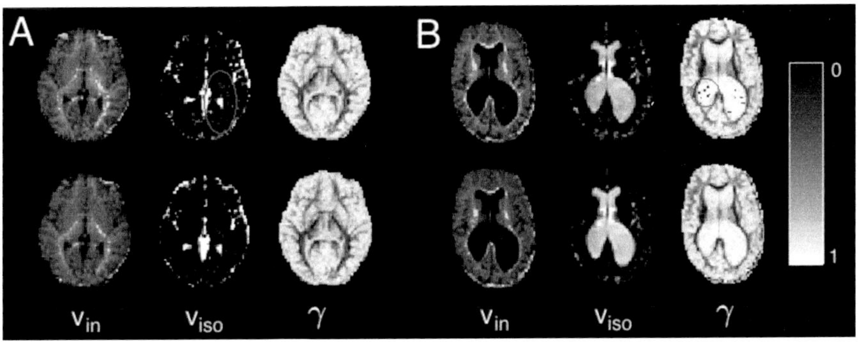

Fig. 1. Comparison of modified (top row) and non-modified (bottom row) DW model-fitting for two cases. Note the suppressed posterior white-matter v_{iso} volume fraction in case A (circled) and the reduced ventricular CSF noise for case B (v_{iso} and γ (circled)).

3.2 Comparison of Quantitative Neuroimaging Parameters

Figure 2 shows example data for a single representative control subject showing the cortical variability of the CBF and the diffusion imaging parameters. Visible is an empirical correlation between CBF and cortical orientation dispersion (γ) but not between CBF and v_{in}. A propagated labelling is also shown [8].

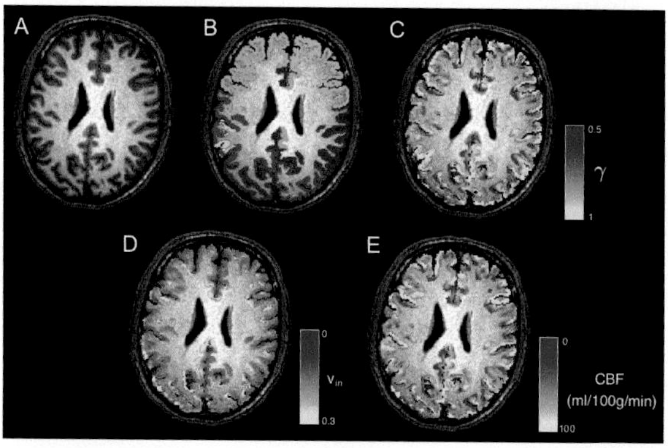

Fig. 2. Example control data. A) T1-weighted slice, B) lobe parcellation, C) cortical CBF D) cortical v_{in} E) cortical orientation dispersion γ.

Figure 3 shows the cortical distribution of diffusion characteristics and CBF. CBF values are found to be lower in the preterm cohort (48.67±5.6ml/100g/min) on average compared to their term-born counterparts (53.9 ± 7.7ml/100g/min). Grey matter volume is also lower in the preterm group with a volume of $0.578 \pm 0.06l$ compared to $0.621 \pm 0.05l$ in the term group. Distributions of parameters from diffusion imaging show increased variability: average values of v_{in} in the term-born cohort are 0.348 ± 0.08 compared to 0.380 ± 0.07 in the preterm cohort; average values of v_{iso} in the term-born cohort are 0.045 ± 0.02 compared to 0.045 ± 0.03 in the preterm cohort; and average values of γ in the term-born cohort are 0.671 ± 0.07 compared to 0.633 ± 0.07 in the preterm cohort. Of these four parameters, only the CBF and GM volume reach a significant difference for $p<0.05$ (p=0.003, p=0.006 respectively) between preterm and term groups.

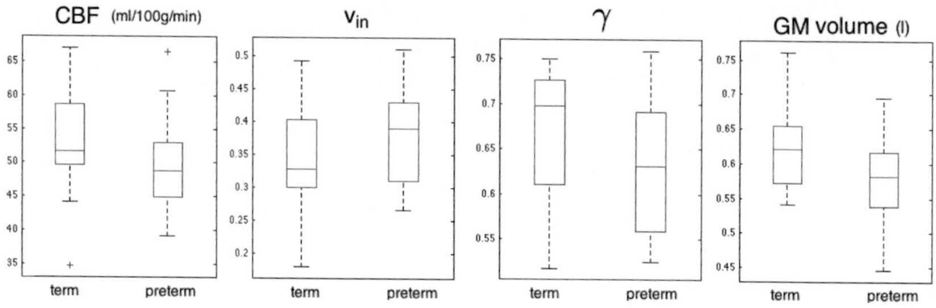

Fig. 3. Group distribution of whole-cortex average grey matter parameter values for a) CBF, b) intra-axonal volume fraction v_{in}, c) grey matter volume (litres), and d) cortical orientation dispersion γ.

3.3 Correlation of Diffusion MRI and Cerebral Blood Flow

In the absence of a known cortical diffusion to blood flow relationship, we investigate the relationship between cortical diffusion properties and CBF by comparing image similarity using Spearman's rank correlation in cortical grey matter. The distribution of correlation values between term and preterm groups is shown in Figure 4. These distributions reveal that the average correlation values are positive for both v_{in} and for γ and slightly negative for v_{iso}. Between term-born and preterm groups, paired t-tests yield insignificance for v_{in} and v_{iso} (p=0.587 and p= 0.644 respectively) and a significant difference between CBF and cortical dispersion (p=0.005). In order to account for volume effects we test for differences while correcting for volume using linear regression with a covariate, correlation for v_{in} and v_{iso} remains insignificant, whilst correlation for CBF and cortical dispersion remains highly significant (p=0.006) a weak correlation (r=0.3, p=0.014) is found between v_{iso} and γ. These results may imply that the relationship between CBF and cortical dispersion could be used as an imaging biomarker.

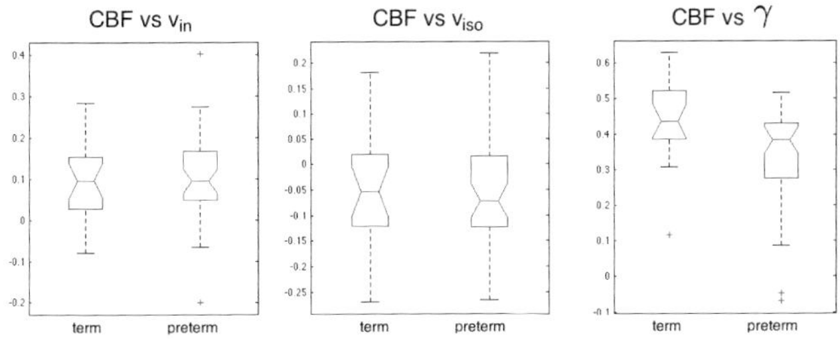

Fig. 4. Group distributions of the single-subject image correlation coefficients between CBF and grey matter parameter values for a) v_{in}, b) v_{iso} and c) γ.

We also investigate differences between frontal, temporal, parietal and occipital lobe regions (both hemispheres combined). Label-based results are shown for the four major lobes in Figure 5. The highest correlations between CBF and γ are seen in the parietal lobe and the pattern is consistent across lobes for both groups. These results are commensurate with a theory of blood delivery governed by the diffusivity of the local environment to extra-capillary oxygen.

4 Discussion

We have shown that advanced diffusion model fitting and arterial spin labelled MRI can be used to investigate the cerebral cortex and that CBF values derived from ASL MRI correlate strongly with measures of cortical orientation dispersion found from DWI. Additionally we have shown that this relationship is different between preterm and term born 19 year olds, which possibly reflects long term

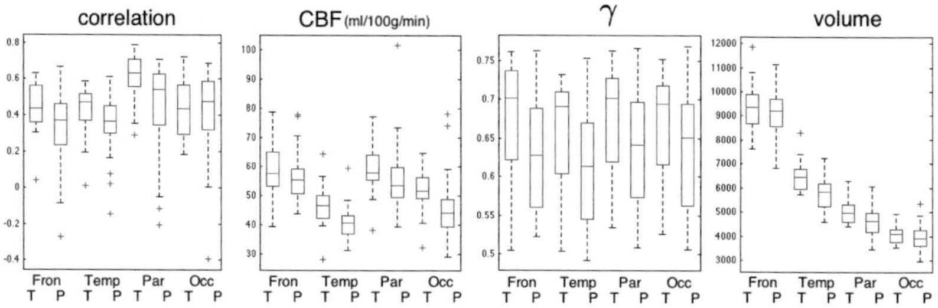

Fig. 5. Group distributions for a) the spatial correlation coefficient between CBF and γ b) CBF, c) γ and d) lobe volume for frontal (fron), temporal (temp), parietal (par) and occipital (occ) lobes (P=preterm, T=term-born).

differences in cortical architecture as a result of being born extremely premature. Including volumetric data we find that subjects in the preterm cohort have significantly reduced GM volume, but that this does not seem to influence the parametric results obtained. This is despite GM volume reduction increasing partial voluming in both the CBF and DWI parameter estimates. This effect is to some extent mitigated by the multi-compartment DWI model and its effect in ASL is unclear and confounded by global volume differences that affect CBF estimates via transit times and tissue type (T1) effects. Erring on the side of caution, the correlations we observe may thus not be causal in nature.

The combination of DWI and multi-echo T2 weighted imaging is novel and allows more robust model-fitting and has the potential to enable new models to be more accurately fitted. Future work will use this model in combination with ASL to make predictions about functional development and develop vascular biomarkers in preterm children. Once again, the combination of measurements in this work: the acquisition of widely available multi-shell DWI, multi-echo T2 imaging and CBF data within clinically feasible time frames is important and will encourage research into the generation of new predictive structural biomarkers that have a tangible physical link to neuronal structure and function.

One interesting observation for fitting of this type is that the v_{iso} estimates fitted from the diffusion model with and without varying echo-time data are complicated slightly by the different treatment of perfusion effects with and without diffusion weighting. If these can be neglected, improved model-fitting performance can be achieved; conversely, if these effects cannot be neglected this methodology opens the door to more elaborate models of MR measurement.

The analysis in this work can be developed further by acquiring more sophisticated, albeit time-consuming, multi inversion-time ASL experiments. Furthermore, although they are notoriously difficult, cortical thickness measurements could be used to assess CBF as a function of cortical tissue volume in addition to local structural differences.

In conclusion, we have shown that MRI measurement of cortical microstructure can be linked to indices of cerebral perfusion. Work of this type, linking functional performance with structural measurement; is particularly salient for preterm-born cohorts for which accurate prediction of function is crucial to providing effective intervention. The investigation of the long term sequelae of extreme prematurity will help inform early support and intervention for those infants being born extremely premature now.

Acknowledgements. We would like to acknowledge the MRC, the National Institute for Health Research (NIHR), the EPSRC (EP/H046410/1) and the UCLH/UCL CBRC Strategic Investment Award (Ref. 168).

References

1. Costeloe, K.L., Hennessy, E.M., Haider, S., Stacey, F., Marlow, N., Draper, E.S.: Short term outcomes after extreme preterm birth in england: comparison of two birth cohorts in, and (the epicure studies). BMJ 345, e7976 (1995)
2. Lewandowski, A.J., Augustine, D., Lamata, P., Davis, E.F., Lazdam, M., Francis, J., McCormick, K., Wilkinson, A.R., Singhal, A., Lucas, A., Smith, N.P., Neubauer, S., Leeson, P.: Preterm heart in adult life: cardiovascular magnetic resonance reveals distinct differences in left ventricular mass, geometry, and function. Circulation 127(2), 197–206 (2013)
3. Alsop, D.C., Detre, J.A., Golay, X., Günther, M., Hendrikse, J., Lu, H., Macintosh, B.J., Parkes, L.M., Smits, M., van Osch, M.J.P., Wang, D.J.J., Wong, E.C., Zaharchuk, G.: Recommended implementation of arterial spin-labeled perfusion mri for clinical applications: A consensus of the ismrm perfusion study group and the european consortium for asl in dementia. Magn. Reson. Med. (April 2014)
4. Eaton-Rosen, Z., Melbourne, A., Orasanu, E., Cardoso, M.J., Modat, M., Bainbridge, A., Kendall, G.S., Robertson, N.J., Marlow, N., Ourselin, S.: Longitudinal measurement of the developing grey matter in preterm subjects using multi-modal mri. Neuroimage 111, 580–589 (2015)
5. Volpe, J.J.: Brain injury in premature infants: a complex amalgam of destructive and developmental disturbances. Lancet Neurol. 8(1), 110–124 (2009)
6. Buxton, R.B., Frank, L.R.: A model for the coupling between cerebral blood flow and oxygen metabolism during neural stimulation. J. Cereb. Blood Flow Metab. 17(1), 64–72 (1997)
7. Hoge, R.D., Atkinson, J., Gill, B., Crelier, G.R., Marrett, S., Pike, G.B.: Linear coupling between cerebral blood flow and oxygen consumption in activated human cortex. Proc. Natl. Acad. Sci. U S A 96(16), 9403–9408 (1999)
8. Cardoso, M.J., Modat, M., Wolz, R., Melbourne, A., Cash, D., Rueckert, D., Ourselin, S.: Geodesic information flows: spatially-variant graphs and their application to segmentation and fusion. IEEE TMI 99 (2015)
9. Zhang, H., Schneider, T., Wheeler-Kingshott, C.A., Alexander, D.C.: Noddi: practical in vivo neurite orientation dispersion and density imaging of the human brain. Neuroimage 61(4), 1000–1016 (2012)
10. Alexander, D.C., Hubbard, P.L., Hall, M.G., Moore, E.A., Ptito, M., Parker, G.J.M., Dyrby, T.B.: Orientationally invariant indices of axon diameter and density from diffusion mri. Neuroimage 52(4), 1374–1389 (2010)

Interactive Whole-Heart Segmentation in Congenital Heart Disease

Danielle F. Pace[1], Adrian V. Dalca[1], Tal Geva[2,3], Andrew J. Powell[2,3], Mehdi H. Moghari[2,3], and Polina Golland[1]

[1] Computer Science and Artificial Intelligence Lab, MIT, Cambridge, MA, USA
[2] Department of Cardiology, Boston Children's Hospital, Boston, MA, USA
[3] Department of Pediatrics, Harvard Medical School, Boston, MA, USA
dfpace@mit.edu

Abstract. We present an interactive algorithm to segment the heart chambers and epicardial surfaces, including the great vessel walls, in pediatric cardiac MRI of congenital heart disease. Accurate whole-heart segmentation is necessary to create patient-specific 3D heart models for surgical planning in the presence of complex heart defects. Anatomical variability due to congenital defects precludes fully automatic atlas-based segmentation. Our interactive segmentation method exploits expert segmentations of a small set of short-axis slice regions to automatically delineate the remaining volume using patch-based segmentation. We also investigate the potential of active learning to automatically solicit user input in areas where segmentation error is likely to be high. Validation is performed on four subjects with double outlet right ventricle, a severe congenital heart defect. We show that strategies asking the user to manually segment regions of interest within short-axis slices yield higher accuracy with less user input than those querying entire short-axis slices.

1 Introduction

Whole-heart segmentation in pediatric cardiac MRI has great potential to improve surgical planning in children with congenital heart defects by enabling creation of patient-specific 3D heart models. In particular, 3D-printed heart models promise to provide surgeons with an anatomically faithful, tactile experience [7]. Building such models requires delineating all of the cardiac structures in a patient's MRI, including the entire blood pool, epicardial surface and the great vessels. Clinically available tools often require 4-8 hours of user interaction to manually segment 100-200 slices covering the entire heart and the great vessels [4,11], which precludes routine clinical use of 3D heart models.

Whole-heart segmentation is challenging even in normal subjects. Previously demonstrated methods typically employ atlas-based segmentation or fit deformable models to the image to be segmented [15]. The substantial changes in heart topology and high anatomical variability in congenital heart disease (CHD) render such model-based methods infeasible without an extremely large database of previously annotated scans. For example, in a subclass of CHD called

N. Navab et al. (Eds.): MICCAI 2015, Part III, LNCS 9351, pp. 80–88, 2015.
DOI: 10.1007/978-3-319-24574-4_10

double outlet right ventricle (DORV), the aorta arises from the right ventricle (instead of the left) and a ventricular septal defect forms a hole in the septum between the two ventricles. Specialized segmentation algorithms have been developed for hearts with infarcts, left ventricular hypertropy, or pulmonary hypertension [1,9]. These methods use probabilistic atlases or point distribution models built for normal subjects by finding some transformation between the abnormal heart and the normal model. These algorithms were designed for segmenting the ventricles, and it is unlikely that such methods will perform well for whole-heart segmentation in CHD. Automatic segmentation in cardiac MRI is also complicated by intensity inhomogeneities, low contrast, and thin heart walls near the atria, valves and great vessels which are barely visible. At the same time, high accuracy is required for creating useful heart models for surgical planning.

We therefore focus on developing efficient interactive segmentation methods. Interactive segmentation fits well into clinical workflows since physicians must validate any segmentation used for decision making and correct the errors that are inevitable in automatic segmentation. We present a patch-based [3,6] interactive segmentation method that provides accurate whole-heart segmentation in CHD. The method uses a small set of manually labeled slices to segment the remaining volume, thus circumventing the challenges of anatomical variability.

Moreover, we examine active learning methods [8] to further reduce the number of interactions. At each step of an active learning session, the algorithm directs the user to manually label part of the data deemed most informative. These methods promise better accuracy with fewer user interactions compared to systems in which the user decides where to provide input. Most active learning methods for interactive medical image segmentation rely on uncertainty sampling with a batch selection query strategy [2,5,10,12,13,14]. In uncertainty sampling, the active learner selects the voxels in which it is least confident. Confidence can be measured using image-based metrics [10,14] or label probabilities [5,13]. Ensemble methods assess the disagreement among votes [2], while SVM classifiers choose data based on distance to the margin [12]. Batch queries ask the user to label multiple voxels in each interaction step. A query can involve annotating sets of the most informative voxels [2,5,12], segmenting entire slice planes [10,14] or deciding whether or not to include an entire hypothesized object [13].

Within our patch-based interactive segmentation framework for high-quality segmentation in CHD, we explore the potential benefits of active learning with batch queries based on uncertainty sampling. We show that methods that select entire slices for manual delineation fail to perform significantly better than a simple strategy based on a uniform distribution of the input slices. In contrast, active learning queries that asks the user to segment regions of interest (ROIs) within short-axis planes are more accurate with less user interaction.

2 Patch-Based Interactive Segmentation

In this section we describe our interactive patch-based segmentation algorithm that incorporates user annotations. The method also provides a baseline for our study of active learning strategies for cardiac MRI segmentation.

Given input image $I : \Omega_I \in \mathbb{R}^3 \to \mathbb{R}$, we seek a label map $L : \Omega_I \to \{l_b, l_m, l_k\}$ that parcellates image I into blood pool, myocardium and background. For the purpose of creating 3D heart models, the myocardium class includes the papillary muscles and the great vessel walls. We let $\mathcal{R}_I = \{r_i : \Omega_i \in \mathbb{R}^2 \to \{l_b, l_m, l_k\}\}$ be a set of manually labeled reference regions, where each subdomain $\Omega_i \in \Omega_I$ is defined on a short-axis plane. We focus on short-axis slices because clinicians are already accustomed to segmenting short-axis views for making cardiac function measurements such as ejection fraction. In the simplest case, a reference domain Ω_i is an entire short-axis slice plane, but it may represent a region of interest within a slice. In our baseline algorithm, the expert segments entire short-axis slices that are uniformly distributed in the MRI volume.

At each step of the interactive segmentation procedure, the user manually segments a provided short-axis region and a patch-based method is used to update the segmentation volume [3,6]. The manually segmented regions provide patient-specific information on the heart's shape and the local appearance of the blood pool, myocardium and surrounding organs, which is exploited by the algorithm to infer labels in the remaining image.

For every target slice t to be segmented, a library of intensity patches with corresponding labels is constructed using the target's set of relevant reference regions $\mathcal{R}_t \in \mathcal{R}_I$. If every reference domain Ω_i is an entire short-axis slice, each remaining target slice in the volume is segmented using the closest reference slice above and below. If $\{\Omega_i\}$ contains smaller ROIs, each target slice is segmented using patches from the two closest entire reference slices plus all of the ROIs between them. An ROI segmentation "shadows" the region behind it so that only the physically closest information is used for each voxel in the target slice.

To segment patch $p_t(x^i)$ centered at voxel position x^i in target slice t, we find the k most similar patches in $\mathcal{R}_t$. We use $x = [x_1, x_2, x_3]$ to denote the three coordinates of position x, where x_1 and x_2 are in-plane (short-axis) coordinates and x_3 is the out-of-plane coordinate. Given a patch $p_r(x^j)$ centered at voxel position x^j in a reference $r \in \mathcal{R}_t$ with domain Ω_r, the distance between patch $p_t(x^i)$ and patch $p_r(x^j)$ depends on the patch intensities, gradients and positions:

$$\begin{aligned} d(p_t(x^i), p_r(x^j)) &= \alpha \|p_t(x^i) - p_r(x^j)\|^2 + \beta \|\nabla p_t(x^i) - \nabla p_r(x^j)\|^2 \\ &+ \delta_{\|}(x^i, \Omega_r)\Big[(x_1^i - x_1^j)^2 + (x_2^i - x_2^j)^2\Big] + \delta_{\perp}(x^i, \mathcal{R}_t)(x_3^i - x_3^j)^2. \end{aligned} \tag{1}$$

Here, α and β are weights on the relative importance of the intensity and gradient terms, respectively, and $\delta_{\|}(x^i, \Omega_r)$ and $\delta_{\perp}(x^i, \mathcal{R}_t)$ are spatially-varying weights on the in-plane and out-of-plane components of the positions, respectively.

The position weighting is higher when a target patch is close to one of its references, to encourage matching to the close reference since it likely contains the same structures. To this end, the out-of-plane position weight $\delta_{\perp}(x^i, \mathcal{R}_t)$ is defined as the distance from x^i to the closest point within any of its references:

$$\begin{aligned} \delta_{\perp}(x^i, \mathcal{R}_t) &= \gamma_1 \exp^{-\gamma_2 \cdot D_{\perp}(x^i, \mathcal{R}_t)} + \gamma_3, \\ D_{\perp}(x^i, \mathcal{R}_t) &= \min_{r \in \mathcal{R}_t} \min_{x^j \in \Omega_r} \|x^i - x^j\|. \end{aligned} \tag{2}$$

Second, we allow a larger effective search area within distant reference slices, which enables matching of structures that might change shape substantially across neighboring slices. In contrast, if the reference slice is very close then the matching structure is probably at a similar position. The in-plane position weight $\delta_{\|}(x^i, \Omega_r)$ is therefore different for each reference r, and is defined as the distance from x^i to the closest point in the reference domain Ω_r:

$$\begin{aligned} \delta_{\|}(x^i, \Omega_r) &= \lambda_1 \exp^{-\lambda_2 \cdot D_{\|}(x^i, \Omega_r)} + \lambda_3, \\ D_{\|}(x^i, \Omega_r) &= \min_{x^j \in \Omega_r} \|x^i - x^j\|. \end{aligned} \tag{3}$$

Given the k most similar reference patches, the labeling for the target patch is determined through majority voting. The reference patch segmentations contribute overlapping votes (i.e., they vote for all voxels in a patch), which smooths the segmentation. This variant removes the need for additional smoothness constraints that could potentially eliminate small walls in the heart and great vessels.

3 Empirical Study: Active Learning for Reference Selection

Here we investigate batch query strategies for automatically choosing the subdomains $\{\Omega_i\}$ to be segmented by the expert. First, we compare interactive workflows that select entire short-axis slices versus those selecting smaller ROIs of a fixed size. To decouple the effect of the reference domain size from that of a specific uncertainty sampling method, we use a gold-standard manual segmentation to identify the next region to be segmented. At each step, the region with the highest segmentation error over its domain spanning $\pm h$ slices is selected for manual segmentation. We refer to this iterative setup as **oracle** uncertainty estimation. We emphasize that our goal is to investigate the effect of the interaction strategy, as this approach is clearly infeasible for segmentation of novel images. In practice, uncertainty can be measured using metrics that locally estimate segmentation accuracy through the entropy of the patch vote distributions, alignment of label boundaries with image gradients, and intensity homogeneity within small regions with the same label [10,14].

We compare the two active learning methods (entire slices vs. smaller ROIs) with several baseline approaches in which the user segments entire slices. First, we test against our baseline algorithm using **uniform** slice distribution. We also compare against **random** slice selection, a common baseline in active learning [10,14]. These two slice selection schemes are not iterative. Finally, we implemented a strategy that exhaustively tries all possible new reference slices at each step and uses the gold-standard segmentation to add the slice that maximally reduces the segmentation error. This represents an iterative **optimal greedy** error reduction strategy with respect to maximizing improvement at each step.

4 Results

Data: Validation was performed using four pediatric cardiac MRI images from patients with DORV. A high resolution isotropic whole-heart image was acquired for each patient as part of surgical planning. The scans were performed without contrast agents on a clinical 1.5T scanner (Philips Achieva), using a free-breathing steady-state free precession (SSFP) pulse sequence with ECG and respiratory nagivator gating (TR $=$ 3.4ms/TE $=$1.7ms/$\alpha = 60°$). All images were cropped to a tight region around the heart, rotated into a short-axis orientation and smoothed slightly using anisotropic diffusion. The final image size was around $120 \times 150 \times 200$ and varied across patients. Voxel size was around 0.9mm^3 and also varied slightly across subjects. A gold-standard manual segmentation of the entire image volume was created in approximately eight hours per scan, and is used to simulate user input in interactive segmentation.

Parameter Selection: For interactive patch-based segmentation, we use 5×5 patches and retrieve $k = 10$ nearest neighbor patches for each target patch. The nearest neighbor search was limited to a 101×101 in-plane bounding box. The weights governing the relative influence of the terms used to calculate patch similarity in Eqs. (1)-(3) were determined empirically using the four datasets: for all patients, $\alpha = 1, \beta = 1, \gamma = [8.49, 0.02, 0.0375]$ and $\lambda = [1.62, 0.2, 1.25]$.

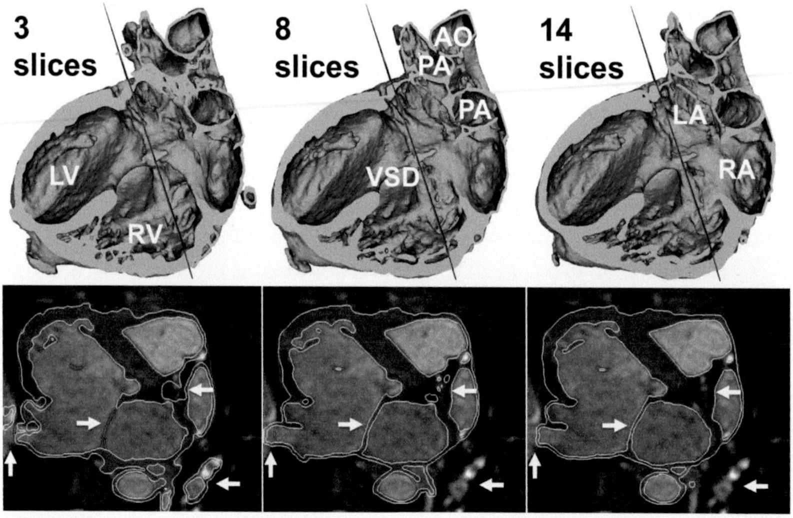

Fig. 1. Example 3D heart models (cut in half to visualize the interior) and segmentation results for a subject with DORV, from patch-based interactive segmentation instantiated with 3, 8 and 14 uniformly distributed reference slices, respectively. Interactive segmentation (yellow) and gold-standard segmentation (red) are shown. LV/RV/LA/RA = left/right ventricle/atrium; VSD = ventricular septal defect; AO = aorta; PA = pulmonary artery. Arrows indicate segmentation errors that are corrected by including more reference slices.

In both oracle strategies, we evaluate errors on regions spanning $\pm h = 2$ slices. In the oracle ROI strategy, we use ROIs of size 39×39. Finally, the oracle and optimal greedy strategies are initialized using three uniformly distributed slices.

Findings: Fig. 1 shows example heart models and segmentations created using interactive patch-based segmentation instantiated with 3, 8 and 14 uniformly distributed reference slices, respectively. The accuracy improvement when more input is provided is clear. A high quality model can be created using only 14 reference short-axis segmentations (out of ~200 slices). Even the model instantiated with 3 reference slices shows roughly correct global structure. Fig. 2 shows segmentation accuracy for uniform slice selection measured as Dice volume overlap for the blood pool and myocardium. The patch-based segmentation method achieves good accuracy using relatively few segmented slices, especially considering the difficulty of whole-heart segmentation in CHD.

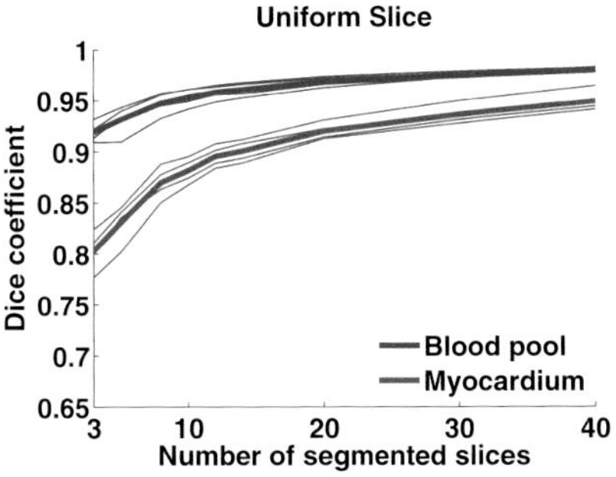

Fig. 2. Accuracy of patch-based interactive segmentation as a function of the number of uniformly distributed reference slices. Thin lines represent each subject and the thick line corresponds to the mean.

Experimental results for active learning are reported in Fig. 3. We observed that the slices selected by active learning are sampled more densely near the base of the heart and less so near the apex, which correlates with the relative difficulty of segmenting these areas. The active learning strategy that selects entire short-axis slices does not achieve a meaningful improvement compared to uniform slice selection. Even the optimal greedy strategy only shows a modest improvement compared to uniform distribution, indicating that there is not much scope for improvement for active learning methods that iteratively choose entire short-axis slices. All methods substantially outperform random slice selection. This suggests that random selection is not necessarily the most appropriate baseline when evaluating new active learning methods, although it is widely used.

Oracle ROI active learning shows substantial improvement (~5 Dice points for the myocardium) using less user input. Having the user label ROIs targets areas of concentrated errors, leading to more efficient interactive segmentation.

Manual delineation of 15 short-axis slices requires less than one hour of an expert's time, vs 4-8 hours for the entire volume. The runtime of our current implementation of patch-based segmentation takes roughly one hour per scan. The computation time associated with adding a new reference region is proportional to the number of affected target slices. Future work will focus on improving the algorithm runtime, e.g., through the use of approximate nearest neighbors.

Our experiments raised an interesting question of what should be used as a surrogate measure for the amount of user interaction. The results reported in Fig. 3 employ the ROI area as such a measure. However, several alternative

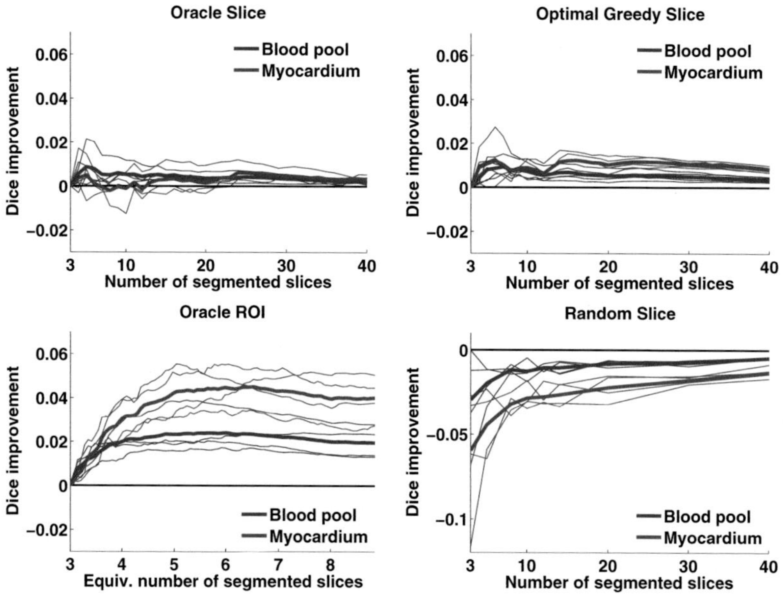

Fig. 3. Segmentation accuracy of alternative reference selection methods, reported as the improvement over uniform slice selection. Negative values indicate that uniform slice selection outperforms the method. For oracle ROI active learning, results are reported as a function of the cumulative area segmented by the user. Random slice selection scores are averages over five trials per subject.

metrics are plausible, depending on whether the user paints the labels or draws curves outlining the different tissue types. We also examined accuracy as a function of the number of edge pixels in the reference label maps. When evaluated this way, the differences between slice and ROI active learning disappear, and simply uniformly distributing the reference slices may be the best choice. In this case, even the optimal greedy strategy, which does not normalize by the effort required to segment each slice, can be worse than uniform slice selection. A user study evaluating the time required to manually segment slices versus ROIs is the best way to determine the most appropriate proxy for interaction time.

5 Conclusions

We presented an accurate interactive method for whole-heart segmentation in congenital heart disease. To the best of our knowledge, this is one of the first demonstrations towards clinically practical image segmentation to enable routine use of 3D heart models for surgical planning in CHD. We also show that active learning approaches in which the user annotates uncertain ROIs have potential to further reduce segmentation time. Future work includes active learning for arbitrarily oriented slices or ROIs. More sophisticated active learning methods that probabilistically model the expected error reduction given a candidate ROI could also yield improved segmentation results with minimal user effort.

Acknowledgements. NSERC CGS-D, the Wistron Corporation, NIH NIBIB NAMIC U54-EB005149, the Boston Children's Hospital Translational Research Program Fellowship and Office of Faculty Development, and Harvard Catalyst.

References

1. Albà, X., Lekadir, K., Hoogendoorn, C., Pereanez, M., Swift, A.J., Wild, J.M., Frangi, A.F.: Reusability of statistical shape models for the segmentation of severely abnormal hearts. In: Camara, O., Mansi, T., Pop, M., Rhode, K., Sermesant, M., Young, A. (eds.) STACOM 2014. LNCS, vol. 8896, pp. 257–264. Springer, Heidelberg (2015)
2. Chyzhyk, D., Dacosta-Aguayo, R., Mataró, M., Graña, M.: An active learning approach for stroke lesion segmentation on multimodal MRI data. Neurocomputing 150(A), 26–36 (2015)
3. Coupé, P., Manjón, J.V., Fonov, V., Pruessner, J., Robles, M., Collins, D.L.: Patch-based segmentation using expert priors: Application to hippocampus and ventricle segmentation. NeuroImage 54(2), 940–954 (2011)
4. Jacobs, S., Grunert, R., Mohr, F.W., Falk, V.: 3D-Imaging of cardiac structures using 3D heart models for planning in heart surgery: A preliminary study. Interact. Cardiovasc. Thorac. Surg. 7(1), 6–9 (2008)
5. Mahapatra, D., Schüffler, P.J., Tielbeek, J.A.W., Vos, F.M., Buhmann, J.M.: Semi-supervised and active learning for automatic segmentation of Crohn's disease. In: Mori, K., Sakuma, I., Sato, Y., Barillot, C., Navab, N. (eds.) MICCAI 2013, Part II. LNCS, vol. 8150, pp. 214–221. Springer, Heidelberg (2013)
6. Rousseau, F., Habas, P., Studholme, C.: A supervised patch-based approach for human brain labeling. IEEE Trans. Med. Imaging 30(10), 1852–1862 (2011)
7. Schmauss, D., Haeberle, S., Hagl, C., Sodian, R.: Three-dimensional printing in cardiac surgery and interventional cardiology: A single-centre experience. Eur. J. Cardio.-Thorac. 47(6), 1044–1052 (2015)
8. Settles, B.: Active Learning. Morgan & Claypool Publishers, San Rafael (2012)
9. Shi, W., Zhuang, X., Wang, H., Duckett, S., Oregan, D., Edwards, P., Ourselin, S., Rueckert, D.: Automatic segmentation of different pathologies from cardiac cine MRI using registration and multiple component EM estimation. In: Metaxas, D.N., Axel, L. (eds.) FIMH 2011. LNCS, vol. 6666, pp. 163–170. Springer, Heidelberg (2011)
10. Top, A., Hamarneh, G., Abugharbieh, R.: Active learning for interactive 3D image segmentation. In: Fichtinger, G., Martel, A., Peters, T. (eds.) MICCAI 2011, Part III. LNCS, vol. 6893, pp. 603–610. Springer, Heidelberg (2011)
11. Valverde, I., Gomez, G., Gonzalez, A., Suarez-Mejias, C., Adsuar, A., Coserria, J.F., Uribe, S., Gomez-Cia, T., Hosseinpour, A.R.: Three-dimensional patient-specific cardiac model for surgical planning in Nikaidoh procedure. Cardiol. Young 25(4), 698–704 (2014)

12. Veeraraghavan, H., Miller, J.: Active learning guided interactions for consistent image segmentation with reduced user interactions. In: IEEE International Symposium on Biomedical Imaging, pp. 1645–1648. IEEE Press, New York (2011)
13. Wang, B., Liu, K.W., Prastawa, K.M., Irima, A., Vespa, P.M., et al.: 4D active cut: An interactive tool for pathological anatomy modeling. In: IEEE International Symposium on Biomedical Imaging, pp. 529–532. IEEE Press, New York (2014)
14. Yifrah, S., Zadicario, E., Ju, T., Cohen-Or, D.: An algorithm for suggesting delineation planes for interactive segmentation. In: IEEE International Symposium on Biomedical Imaging, pp. 361–364. IEEE Press, New York (2014)
15. Zhuang, X.: Challenges and methodologies of fully automatic whole heart segmentation: A review. J. Healthc. Eng. 4(3), 371–408 (2013)

Automatic 3D US Brain Ventricle Segmentation in Pre-Term Neonates Using Multi-phase Geodesic Level-Sets with Shape Prior

Wu Qiu[1,⋆], Jing Yuan[1,⋆], Jessica Kishimoto[1], Yimin Chen[2], Martin Rajchl[3], Eranga Ukwatta[4], Sandrine de Ribaupierre[5], and Aaron Fenster[1]

[1] Robarts Research Institute, University of Western Ontario, London, ON, CA
[2] Department of Electronic Engineering, City University of Hong Kong, CN
[3] Department of Computing, Imperial College London, London, UK
[4] Sunnybrook Health Sciences Centre, Toronto, CA,
Department of Biomedical Engineering, Johns Hopkins University, MD, USA
[5] Neurosurgery, Department of Clinical Neurological Sciences,
University of Western Ontario, London, ON, CA

Abstract. Pre-term neonates born with a low birth weight ($< 1500g$) are at increased risk for developing intraventricular hemorrhage (IVH). 3D ultrasound (US) imaging has been used to quantitatively monitor the ventricular volume in IVH neonates, instead of typical 2D US used clinically, which relies on linear measurements from a single slice and visually estimates to determine ventricular dilation. To translate 3D US imaging into clinical setting, an accurate segmentation algorithm would be desirable to automatically extract the ventricular system from 3D US images. In this paper, we propose an automatic multi-region segmentation approach for delineating lateral ventricles of pre-term neonates from 3D US images, which makes use of multi-phase geodesic level-sets (MP-GLS) segmentation technique via a variational region competition principle and a spatial shape prior derived from pre-segmented atlases. Experimental results using 15 IVH patient images show that the proposed GPU-implemented approach is accurate in terms of the Dice similarity coefficient (DSC), the mean absolute surface distance (MAD), and maximum absolute surface distance (MAXD). To the best of our knowledge, this paper reports the first study on automatic segmentation of ventricular system of premature neonatal brains from 3D US images.

Keywords: 3D ultrasound, pre-term neonatal ventricle segmentation, multi-phase geodesic level-sets, shape prior, convex optimization.

1 Introduction

Pre-term neonates born with a low birth weight ($< 1500g$) are at increased risk of intraventricular hemorrhage (IVH). The blood within the ventricles and surrounding brain can cause an abnormal accumulation of cerebral spinal fluid

⋆ Contributed equally.

N. Navab et al. (Eds.): MICCAI 2015, Part III, LNCS 9351, pp. 89–96, 2015.
DOI: 10.1007/978-3-319-24574-4_11

(CSF), a condition is called post hemorrhagic ventricle dilatation (PHVD). The progressive dilatation of the ventricles will then cause raised increased intracranial pressure (ICP), leading to potential neurological damage, such as cerebral palsy and neurodevelopmental delay [1]. Trans-fontanel 2D cranial ultrasound (US) is routinely used to monitor any patient born $< 1500g$. Even though IVH is relatively easy to detect using 2D US, it is difficult to assess the progression of ventricle dilatation over time from 2D US planes due to the high user dependency. Clinically, the ventricular size is often estimated qualitatively with 2D US. Because of this inaccurate method of measurement, there is no clinical consensus as to when to perform an interventional therapy (such as a ventricle tap) and how much CSF should be drained [2]. 3D US can be used to quantitatively monitor the ventricular volume in neonates [3,4], and can be done at the bedside. However, to incorporate 3D US into clinical setting, an accurate and efficient segmentation algorithm is highly desirable to extract the ventricular system from the 3D US images.

Previous cerebral ventricle segmentation algorithms have been used extensively for CT [5] and MR images [6], but mainly for adult populations. There are a few studies focusing on neonatal ventricle segmentation [7,8], however, most of them dealt with healthy neonatal MR images. Unlike healthy neonatal MR images, the segmentation of 3D IVH neonate US images poses many more unique challenges, such as US image speckle, low soft tissue contrast, fewer image details of structures, and dramatic inter-subject shape deformation [4,9]. While studies have quantified 3D US ventricle volumes in neonates, all have used manual contouring [3] or user-initialized semi-automatic segmentation [9] in lieu of an automatic approach. In particular, we previously proposed a semi-automatic segmentation approach [10], initialized by a single subject-specific atlas based on user-manual-selected anatomic landmarks. Then, a single-phase level set image segmentation method was used to partition the image into two parts: the background and whole ventricle region. Although a low observer variability was reported in [10], the initial landmark selection was still user dependant, labor intensive and time consuming. Thus, an accurate and efficient automatic ventricle segmentation approach from 3D US images would be required in clinical practice.

Contributions: In this study, we propose an automatic convex optimization based approach for delineating lateral ventricles of pre-term neonates from 3D US images, which makes use of multi-phase geodesic level-sets (MP-GLS) segmentation technique via a variational region competition principle and a spatial prior derived from pre-segmented atlases. In particular, the proposed multi-region segmentation has been parallelized and implemented on a GPU to achieve a speed-up in computation. To the best of our knowledge, this paper reports the first study on automatic segmentation of ventricular system of premature neonatal brains from 3D US images.

2 Method

Segmentation Pipeline: Multiple manually pre-segmented patient images from the training dataset are initially registered to the subject image using affine registration followed by a deformable registration. The multiple registered labels are averaged to acquire a probabilistic labeling map, which serves as a spatial prior for a subsequent segmentation procedure. A thresholding procedure of the probabilistic labeling map follows to generate the initial guess and to approximate intensity appearance model (*i.e.*, the probability density function (PDF)) for each individual sub-region: the left, right ventricle, and background regions respectively. Finally, a MP-GLS based multi-region contour evolution approach is proposed to minimize an introduced energy function, which incorporates the information including the shape prior, the constraints to avoid intersections among structures, the image intensity model, as well as a gradient edge map.

Construction of Spatial Priors: Each training image of $(I_i(x), i = 1, 2, ..., n)$ is registered by $\mathbf{u}_i^{affine}(x)$ to the subject image $I_s(x)$ using an affine block-matching approach with default parameters, which is implemented in the Nifty Reg package [11]. Following the affine registration, a recently developed deformable registration algorithm (RANCOR) [12] is used to non-linearly register each pre-segmented image I_i to the subject image I_s by $\mathbf{u}_i^{non-linear}(x)$, $i = 1, 2, ..., n$. Let $L(x) \in \{0, 1, 2\}$ $i = 1, 2, ..., n$, be the label function of each pre-segmented image $I_i(x)$, where $\{0, 1, 2\}$ denotes {background, left, right ventricle}. For the simplicity, the average of each label $L(x)$ is used as the probabilistic label function $P_L(x)$, which is used as a probabilistic shape prior and provides a global shape-associated energy cost term in the applied multi-region segmentation. Thresholding $P_L(x)$ using a value of 0.8 generates a binary label image for each sub-region, which provides a proper initial guess to the ventricle segmentation agreed by all the training images. The completely consensus of all the training images is not used in case of an empty set of the intersections of all deformed labels. Therefore, the voxels labeled by this binary image are sampled to approximate the intensity PDF prior $F_L(I(x))$ for each ventricle sub-region.

MP-GLS Segmentation with Spatial Priors: We study the evolution of multiple mean-curvature-driven contours with respect to a disjoint region constraint, for which we propose a novel variational principle, *i.e.*, the *variational region competition*. The proposed *variational region competition* generalizes recent developments in level-set methods and establishes a variational basis for simultaneously propagating multiple disjoint level-sets by means of minimizing costs w.r.t. region changes. In addition, the proposed principle can be reformulated as a spatially continuous Potts problem [13], *i.e.*, a continuous multi-region min-cut problem, which can be solved via convex relaxation under a continuous max-flow perspective [14].

We consider the evolution of n disjoint regions/geodesic level-sets $\mathcal{C}_i$, $i = 1 \dots n$, under the constraint:

$$\Omega = \cup_{i=1}^n \mathcal{C}_i \,, \quad \mathcal{C}_k \cap \mathcal{C}_l = \emptyset \,, \quad \forall k \neq l \,. \tag{1}$$

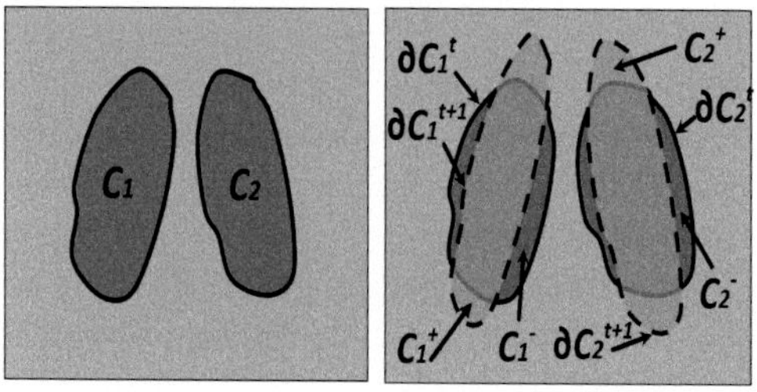

(a) (b)

Fig. 1. An example of the evolution of 2 disjoint regions.(a) 2 disjoint regions at the current time frame t; (b) evolution of two contours from discrete time t to $t+1$, where $\mathcal{C}^{t+1}$ is the evoluted contour at the time frame $t+1$, and $\mathcal{C}^{+}$ and $\mathcal{C}^{-}$ show region expansion and shrinkage, respectively.

Let $\mathcal{C}_i^t$, $i = 1 \ldots n$, be the i-th region at the current time frame t, which moves to position $\mathcal{C}_i^{t+1}$ at the next time frame $t+1$. For each region $\mathcal{C}_i^t$, $i = 1 \ldots n$, at time t, we define two types of difference regions with respect to $\mathcal{C}_i^{t+1}$ (see Fig.1 for an illustration):

1. $\mathcal{C}_i^+$ indicates expansion of $\mathcal{C}_i^t$ w.r.t. $\mathcal{C}_i^{t+1}$: for $\forall x \in \mathcal{C}_i^+$, it is outside $\mathcal{C}_i^t$ at time t, but inside $\mathcal{C}_i^{t+1}$ at $t+1$; for such an expansion, x is assinged with a cost $c_i^+(x)$.
2. $\mathcal{C}_i^-$ indicates shrinkage of $\mathcal{C}_i^t$ w.r.t. $\mathcal{C}_i^{t+1}$: for $\forall x \in \mathcal{C}_i^-$, it is inside $\mathcal{C}_i^t$ at time t, but outside $\mathcal{C}_i^{t+1}$ at $t+1$; for such a shrinkage, x is assinged with a cost $c_i^-(x)$.

With these definitions, we propose the variational principle as: Given n disjoint regions $\mathcal{C}_i$, $i = 1 \ldots n$, the evolution of each region over the discrete time frame from t to $t+1$ minimizes total cost of region changes. That is, the new *optimal* contours $\mathcal{C}_i^{t+1}$, $i = 1 \ldots n$, minimize the energy:

$$\min_{\mathcal{C}_i} \sum_{i=1}^{n} \Big\{ \int_{\mathcal{C}_i^-} c_i^-(x)\, dx + \int_{\mathcal{C}_i^+} c_i^+(x)\, dx \Big\} + \sum_{i=1}^{n} \int_{\partial \mathcal{C}_i} g(s)\, ds \tag{2}$$

subject to (1), where $g(s)$ is the weighting function along the contour boundaries.

For the mean-curvature-driven evolution of multiple disjoint level-sets $\mathcal{C}_i$, $i = 1 \ldots n$, we define the cost functions $c_i^-(x)$ and $c_i^+(x)$, $i = 1 \ldots n$, to be proportional to the geodesic distance function from x to the current boundary $\partial \mathcal{C}_i^t$ such that $c_i^-(x) = c_i^+(x) = \mathrm{gdist}(x, \partial \mathcal{C}_i^t)/h\,, \quad i = 1 \ldots n$. Using the *variational region competition* principle (2), we have: The mean-curvature-driven evolution of multiple disjoint level-sets $\mathcal{C}_i$, $i = 1 \ldots n$, during time frame t to $t+1$ minimizes the cost w.r.t. region changes. The optimal new regions $\mathcal{C}_i^{t+1}$, $i = 1 \ldots n$, therefore minimize:

$$\min_{\mathcal{C}_i} \sum_{i=1}^{n} \int_{\mathcal{C}_i \triangle \mathcal{C}_i^t} \frac{1}{h} \mathrm{gdist}(x, \partial \mathcal{C}_i^t)\, dx + \sum_{i=1}^{n} \int_{\partial \mathcal{C}_i} ds \tag{3}$$

subject to the constraint (1), where $\mathcal{C}_t \triangle \mathcal{C}_{t+h}$ denotes the symmetric difference between $\mathcal{C}_t$ and $\mathcal{C}_{t+h}$. For multi-region segmentation in this study, the level-set evolution is driven not only by the geodesic distance functions as above, but also by image features. In general, the cost functions $c_i^-(x)$ and $c_i^+(x)$, $i = 1 \ldots n$, w.r.t. region changes are given by the combination of the image feature costs and the geodesic distance functions. In this application, we define the cost functions as follows:

$$c_i^+(x) = c_i^-(x) = -\,\omega_1 \log F_L(I(x)) - \omega_2 \log \big(P_L(x) * G_\sigma(x)\big) + \omega_3 \frac{1}{h} \operatorname{gdist}(x, \partial\mathcal{C}_i^t) \quad \forall x \in \mathcal{C}_i^t$$

where the weighting parameters $\omega_1, \omega_2, \omega_3 > 0$, $\omega_1 + \omega_2 + \omega_3 = 1$ weight the contributions from the intensity, shape priors and geodesic distance for each voxel, respectively, and $G_\sigma(x)$ is the Gaussian smoothing function. $\omega_1 = 0.3, \omega_2 = 0.4, \omega_3 = 0.3$ were used in our experiments. The corresponding optimization formulation is then given by the *variational region competition* principle (2) directly. We show that the variational problem (2) introduced by the *variational region competition* principle can be equally reformulated as the Potts problem [13]. For this purpose, we define two cost functions $D_i^s(x)$ and $D_i^t(x)$ w.r.t. the current contour $\mathcal{C}_i^t$, $i = 1 \ldots n$, at time t:

$$D_i^s(x) := \begin{cases} c_i^-(x)\,, & \text{where } x \in \mathcal{C}_i^t \\ 0\,, & \text{otherwise} \end{cases} \tag{4}$$

$$D_i^t(x) := \begin{cases} c_i^+(x)\,, & \text{where } x \notin \mathcal{C}_i^t \\ 0\,, & \text{otherwise} \end{cases}\,. \tag{5}$$

Let $u_i(x) \in \{0, 1\}$, $i = 1 \ldots n$, be the indicator function of the region $\mathcal{C}_i$. Therefore, the disjoint constraint in (1) can be represented by $\sum_{i=1}^n u_i(x) = 1$; $u_i(x) \in \{0, 1\}$, $\forall x \in \Omega$. Via the cost functions (4) and (5), we can prove that the variational formulation (2) associated with the *variational region competition* principle can be expressed as the Potts problem:

$$\min_{u_i(x) \in \{0,1\}} \sum_{i=1}^n \langle u_i, D_i^t - D_i^s \rangle + \sum_{i=1}^n \int_\Omega g(x)\, |\nabla u_i|\, dx \tag{6}$$

subject to the contour disjointness constraint (1), where the weighted length term in (2) is encoded by the weighted total-variation functions. The resulting formulation (6) gives rise to a challenging combinatorial optimization problem. From recent developments of convex optimization, its global optimum can be approximated efficiently through convex relaxation [15,16].

3 Experiments and Results

Image Acquisition: A motorized 3D US system developed for cranial US scanning of pre-term neonates was used to acquire the images [4]. Following the routine cranial US exam, the 2D US transducer (Phillips C8-5 broadband curved

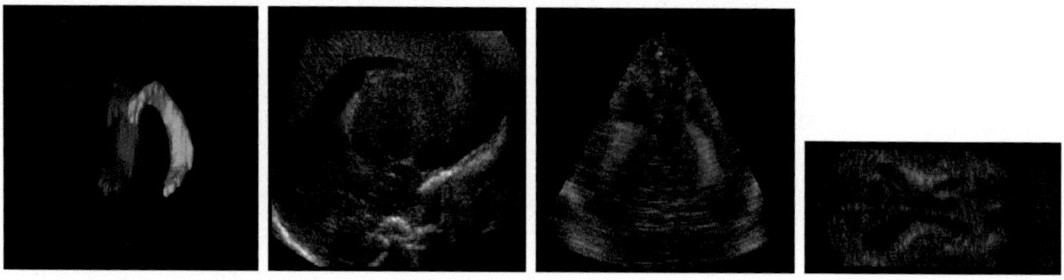

Fig. 2. An example of segmented ventricles. (a) segmented surface, (b) sagittal, (c) coronal, and (d) transverse views

array) was placed into the motorized housing and the 3D US image was acquired. The acquired 3D US image sizes ranged from $300 \times 300 \times 300$ to $450 \times 450 \times 450$ voxels at the same voxel spacing of $0.22 \times 0.22 \times 0.22\, mm^3$. Fifteen patient (with the gestation from 37 to 42 weeks) with different IVH grades were involved in this study. The proposed segmentation approach was evaluated with the 15 patient images using leave-one-out cross validation strategy.

Evaluation Metrics: The proposed segmentation approach was evaluated by comparing the algorithm to manual segmentation results using the Dice similarity coefficient (DSC), the mean absolute surface distance (MAD), and maximum absolute surface distance (MAXD) [17,18].

Results: Figure. 2 shows one example of the algorithm segmented lateral ventricles from an IVH neonate. Quantitative results for the 15 patient images were demonstrated in Table. 1. The proposed approach was implemented using parallel computing architecture (CUDA, NVIDIA Corp., Santa Clara, CA) and the user interface in Matlab (Natick, MA). The experiments were conducted on a Windows desktop with an Intel i7-2600 CPU (3.4 GHz) and a GPU of NVIDIA Geforce 5800X. The mean run time of three repeated segmentations for each 3D US image was considered as the segmentation time to assess the algorithm's efficiency. Each computation of convex optimization required approximately 2 minutes, and each pairwise registration from one training image to the target subject was composed of an affine registration (no GPU acceleration: 3 minutes) and deformable registration (GPU: 50 seconds). Thus, an average of 54 minutes was required for each subject image.

Table 1. Segmentation results of fifteen 3D US images in terms of DSC, MAD, and MAXD, represneted as mean ± standard deviation.

	DSC (%)	MAD (mm)	MAXD (mm)
Left ventricle	72.5 ± 2.8	0.67 ± 0.2	4.1 ± 1.3
Right ventricle	74.0 ± 3.3	0.63 ± 0.3	3.5 ± 1.6
In all	73.2 ± 3.0	0.64 ± 0.3	3.8 ± 1.5

4 Discussion and Conclusion

This paper proposes a GPU-implemented automatic multi-region segmentation approach to extract the lateral ventricles of pre-term neonates from 3D US images, which formulates a MP-GLS segmentation technique via variational region competition, in combination with a spatial prior obtained from pre-segmented atlases. The experimental results using 15 IVH patient images show that the proposed method is accurate and efficient in terms of metrics of DSC, MAD, and MAXD. There were only a few previous studies focusing on 3D US lateral ventricle segmentation problem [9,10]. The DSC of 73.2 ± 3.0 yielded by the proposed approach is higher than the DSC of $72.4 \pm 2.5\%$ reported in [10]. Although [9] reported a higher DSC of $78.4 \pm 4.4\%$, it required careful initialization to the algorithm, which introduced observer variability. Compared to the semi-automatic methods [9,10], the proposed segmentation approach is capable of extracting lateral ventricles in a fully automatic fashion, which does not require any user interactions as input, avoiding observer dependency. The proposed MP-GLS segmentation approach is compared with several other methods using the 15 patient images, including STAPLE, majority voting (MV), single classic level set (SLS), single geodesic level set (SGLS), and multi-phase classic level-sets (MLS). The results show that a mean DSC of 65.5% for STAPLE, 58.3% for MV, 67.4% for SLS, 68.5% for SGLS, and 69.7% for MLS were generated, lower than 73.2% obtained by the proposed method.

The computational time required by the proposed method limits this technique for application at the bedside, where clinicians need to know the ventricle volume immediately after the image acquisition is finished. However, as an off-line processing technique, the proposed technique may be used for the longitudinal analysis of ventricle changes, which could affect specific white matter bundles, such as in the motor or visual cortex, and could be linked to specific neurological problems often seen in this patient population later in life. Considering the small number of images in the employed database, further evaluation experiments are required to cover the anatomical and pathological variation in data.

Acknowledgments. The authors are grateful for the funding support from the Canadian Institutes of Health Research (CIHR) and Academic Medical Organization of Southwestern Ontario (AMOSO).

References

1. Adams-Chapman, I., Hansen, N.I., Stoll, B.J., Higgins, R., et al.: Neurodevelopmental outcome of extremely low birth weight infants with posthemorrhagic hydrocephalus requiring shunt insertion. Pediatrics 121(5), e1167–e1177 (2008)
2. Klebermass-Schrehof, K., Rona, Z., Waldhör, T., Czaba, C., Beke, A., Weninger, M., Olischar, M.: Can neurophysiological assessment improve timing of intervention in posthaemorrhagic ventricular dilatation? Archives of Disease in Childhood-Fetal and Neonatal Edition 98(4), F291–F297 (2013)

3. McLean, G., Coombs, P., Sehgal, A., Paul, E., Zamani, L., Gilbertson, T., Ptasznik, R.: Measurement of the lateral ventricles in the neonatal head: Comparison of 2-d and 3-d techniques. Ultrasound in Medicine & Biology (2012)
4. Kishimoto, J., de Ribaupierre, S., Lee, D., Mehta, R., St Lawrence, K., Fenster, A.: 3D ultrasound system to investigate intraventricular hemorrhage in preterm neonates. Physics in Medicine and Biology 58(21), 7513 (2013)
5. Liu, J., Huang, S., Ihar, V., Ambrosius, W., Lee, L.C., Nowinski, W.L.: Automatic model-guided segmentation of the human brain ventricular system from CT images. Academic Radiology 17(6), 718–726 (2010)
6. Liu, J., Huang, S., Nowinski, W.L.: Automatic segmentation of the human brain ventricles from MR images by knowledge-based region growing and trimming. Neuroinformatics 7(2), 131–146 (2009)
7. Wang, L., Shi, F., Lin, W., Gilmore, J.H., Shen, D.: Automatic segmentation of neonatal images using convex optimization and coupled level sets. NeuroImage 58(3), 805–817 (2011)
8. Shi, F., Fan, Y., Tang, S., Gilmore, J.H., Lin, W., Shen, D.: Neonatal brain image segmentation in longitudinal MRI studies. NeuroImage 49(1), 391–400 (2010)
9. Qiu, W., Yuan, J., Kishimoto, J., McLeod, J., de Ribaupierre, S., Fenster, A.: User-guided segmentation of preterm neonate ventricular system from 3d ultrasound images using convex optimization. Ultrasound in Medicine & Biology 41(2), 542–556 (2015)
10. Qiu, W., Yuan, J., Kishimoto, J., Ukwatta, E., Fenster, A.: Lateral ventricle segmentation of 3D pre-term neonates US using convex optimization. In: Mori, K., Sakuma, I., Sato, Y., Barillot, C., Navab, N. (eds.) MICCAI 2013, Part III. LNCS, vol. 8151, pp. 559–566. Springer, Heidelberg (2013)
11. Ourselin, S., Stefanescu, R., Pennec, X.: Robust registration of multi-modal images: towards real-time clinical applications. In: Dohi, T., Kikinis, R. (eds.) MICCAI 2002, Part II. LNCS, vol. 2489, pp. 140–147. Springer, Heidelberg (2002)
12. Rajchl, M., Baxter, J.S., Qiu, W., Khan, A.R., Fenster, A., Peters, T.M., Yuan, J.: Rancor: Non-linear image registration with total variation regularization. arXiv preprint arXiv:1404.2571 (2014)
13. Potts, R.B.: Some generalized order-disorder transformations. Proceedings of the Cambridge Philosophical Society 48, 106–109 (1952)
14. Yuan, J., Ukwatta, E., Tai, X.C., Fenster, A., Schnoerr, C.: A fast global optimization-based approach to evolving contours with generic shape prior. Technical report CAM-12-38, UCLA (2012)
15. Yuan, J., Bae, E., Tai, X.-C., Boykov, Y.: A continuous max-flow approach to potts model. In: Daniilidis, K., Maragos, P., Paragios, N. (eds.) ECCV 2010, Part VI. LNCS, vol. 6316, pp. 379–392. Springer, Heidelberg (2010)
16. Lellmann, J., Breitenreicher, D., Schnörr, C.: Fast and exact primal-dual iterations for variational problems in computer vision. In: Daniilidis, K., Maragos, P., Paragios, N. (eds.) ECCV 2010, Part II. LNCS, vol. 6312, pp. 494–505. Springer, Heidelberg (2010)
17. Qiu, W., Yuan, J., Ukwatta, E., Sun, Y., Rajchl, M., Fenster, A.: Dual optimization based prostate zonal segmentation in 3D MR images. Medical Image Analysis 18(4), 660–673 (2014)
18. Qiu, W., Yuan, J., Ukwatta, E., Sun, Y., Rajchl, M., Fenster, A.: Prostate segmentation: An efficient convex optimization approach with axial symmetry using 3D TRUS and MR images. IEEE Trans. Med. Imag. 33(4), 947–960 (2014)

Multiple Surface Segmentation Using Truncated Convex Priors

Abhay Shah[1], Junjie Bai[1], Zhihong Hu[3], Srinivas Sadda[1], and Xiaodong Wu[1,2]

[1] Department of Electrical and Computer Engineering
[2] Radiation Oncology, University of Iowa, Iowa City, USA
[3] Doheny Eye Institute, Los Angeles, USA

Abstract. Multiple surface segmentation with mutual interaction between surface pairs is a challenging task in medical image analysis. In this paper we report a fast multiple surface segmentation approach with truncated convex priors for a segmentation problem, in which there exist abrupt surface distance changes between mutually interacting surface pairs. A 3-D graph theoretic framework based on *local range search* is employed. The use of truncated convex priors enables to capture the surface discontinuity and rapid changes of surface distances. The method is also capable to enforce a minimum distance between a surface pair. The solution for multiple surfaces is obtained by iteratively computing a maximum flow for a subset of the voxel domain at each iteration. The proposed method was evaluated on simultaneous intraretinal layer segmentation of optical coherence tomography images of normal eye and eyes affected by severe drusen due to age related macular degeneration. Our experiments demonstrated statistically significant improvement of segmentation accuracy by using our method compared to the optimal surface detection method using convex priors without truncation (OSDC). The mean unsigned surface positioning errors obtained by OSDC for normal eyes $(4.47 \pm 1.10)\mu m$ was improved to $(4.29 \pm 1.02)\mu m$, and for eyes with drusen was improved from $(7.98 \pm 4.02)\mu m$ to $(5.12 \pm 1.39)\mu m$ using our method. The proposed approach with average computation time of 539 sec is much faster than 10014 sec taken by OSDC.

Keywords: Local range search, segmentation, truncated convex.

1 Introduction

The surface detection methods [6][10] with a global optimization property have been used for various image segmentation applications but they may have a problem in cases with presence of steep surface smoothness changes (surface discontinuity) and abrupt surface separation (distance) changes between a pair of interacting surfaces. Some examples are spectral-domain optical coherence tomography (SD-OCT) volumes of subjects with severe glaucoma [9], and drusen due to age-related macular degeneration (AMD) [1] (Fig. 1). The optimal surface detection method [6][10] uses hard smoothness constraints that are a constant in each direction to specify the maximum allowed "jump" of any two adjacent

N. Navab et al. (Eds.): MICCAI 2015, Part III, LNCS 9351, pp. 97–104, 2015.
DOI: 10.1007/978-3-319-24574-4_12

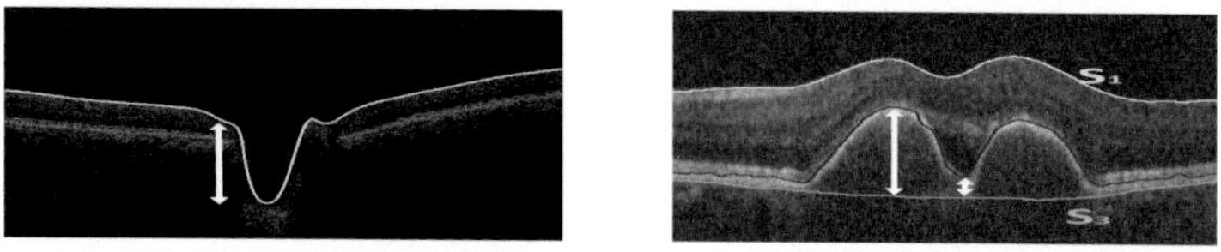

Fig. 1. Steep change in surface smoothness can be seen in SD-OCT image of an eye with severe glaucoma (*left*). Abrupt changes in surface separation between surface 2 (S_2) and surface 3 (S_3) can be seen in SD-OCT image of an eye with AMD (*right*).

voxels on a feasible surface. It uses surface separation constraints to specify the maximum and minimum allowed distances between a pair of surfaces. This does not allow for flexibility in constraining surfaces. Methods employing trained hard and soft constraints [2][8], use prior terms to penalize local changes in surface smoothness and surface separation. The prior term requires learning and may give inaccurate results when there is plenty of variations within the data. Approaches using multiple resolution technique [5] for reduction of time and memory consumption, need to define the region of interest at each iterative scale. Identifying a region of interest for cases with abrupt surface smoothness or separation changes due to presence of pathology is challenging, and may result in suboptimal solutions. In this paper, we consider using truncated convex priors for surface smoothness and surface separation. We also ensure the enforcement of a minimum separation between a surface pair. A truncated convex prior is discontinuity preserving with a bound on the largest possible penalty for surface discontinuity. The main idea is to take advantage of a local search technique which allows for enforcement of truncated convex priors, and is much faster than optimal surface detection methods for large data volumes in a high resolution. Such a method is used for single surface segmentation[7]. We further extend this framework to simultaneously segment multiple surfaces using truncated convex penalties and ensuring a minimum separation between a given surface pair.

2 Method

Our method segments the surfaces from the 3-D volumes directly, not slice by slice. Consider a volumetric image $I(x, y, z)$ of size $X \times Y \times Z$. A surface is defined as a function $S(x, y)$, where $x \in \mathbf{x} = \{0, 1, ...X-1\}$, $y \in \mathbf{y} = \{0, 1, ...Y-1\}$ and $S(x, y) \in \mathbf{z} = \{0, 1, ...Z-1\}$. Each (x, y)-pair corresponds to a *column* of voxels $\{(I(x, y, z)|z = 0, 1, \ldots, Z-1\}$, denoted by $col(x, y)$. We use a and b to denote two neighboring (x, y)-pairs in the image domain $\mathbf{x} \times \mathbf{y}$ and N_s to denote the neighborhood setting in the image domain. The function $S(a)$ can be viewed as labeling for a with the label set $\mathbf{z}$ ($S(a) \in \mathbf{z}$). For simultaneously segmenting $\lambda (\lambda \geq 2)$ surfaces, the goal of the problem is to seek the "best" surfaces $S_i(a)$ $(i = 1, 2, ...\lambda)$ in I with minimum separation $d_{i,i+1}$ $(i = 1, 2, ...\lambda - 1)$ between each adjacent pair of surfaces S_i and S_{i+1}. The problem is transformed into an energy minimization problem. The energy function $E(S)$ takes the following form in Eqn. (1):

$$E(S) = \sum_{i=1}^{\lambda} \Big(\sum_{a \in \mathbf{x} \times \mathbf{y}} D_i(S_i(a)) + \sum_{(a,b) \in N_s} V_{ab}(S_i(a), S_i(b)) \Big) + \sum_{i=1}^{\lambda-1} \sum_{a \in \mathbf{x} \times \mathbf{y}} H_a(S_i(a), S_{i+1}(a)) \tag{1}$$

The data cost term $\sum_{a \in \mathbf{x} \times \mathbf{y}} D_i(S_i(a))$ measures the total cost of all voxels on a surface S_i, while the surface smoothness term $\sum_{(a,b) \in N_s} V_{ab}(S_i(a), S_i(b))$ measures the extent to which S_i is not piecewise smooth. A truncated convex $V_{ab}(.)$ is used to preserve discontinuity of the target surfaces and is computed on the height changes of two adjacent surface voxels. The surface separation term $H_a(S_i(a), S_{i+1}(a))$ incorporates a truncated convex penalty[7] for the separation between two adjacent surfaces, and ensures a minimum separation between them, which takes the following form in Eqn. (2):

$$H_a(S_i(a), S_{i+1}(a)) = \begin{cases} \infty, & \text{if } (S_{i+1}(a) - S_i(a)) < d_{i,i+1}, \\ w_a \min(f(S_{i+1}(a) - S_i(a)), M_{i,i+1}), & \text{otherwise} \end{cases} \tag{2}$$

where $f(.)$ is a convex function, $M_{i,i+1} > 0$ is the truncation factor, and $w_a \geq 0$.

Overview of the method: Our method is iterative in nature. The pipeline for our method is shown in Fig. 2. At each iteration, it searches a small subset of the

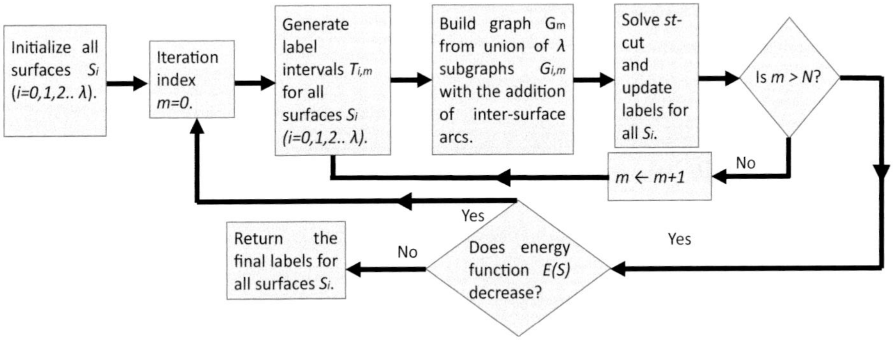

Fig. 2. Pipeline for our method. N is the maximum iteration index.

solution space defined by a label interval, consisting of a set of consecutive possible surface heights for each point in the image domain along the z-dimension. For each surface S_i, a subgraph $G_{i,m}$ (m is the index for iteration and i is the index of the sought surface) is then constructed using the technique for single surface detection[4][7]. In addition, inter-surface arcs are added between each pair of subsequent subgraphs, to construct the graph G_m for the simultaneous search of all λ surfaces at the iteration m. The inter-surface arcs incorporate the truncated convex penalty for the point-wise surface distance changes between two surfaces. The graph G_m is then solved by computing a minimum *st*-cut which minimizes the energy function $E(S)$. The labeling of each target surface is then updated according to the computed *st*-cut at the end of each iteration m. The iterations are continued until all the defined label intervals for each surface S_i has been iterated over, at the end of which the total energy $E(S)$ of the segmented λ surfaces is compared to the previous solution. If the energy is found to have decreased, the entire defined label intervals are iterated over again for each surface S_i, initialized with the current solution obtained. The method terminates while $E(S)$ converges.

Graph construction: A constant interval length L is defined to determine a subset of consecutive labels to be considered for all λ surfaces. An interval of consecutive labels for surface S_i is defined as $T_i \subset \mathbf{z}$ where $\mathbf{z} = \{0, 1, ...Z-1\}$. Denote $T_{i,m}$ shown in Eqn.(3) as the label interval for S_i at iteration m, where $m = 0, 1, ...Z-2-\sum_{i=1}^{\lambda-1} d_{(i,i+1)}$. Interval $T_{i+1,m}$ is displaced by $d_{i,i+1}$ from $T_{i,m}$ to ensure the minimum separation constraint between each pair of adjacent surfaces S_i and S_{i+1}. Since each pair of adjacent intervals are displaced from each other, the maximum of iteration index(m) is calculated by subtracting the sum of the minimum separation for each pair of adjacent surfaces from Z, thus ensuring no undefined interval is formed.

$$T_{i,m} = \{l \mid m + \sum_{j=1}^{i} d_{(j-1,j)} \leq l \leq \min(m + \sum_{j=1}^{i} d_{(j-1,j)} + (L-1),\ Z-1)\} \quad (3)$$

In iteration m, we search for each surface S_i in the sub-volume $\mathbf{x} \times \mathbf{y} \times T_{i,m}$ of I using the subgraph $G_{i,m}$. Each subgraph $G_{i,m}$ incorporates all intra-column arcs for surface monotonicity for data cost volume $D_{i,m}$(for searching S_i at iteration m) and inter-column arcs for surface smoothness(truncated convex penalty) to search a single surface S_i[4][7]. At iteration m, denote the set of labels given by Eq.(3) for corresponding columns $col(a,i)$(resp., $col(a,i+1)$) is $T_{i,m} = [q_{a,i}, q_{a,i}+1, \ldots q_{a,i}+L-1]$ (resp., $T_{i+1,m} = [q_{a,i+1}, q_{a,i+1}+1, \ldots q_{a,i+1}+L-1]$), i.e., $T_{i,m}$(resp.,$T_{i+1,m}$) includes all possible surface positions that S_i(resp.,S_{i+1}) can change into at iteration m. We refer each node in the graph with its corresponding label. Inter-surface arcs are added between corresponding columns of subgraphs $G_{i,m}$'s to construct the graph G_m. Denote the initial surface position of S_i on column $col(a,i)$ at the beginning of iteration m as $S_{i,m-1}(a)$. At each iteration m, a labeling can either retain its current label $S_{i,m-1}(a)$ or can be changed to a label in interval $T_{i,m}$. We distinguish four such cases for a given pair of corresponding columns. Case 1: $S_{i,m-1}(a) \in T_{i,m}$ and $S_{i+1,m-1}(a) \in T_{i+1,m}$, Case 2: $S_{i,m-1}(a) \notin T_{i,m}$ and $S_{i+1,m-1}(a) \in T_{i+1,m}$, Case 3: $S_{i,m-1}(a) \in T_{i,m}$ and $S_{i+1,m-1}(a) \notin T_{i+1,m}$, Case 4: $S_{i,m-1}(a) \notin T_{i,m}$ and $S_{i+1,m-1}(a) \notin T_{i+1,m}$.

Case 1 is the base case where the current labels of both the columns belong to the given interval and encodes the convex penalty using the second derivative of the convex function $f(.)$. These convex penalty arcs are also common for the remaining three cases and additional arcs are added to truncate this convex penalty. Case 2 and Case 3 are symmetric cases where one of the current labels

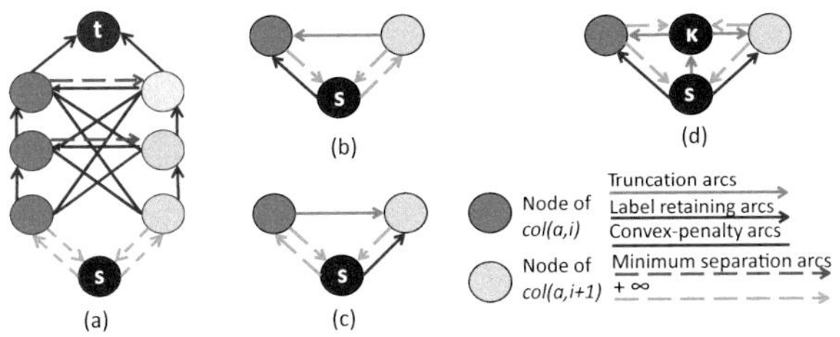

Fig. 3. (a)Example graph construction for Case 1. Additional arcs added to (a) for (b)Case 2, (c) Case 3, (d) Case 4. Length of interval $L = 3$

does not belong to the given interval. Case 4 is the combination of case 2 and case 3 when both the current labels do not belong to the interval in consideration.

Case 1 (base case): The convex penalty is enforced by adding the following arcs. For all $k \in [0, L-1]$, $k' \in [0, L-1]$ and $k \neq k'$, we add an arc with a weight of $\frac{w_a}{2}(f(k-k'+1)-2f(k-k')+f(k-k'-1))$ between nodes $q_{a,i}+k$ and $q_{a,i+1}+k'$ in both directions. For all $k = k'$ except when $k = k' = 0$, we put in an arc of weight $\frac{w_a}{2}(f(1) + f(-1))$ from node $q_{a,i+1} + k'$ to $q_{a,i} + k$, and a *minimum separation arc* of weight $+\infty$ in opposite direction (These $+\infty$ arcs ensure that minimum separation constraint is not violated within the interval). For each $k \in [0, L-2]$, a weighted arc with a weight of $\frac{w_a}{2}(f(L-k-1) + f(k+1)$ is added from node $q_{a,i}+k$ (resp., $q_{a,i+1}+k$) to $q_{a,i}+k+1$ (resp., $q_{a,i+1}+k+1$). Furthermore, we put in an arc with a weight of $\frac{w_a}{2}f(L)$ from each node of q_a+L-1 and $q_{a,i+1}+L-1$ to the terminal node t. Using the similar techniques in Ref. [4], we can prove that these arcs ensure the cost of any finite st-cut to be $w_a f(k-k') + w_a f(L)$, where $w_a f(L)$ is an overestimation constant for approximation. No finite st-cut shall be possible when $S_{i+1,m}(a) - S_{i,m}(a) < d_{i,i+1}$ within the interval at iteration m due to the minimum separation arcs. Thus minimum separation constraints are not violated within the interval. An example is shown in Fig. 3(a).

Case 2 , Case 3 (symmetric cases): For case 2, we additionally introduce following arcs to the construction shown in Fig. 3(a):(1) a *truncation arc* from node $q_{a,i+1}$ to node $q_{a,i}$ whose weight is $w_a M + \frac{w_a}{2} f(L)$ if $(q_{a,i+1} - S_{i,m-1}(a)) \geq d_{i,i+1}$ and is $+\infty$ if $(q_{a,i+1} - S_{i,m-1}(a)) < d_{i,i+1}$, to encode the truncated penalty and minimum separation constraint, (2) a *label retaining arc* $(s, q_{a,i})$ with weight $D_i(S_{i,m-1}(a))$ to allow surface S_i retain its current label($S_{i,m-1}(a)$). Any finite st-cut including the label retaining arc must also include the truncation arc (Fig. 3(b)), hence enforcing the truncated convex penalty with possible overestimation. For Case 3, we symmetrically add arcs as discussed for Case 2 (Fig. 3(c)).

Case 4 (combination case): We include all arcs of case 1, case 2 and case 3. We additionally introduce a new node κ and a truncation arc from source node s to κ with a weight of $H_a(S_{i,m-1}(a), S_{i+1,m-1}(a))$ (Fig. 3(d)). Note that any finite st cut including both the label retaining arcs $((s, q_{a,i}), (s, q_{a,i+1}))$, must also include the truncation arc (s, κ), hence enforcing the truncated convex penalty.

3 Experimental Methods

The experiment compares segmentation accuracy of the proposed method (truncated convex prior) and OSDC [8]. The three surfaces simultaneously segmented in this study are S_1-Internal Limiting Membrane (ILM), S_2-inner aspect of retinal pigment epithelium drusen complex (IRPEDC), S_3-outer aspect of Bruch's membrane (OBM) as shown in Fig. 1.

Comparison was done by calculating the unsigned surface positioning errors (USPE) as absolute distances between the computed surfaces and the expert manual tracings in each column of the image. Statistical significance of observed differences was determined by paired Student t-tests for which p value of 0.05 were considered significant. Experiments were carried out on a Linux workstation (3.4 GHz, 16 GB memory).

20 SD-OCT scans of normal eyes (Type I), 20 SD-OCT scans of eyes with AMD (Type II) and their respective expert manual tracings were obtained from the publicly available repository of datasets Ref. [3]. The 3-D volumes ($1000 \times 100 \times 512$ voxels with voxel size $6.54 \times 67 \times 3.23$ μm^3) for our study were randomly selected from the repository. Segmenting the surfaces simultaneously using OSDC [8] on original resolution is not efficient enough for large data volumes. To make fair comparisons, we first downsample the image by a factor of four in the x direction to reduce the computation time. The datasets were segmented in both their original resolution and down-sampled version by our method to demonstrate the performance and capacity of our method for large clinical datasets. For cases where segmentation was done in the down-sampled version, the resulting segmentation was up-sampled to original resolution for comparison purposes. The data cost volumes (data cost term) were generated (computed) as follows. First, a $11 \times 11 \times 11$ Gaussian filter with a standard deviation of 11 was applied. To detect S_1 and S_3, a 3-D Sobel filter ($3 \times 3 \times 3$) emphasizing the vertical edges for the dark to bright and bright to dark transitions respectively were applied. To detect S_2, we apply the following operations to each slice of the volume. Edges are extracted using a high pass filter; image is normalized to range from 0 to 1; a binary mask is generated for the region containing S_2 by thresholding of 0.5 and finally mask is applied to the data cost volume for S_1.

Parameters are reported for downsampled version of the datasets and are summarized in Table 1. For both the methods, we use a linear convex function $f(x) = |x|$. For our method, an interval length $L = 2$ was used and surface S_1 (resp., S_2, S_3) was initialized as 0 (resp., $d_{1,2}$, $d_{1,2}+d_{2,3}$). The parameters and the weight coefficients (w_{ab}, w_a) were experimentally determined by testing on a similar group of datasets (with the same data size) obtained from the same repository [3] for best results.

4 Results

Illustrative results of our proposed method and the OSDC for downsampled data can be seen in Fig. 4. Quantitative comparison between our method and

Table 1. M_x, M_y - truncation factors in x, y directions. M - truncation factor for surface separation of a surface pair, d - minimum separation between a surface pair.

		Our method			OSDC	Our method	
Surface	Dataset	M_x	M_y	Surface pair	d	M	d
S_1	Type I	30	5	S_1-S_2	30	15	30
S_2	Type I	30	5	S_2-S_3	3	3	3
S_3	Type I	10	2				
S_1	Type II	30	5	S_1-S_2	20	10	20
S_2	Type II	10	5	S_2-S_3	3	5	3
S_3	Type II	5	2				

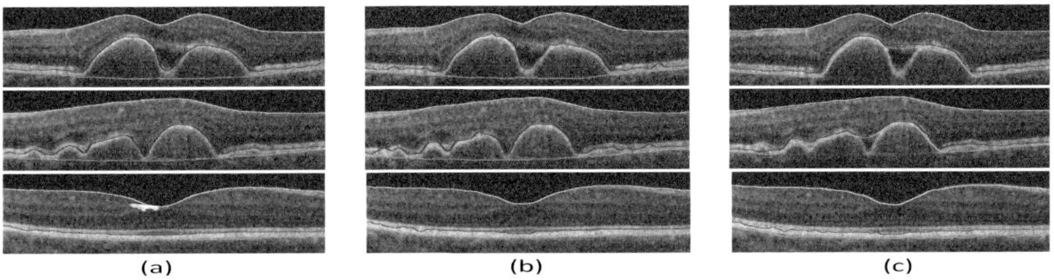

Fig. 4. Top two rows - image slices of Type II, bottom row - image slice of Type I. Yellow - ILM, Red - IRPEDC and Blue - OBM. (a)Expert manual tracing, segmentation using (b)our method, (c)OSDC.

OSDC is summarized in Table 2. For the downsampled version of the datasets, our method produced significantly lower USPE for surfaces S_1 ($p < 0.05$), S_2 ($p < 0.03$) and S_3 ($p < 0.002$) in Type II datasets. In type I datasets, our method significantly lowered USPE for surface S_3 ($p < 0.05$). Comparisons were also made between the segmentations using our method in original resolution and OSDC in downsampled version. Our method significantly improved the USPE for S_1 ($p < 0.001$), S_2 ($p < 0.006$) and S_3 ($p < 0.001$) in both types of the datasets. For the downsampled version of the datasets, our method with average computation time of 539 seconds is much faster than OSDC with average computation time of 10014 seconds. Average computation time using our method was 3394 seconds for datasets in original resolution.

Table 2. Unsigned surface positioning errors (USPE) (mean ± standard deviation)μm. Obsv - Expert manual tracing.

	Data in downsampled resolution				Data in original resolution	
	Normal eye (Type I)		Eye with AMD (Type II)		Type I	Type II
Surface	Our method vs. Obsv	OSDC vs. Obsv	Our method vs. Obsv	OSDC vs. Obsv	Our method vs. Obsv	Our method vs. Obsv
S_1	3.62 ± 0.23	3.67 ± 0.30	3.95 ± 0.72	4.24 ± 0.56	1.99 ± 0.36	2.07 ± 0.38
S_2	5.56 ± 2.13	5.77 ± 2.41	6.86 ± 2.04	8.06 ± 2.79	4.72 ± 1.68	6.49 ± 2.46
S_3	3.69 ± 0.70	3.98 ± 0.60	4.56 ± 1.40	11.65 ± 8.72	2.95 ± 0.41	3.64 ± 0.62
Overall	4.29 ± 1.02	4.47 ± 1.10	5.12 ±1.39	7.98 ± 4.02	3.32 ± 0.82	4.06 ± 1.15

5 Discussion and Conclusion

A novel approach for segmentation of multiple surfaces with usage of truncated convex surface smoothness and surface separation constraints was proposed. Our method demonstrated significant improvement in segmentation accuracy and computation time compared to OSDC, thus making our method useful for segmenting datasets in high resolution without using a multiple resolution approach. Our method also demonstrated efficient and improved simultaneous segmentation of surfaces with surface discontinuity and abrupt surface separation changes.

Our algorithm does not guarantee a globally optimal solution since a truncated convex function is submodular in nature and hence is optimized using an approximate algorithm. The difference between the results on different resolutions are partially due to sampling technique. More advanced automated techniques may be used for training of the parameters.

References

1. Bressler, N.M.: Age-related macular degeneration is the leading cause of blindness. Jama 291(15), 1900–1901 (2004)
2. Dufour, P.A., Ceklic, L., Abdillahi, H., Schroder, S., De Dzanet, S., Wolf-Schnurrbusch, U., Kowal, J.: Graph-based multi-surface segmentation of data using trained hard and soft constraints. IEEE Transactions on Medical Imaging 32(3), 531–543 (2013)
3. Farsiu, S., Chiu, S.J., O'Connell, R.V., Folgar, F.A., Yuan, E., Izatt, J.A., Toth, C.A.: Quantitative classification of eyes with and without intermediate age-related macular degeneration using optical coherence tomography. Ophthalmology 121(1), 162–172 (2014)
4. Kumar, M.P., Veksler, O., Torr, P.H.: Improved moves for truncated convex models. J. Mach. Learn. Res. 12, 31–67 (2011)
5. Lee, K., Niemeijer, M., Garvin, M.K., Kwon, Y.H., Sonka, M., Abràmoff, M.D.: Segmentation of the optic disc in 3-d scans of the optic nerve head. IEEE Transactions on Medical Imaging 29(1), 159–168 (2010)
6. Li, K., Wu, X., Chen, D., Sonka, M.: Optimal surface segmentation in volumetric images-a graph-theoretic approach. IEEE Transactions on Pattern Analysis and Machine Intelligence 28(1), 119–134 (2006)
7. Shah, A., Wang, J.K., Garvin, M.K., Sonka, M., Wu, X.: Automated surface segmentation of internal limiting membrane in spectral-domain optical coherence tomography volumes with a deep cup using a 3-d range expansion approach. In: 2014 IEEE 11th International Symposium on Biomedical Imaging (ISBI), pp. 1405–1408. IEEE (2014)
8. Song, Q., Bai, J., Garvin, M.K., Sonka, M., Buatti, J.M., Wu, X.: Optimal multiple surface segmentation with shape and context priors. IEEE Transactions on Medical Imaging 32(2), 376–386 (2013)
9. Tielsch, J.M., Sommer, A., Katz, J., Royall, R.M., Quigley, H.A., Javitt, J.: Racial variations in the prevalence of primary open-angle glaucoma: The baltimore eye survey. JAMA 266(3), 369–374 (1991)
10. Wu, X., Chen, D.Z.: Optimal net surface problems with applications. In: Widmayer, P., Triguero, F., Morales, R., Hennessy, M., Eidenbenz, S., Conejo, R. (eds.) ICALP 2002. LNCS, vol. 2380, pp. 1029–1042. Springer, Heidelberg (2002)

Statistical Power in Image Segmentation: Relating Sample Size to Reference Standard Quality

Eli Gibson[1,2], Henkjan J. Huisman[1], and Dean C. Barratt[2]

[1] Radboud University Medical Center, Nijmegen, The Netherlands
[2] University College London, London, UK

Abstract. Ideal reference standards for comparing segmentation algorithms balance trade-offs between the data set size, the costs of reference standard creation and the resulting accuracy. As reference standard quality impacts the likelihood of detecting significant improvements (i.e. the statistical power), we derived a sample size formula for segmentation accuracy comparison using an imperfect reference standard. We expressed this formula as a function of algorithm performance and reference standard quality (e.g. measured with a high quality reference standard on pilot data) to reveal the relationship between reference standard quality and statistical power, addressing key study design questions: (1) How many validation images are needed to compare segmentation algorithms? (2) How accurate should the reference standard be? The resulting formula predicted statistical power to within 2% of Monte Carlo simulations across a range of model parameters. A case study, using the PROMISE12 prostate segmentation data set, shows the practical use of the formula.

Keywords: Segmentation accuracy, statistical power, reference standard.

1 Introduction

Segmentation of anatomy and pathology on medical images plays a key role in many clinical scenarios, such as the delineation of the prostate to plan radiotherapy [2]. As a result, many algorithms for supporting or automating segmentation have been developed, and segmentation remains an active area of research [5].

Selecting reference standards (e.g. expert manual segmentations) to evaluate and compare segmentation algorithms involves balancing trade-offs between sample size, quality, and cost. An ideal reference standard would match the anatomy (or pathology) perfectly; however, anatomic/pathologic variation, ambiguous anatomical definitions, clinical constraints, and interobserver variability can introduce errors into the reference standard [8]. The quality and cost of the reference standard may be affected by the time and effort devoted to segmentation accuracy, the number of observers and the expertise of the observer(s). For example, the PROMISE12 prostate segmentation challenge [5] used two reference standards (see Fig. 1), a *high quality* one created by one experienced clinical reader and verified by another independent one, and a *low quality* one created

N. Navab et al. (Eds.): MICCAI 2015, Part III, LNCS 9351, pp. 105–113, 2015.
DOI: 10.1007/978-3-319-24574-4_13

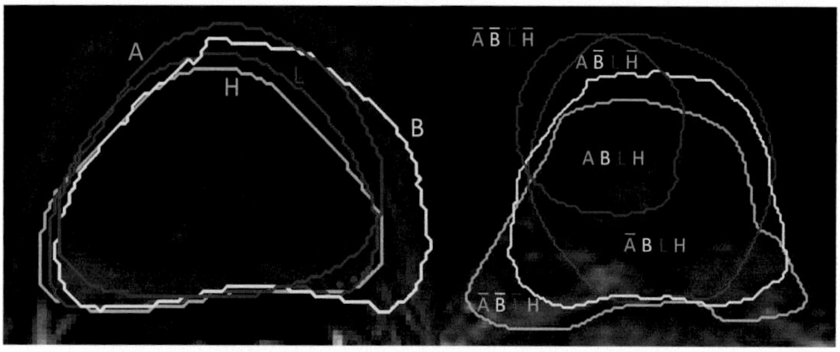

Fig. 1. Left: Prostate MRI segmentations by algorithms A (blue) and B (yellow), and low (L; red) and high (H; green) quality reference standards from the PROMISE12 data [5]. Relative to H, L oversegmented anteriorly, affecting accuracy measurements of A and B using L. Right: Apical segmentations showing regions of different segmentation outcomes ABLH (overbar denotes negative classifications). The statistical power of segmentation evaluation studies are modeled using outcome probability distributions.

by an inexperienced nonclinical observer. Due to the high costs of creating high quality reference standards, affordable lower quality ones are commonly used.

Reference standard errors can introduce uncertainty into performance measures, and impact the probability of detecting a significant difference (i.e. the statistical power) in validation studies [1]. Thus, there are trade-offs between generating large (and expensive) data sets to mitigate the uncertainty from imperfect reference standards, generating highly accurate reference standards (requiring substantial clinician time and expertise), and successfully finding significant differences. To balance these trade-offs, it is important to quantify the impact of reference standard quality on the statistical power of experiments comparing segmentation algorithm performance.

In the first steps towards this goal, we present the derivation of a new segmentation sample size formula that relates the statistical power to reference standard quality and algorithm performance measured with respect to a higher quality reference standard. After estimating the reference standard and algorithm performance (e.g. in a pilot study), this formula can inform key questions affecting study design: **(1) How many validation images are needed to evaluate a segmentation algorithm?** (i.e. given a reference standard with an estimated error rate, what is the sample size needed to show a clinically important improvement? **(2) How accurate does the reference standard need to be?** (i.e. given a data set of a fixed sample size, what level of reference standard accuracy must be attained to show a clinically important improvement)

2 Derivation of the Sample Size Formula

Since sample size formulae are analysis-specific, this paper focuses on one performance metric (differences in the mean segmentation accuracy between a pair of algorithms), and one statistical analysis comparing the performance of two algorithms using a paired T test on the same data set of images. The sample size formula can then be expressed in a generic form as

$$N = \left(T_{\alpha/2}\sigma_0 + T_\beta \sigma_{Alt}\right)^2 / \delta_R^2, \tag{1}$$

where N is the number of images needed to detect a population difference in accuracy δ_R with respect to the reference standard R, σ_0^2 and σ_{Alt}^2 are the variances of the differences in accuracies under the null hypothesis ($\delta_R = 0$) and alternate hypothesis ($\delta_R \neq 0$), respectively, and $T_{\alpha/2}$ and T_β are N – 1-degree-of-freedom Student T quantiles controlling type I and type II study error rates, respectively. A segmentation-specific sample size formula is derived in Section 2.1.

If the clinical goal requires true improvements in accuracy, these may be better reflected by specifying the minimal detectable difference δ_R with respect to the high quality reference standard, even if the actual study will use a lower quality reference study. In Section 2.2, this concept is used to relate the impact of reference standard quality on statistical power by expressing the sample size in terms of the performance of the algorithms and a low quality reference standard, measured against a higher quality reference standard (e.g. in a pilot study).

2.1 Sample Size for Segmentation Accuracy

We model the segmentation of an image as a set of binary classifications of n segmentation elements (such as voxels or superpixels). For each element, these classifications are modeled as independent samples from random variables representing the high (H) and low (L) quality reference standards and the algorithms (A and B). The classification outcome from all four is denoted $ABLH$ (see Fig. 1). One image event in a segmentation study can be represented as a scaled contingency table denoting the proportion of each type of classification outcome. If the outcome probabilities were fixed and known, this could be represented as a sample from a 16-element multinomial distribution with n trials, scaled by $\frac{1}{n}$. To model variability in the multinomial probability, the conjugate Dirichlet prior is commonly used [3], parameterized by the mean probability vector p and precision ω [7]. With this prior, the resulting image events are distributed as a 16-element Dirichlet-multinomial (Pólya) distribution P with n trials, scaled by $\frac{1}{n}$, with mean p and covariance $\frac{(n+\omega)}{n(\omega+1)}\left(diag(p) - p^T p\right)$. The differences in accuracy are then distributed as a linear transformation D of P, weighting outcomes where A outperforms B (event $C_A : A = L \neq B$) by 1, outcomes where B outperforms A (event $C_B : A \neq L = B$) by -1, and other outcomes ($A = B$) by 0. This distribution has a mean $\delta_L = p(C_A) - p(C_B)$ and a variance $\sigma_{Alt}^2 = \frac{(n+\omega)}{n(\omega+1)}(\psi - \delta_L^2)$, where $\psi = p(C_A) + p(C_B)$. Under the null hypothesis, $\delta_L = 0$, therefore $\sigma_0^2 = \frac{(n+\omega)}{n(\omega+1)}\psi$. Substituting σ_0 and σ_{Alt} into Eq. 1 and factoring out $\frac{(n+\omega)}{n(\omega+1)}$, the sample size for accuracy difference with respect to reference standard L is

$$N = \frac{(n+\omega)}{n(\omega+1)} \frac{\left(T_{\alpha/2}\sqrt{\psi} + T_\beta\sqrt{\psi - \delta_L^2}\right)^2}{\delta_L^2}. \tag{2}$$

2.2 Sample Size in Terms of the High Quality Reference Standard

Eq. 2 with δ_L measured with respect to the low quality reference standard can be expressed in terms of the performance of the algorithms and the low quality reference standard with respect to the high quality reference. As ψ can be expressed as $p(A\bar{B} \cup \bar{A}B)$ which is independent of the reference standard, only δ_L needs to be rewritten. For tractability, it is furthermore assumed that A, B and L are conditionally independent given H. For brevity, for $X \in \{A, B, L\}$, we denote conditional probabilities $p(X|H)$ using an overbar for $X = 0$, and an underline for $H = 0$: sensitivity $x = p(X = 1|H = 1)$, false negative rate $\bar{x} = p(X = 0|H = 1)$, false positive rate $\underline{x} = p(X = 1|H = 0)$, and specificity $\bar{\underline{x}} = p(X = 0|H = 0)$. Additionally, we use the following notation: $h = p(H = 1)$; and $\bar{h} = p(H = 0)$. Since outcomes where $A = B$ do not affect the *difference* in accuracy, δ_L is the probability of classification outcomes where $A = L$ and $B \neq L$ minus the probability of those where $A \neq L$ and $B = L$ (Eq. 3). By assuming conditional independence (Eq. 4), this can be rearranged algebraically (Eq. 5) to express δ_L in terms of the difference in accuracy ($\delta_a = (a-b)h + (\underline{a} - \underline{b})\bar{h}$) and sensitivity ($\delta_s = a - b$) with respect to the high quality reference, the sensitivity (l) and specificity ($\bar{\underline{l}}$) of the low quality reference standard, and the probability of positive outcomes (h) according to the high quality reference standard (Eq. 6). Placing this term in Eq. 2 yields the sample size formula in Eq. 7.

$$\begin{aligned}
\delta_L = \;& p(A\bar{B}LH) + p(A\bar{B}L\bar{H}) + p(\bar{A}B\bar{L}H) + p(\bar{A}B\bar{L}\bar{H}) \\
& - p(\bar{A}BLH) - p(\bar{A}BL\bar{H}) - p(A\bar{B}\bar{L}H) - p(A\bar{B}\bar{L}\bar{H}) && (3)\\
= \;& a\bar{b}lh + \underline{a\bar{b}l}\bar{h} + \bar{a}b\bar{l}h + \underline{\bar{a}b\bar{l}}\bar{h} - \bar{a}blh - \underline{\bar{a}bl}\bar{h} - a\bar{b}\bar{l}h - \underline{a\bar{b}\bar{l}}\bar{h} && (4)\\
= \;& \left((a-b)h + (\underline{a} - \underline{b})\bar{h}\right)(2\bar{\underline{l}} - 1) - 2\,(a-b)\,(\bar{\underline{l}} - l)h && (5)\\
= \;& \delta_a(2\bar{\underline{l}} - 1) - 2\delta_s(\bar{\underline{l}} - l)h. && (6)
\end{aligned}$$

$$N = \frac{(n+\omega)}{n(\omega+1)} \frac{\left(T_{\alpha/2}\sqrt{\psi} + T_{\beta}\sqrt{\psi - \left(\delta_a(2\bar{\underline{l}} - 1) - 2\delta_s(\bar{\underline{l}} - l)h\right)^2}\right)^2}{\left(\delta_a(2\bar{\underline{l}} - 1) - 2\delta_s(\bar{\underline{l}} - l)h\right)^2}. \quad (7)$$

3 Simulations

We performed Monte Carlo simulations to assess the accuracy of the sample size formula. In each simulation, we instantiated a parametric model (described below) representing a segmentation validation experiment with an underlying difference in accuracy, and repeatedly simulated the experiment to estimate the simulated power (i.e. the proportion of simulations yielding true positive outcomes) and compared it to the specified power. To exclude error due to using $\lceil N \rceil$ instead of N (because N must be a natural number), we determined $\lceil N \rceil$ using a specified power $1-\beta = 0.8$, but compared the resulting power to $1-\beta_{\lceil N \rceil}$

Table 1. Parameters used to estimate the accuracy of the model

	n	h	A_a	δ_a	a/A_a	δ_s	l	$\underline{l}$	ω
Baseline	10000	0.4	0.8	0.05	1	0.05	0.8	0.8	100
Minimum	100	0.1	0.6	0.01	0.75	0.01	0.6	0.6	16
Maximum	100000	0.9	0.99	0.25	1.25	0 .30	1	1	1024

computed by solving Eq. 7 for $N = \lceil N \rceil$. We used 25,000 repetitions, yielding a 1% wide 95% confidence interval on the error in predicted power.

To assess the accuracy of Eq. 7, we used a parametric model with random variables A, B, L and H, for the two algorithms and the low and high quality reference standards. A, B and L could be defined by mean sensitivities and specificities with respect to H; however, to independently manipulate δ_a and δ_s in Eq. 7, A and B were redefined in terms of δ_a, δ_s, the accuracy of A (A_a) and a sensitivity factor a/A_a. H was parameterized by a mean probability of positive outcomes, and parameter n specified the number of segmentation elements. Type I and II error rates were fixed to be 0.05 and 0.2, respectively. A precision parameter ω was used to model inter-image variability and variability in positive outcomes. The segmentation outcomes were sampled from a Dirichlet-Multinomial distribution parameterized by ω and $p = p(ABLH) = p(A|H)p(B|H)p(L|H)p(H)$. Model parameters were initialized with baseline values given in the first row of Table 1, and were varied independently through the ranges given in rows 2-3.

4 Results

The error in the power predicted by the model over a range of parameters are shown in Fig. 4; the 95% confidence interval bounds on prediction error were within 2% throughout. To ensure high sensitivity to all parameter values where the model has prediction error, multiple comparison correction, which would widen the intervals and hide model errors, was not used. Thus, the 95% confidence intervals for a perfect model would include 0% error for 95% of parameter sets; for our model, the confidence intervals included 0% error for 89% of the parameter sets. Three regions showed notable deviation from the simulations: high accuracy ($A_a > 0.975$), large differences in accuracy ($\delta_a \geq 0.2$) and high precision ($\omega = 1024$), although these errors did not exceed 2% (95% confidence).

5 Case Study

Using data from the PROMISE12 prostate MRI segmentation challenge [5], this case study demonstrates how to apply Eq. 7. In this data set, two experienced clinicians generated a high quality reference standard, and a graduate student generated a low quality reference standard. Although, in the challenge, algorithms were compared to the high quality reference standard, this case study considers comparing segmentation algorithms using the graduate-student reference

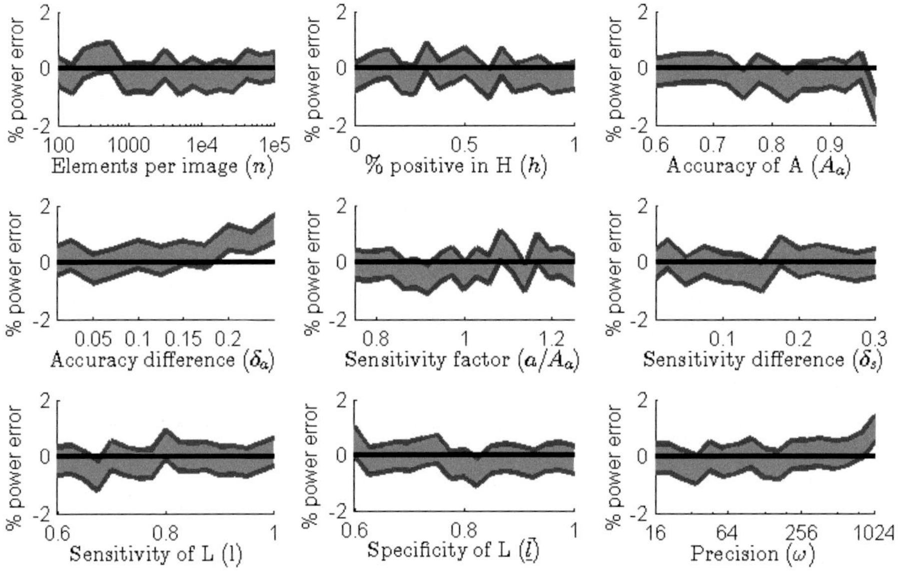

Fig. 2. Model accuracy: 95% confidence regions on the power prediction error (%). Values where the region does not contain the 0% error line suggest prediction error.

standard. To apply Eq. 7, one must estimate, from literature or pilot data, the algorithm and reference performance with respect to the high quality reference standard (a, b, l, $\underline{\bar{a}}$, $\underline{\bar{b}}$, and $\underline{\bar{l}}$), the probability of positive outcomes (h), the precision ω, the probability of disagreement between A and B (ψ), and the desired (or observed) performance differences (δ_L, δ_a and δ_s). In this case study, image events (i.e. 16-element contingency tables) were computed for 30 cases from the segmentations of the high and low quality reference standards and two algorithms submitted for the challenge. If such a data set is not available, a high quality reference standard on a small pilot data set could be generated to make these estimates. Precision was estimated by setting $\frac{n+\omega}{n(\omega+1)}$ to $s^2/(D^T(diag(\tilde{p})-\tilde{p}^T\tilde{p})D)$, where s^2 was the observed variance in accuracy difference and $\tilde{p}$ was the vector of observed probabilities: $\omega_L = 1600$ (low quality reference standard), and $\omega_H = 1900$ (high quality). Other parameters were estimated by combining the counts of classification outcomes (e.g. $\underline{\bar{a}} = p(\bar{A}|\bar{H}) = \frac{||\bar{A}\cap\bar{H}||}{||\bar{H}||}$) and averaging over the images: $a = 0.892$, $b = 0.899$, $l = 0.892$, $\underline{\bar{a}} = 0.998$, $\underline{\bar{b}} = 0.997$, and $\underline{\bar{l}} = 0.999$, $h = 0.171$, $\delta_L = 0.0016$, $\delta_a = 0.0016$, $\delta_s = -0.0066$, $\psi = 0.0047$. Substituting ψ, δ_a and ω_T into Eq. 2 yielded a sample size of $N = 7.2$ to detect a difference of δ_a using the high quality reference standard. Substituting the parameters (except δ_L) into Eq. 7 yielded $N = 8.4$ to detect a difference of δ_a (as measured with a high quality reference standard) using the low quality reference standard. For comparison, $N = 8.5$ when substituting ψ, δ_L and ω_T into Eq. 2 directly, suggesting that assuming conditional independence introduced minimal error.

In this case study, the low quality reference standard required only a slightly larger sample size, and could be a suitable approach.

6 Discussion

This paper derived a sample size formula for comparisons of segmentation accuracy between two algorithms, and expressed it as a function of performance of the algorithms and a low quality reference standard performance measured against a higher quality reference standard. This relationship can be used to address central questions in the design of segmentation validation experiments: **(1) How many validation images are needed to evaluate a segmentation algorithm? (2) How accurate does my reference standard need to be?** The relationship can be used in several contexts. For researchers designing novel segmentation algorithms, the relationship can inform the selection of validation data sets and reference standards needed to evaluate the algorithms. For researchers involved in creating validation data sets and reference standard segmentations, the relationship can guide the trade-offs between the costs of generating large data sets and those of generating highly accurate reference standards.

While this paper considers the common approach of using low quality reference standards directly, other approaches have been proposed to leverage lower quality reference standards. Most notably, label fusion algorithms, such as STAPLE [8] aim to infer a high quality reference standard from multiple low quality reference standards. This has even been extended to use *crowd-sourced* segmentations by minimally trained users [4]. These methods may be preferable, when feasible, to using low quality reference standards; however, the need to create multiple reference standards may increase the cost/complexity of such studies.

The predicted power was within 2% of the simulations over the tested parameters. Three conditions showed measurable deviations from 0% error. With high accuracies, the algorithms disagreed on few classifications and accuracy differences were not normally distributed as assumed by the T-test; this was compounded by the low sample size ($N = 11$) where the T-test is more sensitive to assumption violations [6]. Thus, statistical comparisons of highly accurate algorithms may be challenging. Large or very consistent (high ω) accuracy differences, yielded even lower sample sizes ($N \leq 6$). Low predicted sample sizes may have higher error, although, even in these cases, it did not exceed 2%.

Sample size formulae are inherently specific to the statistical analysis being performed. The presented formula is specific to studies comparing the accuracy of two algorithms using one reference standard. As illustrated by the PROMISE12 challenge, many segmentation evaluation studies compare multiple measures (e.g. Dice coefficients and boundary distances) between >2 algorithms using multiple reference standards. Deriving analogous sample size formulae for these studies would be a valuable direction for future work.

Two key derivational assumptions may constrain the use of the formula. First, we assumed that given the high quality reference standard outcome, the low quality reference standard and algorithm segmentations are conditionally independent (i.e. do not make the same error more than predicted by chance). In practice, segmentation elements with confounding image features (e.g. low contrast or artifacts) may induce similar errors in the segmentations, potentially violating conditional independence. In the case study, any such correlation did not substantially impact the calculation; however, other data sets may be more prone to violations of this assumption. Additionally, segmentation algorithms trained using the low quality reference standard may make the same types of error as the reference standard potentially violating conditional independence. This was not a factor in the PROMISE12 data set, as algorithms were trained using the high quality reference standard. Using pilot data to test for conditional independence or to evaluate the impact of such correlation (as in the case study) may identify such situations. Second, we modelled segmentation as a set of independent decisions on segmentation elements, such as voxels or superpixels. In practice, regularization (e.g. enforcing smooth segmentations), clinical knowledge (e.g. anatomical constraints) or image features (e.g. artifacts) may cause correlated segmentation outcomes. It is unclear to what extent the aggregation of these outcomes in the multinomial and the variance in the Dirichlet prior mitigate violations of this assumption. Characterizing the sensitivity of the model to violations of these assumptions would be a valuable direction for future work.

In conclusion, this paper derived a sample size formula for comparing the accuracy of two segmentation algorithms using an imperfect reference standard, expressed as a function of algorithm and reference standard performance (measured against a higher quality reference standard). The model was accurate to within 2% across the tested range of model parameters, although it began to deviate measurably from simulations when N was low. We also showed a case study where using a low quality reference standard could cause little increase in sample size, and where assuming conditional independence for the algorithms and low quality reference standard introduced little error. The Medical Research Council and the Canadian Institutes of Health Research supported this work.

References

1. Beiden, S.V., Campbell, G., Meier, K.L., Wagner, R.F.: The problem of ROC analysis without truth: The EM algorithm and the information matrix. In: SPIE Medical Imaging, pp. 126–134 (2000)
2. Boehmer, D., Maingon, P., Poortmans, P., Baron, M.H., Miralbell, R., Remouchamps, V., Scrase, C., Bossi, A., Bolla, M.: Guidelines for primary radiotherapy of patients with prostate cancer. Radiother. Oncol. 79(3), 259–269 (2006)
3. Gelman, A., Carlin, J.B., Stern, H.S., Rubin, D.B.: Bayesian data analysis, vol. 2. Taylor & Francis (2014)
4. Landman, B.A., Asman, A.J., Scoggins, A.G., Bogovic, J.A., Stein, J.A., Prince, J.L.: Foibles, follies, and fusion: Web-based collaboration for medical image labeling. NeuroImage 59(1), 530–539 (2012)

5. Litjens, G., Toth, R., van de Ven, W., Hoeks, C., Kerkstra, S., van Ginneken, B., Vincent, G., Guillard, G., et al.: Evaluation of prostate segmentation algorithms for MRI: the PROMISE12 challenge. Med. Image Anal. 18(2), 359–373 (2014)
6. Lumley, T., Diehr, P., Emerson, S., Chen, L.: The importance of the normality assumption in public health data sets. Ann. Rev. Pub. Health 23(1), 151–169 (2002)
7. Minka, T.P.: Estimating a Dirichlet distribution. Tech. rep., M.I.T. (2000)
8. Warfield, S.K., Zou, K.H., Wells, W.M.: Simultaneous truth and performance level estimation (STAPLE): an algorithm for the validation of image segmentation. IEEE Trans. Med. Imag. 23(7), 903–921 (2004)

Joint Learning of Image Regressor and Classifier for Deformable Segmentation of CT Pelvic Organs

Yaozong Gao[1,2], Jun Lian[3], and Dinggang Shen[1]

[1] Departments of Radiology, Chapel Hill, USA
[2] Computer Science, Chapel Hill, USA
[3] Radiation Oncology, University of North Carolina at Chapel Hill, Chapel Hill, USA

Abstract. The segmentation of pelvic organs from CT images is an essential step for prostate radiation therapy. However, due to low tissue contrast and large anatomical variations, it is still challenging to accurately segment these organs from CT images. Among various existing methods, deformable models gain popularity as it is easy to incorporate shape priors to regularize the final segmentation. Despite this advantage, the sensitivity to the initialization is often a pain for deformable models. In this paper, we propose a novel way to guide deformable segmentation, which could greatly alleviate the problem caused by poor initialization. Specifically, random forest is adopted to jointly learn image regressor and classifier for each organ. The image regressor predicts the 3D displacement from any image voxel to the organ boundary based on the local appearance of this voxel. It is used as an external force to drive each vertex of deformable model (3D mesh) towards the target organ boundary. Once the deformable model is close to the boundary, the organ likelihood map, provided by the learned classifier, is used to further refine the segmentation. In the experiments, we applied our method to segmenting prostate, bladder and rectum from planning CT images. Experimental results show that our method can achieve competitive performance over existing methods, even with very rough initialization.

1 Introduction

Prostate cancer is the second leading cause of cancer death in American men. External beam radiation therapy (EBRT) is an effective treatment option to control prostate cancer. In the planning stage of EBRT, a planning CT image is acquired. Physicians need to segment major structures such as the prostate, bladder and rectum from this CT image to design a radiation treatment plan. The efficacy of EBRT depends heavily on the quality of segmentation. As manual segmentation is time-consuming and often suffers from large inter-observer variability, it is clinically desirable to develop accurate automatic methods for segmenting CT pelvic organs.

Among various existing methods, deformable models have gained the most popularity, as it is easy to impose shape regularization. For example, Lay et al. [1] adopted the active shape model with boundary detectors to segment pelvic

N. Navab et al. (Eds.): MICCAI 2015, Part III, LNCS 9351, pp. 114–122, 2015.
DOI: 10.1007/978-3-319-24574-4_14

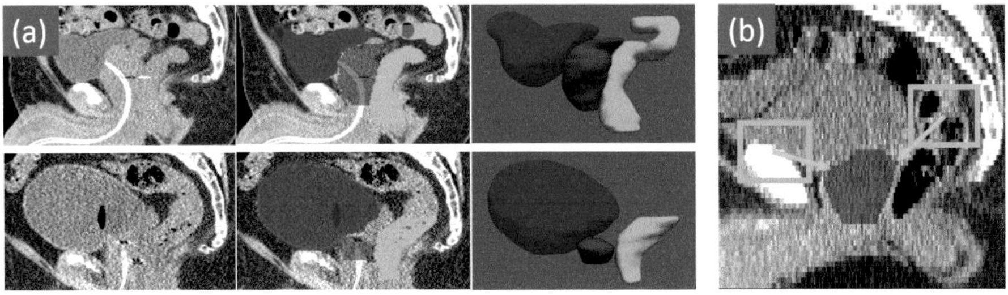

Fig. 1. (a) Two planning CTs and their segmentations of prostate (red), bladder (blue) and rectum (green). The 1st, 2nd, and 3rd columns show sagittal CT slices, the same slices overlaid with segmentations, and 3D views of segmentations, respectively. (b) 3D displacements (cyan arrows) to the organ boundary, where green boxes indicate the local patches of voxels.

organs from CT images. Chen et al. [2] used a Bayesian framework that integrates anatomical constraints from pelvic bones to segment the prostate and rectum. Costa et al. [3] proposed coupled deformable models to segment the prostate and bladder. Despite the popularity, deformable models are known to be sensitive to the initialization. If the initial shape model (e.g., 3D mesh) is not close to the target boundary, deformable models are likely to fail.

However, it is difficult to robustly initialize the shape model for CT pelvic organ segmentation due to two reasons: 1) pelvic organs show poor contrast (Fig. 1(a)), especially on their touching boundaries, and 2) the shape variations of pelvic organs are large across patients. These two factors hinder robust initialization, hence limiting the segmentation accuracy of deformable models.

In this paper, we propose a novel way to guide deformable models by jointly learning image regressor and classifier, which can greatly alleviate the problem caused by poor initialization. In the conventional learning-based deformable models, classifier is often used to guide deformable segmentation by producing an organ likelihood map, based on which each vertex of deformable model locally deforms along its normal direction to the position with the maximum boundary response. If the shape model is initialized far away from the true boundary, the conventional deformable models could suffer, as the local search will not be able to find the target boundary. To address this issue, in addition to classifier, we utilize random forest to jointly learn an image regressor. The image regressor predicts the 3D displacement from each image voxel to its nearest point on the organ boundary based on the local image appearance (Fig. 1(b)). It is used to drive each vertex of the deformable model towards the target boundary, thus relieving the problem caused by poor initialization. Once the deformable model is close to the boundary, the conventional local search strategy can be used to further refine the segmentation based on the organ likelihood map produced by the learned classifier. Validated on a CT dataset, experimental results show the robustness of our deformable model to the initialization as well as the effectiveness of our method in CT pelvic organ segmentation.

2 Method

2.1 Joint Learning of Image Regressor and Classifier

Random forest has been widely used in medical image analysis [1,5] due to its efficiency and effectiveness. In this paper, we use random forest to learn image regressor and classifier for each organ. The image regressor predicts the 3D displacement from any image voxel to its nearest point on the target organ boundary. The image classifier predicts the class label of each image voxel (i.e., target organ versus background). Both the image regressor and classifier make predictions according to the local appearance of image voxel. Considering that 3D displacement of a voxel is often correlated with its label, we propose to use random forest to learn image regressor and classifier jointly.

Joint Regression and Classification. Since both continuous variables (3D displacement) and discrete label need to be predicted together, we consider joint learning to be a joint regression and classification problem. Motivated by [5], we modify the objective function of random forest to consider both regression and classification in the tree optimization:

$$\{f^*, t^*\} = \max_{f,t}\{\frac{1}{Z_v}(v - \sum_{j\in\{L,R\}} \frac{N^j}{N} v^j) + \frac{1}{Z_c}(e - \sum_{j\in\{L,R\}} \frac{N^j}{N} e^j)\} \quad (1)$$

where f and t are a feature and threshold, respectively. Here, 3D Haar-like features [4] are used to represent the local appearance of each voxel. v, e and N denote average variance, entropy and the number of training samples arriving at one node, respectively. The superscript $j \in \{L, R\}$ indicates the measurements computed after being split into the left or right child node. The first term of Eq. 1 computes variance reduction for regression, which is different from the differential entropy used in [5]. The second term of Eq. 1 computes entropy reduction for classification. Since the magnitudes of variance and entropy reductions are not of the same scale, we normalize both magnitudes by dividing the average variance and entropy at the root node (Z_v and Z_c), respectively.

Iterative Auto-Context Refinement. With the above modification, random forest can be learned to jointly predict the 3D displacement and class label for each voxel in the image. However, since both the displacement and label of each voxel are predicted independently from those of nearby voxels, the obtained 3D displacement field and label likelihood map are often spatially inconsistent, as shown in the first row of Fig. 2. To ensure the spatial consistency, it is necessary to consider the predictions of neighboring voxels during the voxel-wise displacement and label estimation.

Auto-context [6] is an iterative scheme that can incorporate the neighboring prediction information to compensate for the limitation of the independent voxel-wise estimation. The first iteration of training in the auto-context is the same as the conventional voxel-wise estimation method, which trains a prediction model according to local appearance features (e.g., Haar-like features) extracted from

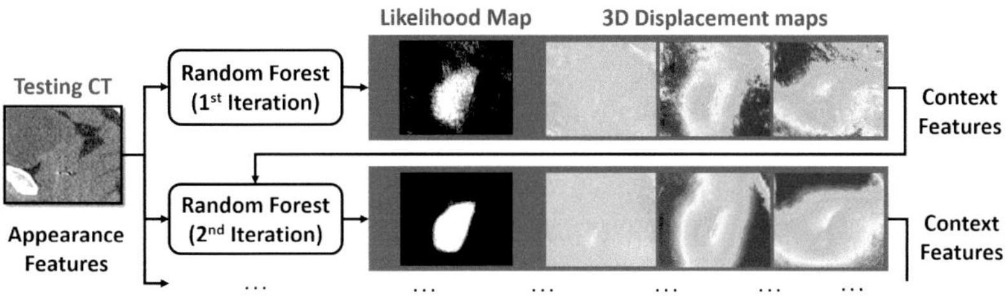

Fig. 2. Illustration of iterative auto-context refinement for prostate. Cold and warm colors in the color maps denote small and large distance values, respectively.

each voxel. In the second iteration, the model, learned in the previous iteration, is first applied to estimate the prediction maps (e.g., likelihood and displacement maps) for each training image. Additional features can be extracted at these prediction maps for each voxel. These features are named "*context features*" in the auto-context. Different from the traditional auto-context, which uses radiation-like context features, we extract Haar-like context features, which shows better performance. By combining appearance features from intensity image and context features from prediction maps, a new prediction model can be trained to update the prediction maps in the previous iteration. Following the same manner, a sequence of prediction models can be trained to iteratively update the prediction maps. Fig. 2 illustrates the testing stage of the auto-context.

Context features, which are extracted from local patches in previous prediction maps, capture the neighboring prediction information for a voxel, making this a significant area for improvement. As the predictions of neighboring voxels are highly correlated, the inclusion of context features in the prediction model could exploit this neighborhood correlation, which will improve the spatial consistency of prediction maps.

2.2 Deformable Segmentation with Regressor and Classifier

For each voxel in the image, the jointly learned image regressor and classifier can be used to estimate 3D displacement to the target organ boundary and organ likelihood. As introduced previously, the conventional learning-based deformable models use only the estimated organ likelihoods of voxels and rely on local search to drive deformable models onto the target organ boundary, causing them to be sensitive to model initialization. To overcome this problem, we utilize both image regressor and classifier to guide deformable models. Specifically, our deformable segmentation consists of two steps, as detailed below:

Pose Adjustment by Image Regressor. Considering that the deformable model may be initialized far from the target organ boundary, we first utilize image regressor to pull deformable model towards the boundary. Specifically, for each vertex of the deformable model, image regressor is used to estimate the 3D displacement of the vertex to the nearest point on the target organ boundary.

The estimated displacement is used as an external force to deform the shape model by sequentially adjusting its position, orientation and scale. Initially, the shape model is only allowed to translate under the guidance of image regressor. Once it is well positioned, we estimate its orientation by allowing it to rigidly deform. Finally, the deformation is relaxed to the affine transformation to estimate the scaling and shearing parameters of the shape model.

Boundary Refinement by Image Classifier. Once the shape model is close to the target organ boundary after pose adjustment, the conventional local search strategy can be used to refine the shape model based on the organ likelihood map provided by the image classifier. Specifically, in the refinement step, each vertex of deformable model locally searches along its normal direction to find its new position with the maximum likelihood gradient. After every vertex has deformed for one step, the entire shape model (3D mesh) is then smoothened prior to the next round of deformation. The vertex-wise deformation and mesh smoothing are iterated until convergence.

To increase the efficiency of our deformable model, we implement our model in multi-resolution. A joint image regressor and classifier is trained independently at two resolutions, such as coarse resolution and fine resolution. In the coarse resolution, the testing image is down-sampled by a factor of 4, which allows fast computation of rough segmentation. In the fine resolution, we need to compute only the 3D displacement field and organ likelihood map near the rough segmentation, which significantly reduces the computation time.

3 Experimental Results

Our dataset consists of 29 prostate cancer patients, each with one planning CT scan available. The prostate, bladder and rectum in all CT scans have been manually segmented by a physician, and serve as ground truth for our segmentation method. The image size is $512 \times 512 \times (400 \sim 500)$, and the image spacing is $1.172 \times 1.172 \times 1$ mm^3. Three-fold cross validation is used to evaluate our method. In random forest training, we prevent overfitting by stopping node splitting if the number of training samples arriving at one node is below 8. We do not limit the tree depth. The number of trees in the forest is 10. Three iterations are used in the auto-context.

Model Initialization. To demonstrate the robustness of our deformable model to the initialization, we initialize mean shape model at the center of every testing image. As shown in Fig. 3(a), the initialized shape model may be far away from the target organ. In such case, the conventional deformable models could fail, as the local search would not be able to find the interested organ boundary. In contrast, with the guidance from image regressor (Fig. 3(b)), the poorly initialized shape model could be effectively driven towards the target organ (Fig. 3(d)), which alleviates the dependency of deformable models on good initialization.

Auto-Context and Joint Model. Fig. 4 shows the magnitude of 3D displacement fields estimated by separately- and jointly- learned image regressors,

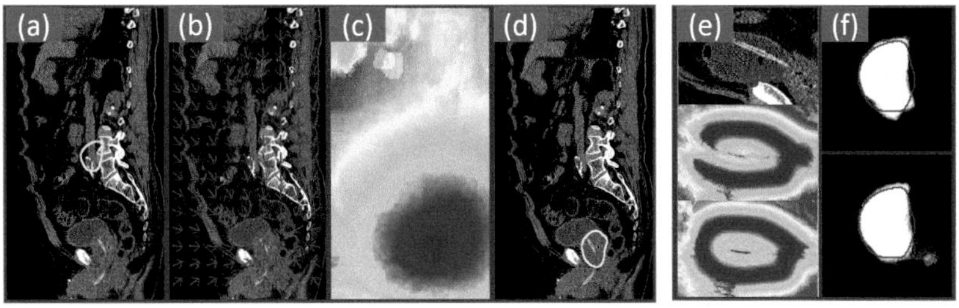

Fig. 3. (a-d) CT prostate segmentation. (a) Model initialization (yellow contour). (b-c) Direction and magnitude of 3D displacement field estimated in the coarse resolution. (d) Final segmentation. (e-f) Bladder displacement magnitude maps and prostate likelihood maps obtained by separate (upper) and joint (lower) models, respectively. Cold and warm colors in (c) and (e) denote small and large distances, respectively. Yellow contour in (d) denotes the automatic segmentation, and red contours in (d) and (f) denote ground truths.

without and with auto-context, respectively. We can see from Fig. 4(b-c) that the estimated 3D displacement field is noisy without auto-context, which makes it unreliable for guiding deformable models. We tested our method without auto-context, and found it failed in most cases. In contrast, with the help of auto-context, the quality of estimated 3D displacement significantly improves. Moreover, by comparing Fig. 4(d) and (e), we noticed that jointly-learned image regressor often obtains better displacement maps than separately-learned image regressor. In several cases (Fig. 3e), the displacement field estimated by separately-learned regressor may not necessarily form a closed surface (2nd row), due to inaccurate predictions for a small region. In such case, the pose adjustment will fail. In contrast, with evidence from classification, the jointly-learned regressor can effectively overcome this problem (3rd row), leading to better segmentation than separately-learned regressor (Table 1).

On the other hand, classification also benefits from regression. Fig. 3(f) gives one example of the prostate. Compared with separately-learned classifier (1st row), the jointly-learned classifier (2nd row) obtains better classification results on the boundary. This boundary difference also contributes to better segmentation accuracy of joint models compared to separated models (Table 1).

Table 2 (left) compares the traditional radiation-like context features with our Haar-like context features, which shows the superiority of Haar-like context features in the auto-context model.

Comparisons with Other Methods. Table 2 (right) compares our pose adjustment strategy with two other methods for model initialization. "Mass" uses the classification mass center from the coarse resolution, and "Box" uses the anatomy bounding box detection method [8]. The performances were obtained by replacing the pose adjustment strategy with respective initialization techniques. By comparing their results with ours in Table 1, we can conclude that the pose adjustment strategy is more effective in initializing deformable models of CT pelvic organs.

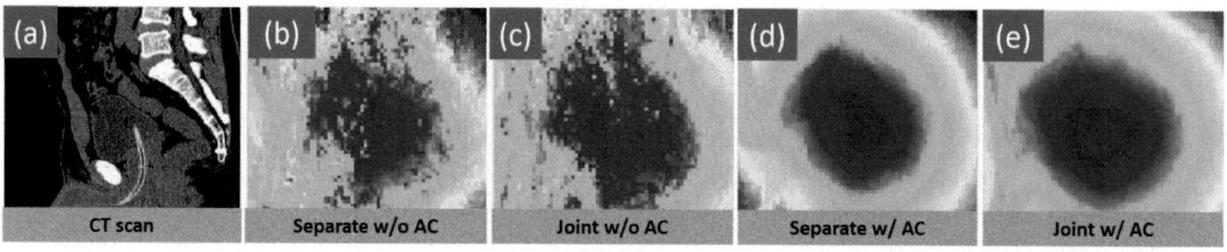

Fig. 4. Displacement magnitude maps of bladder obtained by different strategies. (b-c) Separately- and jointly- learned image regressors without auto-context. (d-e) Separately- and jointly- learned image regressors with auto-context.

Table 1. Quantitative comparison between separately-learned image regressor and classifier (Separate), and jointly-learned image regressor and classifier (Joint). Both of them use auto-context. DSC: Dice Similarity Coefficient for measuring overlap ratio. ASD: average surface distance for measuring boundary difference. Bold numbers indicate the best performance.

Organ		Prostate		Bladder		Rectum	
Resolution		Coarse	Fine	Coarse	Fine	Coarse	Fine
Separate	DSC(%)	72.7 $\pm$11.3	84.8 $\pm$3.97	79.0 $\pm$15.3	92.1 $\pm$13.3	70.9 $\pm$7.05	84.3 $\pm$6.25
	ASD(mm)	4.19 $\pm$1.60	2.28 $\pm$0.55	4.15 $\pm$2.12	1.38 $\pm$1.02	3.23 $\pm$0.69	1.97 $\pm$0.97
Joint	DSC(%)	73.0 $\pm$8.99	**85.2 $\pm$3.74**	82.7 $\pm$5.74	**94.9 $\pm$1.62**	69.3 $\pm$7.52	**84.7 $\pm$5.22**
	ASD(mm)	4.20 $\pm$1.32	**2.23 $\pm$0.53**	3.78 $\pm$1.26	**1.15 $\pm$0.29**	3.51 $\pm$0.82	**1.97 $\pm$0.92**

Table 3 quantitatively compares our method with other existing segmentation methods. Since different methods use different metrics to measure their performance, we separate the comparisons into two tables. We can see from Table 3 that our method achieves better accuracy than the existing methods under comparison. It is worth noting that most previous works use either sophisticated methods for model initialization [1,3,7], or rely on shape priors to regularize the segmentation [1,2,3,7]. In contrast, our method uses a fairly simple initialization method (i.e., initialize the mean shape model at image center), and does not rely on shape priors (e.g., PCA shape analysis, or sparse shape model [9]). It is interesting to observe that even with this setup, our method still results in more competitive results, when compared to previous methods. This demonstrates the robustness of our method in the initialization and effectiveness of our method for CT pelvic organ segmentation.

Table 2. Quantitative comparisons (left) between radiation-like (RADI) and Haar-like (Haar) context features in the auto-context, and (right) between different deformable initialization methods, where "Mass" uses the classification mass center from the coarse resolution to initialize deformable models.

DSC(%)	Prostate	Bladder	Rectum
RADI	84.5$\pm$4.4	94.0$\pm$6.1	82.7$\pm$8.5
Haar	85.2$\pm$3.7	94.9$\pm$1.6	84.3$\pm$6.2

DSC (%)	Prostate	Bladder	Rectum
Mass	81.5$\pm$12.0	82.9$\pm$18.1	46.0$\pm$26.8
Box[8]	74.4$\pm$21.2	71.7$\pm$26.0	66.4$\pm$20.3

Table 3. Comparisons of our method with other existing works. Left panel shows the comparison based on average surface distance (ASD). Right panel shows the comparison based on sensitivity (Sen) and positive predictive value (PPV). Good segmentation results have small ASD, and large Sen and PPV.

	Prostate	Bladder	Rectum
Mean±Std	ASD(mm)	ASD(mm)	ASD(mm)
Lay [1]	3.57±2.01	2.59±1.70	4.36±1.70
Lu [7]	2.37±0.89	2.81±1.86	4.23±1.46
Proposed	**2.23±0.53**	**1.15±0.29**	**1.97±0.92**

	Prostate		Bladder		Rectum	
Median	Sen	PPV	Sen	PPV	Sen	PPV
Costa [3]	0.79	0.86	0.87	0.93	N/A	N/A
Chen [2]	**0.84**	0.87	N/A	N/A	0.71	0.76
Proposed	0.82	**0.91**	**0.94**	**0.97**	**0.88**	**0.84**

4 Conclusion

In this paper, we propose a novel way to guide deformable segmentation by jointly learning image regressor and classifier for each organ. The image regressor is used to initially drive deformable model towards the organ boundary, while the image classifier is used to refine the segmentation once the pose (i.e., position, orientation and scale) of the deformable model has been adjusted by image regressor. Experimental results, based on a CT pelvic dataset, demonstrate the robustness of our deformable model to initialization, as well as the competitive performance of our method to other existing methods.

References

1. Lay, N., Birkbeck, N., Zhang, J., Zhou, S.K.: Rapid multi-organ segmentation using context integration and discriminative models. In: Gee, J.C., Joshi, S., Pohl, K.M., Wells, W.M., Zöllei, L. (eds.) IPMI 2013. LNCS, vol. 7917, pp. 450–462. Springer, Heidelberg (2013)
2. Chen, S., Lovelock, D.M., Radke, R.J.: Segmenting the prostate and rectum in CT imagery using anatomical constraints. Medical Image Analysis 15(1), 1–11 (2011)
3. Costa, M.J., Delingette, H., Novellas, S., Ayache, N.: Automatic segmentation of bladder and prostate using coupled 3D deformable models. In: Ayache, N., Ourselin, S., Maeder, A. (eds.) MICCAI 2007, Part I. LNCS, vol. 4791, pp. 252–260. Springer, Heidelberg (2007)
4. Gao, Y., Wang, L., Shao, Y., Shen, D.: Learning distance transform for boundary detection and deformable segmentation in CT prostate images. In: Wu, G., Zhang, D., Zhou, L. (eds.) MLMI 2014. LNCS, vol. 8679, pp. 93–100. Springer, Heidelberg (2014)
5. Glocker, B., Pauly, O., Konukoglu, E., Criminisi, A.: Joint classification-regression forests for spatially structured multi-object segmentation. In: Fitzgibbon, A., Lazebnik, S., Perona, P., Sato, Y., Schmid, C. (eds.) ECCV 2012, Part IV. LNCS, vol. 7575, pp. 870–881. Springer, Heidelberg (2012)
6. Tu, Z., Bai, X.: Auto-context and its application to high-level vision tasks and 3D brain image segmentation. TPAMI 32(10), 1744–1757 (2010)

7. Lu, C., Zheng, Y., Birkbeck, N., Zhang, J., Kohlberger, T., Tietjen, C., Boettger, T., Duncan, J.S., Zhou, S.K.: Precise segmentation of multiple organs in CT volumes using learning-based approach and information theory. In: Ayache, N., Delingette, H., Golland, P., Mori, K. (eds.) MICCAI 2012, Part II. LNCS, vol. 7511, pp. 462–469. Springer, Heidelberg (2012)
8. Criminisi, A., et al.: Regression forests for efficient anatomy detection and localization in computed tomography Scans. MedIA 17(8), 1293–1303 (2013)
9. Zhang, S., et al.: Towards robust and effective shape modeling: Sparse shape composition. MedIA 16(1), 265–277 (2012)

Corpus Callosum Segmentation in MS Studies Using Normal Atlases and Optimal Hybridization of Extrinsic and Intrinsic Image Cues

Lisa Y.W. Tang[1], Ghassan Hamarneh[2], Anthony Traboulsee[1], David Li, and Roger Tam[1]

[1] University of British Columbia, Vancouver, British Columbia, Canada
[2] Medical Image Analysis Lab., Simon Fraser University, Burnaby, Canada

Abstract. The corpus callosum (CC) is a key brain structure and change in its size and shape is a focal point in the study of neurodegenerative diseases like multiple sclerosis (MS). A number of automatic methods have been proposed for CC segmentation in magnetic resonance images (MRIs) that can be broadly classified as intensity-based and template-based. Imaging artifacts and signal changes due to pathology often cause errors in intensity-based methods. Template-based methods have been proposed to alleviate these problems. However, registration inaccuracies (local mismatch) can occur when the template image has large intensity and morphological differences from the scan to be segmented, such as when using publicly available normal templates for a diseased population. Accordingly, we propose a novel hybrid segmentation framework that performs optimal, spatially variant fusion of multi-atlas-based and intensity-based priors. Our novel *coupled* graph-labeling formulation effectively optimizes, on a per-voxel basis, the weights that govern the choice of priors so that intensity priors derived from the subject image are emphasized when spatial priors derived from the registered templates are deemed less trustworthy. This stands in contrast to existing hybrid methods that either ignore local registration errors or alternate between the optimization of fusion weights and segmentation results in an expectation-maximization fashion. We evaluated our method using a public dataset and two large in-house MS datasets and found that it gave more accurate results than those achieved by existing methods for CC segmentation.

1 Introduction

The corpus callosum (CC) is the largest white matter structure in the brain and plays the crucial role of relaying communication signals between the cerebral hemispheres. A growing body of recent literature [1–3] has shown that the change in its size as measured in structural MRIs[1] is a sensitive measure of regional brain atrophy that is effective for the monitoring of multiple sclerosis (MS) progression. However, in all of the aforementioned clinical studies [1–3], the CC structures were manually segmented by clinical experts. While various methods [4–6] have been proposed to segment the CC, these

[1] We focus on structural MRIs as it is a more common modality than the others.

N. Navab et al. (Eds.): MICCAI 2015, Part III, LNCS 9351, pp. 123–131, 2015.
DOI: 10.1007/978-3-319-24574-4_15

methods either perform segmentation in 2D [4–8], which is confounded by the selection of the appropriate plane of measurement [9] and hinders 3D shape analyses [9], or require human intervention ([4]), which makes large-scale analyses infeasible.

Existing automatic methods for 2D segmentation of the CC in structural MRIs may generally be classified [4] into two categories. In *intensity-based* methods [4–6, 8], segmentation is mostly driven by intrinsic data from the subject image. Both [5, 6] require a midsagittal plane extraction tool. Other methods [4, 8] require tissue segmentation, which makes them susceptible to partial volume effects and errors in segmentation. For example, it was noted in [4] that the method should not be used for MR images of patients with demyelinating diseases (e.g. MS) because significant alterations in image intensities tend to occur in these images. In *template-based* methods (e.g. [4, 10] and references therein), labels of pre-segmented template images are propagated and fused, in the case of multiple templates, to obtain the final segmentation. This approach, more generally known as multi-atlas segmentation (MAS) [11], is more robust than intensity-based methods due to the spatial constraints implicitly imposed by registration. However, segmentation accuracy not only depends on registration, but also on the choice of the template images ([4]). When there exists large intensity and morphological variability between the template(s) and the subject image, registration accuracy suffers, which in turn limits segmentation accuracy. Hence, one should use templates drawn from the population of the target image, which is often not publicly available (e.g. in case of pathology such as MS) nor easy to create without introducing biases (i.e. one with templates that span the whole population without favoring any subset).

In addition to the above problems, two issues particular to MS datasets bring further challenges: 1) retrospective studies can span over a decade, and older data tends to have low resolution, poor image contrast, and low signal-to-noise ratio (SNR); and 2) the possible use of gadolinium contrast in T1-weighted scans results in hyper-intensities in the CC periphery. These factors render the publicly available algorithms [4, 6] largely inapplicable in our two MS datasets.

To overcome the aforementioned problems, a hybrid approach may be adopted where MAS results are incorporated into an intensity-based segmentation framework in the form of spatial priors and the segmentation problem is then solved via energy minimization, as done in [12]. This approach was applied to the cerebellum and other structures but, to the best of our knowledge, has never been applied to the CC. More importantly, most hybrid methods, e.g. [12], employ spatial priors without accounting for *local* mismatches between the registered images. Hence, registration errors can be large in some regions, yielding spatial prior information that is misleading at these regions.

Accordingly, we propose a novel graph-based formulation that explicitly accounts for registration errors and spatially adapts fusion of priors accordingly by coupling the tasks of optimal locally adaptive label fusion and segmentation. This stands in contrast with existing MAS methods [11–13] in that we optimize the fusion of all data priors based on available information (as opposed to criteria derived from additional learning with training data [13] or "labeling unanimity" [11]) so that we can handle local mismatches that may occur in *all* templates due to inherent incompatibility between the diseased and normal images. In summary, unlike existing CC segmentation algorithms, our method 1) performs the segmentation in 3D; 2) requires no tissue segmentation nor training data from diseased-subjects; 3) is more robust to registration errors than existing methods, as we show in our results involving two large MS datasets; and 4) is robust even when a small template set is used, unlike existing methods.

2 Methods

Preliminaries. Let there be a set of N template images with corresponding expert segmentations of the CC. For a given subject image $I : \Omega \subset \mathbb{R}^d \mapsto \mathbb{R}$ which we aim to find the segmentation label field $\mathbf{S}$ of the CC, we register each template image to I and apply the resolved spatial transformation to its corresponding label field, resulting in pairs of template images and corresponding labels, denoted as $\mathcal{T}{=}\{T\}_{n=1}^{N}$ and $\mathcal{S}{=}\{S\}_{n=1}^{N}$ respectively, all approximately[2] aligned to I via spatial transforms $\tau{=}\{\tau\}_{n=1}^{N}$. These can then be used to generate a rough fuzzy segmentation $\hat{S}$ for I in the form of majority voting (MV) [14]; i.e. $\hat{\mathbf{S}}(\mathbf{x}) = \frac{1}{N}\sum_{n=1}^{N} S_n(\mathbf{x})$, followed by thresholding.

In weighted majority voting (WMV), labels of the aligned templates are fused in a locally adaptive manner, where the normalized weight of template T_n at voxel $\mathbf{x}$ may be determined based on a patch-based image similarity measure Θ, i.e.

$$w(\mathbf{x}, n) = \frac{1}{\eta}\Theta(\mathbf{x}; I, T_n), \tag{1}$$

where $\eta{=}\sum_{n=1}^{N}\Theta(\mathbf{x}; I, T_n)$. Spatial regularization on w (e.g. via smoothing as done in [15]) may further be imposed to encourage smoothness of $\hat{\mathbf{S}}$, leading to a more general approach that we denote here as optimized label fusion (OLF). A fuzzy label assignment is then computed as $\Phi(\mathbf{x}){=}\sum_{n=1}^{N} w(\mathbf{x}, n)S_n(\mathbf{x})$, which is then binarized so that the final segmentation is computed as $\hat{\mathbf{S}}(\mathbf{x}){=}1$, if $\Phi(\mathbf{x}) > 0.5$ or $\hat{\mathbf{S}}(\mathbf{x}) = 0$ otherwise.

Rather than calculating w as a post-processing step that is independent of calculating $\mathbf{S}$, or as part of an expectation-maximization framework [11] that alternates between calculations of the two, we herein propose to optimize w *jointly* with $\mathbf{S}$ so that the segmentation process explicitly accounts for registration errors and performs spatially variant prior-selection accordingly. In doing so, we formulate CC segmentation as a graph-labeling task with a *coupled* label set $\mathcal{L}$, consisting of a segmentation label field for I and labels indexing elements of $\mathcal{T}$, i.e. $\mathcal{L}{=}\{0, 1\}\bigcup\mathcal{L}_{corr}$, where $\mathcal{L}_{corr}{=}\{1, 2, \ldots, N\}$ defines a set of labels indexing the n-th template that best corresponds to I at $\mathbf{x}$. As we explain in the next section, by employing the random walker (RW) formulation [16] that generates fuzzy label assignments, we perform segmentation and optimal label fusion simultaneously, with a byproduct of an optimized spatially variant fusion of priors.

Joint Optimal Label Fusion and Segmentation via RW. Coupling the two problems allows us to take the new perspective of viewing all available images simply as an augmented set of information *sources* $\mathcal{I}{:=}\{T_1, \cdots T_N, I\}{=}\ \{\mathcal{I}\}_{k=1}^{K}$, where $K{=}N{+}1$, such that *intrinsic* information from I and *extrinsic* information from T together guide the labeling of I. Furthermore, each source shall be accompanied by a function f_k that outputs an estimate of the class-likelihood given the observations made on that source.

[2] We will examine the impact of registration accuracy on segmentation results in Sec. 3.

In this paper, for the intrinsic source, its corresponding function, f_K, is a naive Bayes classifier [17] while those of the extrinsic sources f_k are given by S_k ($k < K$). With this perspective, our task thus becomes optimizing the fusion of the outputs of f_k that have high confidence in casting label predictions correctly so that we can tune weights on the priors accordingly.

In this work, we propose to quantify the confidence of each source f_k in a spatially adaptive manner via the use of a function $\mathbf{C} : \Omega \mapsto \Delta^K$, where Δ^K refers to a K-dimensional unit simplex. In absence of training data that would allow us to estimate the confidence of each f_k based on some performance criteria (e.g. [13]), we infer confidence by quantifying its strength of belief on the CC class label. As similarly done in [17], for the intrinsic source, we infer confidence of its predictive function f_K by estimating the data-likelihood at $\mathbf{x}$ as:

$$\mathbf{C}_K(\mathbf{x}) = Pr(\mathbf{S}(\mathbf{x}) = 1|I(\mathbf{x})) = \frac{1}{a}\exp\left(\frac{-||I(\mathbf{x}) - \mu||^2}{\sigma^2}\right), \tag{2}$$

where μ and σ respectively represent the mean and standard deviation of the intensity values of the CC estimated using $\hat{\mathbf{S}}$, and a rescales the data-likelihood to [0,1]. For $k < K$, the confidence of f_k that uses extrinsic source T_k depends on how well T_k and I are registered at $\mathbf{x}$ and thus is estimated from information available from the registration results (e.g. quality of alignment as estimated by the regularity of τ_n and/or Θ measured between the registered image pair). Based on preliminary experiments, we found that examining only Θ was sufficient (i.e. required least computation without compromising accuracy). Hence, we estimated the confidence of each f_k ($k < K$) as:

$$\mathbf{C}_k(\mathbf{x}) = \frac{1}{b}\Theta(I(\mathbf{x}), T_k(\mathbf{x})), \tag{3}$$

where $b = \sum_{k=1}^{N} \Theta(I(\mathbf{x}), T_k(\mathbf{x}))$ is a normalization constant and Θ is based on the Modality-Independent Neighbourhood Descriptor (MIND) [18] (with its default parameters) to ensure robustness to variations in image contrast.

Without other *a priori* knowledge, $\mathbf{C}$ may be used directly for fuzzy label assignment (as in WMV noted above), i.e.:

$$\Phi(\mathbf{x}) = \alpha\mathbf{C}_K(\mathbf{x})\mathbf{S}_{init}(\mathbf{x}) + (1-\alpha)\sum_{k=1}^{N}\mathbf{C}_k(\mathbf{x})S_k(\mathbf{x}) \tag{4}$$

where α is a constant governing global preference for intensity-based priors and $\mathbf{S}_{init}(\mathbf{x})$=1 if $\hat{\mathbf{S}}(\mathbf{x}) > 0.5$, or $\mathbf{S}_{init}(\mathbf{x})$=0 otherwise. However, as shown in the literature [11], the desired spatial smoothness of the segmentation is directly influenced by smoothness of the weights. We thus search for a function $\mathbf{W}$ surrogate of $\mathbf{C}$ that is spatially smooth but remains similar to $\mathbf{C}$, thus leading to this energy minimization:

$$\mathbf{W}^* = \arg\min_{\mathbf{W}} \int_\Omega ||\mathbf{W}(\mathbf{x}) - \mathbf{C}(\mathbf{x})||d\mathbf{x} + \beta\sum_{k=1}^{K}\int_\Omega (\nabla\mathbf{W}_k(\mathbf{x}))^T\nabla\mathbf{W}_k(\mathbf{x})d\mathbf{x}, \tag{5}$$

where β is a constant governing the strength of diffusion-based regularization [16]; $\mathbf{W}_k$ and $\mathbf{C}_k$ denote the k-th components of $\mathbf{W}$ and $\mathbf{C}$, respectively.

As presented in [16], we can obtain a unique, globally optimal solution to (5) by adopting a graph-based approach. Specifically, if we let $\mathcal{G}(\mathcal{V}, \mathcal{E})$ be a graph representing the subject image I, where each graph node $p \in \mathcal{V}$ represents a spatial coordinate $\mathbf{x}_p \in \Omega$, and let L be the Laplacian matrix encoding $\mathcal{E}$, then (5) is equivalent [16] to:

$$\mathbf{W}^* = \arg\min_{\mathbf{W}} \sum_{j=1, j \neq k}^{K} \mathbf{W}_k^T \Lambda_j \mathbf{W}_k + (1 - \mathbf{W}_k)^T \Lambda_k (1 - \mathbf{W}_k) + \beta (\mathbf{W}_k)^T L \mathbf{W}_k, \quad (6)$$

where Λ_k is a diagonal matrix with entries $[\mathbf{C}_{1k}, \cdots, \mathbf{C}_{Vk}]$ where $\mathbf{C}_{pk}$ denotes the normalized[3] confidence value of source k as estimated at $\mathbf{x}_p$. In this work, we set the edge weights in same manner as we have done in [19]. The minimum of the energy (6) is obtained when $\mathbf{W}_k$ is the solution to a combinatorial Laplace equation, which can be solved in closed-form as shown in [16]. Once (6) is solved, we compute $\mathbf{S}$ by using (4), with $\mathbf{C}$ now replaced by $\mathbf{W}^*$.

3 Evaluation Results

Materials. Our template set ($\mathcal{T}$) is derived from the publicly available MRI dataset of normal subjects from [20]; this set is hereafter denoted as HAMMERS. Various registration settings were explored for finding the registration solutions (τ); these include affine and deformable registration using free-form-deformation (FFD) and SyN [21], all of which used cross-correlation (CrCo) as the image similarity measure, as well as the method of [22] that computed the image similarity measure based on MIND [18]. Except when varying N to determine its effect, we set N=6 based on experiments in [10], which showed that N=6 using STAPLE yielded high accuracy. Note that minimizing N is advantageous by requiring fewer registrations and thus reducing computations. As our experiments below show, our method is relatively insensitive to the choice of N when compared to other MAS-based methods.

To assess the performance of our method on images acquired from subjects with MS, we further collected T1-weighted brain MRIs originally acquired using different imaging protocols for two independent MS clinical trials. We denote these as MS Dataset1 and MS Dataset2 (sizes of 85 and 187, respectively). Automatic CC segmentation of these MS images is much more challenging due to the reasons highlighted in Sec. 1. In addition, these images were acquired from multiple imaging centers, leading to large intensity and anatomical variations within and across these image sets. The latter is the most challenging of all datasets examined in this paper due to the additional use of contrast agent during image acquisition. In both MS datasets, only 2D segmentations are available. These were manually prepared by a clinical expert using the ITK-SNAP® software, subsequent to 2D midsagittal plane extraction (see [2] for further details).

Experiment I: Effect of combined intensity and spatial priors on accuracy. As conventional baselines, we compared our proposed method with MV and WMV, which do not employ intrinsic information from I, i.e. intensity-based priors. To specifically

[3] $\mathbf{C}$ is normalized to rows with unity sum.

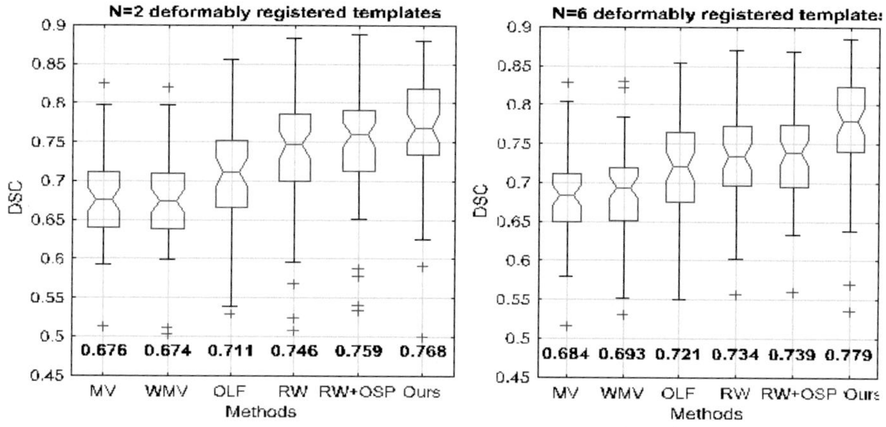

Fig. 1. Accuracy as measured with DSC of various methods compared (bolded numbers indicate the medians of DSC). Note that even for the case when N=2, our method achieved results better than (weighted) majority voting (MV/WMV), optimal label fusion (OLF), and hybrid random walker (RW) with/without optimized spatial priors (OSP).

determine the effect of spatially adaptive, optimized fusion of priors that our proposed method uses, we also tested random walker segmentation [16] using constant weight (α) between the intensity and spatial priors constructed from $\mathcal{T}$ which we denote as RW. For reference, we also examined the case of constructing spatial priors optimized for I where results from OLF were used in RW. We denote this approach as RW with optimized spatial priors (RW+OSP).

Fig. 1 compares the results of segmentation accuracy of each method on a subset of the MS Dataset2 (60 randomly selected images) when evaluated in a leave-one-out cross validation experiment, where we optimized the hyper-parameters for each method by performing a grid-search over $\alpha = \{.1, .3, .4, .5, .6, .7, .9\}$ and $\beta = \{0.01, 0.1, 1\}$. Firstly, from the figure, where accuracy was measured with the Dice coefficient (DSC), we see that optimal label fusion (OLF) achieved better results than both MV and WMV, which supports the use of spatially regularized fusion weights as suggested in the literature [11]. Secondly, we see the advantage of jointly examining both spatial and intensity-based priors in RW, which performed better than MV, WMV, and OLF, which disregard intrinsic information. However, due to registration errors, the constructed spatial priors are not trustworthy everywhere in the image. With our proposed spatially variant prior-selection, our method was able to outperform RW with non-adaptive priors. Note also that because RW+OSP does not perform prior-selection in a spatially adaptive manner, it did not produce an improvement similar to ours.

Experiment II: 3D Validation Using the HAMMERS Dataset [20]. We next validated our method using 14 images in the HAMMERS dataset (exclusive of the aforementioned $N = 6$ randomly chosen template images). Table 1a reports the performance (median of DSC) of our proposed method with respect to MV, WMV, RW+OSP, and STAPLE [10]. We also examined the effects of registration accuracy (and thus the qual-

Table 1. Evaluation on (a) HAMMERS and (b) two MS datasets using N=6 templates aligned by different registration algorithms. MS Dataset2 contains images with contrast agent and thus presents more challenging cases.

(a)	HAMMERS					(b) MS Dataset1				MS Dataset2			
Spatial priors	MV	WMV	STAPLE [10]	RW+OSP	Ours	MV	WMV	STAPLE [10]	Ours	MV	WMV	STAPLE [10]	Ours
Affine+CrCo [21]	.586	.699	.499	.824	**.825**	.708	.719	.710	**.812**	.617	.630	.617	**.658**
Affine/FFD+CrCo [21]	.662	.712	.513	.832	**.837**	.871	.878	.824	**.901**	.689	.690	.614	**.713**
Affine/FFD [22]+MIND	.831	.831	.822	.842	**.865**	.838	.838	.796	**.860**	.729	.729	.702	**.763**
Affine/SyN+CrCo [21]	.740	.733	.556	.833	**.852**	.898	.898	.863	**.926**	.718	.724	.666	**.751**

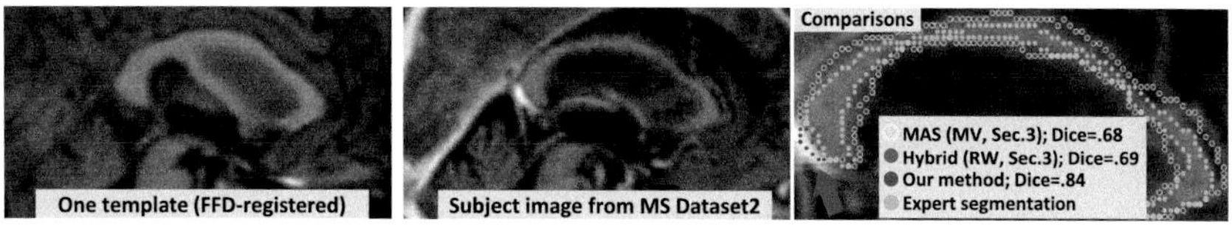

Fig. 2. An example segmentation for an image from the MS Dataset2. As noted by the red arrow in the zoomed-up view (right subfigure), due to local misregistration between the subject and template images (as contrast enhanced vessels in the subject are not visible in any of the templates used), non-adaptive methods cannot segment the noted region accurately. Our hybrid method with optimized spatially adaptive fusion of priors placed greater weights on intensity-based priors in this region, and thus could segment this region properly.

ity of the spatial priors) on segmentation accuracy. As shown in the table, our method achieved the best accuracy regardless of how the templates were registered.

Experiment III: Accuracy Evaluated on two MS-specific Datasets. We also compared our method with several published methods examined in [10] (MW/WMV/STAPLE), using all of the MS images not used in Experiment I. Table 1b summarizes the results. Dataset2 consists of MRIs with contrast agent, so that segmentation of these images was especially challenging (mismatch between the templates and I around the CC periphery occurred more often. As illustrated in Fig. 2, our proposed use of spatially adaptive optimized fusion of priors enables our method to handle these problem regions better than the other methods. Overall, our method achieved the best accuracy in all cases tested. Lastly, performing a comparison to the state-of-art algorithm STEPS [23] using MS Dataset2 showed that our proposed method remains highly competitive: using N=20 atlases randomly selected from the HAMMERS dataset, our method achieved a mean Dice of 0.798, while that of STEPS [23] is 0.775. When N=15, our method still maintained a mean Dice of 0.798, while that of STEPS [23] dropped to 0.751.

4 Conclusions

We introduced a novel framework that performs automatic volumetric CC segmentation in MRIs without the use of disease-specific brain templates. Experiments on 3 datasets show that our method can perform robustly, even in presence of large intensity and morphological variability, thanks to our coupled framework that explicitly accounts for local registration errors and weighs down untrusted spatial priors in a spatially varying manner. For $N \leq 6$, our method took $\approx$5 minutes to solve (6) (as executed on a dual-core 2.4 GHz CPU) in addition to the time needed to register the templates. Future work will involve evaluating the proposed method on other brain structures, including thalamus and putamen, which also have relevance to MS as shown in recent clinical studies.

Acknowledgements. We wish to thank NSERC, Engineers-in-Scrubs of UBC, and the Milan and Maureen Ilich Foundation for partially funding this work.

References

1. Wang, et al.: 3D vs. 2D surface shape analysis of the corpus callosum in premature neonates. In: MICCAI: Workshop on Paediatric and Perinatal Imaging (2012)
2. Kang, et al.: Corpus callosum atrophy in a large SPMS cohort and its correlation with PASAT as a cognitive marker. In: ECTRIMS (2013)
3. Mitchell, et al.: Reliable callosal measurement: population normative data confirm sex-related differences. American Journal of Neuroradiology 24(3), 410–418 (2003)
4. Herron, et al.: Automated measurement of the human corpus callosum using MRI. Frontiers in neuroinformatics 6 (2012)
5. Ardekani, et al.: Multi-atlas corpus callosum segmentation with adaptive atlas selection. In: Proc. Int. Soc. Magn. Reson. Med. Melbourne, Australia, Abstract, vol. 2564 (2012)
6. Adamson, et al.: Software pipeline for midsagittal corpus callosum thickness profile processing. Neuroinformatics, 595–614 (2014)
7. McIntosh, Hamarneh: Medial-based deformable models in nonconvex shape-spaces for medical image segmentation. IEEE Trans. Medical Imaging 31(1), 33–50 (2012)
8. Vachet, et al.: Automatic corpus callosum segmentation using a deformable active Fourier contour model. In: SPIE Medical Imaging, pp. 831707–831707 (2012)
9. Changizi, N., Hamarneh, G., Ishaq, O., Ward, A., Tam, R.: Extraction of the Plane of Minimal Cross-Sectional Area of the Corpus Callosum Using Template-Driven Segmentation. In: Jiang, T., Navab, N., Pluim, J.P.W., Viergever, M.A. (eds.) MICCAI 2010, Part III. LNCS, vol. 6363, pp. 17–24. Springer, Heidelberg (2010)
10. Meyer: Multi-atlas Based Segmentation of Corpus Callosum on MRIs of Multiple Sclerosis Patients. In: Pattern Recognition: 36th German Conference, pp. 729–735 (2014)
11. Wu, et al.: A generative probability model of joint label fusion for multi-atlas based brain segmentation. Medical Image Analysis, 881–890 (2014)
12. Lötjönen, et al.: Fast and robust multi-atlas segmentation of brain magnetic resonance images. NeuroImage, 2352–2365 (2010)
13. Sanroma, et al.: Learning-based atlas selection for multiple-atlas segmentation. In: IEEE CVPR, pp. 3111–3117 (2014)
14. Aljabar, et al.: Multi-atlas based segmentation of brain images: atlas selection and its effect on accuracy. NeuroImage 46, 726–738 (2009)
15. Wang, et al.: Multi-atlas segmentation with joint label fusion. TPAMI, 611–623 (2013)
16. Grady, L.: Multilabel random walker image segmentation using prior models. In: CVPR, vol. 1, pp. 763–770. IEEE (2005)
17. Zhang, Z., Zhu, Q., Xie, Y.: A novel image matting approach based on naive Bayes classifier. In: Huang, D.-S., Jiang, C., Bevilacqua, V., Figueroa, J.C. (eds.) ICIC 2012. LNCS, vol. 7389, pp. 433–441. Springer, Heidelberg (2012)
18. Heinrich, et al.: MIND: Modality independent neighbourhood descriptor for multi-modal deformable registration. Medical Image Analysis 16, 1423–1435 (2012)

19. Tang, L.Y.W., Hamarneh, G.: Random walks with efficient search and contextually adapted image similarity for deformable registration. In: Mori, K., Sakuma, I., Sato, Y., Barillot, C., Navab, N. (eds.) MICCAI 2013, Part II. LNCS, vol. 8150, pp. 43–50. Springer, Heidelberg (2013)
20. Hammers, et al.: Three-dimensional maximum probability atlas of the human brain, with particular reference to the temporal lobe. Human Brain Mapping 19, 224–247 (2003)
21. Avants, et al.: A reproducible evaluation of ANTs similarity metric performance in brain image registration. NeuroImage 52, 2033–2044 (2011)
22. Heinrich, M.P., Jenkinson, M., Brady, S.M., Schnabel, J.A.: Globally optimal deformable registration on a minimum spanning tree using dense displacement sampling. In: Ayache, N., Delingette, H., Golland, P., Mori, K. (eds.) MICCAI 2012, Part III. LNCS, vol. 7512, pp. 115–122. Springer, Heidelberg (2012)
23. Cardoso, et al.: STEPS: Similarity and Truth Estimation for Propagated Segmentations and its application to hippocampal segmentation and brain parcelation. Medical Image Analysis 17(6), 671–684 (2013)

Brain Tissue Segmentation Based on Diffusion MRI Using ℓ_0 Sparse-Group Representation Classification

Pew-Thian Yap[1], Yong Zhang[2], and Dinggang Shen[1]

[1] Department of Radiology and Biomedical Research Imaging Center,
The University of North Carolina at Chapel Hill, USA
[2] Department of Psychiatry and Behavioral Sciences,
Stanford University, USA
ptyap@med.unc.edu

Abstract. We present a method for automated brain tissue segmentation based on diffusion MRI. This provides information that is complementary to structural MRI and facilitates fusion of information between the two imaging modalities. Unlike existing segmentation approaches that are based on diffusion tensor imaging (DTI), our method explicitly models the coexistence of various diffusion compartments within each voxel owing to different tissue types and different fiber orientations. This results in improved segmentation in regions with white matter crossings and in regions susceptible to partial volume effects. For each voxel, we tease apart possible signal contributions from white matter (WM), gray matter (GM), and cerebrospinal fluid (CSF) with the help of diffusion exemplars, which are representative signals associated with each tissue type. Each voxel is then classified by determining which of the WM, GM, or CSF diffusion exemplar groups explains the signal better with the least fitting residual. Fitting is performed using ℓ_0 sparse-group approximation, circumventing various reported limitations of ℓ_1 fitting. In addition, to promote spatial regularity, we introduce a smoothing technique that is based on ℓ_0 gradient minimization, which can be viewed as the ℓ_0 version of total variation (TV) smoothing. Compared with the latter, our smoothing technique, which also incorporates multi-channel WM, GM, and CSF concurrent smoothing, yields marked improvement in preserving boundary contrast and consequently reduces segmentation bias caused by smoothing at tissue boundaries. The results produced by our method are in good agreement with segmentation based on T_1-weighted images.

1 Introduction

Brain tissue segmentation is most commonly performed using T_1-weighted images, which are typically rich with anatomical details thanks to their higher spatial resolution ($1 \times 1 \times 1\,\mathrm{mm}^3$). However, the recent availability of high spatial resolution ($1.25 \times 1.25 \times 1.25\,\mathrm{mm}^3$) diffusion MRI data from the Human Connectome Project[1] begs the following questions: 1) Can tissue segmentation be performed equally well solely based on diffusion data, therefore making it possible to avoid the technical difficulties involved in transferring segmentation information from T_1-weighted images,

[1] http://www.humanconnectome.org/

N. Navab et al. (Eds.): MICCAI 2015, Part III, LNCS 9351, pp. 132–139, 2015.
DOI: 10.1007/978-3-319-24574-4_16

such as geometric distortion and cross-modality registration? 2) Can diffusion data, acquired based on a totally different contrast mechanism, provide information complementary to T_1-weighted images for further improving segmentation?

In this paper, we attempt to address these questions by introducing a segmentation method that works directly with diffusion MRI data. In contrast to existing segmentation methods that are based on diffusion tensor imaging (DTI) [1,8,9], our method explicitly models the coexistence of various diffusion compartments within each voxel owing to different tissue types and different fiber orientations. This improves segmentation in regions with white matter crossings and in regions susceptible to partial volume effects. For each voxel, we tease apart possible signal contributions from white matter (WM), gray matter (GM), and cerebrospinal fluid (CSF) with the help of diffusion exemplars, which are representative signals associated with each tissue type. More specifically, the WM diffusion exemplars are sampled from diffusion tensors oriented in different directions with different axial and radial diffusivities; GM from isotopic tensors of low diffusivities; and CSF from isotropic tensors of high diffusivities. Each voxel is then classified by determining which of the WM, GM, or CSF diffusion exemplars explain the signal better with the least fitting residual.

Fitting is performed using ℓ_0 sparse-group approximation, circumventing various reported limitations of ℓ_1 fitting. The use of ℓ_0 penalization is motivated by the observations reported in [5], where the authors have shown that the commonly used ℓ_1-norm penalization [11,18] conflicts with the unit sum requirement of the volume fractions and hence results in suboptimal solutions. To overcome this problem, the authors propose to employ the reweighted ℓ_1 minimization approached described by Candès et al. [4] to obtain solutions with enhanced sparsity, approximating solutions given by ℓ_0 minimization. However, despite giving improved results, this approach is still reliant on the suboptimal solution of the unweighted ℓ_1 minimization problem that has to be solved in the first iteration of the reweighted minimization scheme. In the current work, we will employ an algorithm that is based directly on ℓ_0 minimization.

To promote spatial regularity, we introduce a smoothing technique that is based on ℓ_0 gradient minimization [16]. This can be viewed as the ℓ_0 version of total variation (TV) smoothing. Compared with the latter, our smoothing technique yields marked improvement in the preservation of boundary contrast. In addition, our method smooths the probability maps of WM, GM, and CSF concurrently. This is achieved by an ℓ_0 adaptation of a multi-channel smoothing algorithm [17], solved using alternating direction method of multipliers (ADMM) [14].

2 Approach

Our approach to tissue segmentation is inspired by the face recognition work of Wright et al. [15]. However, instead of the ℓ_1 sparse approximation used in [15], we use a sparse-group ℓ_0 minimization approach that circumvents the problems mentioned in [5]. To promote spatial regularity, we also propose a multi-channel gradient minimization algorithm for smoothing of the tissue probability maps, producing edge-preserving effect better than smoothing based on TV regularization [12].

Linear Subspaces: We assume that the signal from each class of tissue lies in a linear subspace. The subspace is spanned by diffusion exemplars, which are hypothetical signal vectors generated using the tensor model, $S(b, \hat{\mathbf{g}}) = S_0 \exp(-b\hat{\mathbf{g}}^{\mathrm{T}}\mathbf{D}\hat{\mathbf{g}})$, with varying diffusion parameters. Here, $\hat{\mathbf{g}}$ is a unit vector representing the gradient direction, S_0 is the baseline signal with no diffusion weighting, and $\mathbf{D}$ is the diffusion tensor. The WM subspace is spanned by multiple groups of diffusion exemplars. Each WM diffusion exemplar group consists of signal vectors sampled from a set of unidirectional axial-symmetric diffusion tensor models with a range of typical axial and radial diffusivities. Multiple groups of WM diffusion exemplars are generated by tensors with principal directions uniformly covering the unit sphere. The GM and CSF diffusion exemplar groups consist of signal vectors sampled from isotropic tensors with GM diffusivities set lower than CSF diffusivities, consistent with what was reported in [7,9]. For each class $c \in \mathcal{C} = \{\text{WM}, \text{GM}, \text{CSF}\}$, we arrange the n_c signal vectors of the diffusion exemplars as columns of a matrix $\mathbf{A}_c = [\mathbf{s}_{c,1}, \mathbf{s}_{c,2}, \ldots, \mathbf{s}_{c,n_c}]$. We then concatenate the exemplar matrices of all tissue classes into a matrix $\mathbf{A} = [\mathbf{A}_{\text{WM}}|\mathbf{A}_{\text{GM}}|\mathbf{A}_{\text{CSF}}]$, where $\mathbf{A}_{\text{WM}} = \left[\mathbf{A}_{\text{WM}_1}|\ldots|\mathbf{A}_{\text{WM}_k}|\ldots|\mathbf{A}_{\text{WM}_{N_{\text{WM}}}}\right]$ and each numerical subscript k of the WM exemplar matrix $\mathbf{A}_{\text{WM}_k}$ denotes the index corresponding to a WM direction.

ℓ_0 Sparse-Group Representation: Given the signal vector s of a voxel that we wish to classify, we first compute its sparse-representation coefficient vector **f** by solving the follow ℓ_0 sparse-group approximation problem:

$$\min_{\mathbf{f}\geq 0} \left\{ \phi(\mathbf{f}) = \|\mathbf{A}\mathbf{f} - \mathbf{s}\|_2^2 + \gamma \left[\alpha\|\mathbf{f}\|_0 + (1-\alpha) \sum_{g\in\mathcal{G}} \mathcal{I}(\|\mathbf{f}_g\|_2) \right] \right\}, \tag{1}$$

where $\mathcal{I}(z)$ is an indicator function returning 1 if $z \neq 0$ or 0 if otherwise. The ℓ_0-"norm" gives the cardinality of the support, i.e., $\|\mathbf{f}\|_0 = |\mathtt{supp}(\mathbf{f})| = |\{k : f_k \neq 0\}|$. Parameters $\alpha \in [0, 1]$ and $\gamma > 0$ are for penalty tuning, analogous to those used in the sparse-group LASSO [13]. Note that $\alpha = 1$ gives the ℓ_0 fit, whereas $\alpha = 0$ gives the group ℓ_0 fit. $\mathbf{f}_g$ denotes the subvector containing the elements associated with group $g \in \mathcal{G} = \{\text{WM}_1, \ldots, \text{WM}_{N_{\text{WM}}}, \text{GM}, \text{CSF}\}$. We solve this problem using an algorithm called non-monotone iterative hard thresholding (NIHT) [19], inspired by [2,10]. Proof of convergence can be obtained by modifying the results shown in [10].

Tissue Classification: Each voxel is classified as the class with diffusion exemplars that best explain the signal. This is achieved, based on [15], by determining the class that gives the least reconstruction residual:

$$\min_{c} \{r(\mathbf{s}|c) = \|\mathbf{A}\boldsymbol{\delta}_c(\mathbf{f}) - \mathbf{s}\|_2\}, \tag{2}$$

where $\boldsymbol{\delta}_c(\mathbf{f})$ is a new vector whose only nonzero entries are the entries in **f** that are associated with class c. We modify the above problem to become a maximum a posteriori (MAP) estimation problem:

$$\max_{c} \{p(c|\mathbf{s}) \propto p(\mathbf{s}|c)p(c)\}, \tag{3}$$

where $p(c)$ is the prior probability and $p(\mathbf{s}|c)$ is the likelihood function defined as

$$p(\mathbf{s}|c) = \frac{1}{\sigma_c\sqrt{2\pi}} \exp\left[-\frac{r^2(\mathbf{s}|c)}{2\sigma_c^2}\right]. \tag{4}$$

The scale σ can be determined from the data via $\sigma_c^2 = \frac{1}{|\Omega_c|}\sum_{i\in\Omega_c} r^2(\mathbf{s}_i|c)$, where $\Omega_c \subset \Omega = \{1,\ldots,N\}$ is the subset of indices of voxels with class c giving the least residuals. N is total number of voxels. This alternative formulation allows us to visualize the posterior probability maps $\{p(c|\mathbf{s}_i)|i \in \Omega, c \in \mathcal{C}\}$ (disregarding constant scaling) for qualitative assessment of tissue segmentation. The prior probabilities can be set according to a pre-computed probabilistic atlas for guided segmentation.

Multi-Channel Gradient Minimization: Tissue classification as discussed in the previous section can be improved in terms of robustness by imposing spatial regularity. To achieve this, we smooth the posterior probability maps of WM, GM, and CSF concurrently prior to MAP estimation. In contrast to the commonly used TV-regularized smoothing, which is essentially an ℓ_1 gradient minimization (L1-GM) algorithm, we will use here ℓ_0 gradient minimization (L0-GM), which has been shown in [16] to be more effective than L1-GM in preserving edges. Moreover, L0-GM is more suitable in our case due to the piecewise constant nature of the segmentation maps. Here, we describe a multi-channel version of L0-GM.

We first define for the i-th voxel a probability vector $\mathbf{p}_i \equiv \mathbf{p}(\mathbf{s}_i) = [p(\text{WM}|\mathbf{s}_i), p(\text{GM}|\mathbf{s}_i), p(\text{CSF}|\mathbf{s}_i)]^{\mathrm{T}}$. We then solve for a smoothed version of the probability map $\{\mathbf{p}_i \in \mathbb{R}^{|\mathcal{C}|}, i \in \Omega\}$, i.e., $\mathbf{u} = \{\mathbf{u}_i \in \mathbb{R}^{|\mathcal{C}|}, i \in \Omega\}$ via the following problem:

$$\min_{\mathbf{u}} \left\{ \psi(\mathbf{u}) = \sum_i \|\mathbf{u}_i - \mathbf{p}_i\|_2^2 + \beta \sum_i \left\| \sqrt{\sum_d \|D_{i,d}\mathbf{u}\|_2^2} \right\|_0 \right\}. \tag{5}$$

We let $D_{i,d}\mathbf{u} \in \mathbb{R}^{1\times|\mathcal{C}|}$, where $\mathbf{u} \in \mathbb{R}^{N\times|\mathcal{C}|}$, be a row vector concatenating the finite difference values of all channels of $\mathbf{u}$ in the d-th spatial dimension. Note that $D_{i,d} \in \mathbb{R}^{1\times N}$ is the finite difference matrix. The first term in (5) maintains data fidelity and the second term penalizes small edges in a multi-channel image. If we replace the ℓ_0-"norm" in the second term with ℓ_1-norm, the above problem become a TV-regularized smoothing problem. Note that the above optimization problem is known to be computationally intractable. We thus implement an approximate solution using ADMM [3] by introducing a number of auxiliary variables. The ADMM formulation amounts to repeatedly performing hard thresholding and spatial convolution/deconvolution [14].

3 Experiments

3.1 Data

Diffusion weighted (DW) datasets from the Human Connectome Project (HCP) [6] were used. DW images with $1.25 \times 1.25 \times 1.25\,\text{mm}^3$ resolution were acquired with diffusion weightings $b = 1000$, 2000, and $3000\,\text{s/mm}^2$, each applied in 90 directions.

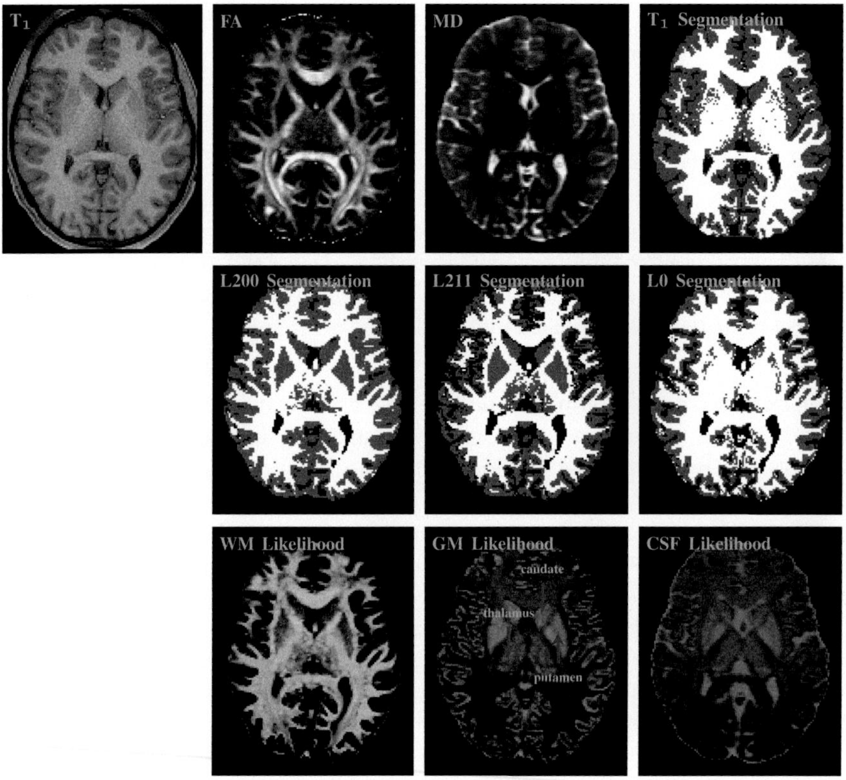

Fig. 1. (Top) T_1-weighted, fractional anisotropy (FA), mean diffusivity (MD), and T_1 segmentation images. **(Middle)** Segmentation maps given by L200 (proposed), L211, and L0. **(Bottom)** Likelihood maps for WM, GM, and CSF given by L200.

18 baseline images with low diffusion weighting $b = 5\,\mathrm{s/mm^2}$ were also acquired. The DW datasets were acquired with reversed phase encoding to correct for EPI distortion. T_1-weighted anatomical images were acquired as anatomical references.

3.2 Diffusion Parameters

The parameters of the tensors used to generate the diffusion exemplars were set to cover the typical values of the diffusivities of the WM, GM, and CSF voxels in the above dataset: $\lambda_{\|}^{\mathrm{WM}} = 1 \times 10^{-3}\,\mathrm{mm}^2/s$, $\lambda_{\perp}^{\mathrm{WM}} = [0.1 : 0.1 : 0.3] \times 10^{-3}\,\mathrm{mm}^2/s$, $\lambda^{\mathrm{GM}} = [0.00 : 0.01 : 0.80] \times 10^{-3}\,\mathrm{mm}^2/s$, and $\lambda^{\mathrm{CSF}} = [1.0 : 0.1 : 3.0] \times 10^{-3}\,\mathrm{mm}^2/s$. The notation $[a : s : b]$ denotes values from a to b, inclusive, with step s. Note that in practice, these ranges do not have to be exact but should however cover possible parameter values. The direction of each group of the WM diffusion exemplars corresponds to one of the 321 points evenly distributed on a hemisphere, generated by the subdivision of the faces of an icosahedron three times.

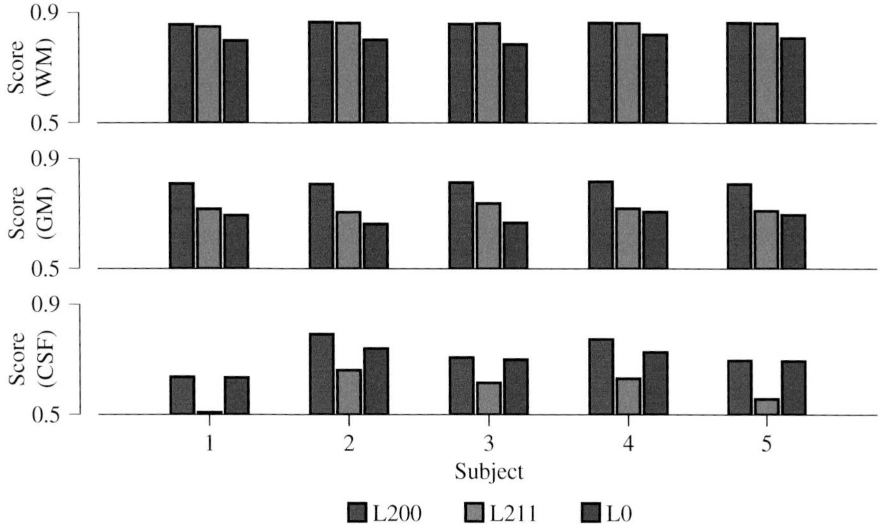

Fig. 2. Accuracy of segmentation outcomes evaluated based on Dice score using T_1 segmentations as the ground truth.

3.3 Comparison Methods

We compared the proposed method (**L200**) with the following methods:

- **L211**: Sparse-group LASSO [13] using diffusion exemplars identical to the proposed method. Similar to [5] and according to [4], we executed sparse-group LASSO multiple times, each time reweighing the ℓ_{21}-norm and the ℓ_1-norm so they eventually approximate their ℓ_0 counterparts.
- **L0**: ℓ_0 minimization using a single diffusion exemplar each for WM, GM, and CSF [7]. Similar to [7], WM-GM-CSF segmentation was used to help determine the parameters for the diffusion exemplars. The axial and radial diffusivities of the WM diffusion exemplars were determined based on WM voxels with fractional anisotropy (FA) greater than 0.7. The diffusivity of the isotropic GM/CSF diffusion exemplar was determined based on GM/CSF voxels with FA less than 0.2.

The tuning parameter γ was set to 1×10^{-4} for all methods. In addition, we set $\alpha = 0.05$, $\beta = 0.001$, $p(\text{WM}) = 0.35$, $p(\text{GM}) = 0.50$, and $p(\text{CSF}) = 0.15$ for the proposed method.

3.4 Results

Qualitative: Figure 1 indicates that the segmentation result of the proposed method, L200, resembles very closely to that produced using the T_1-weighted image with the FSL FAST algorithm [20]. L211 produces WM segmentation result that is similar to L200, but underestimates GM. Note that these two methods are able to separate the deep GM structures, such as caudate and putamen, from the surrounding WM. The segmentation of the thalamus is more challenging because it is a mixture of GM and WM (see likelihood maps in the bottom row of Fig. 1).

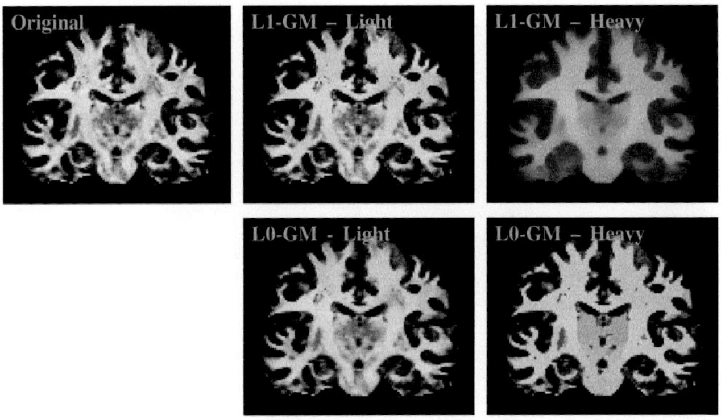

Fig. 3. Effects of light and heavy smoothing using L1-GM and L0-GM. The WM, GM, CSF posterior probability maps are smoothed concurrently. However, due to space limitation, only the WM probability maps are shown here.

Quantitative: Figure 2 shows the Dice scores for WM-GM-CSF segmentation of 5 subjects from the HCP data repository, confirming again that the proposed method produces segmentation results that agree most with segmentation based on T_1-weighted images. The average Dice scores for L200/L211/L0 are 0.8603/0.8581/0.8019 (WM), 0.8105/0.7177/0.6844 (GM), and 0.7204/0.5941/0.6985 (CSF).

Smoothing: Figure 3 shows the effects of smoothing with different strengths using L1-GM and L0-GM. The results confirm that despite the increased smoothing strength, L0-GM can still preserve edges effectively. On the other hand, L1-GM blurs the edges when the smoothing strength is increased.

4 Conclusion

In this paper, we have presented a tissue segmentation method that works directly with diffusion MRI data. We demonstrated that the proposed method is able to produce segmentation results that are in good agreement with the more conventional T_1-based segmentation. We also showed that diffusion MRI provides additional information for segmentation of deep gray matter structures, complementary to T_1-weighted imaging, where image contrast in this region is typically low. Future research will be directed to further improving the segmentation of deep gray matter.

Acknowledgment. This work was supported in part by a UNC BRIC-Radiology start-up fund and NIH grants (EB006733, EB009634, AG041721, MH100217, AA010723, and 1UL1TR001111).

References

1. Awate, S.P., Zhang, H., Simon, T.J., Gee, J.C.: Multivariate segmentation of brain tissues by fusion of MRI and DTI data. In: IEEE International Symposium on Biomedical Imaging (ISBI), pp. 213–216 (2008)

2. Blumensath, T., Davies, M.E.: Iterative thresholding for sparse approximations. Journal of Fourier Analysis and Applications 14(5-6), 629–654 (2008)
3. Boyd, S., Parikh, N., Chu, E., Peleato, B., Eckstein, J.: Distributed optimization and statistical learning via the alternating direction method of multipliers. Foundations and Trend in Machine Learning 3(1), 1–122 (2010)
4. Candès, E.J., Wakin, M.B., Boyd, S.P.: Enhancing sparsity by reweighted ℓ_1 minimization. Journal of Fourier Analysis and Applications 14(5), 877–905 (2008)
5. Daducci, A., Ville, D.V.D., Thiran, J.P., Wiaux, Y.: Sparse regularization for fiber ODF reconstruction: From the suboptimality of ℓ_2 and ℓ_1 priors to ℓ_0. Medical Image Analysis 18, 820–833 (2014)
6. Essen, D.C.V., Smith, S.M., Barch, D.M., Behrens, T.E., Yacoub, E., Ugurbil, K.: The WU-Minn human connectome project: An overview. NeuroImage 80, 62–79 (2013)
7. Jeurissen, B., Tournier, J.D., Dhollander, T., Connelly, A., Sijbers, J.: Multi-tissue constrained spherical deconvolution for improved analysis of multi-shell diffusion MRI data. NeuroImage (2014)
8. Lenglet, C., Rousson, M., Deriche, R.: A statistical framework for DTI segmentation. In: International Symposium on Biomedical Imaging, pp. 794–797 (April 2006)
9. Liu, T., Li, H., Wong, K., Tarok, A., Guo, L., Wong, S.T.: Brain tissue segmentation based on DTI data. NeuroImage 38(1), 114–123 (2007)
10. Lu, Z.: Iterative hard thresholding methods for ℓ_0 regularized convex cone programming. Mathematical Programming, 1–30 (2013)
11. Ramirez-Manzanares, A., Rivera, M., Vemuri, B.C., Carney, P., Mareci, T.: Diffusion basis functions decomposition for estimating white matter intra-voxel fiber geometry. IEEE Transactions on Medical Imaging 26(8), 1091–1102 (2007)
12. Rudin, L.I., Osher, S., Fatemi, E.: Nonlinear total variation based noise removal algorithms. Physica D 60, 259–268 (1992)
13. Simon, N., Friedman, J., Hastie, T., Tibshirani, R.: A sparse-group lasso. Journal of Computational and Graphical Statistics 22(2), 231–245 (2013)
14. Tao, M., Yang, J.: Alternating direction algorithms for total variation deconvolution in image reconstruction. Tech. rep., Department of Mathematics, Nanjing University (2009)
15. Wright, J., Yang, A.Y., Ganesh, A., Sastry, S.S., Ma, Y.: Robust face recognition via sparse representation. IEEE Transactions on Pattern Analysis and Machine Intelligence 31(2), 1–18 (2009)
16. Xu, L., Lu, C., Xu, Y., Jia, J.: Image smoothing via ℓ_0 gradient minimization. ACM Transactions on Graphics 30(5) (2011)
17. Yang, J., Yin, W., Zhang, Y., Wang, Y.: A fast algorithm for edge-preserving variational multichannel image restoration. SIAM Journal on Imaging Sciences 2(2), 569–592 (2009)
18. Yap, P.T., Shen, D.: Spatial transformation of DWI data using non-negative sparse representation. IEEE Transactions on Medical Imaging 31(11), 2035–2049 (2012)
19. Yap, P.T., Zhang, Y., Shen, D.: Diffusion compartmentalization using response function groups with cardinality penalization. In: A. Frangi et al. (eds.) MICCAI 2015, Part I, LNCS 9349, pp. 183–190. Springer, Heidelberg (2013)
20. Zhang, Y., Brady, M., Smith, S.: Segmentation of brain MR images through a hidden Markov random field model and the expectation-maximization algorithm. IEEE Transactions on Medical Imaging 20(1), 45–57 (2001)

A Latent Source Model for Patch-Based Image Segmentation

George H. Chen, Devavrat Shah, and Polina Golland

Massachusetts Institute of Technology, Cambridge MA 02139, USA

Abstract. Despite the popularity and empirical success of patch-based nearest-neighbor and weighted majority voting approaches to medical image segmentation, there has been no theoretical development on when, why, and how well these nonparametric methods work. We bridge this gap by providing a theoretical performance guarantee for nearest-neighbor and weighted majority voting segmentation under a new probabilistic model for patch-based image segmentation. Our analysis relies on a new local property for how similar nearby patches are, and fuses existing lines of work on modeling natural imagery patches and theory for nonparametric classification. We use the model to derive a new patch-based segmentation algorithm that iterates between inferring local label patches and merging these local segmentations to produce a globally consistent image segmentation. Many existing patch-based algorithms arise as special cases of the new algorithm.

1 Introduction

Nearest-neighbor and weighted majority voting methods have been widely used in medical image segmentation, originally at the pixel or voxel level [11] and more recently for image patches [2,6,10,12]. Perhaps the primary reason for the popularity of these nonparametric methods is that standard label fusion techniques for image segmentation require robust nonrigid registration whereas patch-based methods sidestep nonrigid image alignment altogether. Thus, patch-based approaches provide a promising alternative to registration-based methods for problems that present alignment challenges, as in the case of whole body scans or other applications characterized by large anatomical variability.

A second reason for patch-based methods' growing popularity lies in their efficiency of computation: fast approximate nearest-neighbor search algorithms, tailored for patches [3] and for high-dimensional spaces more generally (e.g., [1,9]), can rapidly find similar patches, and can readily parallelize across search queries. For problems where the end goal is segmentation or a decision based on segmentation, solving numerous nonrigid registration subproblems required for standard label fusion could be a computationally expensive detour that, even if successful, might not produce better solutions than a patch-based approach.

Many patch-based image segmentation methods can be viewed as variations of the following simple algorithm. To determine whether a pixel in the new image should be foreground (part of the object of interest) or background, we consider

N. Navab et al. (Eds.): MICCAI 2015, Part III, LNCS 9351, pp. 140–148, 2015.
DOI: 10.1007/978-3-319-24574-4_17

the patch centered at that pixel. We compare this image patch to patches in a training database, where each training patch is labeled either foreground or background depending on the pixel at the center of the training patch. We transfer the label from the closest patch in the training database to the pixel of interest in the new image. A plethora of embellishments improve this algorithm, such as, but not limited to, using K nearest neighbors or weighted majority voting instead of only the nearest neighbor [6,10,12], incorporating hand-engineered or learned feature descriptors [12], cleverly choosing the shape of a patch [12], and enforcing consistency among adjacent pixels by assigning each training intensity image patch to a label patch rather than a single label [10,12], or by employing a Markov random field [7].

Despite the broad popularity and success of nonparametric patch-based image segmentation and the smorgasbord of tricks to enhance its performance, the existing work has been empirical with no theoretical justification for when and why such methods should work and, if so, how well and with how much training data. In this paper, we bridge this gap between theory and practice for nonparametric patch-based image segmentation algorithms. We propose a probabilistic model for image segmentation that draws from recent work on modeling natural imagery patches [13,14]. We begin in Section 2 with a simple case of our model that corresponds to inferring each pixel's label separately from other pixels. For this special case of so-called pointwise segmentation, we provide a theoretical performance guarantee for patch-based nearest-neighbor and weighted majority voting segmentation in terms of the available training data. Our analysis borrows from existing theory on nonparametric time series classification [5] and crucially relies on a new structural property on neighboring patches being sufficiently similar. We present our full model in Section 3 and derive a new iterative patch-based image segmentation algorithm that combines ideas from patch-based image restoration [13] and distributed optimization [4]. This algorithm alternates between inferring label patches separately and merging these local estimates to form a globally consistent segmentation. We show how various existing patch-based algorithms are special cases of this new algorithm.

2 Pointwise Segmentation and a Theoretical Guarantee

For an image A, we use $A(i)$ to denote the value of image A at pixel i, and $A[i]$ to denote the patch of image A centered at pixel i based on a pre-specified patch shape; $A[i]$ can include feature descriptors in addition to raw intensity values. Each pixel i belongs to a finite, uniformly sampled lattice $\mathcal{I}$.

Model. Given an intensity image Y, we infer its label image L that delineates an object of interest in Y. In particular, for each pixel $i \in \mathcal{I}$, we infer label $L(i) \in \{+1, -1\}$, where $+1$ corresponds to foreground (object of interest) and -1 to background. We make this inference using patches of image Y, each patch of dimensionality d (e.g., for 2D images and 5-by-5 patches, $d = 5^2 = 25$). We model the joint distribution $p(L(i), Y[i])$ of label $L(i)$ and image patch $Y[i]$ as a generalization of a Gaussian mixture model (GMM) with diagonal covariances, where each mixture component corresponds to either $L(i) = +1$ or $L(i) = -1$. We define this generalization, called a *diagonal sub-Gaussian mixture model*, shortly.

First, we provide a concrete example where label $L(i)$ and patch $Y[i]$ are related through a GMM with $\mathcal{C}_i$ mixture components. Mixture component $c \in \{1, \ldots, \mathcal{C}_i\}$ occurs with probability $\rho_{ic} \in [0, 1]$ and has mean vector $\mu_{ic} \in \mathbb{R}^d$ and label $\lambda_{ic} \in \{+1, -1\}$. In this example, we assume that all covariance matrices are $\sigma^2 \mathbf{I}_{d\times d}$, and that there exists constant $\rho_{\min} > 0$ such that $\rho_{ic} \geq \rho_{\min}$ for all i, c. Thus, image patch $Y[i]$ belongs to mixture component c with probability ρ_{ic}, in which case $Y[i] = \mu_{ic} + W_i$, where vector $W_i \in \mathbb{R}^d$ consists of white Gaussian noise with variance σ^2, and $L(i) = \lambda_{ic}$. Formally,

$$p(L(i), Y[i]) = \sum_{c=1}^{\mathcal{C}_i} \rho_{ic} \mathcal{N}(Y[i]; \mu_{ic}, \sigma^2 \mathbf{I}_{d\times d}) \delta(L(i) = \lambda_{ic}),$$

where $\mathcal{N}(\cdot; \mu, \Sigma)$ is a Gaussian density with mean μ and covariance Σ, and $\delta(\cdot)$ is the indicator function.

The *diagonal sub-Gaussian mixture model* refers to a generalization where noise vector W_i consists of zero-mean i.i.d. random entries whose distribution has tails that decay at least as fast as that of a Gaussian random variable. Formally, a zero-mean random variable X is sub-Gaussian with parameter σ if its moment generating function $\mathbb{E}[e^{sX}]$ satisfies $\mathbb{E}[e^{sX}] \leq e^{s^2\sigma^2/2}$ for all $s \in \mathbb{R}$. Examples of such random variables include $\mathcal{N}(0, \sigma^2)$ and Uniform$[-\sigma, \sigma]$.

Every pixel is associated with its own diagonal sub-Gaussian mixture model whose parameters $(\rho_{ic}, \mu_{ic}, \lambda_{ic})$ for $c = 1, \ldots, \mathcal{C}_i$ are fixed but unknown. Similar to recent work on modeling generic natural image patches [13,14], we do not model how different overlapping patches behave jointly and instead only model how each individual patch, viewed alone, behaves. We suspect that medical image patches have even more structure than generic natural image patches, which are very accurately modeled by a GMM [14].

Rather than learning the mixture model components, we instead take a nonparametric approach, using available training data in nearest-neighbor or weighted majority voting schemes to infer label $L(i)$ from image patch $Y[i]$. To this end, we assume we have access to n i.i.d. training intensity-label *image* pairs $(Y_1, L_1), \ldots, (Y_n, L_n)$ that obey our probabilistic model above.

Inference. We consider two simple segmentation methods that operate on each pixel i separately, inferring label $L(i)$ only based on image patch $Y[i]$.

Pointwise nearest-neighbor segmentation first finds which training intensity image Y_u has a patch centered at pixel j that is closest to observed patch $Y[i]$. This amounts to solving $(\widehat{u}, \widehat{j}) = \text{argmin}_{u\in\{1,2,\ldots,n\}, j\in N(i)} \|Y_u[j] - Y[i]\|^2$, where $\|\cdot\|$ denotes Euclidean norm, and $N(i)$ refers to a user-specified finite set of pixels that are neighbors of pixel i. Label $L(i)$ is estimated to be $L_{\widehat{u}}(\widehat{j})$.

Pointwise weighted majority voting segmentation first computes the following weighted votes for labels $\ell \in \{+1, -1\}$:

$$V_\ell(i|Y[i];\theta) \triangleq \sum_{u=1}^{n} \sum_{j \in N(i)} \exp\big(-\theta\|Y_u[j] - Y[i]\|^2\big)\delta(L_u(j) = \ell),$$

where θ is a scale parameter, and $N(i)$ again refers to user-specified neighboring pixels of pixel i. Label $L(i)$ is estimated to be the label ℓ with the higher vote $V_\ell(i|Y[i];\theta)$. Pointwise nearest-neighbor segmentation can be viewed as this weighted voting with $\theta \to \infty$. Pointwise weighted majority voting has been used extensively for patch-based segmentation [2,6,10,12], where we note that our formulation readily allows for one to choose which training image patches are considered neighbors, what the patch shape is, and whether feature descriptors are part of the intensity patch vector $Y[i]$.

Theoretical Guarantee. The model above allows nearby pixels to be associated with dramatically different mixture models. However, real images are "smooth" with patches centered at two adjacent pixels likely similar. We incorporate this smoothness via a structural property on the sub-Gaussian mixture model parameters associated with nearby pixels. We refer to this property as the *jigsaw condition*, which holds if for every mixture component $(\rho_{ic}, \mu_{ic}, \lambda_{ic})$ of the diagonal sub-Gaussian mixture model associated with pixel i, there exists a neighbor $j \in N^*(i)$ such that the diagonal sub-Gaussian mixture model associated with pixel j also has a mixture component with mean μ_{ic}, label λ_{ic}, and mixture weight at least $\rho_{\min}$; this weight need not be equal to ρ_{ic}. The shape and size of neighborhood $N^*(i)$, which is fixed and unknown, control how similar the mixture models are across image pixels. Note that $N^*(i)$ affects how far from pixel i we should look for training patches, i.e., how to choose neighborhood $N(i)$ in pointwise nearest-neighbor and weighted majority voting segmentation, where ideally $N(i) = N^*(i)$.

Separation gap. Our theoretical result also depends on the separation "gap" between training intensity image patches that correspond to the two different labels:

$$\mathcal{G} \triangleq \min_{\substack{u,v \in \{1,\ldots,n\}, \\ i \in \mathcal{I}, j \in N(i) \text{ s.t. } L_u(i) \neq L_v(j)}} \|Y_u[i] - Y_v[j]\|^2.$$

Intuitively, a small separation gap corresponds to the case of two training intensity image patches that are very similar but one corresponds to foreground and the other to background. In this case, a nearest-neighbor approach may easily select a patch with the wrong label, resulting in an error.

We now state our main theoretical guarantee. The proof is left to the supplementary material and builds on existing time series classification analysis [5].

Theorem 1. *Under the model above with n training intensity-label image pairs and provided that the jigsaw condition holds with neighborhood N^*, pointwise nearest-neighbor and weighted majority voting segmentation (with user-specified* *neighborhood N satisfying $N(i) \supseteq N^*(i)$ for every pixel i and with parameter $\theta = \frac{1}{8\sigma^2}$ for weighted majority voting) achieve expected pixel labeling error rate*

$$\mathbb{E}\Big[\frac{1}{|\mathcal{I}|}\sum_{i\in\mathcal{I}}\delta(\textit{mislabel pixel } i)\Big] \le |\mathcal{I}|\mathcal{C}_{\max}\exp\Big(-\frac{n\rho_{\min}}{8}\Big) + |N|n\exp\Big(-\frac{\mathcal{G}}{16\sigma^2}\Big),$$

where $\mathcal{C}_{\max}$ is the maximum number of mixture components of any diagonal sub-Gaussian mixture model associated with a pixel, and $|N|$ is the largest user-specified neighborhood of any pixel.

To interpret this theorem, we consider sufficient conditions for each term on the right-hand side bound to be at most $\varepsilon/2$ for $\varepsilon \in (0,1)$. For the first term, the number of training intensity-label image pairs n should be sufficiently large so that we see all the different mixture model components in our training data: $n \ge \frac{8}{\rho_{\min}}\log(2|\mathcal{I}|\mathcal{C}_{\max}/\varepsilon)$. For the second term, the gap $\mathcal{G}$ should be sufficiently large so that the nearest training intensity image patch found does not produce a segmentation error: $\mathcal{G} \ge 16\sigma^2\log(2|N|n/\varepsilon)$. There are different ways to change the gap, such as changing the patch shape and including hand-engineered or learned patch features. Intuitively, using larger patches d should widen the gap, but using larger patches also means that the maximum number of mixture components $\mathcal{C}_{\max}$ needed to represent a patch increases, possibly quite dramatically.

The dependence on n in the second term results from a worst-case analysis. To keep the gap from having to grow as $\log(n)$, we could subsample the training data so that n is large enough to capture the diversity of mixture model components yet not so large that it overcomes the gap. In particular, treating $\mathcal{C}_{\max}$, σ^2, and $\rho_{\min}$ as constants that depend on the application of interest and could potentially be estimated from data, collecting $n = \Theta(\log(|\mathcal{I}|/\varepsilon))$ training image pairs and with a gap $\mathcal{G} = \Omega\big(\log((|N|\log|\mathcal{I}|)/\varepsilon)\big)$, both algorithms achieve an expected error rate of at most ε. The intuition is that as n grows large, if we continue to consider all training subjects, even those that look very different from the new subject, we are bound to get unlucky (due to noise in intensity images) and, in the worst case, encounter a training image patch that is close to a test image patch but has the wrong label. Effectively, outliers in training data muddle nearest-neighbor inference, and more training data means possibly more outliers.

3 Multipoint Segmentation

Model. We generalize the basic model to infer label patches $L[i]$ rather than just a single pixel's label $L(i)$. Every label patch $L[i]$ is assumed to have dimensionality d', where d and d' need not be equal. For example, for 2D images, $Y[i]$ could be a 5-by-5 patch ($d = 25$) whereas $L[i]$ could be a 3-by-3 patch ($d' = 9$). When $d' > 1$, estimated label patches must be merged to arrive at a globally consistent estimate of label image L. This case is referred to as multipoint segmentation.

In this general case, we assume there to be k latent label images $\Lambda_1,\dots,\Lambda_k$ that occur with probabilities $\pi_1,\dots,\pi_k$. To generate intensity image Y, we first sample label image $\Lambda \in \{\Lambda_1,\dots,\Lambda_k\}$ according to probabilities $\pi_1,\dots,\pi_k$. Then we sample label image L to be a perturbed version of Λ such that $p(L|\Lambda) \propto \exp(-\alpha \mathbf{d}(L, \Lambda))$ for some constant $\alpha \geq 0$ and differentiable "distance" function $\mathbf{d}(\cdot, \cdot)$. For example, $\mathbf{d}(L, \Lambda)$ could relate to volume overlap between the segmentations represented by label images L and Λ with perfect overlap yielding distance 0. Finally, intensity image Y is generated so that for each pixel $i \in \mathcal{I}$, patch $Y[i]$ is a sample from a mixture model patch prior $p(Y[i]|L[i])$. If $\alpha = 0$, $d' = 1$, and the mixture model is diagonal sub-Gaussian, we get our earlier model.

We refer to this formulation as a *latent source model* since the intensity image patches could be thought of as generated from the latent "canonical" label images $\Lambda_1, \ldots, \Lambda_k$ combined with the latent mixture model clusters linking label patches $L[i]$ to intensity patches $Y[i]$. This hierarchical structure enables local appearances around a given pixel to be shared across the canonical label images.

Inference. We outline an iterative algorithm based on the expected patch log-likelihood (EPLL) framework [13], deferring details to the supplementary material. The EPLL framework seeks a label image L by solving

$$\widehat{L} = \underset{L \in \{+1,-1\}^{|\mathcal{I}|}}{\operatorname{argmax}} \left\{ \log\left(\sum_{g=1}^{k} \pi_g \exp(-\alpha \mathbf{d}(L, \Lambda_g)) \right) + \frac{1}{|\mathcal{I}|} \sum_{i \in \mathcal{I}} \log p(Y[i]|L[i]) \right\}.$$

The first term in the objective function encourages label image L to be close to the true label images $\Lambda_1, \ldots, \Lambda_k$. The second term is the "expected patch log-likelihood", which favors solutions whose local label patches agree well on average with the local intensity patches according to the patch priors. Since latent label images $\Lambda_1, \ldots, \Lambda_k$ are unknown, we use training label images $L_1, \ldots, L_n$ as proxies instead, replacing the first term in the objective function with $F(L; \alpha) \triangleq \log\left(\frac{1}{n} \sum_{u=1}^{n} \exp(-\alpha \mathbf{d}(L, L_u))\right)$. Next, we approximate the unknown patch prior $p(Y[i]|L[i])$ with a kernel density estimate

$$\widetilde{p}(Y[i]|L[i]; \gamma) \propto \sum_{u=1}^{n} \sum_{j \in N(i)} \mathcal{N}\left(Y[i]; Y_u[j], \frac{1}{2\gamma} \mathbf{I}_{d \times d}\right) \delta(L[i] = L_u[j]),$$

where the user specifies a neighborhood $N(i)$ of pixel i, and constant $\gamma > 0$ that controls the Gaussian kernel's bandwidth. We group the pixels so that nearby pixels within a small block all share the same kernel density estimate. This approximation assumes a stronger version of the jigsaw condition from Section 2 since the algorithm operates as if nearby pixels have the same mixture model as a patch prior. We thus maximize objective $F(L; \alpha) + \frac{1}{|\mathcal{I}|} \sum_{i \in \mathcal{I}} \log \widetilde{p}(Y[i]|L[i]; \gamma)$.

Similar to the original EPLL method [13], we introduce an auxiliary variable $\xi_i \in \mathbb{R}^{d'}$ for each patch $L[i]$, where ξ_i acts as a local estimate for $L[i]$. Whereas two patches $L[i]$ and $L[j]$ that overlap in label image L must be consistent across the overlapping pixels, there is no such requirement on their local estimates ξ_i and ξ_j. In summary, we maximize the objective $F(L; \alpha) + \frac{1}{|\mathcal{I}|} \sum_{i \in \mathcal{I}} \log \widetilde{p}(Y[i]|\xi_i; \gamma) - \frac{\beta}{2} \sum_{i \in \mathcal{I}} \|L[i] - \xi_i\|^2$ for $\beta > 0$, subject to constraints $L[i] = \xi_i$ that are enforced using Lagrange multipliers. We numerically optimize this cost function using the Alternating Direction Method of Multipliers for distributed optimization [4].

Given the current estimate of label image L, the algorithm produces estimate ξ_i for $L[i]$ given $Y[i]$ in parallel across i. Next, it updates L based on ξ_i via a gradient method. Finally, the Lagrange multipliers are updated to penalize large discrepancies between ξ_i and $L[i]$.

Fixing ξ_i and updating L corresponds to merging local patch estimates to form a globally consistent segmentation. This is the only step that involves expression $F(L;\alpha)$. With $\alpha = 0$ and forcing the Lagrange multipliers to always be zero, the merging becomes a simple averaging of overlapping label patch estimates ξ_i. This algorithm corresponds to existing multipoint patch-based segmentation algorithms [6,10,12] and the in-painting technique achieved by the original EPLL method. Setting $\alpha = \beta = 0$ and $d' = 1$ yields pointwise weighted majority voting with parameter $\theta = \gamma$. When $\alpha > 0$, a global correction is applied, shifting the label image estimate closer to the training label images. This should produce better estimates when the full training label images can, with small perturbations as measured by $\mathbf{d}(\cdot,\cdot)$, explain new intensity images.

Experimental Results. We empirically explore the new iterative algorithm on 20 labeled thoracic-abdominal contrast-enhanced CT scans from the Visceral ANATOMY3 dataset [8]. We train the model on 15 scans and test on the remaining 5 scans. The training procedure amounted to using 10 of the 15 training scans to estimate the algorithm parameters in an exhaustive sweep, using the rest of the training scans to evaluate parameter settings. Finally, the entire training dataset of 15 scans is used to segment the test dataset of 5 scans using the best parameters found during training. For each test scan, we first use a fast affine registration to roughly align each training scan to the test scan. Then we apply four different algorithms: a baseline majority voting algorithm (denoted "MV") that simply averages the training label images that are now roughly aligned to the test scan, pointwise nearest neighbor (denoted "1NN") and weighted majority voting (denoted "WMV") segmentation that both use approximate nearest patches, and finally our proposed iterative algorithm (denoted "ADMM"), setting distance $\mathbf{d}$ to one minus Dice overlap. Note that Dice overlap can be reduced to a differentiable function by relaxing our optimization to allow each label to take on a value in $[-1, 1]$. By doing so, the Dice overlap of label images L and Λ is given by $2\langle\widetilde{L},\widetilde{\Lambda}\rangle/(\langle\widetilde{L},\widetilde{L}\rangle+\langle\widetilde{\Lambda},\widetilde{\Lambda}\rangle)$, where $\widetilde{L} = (L + 1)/2$ and $\widetilde{\Lambda} = (\Lambda + 1)/2$.

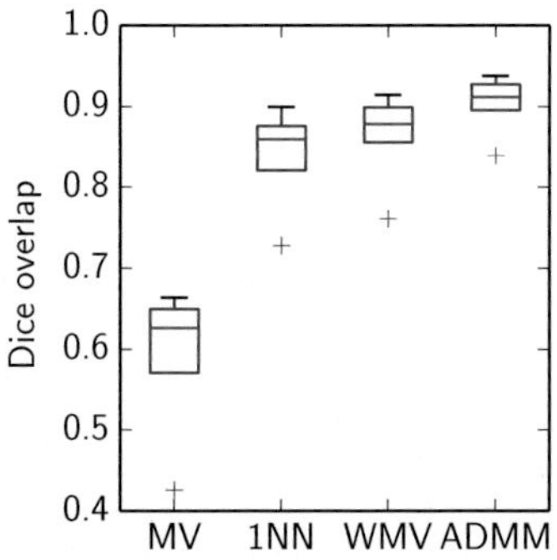

Fig. 1. Liver segmentation results.

We segmented the liver, spleen, left kidney, and right kidney. We report Dice overlap scores for the liver in Fig. 1 using the four algorithms. Our results for segmenting the other organs follow a similar trend where the proposed algorithm outperforms pointwise weighted majority voting, which outperforms both pointwise nearest-neighbor segmentation and the baseline majority voting. For the organs segmented, there was little benefit to having $\alpha > 0$, suggesting the local patch estimates to already be quite consistent and require no global correction.

4 Conclusions

We have established a new theoretical performance guarantee for two nonparametric patch-based segmentation algorithms, uniting recent lines of work on modeling patches in natural imagery and on theory for nonparametric time series classification. Our result indicates that if nearby patches behave as mixture models with sufficient similarity, then a myopic segmentation works well, where its quality is stated in terms of the available training data. Our main performance bound provides insight into how one should approach building a training dataset for patch-based segmentation. The looseness in the bound could be attributed to outliers in training data. Detecting and removing these outliers should lead to improved segmentation performance.

From a modeling standpoint, understanding the joint behavior of patches could yield substantial new insights into exploiting macroscopic structure in images rather than relying only on local properties. In a related direction, while we have modeled the individual behavior of patches, an interesting theoretical problem is to find joint distributions on image pixels that lead to such marginal distributions on patches. Do such joint distributions exist? If not, is there a joint distribution whose patch marginals approximate the mixture models we use? These questions outline rich areas for future research.

Acknowledgments. This work was supported in part by the NIH NIBIB NAC P41EB015902 grant, MIT Lincoln Lab, and Wistron Corporation. GHC was supported by an NDSEG fellowship.

References

1. Ailon, N., Chazelle, B.: Approximate nearest neighbors and the fast johnson-lindenstrauss transform. In: Symposium on Theory of Computing (2006)
2. Bai, W., et al.: A probabilistic patch-based label fusion model for multi-atlas segmentation with registration refinement: Application to cardiac MR images. Transactions in Medical Imaging (2013)
3. Barnes, C., et al.: Patchmatch: a randomized correspondence algorithm for structural image editing. Transactions on Graphics (2009)
4. Boyd, S., et al.: Distributed optimization and statistical learning via the alternating direction method of multipliers. Foundations & Trends in Machine Learning (2011)
5. Chen, G.H., Nikolov, S., Shah, D.: A latent source model for nonparametric time series classification. In: Neural Information Processing Systems (2013)
6. Coupé, P., et al.: Patch-based segmentation using expert priors: Application to hippocampus and ventricle segmentation. NeuroImage (2011)
7. Freeman, W.T., Liu, C.: Markov random fields for super-resolution and texture synthesis. In: Advances in Markov Random Fields for Vision and Image Proc. (2011)

8. Hanbury, A., Müller, H., Langs, G., Weber, M.A., Menze, B.H., Fernandez, T.S.: Bringing the algorithms to the data: Cloud–based benchmarking for medical image analysis. In: Catarci, T., Forner, P., Hiemstra, D., Peñas, A., Santucci, G. (eds.) CLEF 2012. LNCS, vol. 7488, pp. 24–29. Springer, Heidelberg (2012)
9. Muja, M., Lowe, D.G.: Fast approximate nearest neighbors with automatic algorithm configuration. In: ICCVTA (2009)
10. Rousseau, F., Habas, P.A., Studholme, C.: A supervised patch-based approach for human brain labeling. Transactions on Medical Imaging (2011)
11. Sabuncu, M.R., et al.: A generative model for image segmentation based on label fusion. Transactions on Medical Imaging (2010)
12. Wachinger, C., et al.: On the importance of location and features for the patch-based segmentation of parotid glands. MIDAS Journal - IGART (2014)
13. Zoran, D., Weiss, Y.: From learning models of natural image patches to whole image restoration. In: International Conference on Computer Vision (2011)
14. Zoran, D., Weiss, Y.: Natural images, gaussian mixtures and dead leaves. In: Neural Information Processing Systems (2012)

Multi-organ Segmentation Using Shape Model Guided Local Phase Analysis

Chunliang Wang[1,2,3] and Örjan Smedby[1,2,3]

[1] Center for Medical Image Science and Visualization (CMIV), Linköping University, Sweden
[2] Department of Radiology and Department of Medical and Health Sciences, Linköping University, Linköping, Sweden
[3] School of Technology and Health (STH), KTH Royal Institute of Technology, Sweden

Abstract. To improve the accuracy of multi-organ segmentation, we propose a model-based segmentation framework that utilizes the local phase information from paired quadrature filters to delineate the organ boundaries. Conventional local phase analysis based on local orientation has the drawback of outputting the same phases for black-to-white and white-to-black edges. This ambiguity could mislead the segmentation when two organs' borders are too close. Using the gradient of the signed distance map of a statistical shape model, we could distinguish between these two types of edges and avoid the segmentation region leaking into another organ. In addition, we propose a level-set solution that integrates both the edge-based (represented by local phase) and region-based speed functions. Compared with previously proposed methods, the current method uses local adaptive weighting factors based on the confidence of the phase map (energy of the quadrature filters) instead of a global weighting factor to combine these two forces. In our preliminary studies, the proposed method outperformed conventional methods in terms of accuracy in a number of organ segmentation tasks.

Keywords: image segmentation, level set, local phase analysis, shape model.

1 Introduction

Automatic segmentation of anatomical structures is often needed for both clinical and epidemiological studies. As an important initial step for quantitative image analysis and data mining, the accuracy of the organ segmentation is usually one of the main factors that determine the quality of the final image analysis results. Many automated organ segmentation methods have been proposed, such as the active shape model (ASM), atlas-based methods and machine-learning-based methods [1]. No matter what framework is chosen, a crucial factor determining the segmentation accuracy is what kind of local features is used to guide the global optimization process. When dealing with medical images, methods based on the conventional image features, such as intensity and gradient, often fail to deliver satisfactory results, as the boundary between two organs may be inadequately defined due to limited resolution and intensity similarity. Even with the help of shape priors, most algorithms have difficulties in

N. Navab et al. (Eds.): MICCAI 2015, Part III, LNCS 9351, pp. 149–156, 2015.
DOI: 10.1007/978-3-319-24574-4_18

discriminating between a different organ and anatomical variation of the same organ. Local phase has been used as a robust image feature in noisy images in various image segmentation and registration applications [2–4]. However, local phase analysis is often performed using the local orientation, yielding identical local phase estimates for black-to-white and white-to-black edges. This ambiguity may mislead the segmentation when two organs' borders are too close. In this paper, we propose a model-guided local phase analysis method, where the global shape model suggests the searching orientation of the local structures. This suppresses the influence from irrelevant structures not aligned with the shape surface. Moreover, by using the gradient of the signed distance map of a statistical shape model, we can distinguish between the aforementioned two types of edges and avoid the segmentation region leaking into another organ. In addition, we propose a level-set based solution that integrates both the local-phase-based and region-based forces. Compared with previously proposed methods, the current method uses local adaptive weighting factors based on the confidence of the phase map (energy of the quadrature filters), instead of a global weighting factor, to combine these two forces. In our preliminary studies, the proposed method outperformed conventional methods in terms of accuracy for brain stripping and liver, spleen and kidney segmentation tasks.

2 Method

2.1 Quadrature Filters and Model Guided Local Phase Analysis

Quadrature filters, originally proposed by Granlund and Knutsson [5], have been successfully applied for various local structure estimation and image enhancement tasks [3, 4, 6]. The principle of these filters is to combine a ridge-picking filter with an edge-picking filter in the spatial domain. Typical 2-dimensional filter kernels are illustrated in Figs. 1a and 1b. A quadrature filter is a band-pass filter over one half of the Fourier domain. The output of this pair of filters is represented by a complex number where the output of the ridge-picking filter is seen as the real part and the output of the edge-picking filter as the imaginary part. When applied to an image, the response of ridge-like structures will be predominantly real, while the response of edge-like structures will be predominantly imaginary. The argument of this complex number in the complex plan is referred to as the *local phase* [5], θ in Fig. 1c. The magnitude (q) of the complex number is called *local energy* [5]. It is worth mentioning that local phase can also be estimated using Gabor filters where the ridge-picking filter is a sine wave multiplied with a Gaussian function, while the edge-picking filter is a cosine wave multiplied with the same Gaussian function. It is easy to see that the local phase varies when the orientation of a quadrature filter changes. To be able to produce a consistent phase map for any given image, the local phase is often estimated using the local orientation that can be estimated using either the local gradient or eigenvector decomposition of the local structure tensor. Another common way of estimating local phase is simply to combine the complex output of a set of quadrature filter pairs that evenly covers all angles in a 2D or 3D coordinate system (e.g. 4 filters in 2D and 6 filters in 3D as suggested in [5]). Notice that the combination of local phases is implicitly weighted by the local energy of those filters, i.e. the filter with highest local energy will dominate the phase estimation. To avoid that filters with opposite relative orientation cancel out in the imaginary part (the output from an edge-picking filter will switch sign when the filter orientation inverts), Läthén et al. suggested to flip the phase along the real axis for all filters that produce a negative imaginary part [6]. This solution, just like using local orientation, will produce the same phase on black-to-white and white-to-black edges. When used for segmentation, this ambiguity could cause the organ contour to snap to the edge of a neighboring organ if the two organs' borders are too close. This scenario can very often be seen in medical images.

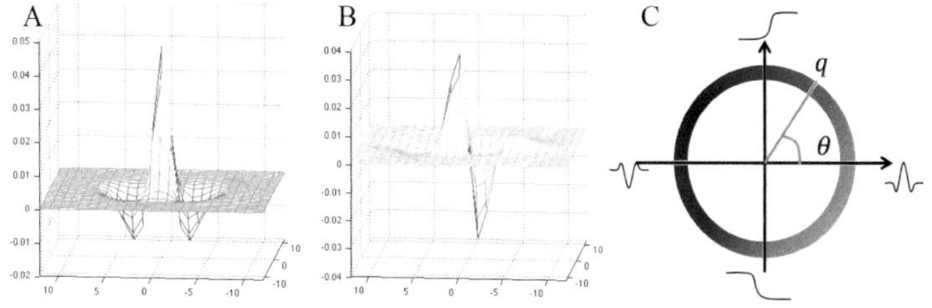

Fig. 1. An example of quadrature filter pairs in 2D. **A**, the ridge-picking filter. **B**, the edge-picking filter. **C**, The quadrature filter's response in the complex plane.

In this study, we propose to use the surface orientation of a given shape model to guide the local phase analysis. Shape models can either be mesh-based or volume-based. A review of various types of statistical shape models can be found in [7]. Nevertheless, all shape models can be converted into a signed distance map. The gradient of the the signed distance map then represents a reference orientation perpendicular to the shape surface. More importantly, the gradient also indicates which direction is inside/outside (here we assume that the distance map is positive inside and negative outside). Local phase is then estimated in the reference direction. Given a white organ on a black background, the local phase of the organ's edge should be –90°, while the local phase of a neighboring organ's edge will be 90°. Fig. 2 shows an example of applying the proposed filtering technique in a brain MRI volume. As compared with the Gaussian gradient (Fig. 2B) and the conventional quadrature filter (Fig. 2C), the energy map from the model-guided quadrature filters focus more on the edges of the skull, which is desired for skull stripping in MRI brain analysis. Compared with the phase map produced by Läthén's method (Fig. 2D), the proposed solution (Fig. 2H) delivers a more distinct pattern for identifying the inner boundary of the skull (blue) from the out surface of the brain (yellow).

As the filter orientation varies across the image, the filtering is made via local resampling by rotating a given kernel grid to align with the local reference direction. This step can also be carried out using a steerable filter, which synthesises a filter with arbitrary orientation from a linear combination of basis filters [8]. The latter may be faster if the local phase analysis needs to be performed for all pixels/voxels. However, in practice, the computation on points that are far away from the model surface can be skipped, as will be further explained in the next section.

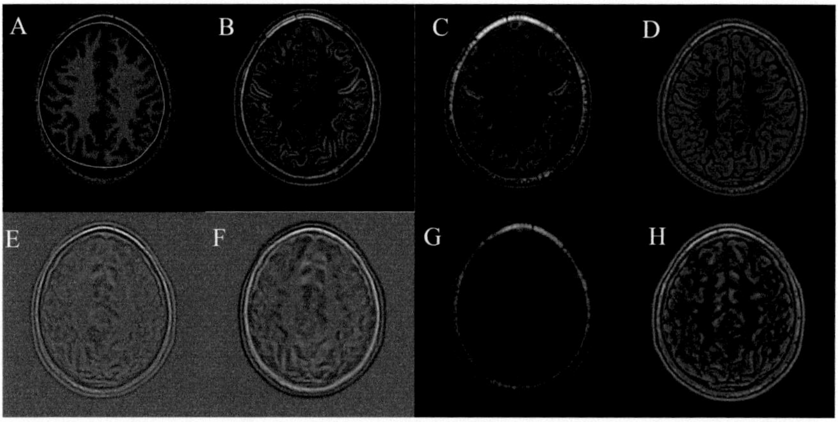

Fig. 2. A: input image, the green contour represents the cross section of the brain model; **B**: the gradient magnitude. **C, D**: local energy and phase maps using Läthén's method [6]. **E, F, G, H**: the real and imaginary parts of the model-guided quadrature filter and corresponding local energy and phase maps. (D, H were created using the color lookup table shown in Fig. 1C)

2.2 Integrating Region-Based and Edge-Based Energy in the Level-Set Method

To incorporate the phase information into the level set framework, we propose an energy function as described in Eq. 1, where I is the input image, and $\mathcal{R}_A$ is the segmented region. The function θ outputs the estimated local phase ($0 \leq \theta < 2\pi$) at any given location. τ is an input parameter defining the targeted phase (e.g. $\pi/2$ for a black-to-white edge and $3\pi/2$ for a white-to-black edge).

$$E(\partial\mathcal{R}) = \int_0^1 g\left[\theta\left(I(\partial\mathcal{R}_A(c))\right) - \tau\right]^2 |\mathcal{R}_A(c)| dc \quad (1)$$

The function g is a simple period-fixing function that ensures that the phase difference between θ and τ is measured in the range from $-\pi$ to π (Eq. 2).

$$g(\delta) = \begin{cases} \delta & if\ -\pi < \delta \leq \pi \\ \delta - 2\pi & if\ \delta > \pi \\ \delta + 2\pi & if\ \delta \leq -\pi \end{cases} \quad (2)$$

Notice that Eq. 1 is very similar to the conventional geodesic active contours, except that $\theta(I)$ replaces∇I, and the period-fixing function g replaces the gradient magnitude inverse function. Similar to the conventional geodesic active contours, the force of this phase-based energy function vanishes in flat areas where the quadrature filters cannot pick up any signals. To overcome this problem and guide the contour's movement even far away from any borders, we propose an integrated energy function that combines the phase-based energy and the region-based energy:

$$E(\partial\mathcal{R}) = \alpha \int_0^1 g\left[\theta\left(I(\partial\mathcal{R}_A(c))\right) - \tau\right]^2 |\mathcal{R}_A(c)| dc - \int_{\mathcal{R}_A}\int w(x,y) \log[p_A(I(x,y))]\, dxdy - \int_{\mathcal{R}_B}\int w(x,y) \log[p_B(I(x,y))]\, dxdy \quad (4)$$

Here, p_A and p_B are the probability functions of a given pixel/voxel falling into region A or B. In the case of medical images, their distributions could be learned either from statistical analysis of image databases, or on the fly using preliminary segmentation results. Function w is a weighting function that weights the fitting energy using the local energy output (q) from the quadrature filter, as described by Eq. 5:

$$w(x,y) = \frac{1}{1+q\left(I(x,y)\right)} \tag{5}$$

Eq. 4 can be minimized by solving the following descent equation:

$$\frac{\partial \phi}{\partial t} = \left[\alpha g(\theta-\tau)^2 \mathrm{div}\left(\frac{\nabla\phi}{|\nabla\phi|}\right) + \alpha g(\theta-\tau) + w\log(p_B) - w\log(p_A)\right]|\nabla\phi| \tag{6}$$

Here, ϕ is the level set function, which is a signed distance map from the contours. The last 3 components on the right side can be seen as a group of external forces. Fig. 3 shows an example of a liver segmentation case, in which the phase-based term, the region-based terms and their combination are visualized side by side. In practice, we simplify the first component on the right side by replacing it with $\beta \mathrm{div}(\nabla\phi/|\nabla\phi|)$, where β is a weighting factor, as it is just a regulation term that corresponds to the curvature force in the conventional level set methods. By plugging the model term into the formulation, we arrive at the final speed function given below:

$$\frac{\partial \phi}{\partial t} = \left[\beta \mathrm{div}\left(\frac{\nabla\phi}{|\nabla\phi|}\right) + \alpha g(\theta-\tau) + w\log(p_B) - w\log(p_A) + m(t)\right]|\nabla\phi| \tag{7}$$

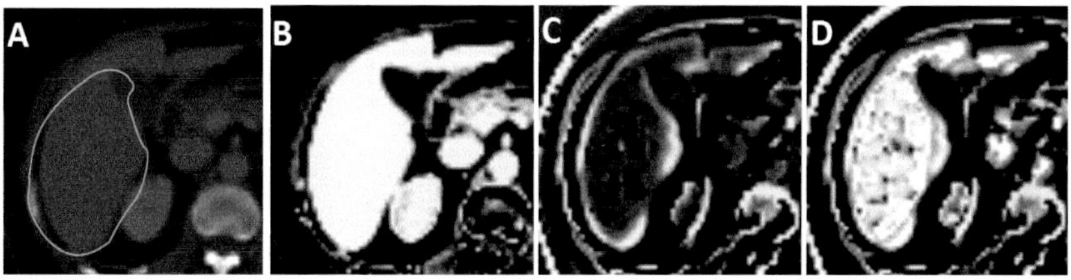

Fig. 3. A. An axial view of an input volume (green contour: the current shape model), **B**. The region-based speed terms based on the image intensity. **C** The phase-based term estimated using the model **D**. The combined external speed map. Notice that the connection between liver and kidney is removed.

To propagate the level set function according to the speed function above, we adapted a coherent propagating level set algorithm proposed in [9, 10]. This method is able to detect the convergence of the level set function. Note that, given a contour starting from the current best fitting model, the statistical model and its corresponding phase map only need to be updated if the contour has moved a certain distance from the current model. As pointed out in [10], it is possible to design a model term that limits the zero level to stay in a narrow band with fixed width (e.g. 3mm) around the previous model. This means that before the contour reaches convergence within this narrow band, the statistical model does not need to be updated. Given a good initialization, the model fitting and the corresponding local phase map regeneration are only repeated a small number of times (<20) throughout the whole segmentation process.

Moreover, since the contour is not allowed to move beyond the narrow band, we only need to compute the local phase map for the points located on the narrow band.

2.3 Hierarchical Segmentation Pipeline and Multi-scale Phase Analysis

To segment multiple organs in full-body CT datasets, we implemented a hierarchical segmentation pipeline, similar to the work of Wang et al. [10]. First, the unseen full body CT volume is registered to a standard patient selected from a set of training data. Then we sequentially segment the ventral cavity, thoracic cavity, abdominal cavity, lungs, liver, spleen, kidneys and bladder. All segmentation steps are made using the proposed method described in section 2.2. The segmentation of the higher-level structures provides an estimated position for the lower level structures for initializing the model-based segmentation. For a non-enhanced CT dataset, the boundary information from higher-level structures, such as the abdominal cavity, also constrains the segmentation of the lower-level structures. However, for enhanced CT, this constraint is removed, thanks to the phase-based energy, which can reliably detect the organ's boundary and avoid the leaking problem in most cases. In addition to the anatomical hierarchy, we also perform the segmentation in a coarse-to-fine resolution hierarchy. All structures are first segmented at 3.5mm isotropic resolution, and then the segmentation of the lower level organs is repeated at 2mm and finally at the input resolution, which is about 0.8×0.8×1.5mm. At each resolution, we used the same 7×7×7voxel quadrature filter, which implies that the local phase analysis is done at different scales (in millimeters). This strategy helps to gradually attract the contour towards the organ border, even if the initial shape model is a bit away from the ideal position.

3 Experiments and Results

To validate the proposed model-guided phase analysis method, we first compared it with the multi-scale phase analysis method proposed in [6] (both put into the integrated phase- and region-based level set framework described in section 2.2) and with the conventional integrated gradient and region-based method [11] for skull stripping in MRI. Publicly available data from the brain segmentation challenge site (http://mrbrains13.isi.uu.nl/) was used. The segmentation accuracy on 5 training datasets is 96.3±1.6% with the gradient- and region-based method, 95.8±2.5% with the multi-scale phase based approach and 97.8±1.4% with the proposed method (mean Dice coefficient ± SD). Results on test datasets are not available as the current implementation cannot provide the white matter and gray matter segmentation required by the website.

The proposed method was further tested for multi-organ segmentation using the data from the Visceral multi-organ segmentation challenge [12]. Our method was trained using 7 non-enhanced CT (CT) and 7 contrast-enhanced CT (CECT) datasets and tested on 8 non-enhanced and 10 enhanced CT datasets. For testing, the participants submitted a virtual machine with their segmentation software installed, and the organizer ran the program against the unseen testing data. This prevents the teams from training their methods on the testing data by visually checking the segmentation results. The proposed method outperformed other methods in liver segmentation and kidney segmentation. Detailed results and comparison with previous leading methods are listed in Table 1. The average processing time for segmenting all 6 major organs is about 30 minutes on a PC with Intel i7 (1.9GHz). A 7×7×7 quadrature filter with a central frequency of $\pi/2$ and a bandwidth of 6 octaves was used for the experiments.

Table 1. Multi-organ segmentation in CT and CECT datasets (mean Dice coefficient)

Data	Method	Liver	Right Kidney	Left Kidney	Spleen	Right Lung	Left Lung
CT (8 cases)	Toro et al.[13]	86.6%	79.0%	78.4%	70.3%	**97.5%**	**97.2%**
	Vincent et al. [12]	93.4%	**92.5%**	86.6%	–	97.0%	97.0%
	Wang et al.[10]	93.4%	90.4%	87.3%	**91.3%**	96.2%	96.0%
	Proposed method	**93.6%**	79.6%	**89.6%**	91.0%	97.0%	96.1%
CECT (10 cases)	Toro et al. [13]	88.7%	88.9%	91.0%	73.0%	96.3%	95.9%
	Vincent et al. [12]	94.2%	92.7%	94.3%	–	**97.4%**	96.9%
	Wang et al.[10]	93.0%	92.9%	93.0%	87.4%	96.6%	96.7%
	Proposed method	**94.9%**	**95.9%**	**94.5%**	**90.9%**	97.1%	**97.2%**

4 Discussion and Conclusion

Shape priors have been adapted in a large variety of image segmentation tasks. However, most existing methods focus on using local image features to update the global shape model and on using the global shape model to regularize the propagation of the segmentation contour/mesh. Very few studies have suggested using the estimated global shape to guide the local feature analysis. To some extent, the proposed method is similar to Zheng et al.'s machine learning based method for heart chamber segmentation [1], where steerable features are used to guide the deformation of an ASM. However, the implementation of using the local phase is more general, as the filter need not be trained for each special type of data, except for choosing a proper target phase τ. In contrast to conventional gradient-based level sets, using model-guided phase analysis can not only attract the contour to the organ edges, but also make it favor a certain type of edges and repel from the edges of a neighboring organ. In addition, local phase is intensity-invariant, which makes it better suited for medical images with inhomogeneity. Although the phase computation is more time-consuming than the gradient, as pointed out in section 2.2, the process needs only to be repeated a small number of times when combined with coherent propagation. Compared to geodesic active contours, which use an advection force (corresponding to the second order derivative of the input image) that needs to be computed in each iteration of the level set propagation, the model-guided local phase analysis could even be favorable in terms of speed.

The integrated energy function presented above is inspired by Paragios' et al. work in [11]. However, instead of using a global weighting factor, we propose a local weighting scheme. This helps to suppress the influence of the intensity-based terms in areas where two organs are close to each other and to let the phase map take more responsibility for delineating the boundary in such cases.

A limitation of the model-guided phase analysis method is that it requires the shape model to be relatively well positioned initially. Large offset from the target may confuse the contour propagation. For example, in our Visceral challenge experiment, the right kidney model initialization was poor in one of the eight CT cases that leading to total failure of the segmentation and explaining the inferior mean Dice coefficient presented in Table 1. It is possible that the machine learning based organ detection and pose estimation proposed in [1] could be a good solution to this issue.

In conclusion, a model-based segmentation framework using model-guided local phase analysis is proposed. By using the surface orientation of the shape model as a reference direction, the proposed method could distinguish between black-to-white and white-to-black edges and avoid the segmentation region leaking into neighboring organs. In our preliminary studies, the proposed method outperformed some conventional methods in a number of single-organ and multi-organ segmentation tasks.

References

1. Zheng, Y., Barbu, A., Georgescu, B., Scheuering, M., Comaniciu, D.: Four-chamber heart modeling and automatic segmentation for 3-D cardiac CT volumes using marginal space learning and steerable features. IEEE Trans. Med. Imaging 27, 1668–1681 (2008)
2. Knutsson, H., Andersson, M.: Morphons: segmentation using elastic canvas and paint on priors. In: IEEE International Conference on Image Processing, pp. II–1226–9 (2005)
3. Belaid, A., Boukerroui, D., Maingourd, Y., Lerallut, J.-F.: Phase-Based Level Set Segmentation of Ultrasound Images. IEEE Trans. Inf. Technol. Biomed. 15, 138–147 (2011)
4. Wang, C., Smedby, Ö.: Model-based left ventricle segmentation in 3d ultrasound using phase image. Presented at the MICCAI Challenge on Echocardiographic Three-Dimensional Ultrasound Segmentation (CETUS), Boston (2014)
5. Granlund, G.H., Knutsson, H.: Signal Processing for Computer Vision. Kluwer Academic Publishers (1994)
6. Läthén, G., Jonasson, J., Borga, M.: Blood vessel segmentation using multi-scale quadrature filtering. Pattern Recognit. Lett. 31, 762–767 (2010)
7. Heimann, T., Meinzer, H.-P.: Statistical shape models for 3D medical image segmentation: A review. Med. Image Anal. 13, 543–563 (2009)
8. Freeman, W.T., Adelson, E.H.: The design and use of steerable filters. IEEE Trans. Pattern Anal. Mach. Intell. 13, 891–906 (1991)
9. Wang, C., Frimmel, H., Smedby, Ö.: Fast Level-set Based Image Segmentation Using Coherent Propagation. Med. Phys. 41, 073501 (2014)
10. Wang, C., Smedby, Ö.: Automatic multi-organ segmentation in non-enhanced CT datasets using Hierarchical Shape Priors. Proceedings of the 22nd International Conference on Pattern Recognition (ICPR). IEEE, Stockholm (2014)
11. Paragios, N., Deriche, R.: Geodesic active regions and level set methods for supervised texture segmentation. Int. J. Comput. Vis. 46, 223–247 (2002)
12. Visceral Benchmark, `http://www.visceral.eu/closed-benchmarks/anatomy2/anatomy2-results/`
13. del Toro, O.A.J., Müller, H.: Hierarchic Multi–atlas Based Segmentation for Anatomical Structures: Evaluation in the VISCERAL Anatomy Benchmarks. In: Menze, B., Langs, G., Montillo, A., Kelm, M., Müller, H., Zhang, S., Cai, W.(T.), Metaxas, D. (eds.) MCV 2014. LNCS, vol. 8848, pp. 189–200. Springer, Heidelberg (2014)

Filling Large Discontinuities in 3D Vascular Networks Using Skeleton- and Intensity-Based Information

Russell Bates[1], Laurent Risser[2], Benjamin Irving[1], Bartłomiej W. Papież[1], Pavitra Kannan[3], Veerle Kersemans[3,⋆], and Julia A. Schnabel[1]

[1] Institute of Biomedical Engineering, Department of Engineering Science, University of Oxford, UK
[2] Institut de Mathématiques de Toulouse (UMR 5219), CNRS, France
[3] Department of Oncology, University of Oxford, UK

Abstract. Segmentation of vasculature is a common task in many areas of medical imaging, but complex morphology and weak signal often lead to incomplete segmentations. In this paper, we present a new gap filling strategy for 3D vascular networks. The novelty of our approach is to combine both skeleton- and intensity-based information to fill *large* discontinuities. Our approach also does not make any hypothesis on the network topology, which is particularly important for tumour vasculature due to the chaotic arrangement of vessels within tumours. Synthetic results show that using intensity-based information, in addition to skeleton-based information, can make the detection of large discontinuities more robust. Our strategy is also shown to outperform a classic gap filling strategy on 3D Micro-CT images of preclinical tumour models.

1 Introduction

Gap filling methods for vascular networks have recently generated significant interest. Many methods for the segmentation of the vasculature rely on the generation of a likelihood or *vesselness* map. To obtain a final segmentation, these maps are usually binarized, meaning that important vessel information may be discarded. Under-segmentation in this sense can lead to discontinuities in the segmentation, which will have implications for any analysis of the branching structure. In this paper, we then propose a novel method to incorporate image intensity information, additional to the final segmentation, to reconnect the gaps in the segmentation. This method is motivated by the extraction of tumour vasculature which is highly leaky and poorly perfused, leading to an irregular distribution of signal within the vasculature (see Fig. 1). No strong hypotheses can therefore be made on their chaotic and highly irregular topology.

⋆ We would like to acknowledge funding from the CRUK/ EPSRC Cancer Imaging Centre in Oxford. JAS and LR also wish to acknowledge the CNRS-INSMI/John Fell Oxford University Press (OUP) Research Fund.

N. Navab et al. (Eds.): MICCAI 2015, Part III, LNCS 9351, pp. 157–164, 2015.
DOI: 10.1007/978-3-319-24574-4_19

Preliminary approaches to perform gap filling or to improve robustness in the segmentation of vascular structures were proposed in [10,13,9]. A gap filling strategy for large 3D images with a discontinuous segmented vasculature, based on a tensor voting strategy [4], was proposed in [11]. This approach, however, only makes use of the skeleton of segmented structures. Another tensor voting strategy was proposed in [7] to segment noisy tubular structures in an iterative fashion. However, this only applies to relatively small gaps. An interesting learning strategy was proposed in [5]. This approach utilizes human interactions to learn appropriate graph connectivity. The decomposition of directional information, *orientation scores*, has been explored [2], but with application to crossing vessels. This high level strategy is complementary to lower level ones like in [11], where only local image features communicate to fill the gaps. In the same vein, the simultaneous reconstruction and separation of multiple interwoven tree structures using high-level representation of the trees was also proposed in [1], and a physiologically motivated strategy based on a simplified angiogenesis model was proposed in [12] to correct the vascular connectivity. Closer to our strategy, [3] derived intensity based information within a tensor model to perform the robust segmentation of tubular structures. However, this strategy is dedicated to robust vessel segmentation in a noisy context, which would typically lead to small discontinuities, and not to the detection of large discontinuities in the segmented network. Note finally that a review of 3D vessels segmentation strategies was recently published in [6].

From a methodological perspective, we define a gap filling strategy adapted to *large discontinuities*. Our approach works on very low level features and places few priors on the structure, distribution and topology of the vessels. Its key novelties are (1) the incorporation of both skeletal and image intensity information whilst enforcing minimal priors on the resultant reconnected morphology, and (2) a new communication model between the different image features, with the clear separation of oriented- and non oriented-information. This paper is structured as follows: Section 2 presents our new gap filling strategy. Results are presented section 3 and discussions are drawn section 4.

2 Methodology

2.1 Method Overview

Suppose we have the following inputs defined on the image domain Ω:

1. A skeletonized vascular network, typically obtained from a segmented vascular network. We denote s_i, $i \in \{1, \cdots, I\}$ the set of network *segments* which contain the set of points between two topological branch points or between a branch point and an end point. The $\mathbf{e}_j$, $j \in \{1, \cdots, J\}$ are the set of *segment ends* connected to any other segment.
2. A list of *uncertain points* $\mathbf{p}_k$, $k \in \{1, \cdots, K\}$ and their intensity w_k, $w_k \in [0, 1]$. Intensities are normalized so that w_k close to 0 means that point $\mathbf{p}_k$ is unlikely to be part of a vessel and w_k close to 1 means that $\mathbf{p}_k$ is very likely

to be part of a vessel. These intensities can be directly extracted from the original image or as the scores of a probabilistic segmentation algorithm.

Fig. 1 illustrates these image features. From each segment end $\mathbf{e}_j$, a path P_j will eventually be generated to fill a gap in the skeleton. To do so, the user has only to define two simple parameters:

1. Characteristic distance σ which represents the typical size of the gaps to fill.
2. Characteristic angle $\theta \in]0, \pi/2[$ of the paths, which permits more or less curvature to an optimal path. A typical value for θ is $\pi/5$.

Based on the segment ends $\mathbf{e}_j$, our strategy first consists of defining a second order tensor field $\mathbf{T}$. This field is used to compute the saliency map to curvilinear shapes S as in [11], plus preferential directions $\mathbf{D}$ for the path search. Based on the segments s_i and intensity based information ($\mathbf{p}_k$,w_k), a so-called enhancement map E is generated to indicate where each path P_j could be found without any clear indication on its local orientation. This differs from [11], where all input information is expressed in the tensor field with preferential directions. Note that we build the two scalar fields S and E so that, for both of them, a value close to 0 at point $\mathbf{p}$ emphasizes that $\mathbf{p}$ should not be part of a path P_j, and values similar to or larger than 1 emphasize that $\mathbf{p}$ is very likely to be part of a path P_j. We describe hereafter how paths P_j are generated using the fields S, E and $\mathbf{D}$. Construction of these fields is described in the following.

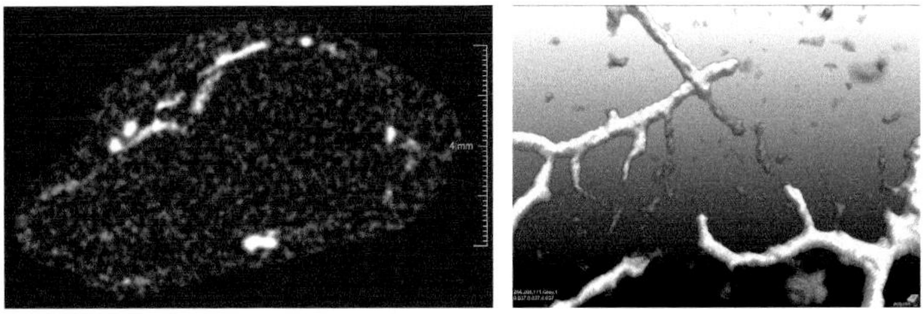

Fig. 1. (left) Slice out of a 3D image of tumour vasculature. **(right)** Primary 3D segmentation shown in white and intensity information shown in gray. In our model, the primary segmentation is skeletonized and intensity information provides an additional guide for reconnection. In the presented ROI, this additional information makes sense to fill skeleton discontinuities.

2.2 Gap Filling

The segment ends $\mathbf{e}_j$ can be linked to other segment ends in case of a gap within a vessel segment, or to other segments s_i in case of a gap at a bifurcation. We use Alg. 1 to generate the paths. Parameter δ is the step length of the recursive path search and is typically similar to the voxel resolution. We define h as equal to 0.05. This is motivated by the fact that the effect of this threshold is largely redundant with respect to σ and θ. Angles θ_1 and θ_2 also ensure that the path search is relatively smooth and follows directions similar to the preferential directions of $\mathbf{D}$. We consider these parameters as secondary here and set them to 20 degrees. However, our tests have shown that they should be contained within $[10, 30]$ degrees to lead to satisfactory results, whatever the network. Note that our algorithm was chosen over a Dijkstra style search algorithm for reasons of computational complexity.

Algorithm 1. Path search from a segment end e_j

$P_j(1) = \text{location}(\mathbf{e}_j)$
$P_j(2) = \text{location}(\mathbf{e}_j) + \delta\text{direction}(\mathbf{e}_j)$
$i = 2$
while [$P_j(i)$ does not reach a segment end or a segment] and $[\max(S(P_j(i)), E(P_j(i))) > h]$ **do**
  List all points $\hat{P}_j(i+1)$ at a distance δ from $P_j(i)$
  Among the $\hat{P}_j(i+1)$, remove those for which the angle between $P_j(i-1)P_j(i)$ and $P_j(i)\hat{P}_j(i+1)$ is higher than θ_1.
  Among the $\hat{P}_j(i+1)$, remove those for which the angle between $\mathbf{D}(P_j(i))$ and $P_j(i)\hat{P}_j(i+1)$ is higher than than θ_2.
  If there remains at least one point in the list $P_j(i+1)$ is the one which have the highest $\max(S(P_j(i)), E(P_j(i)))$
  i++
end while
If $P_j(i)$ reaches a segment end or a segment, then join $\mathbf{e}_j$ with this token using P_j
end

2.3 Generating the Second-Order Tensor Field T

A second-order tensor field constructed from the dyadic products of a vector field allows for a simple mechanism of communication between vector fields. We use a very similar technique as in [11] to define the tensor field $\mathbf{T}$. Let l_j be the location of the segment end $\mathbf{e}_j$ and $\mathbf{d}_j$ be its (normalized) direction. For each point $\mathbf{p}$ close to l_j, a vector $\mathbf{w}_j(p)$ is first generated as:

$$\mathbf{w}_j(\mathbf{p}) = e^{\frac{r^2 + c\varphi^2}{\sigma^2}} (2\mathbf{e}_j\mathbf{p}(\mathbf{e}_j\mathbf{p} \cdot \mathbf{d}_j) - \mathbf{d}_j) \ , \tag{1}$$

where c equals $\sigma^3/(4\sin^2\theta)$ and $(\mathbf{e}_j\mathbf{p} \cdot \mathbf{d}_j)$ is the scalar product between $\mathbf{e}_j\mathbf{p}$ and $\mathbf{d}_j$. Scalars r and φ are, respectively, the length and the curvature of an arc of circle going through $\mathbf{e}_j$ and $\mathbf{p}$ and parallel to $\mathbf{d}_j$ at point $\mathbf{e}_j$ (as in [11]). At each point $\mathbf{p}$, the communication between all segment ends is simply performed by computing the sum of all *tensorized* vector fields $\mathbf{w_j}$:

$$\mathbf{T}(\mathbf{p}) = \sum_{j=1}^{J} \mathbf{w}_j(\mathbf{p}) \otimes \mathbf{w}_j(\mathbf{p}) \, , \tag{2}$$

where $\otimes$ is the tensor product between two vectors. This strategy will allow us to evaluate whether all vectors $\mathbf{w}_j(\mathbf{p})$ have similar directions, by computing the eigenvalues and eigenvectors of $\mathbf{T}(\mathbf{p})$.

2.4 Deriving a Saliency Map S and Preferential Directions $\mathbf{D}$ from $\mathbf{T}$

Our method works on the hypothesis that segments are connected when both ends agree on some path between them. The saliency map is a measure for this agreement by quantifying the degree to which votes from different segments at a given point agree on a preferential direction. As in [4,11,7], each point of $\mathbf{T}$ can be decomposed into eigenvectors and eigenvalues, which describe the principal directions of $\mathbf{T}$ and their strength at each point p: $\mathbf{T}(\mathbf{p}) = \sum_{i=1}^{3} \sigma_i(\mathbf{p})\mathbf{v}_i(\mathbf{p}) \otimes \mathbf{v}_i(\mathbf{p})$. Decomposition can be performed using the Jacobi algorithm. The saliency to a curvilinear shape $S(\mathbf{p})$, defining how likely each point of the domain is to be part of a curve, is defined by $S(\mathbf{p}) = \sigma_1(\mathbf{p}) - \sigma_2(\mathbf{p})$. As the weights given to each vector field $\mathbf{w}_j(\mathbf{p})$ expressing a single segment end in Eq. (1) are contained between 0 and 1, we assume that $S(\mathbf{p})$ higher than 1 means that the saliency of $\mathbf{p}$ to a curve is very high.

Preferential directions $\mathbf{D}$ to join two segment ends can simply be the eigenvector $\mathbf{v}_1$ corresponding to the largest eigenvalue. Note that these eigenvectors are defined on a larger domain than where $S(\mathbf{p}) > h$, which will be the key for the use of the enhancement field E.

2.5 Generating the Enhancement Map E

We first enhance segment surroundings in E: at a point $\mathbf{p}$ close to a segment s_i, we set $E(\mathbf{p}) = \exp\left(-4c^2/\sigma^2\right)$, where c is the distance between $\mathbf{p}$ and s_i.

Then, in order to estimate how uncertain points $\mathbf{p}_k$ and their intensities w_k are expressed in E, we first copy them in a temporary image R_1. All other points of R_1 are null. We then define the temporary images R_2 and R_3 by smoothing R_1 with a kernel $\exp\left(-4d^2/\sigma^2\right)$ and a larger kernel $\exp\left(-d^2/\sigma^2\right)$ respectively, where d is the distance to the kernel origin. Each point $\mathbf{p}$ of E is then influenced by the uncertain points $E(\mathbf{p}) = E(\mathbf{p}) + R_2(\mathbf{p})/R_3(\mathbf{p})$. This approach ensures that a locally isolated point $\mathbf{p}_k$ or a local cluster of uncertain points with the same intensities w_k will be similarly spread in R_2/R_3 (close to Gaussian smoothing) with a maximum value of w_k. As the intensities are sampled within $[0, 1]$, the influence of isolated uncertain points or groups of uncertain points is then similar to the influence of the segments s_i in E and the influence of the segment ends $\mathbf{c}_j$ in S. All non-oriented information for the path search is then sampled on the same scale, which facilitates the communication between skeleton- and intensity-based information in the path search of section 2.2.

3 Results

3.1 Synthetic Data

A synthetic example and two sets of results are presented in Fig. 2. Although this network has no physiological meaning, it represents different configurations which may occur in our application: (top) two segment ends, one in front of the other; (left) segment end pointing a segment; (bottom-right) two segment ends which are relatively close to a segment but with intensity based information indicating that they should be linked together and not linked to the segment. The two first cases can be easily merged using skeleton information only (right illustrations of Fig. 2) but the third one requires intensity information (central illustrations of Fig. 2). A comparison with [11] also led to the same results as our strategy without intensity information. Using large values of σ a false positive junction would be made. Using reasonable σ, as well as intensity information, the two segment ends are properly merged (illustrations on the central column of Fig. 2).

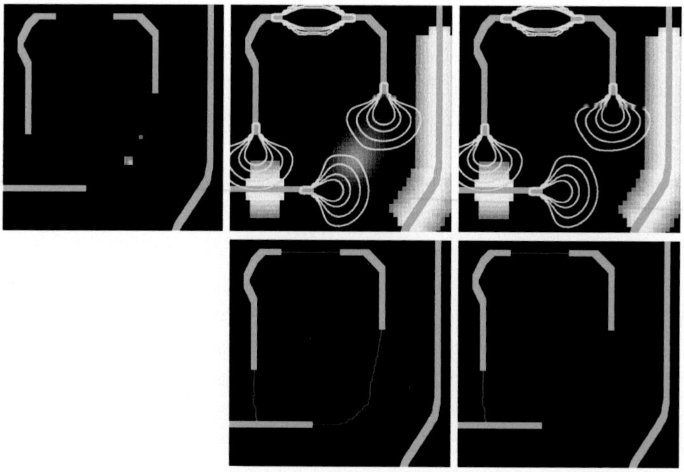

Fig. 2. Gap filling in a synthetic 2D network. Large blue curves represent the initial skeleton. Gray levels represent initial intensities in the top-left image and the enhancement field E in other images. They are sampled between 0 and 1. Yellow curves are the isolines [0.3, 0.2, 0.1, 0.05] of the saliency map S. Thin red curves are the paths P_j filling discontinuities.

3.2 3D Images of Tumour Vasculature

10 volumes of a preclinical tumour model were acquired using the CT component of an Inveon PET/CT system (Siemens Healthcare) with an isotropic voxel size of 32.7μm on a 300×200×170 grid size. The images were derived from a female CBA mouse with murine adenocarcinoma NT (CaNT) implanted subcutaneously on the right flank. For contrast enhanced micro-CT scanning, the

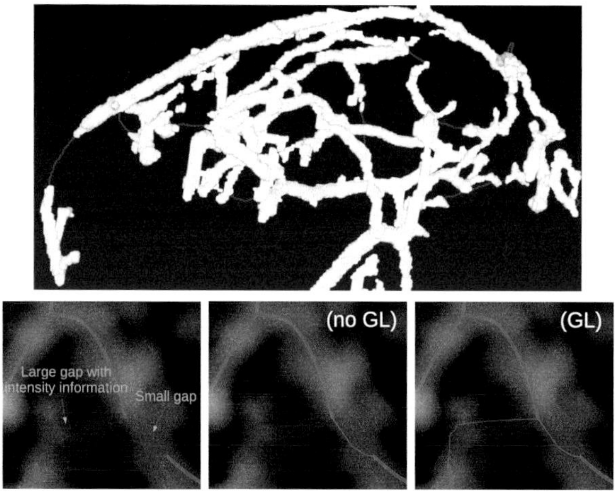

Fig. 3. Result obtained on a 3D tumour vasculature using the proposed strategy. **(Top)** Segmented network is in white and the red curves are the paths P_j filling discontinuities. **(Bottom)** ROI in which intensity information made it possible to fill a gap.

contrast agent Exitron^{TM} nano 12000 (Miltenyi Biotec) was injected into the lateral tail vein and segmentations were performed on the subtraction of pre- and post-contrast agent scans with a vesselness measure derived from [14]. Our primary segmentation was performed using a Markov Random Field approach which leads to a largely contiguous segmentation. The skeletonization algorithm of [8] was used on this segmentation. The secondary segmentation, from which the guiding intensity values were drawn, was formed from a simple thresholding operation which is slightly more permissive than the MRF technique. We compared our strategy to [11], which does not make use of intensity-based information and uses a different communication strategy between the different skeleton elements. We tested our model with (referred by (GL)) and without (referred by (no GL)) intensity information to measure its benefit. The same gap filling parameters were used for all methods ($\sigma = 400\mu$m and $\theta = 25$ degrees).

In total 60 gaps were filled using [11] whereas 75 and 95 gaps were filled using strategies (no GL) and (GL) respectively. None of them are obvious false positives.

4 Discussion

We have presented a new gap filling model using skeleton- and intensity-based information simultaneously, which separates non-oriented (in E and S) and oriented (in $\mathbf{D}$) communication between the different skeleton elements. Here, the oriented information $\mathbf{D}$ is only derived from the segment ends and gives soft preferential directions to fill the gaps. Therefore, it prevents unrealistic junctions.

Saliency to curvilinear structures S is only considered in a reasonable neighborhood around the segment ends, as it may make little sense at a large distance. Finally, the enhancement maps E can help to perform long distance connections with the soft constrains given by $\mathbf{D}$. In our results, obtained on real 3D tumour vasulature, the use of E in addition to S allowed us to fill additional large gaps and did not generate obvious false positive junctions. We believe this to be an encouraging result.

References

1. Bauer, C., Pock, T., Sorantin, E., Bischof, H., Beichel, R.: Segmentation of interwoven 3d tubular tree structures utilizing shape priors and graph cuts. Medical Image Analysis 14, 172–184 (2010)
2. Bekkers, E., Duits, R., Berendschot, T., ter Haar Romeny, B.: A Multi-Orientation Analysis Approach to Retinal Vessel Tracking. J. Math. Imaging and Vision 49, 583–610 (2014)
3. Cetin, S., Demir, A., Yezzi, A.J., Degertekin, M., Ünal, G.B.: Vessel Tractography Using an Intensity Based Tensor Model With Branch Detection. IEEE Trans. Med. Imaging 32, 348–363 (2013)
4. Guy, G., Medioni, G.: Inference of surfaces, 3-D curves, and junctions from sparse, noisy, 3-D data. IEEE Trans. Pat. Anal. Mach. Int. 26, 1265–1277 (1997)
5. Kaufhold, J.P., Tsai, P.S., Blinder, P., Kleinfeld, D.: Vectorization of optically sectioned brain microvasculature: Learning aids completion of vascular graphs by connecting gaps and deleting open-ended segments. Medical Image Analysis 16, 1241–1258 (2012)
6. Lesage, D., Angelini, E.D., Bloch, I., Funka-Lea, G.: A review of 3D vessel lumen segmentation techniques: Models, features and extraction schemes. Medical Image Analysis 13, 819–845 (2009)
7. Loss, L.A., Bebis, G., Parvin, B.: Iterative Tensor Voting for Perceptual Grouping of Ill-Defined Curvilinear Structures. IEEE Trans. Med. Imaging 30, 1503–1513 (2011)
8. Palágyi, K., Kuba, A.: A 3-D 6-subiteration thinning algorithm for extracting medial lines. Pattern Recogn. Lett. 19, 613–627 (1998)
9. Pock, T., Janko, C., Beichel, R., Bischof, H.: Multiscale medialness for robust segmentation of 3-d tubular structures. In: Proc. CVW Workshop (2005)
10. Quek, F.K.H., Kirbas, C.: Vessel extraction in medical images by wave-propagation and traceback. IEEE Trans. Med. Imaging 20, 117–131 (2001)
11. Risser, L., Plouraboué, F., Descombes, X.: Gap Filling in Vessel Networks by Skeletonization and Tensor Voting. IEEE Trans. Med. Imaging 27, 674–687 (2008)
12. Schneider, M., Hirsch, S., Weber, B., Székely, G., Menze, B.H.: TGIF: Topological Gap In-Fill for Vascular Networks. In: Golland, P., Hata, N., Barillot, C., Hornegger, J., Howe, R. (eds.) MICCAI 2014, Part II. LNCS, vol. 8674, pp. 89–96. Springer, Heidelberg (2014)
13. Szymczak, A., Tannenbaum, A., Mischaikow, K.: Coronary vessel cores from 3-d imagery: A topological approach. In: Proc. SPIE Med. Imag. (2005)
14. Xiao, C., Staring, M., Shamonin, D., Reiber, J.H., Stolk, J., Stoel, B.C.: A strain energy filter for 3D vessel enhancement with application to pulmonary CT images. Medical Image Analysis 15, 112–124 (2011)

A Continuous Flow-Maximisation Approach to Connectivity-Driven Cortical Parcellation

Sarah Parisot, Martin Rajchl,
Jonathan Passerat-Palmbach, and Daniel Rueckert

Biomedical Image Analysis Group, Department of Computing,
Imperial College London, UK

Abstract. Brain connectivity network analysis is a key step towards understanding the processes behind the brain's development through ageing and disease. Parcellation of the cortical surface into distinct regions is an essential step in order to construct such networks. Anatomical and random parcellations are typically used for this task, but can introduce a bias and may not be aligned with the brain's underlying organisation. To tackle this challenge, connectivity-driven parcellation methods have received increasing attention. In this paper, we propose a flexible continuous flow maximisation approach for connectivity driven parcellation that iteratively updates the parcels' boundaries and centres based on connectivity information and smoothness constraints. We evaluate the method on 25 subjects with diffusion MRI data. Quantitative results show that the method is robust with respect to initialisation (average overlap 82%) and significantly outperforms the state of the art in terms of information loss and homogeneity.

1 Introduction

Brain connectivity network analysis can provide key insights into the brain's organisation and its evolution through disease and ageing. Building these networks from functional (fMRI) or diffusion (dMRI) MR imaging is a challenge in itself due to the high dimensionality of the data. Therefore, network construction requires an initial parcellation stage of the cortical surface into distinct regions. While anatomical or random parcellations are used in most existing studies, they do not necessarily represent the brain's underlying connectivity accurately and can introduce a strong bias in the constructed network and its subsequent analysis [14].

In order to address the shortcomings of anatomical and random parcellations, connectivity driven brain parcellation has received an increasing amount of attention. In addition to providing a sensible basis for constructing connectivity networks, it can enable the identification of functionally specialised brain regions. The problem is typically cast as a clustering problem of the cortical surface vertices, where the goal is to maximise the correlation between connectivity profiles (dMRI) or time series (fMRI). While common clustering techniques can be used when parcellating a subset of the brain [1,8], the problem becomes more difficult

N. Navab et al. (Eds.): MICCAI 2015, Part III, LNCS 9351, pp. 165–172, 2015.
DOI: 10.1007/978-3-319-24574-4_20

when the aim is to parcellate the whole cortical surface. Hierarchical [3,10] and spectral clustering [5,13] based methods are the most popular approaches. However, the latter tends to create homogeneous parcel sizes, which can disagree with the brain's structure, while hierarchical clustering implies that regions boundaries are the same at different granularity levels. This can propagate errors from low to high resolution.

A Markov Random Field (MRF) based method for fMRI driven parcellation was proposed in [7]. It maximises the correlation between nodes and a parcel centre subject to smoothness constraints. The method considers all nodes (vertices on the cortical surface) as potential parcel centres and adds a penalty term at the introduction of a new label. The use of all nodes as parcel centres makes the method sensitive to noise and computationally very demanding. At the same time, there is no direct control on the number of parcels obtained.

In this paper, we propose an iterative MRF formulation to the parcellation problem based on the continuous flow-maximisation solver introduced in [15]. Each iteration consists of maximising the correlation between the nodes and parcel centres, as well as a smart update of the centres based on the cluster's homogeneity. A coarse to fine multi-resolution implementation allows to reduce the influence of noise while efficiently exploring the space for updates of the parcel centres. The experimental evaluation is performed on 25 subjects from the Human Connectome Project (HCP) database for dMRI driven parcellation. We show that the method is robust with respect to initialisation, and significantly outperforms existing methods in terms of information loss and parcel homogeneity.

2 Methodology

We consider a subject whose cortical surface is to be parcellated into a set of K parcels. The surface is represented as a mesh graph $\mathcal{S} = \{\mathcal{V}, \mathcal{E}\}$, where $\mathcal{V}$ corresponds to a set of N vertices and $\mathcal{E}$ to the edges between neighbouring vertices. The problem is simplified by inflating the cortical mesh to a sphere on which computations are performed. The graph is associated with an affinity matrix describing how dissimilar two nodes are in terms of connectivity. The correlation ρ between the vertices' connectivity profiles obtained from tractography (dMRI-driven) or times series (fMRI-driven) is a commonly employed measure.

2.1 Iterative Markov Random Field Formulation

We cast the connectivity driven parcellation task as a vertex labelling problem, where each graph node $\mathbf{v}$ is to be assigned a label $l \in [\![1, K]\!]$ based on its affinity with a predefined parcel centre c_l. We adopt a coarse to fine multi-level MRF formulation that iteratively evaluates the label assignments of the vertices and updates the parcel centres based on the current parcellation configuration.

We initialise each resolution level R with the construction of a regular icosahedron $\mathcal{S}^R$ of constant radius RAD and the smooth resampling of the data term D to the new resolution.

Assignment Stage: Given a set of parcel centres $C^t = \{\mathbf{c}_1^t, \cdots, \mathbf{c}_K^t\} \subset \mathcal{V}$, the first stage of each iteration t consists of minimising the following energy:

$$\begin{aligned} E^t(\mathbf{l}) &= \sum_{i=1}^{K} \int_{\mathcal{S}} D(\mathbf{c}_i^t, \mathbf{v}) dx + \alpha(\mathbf{v}) \sum_{i=1}^{K} |\partial \mathcal{S}_i| \\ \text{s.t.} \quad & \cup_{i=1}^{K} \mathcal{S}_i = \mathcal{S}, \quad \mathcal{S}_i \cap \mathcal{S}_j = \emptyset, \forall i \neq j \end{aligned} \tag{1}$$

where $\mathcal{S}_i = \{\mathbf{v} \in \mathcal{V} | l(\mathbf{v}) = i\}$ corresponds to the subdomain of $\mathcal{S}$ assigned to label l_i and $D(\mathbf{c}_i, \mathbf{v})$ is the distance between a vertex and a parcel centre. The first term of the equation assigns nodes to the parcel based on how similar they are to its centre, while the second term enforces smoothness of the parcellation by minimising the length of the boundary of each subdomain. The strength of the smoothness term is defined by the position dependent cost $\alpha(\mathbf{v})$.

Centre Update Stage: For each parcel $\mathcal{S}_i$ obtained during the assignment stage, the centre is defined based on the correlation between nodes within the parcel. The parcel centre should have strong connectivity information and be the most similar to the rest of the parcel:

$$\mathbf{c}_i^{t+1} = \arg\max_{\mathbf{v} \in \mathcal{S}_i} \sum_{\mathbf{w} \in \mathcal{S}_i} \rho(\mathbf{v}, \mathbf{w}) \tag{2}$$

This smart centre update enables to guide the parcels' position based on connectivity information. The coarse to fine approach enables to explore the centre space efficiently and to avoid local minima due to the presence of noise. Centres are propagated from one resolution level to the next by minimising the geodesic distance d_g between the parcel centre and the new resolution's vertices on the inflated mesh: $\mathbf{c}_i^{R+1} = \arg\min_{\mathbf{v} \in \mathcal{S}^{R+1}} d_g(\mathbf{v}, \mathbf{c}_i^R)$.

2.2 Continuous Max-Flow Optimisation

We minimise the assignment stage's MRF energy using the recently proposed Continuous MaxFlow (CMF) algorithm [15] that we adapt to triangular spherical meshes. This solver offers two significant advantages over discrete MRF optimisation approaches. First, it is highly paralellisable, and as a result very scalable with respect to the mesh size and number of desired parcels. Second, it provides a continuous labelling, which results in smoother parcel boundaries and a better exploration of the solution space.

Similarly to discrete s-t-mincut/maxflow MRF optimisation methods [4], the continuous maxflow model constructs a directed graph through the introduction of two terminal nodes (source s and sink t). The state of a mesh vertex $\mathbf{v}$ is given by three flows: the source $p^s(\mathbf{v})$ and sink flows $p^t(\mathbf{v})$ connecting $\mathbf{v}$ to both terminal nodes, and a spatial flow field $\mathbf{q}(\mathbf{v})$ connecting neighbouring vertices. In the multi-label setting, K copies of the surface mesh are constructed in parallel, each associated with label-wise spatial and sink flows $\mathbf{q}_i(\mathbf{v}), p_i^t(\mathbf{v}), i \in [\![1, K]\!]$, while $p^s(\mathbf{v})$ remains unique. The multi-label configuration is illustrated in Fig.1a.

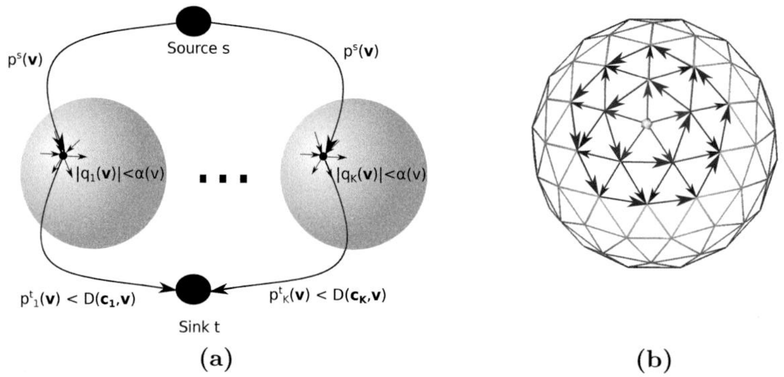

Fig. 1. (a) Configuration of the spherical CMF algorithm with K labels. (b) Spatial flow computation: from a starting vertex (marked), alternation between longitudinal (red arrows) and latitudinal (blue arrows) computation.

The three flows are subject to capacity and conservation constraints:

$$\begin{aligned} \forall i \in [\![1, K]\!], \quad |\mathbf{q}_i(\mathbf{v})| < \alpha(\mathbf{v}), \quad p_i^t(\mathbf{v}) < D(\mathbf{c}_i, \mathbf{v}) \\ \forall i \in [\![1, K]\!], \quad (\nabla \cdot \mathbf{q}_i - p^s + p_i^t)(\mathbf{v}) = 0 \end{aligned} \tag{3}$$

As a result, the CMF algorithm consists of maximising the total flow $p^s(\mathbf{v})$ from the source under the aforementioned constraints. The optimisation is based on the augmented Lagrangian method through the introduction of the indicator function $u_i(\mathbf{v}), i \in [\![1, K]\!]$, that have been shown to correspond to the optimal continuous labelling functions [15].

One of the main challenges associated to the new mesh space is to adapt the spatial flow computation task from a rectangular grid (image pixels and neighbours) to a triangular mesh with different neighbourhood configurations. We split the spatial flow into two components (see Fig.1b): a latitudinal and a longitudinal one (with varying number of components) that are computed alternatingly. This ensures that the flow can be computed in parallel in a consistent flow direction. The CMF optimisation is performed at each iteration until convergence. After convergence, the parcellation is obtained by selecting for each node the label that maximises the labelling function u_i. This iterative process is then repeated until convergence of the labelling function (minimal label update).

3 Results

We evaluated our method on 25 different subjects from the latest release of HCP, which were preprocessed following the HCPs minimum processing pipeline [6]. The cortical surfaces are represented as a triangular mesh of 32k vertices per hemisphere. Vertices corresponding to the medial wall are excluded from parcellations due to the lack of reliable connectivity information in this region. We tested the method on structural connectivity based parcellation obtained from

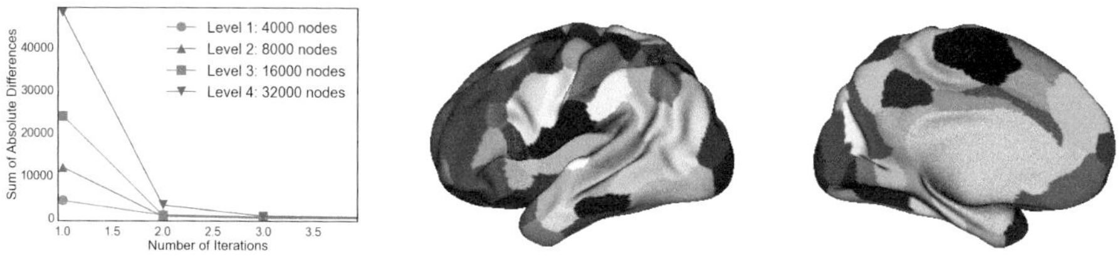

(a) (b)

Fig. 2. (a) Convergence of the labelling update at each resolution level: sum of absolute differences between the continuous labelling functions u_i of two consecutive iterations. (b) Associated parcellation after convergence.

20 different random initialisations via Poisson disc sampling, and four different number of labels (50, 100, 150 and 200 labels). We set the smoothness parameter $\alpha(\mathbf{v})$ to a constant to 0.1 over all vertices $\mathbf{v}$. Structural connectivity information is obtained from dMRI and tractography. The data term D is defined as $D(\mathbf{c}_i, \mathbf{v}) = 1 - \rho(\mathbf{c}_i, \mathbf{v})$, where ρ is the correlation between the vertices' connectivity profiles. The tractography matrix is obtained using FSLs bedpostX and probtrackX methods [2,9] which estimate the fibres orientation at each voxel with a ball and stick model, and perform probabilistic tractography respectively. Following [9], we fitted three fibre compartments per voxel. 5000 streamlines were sampled from each of the vertices. Each entry of the tractography matrix counts the number of streamlines sampled from vertex $\mathbf{v}$ that reach vertex $\mathbf{q}$.

Our framework consists of four resolution levels (32k, 16k, 8k and 4k nodes). The convergence at each level was monitored by computing the sum of absolute differences between two consecutive labellings functions u_i. As illustrated in Fig.2 for a randomly selected experiment, all four resolution levels converge through the different centres updates. As expected, the convergence rates vary with respect to the quality of the initialisation and number of nodes.

The reproducibility with respect to initialisation is evaluated by computing the Dice similarity coefficient (DSC) between same subject parcellations. Depending on the initialisation, certain parcels can be split in several subparcels but have the same overall boundary. To find correspondences between parcellations, we consider a pair of parcellations P_1 and P_2 obtained from different initialisations. Each parcel of P_1 is assigned to the parcel in P_2 that has the highest overlap. Parcels in P_1 are merged if they are assigned to the same parcel in P_2 (split parcel case). The same process is repeated for P_2 with respect to the updated parcellation P_1^*. The DSC between the matched parcellations is computed for all subjects, numbers of labels and initialisations. The values are compared to the DSC between the random initialisations as a baseline. For all numbers of labels, we consistently obtain an average DSC of 0.82 ± 0.01, while random initialisation only reaches 0.64 ± 0.02 on average. Figure 3 shows the comparison between example parcellations after matching, and the local average reproducibility of parcels. We can see that parcels boundaries are very similar

Table 1. Mean Kullback Leibler divergence (a) and parcel homogeneity (b) for all tested labels and methods. The best value is shown in bold. Statistically significant results: $^{*}p < 0.01$.

(a) Kullback Leibler divergence

Method	50 labels	100 labels	150 labels	200 labels
Random	2.67 ± 0.08	2.33 ± 0.08	2.09 ± 0.08	1.96 ± 0.08
Hierarchical	2.55 ± 0.08	2.15 ± 0.08	1.92 ± 0.07	1.80 ± 0.06
Spectral	2.54 ± 0.08	**2.10*** ± 0.08	1.89 ± 0.07	1.80 ± 0.07
Proposed	**2.50*** ± 0.09	2.16 ± 0.1	**1.87** ± 0.09	**1.74*** ± 0.07

(b) Homogeneity

Method	50 labels	100 labels	150 labels	200 labels
Random	0.11 ± 0.005	0.16 ± 0.008	0.19 ± 0.011	0.22 ± 0.015
Hierarchical	0.11 ± 0.006	0.16 ± 0.009	0.21 ± 0.013	0.24 ± 0.016
Spectral	0.11 ± 0.006	0.16 ± 0.009	0.20 ± 0.013	0.24 ± 0.015
Proposed	**0.12*** ± 0.006	**0.18*** ± 0.011	**0.22*** ± 0.015	**0.26*** ± 0.017

despite different initialisations. Figure 3b shows that some regions have consistently matching boundaries while others are more variable across initialisations. This could be due to the fact that the connectivity information in these regions is too weak or that the differences are too subtle to drive the parcellation task.

The quality of the parcellation is evaluated through computation of the average intra-cluster connectivity homogeneity [5], and the Kullback Leibler divergence (KLD) between the normalised tractography matrix and its approximation obtained after parcellation. The KLD evaluates the information loss caused by such approximation. KLD and homogeneity values are compared to the ones obtained by Poisson disc sampling (random parcellations), multi-scale spectral clustering (SC) [11], and hierarchical clustering (HC). Both spectral and hierarchical clustering are spatially constrained and based on an initial connectivity-driven oversegmentation of the cortical surface to adjust for the noise (2000 regions for HC; 500, 1000 and 2000 regions for the multi-scale SC). For each subject, we compute the average KLD for parcellations obtained from the different initialisations. As illustrated in Table 1a, we can observe that the average KLD outperforms spectral and hierarchical clustering at most resolutions. Paired T-tests of our proposed method with the three different methods (random, SC, HC) show that we obtain significantly better results ($p \leq 0.01$) for most label configurations. Furthermore, homogeneity measures show that we consistently obtain significantly better values for all label configurations ($p \leq 0.01$). Average homogeneity and KLD results are shown in Table 1b. Correspondences between our obtained parcel boundaries and cortical myelination are shown in Fig. 3c.

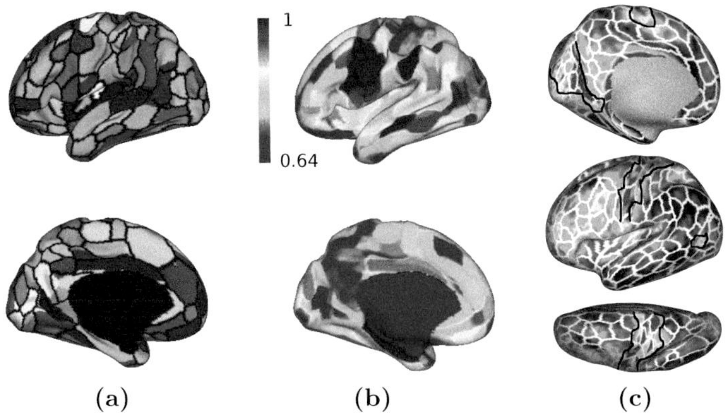

Fig. 3. (a,b) Reproducibility between initialisations: (a) A parcellation result is superimposed to the boundaries of a parcellation obtained with a different initialisation. (b) Local average DSC over all initialisations for the same subject. (c) Comparison of parcellation borders with cortical myelination. Parcel boundaries matching high myelin variations are highlighted.

4 Discussion

In this paper, we propose a continuous MRF model for connectivity-driven cortex parcellation. We develop a coarse to fine approach that iteratively updates parcel centres and the remaining nodes assignments. The inference is performed using a Continuous MaxFlow algorithm that is adapted to spherical meshes. We demonstrate the method's robustness with respect to initialisation and show that it significantly outperforms state-of-the-art clustering methods both in terms of information loss and homogeneity for most tested label configurations. The method is generalisable and can be applied to both fMRI and dMRI data. Furthermore, it is very flexible with respect to the definition of the cost function and smoothness term. For instance, it is straightforward to implement data-driven or inter-subject pairwise costs for groupwise parcellation. Other applications could also be considered, such as MRF based cortical registration [12]. The continuous solver could prove very useful in this kind of set up for finding a smooth deformation field. In order to show the robustness of the method, we have presented parcellation results obtained with a poor initialisation that has no correlation with the underlying connectivity. A smart centre initialisation would provide faster convergence, and potentially better consistency in less reproducible regions where the information from the tractography matrix is not strong enough. Identifying the regions that are the most reproducible also enables to identify where the connectivity information can be relied upon. This could provide interesting insight into multi-modal analysis of functional and structural data.

Acknowledgments. Data were provided by the Human Connectome Project, WU-Minn Consortium (Principal Investigators: David Van Essen and Kamil Ugurbil; 1U54MH091657). The research leading to these results has received funding from the European Union's Seventh Framework Programme (FP/2007-2013) / ERC Grant Agreement no. 319456.

References

1. Anwander, A., Tittgemeyer, M., von Cramon, D.Y., Friederici, A.D., Knösche, T.R.: Connectivity-based parcellation of Broca's area. Cereb. Cortex 17(4), 816–825 (2007)
2. Behrens, T., Berg, H.J., Jbabdi, S., Rushworth, M., Woolrich, M.: Probabilistic diffusion tractography with multiple fibre orientations: What can we gain? NeuroImage 34(1), 144–155 (2007)
3. Blumensath, T., Jbabdi, S., Glasser, M.F., Van Essen, D.C., Ugurbil, K., Behrens, T.E., Smith, S.M.: Spatially constrained hierarchical parcellation of the brain with resting-state fMRI. NeuroImage 76, 313–324 (2013)
4. Boykov, Y., Funka-Lea, G.: Graph cuts and efficient ND image segmentation. International Journal of Computer Vision 70(2), 109–131 (2006)
5. Craddock, R.C., James, G.A., Holtzheimer, P.E., Hu, X.P., Mayberg, H.S.: A whole brain fMRI atlas generated via spatially constrained spectral clustering. Hum. Brain Mapp. 33, 1914–1928 (2012)
6. Glasser, M.F., Sotiropoulos, S.N., Wilson, J.A., Coalson, T.S., Fischl, B., Andersson, J.L., Xu, J., Jbabdi, S., Webster, M., Polimeni, J.R., Essen, D.C.V., Jenkinson, M.: The minimal preprocessing pipelines for the Human Connectome Project. NeuroImage 80, 105–124 (2013)
7. Honnorat, N., Eavani, H., Satterthwaite, T., Gur, R., Gur, R., Davatzikos, C.: GraSP: Geodesic Graph-based Segmentation with Shape Priors for the functional parcellation of the cortex. NeuroImage 106, 207–221 (2015)
8. Jbabdi, S., Woolrich, M.W., Behrens, T.E.: Multiple-subjects connectivity-based parcellation using hierarchical Dirichlet process mixture models. NeuroImage 44, 373–384 (2009)
9. Jbabdi, S., Sotiropoulos, S.N., Savio, A.M., Graña, M., Behrens, T.E.J.: Model-based analysis of multishell diffusion MR data for tractography: How to get over fitting problems. Magn. Reson. Med. 68(6), 1846–1855 (2012)
10. Moreno-Dominguez, D., Anwander, A., Knösche, T.R.: A hierarchical method for whole-brain connectivity-based parcellation. Hum. Brain Mapp. 35, 5000–5025 (2014)
11. Parisot, S., Arslan, S., Passerat-Palmbach, J., Wells III, W.M., Rueckert, D.: Tractography-driven groupwise multi-scale parcellation of the cortex. In: IPMI (2015, in press)
12. Robinson, E.C., Jbabdi, S., Glasser, M.F., Andersson, J., Burgess, G.C., Harms, M.P., Smith, S.M., Van Essen, D.C., Jenkinson, M.: MSM: A new flexible framework for Multimodal Surface Matching. Neuroimage 100, 414–426 (2014)
13. Shen, X., Tokoglu, F., Papademetris, X., Constable, R.: Groupwise whole-brain parcellation from resting-state fMRI data for network node identification. NeuroImage 82, 403–415 (2013)
14. Sporns, O.: The human connectome: a complex network. Ann. NY Acad. Sci. 1224, 109–125 (2011)
15. Yuan, J., Bae, E., Tai, X.C., Boykov, Y.: A continuous max-flow approach to potts model. In: Daniilidis, K., Maragos, P., Paragios, N. (eds.) ECCV 2010, Part VI. LNCS, vol. 6316, pp. 379–392. Springer, Heidelberg (2010)

A 3D Fractal-Based Approach towards Understanding Changes in the Infarcted Heart Microvasculature*

Polyxeni Gkontra[1], Magdalena M. Żak[1], Kerri-Ann Norton[2], Andrés Santos[3], Aleksander S. Popel[2], and Alicia G. Arroyo[1]

[1] Centro Nacional de Investigaciones Cardiovasculares Carlos III (CNIC), Madrid, Spain
[2] Department of Biomedical Engineering, School of Medicine, Johns Hopkins University, Baltimore, MD, US
[3] Universidad Politécnica de Madrid and CIBERBBN, Spain

Abstract. The structure and function of the myocardial microvasculature affect cardiac performance. Quantitative assessment of microvascular changes is therefore crucial to understanding heart disease. This paper proposes the use of 3D fractal-based measures to obtain quantitative insight into the changes of the microvasculature in infarcted and non-infarcted (remote) areas, at different time-points, following myocardial infarction. We used thick slices ($\sim 100\mu$m) of pig heart tissue, stained for blood vessels and imaged with high resolution microscope. Firstly, the cardiac microvasculature was segmented using a novel 3D multi-scale multi-thresholding approach. We subsequently calculated: i) fractal dimension to assess the complexity of the microvasculature; ii) lacunarity to assess its spatial organization; and iii) succolarity to provide an estimation of the microcirculation flow. The measures were used for statistical change analysis and classification of the distinct vascular patterns in infarcted and remote areas, demonstrating the potential of the approach to extract quantitative knowledge about infarction-related alterations.

1 Introduction

Cardiovascular diseases (CVDs) result in the alteration of microvasculature [14]. Therefore, there is increased interest in gaining deeper knowledge of the microvascular patterns and their changes during the development of CVDs in an effort to identify the underlying biological mechanisms and develop more efficient therapeutic approaches. Advances in imaging systems, particularly in high

* This research is funded by the European Commission (FP7-PEOPLE-2013-ITN 'CardioNext', No. 608027) and La Marató de TV3 Foundation. CNIC is supported by the MINECO and the Pro-CNIC Foundation. Kerri-Ann Norton is funded by the American Cancer Society Postdoctoral Fellowship. The authors would like to thank Jaume Agüero for performing the infarction in the pigs.

N. Navab et al. (Eds.): MICCAI 2015, Part III, LNCS 9351, pp. 173–180, 2015.
DOI: 10.1007/978-3-319-24574-4_21

resolution microscopy, allow visualization at sub-micrometer resolution and increasing depths of the three-dimensional (3D) microvasculature [13], which is inaccessible by other imaging technologies.

However, understanding and identifying changes in the 3D structure of the microvasculature not only requires the use of state-of-the-art imaging techniques, but also the use of unbiased image analysis methods that allow the translation of qualitative biological observations into quantitative knowledge. Furthermore, automatic 3D image analysis allows extracting information not attainable from traditional manual analysis, and at the same time, diminishes subjectivity problems, time and labor requirements, of both manual and supervised analysis.

Nevertheless, even in the case of automatic analysis, the problem of identifying measures that can optimally describe highly complex structures, their changes and structural-function relations remains a challenging task. Traditional analysis provide information of paramount importance regarding vessel structure and function, but is insufficient when dealing with complex objects [7], such as biological samples, which can be self -similar, i.e. fractals. The concept of fractals was introduced by [10] and ever since they have been applied in a variety of image analysis and pattern recognition problems. In the biomedical field, they found great appeal in the study of vascular networks [9].

This paper provides a quantitative approach of describing changes that occur to the cardiac microvasculature at different time-points, after myocardial infarction (MI), at remote and infarcted regions. To achieve this, while also accommodating the complex and multi-scale properties of the microvasculature, a 3D fractal-based approach was followed. To the best of our knowledge this is the first effort made to apply a complete 3D fractal-based analysis (fractal dimension, lacunarity, succolarity) to quantitatively assess progressive MI-related changes of the microvascular patterns. In biological terms, the higher the fractal dimension, the higher the morphological complexity is, i.e. the number of microvessels. The higher the lacunarity, the more heterogeneous the gap distribution and as a result the blood supply within the tissue is. The higher the succolarity, the larger the amount of blood that can flow in the vessels, thus the better the oxygenation. Furthermore, a simple, but efficient, 3D method is proposed for the segmentation of vascular structures from images stained for blood vessels.

2 Methods

2.1 Data Acquisition and Pre-processing

All experiments were approved by the Institutional Animal Research Committee. Three adult male Large-White pigs were anesthetized and acute MI was induced using an angioplasty balloon with 30-minute occlusion of the left anterior descending coronary artery followed by reperfusion. The pigs were sacrificed 1, 3 and 7 days after reperfusion.

Tissue samples from both infarcted and remote areas from each left ventricle were collected. Samples were fixed with 0.4% paraformaldehyde, embedded in

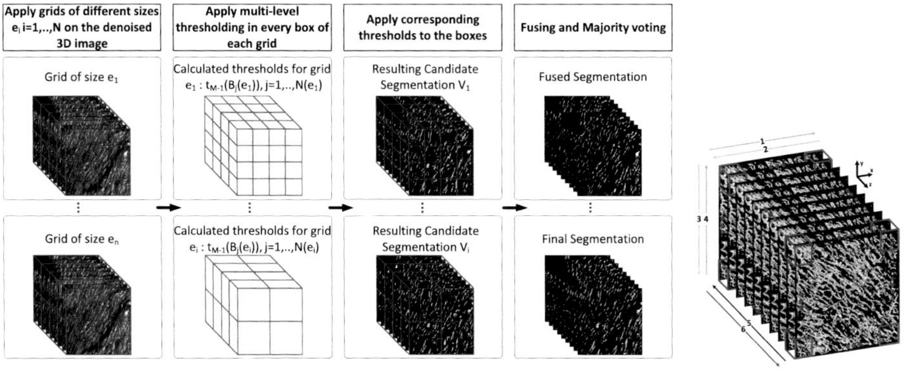

(a) (b)

Fig. 1. (a) Overview of MMT method. (b) Possible directions of blood flow through the segmented microvasculature; horizontal flow from left to right (arrow 1) and vice versa (arrow 2), vertical flow from up to down (arrow 3) and vice versa (arrow 4), and in depth blood flow from upper to lower slices (arrow 5) and vice versa (arrow 6).

OCT and frozen down. Thick sections ($\sim 100\mu$m) were obtained in the cryostat, stained in flotation for the microvasculature with primary antibody anti-VE-Cadherin (Santa Cruz) 1:100, and incubated with secondary antibodies, Alexa-Fluor 568 (Molecular probes) 1:500 and Hoechst (Life Technologies) 1:10000.

Spectral imaging was performed with a Leica SP5 confocal microscopy using emission from a $561nm$ laser and $40\times/1.25$N.A. oil immersion lens. Z-stack slices (1024×1024 pixels) were acquired every $1\mu m$ by applying the deepness correction setup. The resulting voxel size was $0.3785\mu m \times 0.3785\mu m \times 1.007\mu m$.

Prior to proceeding with the analysis, Non-Local Means Filtering [4], was adapted for enhancing the quality of the images.

2.2 Segmentation

A 3D multi-scale multi-level thresholding approach (MMT) was developed for the segmentation of the labeled vessels from confocal images, inspired by the box counting (BC) method [3] and Otsu's multi-level thresholding method [12].

Grids of varying size e were overlaid onto the image under investigation. Subsequently, the multi-level thresholding was applied to each box $B_j(e), j = 1, ..., N(e)$ of the grid with size e in order to calculate the M intensity classes that maximize the inter-class variance within the box. For every grid, $N(e)$ thresholds (t_M), as many as the boxes that composed it, were therefore calculated and applied to the corresponding box. In total, k candidate segmentations $V_i, i = 1, .., k$ were produced, one per grid size e, as a mosaic of the application of the $N(e)$ thresholds on the boxes. Only voxels that belong to the two classes with higher intensity $(M-1, M)$ were considered as parts of the microvasculature. Thus,

$$V_i(u) = \begin{cases} 1, I(u) \geq t_{(M-1)}(B_j(e)) \\ 0, I(u) < t_{(M-1)}(B_j(e)) \ . \end{cases} \qquad (1)$$

where voxel $u = (x, y, z) \in B_j(e)$ and I the original image.

Subsequently, candidate segmentations $V_i, i = 1, .., k$ had to be fused into a single segmentation. To achieve this, majority rule voting applied:

$$V(u) = \frac{\sum_{i=1,..,k} w_i V_i(u)}{\sum_{i=1,..,k} w_i} , \tag{2}$$

where w_i are the weights that define the degree to which candidate segmentation V_i will contribute to the final segmentation and were set to 1 considering equal contribution of all candidate segmentations.

An overview of the MMT method is presented in Fig. 1 (a). It is worth mentioning that in the traditional BC, cubic boxes compose the grid. However, here, boxes of size $e \times e \times e_z$ with $e_z = 10 < e = 2^5, .., N$, were used in order to accommodate for the smaller size of our images along z-direction and to cover a wide range of scales while ignoring the smaller ones that provide a very limited region for variance calculation.

2.3 Fractal-Based Methods

Fractal Dimension. A variety of methods have been proposed for the calculation of fractal dimension [8]. Among them, the box-counting method (BC), which is the most popular and widely used approach, was applied in this work. Grids of cubic boxes of size e are overlaid on the original image. Subsequently, the fractal dimension(F_d) is defined as the negative slope of the bi-logarithmic plot of the number of boxes N_e needed to cover the microvasculature as a function of the box size e. Thus,

$$F_d = -\lim_{e \to 0} \frac{\log(N_e)}{\log(e)} . \tag{3}$$

However, real-life objects might not present self-similarity over an infinite range of scales but rather over finite [9,2]. To deal with this limitation, we followed the procedure presented in [2] to identify cut-offs scales for which the microvasculature can no longer be considered as fractal. However, no statistically significant difference was observed between the calculation of fractal dimension with and without cut-offs and the former is presented in this document.

Lacunarity. The gliding box (GB) method [1] was used for the calculation of lacunarity L. According to the GB method, boxes of different sizes are glided every 1 voxel over the image and the number of voxels inside the boxes belonging to the structure of interest, i.e. voxels with value 1, are calculated and represent box mass M. Therefore, for each box size e, lacunarity is calculated by the first and second moments of inertia of mass distribution

$$L(e) = \frac{\sum_{e=1,..,N} M(e)P(M,e)}{\sum_{e=1,..,N} M(e)^2 P(M,e)} , \tag{4}$$

where $P(M,e) = \frac{n(M,e)}{N(e)}$, $n(M,e)$ stands for the number of boxes with mass M and $N(e)$ for the number of boxes of size e.

When comparing images with different densities, one limitation presented by lacunarity is its dependence on image density. To tackle this incompatibility, we used the normalized lacunarity (L_{norm}) as proposed by [5],

$$L_{norm}(e) = 2 - (\frac{1}{L(e)} + \frac{1}{cL(e)}) , \quad (5)$$

where $cL(e)$ is the lacunarity the complemented image ($cL(e)$). This formulation results in lacunarity values that are in the range $[0, 1]$, allowing comparison among images with different densities. The lacunarity over all scales is defined by the mean along all scales.

Succolarity. Although succolarity (S) was firstly described by Mandelbrot [10], the first formal definition and method for its calculation, based on an adaption of BC method, was proposed recently by [11]. In brief, regions, i.e. blood vessels in the case of this study, that a fluid, i.e. blood, can flow are represented by 1 while obstacles to the fluid with 0. For the 3D case, 6 different directions that the blood can flow through the vascular structure are defined as shown in Fig. 1(b).

A segmented image V is therefore decomposed in six 3D images V_d one per direction $d = 1,..,6$. Subsequently, the BC method is applied to each V_d. The number of voxels with value 1 is calculated $n(e)$, as well as the pressure (P) of the flow in each box by the coordinates of the centroid of the box, following the direction under investigation. The normalized succolarity is given by

$$S(d, e) = \frac{\sum_{e=1,..,N} O(e)P(e)}{\sum_{e=1,..,N} P(e)} , \quad (6)$$

where $O = \frac{n(e)}{e}$ stands for the occupation percentage of boxes of size e.

Ultimately, in this work, overall succolarity was approximated by its maximum value among all 6 directions, i.e. the dominant direction of blood flow.

3 Results

Fifty-four 3D confocal images, nine for each tissue category, were used for the analysis of the infarcted heart microvasculature. For simplicity, images corresponding to tissue from infarcted and remote areas, 1 day, 3 and 7 days post MI were abbreviated as I1MI, R1MI, I3MI, R3MI, I7MI, and R7MI.

Firstly, the outcome of the multi-scale multi-thresholding method was visually evaluated by an experienced biologist in order to avoid bias in the analysis due to erroneously segmented images. In solely one case out of fifty-five the segmentation outcome was considered unsatisfactory.

In order to quantify alterations in the complexity, gap distribution and/or microcirculation of the microvasculature, as expressed quantitatively by fractal dimension, lacunarity and succolarity, statistical change analysis was performed. To achieve this, we applied Wilcoxon rank sum tests and Multi-variate analysis of variances (MANOVA) to perform pairwise comparisons of the characteristics

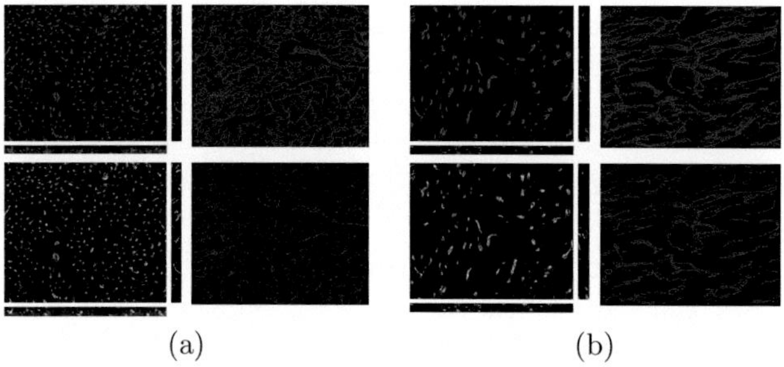

Image	(a)	(b)
Fd	2.3	2.1
L_{norm}	0.7	0.8
S	0.008	0.003

Fig. 2. Example segmentations by means of MMT method (first row) and of traditional multi-level thresholding (second row) from remote (a) and from infarcted area (b) along with the corresponding 3D fractal measures. The segmented vessels are presented with red on the slices along x-y,y-z,x-z (right) and on the 3D reconstructions (left).

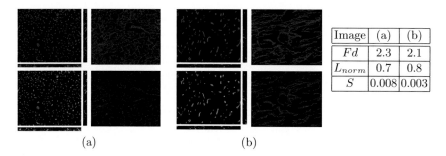

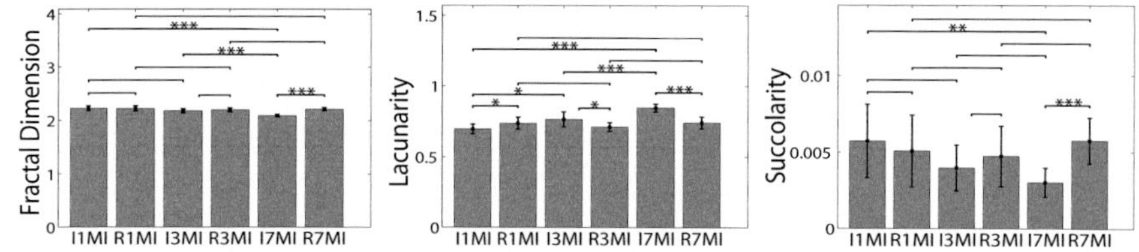

Fig. 3. Statistical comparison by means of (i) Fractal Dimension, (ii) Lacunarity, (iii) Succolarity, where *, ** and *** represent p-value< 0.05, 0.01 and 0.001 respectively.

Table 1. Multivariate Anova. P-values for cases that the null hypotheses is rejected at the 1 % significance level are shown in bold.

I1MI - R1MI	$\mathbf{p = 0.0039}$	I1MI - I3MI	$p = 0.056$	R1MI - R3MI	$p = 0.0122$
I3MI - R3MI	$p = 0.0702$	**I1MI - I7MI**	$\mathbf{p < 10^{-9}}$	R1MI - R7MI	$p = 0.0367$
I7MI - R7MI	$\mathbf{p = 10^{-6}}$	**I3MI - I7MI**	$\mathbf{p < 10^{-7}}$	R3MI - R7MI	$p = 0.2383$

Table 2. Accuracy (%) in classifying the distinct vascular patterns using different classifiers: (1) Knn, (2) SVM, (3) Adaboost.

Classifier	1	2	3	Classifier	1	2	3	Classifier	1	2	3
I1MI - R1MI	58	73	75	**I1MI - I3MI**	58	75	83	**R1MI - R3MI**	68	73	79
I3MI - R3MI	64	71	57	**I1MI - I7MI**	100	100	100	**R1MI - R7MI**	52	57	72
I7MI - R7MI	100	100	100	**I3MI - I7MI**	79	100	86	**R3MI - R7MI**	53	60	65

of the microvasculature from infarcted vs remote areas at all time-points, and of the same tissue area progressively in time.

Fig. 2 provides examples of the performances of MMT method and traditional multi-level thresholding on two images of our dataset, along with the calculated metrics for comparison purposes.

Table 1 provides the p-values for all pairwise comparisons performed by means of MANOVA. The null hypothesis, that there is no statistically significant differences between the infarct and remote areas, was rejected in the case of I1MI vs R1MI and in that of I7MI vs R7MI. This implies significant differences regarding the space filling properties of the microvessels (fractal dimension, lacunarity) and microcirculation. Of particular interest is the fact that 3 days after MI the null hypothesis is not rejected. This, in conjunction with recent work by [6] on the bimodal pattern of edema after MI, makes the study of changes at 3 days post MI a point for further investigation. I1MI and I3MI differ significantly from I7MI, but not among them, while remote areas at different time-points present no significant differences.

Fig. 3 presents plots which indicate mean values, standard deviations and p-values, resulting from Wilcoxon rank sum tests, for the statistical change comparison in terms of each fractal measure independently. A statistically significant decreased complexity, expressed by fractal dimension, was observed between I1MI and I3MI, when compared with I7MI. In contrast, a progressively increased varying distribution of gaps was observed by means of lacunarity. This inversely proportional relation between fractal dimension and lacunarity might be related to a wider range of sizes of microvessels. In fact, 7 days post MI apart from capillaries, larger vessels were observed, as also reported in the canine MI model [15]. Moreover, by comparing succolarity in infarcted areas 1 and 7 days post MI, functional changes related with microcirculation were added to the structural, expressed by fractal dimension and lacunarity. As it might have been expected, there was no measure that presented significant differences for remote areas at progressing time-points. As far as between infarcted and remote areas comparisons are concerned, gap distribution, presented statistically significant differences at all time-points under comparison, which makes lacunarity the most sensitive among the measures compared. Differences between remote and infarcted areas became clear in terms of all metrics only 7 days post MI.

Ultimately, we incorporated the metrics into a classification scheme. The classifiers used are, (i) K-nearest neighbor classifier (knn), (ii) Support Vector Machines (SVM), and (iii) Adaboost [17]. In all cases, 9-fold cross validation repeated 100 times was used. Accuracy rates (%) are presented in Table 2. The classifiers demonstrated similar behavior with higher accuracy in those pairs of comparisons for which MANOVA had demonstrated differences. In addition, Adaboost and SVM classifiers achieved more than 70 and 75 % accuracy respectively, for all of those cases. This demonstrates the power of fractal measures to describe and identify between different microvascular patterns post infarction.

4 Conclusions

We proposed the use of a 3D fractal-based approach to quantify infarction-related changes of the microvasculature at three different time-points after MI. 3D confocal images stained for blood vessels of both infarcted and remote areas were used. The animal model chosen was the pig due to its high translational value related with the similarity of its coronary artery anatomy and distribution to those of humans [16].

Statistically significant changes in terms of structure (fractal dimension and lacunarity) and function (succolarity) were detected by means of significance tests and MANOVA. Furthermore, relatively high rates of correct classification of unseen 3D microvascular images into distinct tissue categories, based on just their complexity, gap distribution and dominant blood flow as expressed by the applied fractal measures, demonstrate their potential to describe and recognize characteristics and changes due to infarction at the microvascular level.

References

1. Allain, C., Cloitre, M.: Characterising the lacunarity of random and deterministic fractal sets. Phys. Rev. Lett. 44, 3552–3558 (1991)
2. Berntson, G.M., Stoll, P.: Correcting for Finite Spatial Scales of Self-Similarity When Calculating Fractal Dimensions of Real-World Structures. Proceedings of the Royal Society B: Biological Sciences 264(1387), 1531–1537 (1997)
3. Block, A., von Bloh, W., Schellnhuber, H.J.: Efficient box-counting determination of generalized Fractal Dimensions. Physical Review A 42, 1869–1874 (1990)
4. Buades, A., Coll, B., Morel, J.-M.: A non-local algorithm for image denoising. In: CVPR (2), pp. 60–65 (2005)
5. Dougherty, G., Henebry, G.M.: Fractal signature and lacunarity in the measurement of the texture of trabecular bone in clinical CT images. Med. Eng. Phys. 23(6), 369–380 (2001)
6. Fernández-Jiménez, R., Sánchez-González, J., Agüero, J., et al.: Myocardial Edema After Ischemia/Reperfusion Is Not Stable and Follows a Bimodal Pattern: Imaging and Histological Tissue Characterization. J. Am. Coll. Cardiol. 65(4), 315–323 (2015)
7. Gould, D.J., Vadakkan, T.J., Poché, R.A., Dickinson, M.E.: Multifractal and Lacunarity Analysis of Microvascular Morphology and Remodeling. Microcirculation 18(2), 136–151 (2011)
8. Lopes, R., Betrouni, N.: Fractal and multifractal analysis: a review. Med. Image Anal. 13(4), 634–649 (2009)
9. Lorthois, S., Cassot, F.: Fractal analysis of vascular networks: insights from morphogenesis. J. Theor. Biol. 262(4), 614–633 (2010)
10. Mandelbrot, B.B.: Fractal geometry of nature. Freeman, New York (1977)
11. Melo, R.H.C., Conci, A.: How Succolarity could be used as another fractal measure in image analysis. Telecommunication Systems 52(3), 1643–1655 (2013)
12. Otsu, N.: A Threshold Selection Method from Gray-Level Histograms. IEEE Transactions on Systems, Man, and Cybernetics 9(1), 62–66 (1979)
13. Pawley, J.B.: Handbook of Biological Confocal Microscopy. Springer (2006)
14. Petersen, J.W., Pepine, C.J.: Microvascular coronary dysfunction and ischemic heart disease: Where are we in 2014? Trends Cardiovasc. Med. 25(2), 98–103 (2015)
15. Ren, G., Michael, L.H., Entman, M.L., Frangogiannis, N.G.: Morphological characteristics of the microvasculature in healing myocardial infarcts. J. Histochem. Cytochem. 50(1), 71–79 (2002)
16. Weaver, M.E., Pantely, G.A., Bristow, J.D., Ladley, H.D.: A quantitative study of the anatomy and distribution of coronary arteries in swine in comparison with other animals and man. Cardiovasc. Res. 20(12), 907–917 (1986)
17. Wu, X., Kumar, V., Quinlan, J.R., et al.: Top 10 algorithms in data mining. Knowledge and Information Systems 14(1), 1–37 (2008)

Segmenting the Uterus in Monocular Laparoscopic Images without Manual Input

Toby Collins, Adrien Bartoli, Nicolas Bourdel, and Michel Canis

ALCoV-ISIT, UMR 6284 CNRS/Université d'Auvergne, Clermont-Ferrand, France

Abstract. Automatically segmenting organs in monocular laparoscopic images is an important and challenging research objective in computer-assisted intervention. For the uterus this is difficult because of high inter-patient variability in tissue appearance and low-contrast boundaries with the surrounding peritoneum. We present a framework to segment the uterus which is completely automatic, requires only a single monocular image, and does not require a 3D model. Our idea is to use a patient-independent uterus detector to roughly localize the organ, which is then used as a supervisor to train a patient-specific organ segmenter. The segmenter uses a physically-motivated organ boundary model designed specifically for illumination in laparoscopy, which is fast to compute and gives strong segmentation constraints. Our segmenter uses a lightweight CRF that is solved quickly and globally with a single graphcut. On a dataset of 220 images our method obtains a mean DICE score of 92.9%.

1 Introduction and Background

The problem of segmenting organs in monocular laparoscopic images without any manual input is important yet unsolved for computer assisted laparoscopic surgery. This is challenging due to multiple factors including inter and intra-patient tissue appearance variability, low-contrast and/or ambiguous organ boundaries, texture inhomogeneity, bleeding, motion blur, partial views, surgical intervention and lens smears. In previous works a manual operator has been needed to identify the organ in one or more training images [3,11]. From these images, models of patient-specific tissue appearance can be learned and used to segment the organ in other images. We present the first methodology to accurately segment an organ in laparosurgery *without any manual input*. Our solution is simple, fast and does not require separate training images, since training and segmentation is performed on the same image. We also do not require patient-specific prior knowledge such as a pre-operative 3D model. Using a 3D model requires registration [11] to give the segmentation (*i.e. segmentation-by-registration*). This shifts the problem burden to registration, which itself is hard to do automatically and reliably for soft organs and monocular laparoscopes [10]. Our approach uses recent work in patient-generic organ detection in laparoscopic images [13]. It was shown that the uterus can be reliably detected in an image *without* patient specific knowledge using a state-of-the-art 2D Deformable Part Model (DPM) detector [8,15] trained on a uterus image database. The problem

N. Navab et al. (Eds.): MICCAI 2015, Part III, LNCS 9351, pp. 181–189, 2015.
DOI: 10.1007/978-3-319-24574-4_22

of segmentation however was not considered, which is a fundamentally different problem.

For a given image our goal is to compute the binary label matrix $\mathcal{L}(\mathbf{x}) \in \{0, 1\}$ where $\mathcal{L}(\mathbf{x}) = 1$ means pixel $\mathbf{x}$ is on the organ and $\mathcal{L}(\mathbf{x}) = 0$ means it is not. We refer to these as the foreground and background labels respectively. We propose an energy minimisation-based approach to solve $\mathcal{L}$ that incorporates information from the DPM detector to define the energy function. The function is a submodular discrete Conditional Random Field (CRF) that is globally optimised with a *single* graphcut. Much inspiration has come from graphcut-based interactive image segmentation methods [2,14,12] where manual strokes or bounding boxes are used to guide the segmentation. Instead of user interaction, we do this using information from the DPM detector, which in contrast to user interaction information is inherently uncertain. A second major difference is that most graphcut-based methods for optical images use the contrast-sensitive Ising prior from [2], which encourages segmentation boundaries at strong intensity step-edges (*i.e.* points with strong first-order intensity derivatives). However step-edges do not accurately model the appearance of an organ's boundary in laparoscopic images. We show that far better segmentations are obtained using a physically-motivated *trough-sensitive Ising prior*, which is computed from the response of a positive Laplacian of Gaussian (LoG^+) filter (*i.e.* a LoG filter with negative responses truncated to zero). This encourages segmentation boundaries at points with strongly positive *second-order* intensity derivatives.

2 Methodology

Segmentation pipeline. The main components of our method are illustrated in Fig. 1, which processes an image in five stages. In stage 1 we detect the presence of the organ with the DPM uterus detector from [13]. We take the detector's highest-confidence detection and if it exceeds the detector's threshold we assume the organ is visible and proceed with segmentation. The highest-confidence detection has an associated bounding box $\mathcal{B}$, which gives a rough localisation of the organ. In stage 2 we use $\mathcal{B}$ to train rough appearance models for the organ and background, which are used in the CRF as colour-based segmentation cues. Similarly to GrabCut [14] we use Gaussian Mixture Models (GMMs) with parameters denoted by θ_{fg} and θ_{bg} respectively. However unlike GrabCut, we do not iteratively recompute the GMM parameters and the segmentation. This is because with our organ boundary model, the first segmentation is usually very accurate even if the appearance parameters are not. This has the advantage of reduced computation time since we only perform one graphcut.

In stage 3 we use the detection's bounding box to extract a Region Of Interest (ROI) $\mathcal{R}$ around the organ, and all pixels outside $\mathcal{R}$ are labelled background. This reduces computation time because pixels outside $\mathcal{R}$ are not included in the CRF. One cannot naively set $\mathcal{R}$ as the detection's bounding box because there is no guarantee that it will encompass the whole organ, as seen in Fig. 2, bottom row. We normalise $\mathcal{R}$ to have a default width of 200 pixels, which gives sufficiently high resolution to accurately segment the uterus. The normalisation step is important because it means the CRF energy is independent of the organ's scale. Therefore we do not need to adapt any parameters depending on the organ's physical size, distance to the camera or camera focal length. In stage 4 we construct the CRF which includes information from three important sources. The first is colour information from the foreground and background colour models. The second is edge information from the response of a LoG$^+$ filter applied to $\mathcal{R}$. The third are spatial priors that give energy to pixels depending on where they are in $\mathcal{R}$. All of the CRF energy terms are submodular which means it can be solved globally and quickly using the maxflow algorithm. In practice this takes between 20-50ms with a standard desktop CPU implementation.

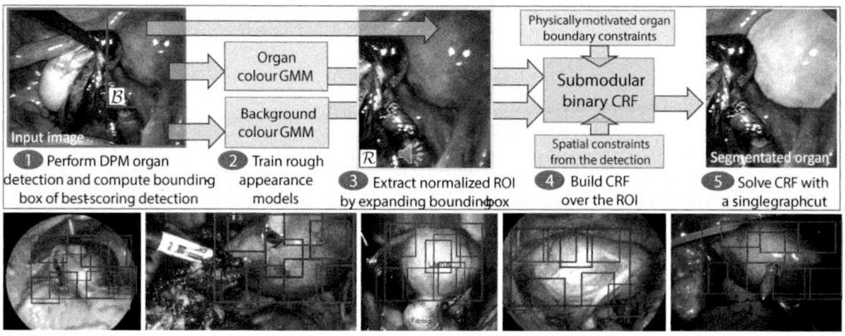

Fig. 1. Proposed framework for segmenting the uterus in a monocular laparoscopic image without manual input. The top row shows the five processing stages and the bottom row shows example uterus detections using the DPM detector [13,8].

The CRF energy function. The CRF is defined over the ROI $\mathcal{R}$, which is computed by enlarging the bounding box to encompass all likely foreground pixels. This is done by scaling the bounding box about its centre $\mathbf{x}_b$ by a factor of $x\%$. We set this very conservatively to $x = 60\%$, which means all foreground pixels will be within $\mathcal{R}$ when the bounding box of the detection overlaps the ground truth bounding box by at least $\approx 40\%$. In practice we do not normally obtain detections with less than 40% overlap with the ground truth bounding box, because the corresponding detection score would normally be too low to trigger a detection. The CRF energy E is conditioned on $\mathcal{R}$ and $\mathcal{B}$ and is as follows:

$$\begin{aligned} E(\mathcal{L};\mathcal{R},\mathcal{B}) &\stackrel{\text{def}}{=} E_{app}(\mathcal{L};\mathcal{R}) + \lambda_{edge}E_{edge}(\mathcal{L};\mathcal{R}) + \lambda_{spatial}E_{spatial}(\mathcal{L};\mathcal{R},\mathcal{B}) \\ E_{app}(\mathcal{L};\mathcal{R}) &\stackrel{\text{def}}{=} \textstyle\sum_{\mathbf{x}\in\mathcal{R}} \mathcal{L}(\mathbf{x})E'_{app}(\mathbf{x};\theta_{fg}) + (1-\mathcal{L}(\mathbf{x}))E'_{app}(\mathbf{x};\theta_{bg}) \end{aligned} \qquad (1)$$

The first term E_{app} denotes the *appearance energy*, which is a standard unary term that encourages pixel labels to agree with the foreground and background GMM models [14]. The term $E'_{app}(\mathbf{x};\theta)$ denotes the negative density of a GMM parameterised by θ. The terms E_{edge} and $E_{spatial}$ denote the edge and spatial energies, which are unary and pairwise clique energies respectively. The terms λ_{edge} and $\lambda_{spatial}$ are weights that govern the relative influence of the energies.

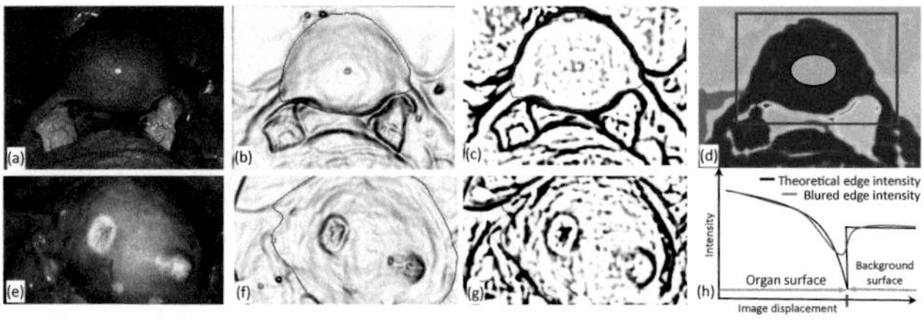

Fig. 2. Laparoscopic images of two uteri with different filter response maps (Sobel: (b,f), LoG$^+$: (c,g)), overlaid with manual segmentations. The LoG$^+$ geodesic distance transform $\mathcal{D}$ for (a) is shown in (d), with the detection's bounding box and central ellipse $\mathcal{S}$ overlaid. An illustration of the edge intensity profile across an organ boundary edge is shown in (h).

A physically-motivated edge energy model based on the LoG$^+$ filter. The purpose of the edge energy is to encourage a smooth segmentation whose boundary is attracted to probable organ boundaries. In nearly all graphcut-based optical image segmentation methods, this is based on the step-edge model, which says that a transition between labels should occur at regions with high first-order intensity derivatives [2]. However this model does not match well with the physical image formation process in laparoscopic images. This is a combination of the fact that the scene is illuminated by a proximal light source centred close to the camera's optical center, and that because organs are smooth, discontinuities in surface orientation are rare. To see this, consider a point $\mathbf{p}$ on the organ's boundary with a normal vector $\mathbf{n}$ in camera coordinates. By definition $\mathbf{n}$ must be orthogonal to the viewing ray, which implies $\mathbf{n}$ is approximately orthogonal to the light source vector, so $\mathbf{p}$ necessarily reflects a very small fraction of direct illumination. Consider now the image intensity profile as we transition from the organ to a background structure (Fig. 2(h)). We observe a smooth intensity fall-off as the boundary is reached, and then a discontinuous jump as we transition to the background. Due to imperfect optics we measure a smooth version of this profile, which is characterised by a smooth intensity trough at a boundary point. *Likely organ boundaries are therefore those image points with strongly positive second-order intensity derivatives*, which can be computed stably with the LoG$^+$ filter. One issue is that edge filters such as LoG$^+$ are also sensitive to superficial texture variation of the organ. An effective way to deal with this is to apply the filter on the red channel only, because red light diffuses deeper into tissue than blue and green light [4]. Fig. 2 illustrates the effectiveness of the LoG$^+$ filter for revealing the uterus boundaries, which we compare to the Sobel step-edge filter.

We define E_{edge} in a similar manner to [2] but replace the intensity difference term by the LoG$^+$ response at the midpoint of two neighbouring pixels $\mathbf{x}$ and $\mathbf{y}$:

$$\begin{aligned} E_{edge}(\mathcal{L}) &\stackrel{\text{def}}{=} \textstyle\sum_{(\mathbf{x},\mathbf{y})\in\mathcal{N}} w_{\mathbf{x},\mathbf{y}}(\mathcal{L}) \exp\left(-\text{LoG}^+((\mathbf{x}+\mathbf{y})/2)/2\sigma\right) \\ w_{\mathbf{x},\mathbf{y}}(\mathcal{L}) &= \begin{cases} 1/d(\mathbf{x},\mathbf{y}) & \text{if } \mathcal{L}(\mathbf{x}) \neq \mathcal{L}(\mathbf{y}) \\ 0 & \text{otherwise} \end{cases} \end{aligned} \tag{2}$$

where $\mathcal{N}$ denotes the set of pixel neighbour pairs (we use the standard 8-way connected neighbours from the pixel grid). The term $w_{\mathbf{x},\mathbf{y}} \in \mathbb{R}$ assigns energy when neighbouring pixels have different labels. The function d gives the Euclidean distance between $\mathbf{x}$ and $\mathbf{y}$, which reduces the influence of neighbours that are further away. Inspired by [2] we set σ automatically as the standard deviation of the LoG$^+$ filter across all pixels in $\mathcal{R}$. The LoG$^+$ filter has a free parameter σ_N that pre-smoothes the image to mitigate noise. We have found that results are not highly sensitive to σ_N, and in all experiments we use $\sigma_N = 3$ pixels with a filter window of 7 pixels.

Hard labels and spatial energy. We assign hard labels to pixels in the image that we are virtually certain of either being on the organ or on the background. The job of this is to prevent complete over or under-segmentation in instances when the organ's appearance is very similar to the background. We assign pixels within a small region around the bounding box center $\mathbf{x}_b$ the foreground label, which is valid because the main body of the uterus is always highly convex. Specifically we define a small elliptical region $\mathcal{S}$ by $\mathbf{x} \in \mathcal{S} \Leftrightarrow s^2(\mathbf{x}-\mathbf{x}_b)^\top \mathrm{diag}(1/w, 1/h)(\mathbf{x}-\mathbf{x}_b) \leq 1$, and assign all pixels in $\mathcal{S}$ the foreground label. This is an ellipse with the same aspect ratio as the bounding box, where w and h are the width and height of the bounding box. The scale of $\mathcal{S}$ is given by s, which is not a sensitive parameter and in all experiments we use $s = 0.2$. To prevent complete over-segmentation we assign pixels very far from the bounding box the background label. We do this by padding $\mathcal{R}$ by a small amount by replication (we use 20 pixels), and assign the perimeter of the padded image the background label.

The spatial energy encodes the fact that pixels near the detection's center are more likely to be on the organ. We measure distances to the detection's center in terms of geodesics $\mathcal{D}(\mathbf{x}) : \mathcal{R} \rightarrow \mathbb{R}^+$ using the LoG$^+$ filter response as a local metric. This is fast to compute and more informative than the Euclidean distance because it takes into account probable organ boundaries in the image. We compute $\mathcal{D}(\mathbf{x})$ by measuring the distance of $\mathbf{x}$ to $\mathcal{S}$ using the fast marching method. We give a visualisation of $\mathcal{D}$ for the image in Fig. 2 (a) in Fig. 2 (d), with the central ellipse overlaid in red. Dark blue indicates lower distances, and the darkest shade corresponds to a distance of zero. One can see that for most pixels either on the uterus body, or connected to the uterus body by ligaments or the Fallopian tubes, the distance is zero, because for these points there exists a path in the image to $\mathcal{S}$ that does cross an organ boundary. We therefore propose a very simple spatial energy function, which works by increasing the energy of a pixel $\mathbf{x}$ if it is labelled background and has $\mathcal{D}(\mathbf{x}) = 0$. We do this for all pixels within the detection's bounding box, and define the spatial energy as

$$E_{spatial}(\mathcal{L}; \mathcal{D}, \mathcal{B}) \stackrel{\text{def}}{=} \sum_{\mathbf{x} \in R} \begin{cases} 1 & \text{if } \mathcal{L}(\mathbf{x}) = 0 \text{ and } \mathcal{D}(\mathbf{x}) = 0 \text{ and } \mathbf{x} \in \mathcal{B} \\ 0 & \text{otherwise} \end{cases} \tag{3}$$

The effect of $E_{spatial}$ is to encourage pixels within the bounding box to be labelled foreground if they can reach the detection's center by a path that does not cross points that are likely to be organ boundaries. To improve the computation speed for $E_{spatial}$ we compute $\mathcal{D}$ on a down-sampled version of $\mathcal{R}$ (by a factor of two). On a standard desktop PC this means $E_{spatial}$ can be computed in approximately 100 to 200ms without significant impact on accuracy.

3 Experimental Results

We have evaluated on a new dataset consisting of 235 uterus images of 126 different individuals, which extends the 39-individual database from [13] (Fig. 3). The dataset includes common difficulties caused by pathological shape, surgical change, partial occlusion, strong light fall-off, low-contrast boundaries and over-saturation. The dataset was gathered from patients at our hospital (12 individuals) and demonstration and tuition images from the web (114 patients). 35.0% of the patients had uteri with pathological shape, caused mostly by uterine fibroids. For each image we computed the best-scoring detection from the uterus detector using the accelerated code of [7]. A detection was considered a true positive if the overlap between the detection's bounding box and the manually-computed bounding box exceeded 55% (which is a typical threshold in object detection literature). In total 220 images had true positive detections. In the other 15 images false positives were caused nearly always by strong tool occlusions. We then segmented all images with true positive detections. Because our method is the first to achieve completely automatic organ segmentation in laparoscopic images, there is not a direct baseline method to compare to. We therefore adapted a number of competitive interactive and seed-based segmentation methods, by replacing manual inputs with the output of the uterus detector. These were as follows. (*i*) *GrabCut-I* [14]: we replaced the user-provided bounding box required in GrabCut with the bounding box from the detection, and replaced hard labels from the user with the same hard labels as described above. (*ii*) *Non-iterative GrabCut* (GrabCut-NI): This was the same as GrabCut-I but terminating after one iteration (*i.e.* the appearance models and segmentation were not iteratively refined). (*ii*) *GrowCut* [15]: we used GrowCut with $\mathcal{S}$ as the foreground seed region and the perimeter of $\mathcal{R}$ as the background seed region. (*ii*) *Edge-based Levelset Region growing* (ELR) [9]: we used a well-known levelset region growing method, using $\mathcal{S}$ as the initial seed region. For GrabCut-I, GrabCut-NI, GrowCut and our method, we tested with RGB and illumination-invariant colourspaces. We found negligible differences between the common illumination-invariant colourspaces, so report results with just one (CrCb). The free parameters of the baseline methods were set by hand to maximise their performance on the dataset. The free parameters of our method (λ_{edge} and $\lambda_{spatial}$) were set manually with 20 training images, giving $\lambda_{edge} = 90$ and $\lambda_{spatial} = 7$. The training images were no included in the 220 image dataset and were of different patients. We did not use separate training images for the baseline methods, so we could measure their best possible performance on the dataset.

DICE coefficient boxplots (from Matlab's `boxplot`) and summary statistics are given in Fig. 4. We report p-values using the two-sample t-test with equal variance. The suffixes (RGB) and (CrCb) indicate running a method with RGB and CrCb colourspaces respectively. We also tested whether our method could

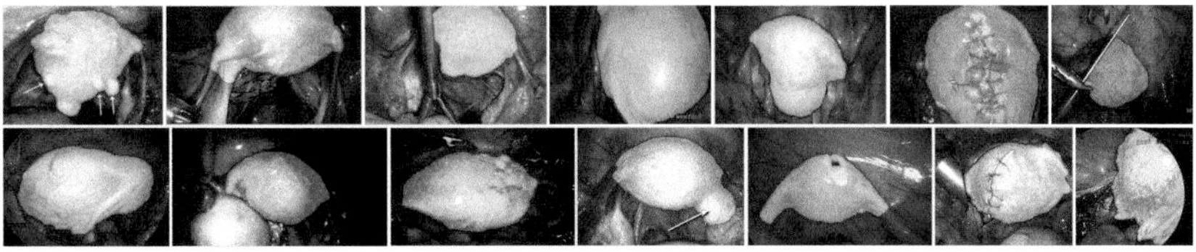

Fig. 3. Example images from the test dataset and segmentations from our method.

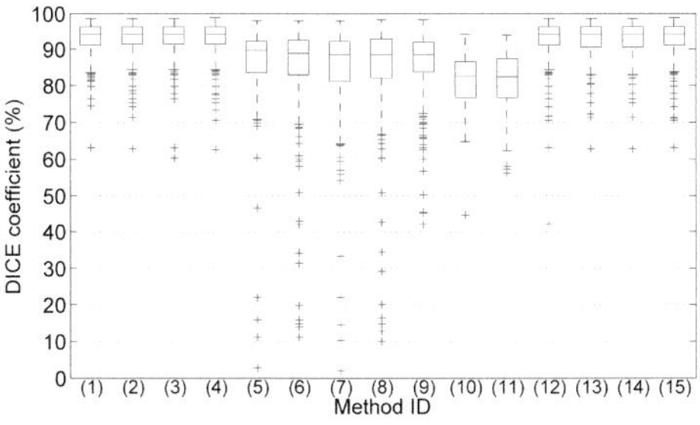

ID	Method	max.	min.	mean	median	s.d.	
(1)	Proposed-NI (RGB)	98,59	**63,04**	92,88	94,32	**4,95**	} p =0.892
(2)	Proposed-NI (CrCb)	98,59	62,75	**92,95**	**94,39**	5,07	
(3)	Proposed-I (RGB)	98,60	60,16	92,95	94,37	5,19	} p =0.974
(4)	Proposed-I (CrCb)	**98,65**	62,56	**92,93**	**94,39**	5,17	
(5)	Grabcut-NI (RGB)	97,93	2,66	86,06	89,67	12,33	} p =0.247
(6)	Grabcut-NI (CrCb)	97,96	11,01	84,46	89,06	15,06	
(7)	Grabcut-I (RGB)	97,85	1,90	84,63	88,72	13,66	} p =0.963
(8)	Grabcut-I (CrCb)	98,12	9,94	84,57	88,74	14,80	
(9)	ELR	98,06	41,92	85,76	88,58	9,76	
(10)	Growcut (RGB)	94,26	44,63	81,21	82,69	7,31	} p =0.836
(11)	Growcut (CrCb)	93,95	56,12	81,06	82,56	7,94	
(12)	(2) with λ_{edge} =112.5 (+25%)	98,59	41,99	92,64	94,37	6,20	} p =0.956
(13)	(2) with λ_{edge} =67.5 (-25%)	98,59	62,78	92,68	94,31	5,13	
(14)	(2) with λ_{smooth} =8.75 (+25%)	98,59	62,76	92,77	94,24	5,07	} p =0.982
(15)	(2) with λ_{smooth} =5.25 (-25%)	98,64	62,93	92,75	94,35	5,42	

Fig. 4. DICE performance statistics of our proposed method in four configurations (1-4), baseline methods (5-11) and a sensitivity analysis of our method (12-15).

be improved by iteratively retraining the appearance models and resegmenting in the same way as GrabCut (denoted by Proposed-I). Finally, we included a sensitivity analysis of our method, by computing results with λ_{edge} and λ_{smooth} perturbed from the default by $\pm 25\%$. We observe the following. The best performing configurations across all statistics are from the proposed method. There are virtually no differences between our method using RGB or CrCb colourspace, which indicates shading variation does not significantly affect segmentation accuracy. There is also no improvement in our method by iteratively updating the appearance models and resegmenting (Proposed (RGB): $p = 0.998$, Proposed (CrCb): $p = 0.941$). We also see that our method is very stable to a considerable perturbation of the parameters. Fig. 3 shows visually the segmentations from our method (Proposed-NI (CrCb)). The images on the far right show two failure cases. These were caused by a tool occlusion that completely bisected the uterus and a uterus significantly occluded by the laparoscope's optic ring.

4 Conclusion

We have presented a method for segmenting the uterus in monocular laparoscopic images that requires no manual input and no patient-specific prior knowledge. We have achieved this using a patient-independent uterus detector to supervise the training of a CRF-based patient-specific segmenter. High accuracy and speed has been obtained by using a physically-motivated organ boundary model based on the LoG^{+} filter. There are several directions for future work. Firstly, we will transfer many functions, such as training the GMMs and evaluating the graph constraints onto the GPU for realtime computation. Secondly we will investigate combining our method with a tool segmentation method such as [1]. In terms of applications, our method can be used as a module for automatic laparoscopic video parsing and content retrieval, and for solving problems that have previously required manual organ segmentation. These include building 3D organ models *invivo* [5] and inter-modal organ registration using occluding contours [6].

References

1. Allan, M., Thompson, S., Clarkson, M.J., Ourselin, S., Hawkes, D.J., Kelly, J., Stoyanov, D.: 2D-3D pose tracking of rigid instruments in minimally invasive surgery. In: Stoyanov, D., Collins, D.L., Sakuma, I., Abolmaesumi, P., Jannin, P. (eds.) IPCAI 2014. LNCS, vol. 8498, pp. 1–10. Springer, Heidelberg (2014)
2. Boykov, Y., Jolly, M.-P.: Interactive graph cuts for optimal boundary amp; region segmentation of objects in N-D images. In: ICCV (2001)
3. Chhatkuli, A., Malti, A., Bartoli, A., Collins, T.: Monocular live image parsing in uterine laparoscopy. In: ISBI (2014)
4. Collins, T., Bartoli, A.: Towards live monocular 3D laparoscopy using shading and specularity information. In: Abolmaesumi, P., Joskowicz, L., Navab, N., Jannin, P. (eds.) IPCAI 2012. LNCS, vol. 7330, pp. 11–21. Springer, Heidelberg (2012)
5. Collins, T., Pizarro, D., Bartoli, A., Canis, M., Bourdel, N.: Realtime wide-baseline registration of the uterus in laparoscopic videos using multiple texture maps. In: MIAR (2013)
6. Collins, T., Pizarro, D., Bartoli, A., Canis, M., Bourdel, N.: Computer-assisted laparoscopic myomectomy by augmenting the uterus with pre-operative MRI data. In: ISMAR (2014)
7. Dubout, C., Fleuret, F.: Exact acceleration of linear object detectors. In: Fitzgibbon, A., Lazebnik, S., Perona, P., Sato, Y., Schmid, C. (eds.) ECCV 2012, Part III. LNCS, vol. 7574, pp. 301–311. Springer, Heidelberg (2012)
8. Felzenszwalb, P., Girshick, R., McAllester, D., Ramanan, D.: Object detection with discriminatively trained part-based models. IEEE PAMI (2010)
9. Li, C., Xu, C., Gui, C., Fox, M.D.: Distance regularized level set evolution and its application to image segmentation. IEEE Trans. Image Process. (2010)
10. Malti, A., Bartoli, A., Collins, T.: Template-based conformal shape-from-motion-and-shading for laparoscopy. In: Abolmaesumi, P., Joskowicz, L., Navab, N., Jannin, P. (eds.) IPCAI 2012. LNCS, vol. 7330, pp. 1–10. Springer, Heidelberg (2012)
11. Nosrati, M., Peyrat, J.-M., Abi-Nahed, J., Al-Alao, O., Al-Ansari, A., Abugharbieh, R., Hamarneh, G.: Efficient multi-organ segmentation in multi-view endoscopic videos using pre-op priors. In: Golland, P., Hata, N., Barillot, C., Hornegger, J., Howe, R. (eds.) MICCAI 2014, Part II. LNCS, vol. 8674, Springer, Heidelberg (2014)
12. Price, B.L., Morse, B.S., Cohen, S.: Geodesic graph cut for interactive image segmentation. In: CVPR (2010)

13. Prokopetc, K., Collins, T., Bartoli, A.: Automatic detection of the uterus and fallopian tube junctions in laparoscopic images. In: Ourselin, S., Alexander, D.C., Westin, C.-F., Cardoso, M.J. (eds.) IPMI 2015. LNCS, vol. 9123, pp. 552–563. Springer, Heidelberg (2015)
14. Rother, C., Kolmogorov, V., Blake, A.: Grabcut - Interactive foreground extraction using iterated graph cuts. ACM Transactions on Graphics (2004)
15. Vezhnevets, V., Konushin, V.: Growcut - Interactive multi-label n-d image segmentation by cellular automata. In: GraphiCon (2005)

Progressive Label Fusion Framework for Multi-atlas Segmentation by Dictionary Evolution

Yantao Song[1,2], Guorong Wu[2], Quansen Sun[1], Khosro Bahrami[2], Chunming Li[3], and Dinggang Shen[2]

[1] School of Computer Science and Engineering, Nanjing University of Science & Technology, Nanjing, Jiangsu, China
[2] Department of Radiology and BRIC, University of North Carolina at Chapel Hill, NC, USA
[3] School of Electronic Engineering, University of Electronic Science & Technology, Chengdu, Sichuan, China

Abstract. Accurate segmentation of anatomical structures in medical images is very important in neuroscience studies. Recently, multi-atlas patch-based label fusion methods have achieved many successes, which generally represent each target patch from an atlas patch dictionary in the image domain and then predict the latent label by directly applying the estimated representation coefficients in the label domain. However, due to the large gap between these two domains, the estimated representation coefficients in the image domain may not stay optimal for the label fusion. To overcome this dilemma, we propose a novel label fusion framework to make the weighting coefficients eventually to be optimal for the label fusion by progressively constructing a dynamic dictionary in a layer-by-layer manner, where a sequence of intermediate patch dictionaries gradually encode the transition from the patch representation coefficients in image domain to the optimal weights for label fusion. Our proposed framework is general to augment the label fusion performance of the current state-of-the-art methods. In our experiments, we apply our proposed method to hippocampus segmentation on ADNI dataset and achieve more accurate labeling results, compared to the counterpart methods with single-layer dictionary.

1 Introduction

Accurate and fully automatic segmentation is in high demand in many imaging-based studies. For instance, hippocampus is known as an important structure related with Alzheimer's disease, temporal lobe epilepsy and schizophrenia. Consequently, many neuroscience and clinical applications aim to seek for the imaging biomarker around hippocampus, which is indispensable of accurate segmentation of hippocampus from the MR brain images.

Recently, multi-atlas patch-based segmentation methods [1-5] have achieved many successes in medical imaging area. In current multi-atlas based methods,

N. Navab et al. (Eds.): MICCAI 2015, Part III, LNCS 9351, pp. 190–197, 2015.
DOI: 10.1007/978-3-319-24574-4_23

a set of patches, collected in a searching neighborhood and across all registered atlases, form a patch dictionary to represent the target image patch. In these methods, the assumption is that the representation profile obtained in the image (continuous) domain can be directly transferred to the (binary) domain of anatomical label. However, there is no evidence that such profile is domain-invariant. As a result, representation coefficients may not guarantee the optimal label fusion results.

To alleviate this issue, we propose a novel label propagation framework to progressively transfer the representation profile from the image domain to the anatomical label domain. To achieve it, we construct a set of intermediate dictionaries, which are eventually a sequence of milestones guiding the above domain transition. Then we apply the label fusion techniques (e.g., non-local mean [1, 2] and sparse representation [3, 6]) in a leave-one-out manner to obtain the representation profile for each atlas patch in each layer dictionary where all other instances are regarded as the atlas patches. Then, we can compute a label probability patch by applying the obtained representation profile to the respective label patches. Repeating the above procedure to all patches, we can iteratively construct the higher layer dictionaries, as the probability map within each label probability patch becomes sharper and shaper, until all label probability patches end up to the binary shapes of the corresponding label patches.

Given the learned multi-layer dictionary at each image point, the final weights for voting the label are also estimated in a progressive way. Starting from the initial layer, we gradually refine the label fusion weights by alternating the following two steps: (1) compute the representation profile of target image patch by using the patch dictionary in the current layer; and (2) refine the label probability map within the target image patch by applying the latest representation profile to the binary label patches, where the new probability patch is used as the new target in the next layer. In this way, we can gradually achieve the optimal weights for determining the anatomical label, under the guidance of the intermediate dictionary at each layer.

The contributions of our proposed multi-layer dictionary method include: (1) Since we harness the multi-layer dictionary to remedy the gap between patch appearance and anatomical label, our label fusion essentially seeks for the best label fusion weights, instead of only the optimal patch-wise representation; (2) The evolution of intermediate dictionaries allows us to use not only appearance features but also structure context information [7], which significantly improves the robustness in patch representation; (3) the framework of progressive patch representation by multi-layer dictionary is general enough to integrate with most of conventional patch-based segmentation methods and improve their segmentation performances instantly. Our proposed method has been evaluated in a specific problem of segmenting hippocampus from elderly brain MR images in the ADNI dataset. More accurate segmentation results have been achieved, with comparison to the state-of-the-art non-local mean [2] and sparse patch-based label fusion methods [6].

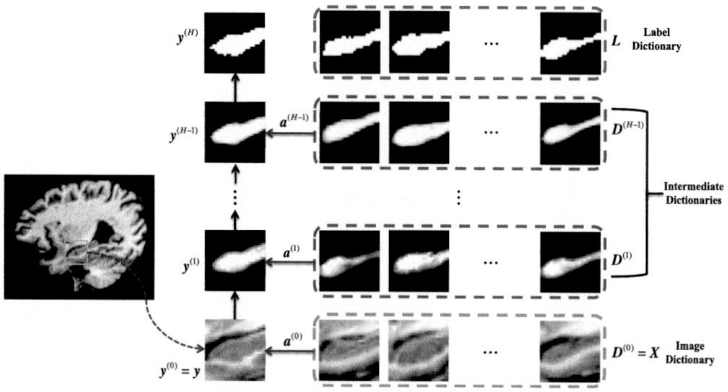

Fig. 1. The framework of proposed method. Given the image dictionary (green dash box) and the label dictionary (blue dash box). In order to overcome the significant gap between two different dictionaries, our method uses a set of intermediate dictionaries (red dash boxes) to gradually encode the transition from the representation coefficients in image domain to the optimal weights for label fusion. In the label fusion stage, we sequentially go through the intermediate dictionaries and obtain the final binary label via a set of probability maps, which become sharper and sharper as the layer increases.

2 Proposed Method

In general, multi-atlas patch-based segmentation aims to determine the label of each point in the target image T by using a set of N registered atlas images I_s as well as the registered label images L_s, $s = 1, \ldots, N$. For each voxel v in the target image, most of patch-based approaches construct a patch dictionary which consists of all patches extracted from the search neighborhood across all atlases. Without loss of generality, we assume there are K candidate atlas patches in the intensity patch dictionary $\boldsymbol{X} = [\boldsymbol{x}_k]_{k=1,\ldots,K}$, where we vectorize each patch into a column vector $\boldsymbol{x}_k$ and turn $\boldsymbol{X}$ into a matrix. Since each atlas patch has the label information, it is straightforward to construct a corresponding label patch dictionary $\boldsymbol{L} = [\boldsymbol{l}_k]_{k=1,\ldots,K}$, where each $\boldsymbol{l}_k$ is the column vector of labels coupled with $\boldsymbol{x}_k$. A lot of label fusion strategies have been proposed to propagate the labels from $\boldsymbol{L}$ to the target image voxel v, mainly driven by the patch-wise similarity α_k between each atlas patch $\boldsymbol{x}_k$ in $\boldsymbol{X}$ and the image patch $\boldsymbol{y}$ extracted at v. For example, non-local mean method [1,2] penalizes patch-wise appearance discrepancy in an exponential way as below

$$\alpha_k = \exp(-||\boldsymbol{y} - \boldsymbol{x}_{\mathrm{k}}||^2/2\sigma^2) \tag{1}$$

where σ controls the penalty strength. Instead of computing α_k independently, sparse patch based label fusion method (SPBL) [3,6] casts the optimization of weighting vector $\boldsymbol{\alpha} = [\alpha_k]_{k=1,\ldots,K}$ into the sparse patch representation scenario by

$$\arg min_{\boldsymbol{\alpha}} ||\boldsymbol{y} - \boldsymbol{X}\boldsymbol{\alpha}||_2^2 + \lambda||\boldsymbol{\alpha}||_1 \tag{2}$$

where λ controls the sparsity strength.

Hereafter, we call the weighting vector $\boldsymbol{\alpha}$ as the *patch representation profile*. Given the profile $\boldsymbol{\alpha}$ optimized based on appearance information, the latent label on v is assigned to the anatomical label which has the largest accumulated weights within $\boldsymbol{\alpha}$. However, there is a large gap between the intensity dictionary $\boldsymbol{X}$ and label dictionary $\boldsymbol{L}$ as shown in Fig.1. In order to make the patch representation profile $\boldsymbol{\alpha}$ eventually to be the optimal weighting vector for the label fusion, we construct a set of intermediate dictionaries to augment the single-layer dictionary $\boldsymbol{X}$ to the H-layer dictionary $\boldsymbol{D} = \{\boldsymbol{D}^{(h)} | h = 0, \ldots, H-1\}$ and gradually transform the representation profile from the purely appearance representation profile $\boldsymbol{\alpha}^{(0)}$ to the final optimal label fusion weighting vector $\boldsymbol{\alpha}^{(H-1)}$, where for each $\boldsymbol{\alpha}^{(h)}$ we get the corresponding probability map $\boldsymbol{y}^{(h)}$. As $\boldsymbol{\alpha}^{(h)}$ getting more and more reliable for label domain, the probability map becomes sharper and shaper, and eventually the probability map ends up to the binary shape $\boldsymbol{y}^{(H)}$ as shown in the top of Fig.1.

2.1 Dictionary Construction

To construct the multi-layer patch dictionary, we use the original image patch dictionary $\boldsymbol{X}$ to form the initial layer dictionary $\boldsymbol{D}^{(0)} = \boldsymbol{X}$ as shown in the bottom of Fig. 1, i.e., $\boldsymbol{D}^{(0)} = [\boldsymbol{d}_k^{(0)}]$, where $\boldsymbol{d}_k^{(0)} = \boldsymbol{x}_k$. From the first layer, we iteratively construct the intermediate dictionaries $\boldsymbol{D}^{(h)} (h = 1, \ldots, H-1)$ by alternating the following three steps.

First, starting from $h = 1$, for each instance $\boldsymbol{d}_k^{(h-1)}$ in the previous dictionary $\boldsymbol{D}^{(h-1)}$, we seek to use all the other instances $\boldsymbol{d}_j^{(h-1)} (j \neq k)$ in $\boldsymbol{D}^{(h-1)}$ to represent the underlying $\boldsymbol{d}_k^{(h-1)}$ by regarding that all instances in $\boldsymbol{D}^{(h-1)}$ form the instance-specific dictionary $\boldsymbol{B}_k^{(h)} = [\boldsymbol{d}_j^{(h-1)}]_{j=1,\ldots,K, j\neq k}$, where $\boldsymbol{B}_k^{(h)}$ has $K-1$ column vectors. Thus, we can obtain the patch representation profile $\boldsymbol{\beta}_k^{(h-1)}$ for $\boldsymbol{d}_k^{(h-1)}$ via current label fusion strategy, e.g., either non-local mean in Eq.(1) or sparse representation technique in Eq.(2). Note, $\boldsymbol{\beta}_k^{(h-1)}$ is the column vector of length $K-1$.

Second, since each atom in $\boldsymbol{B}_k^{(h)}$ is associated with one label patch in $\boldsymbol{L}$, we can build the surrogate label patch dictionary $\boldsymbol{L}_k = [\boldsymbol{l}_j]_{j=1,\ldots,K,j\neq k}$ by arranging the label patches with the same order as in $\boldsymbol{B}_k^{(h)}$. Then, we compute the label probability patch $\boldsymbol{p}_k^{(h)}$ by $\boldsymbol{p}_k^{(h)} = \boldsymbol{L}_k \cdot \boldsymbol{\beta}_k^{(h-1)}$.

Third, after repeating the above two steps for all instances $\boldsymbol{d}_k^{(h-1)}$, we evolve the intermediate patch dictionary $\boldsymbol{D}^{(h-1)}$ to the next level $\boldsymbol{D}^{(h)}$ by letting $\boldsymbol{D}^{(h)} = [\boldsymbol{d}_k^{(h)}]$, where $\boldsymbol{d}_k^{(h)} = \boldsymbol{p}_k^{(h)}$.

2.2 Multi-layer Label Fusion

Given the multi-layer dictionary $\boldsymbol{D}$, the conventional single-layer patch representation turns to the progressive patch representation where the weighting vector

$\boldsymbol{\alpha}$ is gradually refined from $\boldsymbol{\alpha}^{(0)}$ at the initial layer (optimal for the patch appearance representation only) to $\boldsymbol{\alpha}^{(H-1)}$ in the last layer (eventually optimal for the label fusion).

In the initial layer, we use the original intensity patch dictionary $\boldsymbol{D}^{(0)}$ to present the target image patch vector $\boldsymbol{y}^{(0)} = \boldsymbol{y}$ located at v and thus obtain the representation profile $\boldsymbol{\alpha}^{(0)}$ of the initial layer. Conventional label fusion methods stop here and then vote for the label via the weights in $\boldsymbol{\alpha}^{(0)}$. Instead, our progressive label fusion method computes the label probability vector $\boldsymbol{y}^{(1)}$ by letting $\boldsymbol{y}^{(1)} = \boldsymbol{L}\boldsymbol{\alpha}^{(0)}$. It is worth noting that the intensity target image vector $\boldsymbol{y}$ turns to the probability vector at this time. After the initial layer, we iteratively refine the probability map within the target image patch until it approaches the binary shape of labels. Specifically, we use $\boldsymbol{y}^{(1)}$ as the new target and continue to represent $\boldsymbol{y}^{(1)}$ by the intermediate dictionary $\boldsymbol{D}^{(1)}$ in the same layer, obtaining the new label probability vector $\boldsymbol{y}^{(2)}$. Then, we continue to represent $\boldsymbol{y}^{(2)}$ in the second layer through the intermediate dictionary $\boldsymbol{D}^{(2)}$, and so on. After repeating the same procedure until we reach the last layer $H-1$, the representation profile $\boldsymbol{\alpha}^{(H-1)}$ is regarded as the best weighting vector to determine the latent label on the target image point v.

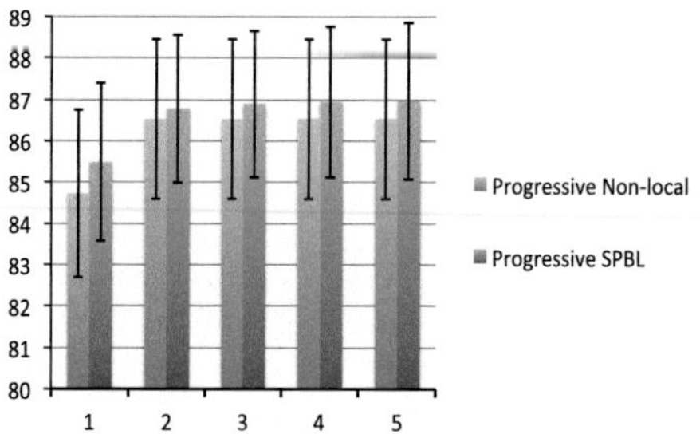

Fig. 2. The evolution curve of Dice ratio as the number of layers in the intermediate dictionary increases.

3 Experiments

In this section, we evaluate the performance of our proposed method on hippocampus segmentation. Specifically, we integrate two state-of-the-art label fusion methods, i.e., non-local [2] and SPBL [6], into our progressive label fusion framework. For comparison, conventional non-local and SPBL methods are used as reference, which only use the single-layer dictionary. Since our method computes the label fusion weights in H layers, the computation time is H times slower than the conventional single-layer method. However, we have used various strategies to speed up our algorithm, such as parallel programming and patch pre-selection.

3.1 Dataset and Parameters

We randomly select 64 normal subjects from the Alzheimer's Disease Neuroimaging Initiative (ADNI) dataset (*www.adni-info.org*), where the hippocampus have been manually labeled for each subject. In our experiments, we regard those manual segmentations as ground truth. To label the target subject, we first aligned all the atlas images to the underlying target subject. In order to improve computational efficiency, atlas selection and patch selection strategies are applied.

In the following experiments, we fix the patch size as $5 \times 5 \times 5$ voxels, where the voxel size is $1mm$ in each direction, and the search window for constructing the dictionary as $5 \times 5 \times 5$ voxels. In non-local mean method, the penalty strength σ is set to 0.5, while in sparse patch based label fusion method the sparse constraint λ is set to 0.1. Here, we use the Dice ratio to measure the overlap between automatic segmentation and ground truth. Also as it is common in evaluation of label fusion method, all testing images were evaluated in a leave-one-out manner. Specifically, in each leave-one-out case, we use FLIRT in the FSL toolbox [8] with 12 degrees of freedom and the search range ± 20 in all directions. For deformable registration, we use diffeomorphic Demons method [9] with smoothing kernel size 1.5. The iteration numbers in diffeomorphic Demons are 15, 10, and 5 in the low, middle, and high resolutions, respectively.

Table 1. The mean and standard deviation of Dice ratio (in %) in hippocampus labeling in the *linear* registration scenario

Method	Left	Right	Overall
Conventional Non-local	85.1±5.7	84.3±5.1	84.7±4.2
*Progressive Non-local	86.8±4.5	86.2±5.1	86.5±3.7
Conventional SPBL	85.8±4.5	85.1±4.8	85.5±3.7
Progressive SPBL	**87.1±3.2**	**86.7±5.3**	**86.9±3.3**

Table 2. The mean and standard deviation of Dice ratio (in %) in hippocampus labeling in the *deformable* registration scenario

Method	Left	Right	Overall
Conventional Non-local	86.8±4.9	86.6±2.9	86.7±3.2
*Progressive Non-local	87.9±4.0	88.1±3.2	88.0±3.0
Conventional SPBL	87.2±3.6	87.1±3.3	87.2±2.9
*Progressive SPBL	**88.2±3.6**	**88.5±3.1**	**88.3±2.8**

The evolution of segmentation accuracy with the number of layers used is shown in Fig.2. We can see that the improvement of our progressive method is obvious after one layer (corresponding to the baseline methods), which offers more than 1% improvement of Dice ratio for both non-local and SPBL methods. Our progressive label fusion framework generally converges after the third layer. Considering the computation time, we use 4 layers ($H = 4$) in the following experiments.

3.2 Hippocampus Segmentation Results

Table 1 and Table 2 show the mean and standard deviation of Dice ratio on hippocampus (left, right and overall) in linear and deformable registration scenarios, respectively. Compared to the baseline methods (i.e., non-local and SPBL methods with single-layer dictionary), our progressive label fusion framework can improve the labeling accuracy with more than **1%** of Dice ratio. Maximum improvement is **1.8%** (conventional non-local vs. progressive non-local in linear registration case). The significant improvement of our method over the baseline method, with p-value less than 0.05 using paired t-test, is indicated with '*' in Table 1 and Table 2, respectively.

Table 3. The surface distance (in mm) on hippocampus labeling between automatic segmentations and ground truth with different number of layers

Number of Layers	H=1	H=2	H=3	H=4	H=5
Maximum Distance	2.83	2.00	1.52	1.22	1.21
Mean Distance	0.27	0.22	0.19	0.18	0.18

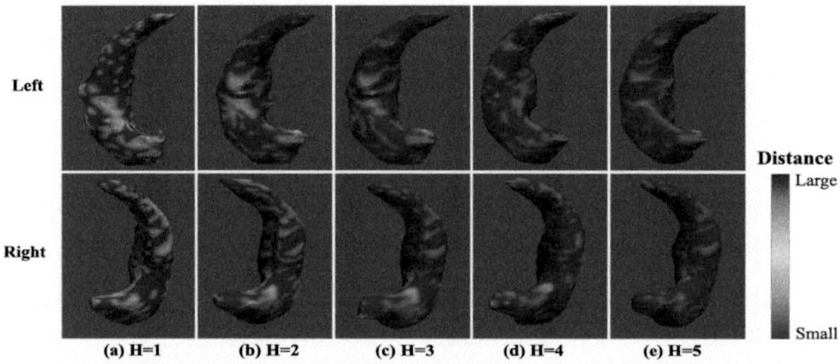

Fig. 3. The evolution of surface distance between the automatic segmentations and ground truth from the initial layer (a) to the last layer (e).

Furthermore, we calculate the surface distance between ground truth and the estimated hippocampus (left and right). SPBL method is used as the example to demonstrate the evolution of surface distance during the progressive label fusion procedure in Fig. 3. According to the color bar shown in the right side of Fig. 3, the surface distances keep decreasing by increasing the number of layers in the intermediate dictionary. Table 3 shows the corresponding surface distance on the whole hippocampus in Fig. 3. In accordance with Fig. 3, as the layer number increases, the mean surface distance becomes smaller and smaller. When $H = 1$, which corresponds to the conventional one-layer SPBL method, the maximum distance is 2.83mm, and it significantly decreases to 1.21mm at $H = 5$ by our method.

4 Conclusion

In this paper, we proposed a progressive label fusion framework for multi-atlas segmentation by dictionary evolution. In our proposed methods, we constructed a set of intermediate dictionaries in a layer-by-layer manner to progressively optimize the weights for label fusion, instead of just using patch-wise representation as used in the conventional label fusion methods. We have applied our new label fusion method to hippocampus segmentation in MR brain images. Promising results were achieved over the state-of-the-art counterpart methods with the single-layer dictionary.

References

1. Coupe, P., Manjon, J.V., Fonov, V., et al.: Patch-based segmentation using expert priors: Application to hippocampus and ventricle segmentation. NeuroImage 54(2), 940–954 (2011)
2. Rousseau, F., Habas, P.A., Studholme, C.: A Supervised Patch-Based Approach for Human Brain Labeling. IEEE Trans. Medical Imaging 30(10), 1852–1862 (2011)
3. Tong, T., Wolz, R., Coupe, P., et al.: Segmentation of MR images via discriminative dictionary learning and sparse coding: application to hippocampus labeling. NeuroImage 76(1), 11–23 (2013)
4. Wang, H., Suh, J.W., Das, S.R., et al.: Multi-atlas segmentation with joint label fusion. IEEE Trans. Pattern Anal. Mach. Intell. 35(3), 611–623 (2013)
5. Wu, G., Wang, Q., Zhang, D., et al.: A Generative Probability Model of Joint Label Fusion for Multi-Atlas Based Brain Segmentation. Medical Image Analysis 18(8), 881–890 (2014)
6. Zhang, D., Guo, Q., Wu, G., Shen, D.: Sparse patch-based label fusion for multi-atlas segmentation. In: Yap, P.-T., Liu, T., Shen, D., Westin, C.-F., Shen, L. (eds.) MBIA 2012. LNCS, vol. 7509, pp. 94–102. Springer, Heidelberg (2012)
7. Tu, Z., Bai, X.: Auto-context and its application to high-level vision tasks and 3D brain image segmentation. IEEE Trans. Pattern Anal. Mach. Intell. 32(10), 1744–1757 (2010)
8. Smith, S.M., Jenkinson, M., Woolrich, M.W., et al.: Advances in functional and structural MR image analysis and implementation as FSL. Neuroimage 23, S208–S219 (2004)
9. Vercauteren, T., Pennec, X., Perchant, A., et al.: Diffeomorphic demons: Efficient non-parametric image registration. NeuroImage 45(1), S61–S72 (2009)

Multi-atlas Based Segmentation Editing with Interaction-Guided Constraints

Sang Hyun Park[1], Yaozong Gao[1,2], and Dinggang Shen[1]

[1] Department of Radiology and BRIC, UNC at Chapel Hill, NC 27599, USA
[2] Department of Computer Science, UNC at Chapel Hill, NC 27599, USA

Abstract. We propose a novel multi-atlas based segmentation method to address the editing scenario, when given an incomplete segmentation along with a set of training label images. Unlike previous multi-atlas based methods, which depend solely on appearance features, we incorporate *interaction-guided constraints* to find appropriate training labels and derive their voting weights. Specifically, we divide user interactions, provided on erroneous parts, into multiple local interaction combinations, and then locally search for the training label patches well-matched with each interaction combination and also the previous segmentation. Then, we estimate the new segmentation through the label fusion of selected label patches that have their weights defined with respect to their respective distances to the interactions. Since the label patches are found to be from different combinations in our method, various shape changes can be considered even with limited training labels and few user interactions. Since our method does not need image information or expensive learning steps, it can be conveniently used for most editing problems. To demonstrate the positive performance, we apply our method to editing the segmentation of three challenging data sets: prostate CT, brainstem CT, and hippocampus MR. The results show that our method outperforms the existing editing methods in all three data sets.

1 Introduction

Automatic segmentation methods have been proposed for various applications. However, these methods often generate erroneous results in some areas of an image caused by difficulties such as unclear target boundaries, large appearance variations and shape changes. If errors can be edited with a few user annotations after automated segmentation, the total segmentation time could be significantly reduced.

Many interactive segmentation methods [1,2] have been proposed to address the editing problem. These methods can generate certain improved results within a few seconds by using distinct user guidance and simple appearance models. However, it is difficult to directly apply these methods to the editing problem, when allowing only limited annotations on a small number of erroneous parts. For example, the appearance model constructed by a few interactions is often limited to obtain the reliable result as shown in Fig. 1(b). Several methods have

N. Navab et al. (Eds.): MICCAI 2015, Part III, LNCS 9351, pp. 198–206, 2015.
DOI: 10.1007/978-3-319-24574-4_24

been proposed to incorporate high-level information from training data into the editing framework to improve performance. Schwarz *et al.* [3] learned active shape model (ASM) and then incorporated it into an editing framework. When any incorrect landmark point is edited by users, the adjacent landmark points are modified accordingly and regularized by the ASM. However, manual editing of landmarks is intractable in the 3D space, and also the ASM with limited training data often fails to capture local shape variations. Park *et al.* [4] proposed an editing method based on a patch model that includes localized classifiers and spatial relationship between neighboring patches. In this method, the patches are transferred to appropriate places in a target image by considering the spatial relationship and the similarity between labels and interactions. Then the localized classifiers are used for segmentation. The process of simple similarity comparison, however, can cause the patches to be positioned in the wrong places, making the final label prediction inaccurate even if good classifiers are trained with elaborate learning methods.

In this paper, we propose a new editing method, focused on reliable estimation of label information without a complex learning. To achieve this, we refer to multi-atlas based segmentation methods [5,6] that consist of two steps: (1) search of training label patches and (2) label fusion of the selected label patches with respective voting weights. So far, most multi-atlas based methods have used appearance features to achieve these two steps, with the basic assumption that similar patches have similar labels. However, it is typically easy to find patches with similar appearance, but distinct label patterns, for medical images, often include weak boundaries and regions with inter-subject appearance variations. Unlike these methods, we use constraints from user interactions to address both label patch selection and label fusion steps. Specifically, we divide user interactions into multiple local interaction combinations and then search for label patches that are well-matched with both the interactions and the previous segmentation for each combination. Next, we estimate new segmentation by label fusion of the selected label patches that have their weights computed with respect to distances to interactions. Specially, we introduce a novel label-based similarity to address the issue in step (1) and new definition of distance-based voting weights to address the issue in step (2). Compared to the case of considering all interactions jointly, the label patches, corresponding to multiple combinations, can generate more reliable results as shown in Figs. 1(c) and 1(d). Also, since our method does not need image information or learning procedures, it is convenient for practice.

2 Multi-atlas Based Editing Method

Our proposed editing procedure begins with an initial segmentation obtained from any existing method, training label images, and user interactions with erroneous parts. We provide an interface to receive user interactions on erroneous parts of an incomplete segmentation result. Intuitively, we assume that foreground (FG)/background (BG) dots or scribbles are inserted into the erroneous

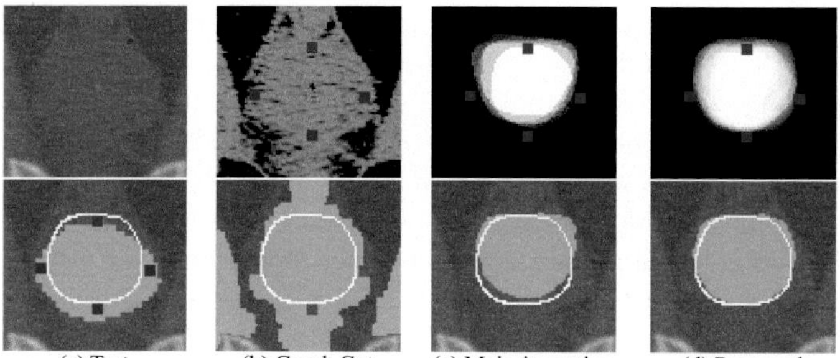

Fig. 1. Editing results for three methods: (b) graph cut, (c) majority voting, and (d) proposed method. Test image, initial segmentation (green), ground-truth (white line), and FG/BG interactions (blue/red dots) are shown in (a). Likelihood maps and editing results (green) are shown in the top and bottom rows of (b), (c), and (d), respectively.

regions near the true object boundary. Specifically, the editing procedure consists of four steps: 1) all training labels are registered to the previous segmentation L^{t-1} for guiding the segmentation update, where t represents the editing iteration and L^0 is the initial segmentation. For the registration, we respectively extract surface points from the training label images and L^{t-1}, and then conduct the iterative closest point method [7]. 2) Local interaction combinations ($\widehat{U}_k^t$ for FG and $\overline{U}_k^t$ for BG) are extracted from the FG / BG user interactions, respectively, where k is the index of combination. For each combination, a region of interest (ROI) is set as a bounding box to include the interactions with a small margin. 3) For each combination, the appropriate training label patches, well-matched with both the interactions and L^{t-1} in the ROI, are searched in the aligned label images, and then averaged to build a local probabilistic likelihood map ($\widehat{P}_k^t$ for FG and $\overline{P}_k^t$ for BG). 4) A global probabilistic likelihood map P^t in the entire image is determined by averaging L^{t-1} and the local probabilistic likelihood maps with their respective distance-based voting weight maps ($\widehat{W}_k^t$ for FG and $\overline{W}_k^t$ for BG) (Fig. 2). Finally, the segmentation is determined by thresholding of P^t. These steps are repeated with inclusion of additional user interactions, if provided, until the segmentation is satisfactory. Note that when repeating each editing procedure, the accumulated user interactions are considered to find the label patches and derive their respective voting weights.

2.1 Extraction of Local Interaction Combinations

In our method, the segmentation is edited by using the information of training labels well-matched with user interactions. If there are many training labels well-matched with all interactions, the segmentation can be edited easily by following the guidance. However, there are few well-matched training labels in most cases. Thus, we separately find the training label patches, which are well-matched with various local interaction combinations, and then aggregate them

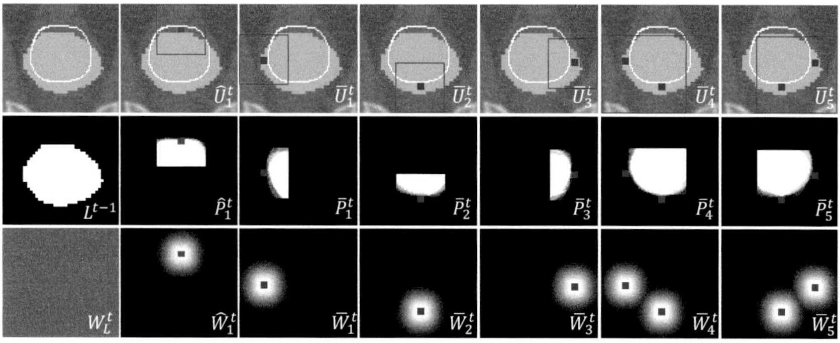

Fig. 2. Interaction combinations, their ROIs (top row), local likelihood maps (middle row), and weight maps (bottom row), obtained from the interactions shown in Fig. 1(a). The initial segmentation, ground-truth, FG/BG interactions, and ROI are shown as green, white line, red/blue dots, and red box, respectively. The global likelihood map in Fig. 1(d) is obtained by fusing L^{t-1} and the local likelihood maps with the weights.

to estimate the voxel likelihood. We extract three types of local combinations for FG and BG interactions, respectively, as follows: 1) *individual interaction* such as a dot or scribble, 2) *pairwise interaction* that includes two individual interactions within a certain distance, and 3) *union interaction* that includes all interactions within the certain distance from each interaction. The combinations are extracted from the interactions provided by the current round of editing, as well as relevant interactions previously. Specifically, if the previous interactions are located within a certain distance from current interactions, the combinations between current and previous interactions are extracted. On the other hand, the previous interactions, far from all the current interactions, will not be used in the current round of editing since the accurate parts of the updated segmentation do not need to be changed. For each kth combination, we set ROI ($\widehat{\varphi}_k^t$ for FG and $\overline{\varphi}_k^t$ for BG) as a bounding box, which covers the interaction combination with a small margin to include possible local variations in the ROI.

2.2 Selection of Training Labels *with respect to* User Interactions

For each interaction combination, we find training label patches well-matched with the interactions and previous segmentation L^{t-1} in ROI. Since training labels are aligned to L^{t-1}, without considering interaction information in the initial registration step, the registration might be inaccurate. To address this issue, we search for the best well-matched label patch in a local search neighborhood for each aligned training label map M with a predefined similarity. Recently, Park *et al.* proposed a label-based similarity [4] that measures the similarity between a label and the interactions. However, since they consider all interactions in ROI to be strong constraints, the number of training label patches well-matched with all interactions is often limited, causing various shape changes to be unable to be well-captured. To avoid this, we define the similarity S_k^t as:

$$S_k^t = \sum_{\substack{v\in\varphi_k^t,\\ U_k^t(v)\neq 0}} \delta(M(v) - U_k^t(v)) + \gamma_O \sum_{\substack{v\in\varphi_k^t,\\ U_k^t(v)=0,\\ U_{\bar{k}}^t(v)\neq 0}} \delta(M(v) - U_{\bar{k}}^t(v)) + \gamma_U \sum_{\substack{v\in\varphi_k^t,\\ U_k^t(v)=0,\\ U_{\bar{k}}^t(v)=0}} \delta(M(v) - L^{t-1}(v)), \tag{1}$$

where δ is the kronecker delta and $U_{\bar{k}}^t$ includes all current and previous user interactions except U_k^t. If v is annotated by users, $U_{\bar{k}}^t(v) = 1$ for FG, and -1 for BG, while if v is not annotated, $U_{\bar{k}}^t(v) = 0$. Here, we assume that a good label patch for U_k^t should be strongly well-matched with U_k^t representing the kth interaction combination (1st term), moderately matched with other interactions except U_k^t (2nd term), and also weakly matched with L^{t-1} on the other voxels (3rd term). γ_O and γ_U denote the parameters for balancing these three terms. In our experiments, γ_O is set as 0.05 to distinguish the strong and moderate constraints for annotated voxels, and γ_U is set as 0.005 to represent the weak constraint for L^{t-1}. The best label patches are found from all the training labels and n_p patches with the highest S_k^t are selected. Finally, the selected patches are averaged to build a local probabilistic likelihood map P_k^t. (2th row in Fig. 2.)

2.3 Label Fusion Based on User Interactions

In the fusion step, local likelihood maps are aggregated to build a global likelihood map P^t for the entire image. Since high emphasis is enforced to the first term of Eq. (1), the local likelihood map is more likely to be accurate near the interaction. In contrast, the confidence of estimated likelihood for a voxel becomes low when its distance from interactions increases. In these low-confidence regions, L^{t-1} is more accurate than the likelihood maps. By considering the distance from interaction and the confidences of $\widehat{P}_k^t$ and $\overline{P}_k^t$, we define $P^t(v)$ as:

$$P^t(v) = \frac{W_L^t(v)L^{t-1}(v) + \sum_{k=1}^{n_f} \widehat{W}_k^t(v)\widehat{P}_k^t(v) + \sum_{k=1}^{n_b} \overline{W}_k^t(v)\overline{P}_k^t(v)}{W_L^t(v) + \sum_{k=1}^{n_f} \widehat{W}_k^t(v) + \sum_{k=1}^{n_b} \overline{W}_k^t(v)}. \tag{2}$$

where n_f, n_b are the numbers of FG and BG combinations. The weight of FG combination $\widehat{W}_k^t(v)$ is defined as:

$$\widehat{W}_k^t(v) = \frac{\alpha_f}{\sqrt{n_f}} \exp(-(\frac{d_k(v) \cdot d_k(v)}{2\sigma^2})), \tag{3}$$

where $d_k(v)$ is the shortest distance between a voxel v and the annotated voxels in U_k^t. σ controls how quickly the emphasis shifts from the probabilistic likelihood maps to L^{t-1} as the voxel is farther from the interactions. If σ is small, only the region close to the user interactions is affected by the probabilistic likelihood maps, while the other regions are affected by L^{t-1}. α_f is the weight for the confidence of voxel likelihood. For example, when many likelihood maps indicate v as BG with low confidence (*e.g.* $P_k^t(v) = 0.2 \sim 0.5$) and less likelihood maps indicate v as FG with high confidence (*e.g.* $P_k^t(v) = 0.8 \sim 1$), we enforce more weight to the latter likelihood maps to follow the high confident likelihood. We set α_f as a value larger than 1, if $P_k^t(v) > 0.8$; otherwise 1. The BG weight $\overline{W}_k^t(v)$ is similarly defined. $W_L^t(v)$ is defined as: $W_L^t(v) = \exp(-(\frac{\beta \cdot \beta}{2\sigma^2}))$, where β controls the importance of L^{t-1}. If β is small, the result is more affected by L^{t-1} compared to P_k^t and vice versa. Finally, we set the label $L^t(v)$ as FG if $P^t(v) > 0.5$ or v is annotated as FG; otherwise, set that as BG.

3 Experimental Result

Our method was evaluated on three data sets: prostate CT, brainstem CT, and hippocampus MR. We first made the automatic segmentation by using the state-of-the-art method [6] and then applied our method to the results with the greatest errors. Specifically, for the prostate set with 73 images, we applied the automatic method using four-fold cross validation and chose 30 images with the lowest DSC. For the brainstem set with 40 images and the hippocampus set with 35 images, we similarly applied the automatic method using the leave-one-out validation and chose 20 and 15 images with the lowest DSC, respectively. For each of these selected prostate, brainstem, and hippocampus images, 12, 30, and 9 dots were inserted on average as the user interactions, depending on the amount of segmentation errors. In our experiments, the ROI margin was set as $13 \times 13 \times 4$ voxels for prostate and brainstem, and $5 \times 5 \times 5$ voxels for hippocampus. Accordingly, the search range was set as $8 \times 8 \times 4$ and $4 \times 4 \times 4$ voxels, respectively. σ and β were set as 7 and 10 for prostate and brainstem, and 3 and 4 for hippocampus. n_p and α_f were set as 7 and 5 for all the experiments.

The proposed method, using the interaction combinations and the weighted voting (ICWV), was compared with 1) initial automatic segmentation, 2) manual editing, 3) a label fusion method using all interactions in the entire image (LFG) for finding training labels, 4) a label fusion method using interactions in local regions (LFL) for finding label patches, 5) a method using the patch model (PM) [4], and 6) a method using the proposed interaction combinations but with the majority voting (ICMV). The performance was measured by DSC between respective results and manual ground-truth labels. The boxplots in Fig. 3 show the distributions of DSC for the three data sets. Fig. 4 shows the qualitative results of LFG, LFL, PM and our proposed methods. In the manual editing method, only the labels of voxels annotated by users were changed. Due to the small amount of interactions, the improvement of manual method was less than DSC of $0.005 - 0.026$. On the other hand, the methods using training labels gave significantly improved scores, *i.e.*, more than DSC of $0.01 - 0.13$ except the LFG method for hippocampus. Since the hippocampus has a non-convex shape with local variations, the number of training labels well-matched with all interactions was very limited, thus the inaccurate training labels that were selected often made the result worse (Fig. 4(c)). The LFL and PM methods had

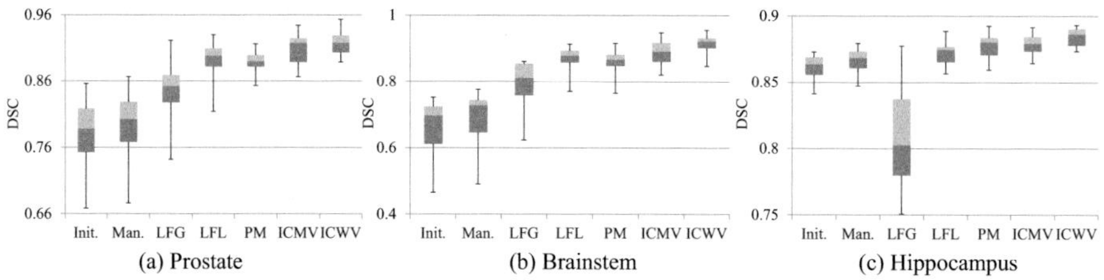

Fig. 3. The distributions of DSC scores for different editing methods. Top, middle, and bottom lines of the box represent upper quartile, median, and lower quartile, respectively. The whiskers represent maximum and minimum values, respectively.

better performances. However, shape variations near the object boundary could not be well-captured in the LFL method due to the limited number of label patches well-matched with all interactions in ROI. The PM method had similar problem near the object boundary due to the patch localization errors and the low intensity contrast between FG and BG. The ICMV method outperformed these methods in terms of accuracy, by finding the well-matched label patches for multiple combinations. Nonetheless, since some inaccurate label patches derived from individual or pairwise combinations still contribute equally to the final result, the large standard deviations were obtained by comparing the proposed ICWV method. On the other hand, the ICWV method outperformed all other editing methods in most cases for both accuracy and robustness.

The procedure of repetitive editing is shown in Fig. 5. In this example, due to the large errors occurred in L^0, there was a lack of good label patches that could cover the large shape change. Thus, the intermediate result (Fig. 5(c)) still included errors on the upper part. In the next round of editing, we inserted additional user dots, re-aligned all training labels to the intermediate result, and further refined the result with additional interaction combinations near the dots. Since the aligned labels were more reliable during the second round of editing, possible shape changes for the erroneous part were covered in the search range, allowing the segmentation to be more accurately demonstrated.

These experiments were performed on a PC with a 3.5 GHz Intel quad-core i7 CPU, and 16GB of RAM. The computational time depended on the number of training labels and interactions, the ROI margin size, and the search range. In our setting, the editing took $1.5 - 7$ min, $2 - 18$ min, and $50 - 80$ seconds for prostate, brainstem, and hippocampus, respectively. Since the editing is conducted with all interactions in the image, our method was unable to promptly produce intermediate results. However, the time issue can be significantly reduced with GPU implementation as the same computation is repeated on every voxel in the search space. The time during the second round of editing was greatly reduced when the number of interaction combinations decreased. In the example of Fig. 5, editing was five times faster than that of the first round.

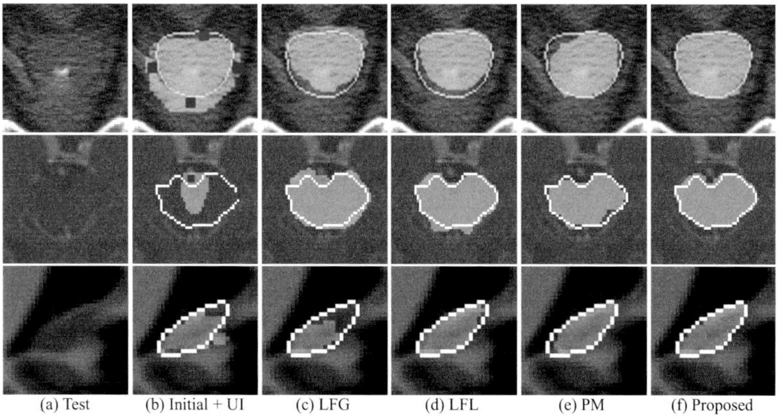

Fig. 4. Segmentation editing results by LFG, LFL, PM, and our proposed methods. Segmentation results, ground-truth, and FG / BG interactions (UI) are shown as green, white lines, and red / blue dots, respectively.

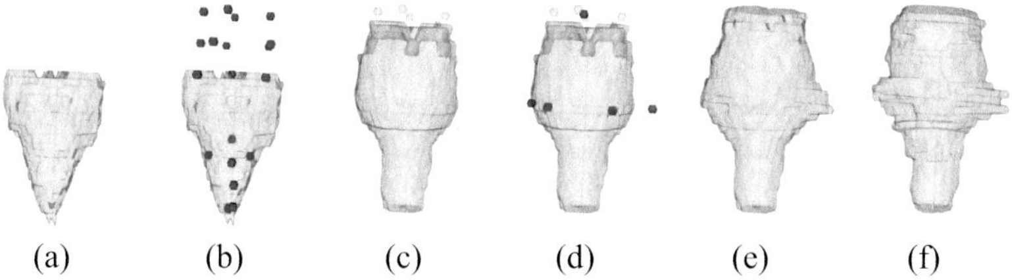

Fig. 5. The procedure of segmentation update with respect to the repetitive user interactions. (a) initial segmentation with large errors, (b) the segmentation with interactions, (c) intermediate segmentation result based on the interactions shown in (b), (d) the segmentation with additional interactions, (e) updated segmentation result based on the interactions shown in (d), and (f) ground-truth.

4 Conclusion

We have proposed a novel multi-atlas based segmentation editing method with interaction-guided constraints to find training label patches and derive voting weights. The proposed method can generate robust editing results in even challenging regions without image information and expensive learning steps. It can help produce accurate segmentations for difficult cases that failed in existing automatic methods. In the future, we will incorporate classifier-based methods into our framework to learn about image features from the label information and eventually release our editing method for public use[1].

[1] `http://www.unc.edu/~tkdgus/`

References

1. Boykov, Y., Funka-Lea, G.: Graph cuts and efficient N-D image segmentation. International Journal of Computer Vision 70(2), 109–131 (2006)
2. Grady, L.: Random walks for image segmentation. IEEE Transactions on Pattern Analysis and Machine Intelligence 28(11), 1768–1783 (2006)
3. Schwarz, T., Heimann, T., Tetzlaff, R., Rau, A.M., Wolf, I., Meinzer, H.P.: Interactive surface correction for 3D shape based segmentation. In: Proc. SPIE (2008)
4. Park, S.H., Lee, S., Yun, I.D., Lee, S.U.: Structured patch model for a unified automatic and interactive segmentation framework. Medical Image Analysis (2015)
5. Coupe, P., Manjon, J.V., Fonov, V., Pruessner, J., Robles, M., Collins, D.L.: Patch-based segmentation using expert priors: Application to hippocampus and ventricle segmentation. NeuroImage 54(2), 940–954 (2011)
6. Wu, G., Wang, Q., Zhang, D., Nie, F., Huang, H., Shen, D.: A generative probability model of joint label fusion for multi-atlas based brain segmentation. Medical Image Analysis 18(6), 881–890 (2014)
7. Besl, P.J., Makay, N.D.: A method of registration of 3-D shapes. IEEE Transactions on Pattern Analysis and Machine Intelligence 14(2), 239–256 (1992)

Quantitative Image Analysis II: Microscopy, Fluorescence and Histological Imagery

Improving Convenience and Reliability of 5-ALA-Induced Fluorescent Imaging for Brain Tumor Surgery

Hiroki Taniguchi[1], Noriko Kohira[1], Takashi Ohnishi[2], Hiroshi Kawahira[2]
Mikael von und zu Fraunberg[3], Juha E. Jääskeläinen[3], Markku Hauta-Kasari[4]
Yasuo Iwadate[5], and Hideaki Haneishi[2]

[1] Graduate School of Engineering, Chiba University, Chiba, Japan
[2] Center for Frontier Medical Engineering, Chiba University, Chiba, Japan
[3] Kuopio University Hospital, University of Eastern Finland
[4] School of Computing, University of Eastern Finland
[5] Graduate School of Medicine, Chiba University, Chiba, Japan
haneishi@faculty.chiba-u.jp

Abstract. This paper presents two features to make neurosurgery with 5-ALA-induced fluorescent imaging more convenient and more reliable. The first one is the concept for a system that switches between white light and excitation light rapidly and allows surgeons to easily locate the tumor region on the normal color image. The second one is the way for color signal processing that yields a stable fluorescent signal without depending on the lighting condition. We developed a prototype system and confirmed that the color image display with the fluorescent region worked well for both the brain of a dead swine and the resected tumor of a human brain. We also performed an experiment with physical phantoms of fluorescent objects and confirmed that the calculated flurophore density-related values were stably obtained for several lighting conditions.

Keywords: neurosurgery, fluorescent imaging, 5-ALA, protoporphyrin, color signal processing, real time processing

1 Introduction

In neurosurgery, fluorescence-based tumor region identification using 5-aminolevulinic acid (5-ALA) is being performed nowadays [1-5]. Within several hours after oral administration of 5-ALA prior to surgery, protoporphyrin IX (PpIX) is induced and it stays predominantly in malignant glioma cells. PpIX is a fluorophore which emits reddish fluorescence with the peak wavelength at 635 nm when it is excited by blue light. While the color of such malignant glioma cells looks similar to that of normal brain tissues under a white light, it is markedly different from the normal tissues under the excitation light.

So lately two kinds of light sources, a normal white light source and an excitation light source, are embedded in commercial operation microscopes (OMs) so that surgeons can change the light according to the operative procedure. Namely, surgeons confirm the fluorescent region in the brain under the excitation light, then they switch to the normal white light and resect the glioma.

N. Navab et al. (Eds.): MICCAI 2015, Part III, LNCS 9351, pp. 209–217, 2015.
DOI: 10.1007/978-3-319-24574-4_25

While this 5-ALA-based neurosurgery results in better identification of glioma in the operating room (OR), there are still two major issues. The first one is that the switching operation between the types of illumination is troublesome. Moreover, the surgeons must memorize where the fluorescent region appears under the excitation light or they must record the image prior to the resection of the glioma under the white light.

The second issue is the lack of quantitativity in the fluorescent images. Ideally, the glioma cell density should be known from the fluorescent image. In fact, currently it is hard to relate the image intensity of the fluorescent image to the glioma cell density. Ando et al. conducted a quantitative evaluation study and reported the relationship between the fluorescent intensities of tumor tissue and its pathological images [6]. Although the report is very informative, further investigation is still needed for practical use. At least, the intensity distribution of fluorescence should be independent of the lighting and imaging geometry. This is the first step to realize the estimation of the glioma cell density.

In this paper, we first propose a system overcoming the first issue. We then formulate the fluorescence imaging and present a processing way to avoid the geometrical effect for quantitative imaging. We then show some experimental results to confirm the performance of the proposed imaging system and the effectiveness of the color signal processing.

2 Concept of the Image Acquisition System

We assume that the OM has two kinds of light sources embedded, excitation light and normal white light, and also a color camera, an image processing unit (IPU) and a display device. Since the fluorescence takes place in the visible range, a conventional color camera can be used. The surgeon does not see the eye lens of the OM, but directly see the display attached on it. There is rapid switching between the two kinds of light sources. The frequency of the switching is typically 30 Hz. The color camera captures the image of the brain under each illumination synchronously. Roughly speaking, each image is captured in 1/60s. Although the surgical field has some flicker due to switching the light sources, it does not cause significant discomfort. Furthermore, by reducing the rate of the excitation light, it may be possible to make this less perceivable.

Obtained images are processed by IPU and displayed in real time. A pair of consecutive two frame images under different lights are processed and the resultant images are displayed. There are some ways to show the images. The simplest way is just to show the two images side by side on a display. In this paper, we implemented another display approach. After capturing the fluorescent image, the fluorescent region is segmented in 1/60s. Such segmented fluorescent regions are overlaid on the normal color image and displayed next to the normal color image. The real time image processing such as the segmentation and image display is computationally possible. Such a system makes the surgical workflow smoother.

As mentioned earlier, a stable processing for the fluorescent images is required for reliable use in OR. In this paper, color image processing to avoid the dependency on the lighting condition is mainly discussed as the first step of quantification.

3 Imaging Formula

Here we formulate the imaging of the object under the excitation light and show how to extract the contribution of the fluorescence. In this formulation, we introduced two assumptions. The first is that the bandwidth of spectral intensity of the excitation light is narrow enough so that the reflectance of the object can be approximated by a certain constant over the bandwidth. The second is that the spectral characteristics of the fluorescence do not change during the experiment. The second assumption should be checked carefully [7]. But to the extent of our experiment, the characteristics stay the same during at least one hour.

Prior to the formulation, we first define some parameters and functions as showing a schematic illustration and some graphs of spectral characteristics in Fig. 1.

$\mathbf{p}$: Position vector of a pixel in an image

$\mathbf{p}_o$: Position vector of the point in the surgical field corresponding to $\mathbf{p}$

$r(\mathbf{p}_o, \lambda)$: Spectral reflectance at $\mathbf{p}_o$

$E(\mathbf{p}_o, \lambda) = G(\mathbf{p}_o)e(\lambda)$: Spectral intensity of excitation light at $\mathbf{p}_o$

$G(\mathbf{p}_o)$: Geometry factor affecting spectral intensity. It includes distance between the light source and the object, normal direction of the object surface, etc.

$e(\lambda)$: Relative spectral characteristics of the excitation light (see Fig. 1(b) left)

$f(\lambda)$: Relative spectral characteristics of the fluorescence (see Fig. 1(b) right)

$h(\mathbf{p}_o)$: Fluorescence-related factor which implicitly includes density of the tumor cell, quantum efficiency, absorbance of the excitation light, etc.

$S_R(\lambda), S_G(\lambda), S_B(\lambda)$: Spectral sensitivities of red, green, blue channels of the color camera, respectively (see Fig. 1(c))

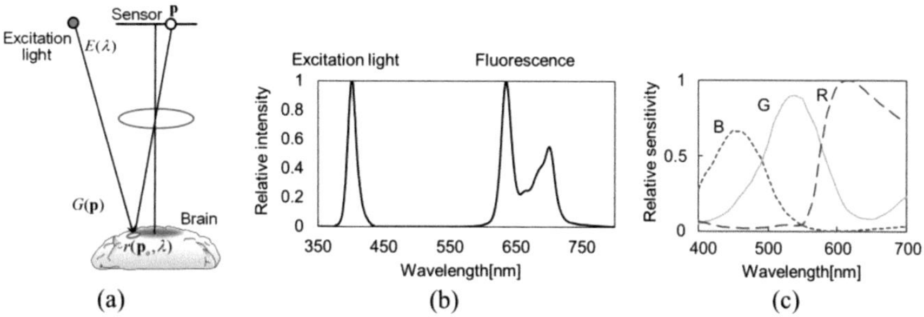

Fig. 1. Schematic illustration of lighting and imaging geometry (a), and relative spectral intensity of the fluorescence of PpIX (b) and spectral sensitivities of RGB camera (c).

Pixel value of the red channel at $\mathbf{p}$ in the image is then approximately modeled by,

$$g_R(\mathbf{p}) = \int [G(\mathbf{p}_o)e(\lambda)r(\mathbf{p}_o, \lambda) + G(\mathbf{p}_o)h(\mathbf{p}_o)f(\lambda)]s_R(\lambda)d\lambda . \quad (1)$$

In this model we assumed the diffuse reflection called Lambertian model. If we take into account the reflection and fluorescent phenomena more exactly, the above equation must be revised. Details will be discussed in the later section.

In Eq. (1), since we assume that the spectral band of the excitation light is narrow enough, the first integral of Eq. (1) is modified and Eq. (1) is expressed as

$$g_R(\mathbf{p}) = G(\mathbf{p}_o)r(\mathbf{p}_o,\lambda_0)\int e(\lambda)s_R(\lambda)d\lambda + G(\mathbf{p}_o)h(\mathbf{p}_o)\int f(\lambda)s_R(\lambda)d\lambda . \tag{2}$$

Here, $\lambda = \lambda_0$ represents the central wavelength of the narrow spectral band. Pixel values of green and blue channels $g_G(\mathbf{p})$ and $g_B(\mathbf{p})$ are given similarly by replacing the sensitivity function $s_R(\lambda)$ by $s_G(\lambda)$ and $s_B(\lambda)$, respectively.

These equations can be represented by a matrix form as

$$\begin{bmatrix} g_R(\mathbf{p}) \\ g_G(\mathbf{p}) \\ g_B(\mathbf{p}) \end{bmatrix} = \begin{bmatrix} a_{eR} & a_{fR} \\ a_{eG} & a_{fG} \\ a_{eB} & a_{fB} \end{bmatrix} \begin{bmatrix} G(\mathbf{p}_o)r(\mathbf{p}_o,\lambda_0) \\ G(\mathbf{p}_o)h(\mathbf{p}_o) \end{bmatrix} = [\mathbf{a}_e \quad \mathbf{a}_f] \begin{bmatrix} G(\mathbf{p}_o)r(\mathbf{p}_o,\lambda_0) \\ G(\mathbf{p}_o)h(\mathbf{p}_o) \end{bmatrix} . \tag{3}$$

Here,

$$a_{ej} = \int e(\lambda)s_j(\lambda)d\lambda, \quad a_{fj} = \int f(\lambda)s_j(\lambda)d\lambda, \quad j = R, G, B$$

The right hand side of equation (3) is a combination of two vectors.

$$\begin{bmatrix} a_{eR} & a_{fR} \\ a_{eG} & a_{fG} \\ a_{eB} & a_{fB} \end{bmatrix} \begin{bmatrix} G(\mathbf{p}_o)r(\mathbf{p}_o,\lambda_0) \\ G(\mathbf{p}_o)h(v) \end{bmatrix} = G(\mathbf{p}_o)r(\mathbf{p}_o,\lambda_0)\mathbf{a}_e + G(\mathbf{p}_o)h(\mathbf{p}_o)\mathbf{a}_f \tag{4}$$

Two vectors can be obtained as follows. The RGB vector of the excitation light $\mathbf{a}_e$ is obtained by capturing the excitation light directly or through the reflection from a perfect reflecting diffuser (no fluorescence). On the other hand, the fluorescent light $\mathbf{a}_f$ can be obtained by capturing the PpIX solution illuminated by excitation light in a manner that the excitation light does not enter the camera. Then, from the RGB pixel values, two factors, $G(\mathbf{p}_o)r(\mathbf{p}_o,\lambda_0)$ and $G(\mathbf{p}_o)h(\mathbf{p}_o)$, can be determined using a least square method.

Next, we calculate the ratio of these two factors and define it as

$$v(\mathbf{p}) \equiv \frac{G(\mathbf{p}_o)h(\mathbf{p}_o)}{G(\mathbf{p}_o)r(\mathbf{p}_o,\lambda_0)} = h(\mathbf{p}_o)/r(\mathbf{p}_o,\lambda_0) \cdot \tag{5}$$

This value is now geometry-independent because the geometry factor $G(\mathbf{p}_o)$ is cancelled. The more important value is $h(\mathbf{p}_o)$. From (5), this value is represented as

$$h(\mathbf{p}_o) = v(\mathbf{p}_o)r(\mathbf{p}_o,\lambda_0) . \tag{6}$$

This means that we need to know the reflectance distribution, $r(\mathbf{p}_o, \lambda_0)$. In fact, it is not easy to obtain $r(\mathbf{p}_o, \lambda_0)$. However, we suppose that the following procedure can provide a good estimation. A perfect reflecting diffuser is illuminated by the excitation light of the OM and its reflected intensity is captured by the color camera of the OM. This is done for many possible distances between the OM and the surgical field prior to the surgery. Intraoperatively, the reflection from the surgical field under the excitation light is recorded by the color camera. The blue channel values are divided by that of the perfect reflecting diffuser obtained at the same distance. These values should give approximately the reflectance $r(\mathbf{p}_o, \lambda_0)$.

4 Experiment

4.1 Prototype System Building

We built an experimental apparatus as shown in Fig. 2(a). It was composed of a white LED (IHRGB-120, IMAC co.), a high intensity blue LED with a peak at 405 nm (LEDH60-405, Hamamatsu Photonics), a CameraLink format color CCD camera (CLB-B1310C-SC, IMPERX), a frame grabber board (PIXCI-E4, EPIX), a handmade switching circuit and a personal computer for controlling the illumination and image capture. Illumination switching is controlled by the strobe signal from the camera. The switching rate of the illumination was set to 30 Hz. The detailed timing chart of the operation is shown in Fig. 2(b).

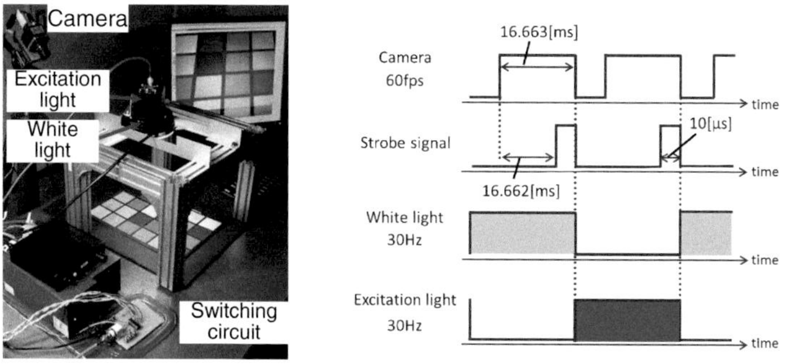

(a) Imaging system (b) Timing chart

Fig. 2. Lighting and imaging system (a) and the timing chart of operation (b).

4.2 Real Time Image Processing and Display

To confirm the performance of the system, a preliminary experiment with the brain of a dead swine was performed. PpIX solution was first made by dissolving PpIX powder (Sigma-Aldrich) with dimethyl sulfoxide. The density of the solution was 25mg/L. A small piece resected from the brain was soaked in the PpIX solution and then put on a fissure of the brain. An operator removed the piece from the brain as its operation was being captured and monitored by the system. Figs. 3 (a) and (b) show the image under the white light and the excitation light, respectively. Here the piece with PpIX was located in the rightmost region in the images. It appeared as slightly reddish in Fig. 3(b).

In the image processing, the image under the excitation light was processed based on the formulas in section 3 to yield $v(\mathbf{p})$ given by Eq. (5). In order to segment the fluorescent region, some pre-processing and a thresholding operation were needed. As pre-processing, the saturated region (halation region) and a very dark region were removed. Then the fluorescent region was extracted by thresholding the $v(\mathbf{p})$ values. The parameters for those processings were determined empirically. Fig. 3(c) shows the segmented PpIX region overlaid on the image under the white light.

We then applied the prototype system to a real human glioma as well. Image acquisition was performed to a resected specimen from the glioma. A resected piece with about 2 cm length was put on a dish and the images were processed as before. Fig. 3 (d)-(f) show the results. We confirmed that the system worked for the resected specimen of a real human glioma as well.

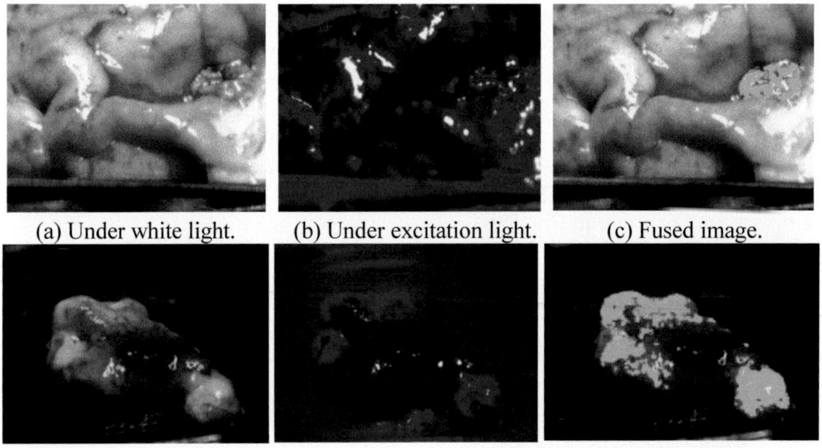

(a) Under white light. (b) Under excitation light. (c) Fused image.

(d) Under white light. (e) Under excitation light. (f) Fused image.

Fig. 3. Captured images in the experiment. (a)-(c): Swine brain. (d)-(f) Resected human glioma.

4.3 Quantitative Imaging Technique

We demonstrated the quantitative imaging technique shown in section 3. We showed that the intensity of the fluorescent image does not depend on the geometry. As shown in Eq. (6), the cell-related value $h(\mathbf{p}_o)$ does not depend on the geometry factor. We examined this formula using physical phantoms. First we measured the relationship between the PpIX density, d, and the h value at a certain lighting condition. That relationship was empirically modeled by an exponential function. Then the model was applied to the other measured images under the different lighting conditions.

In the experiment, PpIX solutions of seven different densities were made and then fixed with agar. The densities of the seven PpIX phantoms were

$$d = kC, \quad \text{where } k = 1,\ldots,7,\ C = 3.0\times10^{-6}\,\text{mol/L}. \tag{7}$$

Fig. 4(a) shows a photo of the PpIX phantoms. Images of each phantom were captured under three different intensities and four different angles of light. As seen in Fig. 4(a), as the density increased, the color became dark. In the images $v(\mathbf{p})$ of these spatially uniform phantoms, a 10x10 pixels area was selected and the mean pixel values of the area $\bar{v}$ were calculated. On the other hand, the corresponding mean reflectance $\bar{r}$ was measured by a spectrophotometer. Fig. 4(b) shows the relationship between the density of the PpIX phantoms and h value in the case that the excitation light intensity was the highest and the illumination angle was 0 deg. Then the density of the PpIX was modeled by the following formula.

$$h(d) = \bar{v}(d)\bar{r}(d) = \alpha \exp(\beta d) \tag{8}$$

We determined two parameters α and β from the data under the highest intensity of the light. Then using the model, we estimated the densities of the phantoms from the images under the different lighting conditions.

Fig. 4(c) shows the results of the density estimation. Circles in the graph represent the mean values of estimated density among three different intensities of excitation light. The top and bottom of the error bars represent the maximum and minimum values of the estimated density, respectively.

Next the lighting angle independency was tested. The phantom of 3C was used and the lighting angle was changed as 15, 30, 45 and 60 deg from the normal direction. The mean, maximum and minimum estimated densities were 2.66C, 2.83C and 2.40C, respectively. In both two examinations, we achieved stable density estimation.

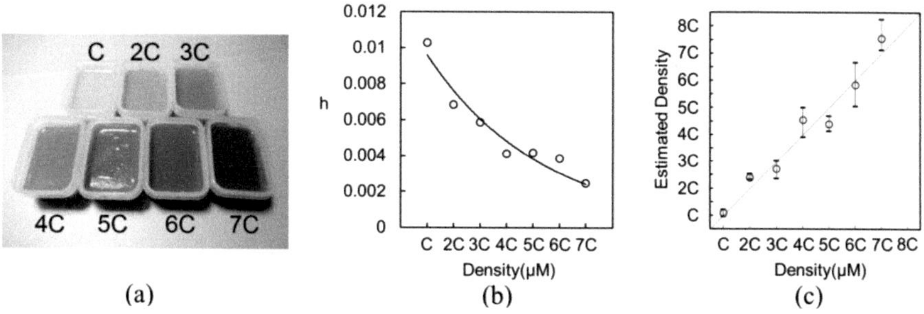

Fig. 4. Experiment for confirming the lighting condition-independent characteristics. (a) PpIX phantoms used. (b) Fitting curve. (c) Estimation result under different light intensities.

5 Discussion and Conclusions

With respect to real time image acquisition under two kinds of light sources, a similar approach was done by Sexton et al [8]. They used pulsed-light for excitation in addition to use of continuous white light. Their system requires an intensified CCD camera to achieve a very short time image acquisition. They did not refer to quantitative analysis. There are respectable works to quantify the fluorescence using fiber optics

[9] or multispectral camera [10]. The former technique measured point-by-point rather than 2D image. Although the latter can get 2D images, the system is bulky and real time processing is not possible. Our approach is a challenge to realize a both convenient and reliable system.

In section 2, we formulated both the value $v(\mathbf{p}_o)$ after cancellation of geometrical factor and the tumor cell density-related function $h(\mathbf{p}_o)$. In the first experiment, we focused on a real time processing and demonstrated the segmentation based on the value of $v(\mathbf{p}_o)$. On the other hand, in the second experiment, $v(\mathbf{p}_o)$ were related to $h(\mathbf{p}_o)$. In the next step, we must establish the real time estimation of $r(\mathbf{p}_o, \lambda_0)$ to get $h(\mathbf{p}_o)$.

In the quantification, we used the Lambertian model for the reflection and assumed that the geometrical factors for the reflection and fluorescence were the same. To be exact, however, more realistic model such as Phong model [11] consisting of the surface reflection and body reflection components. For example, direct reflection of the organ surface like mirror takes place in some parts. In such cases, a different image processing is required.

In this study, we proposed a method for real time image display with tumor location and built an experimental apparatus to confirm the performance. The apparatus was applied to a dead swine brain first then to a resected human brain tumor in OR. A neurosurgeon gave us a positive evaluation of this system. As future works, we need to clarify what is the appropriate switching rate, what are appropriate ways to carry out image processing and displaying. In the quantification of fluorescence, real mapping of the image values to the density of glioma cells is also needed.

Acknowledgments. This study is supported by MEXT/JSPS KAKENHI Grant Number 15H01106 in part.

References

1. Stummer, W., et al.: Intraoperative detection of malignant gliomas by 5-aminolevulinic acid-induced porphyrin fluorescence. Neurosurgery 42, 518–525 (1998)
2. Stummer, W., et al.: Fluorescence-guided surgery with 5-aminolevulinic acid for resection of malignant glioma: a randomised controlled multicentre phase III trial. Lancet Oncology 7(5), 392–401 (2006)
3. Widhalm, G., et al.: 5-Aminolevulinic acid induced fluorescence is a powerful intraoperative marker for precise histopathological grading of gliomas with non-significant contrast-enhancement. PLOS ONE 8(10), e76988 (2013)
4. Tonn, J.C., Stummer, W.: Fluorescence-guided resection of malignant gliomas using 5-aminolevulinic acid: practical use, risks, and pitfalls. Clinical Neurosurgery 55, 20–26 (2008)
5. Liao, H., et al.: An integrated diagnosis and therapeutic system using intraoperative 5-aminolevulinic-acid-induced fluorescence guided robotic Laser ablation for pre-cision neurosurgery. Medical Image Analysis 16(3), 754–766 (2012)
6. Ando, T., et al.: Precise comparison of protoporphyrin IX fluorescence spectra with pathological results for brain tumor tissue identification. Brain Tumor Path. 28, 43–51 (2011)
7. Ericson, M.B., et al.: A spectroscopic study of the photobleaching of protoporphyrin IX in solution. Lasers in Medical Science 18(1), 56–62 (2003)

8. Sexton, K., et al.: Pulsed-light imaging for fluorescence guided surgery under normal room lighting. Optics Letters 38(17), 3249 (2013)
9. Kim, A., et al.: Quantification of in vivo fluorescence decoupled from the effects of tissue optical properties using fiber-optic spectroscopy measurements. Journal of Biomedical Optics 15(6) (2010)
10. Valdés, P.A., et al.: Quantitative, spectrally-resolved intraoperative fluorescence imaging. Scientific Reports 2, Article number 798 (2012)
11. Phong, B.T.: Illumination for computer generated pictures. Communications of ACM 18(6), 311–317 (1975)

Analysis of High-throughput Microscopy Videos: Catching Up with Cell Dynamics

A. Arbelle[1], N. Drayman[2], M. Bray[3], U. Alon[2], A. Carpenter[3], and T. Riklin Raviv[1]

[1] Ben-Gurion University of the Negev
[2] Weizmann Institute of Science
[3] Broad Institute of MIT and Harvard

Abstract. We present a novel framework for high-throughput cell lineage analysis in time-lapse microscopy images. Our algorithm ties together two fundamental aspects of cell lineage construction, namely cell segmentation and tracking, via a Bayesian inference of dynamic models. The proposed contribution exploits the Kalman inference problem by estimating the time-wise cell shape uncertainty in addition to cell trajectory. These inferred cell properties are combined with the observed image measurements within a fast marching (FM) algorithm, to achieve posterior probabilities for cell segmentation and association. Highly accurate results on two different cell tracking datasets are presented.

1 Introduction

High-throughput live cell imaging is an excellent and versatile platform for quantitative analysis of biological processes, such as cell lineage reconstruction. However, lineage analysis poses a difficult problem, as it requires spatiotemporal tracing of multiple cells in a dynamic environment. Since addressing this challenge manually is not feasible for large data sets, numerous cell tracking algorithms have been developed. Forming complete cell tracks based on frame-to-frame cell association is commonly approached by finding correspondences between cell features in consecutive frames. Typical cell properties used for this purpose are cell pose, location and appearance e.g. center of mass (COM), intensity, and shape. As a result, cell segmentation is therefore inevitable, and is thus typically an integral part of the tracking process.

Cell association becomes complicated when the feature similarity of a cell and its within-frame neighbors is comparable to the similarity of the same cell in consecutive frames. When cells cannot be easily distinguished, a more elaborate cell matching criterion is needed, for example, considering cell dynamics [21], solving sub-optimal frame-to-frame assignment problems, via linear programming optimization[8] or by using multiple hypothesis testing (MHT) [17] and its relaxations [7]. In these cases, a two-step approach in which cell segmentation and cell association are treated as independent processes is feasible, provided that the segmentation problem is well-posed and addressed [10,11,12,16,20].

N. Navab et al. (Eds.): MICCAI 2015, Part III, LNCS 9351, pp. 218–225, 2015.
DOI: 10.1007/978-3-319-24574-4_26

Nevertheless, the accurate delineation of cell boundaries is often a challenging task. A high degree of fidelity is required for cell segmentation, even in instances where the cells are far apart and hence can be easily distinguished, especially in cases where the extracted features (e.g. shape or intensity profile) are also the intended subject of the biological experiment. Therefore, several recent methods attempt to support segmentation through solving the cell association problem. For example, the initial cell boundaries in the active contour (AC) framework can be derived from the contours of the associated cells in the previous frame [4]. An alternative AC strategy is to segment a series of time-lapse images as a 3D volume [13]. More recent methods successfully deal with complex data sets using probabilistic frameworks. In the graphical model suggested by [19] cell segments are merged by solving MHT subject to inter-frame and intra-frame constraints. The Gaussian mixture model of [1] is based on the propagation of cell centroids and their approximated Gaussian shape to the following frame in order to combine super-voxels into complete cell regions.

In this paper, cell tracking and segmentation are jointly solved via two intertwined estimators, the Kalman filter and maximum a posteriori probability (MAP). The key idea is a dynamic shape modeling (DSM) by extending the commonly-used Kalman state vector to account for shape fluctuations. Shape inference requires a probabilistic modeling of cell morphology, which is not mathematically trivial. We address this challenge by applying a sigmoid function to the signed distance function (SDF) of the cell boundaries in which the slope of the sigmoid models the shape uncertainty. Given the estimated cell poses, shape models and velocity maps generated from the observed image measurements, we calculate the posterior probabilities of the image pixels via a fast marching (FM) algorithm. Partitioning the image into individual cells and background is defined by the MAP estimates.

The proposed method is mathematically elegant and robust, with just a few parameters to tune. The algorithm has numerous advantages: Estimating the cell temporal dynamics facilitates accurate frame-to-frame association, particularly in the presence of highly cluttered assays, rapid cell movements or sequences with low frame rates. Therefore, unlike the active contour approach, the usability of the segmentation priors is not limited by large displacements or crossing cell tracks. Moreover, the motion estimation allows for lineage recovery in the case of disappearing and reappearing cells, which would otherwise disrupt accurate tracking. The DSM serves as a prior for the consecutive frame segmentation without imposing any predetermined assumptions, in contrast to [1] which implicitly assumes ellipsoidal structures. Furthermore, introducing the boundary uncertainty estimate to the shape model makes our algorithm robust against temporal, morphological fluctuations. Lastly, we note that mitotic events (i.e., cell division) significantly complicate cell tracking. We address this issue by initiating tracks for the daughter cells, using the probabilistic framework to naturally assign a mother cell to its children.

The rest of the paper is organized as follows. In Section 2, we introduce our novel approach which consists of four main components: (1) Extended state vector estimation via Kalman filter; (2) probabilistic DSM based on previous frame segmentation and the estimated boundary uncertainty; (3) FM algorithm for the calculation of the posterior probabilities; and (4) MAP estimation. Section 3 presents highly accurate experimental results for two different datasets of over 70 frames each, and we conclude and outline future directions in Section 4.

2 Methods

2.1 Problem Formulation

Let $\mathcal{C} = \{C^{(1)}, ..., C^{(K)}\}$ denote K cells in a time lapse microscopy sequence, containing $\mathcal{T}$ frames. Let $I_t : \Omega \rightarrow \mathbb{R}^+$ be the t-th frame, in that sequence, where Ω defines the 2D image domain of I_t, and $t = 1, ..., \mathcal{T}$. We assume that each I_t is a gray-level image of $\mathcal{K}_t$ cells which form a subset of $\mathcal{C}$. Our objective is twofold and consists of both cell segmentation and frame-to-frame cell association defined as follows:

Segmentation: For every frame I_t, find a function $f_t \colon \Omega \rightarrow L_t$, (where L_t is a subset of $\mathcal{K}_t + 1$ integers in $[0, \ldots, K]$) that assigns a label $l_t \in L_t$ to each pixel $\mathbf{x} = [x, y] \in \Omega$. The function f_t partitions the t-th frame into $\mathcal{K}_t + 1$ regions, where each segment $\Gamma_t^{(k)} = \{\mathbf{x} \in \Omega | f_t(\mathbf{x}) = l_t = k, \}$ forms a connected component of pixels, in frame I_t, that belongs to either a specific cell in $\mathcal{C}$ or to the background, i.e. $\Gamma_t^{(0)}$.

Association: For every frame I_t find an injective function $h_t : L_{t-1} \rightarrow L_t$ that corresponds cell segments in frame $t - 1$ and frame t. As we will show in the following, the segmentation and association steps are merged and $\Gamma_t^{(k)}, k \geq 1$ defines the segmentation of cell $C^{(k)}$ in frame t.

2.2 Time Series Analysis

For every cell $C^{(k)}$ there exist a number of properties that describe its state at a given time t. Let $\xi_t^{(k)}$ denote the hidden state vector that holds the true, unknown, state of the cell. In the following discussion the superscript (k) is removed for clarity. In our case the state vector holds the following features:

$$\xi_t = [c_{x_t}, c_{y_t}, v_{x_t}, v_{y_t}, \epsilon_t]^T = [\mathbf{c}_t^T, \mathbf{v}_t^T, \epsilon_t]^T \quad (1)$$

where $\mathbf{c}_t = [c_{x_t}, c_{y_t}]^T$ denote the COM of the cell at time t and $\mathbf{v}_t = [v_{x_t}, v_{y_t}]^T$ denote the COM velocities. The variable ϵ_t is the shape uncertainty variable, which will be explained in section 2.3. We assume that the state vector approximately follows a linear time step evolution as follows: $\xi_t = \mathrm{A}\xi_{t-1} + w_{t-1}$, where $\mathrm{A} \in \mathbb{R}^{5 \times 5}$ is the state transition model, and $w_t \in \mathbb{R}^5$ is the process noise drawn i.i.d from $\mathcal{N}(\mathbf{0}, \mathrm{Q}_t)$. In our case: $A_{i,i} = 1, i = 1 \ldots 5$; $A_{1,3} = A_{2,4} = 1$. Since the true state is hidden, the observed state is $\zeta_t = \xi_t + r_t$, where $r_t \in \mathbb{R}^5$ is the measurement noise drawn i.i.d from $\mathcal{N}(\mathbf{0}, \mathrm{R}_t)$. The process and measurement noise covariance matrices $\mathrm{Q}_t, \mathrm{R}_t$ are assumed to be known.

In order to predict the state of a cell at t we utilize the Kalman Filter [9]. The predicted (a priori) state vector estimation and error covariance matrix at t given measurements up to time $t-1$ are: $\hat{\xi}_{t|t-1} = \mathrm{A}\hat{\xi}_{t-1|t-1}$; $\Sigma_{t|t-1} = \mathrm{A}\Sigma_{t-1|t-1}\mathrm{A}^T + \mathrm{Q}_t^T$

The a posteriori state estimate and error covariance matrix at time t given measurements up to and including time t are: $\hat{\xi}_{t|t} = \hat{\xi}_{t|t-1} + G_t\left(\zeta_t - \hat{\xi}_{t|t-1}\right)$; $\Sigma_{t|t} = (\mathrm{I} - G_t\mathrm{B})\,\Sigma_{t|t-1}$

where the Kalman Gain matrix is given as: $\mathrm{G}_t = \Sigma_{t|t-1}\left(\Sigma_{t|t-1} + \mathrm{R}_t\right)^{-1}$.

2.3 Dynamic Shape Model

The estimated segmentation of a cell $C^{(k)}$ in frame t, i.e. $\hat{\Gamma}_{t|t-1}^{(k)}$ is obtained by a translation of the cell segmentation in frame $t-1$:
$\hat{\Gamma}_{t|t-1}^{(k)} = \left\{\mathbf{x}|\left(\mathbf{x} - \hat{\mathbf{v}}_{t|t-1}^{(k)}\right) \in \Gamma_{t-1}^{(k)}\right\}$, where, $\hat{\mathbf{v}}_{t|t-1}^{(k)} \cdot 1$, is the estimated cell displacement. The respective signed distance function (SDF) $\hat{\phi}_{t|t-1}^{(k)} : \Omega \rightarrow \mathbb{R}$ is constructed as follows:

$$\hat{\phi}_{t|t-1}^{(k)}(\mathbf{x}) = \begin{cases} \min_{\mathbf{x}' \in \partial\hat{\Gamma}_{t|t-1}^{(k)}} d_E(\mathbf{x}, \mathbf{x}') & \mathbf{x} \in \hat{\Gamma}_{t|t-1}^{(k)} \\ -\min_{\mathbf{x}' \in \partial\hat{\Gamma}_{t|t-1}^{(k)}} d_E(\mathbf{x}, \mathbf{x}') & \mathbf{x} \notin \hat{\Gamma}_{t|t-1}^{(k)} \end{cases} \tag{2}$$

where $d_E(\cdot,\cdot)$ denotes the Euclidian distance and $\partial\hat{\Gamma}_{t|t-1}$ denotes the estimated segmentation boundary. In the spirit of [18,15], we define the probability that a pixel $\mathbf{x}$ belongs to the domain of cell k by a logistic regression function (LRF):

$$\hat{\Phi}_{t|t-1}^{(k)}(\mathbf{x}) = P\left(\mathbf{x} \in \Gamma_t^{(k)}\right) \triangleq \left(1 + \exp\left\{-\frac{\hat{\phi}_{t|t-1}^{(k)}(\mathbf{x})}{\hat{\epsilon}_{t|t-1}^{(k)}}\right\}\right)^{-1} \tag{3}$$

where, $\hat{\epsilon}_{t|t-1}^{(k)}$ is the estimation of $\epsilon_t^{(k)} \triangleq d_H\left(\partial\Gamma_{t-1}^{(k)}, \partial\Gamma_t^{(k)}\right) \cdot \frac{\sqrt{3}\pi}{2}$ which denotes the calculated[1] boundary uncertainty. The LRF slope is determined by $\epsilon_t^{(k)}$. We set $\epsilon_t^{(k)}$ such that the standard deviation of the probability density function (PDF) corresponding to $P\left(\mathbf{x} \in \Gamma_t^{(k)}\right)$ is equal to the Hausdorff distance between the aligned cell boundaries i.e. $d_H\left(\partial\Gamma_{t-1}^{(k)}, \partial\Gamma_t^{(k)}\right)$. Note, that large temporal fluctuations in a cell boundary, increase d_H, which in turn smooth the LRF slope and increase the shape uncertainty. Eq.3 defines our dynamic shape model.

2.4 MAP Segmentation and Association

We now present the flow of the proposed segmentation algorithm given the state vector estimation $\hat{\xi}_{t|t-1}$ and cell segmentation of the previous frame. Fig.1 illustrates the main concepts to be discussed. Consider the image I_t with $\mathbf{c}_t^{(k)}$ marked

[1] Derived from an analytic expression. See appendix A.1.

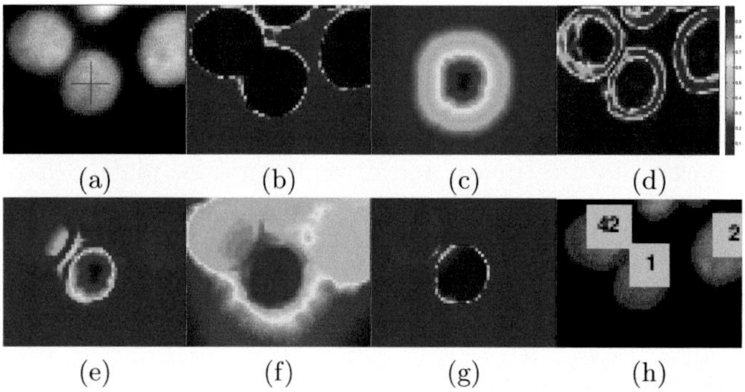

Fig. 1. Segmentation flow of a specific cell. (a) Original image. The estimated COM of the specific cell k is marked by red cross. (b) Intensity probability of the foreground P_{FG}. (c) DSM (Spatial probability). (d) Traversability image $g\left(\nabla_{\mathbf{x}} I_t\right)$. (e) Speed image $\hat{S}^{(k)}_{t|t-1}$, the product of (b-d). (f) FM distance. (g) DSM posterior $P_t^{(k)}$ (h) Labeled segmentation.

by a red cross, shown in Fig.1.a. We model the PDFs of the foreground and background intensities, $f_{FG}(\cdot)$ and $f_{BG}(\cdot)$ respectively by a mixture of Gaussians. The intensity based probability of being a cell or background (Fig.1.b) is defined as follows:

$$P_t^{(BG)}(\mathbf{x}) = \frac{\alpha f_{BG}\left(I_t(\mathbf{x})\right)}{\alpha f_{BG}\left(I_t(\mathbf{x})\right) + (1-\alpha) f_{FG}\left(I_t(\mathbf{x})\right)}; \; P_t^{(FG)}(\mathbf{x}) = 1 - P_t^{(BG)}(\mathbf{x}) \tag{4}$$

where $0 < \alpha < 1$ is a predetermined weight (we set $\alpha = 0.5$).

For each cell segment, in frame t, we construct a DSM, $\hat{\Phi}^{(k)}_{t|t-1}$, as explained in section 2.3 (Fig.1.c). We use the FM algorithm [6] to find the shortest path from each pixel $\mathbf{x}$ to the estimated COM of a cell k s.t. a speed image $\hat{S}^{(k)}_{t|t-1} : \Omega \rightarrow [0,1]$ (Fig.1.e). The FM distance, $d_{FM}\left(\mathbf{x}, \hat{\mathbf{c}}^{(\mathbf{k})}_{t|t-1} | \hat{S}^{(k)}_{t|t-1}\right)$, is the minimal geodesic distance from $\mathbf{x}$ to $\hat{\mathbf{c}}^{(\mathbf{k})}_{t|t-1}$ (Fig.1.f). In other words, the value of $\hat{S}^{(k)}_{t|t-1}(\mathbf{x})$ is the speed of a pixel $\mathbf{x}$ along the shortest path to $\hat{\mathbf{c}}^{(\mathbf{k})}_{t|t-1}$. For each pixel $\mathbf{x}$ in frame t we define its speed $\hat{S}^{(k)}_{t|t-1}(\mathbf{x})$ as the product of three terms: 1. The intensity based probability of belonging to the foreground (Eq.4). 2. The spatial prior of being part of a specific cell i.e. the DSM (Eq.3). 3. The "traversability" (Fig.1.d) which is inverse proportional to the image edges in frame I_t and defined by $g\left(\nabla_{\mathbf{x}} I_t\right) = \left(1 + \frac{|\nabla_{\mathbf{x}} I_t|}{\|\nabla_{\mathbf{x}} I_t\|_2}\right)^{-2}$:

$$\hat{S}^{(k)}_{t|t-1} = P_t^{(FG)} \cdot \hat{\Phi}^{(k)}_{t|t-1} \cdot g\left(\nabla_{\mathbf{x}} I_t\right) \tag{5}$$

The absolute value of the spatial gradient, i.e. $|\nabla_{\mathbf{x}} I_t|$, can be interpreted as "speed bumps" which make the "FM journey" more difficult across edges.

The posterior probability that $\mathbf{x}$ belongs to C_k is inverse proportional[2] to the difference between its geodesic and Euclidean distances to $\hat{\mathbf{c}}^{(\mathbf{k})}_{t|t-1}$ (Fig.

$$P_t^{(k)}(\mathbf{x}) \propto \left(d_{FM}\left(\mathbf{x},\hat{\mathbf{c}}^{(k)}_{t|t-1}|\hat{S}^{(k)}_{t|t-1},\right) - d_E\left(\mathbf{x},\hat{\mathbf{c}}^{(k)}_{t|t-1}\right)+1\right)^{-1} \tag{6}$$

The final segmentation is given as the MAP of (6)(Fig.1.h): $\Gamma_t^{(k)} = \left\{\mathbf{x}|\arg\max_{k'\in L_t} P_t^{(k')}(\mathbf{x}) = k\right\}$. In fact, we see that cell association is inherent to the defined segmentation problem, since each cell is segmented using its estimated properties from the previous frame. The detection of new cells is explained in appendix A.3.

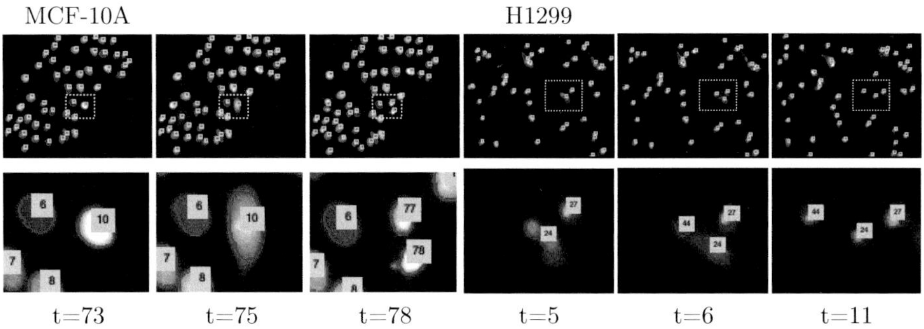

Fig. 2. Top row: A full-frame temporal sequence. Bottom row: Enlargement of inset shown in the top row. Note that mitosis of cells 10 and 24.

3 Experimental Results

We examined two different sequences: (1) MCF-10A cells, expressing RFP- Geminin and NLS- mCerulean, rate: 3fph, 142 frames. (2) H1299 cells, expressing eYFP-DDX5 in the background of an mCherry tagged nuclear protein, rate: 3fph, 72 frames [3]. The input to the algorithm is a manual segmentation of the first two frames of each sequence. We tested our method based on manual annotation generated by an expert. We then compared precision, recall and F-measure scores to those obtained by the maximum correlation thresholding segmentation [14] and linear-assignment problem tracking [7] method as implemented in CellProfiler [2] which is a publicly-available, state of the art, cell analysis tool.

Figure 2 present two sets of sampled frames from the examined data sets. The cell numbers along with the segmentation boundaries are marked. We use purple and red for new and existing tracks, respectively. The upper rows show the full frames, the marked rectangle is magnified in the lower rows. The detected cell trajectories of both data sets can be visualized in Fig.1 in the supplementary material. We note that the noisy linear motion of the cells supports the use of

[2] $P_t^{(k)}(\mathbf{x})$ is normalized such that $\sum_{k'} P_t^{(k')}(\mathbf{x}) = 1$. See appendix A.2.

Table 1. Segmentation and Tracking Results.C.P. is CellProfiler [2] Prc. is Precision, Rcl. is Recall, F is F-measure. Further details can be found in the supp. material.

Data	Method	Segmentation			Full Tracks	Divisions		
		Prc.	Rcl.	F	Success Rate	Prc.	Rcl.	F
H1299	Ours	**0.98**	**0.89**	**0.93**	**0.95**	0.84	0.89	0.86
	C.P	0.93	0.81	0.87	0.86	0.84	0.94	0.88
MCF-10A	Ours	**1**	**0.94**	**0.97**	**0.99**	**0.96**	**0.98**	**0.97**
	C.P	0.98	0.82	0.89	0.94	0.86	0.94	0.90

the Kalman filter. We urge the reader to refer to our live cell segmentation and tracking videos at http://youtu.be/ORx82dCKWlA and in the supplementary material. We quantitatively evaluate our segmentation and mitosis detection as described in [19]. The tracking success was calculated as percentage of full, errorless tracks which were manually counted by an expert. An error was defined as early termination of a track, a split or a merge of tracks. See Table 1 for results.

4 Summary and Conclusions

We address cell segmentation and tracking by jointly solving MAP and Kalman filtering estimation problems. A key contribution is a DSM which accommodates versatile cell shapes with varying levels of uncertainty. The DSM is inferred via time-series analysis and is exploited as a shape prior in the segmentation process. The proposed model can handle long sequences in an elegant and robust manner, requiring minimal input. While the daughters of divided cells are accurately detected, mitotic events are not yet labeled as such. Future work will aim to complete the missing link for cell lineage reconstruction in the spirit of [5] .

Acknowledgments. This work was supported in part by Human Frontiers in Science Program RGP0053/2010 (Carpenter), and NSF RIG DBI 1119830 (Bray) and the Human Frontiers in Science Program RGP0020/2012 (Alon).

References

1. Amat, F., Lemon, W., Mossing, D.P., McDole, K., Wan, Y., Branson, K., Myers, E.W., Keller, P.J.: Fast, accurate reconstruction of cell lineages from large-scale fluorescence microscopy data. Nature Methods (2014)
2. Carpenter, A.E., Jones, T.R., Lamprecht, M.R., Clarke, C., Kang, I.H., Friman, O., Guertin, D.A., Chang, J.H., Lindquist, R.A., Moffat, J., et al.: Cellprofiler: image analysis software for identifying and quantifying cell phenotypes. Genome Biology 7(10), R100 (2006)
3. Cohen, A.A., Geva-Zatorsky, N., Eden, E., Frenkel-Morgenstern, M., Issaeva, I., Sigal, A., Milo, R., Cohen-Saidon, C., Liron, Y., Kam, Z., et al.: Dynamic proteomics of individual cancer cells in response to a drug. Science 322(5907), 1511–1516 (2008)
4. Dzyubachyk, O., van Cappellen, W.A., Essers, J., Niessen, W.J., Meijering, E.: Advanced level-set-based cell tracking in time-lapse fluorescence microscopy. IEEE Trans. on Medical Imaging 29(3), 852–867 (2010)

5. Gilad, T., Bray, M., Carpenter, A., Riklin-Raviv, T.: Symmetry-based mitosis detection in time-lapse microscopy. In: IEEE International Symposium on Biomedical Imaging: From Nano to Macro (2015)
6. Hassouna, M.S., Farag, A.A.: Multistencils fast marching methods: A highly accurate solution to the eikonal equation on cartesian domains. IEEE Trans. on Pattern Analysis and Machine Intelligence 29(9), 1563–1574 (2007)
7. Jaqaman, K., Loerke, D., Mettlen, M., Kuwata, H., Grinstein, S., Schmid, S.L., Danuser, G.: Robust single-particle tracking in live-cell time-lapse sequences. Nature Methods 5(8), 695–702 (2008)
8. Kachouie, N.N., Fieguth, P.W.: Extended-hungarian-jpda: Exact single-frame stem cell tracking. IEEE Trans. Biomed. Eng. 54(11), 2011–2019 (2007)
9. Kalman, R.E.: A new approach to linear filtering and prediction problems. J. of Fluids Engineering 82(1), 35–45 (1960)
10. Kanade, T., Yin, Z., Bise, R., Huh, S., Eom, S., Sandbothe, M.F., Chen, M.: Cell image analysis: Algorithms, system and applications. In: 2011 IEEE Workshop on Applications of Computer Vision (WACV), pp. 374–381. IEEE (2011)
11. Maška, M., Ulman, V., Svoboda, D., Matula, P., Matula, P., Ederra, C., Urbiola, A., España, T., Venkatesan, S., Balak, D.M., et al.: A benchmark for comparison of cell tracking algorithms. Bioinformatics 30(11), 1609–1617 (2014)
12. Meijering, E., Dzyubachyk, O., Smal, I., et al.: Methods for cell and particle tracking. Methods Enzymol. 504(9), 183–200 (2012)
13. Padfield, D., Rittscher, J., Roysam, B.: Spatio-temporal cell segmentation and tracking for automated screening. In: IEEE International Symposium on Biomedical Imaging: From Nano to Macro, pp. 376–379. IEEE (2008)
14. Padmanabhan, K., Eddy, W.F., Crowley, J.C.: A novel algorithm for optimal image thresholding of biological data. J. of Neuroscience Methods 193(2), 380–384 (2010)
15. Pohl, K.M., Fisher, J., Shenton, M.E., McCarley, R.W., Grimson, W.E.L., Kikinis, R., Wells, W.M.: Logarithm odds maps for shape representation. In: Larsen, R., Nielsen, M., Sporring, J. (eds.) MICCAI 2006. LNCS, vol. 4191, pp. 955–963. Springer, Heidelberg (2006)
16. Rapoport, D.H., Becker, T., Mamlouk, A.M., Schicktanz, S., Kruse, C.: A novel validation algorithm allows for automated cell tracking and the extraction of biologically meaningful parameters. PloS One 6(11), e27315 (2011)
17. Reid, D.B.: An algorithm for tracking multiple targets. IEEE Transactions on Automatic Control 24(6), 843–854 (1979)
18. Riklin-Raviv, T., Van Leemput, K., Menze, B.H., Wells, W.M., Golland, P.: Segmentation of image ensembles via latent atlases. Medical Image Analysis 14(5), 654–665 (2010)
19. Schiegg, M., Hanslovsky, P., Haubold, C., Koethe, U., Hufnagel, L., Hamprecht, F.A.: Graphical model for joint segmentation and tracking of multiple dividing cells. Bioinformatics, page btu764 (2014)
20. Su, H., Yin, Z., Huh, S., Kanade, T.: Cell segmentation in phase contrast microscopy images via semi-supervised classification over optics-related features. Medical Image Analysis 17(7), 746–765 (2013)
21. Yang, X., Li, H., Zhou, X.: Nuclei segmentation using marker-controlled watershed, tracking using mean-shift, and kalman filter in time-lapse microscopy. IEEE Trans. Circuits Syst. I, Reg. Papers 53(11), 2405–2414 (2006)

Neutrophils Identification by Deep Learning and Voronoi Diagram of Clusters *

Jiazhuo Wang[1], John D. MacKenzie[2], Rageshree Ramachandran[3], and Danny Z. Chen[1]

[1] Department of Computer Science and Engineering, University of Notre Dame, USA
[2] Department of Radiology and Biomedical Imaging, UCSF, USA
[3] Department of Pathology, UCSF, USA

Abstract. Neutrophils are a primary type of immune cells, and their identification is critical in clinical diagnosis of active inflammation. However, in H&E histology tissue slides, the appearances of neutrophils are highly variable due to morphology, staining and locations. Further, the noisy and complex tissue environment causes artifacts resembling neutrophils. Thus, it is challenging to design, in a hand-crafted manner, computerized features that help identify neutrophils effectively. To better characterize neutrophils, we propose to extract their features in a learning manner, by constructing a deep convolutional neural network (CNN). In addition, in clinical practice, neutrophils are identified not only based on their individual appearance, but also on the context formed by multiple related cells. It is not quite straightforward for deep learning to capture precisely the rather complex cell context. Hence, we further propose to combine deep learning with Voronoi diagram of clusters (VDC), to extract needed context. Experiments on clinical data show that (1) the learned hierarchical representation of features by CNN outperforms hand-crafted features on characterizing neutrophils, and (2) the combination of CNN and VDC significantly improves over the state-of-the-art methods for neutrophil identification on H&E histology tissue images.

1 Introduction

Identification of a primary type of immune cells, neutrophils, is of great medical importance. Because the number and the locations are key features for acute inflammation diagnosis [6]; further, quantitative analysis of the distribution patterns of neutrophils may help provide deep insight into acute inflammation.

In H&E histology tissue images (Fig. 1(a)), neutrophils are characterized as having multiple lobes in their nuclei, and almost invisible cytoplasms (Fig. 1(b)). But, in practice, it is highly challenging to identify them for the following reasons. First, there are lots of variations in neutrophil appearances due to, e.g., staining, shape, and size. In fact, large portions of neutrophils do not show common

* This research was supported in part by NSF Grant CCF-1217906, a grant of the National Academies Keck Futures Initiative (NAKFI), and NIH grant K08-AR061412-02 Molecular Imaging for Detection and Treatment Monitoring of Arthritis.

N. Navab et al. (Eds.): MICCAI 2015, Part III, LNCS 9351, pp. 226–233, 2015.
DOI: 10.1007/978-3-319-24574-4_27

"textbook" characteristics (Fig. 1(c)). Second, the background is quite noisy and complex with a mixture of different biological structures, such as other types of immune cells (e.g., lymphocytes, eosinophils, and plasma cells, see Fig. 1(d)) and some tissue layers (e.g., glands and villi). These structures greatly complicate the neutrophils identification task. For example, each lobe of a neutrophil could be classified incorrectly as a single lymphocyte. Artifacts resembling neutrophils are often created by other structures in H&E histology tissue images (Fig. 1(e)).

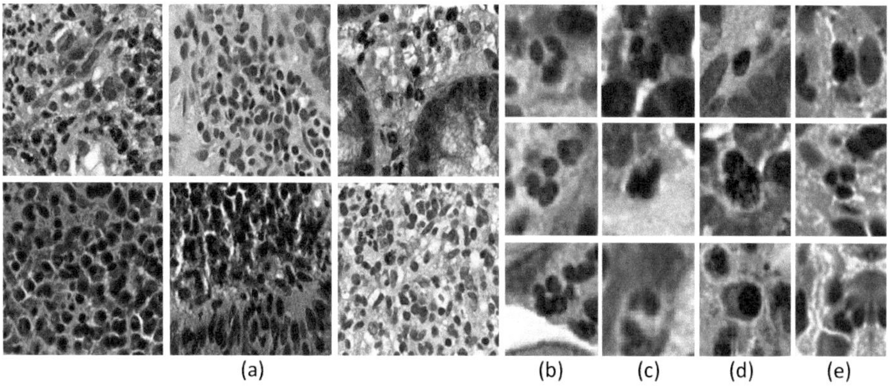

Fig. 1. (a) H&E histology tissue image examples; (b) neutrophils; (c) neutrophils without obvious "textbook" appearances; (d) a lymphocyte (top), an eosinophil (middle), and a plasma cell (bottom); (e) artifacts resembling neutrophils.

The first and state-of-the-art method for neutrophils identification on H&E histology tissue images was proposed very recently in [8]. But further improvements can be made as illustrated below.

One key to effective identification of neutrophils is to well capture the features of individual cells (such features should be invariant to different factors). The method in [8] conducted feature engineering in a hand-crafted manner, which is quite challenging, since the characteristics of neutrophils become highly subtle in the noisy and complex tissue environment. Hence, we advocate to automatically learn features in such settings. In computer vision literature, deep learning [2,1,7] was recently shown to outperform highly-tuned state-of-the-art methods on many problems (e.g., recognition, detection) using the automatically learned hierarchical low, mid, and high level representations of features.

Another key to effective identification of neutrophils is to model cell context, i.e., related cells in a certain neighborhood help determine cell types on one another. In fact, cell context is commonly utilized by pathologists, especially when identifying neutrophils without obvious "textbook" appearances. Therefore, the method in [8] proposed to exploit such cell context, extracted based on Voronoi diagram of clusters (VDC) [3] of "trustable" neutrophils. However, because their "trustable" neutrophils are identified based on hand-crafted features and Random Forest, it is likely that some of the "trustable" neutrophils thus identified are actually not neutrophils. Clearly, using context built on a not so "trustworthy" version of "trustable" neutrophils means propagating noisy or even wrong information on the appearances of neutrophils to the neighborhood.

Motivated by the above two keys, we propose to combine deep learning and Voronoi diagram of clusters (VDC) into one framework for identifying neutrophils in H&E histology tissue images. Our main idea is to first model the appearances of individual cells by a convolutional neural network (CNN) [5] and identify the "trustable" portion of neutrophils, and then model context by constructing the VDC of the "trustable" neutrophils and utilize the context to resolve the ambiguous cases (evaluated on merely individual cell appearances).

Experimental results on clinical data validate that deep learning and VDC are efficacious complements to each other. Also, the general idea of combing deep learning (for modeling individual object appearances) and VDC (for modeling context) can be applicable to other similar identification problems.

2 Modeling Individual Cell Appearances by CNN

Overview. Assume that the cells (regardless of their types) have been segmented and detected (we actually apply the iterative edge labeling method [8] to segment and detect cells). For each segmented and detected cell, we crop a small image patch containing it. Our goal is to capture the subtle characteristics of individual cells, so that we can subsequently classify the image patches into neutrophils and non-neutrophils.

Our main idea is to apply supervised deep neural networks to learn a hierarchical representation of the low, mid, and high level features of the cells. Such a network maps each input image (patch), via a series of parameterized layers, into probabilities of the target classes (in our case, neutrophils and non-neutrophils). The parameters of the layers are learned during training, and some of them can be viewed as filters. Responses to the filters in lower layers (i.e., closer to the input image) usually contain low (e.g., edges, corners) or mid (e.g., correlations between edges) level features, and responses in higher layers contain high level semantic features related to the target classes.

Deep Learning Model Design. We construct a deep convolutional neural network (CNN) [5]. The overall architecture of our CNN (shown in Fig. 2) basically follows that in [5], but with some important modifications to the hyper parameters, as described below. Our modifications to the hyper parameters are motivated mainly by two considerations. First, the size of our input image patch is quite different from that in [5] (256 pixels). Thus, using the same set of hyper parameters cannot describe well the characteristics of our target objects. For example, the size of the filters in the first convolutional layer of [5] is 11×11, which appears seemingly too big for the first layer filters in our case, which are supposed to capture low level features (e.g., edges and corners). Because the layers are closely related, an inappropriate first layer not functioning well could impose negative influence on the subsequent layers. Second, as stated in [10], by visualizing the network of [5] using the method in [10], some hyper parameters do not have appropriate values. For example, the large stride 4 of the filters in the first layer causes aliasing artifacts in the second layer. We set the stride to 1, taking into consideration of such aliasing artifacts, our input image size, and the influence to the subsequent layers.

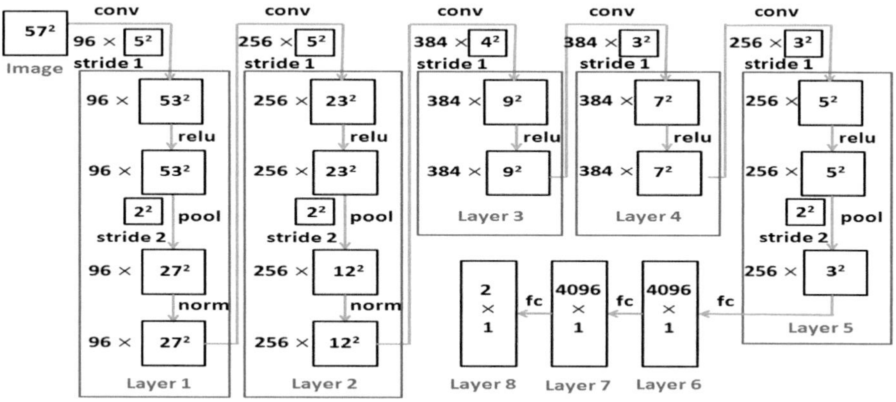

Fig. 2. Our CNN structure. Our CNN has 8 layers. The first 5 layers are convolutional. For example, the input image patch of size 57 × 57 to the first convolutional layer is first convolved (conv) by a set of 96 learned filters of size 5 × 5; the resulting 96 feature maps of size 53 × 53 then pass through a rectified linear function (relu), go through max pooling with stride 2 on each direction, and finally are locally normalized before output to the next layer. The rest 3 layers are fully connected (fc). We minimize the softmax cost function at the last layer. Please see [5] for the roles played by layers.

Training. *Learning Algorithm.* We apply stochastic gradient descent with a batch size of 512 to learn parameters in CNN. We initialize learning rate as 0.01, momentum as 0.9, and weight decay as 0.0005. We also decrease learning rate three times before termination. We iterate 30000 times over the batches.

Overfitting. To combat overfitting, we apply data augmentation [5] and drop out [4]. For data augmentation, we sub-crop 10 images (corners and centers with or without horizontal flips) of size 57 × 57 from the original image patch of size 64 × 64. We apply drop out at the fully connected layers (6 and 7) and set the drop out rate as 0.5. Please see [5,4] for more details of these techniques.

Conservativeness. In our clinical setting of studying inflammatory bowl diseases, neutrophils are usually rare (but important) comparing to other types of immune cells (such as lymphocytes and plasma cells). But, the noisy and complex environment of histology tissue images may cause many artifacts that look similar to neutrophils. Hence, we adopt a conservative strategy to identify neutrophils, by penalizing more when a non-neutrophil is misclassified as a neutrophil than when a neutrophil is misclassified as a non-neutrophil, during the training of CNN. We did so via multiplying by two the computed softmax loss when a non-neutrophil is misclassified as a neutrophil.

3 Modeling Cell Context by VDC

Overview. In clinical practice, when pathologists identify neutrophils, clusters of neutrophils usually attract their attention (bigger clusters may attract more attention), because such clusters can provide some cues about the local appearances difference between neutrophils and non-neutrophils in the neighborhood of the clusters, and help identify near by neutrophils that may appear ambiguous individually. To our best knowledge, no straightforward way is known for deep learning to model precisely such context information. Thus, to complement deep learning and capture cell context, our main idea is to apply the model of Voronoi diagram of clusters (VDC) [8,3], based on the "trustable" portion of neutrophils. Note that, different from [8], we incorporate and utilize the high quality CNN features and CNN probabilities in VDC (as described later in detail below), which make the extracted context information more robust.

Voronoi Diagram of Clusters. We first discuss general concepts for VDC. Different from the common Voronoi diagram, in which each site is a single point, every site of VDC can also be a cluster of points. Due to this feature, VDC can capture the influence of each cluster (i.e., the collective influence of all site points belonging to the cluster) to the neighborhood regions. The tessellation of VDC is built based on the influence function $D(\cdot, \cdot)$, of each cluster C (with site points $\{p_1, p_2, \ldots, p_m\}$) on any point p, which is defined as

$$D(C,p) = \sum_{i=1}^{m} F(p, p_i), \qquad F(p,p_i) = \begin{cases} \frac{w(p_i)}{d(p,p_i)^2}, & \text{if } d(p,p_i) \leq dist_T \\ 0, & \text{otherwise} \end{cases} \tag{1}$$

where $F(p, p_i)$ measures the influence of a single point $p_i \in C$ to the point p, which depends on both the weight $w(p_i)$ (for the "importance" of p_i) and the Euclidean distance $d(p, p_i)$ between p and p_i. Note that we truncate $F(p, p_i)$ using a distance threshold $dist_T$ to reflect that a point p which is too far away from a cluster C is not influenced by C. In this way, a point p would be influenced more by a cluster C whose size is big, and/or its site points have larger weights, and are closer to p. Thus p belongs to the geometric VDC cell of C (i.e., this is not a biological cell) in the tessellation of VDC.

Extracting Cell Context. We extract the cell context to classify individually ambiguous cases by taking the following steps.

(1) Obtain a set of "trustable" neutrophils by thresholding the neutrophil probability of each cell produced by CNN. (Actually, we also obtain a set of "trustable" non-neutrophils for the non-neutrophil probability, based on the same threshold value.) All the remaining cells (i.e., not "trustable" neutrophils nor "trustable" non-neutrophils) are taken as individually ambiguous cells (thus to be classified later on by context). Note that since the learned hierarchical feature representation can capture well the characteristics of individual cells, the "trustable" ones produced by CNN are actually more "trustable" than those produced using hand-crafting features and simple classifier as in [8], even with

similar thresholding. This reduces the chance of propagating noisy or wrong information when we resolve ambiguous cases based on the influence of clusters of "trustable" neutrophils later on.

(2) Apply density-based clustering [9] to the "trustable" neutrophils to capture their potential clustering behaviors.

(3) Compute VDC: Each site of VDC is either a cluster of "trustable" neutrophils found in Step (2), or an individual "trustable" neutrophil that does not belong to any such cluster. Assign the weight of each "trustable" neutrophil as the neutrophil probability computed by CNN (as opposed to 1 in [8]), in the influence function $F(\cdot,\cdot)$ defined above. By doing so, clusters of neutrophils that are more likely to contain correct information would have larger influence to the neighborhood. Set $dist_T = 160$ pixels. Some examples are given in Fig. 3.

(4) For each geometric VDC cell, build a Random Forest classifier, using the "trustable" neutrophils and non-neutrophils within this VDC cell as respectively the "+" and "-" training examples. Here, we simply use the filters' responses in layer 7 of our CNN as the features, because they contain high level semantic information on the cell types. Such a classifier captures locally what neutrophils and non-neutrophils look like in the neighborhood, and thus is referred to as the *LocalExpert* (LE) for the corresponding geometric VDC cell.

(5) For each ambiguous cell c, define its *context* as all the geometric VDC cells overlapping with the circle of radius R centered at c. (Note that if the context is empty, then it essentially means that likely no neutrophil cluster or single neutrophil is around c, and thus we simply take c as a non-neutrophil.) We use the weighted average probabilities of the LEs of these geometric VDC cells to determine whether c is a neutrophil. We set the weight of an LE as the collective influence from the corresponding cluster to c, to reflect that the decision on c's cell type favors more the "opinion" from a cluster with a larger influence to c.

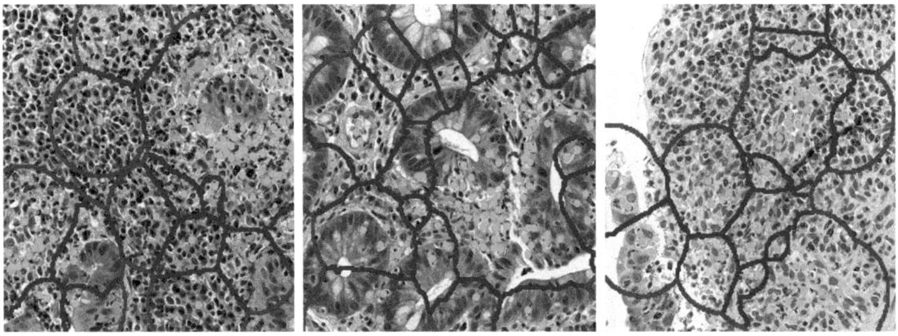

Fig. 3. Some examples of VDC tessellation: The green points are "trustable" neutrophils; the blue curves are boundaries between adjacent geometric VDC cells; the red curves are boundaries between adjacent geometric VDC cells and regions that exceed the distance threshold $dist_T$ based on the influence function $F(\cdot,\cdot)$.

4 Experiments and Evaluation

We collected histology tissue slides (scanned at 40X magnification, which pathologists commonly use to identify cell types) from patients suspected of having inflammatory bowl diseases (the study was performed under an IRB and in compliance with the privacy provisions of HIPPA of 1996). We manually marked 810 neutrophils (we automatically detected the cells regardless of their types; the detected cells that are not marked as neutrophils are taken as non-neutrophil ground truth), from 53 images as ground truth. This a larger and more challenging dataset than that in [8]. Each time, we randomly selected 21 images for training, and the rest images for testing (we repeat 5 times to obtain the average performance). To measure the performance quantitatively, we compute two metrics, $precision = \frac{TP}{TP+FP}$ and $recall = \frac{TP}{TP+FN}$, for neutrophils.

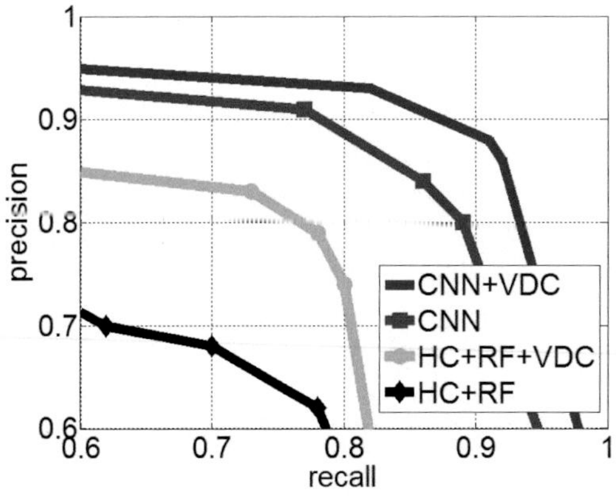

Fig. 4. The precision and recall curves.

Evaluation on Modeling Individual Cell Appearances. To demonstrate the effectiveness of deep learning on capturing the characteristics of cells, we compare the performance based on merely thresholding the probabilities output by CNN (i.e., without VDC), and two versions of the state-of-the-art method [8]: Hand-crafted features (color, texture, etc) + Random Forest (HC + RF), and HC + RF + VDC. The precision and recall curves (obtained by varying the probability threshold for both CNN and HC + RF, and varying the threshold for determining "trustable" neutrophils for HC + RF + VDC) are shown in Fig. 4.

One can see that the combination of hand-crafted features and simple classifier, even after using the additional context information extracted based on VDC, is outperformed by CNN. This validates that the learned hierarchical representation of features by CNN captures well the subtle characteristics of individual cells, which are often further complicated by the noisy and complex environment of H&E histology tissue images.

Evaluation on Modeling Cell Context. The precision and recall curve (obtained by varying the threshold for determining "trustable" neutrophils) of combining CNN and VDC is also shown in Fig. 4. One can see that although CNN alone already performs well, using additional context information extracted from VDC further improves the performance. This validates that VDC is a good complement to CNN, and modeling cell context can considerably help neutrophils identification.

5 Conclusions

In this paper, we present a robust new method that significantly improves the state-of-the-art for neutrophil identification in clinical tissue samples. Our method constructs a CNN to characterize the features of neutrophils, which are subtle and complicated given the cells are embedded in the noisy and complex tissue environment. It also combines CNN with VDC to extract needed cell context that helps identify neutrophils more effectively.

References

1. Bengio, Y.: Learning deep architectures for AI. Foundations and Trends in Machine Learning 2(1), 1–127 (2009)
2. Bengio, Y., Courville, A.C., Vincent, P.: Unsupervised feature learning and deep learning: A review and new perspectives. IEEE Trans. PAMI, special issue Learning Deep Architectures (2012)
3. Chen, D.Z., Huang, Z., Liu, Y., Xu, J.: On clustering induced Voronoi diagrams. In: FOCS, pp. 390–399 (2013)
4. Hinton, G.E., Srivastava, N., Krizhevsky, A., Sutskever, I., Salakhutdinov, R.: Improving neural networks by preventing co-adaptation of feature detectors. CoRR abs/1207.0580 (2012)
5. Krizhevsky, A., Sutskever, I., Hinton, G.E.: Imagenet classification with deep convolutional neural networks. In: NIPS, pp. 1106–1114 (2012)
6. Naini, B.V., Cortina, G.: A histopathologic scoring system as a tool for standardized reporting of chronic (ileo) colitis and independent risk assessment for inflammatory bowel disease. Human Pathology 43, 2187–2196 (2012)
7. Schmidhuber, J.: Deep learning in neural networks: An overview. Neural Networks 61, 85–117 (2014)
8. Wang, J., MacKenzie, J.D., Ramachandran, R., Chen, D.Z.: Identifying neutrophils in H&E staining histology tissue images. In: Golland, P., Hata, N., Barillot, C., Hornegger, J., Howe, R. (eds.) MICCAI 2014, Part I. LNCS, vol. 8673, pp. 73–80. Springer, Heidelberg (2014)
9. Xu, B., Chen, D.Z.: Density-based data clustering algorithms for lower dimensions using space-filling curves. In: Zhou, Z.-H., Li, H., Yang, Q. (eds.) PAKDD 2007. LNCS (LNAI), vol. 4426, pp. 997–1005. Springer, Heidelberg (2007)
10. Zeiler, M.D., Fergus, R.: Visualizing and understanding convolutional networks. In: Fleet, D., Pajdla, T., Schiele, B., Tuytelaars, T. (eds.) ECCV 2014, Part I. LNCS, vol. 8689, pp. 818–833. Springer, Heidelberg (2014)

U-Net: Convolutional Networks for Biomedical Image Segmentation

Olaf Ronneberger, Philipp Fischer, and Thomas Brox

Computer Science Department and BIOSS Centre for Biological Signalling Studies, University of Freiburg, Germany
ronneber@informatik.uni-freiburg.de
http://lmb.informatik.uni-freiburg.de/

Abstract. There is large consent that successful training of deep networks requires many thousand annotated training samples. In this paper, we present a network and training strategy that relies on the strong use of data augmentation to use the available annotated samples more efficiently. The architecture consists of a contracting path to capture context and a symmetric expanding path that enables precise localization. We show that such a network can be trained end-to-end from very few images and outperforms the prior best method (a sliding-window convolutional network) on the ISBI challenge for segmentation of neuronal structures in electron microscopic stacks. Using the same network trained on transmitted light microscopy images (phase contrast and DIC) we won the ISBI cell tracking challenge 2015 in these categories by a large margin. Moreover, the network is fast. Segmentation of a 512x512 image takes less than a second on a recent GPU. The full implementation (based on Caffe) and the trained networks are available at http://lmb.informatik.uni-freiburg.de/people/ronneber/u-net.

1 Introduction

In the last two years, deep convolutional networks have outperformed the state of the art in many visual recognition tasks, e.g. [7]. While convolutional networks have already existed for a long time [8], their success was limited due to the size of the available training sets and the size of the considered networks. The breakthrough by Krizhevsky et al. [7] was due to supervised training of a large network with 8 layers and millions of parameters on the ImageNet dataset with 1 million training images. Since then, even larger and deeper networks have been trained [12].

The typical use of convolutional networks is on classification tasks, where the output to an image is a single class label. However, in many visual tasks, especially in biomedical image processing, the desired output should include localization, i.e., a class label is supposed to be assigned to each pixel. Moreover, thousands of training images are usually beyond reach in biomedical tasks. Hence, Ciresan et al. [2] trained a network in a sliding-window setup to predict the class label of each pixel by providing a local region (patch) around that pixel

N. Navab et al. (Eds.): MICCAI 2015, Part III, LNCS 9351, pp. 234–241, 2015.
DOI: 10.1007/978-3-319-24574-4_28

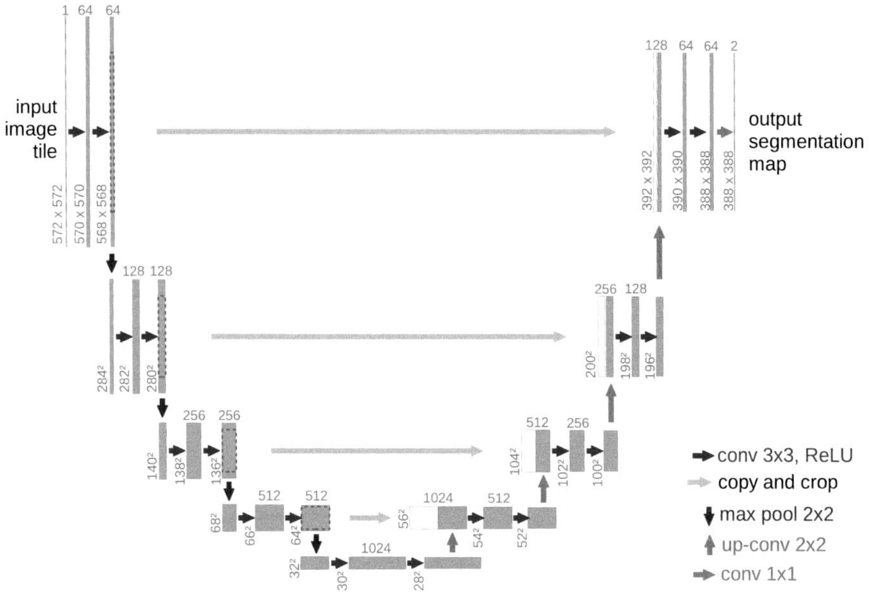

Fig. 1. U-net architecture (example for 32x32 pixels in the lowest resolution). Each blue box corresponds to a multi-channel feature map. The number of channels is denoted on top of the box. The x-y-size is provided at the lower left edge of the box. White boxes represent copied feature maps. The arrows denote the different operations.

as input. First, this network can localize. Secondly, the training data in terms of patches is much larger than the number of training images. The resulting network won the EM segmentation challenge at ISBI 2012 by a large margin.

Obviously, the strategy in Ciresan et al. [2] has two drawbacks. First, it is quite slow because the network must be run separately for each patch, and there is a lot of redundancy due to overlapping patches. Secondly, there is a trade-off between localization accuracy and the use of context. Larger patches require more max-pooling layers that reduce the localization accuracy, while small patches allow the network to see only little context. More recent approaches [11,4] proposed a classifier output that takes into account the features from multiple layers. Good localization and the use of context are possible at the same time.

In this paper, we build upon a more elegant architecture, the so-called "fully convolutional network" [9]. We modify and extend this architecture such that it works with very few training images and yields more precise segmentations; see Figure 1. The main idea in [9] is to supplement a usual contracting network by successive layers, where pooling operators are replaced by upsampling operators. Hence, these layers increase the resolution of the output. In order to localize, high resolution features from the contracting path are combined with the upsampled output. A successive convolution layer can then learn to assemble a more precise output based on this information.

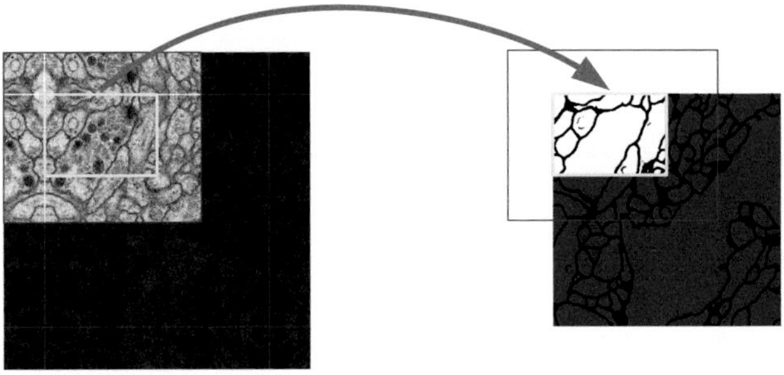

Fig. 2. Overlap-tile strategy for seamless segmentation of arbitrary large images (here segmentation of neuronal structures in EM stacks). Prediction of the segmentation in the yellow area, requires image data within the blue area as input. Missing input data is extrapolated by mirroring

One important modification in our architecture is that in the upsampling part we have also a large number of feature channels, which allow the network to propagate context information to higher resolution layers. As a consequence, the expansive path is more or less symmetric to the contracting path, and yields a u-shaped architecture. The network does not have any fully connected layers and only uses the valid part of each convolution, i.e., the segmentation map only contains the pixels, for which the full context is available in the input image. This strategy allows the seamless segmentation of arbitrarily large images by an overlap-tile strategy (see Figure 2). To predict the pixels in the border region of the image, the missing context is extrapolated by mirroring the input image. This tiling strategy is important to apply the network to large images, since otherwise the resolution would be limited by the GPU memory.

As for our tasks there is very little training data available, we use excessive data augmentation by applying elastic deformations to the available training images. This allows the network to learn invariance to such deformations, without the need to see these transformations in the annotated image corpus. This is particularly important in biomedical segmentation, since deformation used to be the most common variation in tissue and realistic deformations can be simulated efficiently. The value of data augmentation for learning invariance has been shown in Dosovitskiy et al. [3] in the scope of unsupervised feature learning.

Another challenge in many cell segmentation tasks is the separation of touching objects of the same class; see Figure 3. To this end, we propose the use of a weighted loss, where the separating background labels between touching cells obtain a large weight in the loss function.

The resulting network is applicable to various biomedical segmentation problems. In this paper, we show results on the segmentation of neuronal structures in EM stacks (an ongoing competition started at ISBI 2012), where we outperformed the network of Ciresan et al. [2]. Furthermore, we show results for cell segmentation in light microscopy images from the ISBI cell tracking challenge 2015. Here we won with a large margin on the two most challenging 2D transmitted light datasets.

2 Network Architecture

The network architecture is illustrated in Figure 1. It consists of a contracting path (left side) and an expansive path (right side). The contracting path follows the typical architecture of a convolutional network. It consists of the repeated application of two 3x3 convolutions (unpadded convolutions), each followed by a rectified linear unit (ReLU) and a 2x2 max pooling operation with stride 2 for downsampling. At each downsampling step we double the number of feature channels. Every step in the expansive path consists of an upsampling of the feature map followed by a 2x2 convolution ("up-convolution") that halves the number of feature channels, a concatenation with the correspondingly cropped feature map from the contracting path, and two 3x3 convolutions, each followed by a ReLU. The cropping is necessary due to the loss of border pixels in every convolution. At the final layer a 1x1 convolution is used to map each 64-component feature vector to the desired number of classes. In total the network has 23 convolutional layers.

To allow a seamless tiling of the output segmentation map (see Figure 2), it is important to select the input tile size such that all 2x2 max-pooling operations are applied to a layer with an even x- and y-size.

3 Training

The input images and their corresponding segmentation maps are used to train the network with the stochastic gradient descent implementation of Caffe [6]. Due to the unpadded convolutions, the output image is smaller than the input by a constant border width. To minimize the overhead and make maximum use of the GPU memory, we favor large input tiles over a large batch size and hence reduce the batch to a single image. Accordingly we use a high momentum (0.99) such that a large number of the previously seen training samples determine the update in the current optimization step.

The energy function is computed by a pixel-wise soft-max over the final feature map combined with the cross entropy loss function. The soft-max is defined as $p_k(\mathbf{x}) = \exp(a_k(\mathbf{x})) / \left(\sum_{k'=1}^{K} \exp(a_{k'}(\mathbf{x}))\right)$ where $a_k(\mathbf{x})$ denotes the activation in feature channel k at the pixel position $\mathbf{x} \in \Omega$ with $\Omega \subset \mathbb{Z}^2$. K is the number of classes and $p_k(\mathbf{x})$ is the approximated maximum-function. I.e. $p_k(\mathbf{x}) \approx 1$ for the k that has the maximum activation $a_k(\mathbf{x})$ and $p_k(\mathbf{x}) \approx 0$ for all other k. The cross entropy then penalizes at each position the deviation of $p_{\ell(\mathbf{x})}(\mathbf{x})$ from 1 using

$$E = \sum_{\mathbf{x} \in \Omega} w(\mathbf{x}) \log(p_{\ell(\mathbf{x})}(\mathbf{x})) \tag{1}$$

where $\ell : \Omega \to \{1, \ldots, K\}$ is the true label of each pixel and $w : \Omega \to \mathbb{R}$ is a weight map that we introduced to give some pixels more importance in the training.

We pre-compute the weight map for each ground truth segmentation to compensate the different frequency of pixels from a certain class in the training

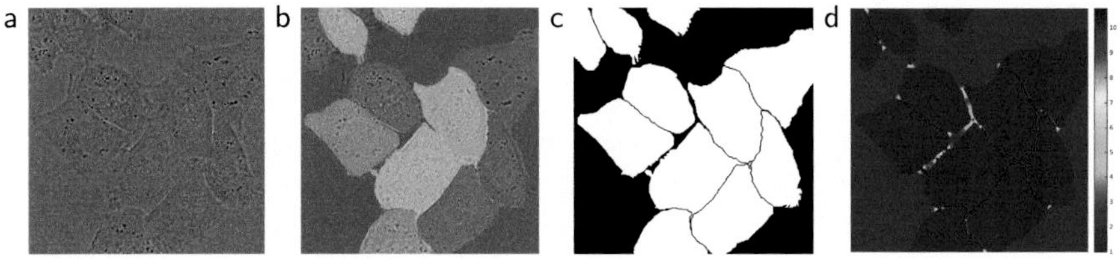

Fig. 3. HeLa cells on glass recorded with DIC (differential interference contrast) microscopy. (**a**) raw image. (**b**) overlay with ground truth segmentation. Different colors indicate different instances of the HeLa cells. (**c**) generated segmentation mask (white: foreground, black: background). (**d**) map with a pixel-wise loss weight to force the network to learn the border pixels.

data set, and to force the network to learn the small separation borders that we introduce between touching cells (See Figure 3c and d).

The separation border is computed using morphological operations. The weight map is then computed as

$$w(\mathbf{x}) = w_c(\mathbf{x}) + w_0 \cdot \exp\left(-\frac{(d_1(\mathbf{x}) + d_2(\mathbf{x}))^2}{2\sigma^2}\right) \tag{2}$$

where $w_c : \Omega \to \mathbb{R}$ is the weight map to balance the class frequencies, $d_1 : \Omega \to \mathbb{R}$ denotes the distance to the border of the nearest cell and $d_2 : \Omega \to \mathbb{R}$ the distance to the border of the second nearest cell. In our experiments we set $w_0 = 10$ and $\sigma \approx 5$ pixels.

In deep networks with many convolutional layers and different paths through the network, a good initialization of the weights is extremely important. Otherwise, parts of the network might give excessive activations, while other parts never contribute. Ideally the initial weights should be adapted such that each feature map in the network has approximately unit variance. For a network with our architecture (alternating convolution and ReLU layers) this can be achieved by drawing the initial weights from a Gaussian distribution with a standard deviation of $\sqrt{2/N}$, where N denotes the number of incoming nodes of one neuron [5]. E.g. for a 3x3 convolution and 64 feature channels in the previous layer $N = 9 \cdot 64 = 576$.

3.1 Data Augmentation

Data augmentation is essential to teach the network the desired invariance and robustness properties, when only few training samples are available. In case of microscopical images we primarily need shift and rotation invariance as well as robustness to deformations and gray value variations. Especially random elastic deformations of the training samples seem to be the key concept to train a segmentation network with very few annotated images. We generate smooth deformations using random displacement vectors on a coarse 3 by 3 grid.

Table 1. Ranking on the EM segmentation challenge [14] (march 6th, 2015), sorted by warping error.

Rank	Group name	Warping Error	Rand Error	Pixel Error
	** human values **	0.000005	0.0021	0.0010
1.	u-net	**0.000353**	0.0382	0.0611
2.	DIVE-SCI	0.000355	0.0305	0.0584
3.	IDSIA [2]	0.000420	0.0504	0.0613
4.	DIVE	0.000430	0.0545	**0.0582**
⋮				
10.	IDSIA-SCI	0.000653	**0.0189**	0.1027

The displacements are sampled from a Gaussian distribution with 10 pixels standard deviation. Per-pixel displacements are then computed using bicubic interpolation. Drop-out layers at the end of the contracting path perform further implicit data augmentation.

4 Experiments

We demonstrate the application of the u-net to three different segmentation tasks. The first task is the segmentation of neuronal structures in electron microscopic recordings. An example of the data set and our obtained segmentation is displayed in Figure 2. We provide the full result as Supplementary Material. The data set is provided by the EM segmentation challenge [14,1] that was started at ISBI 2012 and is still open for new contributions. The training data is a set of 30 images (512x512 pixels) from serial section transmission electron microscopy of the Drosophila first instar larva ventral nerve cord (VNC). Each image comes with a corresponding fully annotated ground truth segmentation map for cells (white) and membranes (black). The test set is publicly available, but its segmentation maps are kept secret. An evaluation can be obtained by sending the predicted membrane probability map to the organizers. The evaluation is done by thresholding the map at 10 different levels and computation of the "warping error", the "Rand error" and the "pixel error" [14].

The u-net (averaged over 7 rotated versions of the input data) achieves without any further pre- or postprocessing a warping error of 0.0003529 (the new best score, see Table 1) and a rand-error of 0.0382.

This is significantly better than the sliding-window convolutional network result by Ciresan et al. [2], whose best submission had a warping error of 0.000420 and a rand error of 0.0504. In terms of rand error the only better performing algorithms on this data set use highly data set specific post-processing methods[1] applied to the probability map of Ciresan et al. [2].

[1] The authors of this algorithm have submitted 78 different solutions to achieve this result.

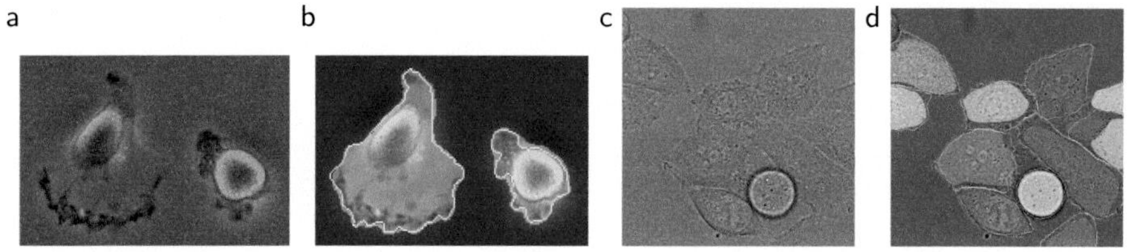

Fig. 4. Result on the ISBI cell tracking challenge. (**a**) part of an input image of the "PhC-U373" data set. (**b**) Segmentation result (cyan mask) with manual ground truth (yellow border) (**c**) input image of the "DIC-HeLa" data set. (**d**) Segmentation result (random colored masks) with manual ground truth (yellow border).

Table 2. Segmentation results (IOU) on the ISBI cell tracking challenge 2015.

Name	PhC-U373	DIC-HeLa
IMCB-SG (2014)	0.2669	0.2935
KTH-SE (2014)	0.7953	0.4607
HOUS-US (2014)	0.5323	-
second-best 2015	0.83	0.46
u-net (2015)	**0.9203**	**0.7756**

We also applied the u-net to a cell segmentation task in light microscopic images. This segmenation task is part of the ISBI cell tracking challenge 2014 and 2015 [10,13]. The first data set "PhC-U373"[2] contains Glioblastoma-astrocytoma U373 cells on a polyacrylimide substrate recorded by phase contrast microscopy (see Figure 4a,b and Supp. Material). It contains 35 partially annotated training images. Here we achieve an average IOU ("intersection over union") of 92%, which is significantly better than the second best algorithm with 83% (see Table 2). The second data set "DIC-HeLa"[3] are HeLa cells on a flat glass recorded by differential interference contrast (DIC) microscopy (see Figure 3, Figure 4c,d and Supp. Material). It contains 20 partially annotated training images. Here we achieve an average IOU of 77.5% which is significantly better than the second best algorithm with 46%.

5 Conclusion

The u-net architecture achieves very good performance on very different biomedical segmentation applications. Thanks to data augmentation with elastic deformations, it only needs very few annotated images and has a very reasonable training time of only 10 hours on a NVidia Titan GPU (6 GB). We provide the

[2] Data set provided by Dr. Sanjay Kumar. Department of Bioengineering University of California at Berkeley. Berkeley CA (USA).

[3] Data set provided by Dr. Gert van Cappellen Erasmus Medical Center. Rotterdam. The Netherlands.

full Caffe[6]-based implementation and the trained networks[4]. We are sure that the u-net architecture can be applied easily to many more tasks.

Acknowlegements. This study was supported by the Excellence Initiative of the German Federal and State governments (EXC 294) and by the BMBF (Fkz 0316185B).

References

1. Cardona, A., et al.: An integrated micro- and macroarchitectural analysis of the drosophila brain by computer-assisted serial section electron microscopy. PLoS Biol. 8(10), e1000502 (2010)
2. Ciresan, D.C., Gambardella, L.M., Giusti, A., Schmidhuber, J.: Deep neural networks segment neuronal membranes in electron microscopy images. In: NIPS, pp. 2852–2860 (2012)
3. Dosovitskiy, A., Springenberg, J.T., Riedmiller, M., Brox, T.: Discriminative unsupervised feature learning with convolutional neural networks. In: NIPS (2014)
4. Hariharan, B., Arbeláez, P., Girshick, R., Malik, J.: Hypercolumns for object segmentation and fine-grained localization (2014), arXiv:1411.5752 [cs.CV]
5. He, K., Zhang, X., Ren, S., Sun, J.: Delving deep into rectifiers: Surpassing human-level performance on imagenet classification (2015), arXiv:1502.01852 [cs.CV]
6. Jia, Y., Shelhamer, E., Donahue, J., Karayev, S., Long, J., Girshick, R., Guadarrama, S., Darrell, T.: Caffe: Convolutional architecture for fast feature embedding (2014), arXiv:1408.5093 [cs.CV]
7. Krizhevsky, A., Sutskever, I., Hinton, G.E.: Imagenet classification with deep convolutional neural networks. In: NIPS, pp. 1106–1114 (2012)
8. LeCun, Y., Boser, B., Denker, J.S., Henderson, D., Howard, R.E., Hubbard, W., Jackel, L.D.: Backpropagation applied to handwritten zip code recognition. Neural Computation 1(4), 541–551 (1989)
9. Long, J., Shelhamer, E., Darrell, T.: Fully convolutional networks for semantic segmentation (2014), arXiv:1411.4038 [cs.CV]
10. Maska, M., et al.: A benchmark for comparison of cell tracking algorithms. Bioinformatics 30, 1609–1617 (2014)
11. Seyedhosseini, M., Sajjadi, M., Tasdizen, T.: Image segmentation with cascaded hierarchical models and logistic disjunctive normal networks. In: 2013 IEEE International Conference on Computer Vision (ICCV), pp. 2168–2175 (2013)
12. Simonyan, K., Zisserman, A.: Very deep convolutional networks for large-scale image recognition (2014), arXiv:1409.1556 [cs.CV]
13. WWW: Web page of the cell tracking challenge, http://www.codesolorzano.com/celltrackingchallenge/Cell_Tracking_Challenge/Welcome.html
14. WWW: Web page of the em segmentation challenge, http://brainiac2.mit.edu/isbi_challenge/

[4] U-net implementation, trained networks and supplementary material available at http://lmb.informatik.uni-freiburg.de/people/ronneber/u-net

Co-restoring Multimodal Microscopy Images*

Mingzhong Li and Zhaozheng Yin

Department of Computer Science, Missouri University of Science and Technology
{ml424,yinz}@mst.edu

Abstract. We propose a novel microscopy image restoration algorithm capable of co-restoring Phase Contrast and Differential Interference Contrast (DIC) microscopy images captured on the same cell dish simultaneously. Cells with different phase retardation and DIC gradient signals are restored into a single image without the halo artifact from phase contrast or pseudo 3D shadow-casting effect from DIC. The co-restoration integrates the advantages of two imaging modalities and overcomes the drawbacks in single-modal image restoration. Evaluated on a datasets of five hundred pairs of phase contrast and DIC images, the co-restoration demonstrates its effectiveness to greatly facilitate the cell image analysis tasks such as cell segmentation and classification.

1 Introduction

Microscopy imaging techniques are critical for biologists to observe, record and analyze the behavior of specimens. Two well-known non-fluorescence microscopy imaging modalities based on light interferences are phase contrast microscopy [1] and differential interference contrast (DIC) microscopy (Chapter 10 in [2]). As non-invasive techniques, phase contrast and DIC have been widely used to observe live cells without staining them.

With the large amount of microscopy image data captured in high-throughput biological experiments, computational algorithms have been developed to analyze cell images automatically [3,4]. In addition to common image processing algorithms [5,6], recently some cell image analysis methods based on microscope optics models have been explored. Due to the specific image formation process, phase contrast microscopy images contain artifacts such as the halo surrounding cells (Fig.1(a)), and DIC microscopy images have the pseudo 3D shadow-cast effect (Fig.1(c)). The computational imaging model of phase contrast microscopy was derived in [8], based on which algorithms have been developed to restore artifact-free images for cell segmentation and detection [10,11]. The computational imaging model of DIC microscopy was derived in [12] and corresponding preconditioning algorithms were developed to preprocess the DIC images to greatly facilitate the cell segmentation [12,13].

However, there are still some challenges which are hard to be conquered by a single microscopy modality. For example, during mitosis (division) or apoptosis (death) events, cells appear brighter than their surrounding medium (a different phenomenon

* This research was supported by NSF CAREER award IIS-1351049, NSF EPSCoR grant IIA-1355406, ISC and CBSE centers at Missouri S&T.

N. Navab et al. (Eds.): MICCAI 2015, Part III, LNCS 9351, pp. 242–250, 2015.
DOI: 10.1007/978-3-319-24574-4_29

compared to halos around dark cells during their migration cell stages, as shown in Fig.1(a)). Since cells become thick during mitotic and apoptotic stages, mitotic and apoptotic cells have different phase retardation compared to migration cells. As a result, mitotic and apoptotic cells are not well restored by the phase contrast microscopy model suitable for migration cells (Fig.1(b)). But, on the other hand, the DIC image has strong gradient response corresponding to mitotic/apoptotic cells (Fig.1(c)), thus they are well restored by the DIC imaging model (Fig.1(d)). However, some flat cells during their migration stages in the DIC image have low gradient signal (regions with shallow optical path slopes produce small contrast and appear in the image at the same intensity level as the background, as shown in Fig.1(c)), which is very challenging for DIC image restoration (Fig.1(d)). But, those flat migration cells can be easily restored in phase contrast models (Fig.1(b)). More detailed comparison on the advantages and disadvantages of phase contrast and DIC microscopy can be found in [15].

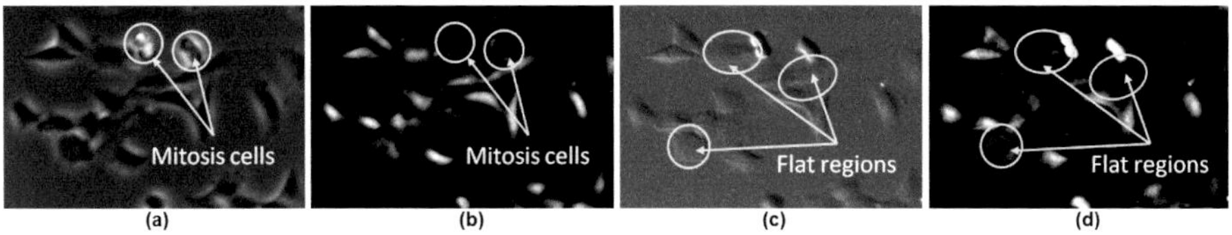

Fig. 1. Challenges. (a) Phase contrast image; (b) Phase contrast image restoration; (c) DIC image; (d) DIC image restoration.

Observing that phase contrast and DIC imaging modalities are complementary to each other, we propose a novel multimodal microscopy image restoration approach via both phase contrast and DIC imaging, with the following contributions:

(1) We capture phase contrast and DIC microscopy images on the specimens simultaneously and develop a co-restoration algorithm such that the two image modalities can be restored into one single image without any artifact from either modality (halo in phase contrast or pseudo 3D relief shading in DIC);

(2) The co-restoration algorithm is adaptive to integrate the advantages of two imaging modalities and overcome the drawback in single-modal image restoration, so regions of mitotic/apoptotic cells rely more on DIC imaging and regions with shallow optical path slopes focus more on phase contrast imaging;

(3) The co-restored images from phase contrast and DIC imaging greatly facilitate cell image analysis tasks such as cell segmentation and cell classification.

2 Data Acquisition

Generating phase contrast and DIC images simultaneously is not an issue on a common motorized microscope. Fig.2(a) is the microscope (Zeiss Axiovert 200M) we used for imaging live cells. The single instrument has multiple microscopy functions including phase contrast and DIC. Different optical components such as the phase plate and DIC analyzer are mounted on a turret. A servo motor in the microscope allows for different optical components to be moved out and into the optical pipeline without any human manipulation. The cells were cultured in an incubation system placed on the top stage of the microscope which didn't move during the entire experiments. Therefore, no image registration was needed.

Switching optical components is very fast (less than 1 second) and the time-lapse images on living cells are taken every 5 minutes. The cell movement within 1 second is very tiny. Thus we can have phase contrast and DIC images "simultaneously" in an automated manner without human interaction, other than setting the time interval and hitting the start button to start image acquisition. For example, Fig.2 (b1) and (b2) show the first DIC and phase contrast images of an experiment, respectively, and Fig.2 (c1) and (c2) show the images after 37 hours (images are taken every 5 minutes).

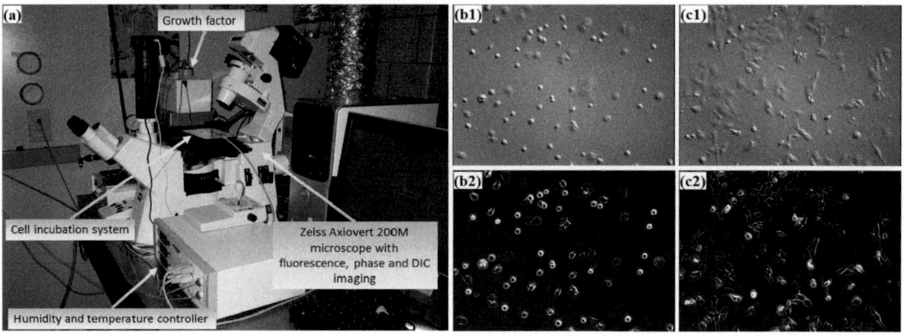

Fig. 2. Zeiss Axiovert 200M microscope with both phase and DIC imaging.

3 Methodology

3.1 Theoretical Foundation of Microscopy Image Restoration

Given cells in a petri dish, we capture their phase contrast microscopy image $\mathbf{g_p}$ and DIC microscopy image $\mathbf{g_d}$, simultaneously. Let $\mathbf{f_p}$ and $\mathbf{f_d}$ be the artifact-free phase contrast and DIC images, respectively, which are related to cell's physical properties such as the optical path length, we adopt the linear imaging models of phase contrast and DIC microscopy [8,12]:

$$\mathbf{g_p} \approx \mathbf{H_p f_p} \tag{1}$$
$$\mathbf{g_d} \approx \mathbf{H_d f_d} \tag{2}$$

where all the images are represented by vectorized $N \times 1$ vectors with N pixels in an image. $\mathbf{H_p}$ and $\mathbf{H_d}$ are two $N \times N$ sparse matrices defined by the Point Spread Function (PSF) of phase contrast [8] and DIC [12], respectively.

Rather than restoring $\mathbf{f_p}$ and $\mathbf{f_d}$ independently, we formulate the following constrained quadratic function to restore a single artifact-free image $\mathbf{f}$ from two microscopy modalities, which is related to cell's physical properties but without any artifacts from either phase contrast or DIC:

$$\mathbf{O(f)} = \|\mathbf{W}_p(\mathbf{H}_p\mathbf{f} - \mathbf{g}_p)\|_2^2 + \|\mathbf{W}_d(\mathbf{H}_d\mathbf{f} - \mathbf{g}_d)\|_2^2 + \omega_s\mathbf{f}^T\mathbf{L}\mathbf{f} + \omega_r\left\|\mathbf{\Lambda f}\right\|_1 \tag{3}$$

where $\mathbf{W}_p$ and $\mathbf{W}_d$ are two $N \times N$ diagonal matrices. $diag(\mathbf{W_p}) = \{w_p(n)\}$ and $diag(\mathbf{W}_d) = \{w_d(n)\}$ where $w_p(n)$ and $w_d(n)$ are the weights for phase contrast and DIC restoration error cost of the nth pixel ($n \in [1, N]$), respectively. $\mathbf{W}_p + \mathbf{W}_d = \mathbf{I}$ where $\mathbf{I}$ is the identity matrix. $\mathbf{L}$ is the Laplacian matrix defining the local smoothness [7]. $\boldsymbol{\Lambda}$ is a diagonal matrix with $diag(\boldsymbol{\Lambda}) = \{\lambda_n\}$ where $\lambda_n > 0$. ω_s and ω_r are the weights for smoothness and sparseness terms, respectively.

Since the objective function in Eq.3 has a l_1 sparseness regularization, there is no closed-form solution on $\mathbf{f}$. We constrain the restored $\mathbf{f}$ to have nonnegative values and convert Eq.3 to a Nonnegative-constrained Quadratic Problem (NQP):

$$\mathbf{f}^* = \arg\min_{\mathbf{f}} \mathbf{f}^T\mathbf{Q}\mathbf{f} + 2(\mathbf{b} + \frac{\omega_r}{2} diag(\boldsymbol{\Lambda}))^T\mathbf{f} + c, \; s.t. \; \mathbf{f} \geq 0 \quad (4)$$

where

$$\mathbf{Q} = \mathbf{H}_p^T\mathbf{W}_p^T\mathbf{W}_p\mathbf{H}_p + \mathbf{H}_d^T\mathbf{W}_d^T\mathbf{W}_d\mathbf{H}_d + \omega_s\mathbf{L} \quad (5)$$

$$\mathbf{b} = -\mathbf{H}_p^T\mathbf{W}_p^T\mathbf{W}_p\mathbf{g}_p - \mathbf{H}_d^T\mathbf{W}_d^T\mathbf{W}_d^T\mathbf{g}_d \quad (6)$$

$$c = \mathbf{g}_p^T\mathbf{W}_p^T\mathbf{W}_p\mathbf{g}_p - \mathbf{g}_d^T\mathbf{W}_d^T\mathbf{W}_d^T\mathbf{g}_d \quad (7)$$

Given $\mathbf{W_d}$ and $\mathbf{W_d}$, we solve the NQP problem in Eq.4 by the following algorithm using the non-negative multiplicative update [9] and re-weighting techniques [14].

3.2 Multimodal Microscopy Image Restoration Algorithm

When solving for the artifact-free image $\mathbf{f}$ in Eq.3 by Algorithm, we need two $N \times N$ diagonal matrices $\mathbf{W_p}$ and $\mathbf{W_d}$, defining the weights of phase contrast and DIC imaging modalities, respectively. Ideally, for each pixel we expect that the imaging modality which has better restoration performance on the pixel has larger weight on that pixel in the objective function. For example, we expect large $w_p(n)$'s on pixel regions with small slopes of optical path length, and large $w_d(n)$'s on pixel regions where mitosis and apoptosis occur. This reasoning leads to a chicken-or-egg problem: restoring $\mathbf{f}$ needs $\mathbf{W_p}$ and $\mathbf{W_d}$ but defining $\mathbf{W_p}$ and $\mathbf{W_d}$ needs the restoration $\mathbf{f}$.

To solve this dilemma, we can initialize the weights ($w_p(n)$ and $w_d(n)$, $w_p(n) + w_d(n) = 1$) randomly between 0 and 1. Then, we restore $\mathbf{f}$ using the weights on two imaging modalities. Based on the restoration result, we update the weights by checking the corresponding restoration errors. The process of restoration and weight updating are iterated until convergence.

Based on the restoration $\mathbf{f}^{(t)}$ at iteration t, the restoration errors of phase contrast and DIC (denoted as $\mathbf{E}_p^{(t)}$ and $\mathbf{E}_d^{(t)}$, respectively) are calculated as:

$$\mathbf{E}_p^{(t)} = \left|(\mathbf{H}_p\mathbf{f}^{(t)} - \mathbf{g}_p)\right| \quad (8)$$

$$\mathbf{E}_d^{(t)} = \left|(\mathbf{H}_d\mathbf{f}^{(t)} - \mathbf{g}_d)\right| \quad (9)$$

where $|\cdot|$ computes the element-wise absolute value of a vector. $\mathbf{E}_p$ and $\mathbf{E}_d$ are two $N \times 1$ vectors with elements defining restoration errors at N pixel locations.

Then, the weighting matrices are updated as:

$$diag(\mathbf{W}_p^{(t+1)}) = diag(\mathbf{W}_p^{(t)}) + 1 - \mathbf{E}_p^{(t)}./(\mathbf{E}_p^{(t)} + \mathbf{E}_d^{(t)}) \quad (10)$$

$$diag(\mathbf{W}_d^{(t+1)}) = diag(\mathbf{W}_d^{(t)}) + 1 - \mathbf{E}_d^{(t)}./(\mathbf{E}_p^{(t)} + \mathbf{E}_d^{(t)}) \quad (11)$$

where './' computes the element-wise division between two vectors. After normalization such that $\mathbf{W}_p + \mathbf{W}_d = \mathbf{I}$, the weight matrices are updated as:

$$diag(\mathbf{W}_p^{(t+1)}) = (diag(\mathbf{W}_p^{(t)}) + \mathbf{E}_d^{(t)}./(\mathbf{E}_p^{(t)} + \mathbf{E}_d^{(t)}))/2 \quad (12)$$

$$diag(\mathbf{W}_d^{(t+1)}) = (diag(\mathbf{W}_d^{(t)}) + \mathbf{E}_p^{(t)}./(\mathbf{E}_p^{(t)} + \mathbf{E}_d^{(t)}))/2 \quad (13)$$

We summarize our iterative co-restoration in Algorithm 1 below.

Algorithm 1. Multimodal microscopy image restoration.

Input: $t = 1$, $\mathbf{W}_p^{(1)}$ and $\mathbf{W}_d^{(1)}$;
Repeat
  Solve for $\mathbf{f}^{(t)}$ in Eq.4 using $\mathbf{W}_p^{(t)}$ and $\mathbf{W}_d^{(t)}$ by **Algorithm1**;
  Calculate the restoration error vectors ($\mathbf{E}_p^{(t)}$ and $\mathbf{E}_d^{(t)}$) in Eq.8 and Eq.9;
  Update $\mathbf{W}_p^{(t)}$ and $\mathbf{W}_d^{(t)}$ using Eq.12 and Eq.13;
  $t \leftarrow t + 1$;
Until the change on $\mathbf{f}$ between two iterations is smaller than a tolerance.

3.3 Build a Look-Up Table for Better Initialization

Good initialization on weight matrices $\mathbf{W}_p$ and $\mathbf{W}_d$ in Algorithm 1 can make the iterative process converge fast and avoid drifting to an undesired local optimum. Hence, we propose to build a look-up table to infer the best initialization on $w_p(n)$ and $w_d(n)$ for every pixel n based on its phase contrast and DIC image values $(\mathbf{g}_p(n), \mathbf{g}_d(n))$.

We offer $M - 1$ different weights for $w_p(n)$: $\{s_1, ..., s_m, ..., s_{M-1}\}$ where $s_m = m/M$. Note that $w_d(n)$ is defined as $w_d(n)$=1 $- w_p(n)$. For example, when $M = 20$, $(0.05, 0.95)$, $(0.1, 0.9)$,..., $(0.95, 0.05)$ are 19 choices of $(w_p(n), w_d(n))$ for pixel n. Based on the phase contrast image $\mathbf{g}_p$ and DIC image $\mathbf{g}_d$, we obtain $M - 1$ restored images $\mathbf{f}_m$ by solving Eq.3 according to the $M - 1$ sets of weight matrices (i.e., $\mathbf{W}_p = s_m\mathbf{I}$ and $\mathbf{W}_d = \mathbf{I} - \mathbf{W}_p$).

Suppose the pixel value ranges of the phase contrast and DIC images are [0,K] and [0,L], respectively. We build a $K \times L$ look-up table $\mathbf{T}$ whose element is defined as [1]:

$$\mathbf{T}(k, l) = s_{m^*} \quad (14)$$

where
$$m^* = \arg\min_m \sum_{n \in \Psi_{k,l}} \{|\mathbf{H}_p\mathbf{f}_m - \mathbf{g}_p|_n + |\mathbf{H}_d\mathbf{f}_m - \mathbf{g}_d|_n\} \quad (15)$$

$$\Psi_{k,l} = \{n | \mathbf{g}_p(n) = k \text{ and } \mathbf{g}_d = l\}.$$

For a pixel location n, if its phase contrast and DIC image values are k and l, respectively, we find all the other pixels with the same value pairs into set $\Psi_{k,l}$. Then, in Eq.15

[1] Practically, the size of the look-up table can be reduced by quantizing the pixel value ranges into a small number of bins.

we search which restored image $\mathbf{f}_m$ has the least total restoration error on the pixel set $\Psi_{k,l}$. Accordingly, the best out of the $M-1$ sets of weights for any pixel with phase contras and DIC image values (k,l) are defined by $w_p(n) = s_{m^*}$ and $w_d(n) = 1 - s_{m^*}$.

Note that the look-up table only needs to be constructed from the first set of phase contrast and DIC images. Afterward, given any pair of phase contrast and DIC images on the same cell dish, for each location n, a weight will be assigned to $w_p(n)$ as the initial value by checking the look-up table $\mathbf{T}(\mathbf{g}_p(n), \mathbf{g}_d(n))$. $\mathbf{W}_p$ is obtained by checking all locations with $n \in [1, N]$, and $\mathbf{W}_d = \mathbf{I} - \mathbf{W}_p$. Fig.3 shows initialization examples of both microscopy modalities via our look-up table. $\mathbf{W}_p$ in Fig.3(b) is large on flat cell regions, and $\mathbf{W}_d$ in Fig.3(d) is large on mitosis/apoptosis cell areas. These initial weight matrices are obtained using the coarse look-up table. Algorithm 1 iteratively updates the weights to a fine optimum, according to their corresponding restoration errors.

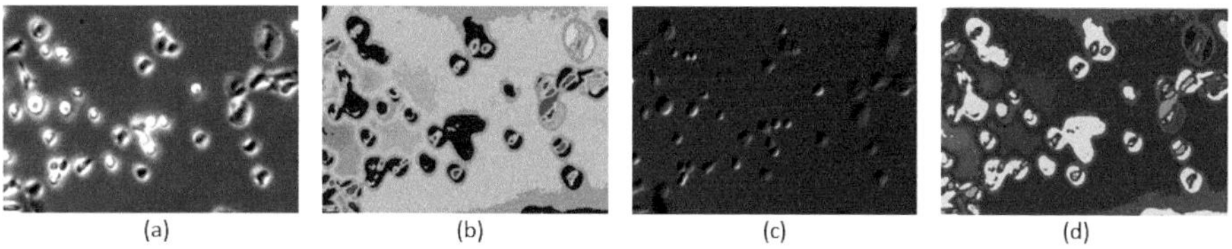

Fig. 3. Initialization via our look-up table. (a) Phase contrast image; (b) Initialization of $\mathbf{W}_p$ by look-up table; (c) DIC image; (d) Initialization of $\mathbf{W}_d$ by look-up table.

3.4 Cell Segmentation and Classification Based on Co-restoration

Fig.4 shows the outline of our segmentation and classification procedure based on co-restoration results. Fig.4(b) shows the restored images by three different approaches from Fig.4(a), where it is noticeable that the non-cell background region has uniform low pixel values, and the contrast between cells and background is high. By simply thresholding the restored images, segmentation results are obtained in Fig.4(c).

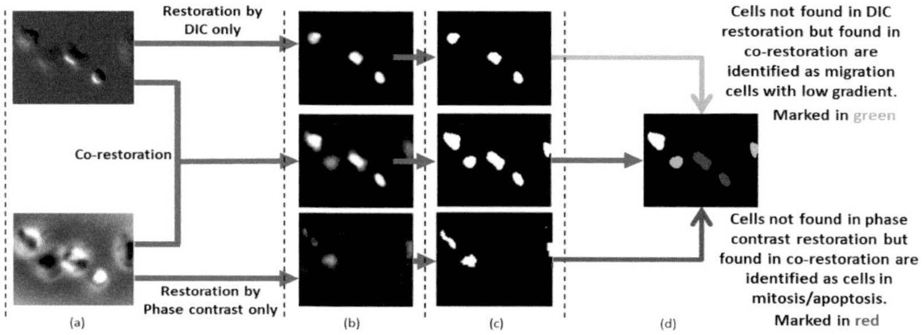

Fig. 4. Cell Segmentation and classification. (a) Original images; (b) Restored images; (c) Segmented images by thresholding; (d) Cell classification.

Then, we classify cells into three classes: (1) mitosis/apoptosis cells (challenging for phase contrast microscopy); (2) flat migration cells (challenging for DIC microscopy); and (3) migration cells before mitosis/apoptosis. By comparing our co-restoration results with the single modality results in Fig.4(c), we define: (1) cells detected through co-restoration but not detected in phase contrast restoration are mitosis/apoptosis cells (shown in Fig.4(d) in red color); (2) cells detected through co-restoration but not detected in DIC restoration are flat migration cells (shown in Fig.4(d) in green color); (3) the rest cells detected through co-restoration are cells before mitosis/apoptosis.

4 Experimental Results

We collected microscopy images from both phase contrast microscopy and DIC microscopy on the same cell dish, and 500 pairs of microscopy images (1040×1388 resolution) with various cell densities were collected to validate our algorithm.

4.1 Qualitative Evaluation

In Fig.5 we show the qualitative comparison between our co-restoration method and previous single-modality microscopy restoration methods. Fig.5(b)(c) show some examples of the phase contrast and DIC microscopy images, respectively. Restoration results of single-modality methods are shown in Fig.5(d)(e), where we can see some cells are not detected. Using our co-restoration approach, the challenging cases are handled well as shown in Fig.5(f). Cell classification is obtained by incorporating both co-restoration result and single-modality results, which is demonstrated in Fig.5(g).(Red: cells in mitosis or apoptosis; Green: cells in migration with flat gradients; White: cells before mitosis/apoptosis)

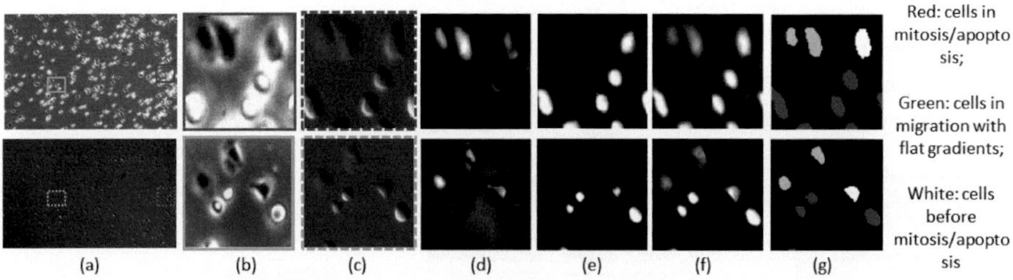

Fig. 5. Comparison with different restoration approaches.

4.2 Quantitative Evaluation

To evaluate the performance of our algorithm quantitatively, we manually labeled cell masks (include mitosis/apoptosis cells, cells before mitosis/apoptosis and flat migrating cells) in all microscopy images as ground truth. We define True Positive (**TP**) as cells segmented correctly, and False Positive (**FP**) as cells segmented mistakenly. Positive (**P**) and negative (**N**) samples are defined as cells and background, respectively. Precision and recall are calculated by: $Precision = \mathbf{TP}/(\mathbf{TP} + \mathbf{FP}), Recall = \mathbf{TP}/\mathbf{P}$, By adjusting different thresholds on the restoration images and comparing with ground

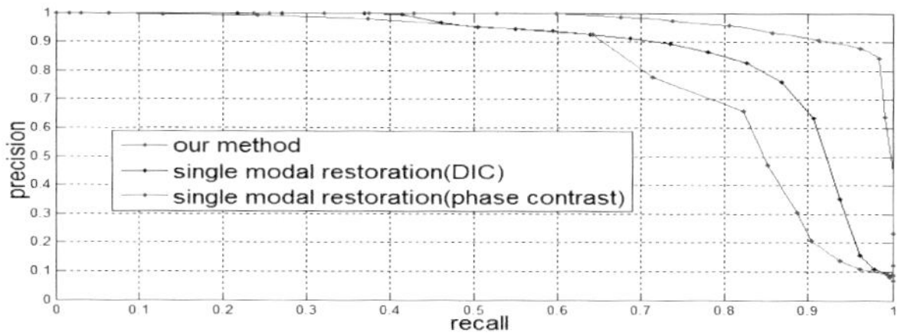

Fig. 6. ROC curve of segmentation results by 3 approaches

truth, we obtain segmentation results with different $precisions$ and $recalls$ for 500 microscopy images, and get a ROC curve. The results are shown in Fig.6 where our co-restoration outperforms single-modal restoration largely.

We also evaluate the mitosis/apoptosis event detection accuracy (EDA), defined as $EDA = (|\mathbf{TP}_e| + |\mathbf{NE}| - |\mathbf{FP}_e|)/(|\mathbf{E}| + |\mathbf{NE}|)$, where True Positive of event detection ($\mathbf{TP}_e$) denotes the mitosis/apoptosis detected correctly, and False Positive of event detection ($\mathbf{FP}_e$) denotes the event detected mistakenly; $\mathbf{E}$ and $\mathbf{NE}$ define the mitotic/apoptotic cells and non-mitotic/apoptotic cells, respectively. By choosing the segmentation threshold at which outputs the best $\mathbf{F}$ score ($\mathbf{F} = 2 \cdot \frac{precision \cdot recall}{precision + recall}$), the EDA of our algorithm is 94.75%, which is also highly reliable considering that we are achieving very high segmentation result at the same time.

5 Conclusion

We propose a novel cell image co-restoration approach by considering Differential Interference Contrast(DIC) and Phase Contrast microscopy images captured on the same cell dish. The challenges in restoring single modular microscopy images is overcome in our algorithm, by leveraging different weighting parameters to cells with different phase retardation and DIC gradient signals. The experimental results show that our approach achieve high quality cell segmentation and accurate event detection.

References

1. Zernike, F.: How I discovered phase contrast. Science 121, 345–349 (1955)
2. Murphy, D.: Fundamentals of Light Microscopy and Electronic Imaging. Wiley (2001)
3. Meijering, E.: Cell Segmentation: 50 Years Down the Road. IEEE Signal Processing Magazine 29(5), 140–145 (2012)
4. Rittscher, J.: Characterization of Biological Processes through Automated Image Analysis. Annual Review of Biomedical Engineering 12, 315–344 (2010)
5. Qu, L., et al.: 3-D Registration of Biological Images and Models: Registration of microscopic images and its uses in segmentation and annotation. IEEE Signal Processing Magazine 32(1), 70–77 (2015)
6. Xu, J., et al.: A Multistaged Automatic Restoration of Noisy Microscopy Cell Images. IEEE Journal of Biomedical and Health Informatics 19(1), 367–376 (2015)
7. Grady, L.: Random Walks for Image Segmentation. IEEE Transaction on Pattern Analysis and Machine Intelligence 28(11), 1768–1783 (2006)

8. Yin, Z., Li, K., Kanade, T., Chen, M.: Understanding the optics to aid microscopy image segmentation. In: Jiang, T., Navab, N., Pluim, J.P.W., Viergever, M.A. (eds.) MICCAI 2010, Part I. LNCS, vol. 6361, pp. 209–217. Springer, Heidelberg (2010)
9. Sha, F., et al.: Multiplicative Updates for Nonnegative Quadratic Programming. Neural Computation 19(8), 2004–2031 (2007)
10. Yin, Z., et al.: Understanding the Phase Contrast Optics to Restore Artifact-free Microscopy Images for Segmentation. Medical Image Analysis 16(5), 1047–1062 (2012)
11. Su, H., et al.: Cell Segmentation in Phase Contrast Microscopy Images via Semi-supervised Classification over Optics-related Features. Medical Image Analysis 17, 746–765 (2013)
12. Li, K., Kanade, T.: Nonnegative mixed-norm preconditioning for microscopy image segmentation. In: Prince, J.L., Pham, D.L., Myers, K.J. (eds.) IPMI 2009. LNCS, vol. 5636, pp. 362–373. Springer, Heidelberg (2009)
13. Yin, Z., Ker, D.F.E., Kanade, T.: Restoring DIC Microscopy Images from Multiple Shear Directions. In: Székely, G., Hahn, H.K. (eds.) IPMI 2011. LNCS, vol. 6801, pp. 384–397. Springer, Heidelberg (2011)
14. Candes, E., et al.: Enhancing Sparsity by Reweighted l_1 Minimization. The Journal of Fourier Analysis and Applications 14(5), 877–905 (2008)
15. `http://www.microscopyu.com/tutorials/java/phasedicmorph/index.html`

A 3D Primary Vessel Reconstruction Framework with Serial Microscopy Images

Yanhui Liang[1], Fusheng Wang[2], Darren Treanor[3,4], Derek Magee[4], George Teodoro[5], Yangyang Zhu[2], and Jun Kong[1⋆]

[1] Emory University, Atlanta, GA, USA
[2] Stony Brook University, Stony Brook, NY, USA
[3] Leeds Teaching Hospitals NHS Trust, Leeds, UK
[4] The University of Leeds, Leeds, UK
[5] University of Brasília, Brasília, DF, Brazil

Abstract. Three dimensional microscopy images present significant potential to enhance biomedical studies. This paper presents an automated method for quantitative analysis of 3D primary vessel structures with histology whole slide images. With registered microscopy images of liver tissue, we identify primary vessels with an improved variational level set framework at each 2D slide. We propose a Vessel Directed Fitting Energy (VDFE) to provide prior information on vessel wall probability in an energy minimization paradigm. We find the optimal vessel cross-section associations along the image sequence with a two-stage procedure. Vessel mappings are first found between each pair of adjacent slides with a similarity function for four association cases. These bi-slide vessel components are further linked by Bayesian Maximum A Posteriori (MAP) estimation where the posterior probability is modeled as a Markov chain. The efficacy of the proposed method is demonstrated with 54 whole slide microscopy images of sequential sections from a human liver.

1 Introduction

Whole slide histological images contain rich information about morphological and pathological characteristics of biological systems, enabling researchers and clinicians to gain insights on the underlying mechanisms of the disease onsets and pathological evolutions of distinct cancers. Although numerous imaging analytical approaches have been proposed to quantitatively analyze the 2D biological structures (such as nuclei and vessels) in microscopy images [1], various clinical applications require 3D modeling of the micro-anatomic objects for better characterization of their biological structures in practice. One such application is liver disease where clinicians and researchers are interested in the 3D structural features of primary vessels from a sequence of 2D images of adjacent liver

⋆ This research was supported in part by National Institute of Health K25CA181503, National Science Foundation ACI 1443054 and IIS 1350885, and CNPq.

N. Navab et al. (Eds.): MICCAI 2015, Part III, LNCS 9351, pp. 251–259, 2015.
DOI: 10.1007/978-3-319-24574-4_30

sections [2,3], as illustrated in Fig. 1(a). Although there are a large suite of methods for vessel structure analysis, they mainly focus on radiology image analysis and are not directly applicable to high resolution whole slide histological images encoding enormous information of complex structures at cellular level.

In this paper, we propose an automated framework for 3D primary vessel reconstruction with a set of registered histological whole slide images of liver sequential tissue sections. To identify vessels, we use an improved variational level set method with a Vessel Directed Fitting Energy (VDFE) as prior information of vessel wall probability for the energy minimization paradigm. We associate the segmented vessel objects across all slides by mapping primary vessels between adjacent slides with four distinct association scenarios, and apply a Bayesian Maximum A Posteriori (MAP) framework to the bi-slide vessel components to recover the global vessel structures across all slides.

2 Methods for 3D Vessel Reconstruction

2.1 Automated 2D Vessel Segmentation

Due to large variations introduced by whole slide microscopy image preparation and strong heterogeneity embedded in tissue anatomical structures, vessels of interest in liver biopsies present distinct staining intensities. Although a number of level set methods have been proposed to solve this issue [4,5], these formulations only work well when a given image has two primary classes of connected regions. In our dataset, each typical liver image consists of primary vessel walls, lumens, small vessel walls, bile ducts, and non-tissue regions, each presenting different intensity characteristics. One solution is to employ multiple fitting functions to reach functional minimum [5]. However, this would inevitably increase the computational complexity. As we focus on identifying primary vessel walls in this work, we propose an improved formulation with directed prior information on vessel wall probability within a variational level set framework based on [5]. Let us denote two 2D vectors $\mathbf{x}$ and $\mathbf{y}$ defined over the image domain Ω of image I. Level set $\phi : \Omega \rightarrow \mathcal{R}$ is a Lipschitz function defined over Ω. Vessel Directed Fitting Energy (VDFE) E_{V} is then defined as follows:

$$\begin{aligned} E_{\mathrm{V}}(\mathbf{x}, f_1, f_2, \phi) =& \lambda_1 \int_{\Omega} G_{\sigma_2}(\|\mathbf{x}-\mathbf{y}\|) Q_{\sigma_3}(\mathbf{y}) |I(\mathbf{y}) * G_{\sigma_1}(\mathbf{y}) - f_1(\mathbf{x})|^2 U_1(\phi(\mathbf{y})) d\mathbf{y} \\ &+ \lambda_2 \int_{\Omega} G_{\sigma_2}(\|\mathbf{x}-\mathbf{y}\|) P(\mathbf{y}) |I(\mathbf{y}) * G_{\sigma_1}(\mathbf{y}) - f_2(\mathbf{x})|^2 U_2(\phi(\mathbf{y})) d\mathbf{y} \end{aligned} \tag{1}$$

where $f_1(\mathbf{x})$ and $f_2(\mathbf{x})$ are two fitting functions for interior and exterior regions of zero level set. G_σ is a bivariate Gaussian filter; $U_i(\phi(\mathbf{x})) = \begin{cases} H(\phi(\mathbf{x})), & \text{if } i=1 \\ 1 - H(\phi(\mathbf{x})), & \text{if } i=2 \end{cases}$ and $H(x)$ is a Heaviside step function; $Q_\sigma(\mathbf{x}) = \exp\left(-\frac{|\nabla \mathbf{x}|^2}{2\sigma^2}\right)$ is a function describing image smoothness. $P(\mathbf{y}) = \max\ p(\mathbf{y}, s_i, \tau, \omega)$ is a pre-computed vessel wall probability map indicating the likelihood of pixel $\mathbf{y}$ belonging to a vessel wall [6] where s_i is the ith scale of a Gaussian filter that convolves with the image channel representing vessel-specific immunohistochemical stain DAB [7]; τ and ω are parameters governing the sensitivity of $P(\mathbf{y})$ to measures of vessel structure similarity and intensity change magnitude. We set $\tau = 0.5$ and $\omega = 15$.

In our formulation, fitting function $f_1(\mathbf{x})$ fits better to $\mathbf{y}$ in close proximity to $\mathbf{x}$ and with large $Q_{\sigma_3}(\mathbf{y})$. Similarly, $f_2(\mathbf{x})$ is biased to image locations $\mathbf{y}$ close to $\mathbf{x}$ and with large $P(\mathbf{y})$. Compared with small vessels, primary vessels have longer edge contours where $Q_{\sigma_3}(\mathbf{y})$ is low. Thus, VDFE minimization guarantees that $f_1(\mathbf{x})$ is automatically elected to fit to primary vessel wall regions where $Q_{\sigma_3}(\mathbf{y})$ is small and that $f_2(\mathbf{x})$ fits to non-primary vessel regions where $P(\mathbf{y})$ is small. Therefore, the proposed VDFE uses joint information derived from image regions, vessel edges, and the prior vessel wall probability map. To regulate zero level set smoothness, and retain signed distance property for stable level set function computation, we use the following accessory energy terms [8]: $E_1(\phi(\mathbf{x})) = \alpha Q_{\sigma_3}(\mathbf{x})|\nabla H(\phi(\mathbf{x}))|$ and $E_2(\phi(\mathbf{x})) = \beta R(|\nabla\phi(\mathbf{x})|)$. In addition, we introduce another energy term to expedite zero level set convergence to vessel walls: $E_3(\phi(\mathbf{x})) = \gamma\,(1 - P(\mathbf{x}))\,H(\phi(\mathbf{x}))$. Combining all energies, we formulate the following functional to be minimized:

$$\mathcal{J}\left(f_1(\mathbf{x}), f_2(\mathbf{x}), \phi\right) = \int_{\Omega}\left[E_{\mathrm{V}}(\mathbf{x}, f_1(\mathbf{x}), f_2(\mathbf{x}), \phi) + \sum_{i=1}^{3} E_i(\phi(\mathbf{x}))\right] d\mathbf{x} \quad (2)$$

We update f_1, f_2, and ϕ in two sequential steps within each iteration as suggested by the local binary fitting model [5]. First, we fix $\phi(\mathbf{x})$ and optimize $f_1(\mathbf{x})$ and $f_2(\mathbf{x})$ to minimize functional by solving the system of Euler-Lagrange equations. Next, we minimize functional $\mathcal{J}$ by optimizing $\phi(\mathbf{x})$ with two updated fitting functions unchanged. Note that we can swap integration variables $\mathbf{x}$ and $\mathbf{y}$, change the integration order for the energy term E_{V}, and re-write the integrand:

$$\begin{aligned}\mathcal{L}(\mathbf{x}, \phi(\mathbf{x})) = {} & \underbrace{\lambda_1 \int_{\Omega} G_{\sigma_2}(\|\mathbf{y}-\mathbf{x}\|)|I(\mathbf{x}) * G_{\sigma_1}(\mathbf{x}) - f_1^*(\mathbf{y})|^2 d\mathbf{y}}_{\text{defined as: } F_1(\mathbf{x})}\, Q_{\sigma_3}(\mathbf{x}) H(\phi(\mathbf{x})) \\ & + \lambda_2 \underbrace{\int_{\Omega} G_{\sigma_2}(\|\mathbf{y}-\mathbf{x}\|)|I(\mathbf{x}) * G_{\sigma_1}(\mathbf{x}) - f_2^*(\mathbf{y})|^2 d\mathbf{y}}_{\text{defined as: } F_2(\mathbf{x})}\, P(\mathbf{x})(1 - H(\phi(\mathbf{x}))) \\ & + \alpha\, Q_{\sigma_3}(\mathbf{x})|\nabla H(\phi(\mathbf{x}))| + \beta\, R(|\nabla\phi(\mathbf{x})|) + \gamma\,(1 - P(\mathbf{x}))H(\phi(\mathbf{x}))\end{aligned}$$

By the Euler-Lagrange equation, we have the final updating equation as:

$$\begin{aligned}\frac{\partial\phi(\mathbf{x};t)}{\partial t} &= -\frac{\partial\mathcal{J}(\phi)}{\partial\phi} = -\frac{\partial\mathcal{L}(\mathbf{x},\phi(\mathbf{x}))}{\partial\phi(\mathbf{x})} + \sum_{i=1}^{2}\frac{\partial}{\partial x_i}\left(\frac{\partial\mathcal{L}(\mathbf{x},\phi(\mathbf{x}))}{\frac{\partial\phi(\mathbf{x})}{\partial x_i}}\right) \\ &= \Big[\lambda_2 F_2(\mathbf{x})P(\mathbf{x}) - \lambda_1 F_1(\mathbf{x})Q_{\sigma_3}(\mathbf{x})\Big]H'(\mathbf{x}) \\ &\quad + \alpha\Big[Q_{\sigma_3}(\mathbf{x})\cdot\frac{\nabla\phi(\mathbf{x})}{|\nabla\phi(\mathbf{x})|} + Q_{\sigma_3}(\mathbf{x})\mathrm{div}\left(\frac{\nabla\phi(\mathbf{x})}{|\nabla\phi(\mathbf{x})|}\right)\Big]H'(\mathbf{x}) \\ &\quad + \beta\,\mathrm{div}\Big(\frac{R'(|\nabla\phi(\mathbf{x})|)}{|\nabla\phi(\mathbf{x})|}\nabla\phi(\mathbf{x})\Big) - \gamma(1 - P(\mathbf{x}))H'(\phi(\mathbf{x}))\end{aligned} \quad (3)$$

2.2 Two-Stage Vessel Association with Vessel Cross-Sections

We perform vessel association by two steps: local bi-slide vessel mapping and global vessel structure association. At each stage, we consider four different association cases: one-to-one (growth), one-to-two (bifurcation), one-to-none (disappearance) and none-to-one (appearance). For local bi-slide vessel mapping, we take into account vessel shape descriptors and spatial features, with the overall similarity function for each association case defined as follows:

(1) One-to-one: $s\left(v_i^t, v_j^{t+1}\right) = \mu_1\, g\left(v_i^t, v_j^{t+1}\right) + \mu_2\, d\left(v_i^t, v_j^{t+1}\right)$
(2) One-to-two: $s\left(v_i^t, v_{j_1}^{t+1}, v_{j_2}^{t+1}\right) = \mu_1\, g\left(v_i^t, v_{j_1}^{t+1} \cup v_{j_2}^{t+1}\right) + \mu_2\, d\left(v_i^t, v_{j_1}^{t+1} \cup v_{j_2}^{t+1}\right)$
(3) One-to-none: $s\left(v_i^t, v_{\varnothing}^{t+1}\right) = d\left(v_i^t, \Omega_t\right)$
(4) None-to-one: $s\left(v_{\varnothing}^{t-1}, v_i^t\right) = d\left(v_i^t, O_t\right)$

where v_i^t is the ith vessel object in slide t; functions $g(\cdot)$ and $d(\cdot)$ are two Gaussian Radial Basis Functions (GRBF) with scale κ_1 and κ_2, representing the similarity of vessel appearance by Fourier shape descriptors and the spatial distance between two vessel objects, respectively; Ω_t and O_t are the boundary and centroid of slide t; $\{\mu_1, \mu_2\}$ with $\mu_1 + \mu_2 = 1$ are constant weights to control the bi-slide vessel mapping smoothness.

The bi-slide vessel mapping is considered as a multi-object tracking problem, and solved by constrained Integer Programming [9] based on the defined similarity functions. This stage generates a set of bi-slide vessel components $\mathbf{B} = \{B_i\}$. Next, we reconstruct the global vessel structures by linking $\{B_i\}$ across all slides within a Bayesian Maximum A Posteriori (MAP) framework [10,11]. Denote $\mathbf{V} = \{V_k\}$ as the set of hypotheses on vessel structures over all slides. Each vessel structure V_k may contain the pre-defined four association cases and can be written as $V_k = \{B_i^k\}$ where B_i^k is the ith bi-slide vessel component in vessel structure V_k. B_i^k can be represented as $B_i^k = (v_{p'}^k \rightarrow v_p^k)$ where $v_{p'}^k$ and v_p^k are the associated vessel objects linked by B_i^k. We maximize the following marginal posterior probability to obtain the best vessel structure hypothesis $\mathbf{V}^*$:

$$\mathbf{V}^* = \arg\max_{\mathbf{V}} P\left(\mathbf{V}|\mathbf{B}\right) = \arg\max_{\mathbf{V}} \prod_{V_k \in \mathbf{V}} P(V_k|\mathbf{B}) = P_{\varnothing\rightarrow 1}\left(B_s^k|B_{\varnothing}\right)_{B_s^k \in V_k}$$
$$\prod_{B_i^k, B_j^k \in V_k} P_{1\rightarrow 1}\left(B_j^k|B_i^k\right) \prod_{B_m^k, B_{n_1}^k, B_{n_2}^k \in V_k} P_{1\rightarrow 2}\left(B_{n_1}^k, B_{n_2}^k|B_m^k\right) \prod_{B_e^k \in V_k} P_{1\rightarrow\varnothing}\left(B_{\varnothing}|B_e^k\right) \tag{4}$$

As no vessel structure in our dataset overlaps with others (i.e., $V_k \cap V_l = \emptyset, \forall k \neq l$), we assume each V_k is conditionally independent given $\mathbf{B}$. We model $P\left(V_k|\mathbf{B}\right)$ as a Markov chain by taking into account the four distinct association cases; B_s^k and B_e^k are the "start" and "end" components of V_k, respectively; B_x^k with $x \in \{i, j, m, n_1, n_2\}$ represents an intermediate vessel component. Probabilities for the four defined association cases are:

$$P_{1\to 1}\left(B_j^k|B_i^k\right) = \omega_1\ g\left(v_p^k, v_q^k\right) + \omega_2\ d\left(v_p^k, v_q^k\right) + \omega_3\ b\left(v_p^k, v_q^k\right)$$
$$P_{1\to 2}\left(B_j^k|B_i^k\right) = \omega_1\ g\left(v_m^k, v_{n_1}^k \cup v_{n_2}^k\right) + \omega_2\ d\left(v_m^k, v_{n_1}^k \cup v_{n_2}^k\right) + \omega_3\ b\left(v_m^k, v_{n_1}^k \cup v_{n_2}^k\right)$$
$$P_{1\to\varnothing}\left(B_\varnothing|B_e^k\right) = L_{const}^{\alpha}, \qquad P_{\varnothing\to 1}\left(B_s^k|B_\varnothing\right) = L_{const}^{\beta}$$

where $B_i^k = (v_{p'}^k \to v_p^k)$ and $B_j^k = (v_q^k \to v_{q'}^k)$; function $b(\cdot)$ indicates the change of a vessel trajectory. L_{const}^{α} and L_{const}^{β} are constant likelihoods of bi-slide vessel components being the last and the first in vessel structure V_k, respectively; $\{\omega_1, \omega_2, \omega_3\}$ $s.t.$ $\omega_1 + \omega_2 + \omega_3 = 1$ are constant weights to adjust the global vessel association smoothness. Function b is defined as:

$$b\left(B_i^k, B_j^k\right) = exp\left(-\left(a\left(v_{p'}^k, v_p^k, v_q^k\right) - a\left(v_p^k, v_q^k, v_{q'}^k\right)\right)/\kappa^2\right) \tag{5}$$

where $a\left(v_{p'}^k, v_p^k, v_q^k\right)$ is defined as $\frac{\langle o(v_{p'}^k)-o(v_p^k),\ o(v_p^k)-o(v_q^k)\rangle}{||o(v_{p'}^k)-o(v_p^k)||\ ||o(v_p^k)-o(v_q^k)||}$, indicating the orientation change when B_i^k is associated with B_j^k. $\boldsymbol{o}(\cdot)$ is a vector pointing to a vessel center. Next, we take logarithm of the objective function and solve the MAP problem by Linear Programming technique. We assume there are M bi-slide vessel components generated from all slides and h possible associations between these bi-slide vessel components. The optimal global vessel structures can be achieved by solving the following problem:

$$\arg\max_{x}\ \mathbf{p}^T\mathbf{x} \quad s.t.\ (R^T x)_i \le 1,\ 0 \le x_j \le 1 \tag{6}$$

where $i = 1, ..., 2M$, $j = 1, ..., h$; $\mathbf{p}$ is a $h \times 1$ vector with each entry representing the likelihood of one bi-slide vessel association; R is a $h \times 2M$ binary matrix with each column indicating the index of bi-slide vessel components on the global association; $(R^T\mathbf{x})_i$ is the ith element of $(R^T\mathbf{x})$ and the constraint $(R^T\mathbf{x})_i \le 1$ guarantees that each bi-slide vessel component can be selected at most once; the optimal solution $\mathbf{x}$ is a $h \times 1$ binary vector where $\mathbf{x}_j = 1$ indicates the jth association is included in the optimal solution. In our tests, the resulting optimal solution by Standard Simplex algorithm [9] is identical to that of the Integer Programming problem.

3 Experimental Results and Validation

We have tested our method on 54 registered whole slide images of sequential liver tissue sections from one human patient, with z-resolution of 50μm. These biopsy sections are stained by Immunohistochemistry (IHC). The resulting images for analysis are down-sampled from the base level by 64:1, with the final resolution of 1530×1373 pixels. We apply our segmentation method to images with parameters: $\sigma_1 = 1, \sigma_2 = 4, \sigma_3 = 1.5, \lambda_1 = \lambda_2 = 1, \alpha = 65, \beta = 2, \gamma = 5$. In general, we can have similar results with reasonable perturbations to this parameter set. The segmentation time cost for each image is 43.65 ± 0.63 seconds in Matlab R2013 with Dual Xeon E5420 CPUs at 2.5Ghz. In Fig. 1, we present vessel segmentation results from a typical image where the detected vessels are marked in green. The final vessel detection results in Fig. 1(e) are produced by

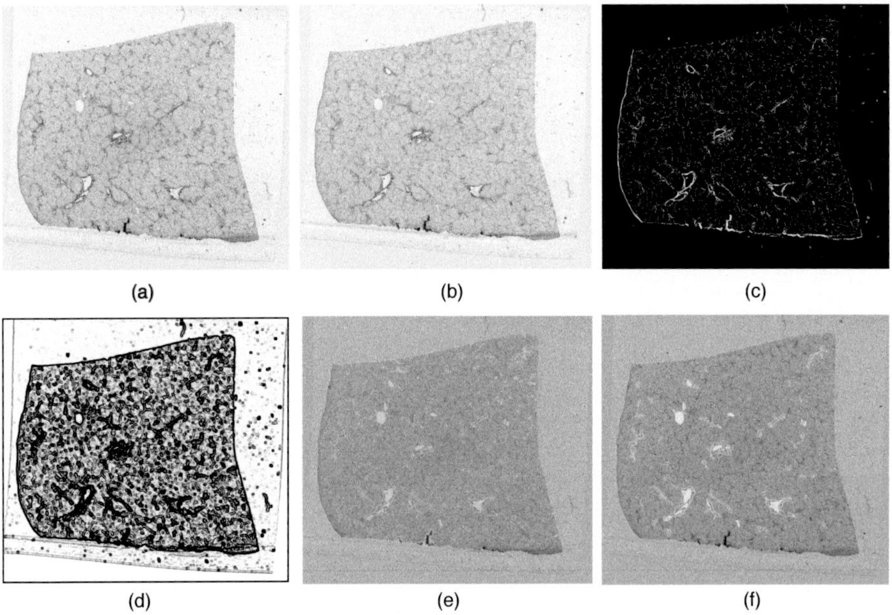

Fig. 1. Representative segmentation result of primary vessels. (a) a typical 2D liver histology image with vessels highlighted in brown; (b) DAB stain image channel derived from color deconvolution; (c) vessel wall probability map $P(\mathbf{x})$; (d) smooth indicator function $Q_{\sigma_3}(\mathbf{x})$; (e) segmented primary vessels after post-processing (in green); and (f) markup image with one-to-one vessel pairs by human (red) and machine (green), with yellow mask resulting from red and green mask.

combining final vessel wall results in Fig. 2(a) with detected lumens after removing candidates with unduly long perimeter length. To further examine the efficacy of VDFE directing level set function to vessel boundaries, we illustrate in Fig. 2 vessel wall segmentation results with and without prior information on vessel wall probability before post-processing. It is apparent that VDFE in Fig. 1(a) navigates zero level set to specific vessel edges in a target segmentation process. By contrast, results without VDFE guidance in Fig. 1(b) show that zero level set partitions the image purely based on fitting error (or homogeneity), with poor selective specificity to primary vessel boundaries. We compare our segmentation results with primary vessel annotations by human. Due to the large number of vessels in presence and variable confidence of vessel recognition by their appearances, only representative primary vessels with high recognition confidence and relatively large size are annotated by human. Table 1 presents the validation results of all one-to-one human-machine vessel pairs measured by Jaccard coefficient, precision, recall, F_1 score, and Hausdorff distance. We also compare our Vessel Directed Level Set (VDLS) method with morphological reconstruction (MR) approach [12] in Table 1. Note that 1336 human-VDLS and 881 human-MR one-to-one vessel pairs from 54 images are found and assessed.

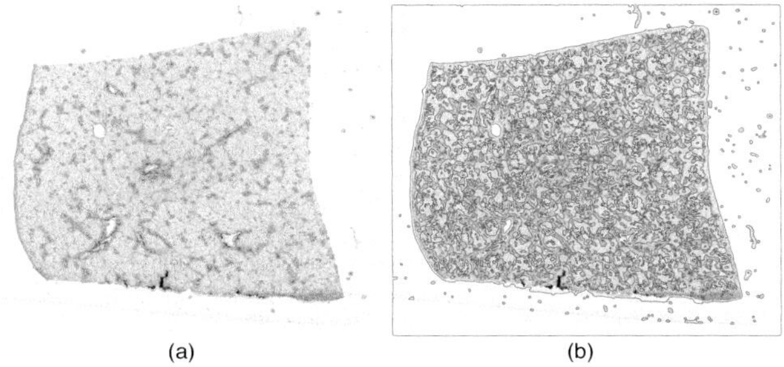

Fig. 2. Primary vessel wall segmentation result of (a) directed and (b) non-directed prior information on vessel wall probability before post-processing.

Table 1. Evaluation of the segmentation results (Mean ± Standard Deviation).

	Jac	Pre	Rec	F_1	*Haus*
MR	0.45 ± 0.21	0.60 ± 0.27	0.77 ± 0.26	0.59 ± 0.22	34.48 ±75.45
VDLS (our method)	0.84 ± 0.10	0.96 ± 0.06	0.87 ± 0.08	0.91 ± 0.07	6.82 ± 30.99

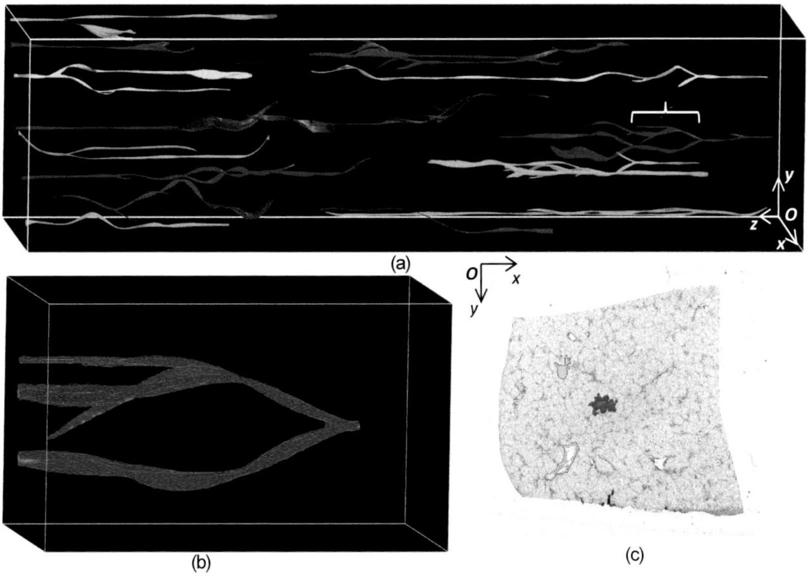

Fig. 3. (a) Panoramic view of 3D reconstructed vessels; (b) a close-up view of a vessel segment indicated by a curly bracket in the panoramic view; (c) color coded vessel candidates in the right most image frame observed from right to left in (a).

To avoid unduly high vessel association complexity and error, we apply our vessel association approach to top 30 candidates by size on each slide. The most expensive computation is linear programming (64.56 ± 3.49 seconds). The parameters are empirically set as $\mu_1 = 0.63$, $\kappa_1^2 = 50000$, $\kappa_2^2 = 50$, $\omega_1 = 0.54$,

$\omega_2 = 0.36$, $\kappa^2 = 500$, $L^{\alpha}_{const} = 0.5$ and $L^{\beta}_{const} = 0.5$. After vessel association, we perform B-Spline interpolation between adjacent associated vessel objects due to low z-axis data resolution, and volumetrically render the 3D vessel structures. In Fig. 3(a), we present a panoramic view of our 3D visualization result for representative primary vessels from our dataset. One close-up view of a vessel segment is illustrated in Fig. 3(b). The right most image frame observed from right to left in the panoramic view is shown in Fig. 3(c), with color-coded 2D vessel candidates for 3D reconstruction. Note that reconstructed vessels with candidates by MR method are generally shorter due to imperfect vessel identification in intermediate image frames. As our analysis focuses on primary vessels, the vessel association result is relatively robust to registration outputs.

4 Conclusion

In this paper, we present an automated framework for 3D primary vessel structure analysis on whole slide histological images of liver tissue sections. For vessel segmentation, we propose an improved variational level set framework with prior information on vessel wall probability. We achieve optimal vessel associations by local bi-slide vessel mapping and global vessel structure association within a MAP framework. Experiments with a real world use case and preliminary evaluations present promising results. In future work, we will assess our method with other larger datasets and extend it to enable micro-vessel analysis.

References

1. Foran, D.J., Chen, W., Yang, L.: Automated Image Interpretation Computer-assisted Diagnosis. Ana. Cell. Path. 34(6), 279–300 (2011)
2. Roberts, N., Magee, D., Song, Y., Brabazon, K., Shires, M., Crellin, D., Orsi, N.M., Quirke, R., Quirke, P., Treanor, D.: Toward Routine Use of 3D Histopathology as a Research Tool. Am. J. of Path. 180(5), 1835–1842 (2012)
3. Schwier, M., Hahn, H.K., Dahmen, U., Dirsch, O.: Reconstruction of Vessel Structures from Serial Whole Slide Sections of Murine Liver Samples. In: Proc. SPIE, Medical Imaging, vol. 8676 (2013)
4. Li, C., Huang, R., Ding, Z., Gatenby, C., Metaxas, D., Gore, J.: A Level Set Method for Image Segmentation in the Presence of Intensity Inhomogeneity With Application to MRI. IEEE Trans. Image Process. 20, 2007–2016 (2011)
5. Li, C., Kao, C., Gore, J.C., Ding, Z.: Implicit Active Contours Driven by Local Binary Fitting Energy. In: IEEE Comp. Vis. and Pat. Rec., pp. 1–7 (2007)
6. Frangi, A.F., Niessen, W.J., Vincken, K.L., Viergever, M.A.: Multiscale Vessel Enhancement Filtering. In: Wells, W.M., Colchester, A.C.F., Delp, S.L. (eds.) MICCAI 1998. LNCS, vol. 1496, pp. 130–137. Springer, Heidelberg (1998)
7. Ruifrok, A.C., Johnston, D.A.: Quantification of Histochemical Staining by Color Deconvolution. Anal. Quant. Cytol. Histol. 23, 291–299 (2001)
8. Li, C., Xu, C., Gui, C., Fox, M.D.: Distance Regularized Level Set Evolution and Its Application to Image Segmentation. IEEE TIP 19, 3243–3254 (2010)

9. Dantzig, G.B.: Linear Programming and Extensions. Princeton Press (1963)
10. Berclaz, J., Fleuret, F., Fua, P.: Multiple Object Tracking using Flow Linear Programming. In: Winter-PETS (2009)
11. Bise, R., Yin, Z., Kanade, T.: Reliable Cell Tracking by Global Data Association. In: ISBI (2011)
12. Vincent, L.: Morphological Grayscale Reconstruction in Image Analysis: Applications and Efficient Algorithms. IEEE TIP 2, 176–201 (1993)

Adaptive Co-occurrence Differential Texton Space for HEp-2 Cells Classification

Xiang Xu[1], Feng Lin[1], Carol Ng[2], and Khai Pang Leong[2]

[1] School of Computer Engineering, Nanyang Technological University, S-639798
[2] Department of Rheumatology, Allergy and Immunology, Tan Tock Seng Hospital, S-308433
{xxu4,asflin}@ntu.edu.sg, {carol_ng,khai_pang_leong}@ttsh.com.sg

Abstract. The occurrence of antinuclear antibodies in patient serum has significant relation to autoimmune disease. But identification of them suffers from serious problems due to human subjective evaluation. In this study, we propose an automatic classification system for HEp-2 cells. Within this system, a Co-occurrence Differential Texton (CoDT) feature is designed to represent the local image patches, and a generative model is built to adaptively characterize the CoDT feature space. We further exploit a more discriminant representation for the HEp-2 cell images based on the adaptive partitioned feature space, then feed the representation into a linear Support Vector Machine classifier for identifying the staining patterns. The experimental results on two benchmark datasets: ICPR12 dataset and ICIP2013 training dataset, verified that our method remarkably outperforms the other contemporary approaches for HEp-2 cells classification.

Keywords: HEp-2 cells, co-occurrence differential texton, generative model, adaptive partitioned feature space.

1 Introduction

Indirect-immunofluorescence (IIF) is the most recommended technique for detecting antinuclear antibodies (ANAs) in patient serum, which can reveal the occurrence of specific autoimmune diseases such as rheumatoid arthritis and multiple sclerosis. In the current clinical practices, IIF slide images are manually inspected by physicians with a fluorescence microscope, therefore it suffers from some intrinsic limitations due to subjective evaluation. Computer Aided Diagnostic (CAD) systems are proposed for automatically supporting the IIF diagnosis. The main technologies investigated in these CAD systems are automated preparation of slides with robotic devices, image acquisition, image segmentation, mitotic cell recognition, fluorescence intensity classification and staining pattern recognition. Staining pattern recognition is proven to be the most challenging task in the research community. In this study, we investigate into the approaches for automatic staining pattern classification of HEp-2 cells.

As a benchmark to evaluate and compare the new methods, a publicly available HEp-2 cells dataset was released at the first edition of the *HEp-2 Cells Classification Contest*. Nosaka et al. [1] propose an extension of Local Binary Pattern (LBP) descriptor (named CoALBP) to extract textural features and win the first prize of the contest. All the participated methods are reported in [2]. Inspired by the contest, Xu et al. [3] improve the coding method of Bag-of-Words (BoW) framework to reduce information loss

N. Navab et al. (Eds.): MICCAI 2015, Part III, LNCS 9351, pp. 260–267, 2015.
DOI: 10.1007/978-3-319-24574-4_31

caused by feature quantization. Shen et al. [4] adopt the BoW framework on intensity order pooling based gradient feature. Theodorakopoulos et al. [5] fuse the distribution of SIFT features [6] and gradient-oriented co-occurrence of LBPs into a dissimilarity space. Then they use a sparse representation-based classification mechanism for classification.

Although considerable progress has been made, research in HEp-2 cell image analysis is still in its early stage. In this study, we first propose a Co-occurrence Differential Texton (CoDT) feature to represent local patches of the HEp-2 cell images. LBP related features have been applied successfully in the HEp-2 cells classification [1], [7]. However, some important information is lost since the LBP represents the local structures with only two quantized levels. Our proposed CoDT feature reduces the information loss by ignoring the quantization. Furthermore, it captures the spatial relations among the differential micro-texton features to increase the discriminative power of features.

Then, we apply a Gaussian Mixture Model (GMM) to adaptively approximate the distribution of the proposed CoDT features. Thus the parameters, adjusted from the training cell images, are better fitting the CoDT feature space.

Last, we utilize the *Fisher Kernel* (FK) principal [8] to improve the BoW framework. The BoW framework is one of the most popular approaches for image classification. However, it suffers from some problems: (i) Information loss in feature quantization process is inevitable [9]; (ii) The cost of histogram computations depends on the number of visual words. Since better performance is always obtained with larger vocabulary, the computational cost is high. The FK based methods can handle these problems. The output image representation is fed into a linear SVM for final classification.

Our proposed framework (AdaCoDT) can exploit the advantages of both generative and discriminative approaches for image classification. Experimental results verify that AdaCoDT can provide remarkable classification performance for HEp-2 cells.

2 Method

2.1 Co-occurrence Differential Texton

LBP [10] can be obtained by thresholding the gray value of the circularly symmetric surrounding pixels with that of the center pixel within a local patch (micro-texton). The LBP at location (x, y) is defined as

$$LBP_{P,R}(x,y) = \sum_{i=1}^{P} 2^{i-1} sign(I(x_i, y_i) - I(x,y)), \tag{1}$$

$$sign(x) = \begin{cases} 1, & \text{if} \quad x \geq 0 \\ 0, & \text{otherwise.} \end{cases} \tag{2}$$

where $I(x, y)$ is a gray value at location (x, y) in image I and $I(x_i, y_i)$ denotes the gray value of P equal spaced pixels on a circle of radius R around center pixel (x, y).

Recently, some improved LBP features [1] have been applied in HEp-2 cells and shown superior performances compared with the conventional LBP. However, one major drawback of the LBP related methods is that they will lose some discriminant

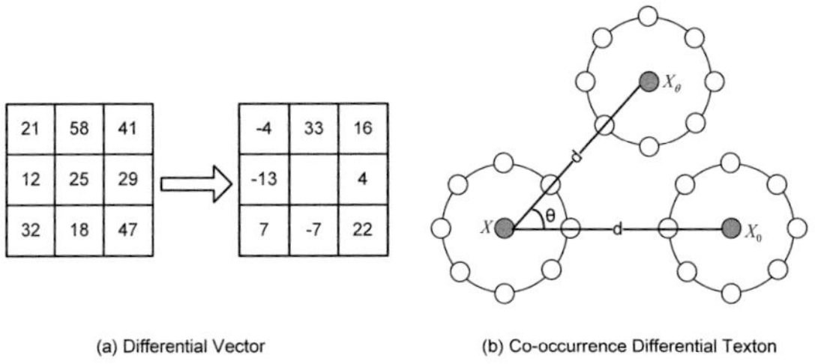

Fig. 1. Illustration of CoDT. (a) an example of Differential Vector (3×3 micro-texton). (b) two pairs of DVs with rotation angles $0°$ and θ respectively.

information since they represent the microstructure with only two quantized levels (i.e. 0 and 1). To reserve more discriminant information, we propose to use *Differential Vectors* (DV) to describe the micro-texton. A DV is a microstructural feature based on the differential domain skipping the quantization procedure, which is formulated as

$$DV_{P,R}(x,y) = (I(x_1,y_1) - I(x,y), ..., I(x_P,y_P) - I(x,y)) \tag{3}$$

To enhance the discriminative power, we further propose a Co-occurrence Differential Texton (CoDT) feature capturing the spatial relation between differential micro-textons. The CoDT feature can provide more information than individual DV since it characterizes more subtle and complex structure. The CoDT feature with one pair of DVs is illustrated in Fig 1 and formulated as

$$CoDT_{P,R,d}(\mathbf{x}) = [DV_{P,R}(\mathbf{x}), DV^{\theta}_{P,R}(\mathbf{x}_\theta)] = [DV_{P,R}(\mathbf{x}), DV_{P,R}(\mathbf{x} + \Delta\mathbf{x}_\theta)] \tag{4}$$

where $\mathbf{x} = (x,y)$ is the position vector in I and $\Delta\mathbf{x}_\theta = (d\cos\theta, d\sin\theta)$ is a replacement vector between a DV pair with interval d and rotation angle θ.

In this study, following the commonly practiced rules, we extract four pairs of DVs, that is $\theta = 0°, 45°, 90°, 135°$ (we find that the classification performance improves very little by using more pairs of DVs). The CoDT feature is a $5P$-dimensional feature vector.

2.2 HEp-2 Cell Image Representation in the Adaptive CoDT Feature Space

To combine the strengths of both generative and discriminative approaches for image classification, we characterize the proposed CoDT features of a HEp-2 cell image by a gradient vector derived from a generative model, then we feed the output image representations into a discriminative classifier for the identification of HEp-2 cells.

Let $X = \{x_n, n = 1,2,...,N\}$ be a set of samples from the CoDT feature space of one HEp-2 cell image. The probability density distribution of the CoDT feature is described by a GMM with parameters $\lambda = \{w_t, \mu_t, \Sigma_t, t = 1,2,...,T\}$, where w_t, μ_t and Σ_t are respectively the mixture weight, mean vector and covariance matrix of Gaussian t. Then we can formulate

$$p(x_n|\lambda) = \sum_{t=1}^{T} w_t p_t(x_n|\lambda), \quad s.t. \quad \sum_{t=1}^{T} w_t = 1 \tag{5}$$

where $p_t(x_n|\lambda) = \frac{exp\{-\frac{1}{2}(x_n-\mu_t)\Sigma_t^{-1}(x_n-\mu_t)\}}{(2\pi)^{D/2}|\Sigma_t|^{1/2}}$. The parameters of GMM can be adaptively estimated by Expectation Maximization (EM) algorithm [11]. Note that we assume that the covariance matrices are diagonal and denoted by $\sigma_t = diag(\Sigma_t)$.

The samples X can be characterized by $G_\lambda(X) = \bigtriangledown_\lambda \log p(X|\lambda)$. The gradient describes how the parameters λ should be modified to best fit X. To measure the similarity between two HEp-2 cell images, a *Fisher Kernel* (FK) [8] is calculated as

$$K_F(X, Y) = G_\lambda^T(X)F_\lambda^{-1}G_\lambda(Y) \tag{6}$$

where $F_\lambda = E_X[G_\lambda(X)G_\lambda^T(X)]$ is the *Fisher Information Matrix* (FIM).

As F_λ is symmetric and positive semi-definite, and F_λ^{-1} has the Cholesky decomposition $F_\lambda^{-1} = L_\lambda^T L_\lambda$, the FK can be re-defined as $K_F(X, Y) = \mathscr{G}_\lambda^T(X)\mathscr{G}_\lambda(Y)$, where $\mathscr{G}_\lambda(X) = L_\lambda \bigtriangledown_\lambda \log p(X|\lambda)$. We only consider the gradients with respect to the mean and covariance since the gradient with respect to the weights brings little additional information [12].

Let $\zeta(t)$ be the occupancy probability of the CoDT feature x_n for the t-th Gaussian:

$$\zeta_n(t) = \frac{w_t p_t(x_n|\lambda)}{\sum_{k=1}^{T} w_k p_k(x_n|\lambda)} \tag{7}$$

The normalized gradients are finally computed as

$$\mathscr{G}_{\mu_t^d}(X) = \frac{1}{\sqrt{w_t}}\sum_{n=1}^{N}\zeta_n(t)(\frac{x_n^d - \mu_t^d}{\sigma_t^d}) \tag{8}$$

$$\mathscr{G}_{\sigma_t^d}(X) = \frac{1}{\sqrt{w_t}}\sum_{n=1}^{N}\zeta_n(t)\frac{1}{\sqrt{2}}[\frac{(x_n^d - \mu_t^d)^2}{(\sigma_t^d)^2} - 1] \tag{9}$$

The Fisher representation is the concatenation of all the gradients $\mathscr{G}_{\mu_t^d}(X)$ and $\mathscr{G}_{\sigma_t^d}(X)$ for $d = 1, 2, ..., D$ dimension of the CoDT feature and for T Gaussians.

The proposed Adaptive CoDT (AdaCoDT) method has several advantages over the BoW framework. First, as a generalization of the BoW framework, the resulting representation is not limited to the number of occurrences of each visual word. It also encodes additional information about the distribution of features. Secondly, it reduces the information loss raised by the coding procedure of the BoW framework. Thirdly, it can be computed from much smaller codebooks therefore it reduces the computational cost. Lastly, with the same size of codebook, it is much larger than the BoW representation. Hence, it assures an excellent performance with a simple linear classifier [12].

3 Experiments and Comparisons

3.1 Datasets

We evaluate the performance of the proposed method for HEp-2 cells classification on two HEp-2 cell datasets. **The ICPR2012 dataset** was released on the ICPR'12 *HEp-2*

Table 1. Parameters for comparative algorithms.

Algorithm	$(\mathbf{P}, \mathbf{R})$ or $(\mathbf{P}, \mathbf{R}, \mathbf{d})$	**T**
FK-SIFT	/	128
CoALBP	(4,1,2),(4,2,4),(4,4,8)	/
RICLBP	(4,1,2),(4,2,4),(4,4,8)	/
LBP	(8,1),(12,2),(16,3)	/

cell classification contest. It consists of 1455 cells, which are manually segmented from 28 slide images. Each cell is identified as one of six patterns: centromere (ce), coarse speckled (cs), cytoplasmic (cy), fine speckled (fs), homogeneous (ho) and nucleolar (nu). According to the experimental protocol of the contest, the dataset is divided into a training set with 721 cells from 14 slide images and a test set with 734 cells from 14 slide images. **The ICIP2013 training dataset** was used as the training dataset in the ICIP'13 *Competition on cells classification by fluorescent image analysis*. It contains 13596 cells which are categorized into six classes: homogeneous (ho), speckled (sp), nucleolar (nu), centromere (ce), nuclear membrane (nm) and golgi (go). We partition the dataset into a training set containing 6842 cells from 42 slide images and a test set containing 6754 cells from 41 slide images. Some examples are shown in Fig 2.

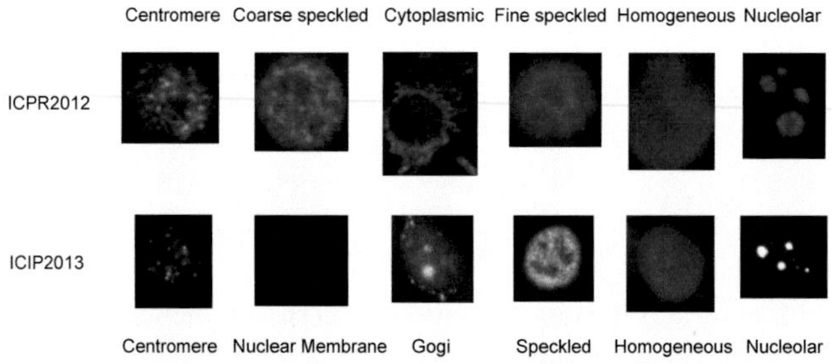

Fig. 2. Sample images of ICPR2012 and ICIP2013 datasets.

3.2 Experimental Results

We quantitatively compare the classification performance achieved by our proposed AdaCoDT framework, with LBP [10], CoALBP [2] (the winner of ICPR'12 contest), RICLBP [1], LSC based on dense SIFT(LSC-SIFT) [13], LSC based on CoDT (LSC-CoDT) and the FK based on dense SIFT (FK-SIFT). The parameters for each method are set as Table 1 which are optimized manually via several trials. With respect to LBP-related features, P is the number of neighbor pixels, R is the the radius and d is the interval between the LBP pair. The number of GMM components T is another parameter to be considered for the FK based methods. The codebook size of LSC method is 1024 due to the trade-off between classification accuracy and computational cost.

Performance Assessment on the ICPR2012 Dataset: We choose parameters $(P, R, d) = (24, 4, 8)$ and $T = 256$ for the proposed AdaCoDT via several trials. We utilize linear SVM due to its effectiveness and efficiency. It is trained using the training set by 10-fold cross validation strategy. The *one-vs-all* approach is used to handle our multi-class problem (the same strategy is used for ICIP2013 training dataset). Table 2(a) shows the classification performance of each method at the cell level. The AdaCoDT method outperforms all the other methods, achieving 75.2% of classification accuracy. The obtained accuracy is even higher than that of a human expert and significantly outperforms CoALBP which is the winner of the contest.

Table 3(a) illustrates the confusion matrices presenting the classification performance for each staining pattern at the cell level. It is obvious that cytoplasmic, centromere and homogeneous patterns are classified more accurately than the others. More particularly, cytoplasmic can achieve 100% of classification accuracy. To evaluate the classification performance at the image level, we report the corresponding confusion matrix in Table 3(b). The prediction for staining pattern of each image is decided by the most frequently assigned pattern of the cells within that image. The proposed AdaCoDT method obtains the classification accuracy of 85.7%, which indicates that 12 images are correctly classified while there are 14 images in the test set.

Table 2. Classification performance at the cell level.

(a) ICPR2012 dataset

Algorithm	Accuracy	Sensitivity
AdaCoDT	**75.2%**	**77.1%**
Human [2]	73.3%	/
LSC-SIFT	68.1%	69.4%
LSC-CoDT	66.9%	66.5%
FK-SIFT	66.6%	66.7%
CoALBP [2]	70.4%	68.7%
RICLBP [1]	68.5%	67.5%
LBP	58.9%	59.2%

(b) ICIP2013 training dataset

Algorithm	Accuracy	Sensitivity
AdaCoDT	**75.8%**	**72.9%**
LSC-SIFT	73.2%	71.9%
LSC-CoDT	70.6%	69.8%
FK-SIFT	69.7%	68.3%
CoALBP	67.1%	65.5%
RICLBP	66.4%	64.4%
LBP	60.7%	54.5%

Table 3. Confusion matrix for the ICPR2012 dataset via our proposed AdaCoDT method.

(a) The cell level (%)

	ce	cs	cy	fs	ho	nu
ce	**85.9**	8.1	0.0	0.0	0.0	6.0
cs	4.0	**75.3**	2.9	17.8	0.0	0.0
cy	0.0	0.0	**100.0**	0.0	0.0	0.0
fs	20.2	3.5	6.2	**52.6**	17.5	0.0
ho	8.3	2.8	0.6	11.1	**73.9**	3.3
nu	2.2	0.0	11.5	3.6	7.9	**74.8**

(b) The image level (%)

	ce	cs	cy	fs	ho	nu
ce	**100.0**	0.0	0.0	0.0	0.0	0.0
cs	0.0	**66.7**	0.0	33.3	0.0	0.0
cy	0.0	0.0	**100.0**	0.0	0.0	0.0
fs	**50.0**	0.0	0.0	**50.0**	0.0	0.0
ho	0.0	0.0	0.0	0.0	**100.0**	0.0
nu	0.0	0.0	0.0	0.0	0.0	**100.0**

Performance assessment on the ICIP2013 training dataset: We choose parameters $(P, R, d) = (16, 5, 10)$ and $T = 128$, which are optimized via several trials, for the proposed AdaCoDT. The classification performance of different methods at the cell level are shown in Table 2(b). Our proposed AdaCoDT method achieves the best performance again. It is also worth noting that the size of codebook for the BoW framework is 1024 while the number of GMM components for the AdaCoDT method is only 128. With the same codebook size (the number of GMM components can be seen as the codebook size), the AdaCoDT method significantly outperforms the BoW framework.

Table 4(a) shows the confusion matrix of the AdaCoDT method at the cell level. Homogeneous pattern gets the highest classification accuracy rate of 89.5%, followed by nuclear membrane as they have distinguished characteristic compared with other patterns. Table 4(b) illustrates the confusion matrix at the image level. The AdaCoDT method obtains the classification accuracy of 87.8% at image level, which means that 36 images are correctly identified while there are 41 images in the test set.

Table 4. Confusion matrix for the ICIP2013 training dataset via our proposed AdaCoDT method.

(a) The cell level (%)

	ho	sp	nu	ce	nm	go
ho	**89.5**	3.4	4.1	0.3	2.4	0.3
sp	11.6	**66.7**	5.6	15.1	0.7	0.3
nu	0.8	8.1	**74.2**	11.7	2.6	2.6
ce	0.5	22.2	2.1	**74.7**	0.0	0.2
nm	1.1	2.4	1.1	0.4	**88.7**	6.3
go	6.6	5.0	38.2	0.8	5.8	**43.6**

(b) The image level (%)

	ho	sp	nu	ce	nm	go
ho	**100.0**	0.0	0.0	0.0	0.0	0.0
sp	12.5	**75.0**	0.0	12.5	0.0	0.0
nu	0.0	0.0	**100.0**	0.0	0.0	0.0
ce	0.0	25.0	0.0	**75.0**	0.0	0.0
nm	0.0	0.0	0.0	0.0	**100.0**	0.0
go	0.0	0.0	**50.0**	0.0	0.0	**50.0**

4 Conclusion

In this study, we have presented a promising framework, AdaCoDT, for automatic staining pattern classification of HEp-2 cells. First, we propose a CoDT feature which directly uses the differential vectors of micro-texton and its neighborhoods to reserve more discriminative information. It further captures the spatial information between neighboring micro-textons to provide strong discriminative and descriptive capability. Then, we approximate the distribution of CoDT feature as a GMM which can adaptively partition the CoDT feature space for the classification task of HEp-2 cells. Finally, we obtain a high discriminative and powerful descriptive HEp-2 cell image representation based on the adaptive CoDT feature space using FK principle. We feed the image representation into a linear SVM classifier to predict staining patterns of the HEp-2 cells. The AdaCoDT method combines the strengths of generative and discriminative approaches for image classification, therefore it can achieve excellent classification performance. Experimental results validate that the proposed AdaCoDT method can provide superior performance for HEp-2 cells classification, compared with the traditional LBP and its extensions. The new feature encoding method also significantly improves the classification performance in comparison of the BoW representation.

Acknowledgment. This work is partially supported by two research grants, MOE2011-T2-2-037 and RG139/14 from Ministry of Education, Singapore.

References

1. Ryusuke, N., Kazuhiro, F.: HEp-2 cell classification using rotation invariant co-occurrence among local binary patterns. Pattern Recogn. 47(7), 2428-2436 (2014)
2. Foggia, P., Percannella, G., Soda, P., Vento, M.: Benchmarking HEp-2 cells classification methods. IEEE Trans. Med. Imaging 32(10), 1878-1889 (2013)
3. Xu, X., Lin, F., Carol, Ng, Leong, K.P.: Linear local distance coding for classification of HEp-2 staining patterns. In: IEEE Winter Conference on Applications of Computer Vision (WACV), pp. 393-400 (2014)
4. Shen, L.L., Lin, J.M., Wu, S.Y., Yu, S.Q.: HEp-2 image classification using intensity order pooling based features and bag of words. Pattern Recogn. 47(7), 2419-2427 (2014)
5. Theodorakopoulos, I., Kastaniotis, D., Economou, G., Fotopoulos, S.: Hep-2 cells classification via sparse representation of textural features fused into dissimilarity space. Pattern Recogn. 47(7), 2367-2378 (2014)
6. Xu, X., Lin, F., Carol, Ng, Leong, K.P.: Staining Pattern Classification of ANA-IIF Based on SIFT Features. J. Medical Imag. Heal. Inform. (2)4, 419-424 (2012)
7. Nanni, L., Paci, M., Brahnam, S.: Indirect immunofluorescence image classification using texture descriptors. Expert Syst. Appl. 41(5), 2463-2471 (2014)
8. Perronnin, F., Dance, C.: Fisher kernels on visual vocabularies for image categorization. In: IEEE Conference on Computer Vision and Pattern Recognition (CVPR), pp. 1-8 (2007)
9. Boiman, O., Shechtman, E., Irani, M.: In defense of nearest-neighbor based image classification. In: IEEE Conference on Computer Vision and Pattern Recognition (CVPR), pp. 1-8 (2008)
10. Ojala, T., Pietikainen, M., Maenpaa, T.: Multiresolution gray-scale and rotation invariant texture classification with local binary patterns. IEEE Trans. Pattern Anal. 24(7), 971-987(2002)
11. Dempster, A.P., Laird, N.M., Rubin, D.B.: Maximum likelihood from incomplete data via the EM algorithm. J. R. Stat. Soc. Series B (Methodological) 1-38 (1977)
12. Sánchez, J., Perronnin, F., Mensink, T., Verbeek, J.: Image classification with the Fisher vector: Theory and practice. Int. J. Comput. Vision 105(3), 222-245 (2013)
13. Liu, L.Q., Wang, L., Liu, X.W.: In defense of soft-assignment coding. In: IEEE International Conference on Computer Vision (ICCV), pp. 2486-2493 (2011)

Learning to Segment: Training Hierarchical Segmentation under a Topological Loss

Jan Funke[1], Fred A. Hamprecht[2], and Chong Zhang[2,3]

[1] Institute of Neuroinformatics UZH/ETHZ, Switzerland
[2] CellNetworks and IWR/HCI, Heidelberg University, Germany
[3] Universitat Pompeu Fabra, Spain

Abstract. We propose a generic and efficient learning framework that is applicable to segment images in which individual objects are mainly discernible by boundary cues. Our approach starts by first hierarchically clustering the image and then explaining the image in terms of a cost-minimal subset of non-overlapping segments. The cost of a segmentation is defined as a weighted sum of features of the selected candidates. This formulation allows us to take into account an extensible set of arbitrary features. The maximally discriminative linear combination of features is learned from training data using a margin-rescaled structured SVM. At the core of our formulation is a novel and simple topology-based structured loss which is a combination of counts and geodesic distance of topological errors (splits, merges, false positives and false negatives) relative to the training set. We demonstrate the generality and accuracy of our approach on three challenging 2D cell segmentation problems, where we improve accuracy compared to the current state of the art.

1 Introduction

Accurately segmenting a large number of objects of similar type in crowded images is challenging, e.g. when cells of interest touch or overlap. Therefore, the development of robust and efficient algorithms, generic enough to be applicable for different scenarios, is of great importance. Since local measurements are usually ambiguous due to noise and imaging artefacts, priors about the objects to be segmented are needed. Two of the main challenges for automatic segmentation are how to reflect those priors in the cost function of the segmentation problem, and how to learn them from training data. Usually, the cost functions are designed "by hand" for a particular segmentation problem, or have user-adjustable tuning parameters like a foreground bias to adapt to different setups [15,14].

In this paper, we propose a generic framework for structured learning of the cost function for cell segmentation. The cost function is defined on *candidate segments*, of which we find a cost-minimal, non-overlapping subset to obtain a final segmentation. The main contributions of our approach are: 1) The novel counting-and-propagating topological loss is simple and generic. 2) Our formulation supports a large set of expressive features on the segment candidates. 3) Optimal feature weights are learned from annotated samples to minimize a

N. Navab et al. (Eds.): MICCAI 2015, Part III, LNCS 9351, pp. 268–275, 2015.
DOI: 10.1007/978-3-319-24574-4_32

topological loss on the final segmentation. The capacity to combine and weigh automatically all features from a large set can reduce the effort previously required to manually select suitable features and tune parameters. 4) By considering candidate segments obtained by iteratively merging superpixels [3,4,7], our method is very efficient while still improving on the current state of the art.

Considering candidates from hierarchy of regions has demonstrated to be an effective method for cell detection and segmentation [3,5,8,7,9]. It has been shown that a globally cost-minimal and non-overlapping set of candidates can efficiently be found, either by ILP or dynamic programming [3,7]. However, the proposed methods differ greatly in the way the candidate costs are obtained. For the cell *detection* proposed by Arteta *et al.* [3], the costs are learned using a structured SVM, taking into account the non-overlap constraint of the inference problem. In the context of cell *segmentation* from candidates obtained from iterative merging [5,8,7,9], the costs are learned by providing samples of positive and negative candidates to a binary classifier.

In the following section, we show how the structured learning framework can be used to learn the candidate costs for segmentation under consideration of the problem structure. For that, we introduce a novel loss function which minimizes the propagated topological errors on the resulting segmentation. In Section 3, we demonstrate the effectiveness of our approach on three datasets.

2 Method

Our method is based on selecting candidates extracted from a hierarchy of segmentations, an approach that has recently attracted attention in a range of computer vision problems [2,3,5,8,7]. The underlying idea is to extract a *merge tree* of candidates (i.e., parent nodes are merged segments of their children, see Fig. 2 for an example) that span the whole range from over- to undersegmentation. A segmentation of the image can now be expressed by a selection of non-overlapping candidates. It remains to rate different segmentations by assigning costs to each candidate, which represent the likelihood of being a correct segment. We propose to train a structured SVM to learn those costs as a linear combination of candidate features. For that, we propose a novel loss function minimizing topological errors during learning.

Candidates Extraction. We perform a watershed transformation on a boundary prediction image, for which we trained a random forest classifier using the open source software ilastik [12], to obtain initial segment candidates. Let $G = (C, E, s)$ be the candidate adjacency graph of the initial segmentation, where $C = \{c_1, \dots, c_N\}$ are the initial candidates and $E \subset C \times C$ is a set of edges representing adjacency, and let $s : E \mapsto \mathbb{R}$ be an edge scoring function. Iteratively, the candidates connected by the edge $\operatorname{argmin}_E s(E)$ with the lowest scores are merged, and the adjacency graph updated accordingly. For the experiments presented in this paper, we use $s(c_i, c_j){=}m(c_i, c_j) \min(|c_i|, |c_j|)$, with $m(c_i, c_j)$ being the median boundary prediction value of all boundary pixels between c_i and c_j, and $|c_i|$ the size of a candidate. Note that this way we obtain a binary merge tree structure, but the candidates extraction is a replaceable part of our pipeline. More sophisticated methods for a general tree like ultrametric contour maps [2], graph-based active learning of agglomeration [9], or hierarchical planar correlation clustering [14] can be used as well.

Inference. Let $T = (C, S, f)$ be a *merge tree* of candidates, where C is the set of all candidates, $S \subset C \times C$ are directed edges indicating superset relations (for an example, see Fig. 2), and let $f : C \mapsto \mathbb{R}$ be a candidate cost function. We introduce binary indicator variables $\mathbf{y} = (y_i, \ldots, y_N)$, where $y_i = 1$ represents the selection of candidate c_i for the final segmentation. To ensure that only non-overlapping candidates are selected, we restrict the possible configurations of $\mathbf{y}$ to select at most one candidate per path in the merge tree and denote the restricted set of configurations by $\mathcal{Y}$. Let $\mathcal{P}$ be the set of all paths in T. We find the cost-optimal selection of candidates with the following LP:

$$\min_{\mathbf{y} \in \mathbb{R}^N} \sum_i f(c_i) y_i, \quad \text{s.t.} \sum_{i \in P} y_i \leq 1 \quad \forall P \in \mathcal{P}; \quad y_i \geq 0 \quad \forall i. \tag{1}$$

Note that there is no need to explicitly express the integrality constraints, here, since the constraint matrix is totally unimodular and the optimization problem is known to have a polynomial-time solution [3].

Structured Learning of Candidate Costs. We propose to learn the candidate cost function f using a structured SVM [13] from labeled training data. For that, we model the costs $f(c_i)$ as a linear combination of features $\boldsymbol{\phi}_i$ extracted for each candidate individually, i.e., $f(c_i) = \langle \boldsymbol{w}, \boldsymbol{\phi}_i \rangle$. Note that here the linearity can be relaxed, as features can also be a function of arbitrary combinations of groups of features. The weights $\boldsymbol{w}$ can be learned to minimize a topological loss on the training data. Let

$$E(\mathbf{y}) = \sum_{i=1}^{N} f(c_i) y_i = \sum_{i=1}^{N} \langle \boldsymbol{w}, \boldsymbol{\phi}_i \rangle \, y_i = \langle \boldsymbol{w}, \boldsymbol{\Phi} \mathbf{y} \rangle \tag{2}$$

be the cost of a segmentation represented by binary indicator variables $\mathbf{y}$, where $\boldsymbol{\Phi}$ is a combined feature matrix for all candidates. In order to learn the weights $\boldsymbol{w}$, the structured SVM framework needs a training sample $(\mathbf{y}', \boldsymbol{\phi})$ with $\mathbf{y}' \in \mathcal{Y}$. Note that multiple training samples can easily be concatenated into a single one. Since the extracted segment candidates may not perfectly correspond to the (human annotated) ground truth (GT), the training sample $\mathbf{y}'$ is obtained by maximizing the spatial overlap to the GT. Therefore, $\mathbf{y}'$ represents the *best-effort* segmentation compared to the GT. Note that since the proposed learning method uses only the best-effort solution for training, small imprecisions in the human generated ground truth are tolerable.

Given a training sample $(\mathbf{y}', \boldsymbol{\Phi})$, we find an optimal set of weights $\boldsymbol{w}^*$ by minimization of the structured SVM objective

$$\boldsymbol{w}^* = \operatorname*{argmin}_{\boldsymbol{w}} \frac{\lambda}{2} |\boldsymbol{w}|^2 + \max_{\mathbf{y} \in \mathcal{Y}} \langle \boldsymbol{w}, \boldsymbol{\Phi}\mathbf{y}' - \boldsymbol{\Phi}\mathbf{y} \rangle + \Delta(\mathbf{y}', \mathbf{y}), \tag{3}$$

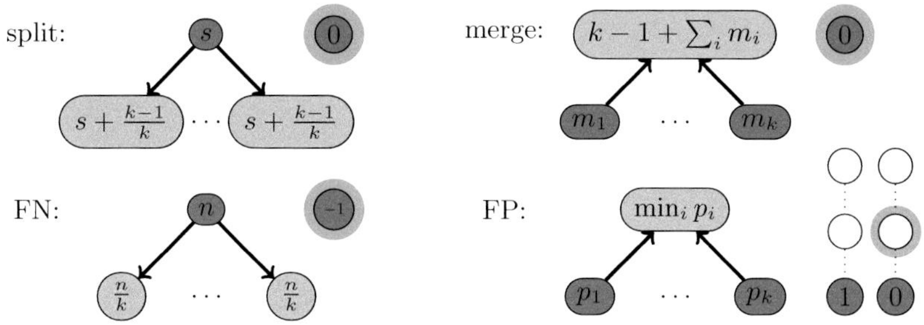

Fig. 1. Illustration of the topological loss used for structured learning: splits, merges, false negatives (FN), and false positives (FP). Starting from nodes with known values (blue): Given the values of parent candidates, split and FN values are propagated downwards; given the values of child candidates, merge and FP values are propagated upwards.

where λ is the weight of the quadratic regularizer and $\Delta(\mathbf{y}', \mathbf{y})$ is an application specific loss function to be minimized. This loss function can be seen as a distance between the desired segmentation $\mathbf{y}'$ and a potential segmentation $\mathbf{y}$. A proper choice of this function is crucial for the success of learning. However, the expressiveness of the loss function is limited by the tractability of the maximization in Eq. 3, which has to be carried out repeatedly during learning.

Here, we propose a topological loss function that directly counts and propagates the number of split, merge, false positive (FP), and false negative (FN) errors of a potential segmentation compared to the best-effort. Due to the tree structure of the candidate subset relations, this loss decomposes into a sum of individual contributions: For each candidate, we determine four values (s, m, p, n), which represent the candidate's contribution to the overall number of split, merge, FN, and FP errors. The distribution of the values is based on the following intuition: Whenever a best-effort candidate is selected, no topological error was made by this selection. If, however, all k children of a best-effort candidate are selected, $k-1$ split errors have been made. In a similar fashion, the selection of a parent of k best-effort candidates causes $k-1$ merge errors. This observation suggests a simple propagation scheme of topological errors: Initial split values of all best-effort candidates and their ancestors are $s = 0$; merge values of all best-effort candidates and their descendants are $m = 0$. In addition to that, the FN value of each best-effort candidate is set to $n = -1$, i.e., as a reward, such that an equivalent amount is payed by not selecting (and therefore missing) the candidate. Initial FP values are set for all leaf nodes in the tree as $p = 0$ if the leaf is a descendant of a best-effort candidate (in this case, selecting the candidate does not cause an FP error), or as $p = 1$ if it is not a descendant of a best-effort candidate. These initial values are then propagated up- and downwards the candidate tree using the rules presented in detail in Fig. 1. For a simple example, see Fig. 2. The sum of the values of a candidate gives the topological error that is caused by selecting this candidate.

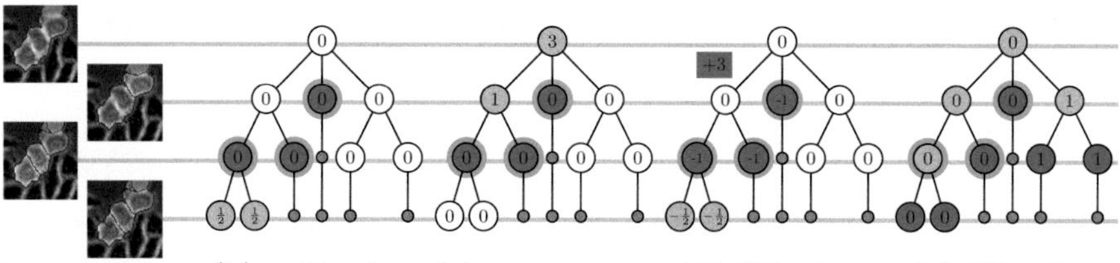

(a) segmentations (b) split values (c) merge values (d) FN values (e) FP values

Fig. 2. Example split, merge, false negative (FN), and false positive (FP) values of candidates in a merge tree. The best-effort solution is highlighted in green.

To combine the topological error values (s, m, p, n) of each candidate into the final topological loss, we suggest a linear combination, i.e.,

$$\Delta(\mathbf{y}', \mathbf{y}) = \sum_{i=1}^{N} (\alpha s_i + \beta m_i + \gamma p_i + \delta n_i)\, y_i + \delta c, \tag{4}$$

where c is the number of best-effort candidates ensuring that the loss is positive. The parameters $(\alpha, \beta, \gamma, \delta)$ can be used to assign different weights to different error types, which can be useful in situations where split errors are preferred over merge errors, since they are usually faster to repair.

The resulting topological loss function is linear in $\mathbf{y}$, which allows us to solve the maximization in Eq. 3 efficiently using the LP formulation in Eq. 1 for any given $\boldsymbol{w}$. It remains to find the minimum of Eq. 3, which is a piece-wise quadratic and convex function of $\boldsymbol{w}$. For that, we use a bundle method [1].

3 Experiments and Results

Datasets. We validate our method on three datasets (see examples in Fig. 3 (a-c)) which present high variabilities in image resolution, microscopy modality, and cell type (shape, appearance and size): 1) phase contrast images of cervical cancer Hela cells from [3] (cells for training/testing: 656/384); 2) bright field images of in-focus Diploid yeast cells from [15] (cells for training/testing: 109/595); 3) bright field images of Fission yeast cells from [10] (cells for training/testing: 1422/240). Challenging problems in general include densely packed and touching cells, intra shape and size variations within the same dataset, weak boundary cues, out-of-focus artifacts, and similar boundaries from other structures.

Experimental Setup. The used intensity- and morphology-based candidate features are: size, intensity (sum, mean, variance, skewness, kurtosis, histogram (20 bins), 7 histogram quantiles), circularity, eccentricity, contour angle histogram (16 bins). The intensity features are extracted from the raw and boundary prediction images, on the whole candidate and on the candidate contours. For each pair of features ϕ_i and ϕ_j, the product $\phi_i * \phi_j$ is also added. All features are normalized

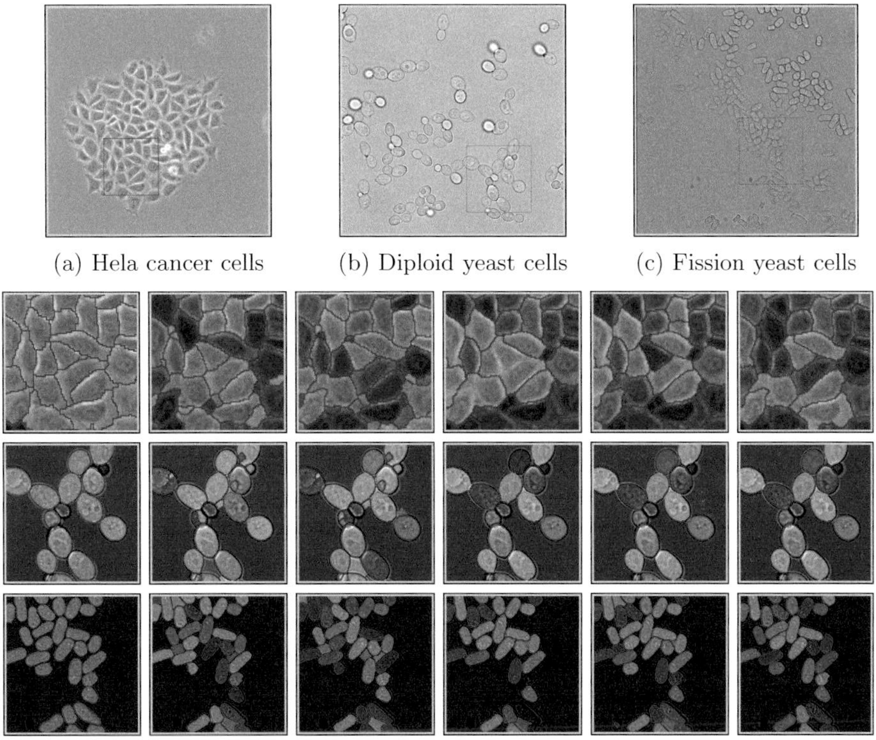

(a) Hela cancer cells (b) Diploid yeast cells (c) Fission yeast cells

ground truth (d) pCC (e) npCC (f) Hamming (g) cover (h) topological

Fig. 3. Example segmentation results on three datasets (a–c). Results (*inset views*) using correlation clustering (d–e) and using our structured learning formulation with different loss functions $\Delta(\mathbf{y}', \mathbf{y})$ (f–h).

to be in the range [0,1]. The weights $(\alpha, \beta, \gamma, \delta)$ for combining the four topological errors are chosen through a Leave-one-out cross-validation, specifically, being (1,2,1,2), (1,2,1,5), and (1,2,1,10), for the three datasets respectively.

Comparison. We compare to the two correlation clustering variants (pCC and npCC) on the investigated datasets [15]. For our structured learning formulation, we also include results from using, as loss $\Delta(\mathbf{y}', \mathbf{y})$, a simple Hamming distance and a cover loss. The latter counts the errors from GT region centroids that are either not covered or wrongly covered by the picked candidates, which is similar to the loss in [3]. As opposed to pCC and npCC, the flexible features enrich learning with boundary and region cues, including e.g. texture and shape priors. This can be seen in Fig. 3, where background regions are correctly identified, owing to concavity or texture. Instead of assigning the same loss to each wrong candidate as in Hamming and cover losses, our topological loss explicitly counts errors proportional to the distance in the merge tree. This is more indicative and robust, which is reflected on less FN and splits in the figure.

Evaluation. We report five quantitative measures: variation of information (VOI) and tolerant edit distance (TED) [6] indicate both detection and segmen-

Table 1. Detection and segmentation results on three datasets. The best value in each column is highlighted.

	VOI			TED [6]					DS			dice	overlap
	split	merge	total	FP	FN	split	merge	total	prec.	rec.	F-sc.		
planarCC	0.33	0.52	0.84	20	43	77	30	170	0.86	0.91	0.89	0.79	69.35
nonplanarCC	0.39	0.43	0.82	31	25	53	41	150	0.89	0.93	0.91	0.80	69.21
Hamming	0.33	0.44	**0.77**	2	41	62	6	111	0.95	0.99	**0.97**	0.83	72.40
cover	0.37	0.43	0.80	9	36	109	3	157	0.82	0.99	0.90	0.81	70.12
topological	0.35	0.42	**0.77**	5	33	49	11	**98**	0.95	0.98	**0.97**	**0.84**	**73.20**

Dataset 1

	VOI			TED [6]					DS			dice	overlap
	split	merge	total	FP	FN	split	merge	total	prec.	rec.	F-sc.		
planarCC	0.72	0.24	0.97	237	36	11	74	358	0.70	0.86	0.77	0.87	79.99
nonplanarCC	1.61	0.21	1.81	402	22	5	59	488	0.59	0.92	0.72	0.86	78.07
Hamming	0.44	0.53	0.97	28	159	3	16	206	0.96	0.72	0.82	0.89	80.91
cover	1.04	0.30	1.34	121	50	2	13	186	0.83	0.91	0.87	0.87	79.51
topological	0.50	0.33	**0.83**	40	69	3	4	**116**	0.93	0.89	**0.91**	**0.90**	**82.22**

Dataset 2

	VOI			TED [6]					DS			dice	overlap
	split	merge	total	FP	FN	split	merge	total	prec.	rec.	F-sc.		
planarCC	0.19	0.07	**0.26**	19	2	8	7	**36**	0.92	0.97	**0.94**	**0.91**	**84.67**
nonplanarCC	0.30	0.07	0.37	56	2	9	6	73	0.82	0.97	0.89	0.91	84.34
Hamming	0.84	0.16	1.00	67	37	1	12	117	0.81	0.86	0.83	0.89	82.05
cover	0.42	0.10	0.52	97	6	12	1	116	0.74	0.99	0.85	0.90	81.84
topological	0.19	0.14	0.33	6	25	1	8	40	0.99	0.90	**0.94**	0.90	82.85

Dataset 3

tation errors; Detection score (DS) measures detection accuracy only; Dice coefficient and area overlap provide segmentation accuracy. For DS, we establish possible matches between found regions and GT regions based on overlap, and find a Hungarian matching using the centroid distance as minimizer. Unmatched GT regions are FN, unmatched segmentation regions are FP. We report precision, recall, and F-score. Area overlap is computed between the true positive (TP) detection regions R_{tpd} and the GT region R_{gt}: $(R_{tpd} \cap R_{gt})/(R_{tpd} \cup R_{gt}) \times 100$. TED measures the minimal number of topological errors under tolerable modifications of the segmentation (here, we tolerated boundary shifts up to 10 pixels for Hela cells, and 25 pixels for two datasets of yeast cells). Results are summarized in Table 1. Our proposed method robustly outperforms for the two more challenging datasets (1 and 2), and achieves amongst the best for dataset 3.

4 Discussion and Conclusions

We have proposed a generic framework for structured learning of the cost function for segmenting cells primarily only with boundary cues (Code available at: `http://github.com/funkey/tobasl`). This reduces the effort previously required for manual feature selection or parameter tuning. The tree-topology based loss from the hierarchical segment regions has demonstrated to be efficient and can improve segmentation. The potential restriction on candidate regions imposed by using only trees can partly be lifted by, e.g., constructing multiple trees, at least in test stage, in the spirit of perturb-and-MAP or as in [11] for user correction. We have validated our approach in the context of biological applications, however we expect that it can be applied in other fields. Also, data which has primarily region rather than boundary cues can be turned into the latter, and hence fit into this mould, by using, e.g., pixel-level classifier to delineate region pixels that are on the border. These form part of our future work.

References

1. sbmrm - Bundle Method for Structured Risk Minimization, `https://github.com/funkey/sbmrm`.
2. Arbeláez, P., Maire, M.L., Fowlkes, C., Malik, J.: Contour Detection and Hierarchical Image Segmentation. IEEE PAMI 33(5), 898–916 (2011)
3. Arteta, C., Lempitsky, V., Noble, J.A., Zisserman, A.: Learning to Detect Cells Using Non-overlapping Extremal Regions. In: Ayache, N., Delingette, H., Golland, P., Mori, K. (eds.) MICCAI 2012, Part I. LNCS, vol. 7510, pp. 348–356. Springer, Heidelberg (2012)
4. Arteta, C., Lempitsky, V., Noble, J.A., Zisserman, A.: Learning to Detect Partially Overlapping Instances. In: CVPR (2013)
5. Funke, J., Andres, B., Hamprecht, F.A., Cardona, A., Cook, M.: Efficient Automatic 3D-Reconstruction of Branching Neurons from EM Data. In: CVPR (2012)
6. Funke, J., Klein, J., Cardona, A., Cook, M.: A Tolerant Edit Distance for Evaluation and Training of Electron Microscopy Reconstruction Algorithms. CoRR (2015)
7. Liu, F., Xing, F., Yang, L.: Robust Muscle Cell Segmentation using Region Selection with Dynamic Programming. In: ISBI, pp. 1381–1384 (2014)
8. Liu, T., Jurrus, E., Seyedhossein, M., Ellisman, M., Tasdizen, T.: Watershed Merge Tree Classification for Electron Microscopy Image Segmentation. In: ICPR (2012)
9. Nunez-Iglesias, J., Kennedy, R., Plaza, S.M., Chakraborty, A., Katz, W.T.: Graph-based Active Learning of Agglomeration (GALA): a Python Library to Segment 2D and 3D Neuroimages. Front. Neuroinform. 8, 34 (2014)
10. Peng, J.Y., Chen, Y.J., Green, M.D., Sabatinos, S.A., Forsburg, S.L., Hsu, C.N.: PombeX: Robust Cell Segmentation for Fission Yeast Transillumination Images. PLoS One 8(12), e81434 (2013)
11. Schiegg, M., Heuer, B., Haubold, C., Wolf, S., Koethe, U., Hamprecht, F.A.: Proofreading Guidance in Cell Tracking by Sampling from Tracking-by-Assignment Models. In: ISBI (2015)
12. Sommer, C., Straehle, C., Koethe, U., Hamprecht, F.A.: ilastik: Interactive Learning and Segmentation Toolkit. In: ISBI (2011)
13. Tsochantaridis, I., Joachims, T., Hofmann, T., Altun, Y., Singer, Y.: Large Margin Methods for Structured and Interdependent Output Variables. J. Mach. Learn. Res. 6, 1453–1484 (2005)
14. Yarkony, J., Zhang, C., Fowlkes, C.C.: Hierarhcical Planar Correlation Clustering for Cell Segmentation. In: Tai, X.-C., Bae, E., Chan, T.F., Lysaker, M. (eds.) EMMCVPR 2015. LNCS, vol. 8932, pp. 492–504. Springer, Heidelberg (2015)
15. Zhang, C., Yarkony, J., Hamprecht, F.A.: Cell Detection and Segmentation using Correlation Clustering. In: Golland, P., Hata, N., Barillot, C., Hornegger, J., Howe, R. (eds.) MICCAI 2014, Part I. LNCS, vol. 8673, pp. 9–16. Springer, Heidelberg (2014)

You Should Use Regression to Detect Cells

Philipp Kainz[1,⋆], Martin Urschler[2,3], Samuel Schulter[2], Paul Wohlhart[2], and Vincent Lepetit[2]

[1] Institute of Biophysics, Medical University of Graz, Austria
[2] Institute for Computer Graphics and Vision, BioTechMed, Graz University of Technology, Austria
[3] Ludwig Boltzmann Institute for Clinical Forensic Imaging, Graz, Austria

Abstract. Automated cell detection in histopathology images is a hard problem due to the large variance of cell shape and appearance. We show that cells can be detected reliably in images by predicting, for each pixel location, a monotonous function of the distance to the center of the closest cell. Cell centers can then be identified by extracting local extremums of the predicted values. This approach results in a very simple method, which is easy to implement. We show on two challenging microscopy image datasets that our approach outperforms state-of-the-art methods in terms of accuracy, reliability, and speed. We also introduce a new dataset that we will make publicly available.

1 Introduction

Analysis of microscopy image data is very common in modern cell biology and medicine. Unfortunately, given the typically huge number of cells contained in microscopic images of histological specimen, visual analysis is a tedious task and can lead to considerable inter-observer variability and even irreproducible results because of intra-observer variability [1].

Automated cell detection and segmentation methods are therefore highly desirable, and have seen much research effort during the previous decades [2]. In histological image analysis, one of the main problems is to count how many cells are present in the captured images, and many automatic methods have already been proposed for this task [3–8]. Some methods are based on simple contour-based cell models [5] or leverage shape and appearance priors [7] in a global optimization strategy. While reasonable success in cell detection may be achieved using conventional image processing, for example based on local symmetry features [4] or using normalized cuts and spectral graph theory to segment cells [3], recently learning based approaches have proven to achieve state-of-the-art results on detection benchmarks like [9]. On this benchmark, the work of [6] currently outperforms other approaches. It is based on extracting a large number of candidate maximally stable extremal cell regions using the MSER detector [10], which are pruned using several, increasingly complex classifiers based

⋆ The authors are grateful to Nasir Rajpoot and Mahonar Kuse for providing the cell data set from the ICPR 2010 Pattern Recognition in Histopathological Images contest, and to Martin Asslaber for providing the bone marrow histology images.

N. Navab et al. (Eds.): MICCAI 2015, Part III, LNCS 9351, pp. 276–283, 2015.
DOI: 10.1007/978-3-319-24574-4_33

on structured SVMs (SSVM). Other approaches apply a classifier densely over the input images in a sliding window fashion [11] or learn regions revealed by the SIFT [12] keypoint detector [8]. A related, but different problem is to count cells without explicitly detecting them by estimating their density [13, 14]. However this approach does not produce the locations of the cells, which are important for example to perform cell type recognition.

We consider here an alternative approach to cell detection. Our method is inspired by the recent [15], which considers the extraction of linear structures in images: Instead of relying on an *ad hoc* model of linear structures such as neurons [16] or a classifier [17], [15] proposes to predict, for each pixel of the input image, a function of the distances to the closest linear structure in a regression step. The local maximums of the predicted function can be extracted easily and correspond to the desired linear structures.

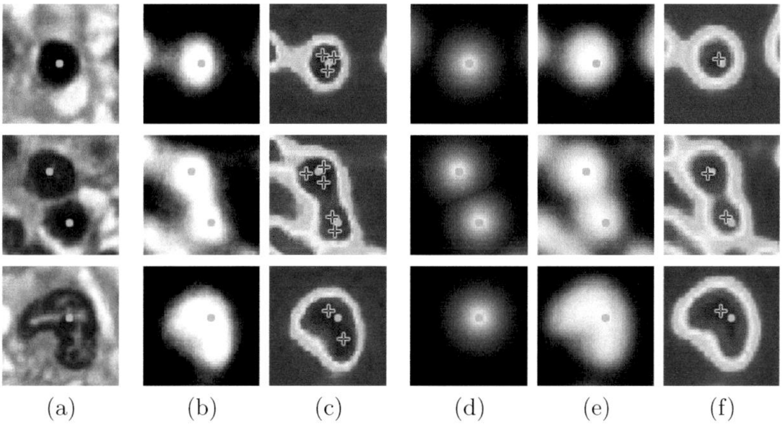

Fig. 1. Comparing classification and regression for cell detection. (a) Several patches of input images from our bone marrow dataset, centered on one or two cells. First row: one fully stained nucleus, second row: two closely located nuclei, third row: one nucleus of anisotropic shape and non-uniform staining. Green dots indicate ground truth annotation of the cell centers. (b) Probability maps provided by a classifier applied to these patches, and (c) the local maximums of these probability maps. They exhibit many local maximums – indicated by crosses – around the actual cell centers while only one maximum is expected. (d) The expected score map that the regressor should predict and (e) the actual predictions. (f) The local maximums of these predictions correspond much better to the cell centers and do not suffer from multiple responses.

As depicted in Fig. 1, we show in this paper that this approach transfers to cell detection, and actually outperforms state-of-the-art approaches over all the standard metrics: Using a standard regression Random Forest [18], we predict for each image location a function of the distance to the closest cell center. We can then identify the cell centers by looking for local maximums of the predictions.

We evaluate our approach on two challenging datasets, illustrated in Fig. 2. For both datasets, the goal is to predict the center of the cells. The first dataset we consider is from the ICPR 2010 Pattern Recognition in Histopathological Images contest [9], consisting of 20 100×100 pixel images of breast cancer tissue. We also introduce a new dataset BM, containing eleven $1,200 \times 1,200$ pixel images of healthy human bone marrow from eight different patients.

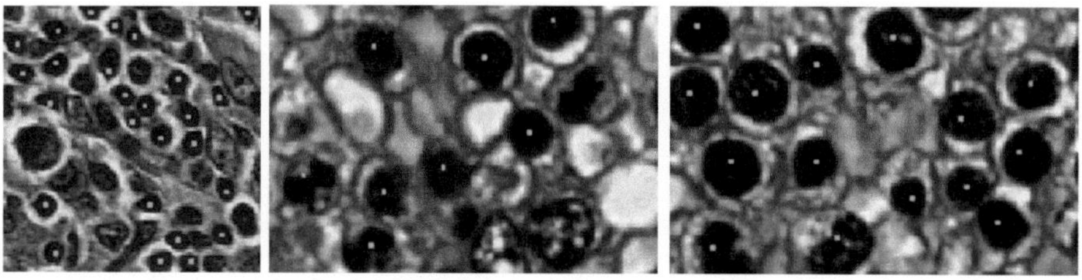

(a) ICPR (b) BM

Fig. 2. Dataset samples: (a) Breast cancer tissue from the ICPR 2010 contest [9] dataset (20× magnification), (b) bone marrow tissue (cropped from full images at 40× magnification). The green dots denote ground truth locations of the cell nuclei.

2 Learning to Localize Cells

Our approach to cell detection is to predict a score map based on the Euclidean distance transform of the cell centers in a given input image. This score map is computed such that each pixel value encodes its distance to the nearest cell center and, ideally, the local extremums correspond to the center of the cells to be detected. The prediction of the score map is performed using a regression method trained from cell images and ground truth cell locations.

2.1 Defining the Proximity Score Map

As shown in Fig. 1(a), our approach is based on statistical learning and relies on a set of annotated images for training. An expert labeled the centers of the cell nuclei in each of these images.

The standard classification approach applied to the cell detection problem would consist of training a classifier to predict whether the center pixel of an input image patch is the center of a cell or is located in the background. Unfortunately, as shown in Fig. 1(c), this often results in multiple peaks for cell nuclei and hence in multiple detections corresponding to a single cell. One option is to apply post-processing to group multiple detections into a single one, for example by smoothing the output of the classifier for each image location with a Gaussian kernel to merge multiple peaks into a single one. However, such a strategy may merge together the responses actually created by multiple cells.

We propose here a better, more principled approach. Inspired by [15], we exploit additional context during the learning phase and define a smooth, continuous prediction target function $d(\mathbf{x})$ expressing the proximity of each pixel $\mathbf{x}$ to the ground truth cell centers, such as the ones shown in Fig. 1(d). This therefore shifts the task from binary classification to regression of the continuous proximity score map.

A straightforward way of defining our proximity score map $d(\mathbf{x})$ is to take the inverted Euclidean distance transform $\mathcal{D}_C$ of the set $C = \{\mathbf{c}_i\}$ of ground truth cell centers: $d(\mathbf{x}) = -\mathcal{D}_C(\mathbf{x})$. However, this approach produces high proximity scores even in background areas. Additionally, it forces the regression model to predict varying scores for different regions of the background. Moreover, cell centers are not well-defined, which exacerbates the learning problem.

Hence, it is better to predict a function of the distance transform that is flat on the background and has better localized, distinctive peaks at cell centers [15]:

$$d(\mathbf{x}) = \begin{cases} e^{\alpha\left(1 - \frac{\mathcal{D}_C(\mathbf{x})}{d_M}\right)} - 1 & \text{if } \mathcal{D}_C(\mathbf{x}) < d_M \\ 0 & \text{otherwise} \end{cases}, \tag{1}$$

where α and d_M control the shape of the exponential function and $\mathcal{D}_C(\mathbf{x})$ is the Euclidean distance transform of the cell centers. In practice, we select d_M such that the maximum width of peaks in $d(\mathbf{x})$ corresponds to the average object size to be detected. We used $\alpha = 5$, $d_M = 16$ for ICPR, and $\alpha = 3$, $d_M = 39$ for BM.

Our goal is now to learn a function g that predicts $d(\mathbf{x})$ given an image patch $I(\mathbf{x})$: By applying g over each $I(\mathbf{x})$, we obtain an entire proximity score map. This is detailed in the next subsection.

2.2 Training and Evaluating a Regression Model

Many options are available for learning function g, and we opted for standard regression Random Forests [18], because they are fast to evaluate, were shown to perform well on many image analysis problems, and are easy to implement.

Instead of directly relying on pixel intensities, we apply the forest on image features extracted from input patches. We use 21 feature channels: RGB channels (3), gradient magnitude (1), first and second order gradients in x- and y-directions (4), Luv channels (3), oriented gradients (9), and histogram equalized gray scale image (1). The split functions in the nodes of the forest include single pixel values, pixel value differences, Haar-like features, and a constrained pixel value difference, where the second patch location for difference computation was chosen within a distance of 10 pixels clamped at the image patch borders. For all the split functions but single pixel values, we randomly select whether to use the values for the same feature channel or across feature channels.

In all experiments, each split was optimized on a random subset of 200 training samples with 1000 random tests and 20 thresholds each. Splitting stops once either maximum tree depth or minimal number of 50 samples per node is reached.

2.3 Detecting the Cells from the Proximity Score Map

Once the forest g is trained, it can predict a proximity score map for unseen images. By construction, the local maximums in this map should correspond to the cell centers. We therefore apply non-maximum suppression, where maximums below a certain threshold κ are discarded. As will be shown, varying κ facilitates optimization of either precision or recall, depending on the task.

3 Experimental Results

We first describe the datasets and protocol used for the evaluation. Then, we provide comparisons of our approach to the current state-of-the-art method of Arteta *et al.* [6], and a standard classification Random Forest based on the same image features as the proposed regression forest.

3.1 Datasets

The ICPR dataset consists of 20 100×100 pixel microscopy images of breast cancer tissue [9] (ICPR). We also introduce a new dataset BM containing eleven $1,200 \times 1,200$ pixel images of healthy human bone marrow from eight different patients[1]. Tissue in both datasets was stained with Hematoxylin and Eosin.

For our BM dataset, all cell nuclei were labeled as *foreground* by providing the location of the center pixel as dot annotation. Debris and staining artifacts were labeled as *background*. Ambiguous parts, for which cell nuclei were not clearly determinable as such, were labeled as *unknown*. Nevertheless, all ambiguous objects are treated as foreground, since the detection method proposed in this work is supposed to identify these objects as candidates for subsequent classification. The resulting 4,205 dot annotations cover *foreground* and *unknown* labels.

3.2 Model Evaluation

To decide if a detection actually corresponds to a cell center, we consider a distance threshold ξ. If the distance between a detection and a ground truth annotation is less or equal ξ, we count the detection as true positive (TP). If more than one detection falls into this area, we assign the most confident one to the ground truth location and consider the others as false positives (FP). Detections farther away than ξ from any ground truth location are FP, and all ground truth annotations without any close detections are false negatives (FN).

Accuracy is evaluated in terms of precision ($= TP/(TP + FP)$), recall ($= TP/(TP + FN)$), F1-score, average Euclidean distance and standard deviation $\mu_d \pm \sigma_d$ between a TP and its correctly assigned ground truth location, as well as the average absolute difference and standard deviation between number of ground truth annotations and detections $\mu_n \pm \sigma_n$. We report results in this section computed with forests composed of 64 trees and a maximum tree depth of 16, an optimal complexity determined in leave-one-out cross validation (LOOCV) on the more complex BM dataset.

[1] The dataset is available from `https://github.com/pkainz/MICCAI2015/`

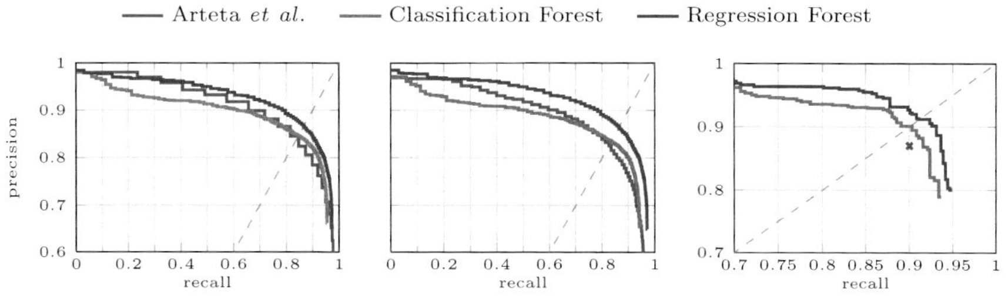

(a) (b) (c)

Fig. 3. Precision-recall curves on the two datasets, obtained by varying the threshold κ on the confidence and recording precision and recall of the resulting detections wrt. the ground truth. (a,b) LOOCV on the *BM dataset*. In (a) the threshold ξ defining the maximum accepted distance between a detection and the ground truth was set to $\xi = 16$, whereas in (b) it was tightened to $\xi = 8$. With the looser bound in (a) the performance of Arteta *et al.* is insignificantly lower than ours (AUC 89.9 vs. 90.7). However, in (b) it drops considerably (AUC 86.9), while for our regression method the curve stays the same (AUC 90.5), demonstrating its capability to localize the cells much more precisely. (c) On the *ICPR benchmark dataset* both classification and regression outperform the current state-of-the-art detector.

Figs. 3(a,b) show precision-recall evaluations on the BM dataset: each curve was obtained in LOOCV by varying κ. Additionally, we assessed the method of Arteta *et al.* [6] in a LOOCV and compared performance measures. Most prominently, the maximum distance threshold between ground truth and detection ξ is responsible for the localization accuracy. In Fig. 3(a), we moderately set $\xi = 16$ and observed that the area under the curve (AUC) is only slightly lower than ours: 89.9 vs. 90.7. As soon as we tighten $\xi = 8$, their AUC measure drops considerably to 86.9, whereas our regression method exhibits the same performance (90.5). This, and the consistent shape of the regression curves strongly indicate our method's superiority over the current state-of-the-art in terms of localization accuracy. Further, by allowing a smaller value of ξ, a more rigorous definition of TP detections is enabled, thus resulting in increased detection confidence. The achieved F1-score on the BM dataset is 84.30 ± 3.28 for Arteta *et al.* [6] vs. 87.17 ± 2.73 for our regression approach.

To assess the stability of our method, which relies on random processes during feature selection, we performed ten independent runs on a predefined, fixed train-test split of the BM dataset. We trained on the first eight and tested on the last three images and achieved a stable F1-score of 88.05 ± 0.06.

Table 1 shows results on the ICPR benchmark dataset [9]. Both our regression approach and the standard classification outperform [6] over all standard metrics, cf. Fig. 3(c). Although [6] state performance values, no value for ξ is mentioned. Given our previous definition, we use a rather strict $\xi = 4$ for both, regression and classification forests. Nevertheless, [6] must have used a value $\xi > 4$ in order to match the numbers reported for $\mu_d \pm \sigma_d$ in Table 1.

Table 1. Performance comparison on the ICPR benchmark dataset [9]. F1-scores for regression and classification were averaged over ten independent iterations and metrics were obtained with $\xi = 4$. Regression outperforms all previously reported competing methods on the standard metrics.

Method	Prec.	Rec.	F1-score	$\mu_d \pm \sigma_d$	$\mu_n \pm \sigma_n$
Regr. Forest	**91.33**	**91.70**	**91.50**	$\mathbf{0.80 \pm 0.68}$	3.26 ± 2.32
Class. Forest	90.66	89.72	90.18	0.86 ± 0.68	4.04 ± 2.26
Arteta *et al.* [6]	86.99	90.03	88.48	1.68 ± 2.55	$\mathbf{2.90 \pm 2.13}$
Bernardis & Yu [3]	-	-	-	2.84 ± 2.89	8.20 ± 4.75
LIPSyM [4]	70.21	70.08	70.14	3.14 ± 0.93	4.30 ± 3.08

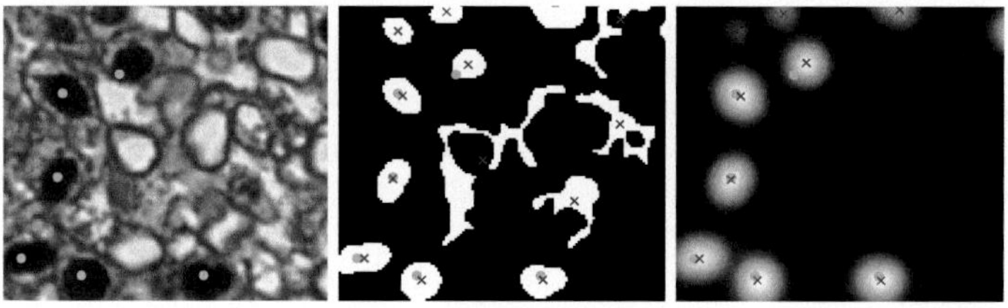

(a) (b) (c)

Fig. 4. Illustration of detection hypotheses on BM data (a): Our regression based detector (c) proposes much more accurate and reliable cell center hypotheses than the detector of Arteta *et al.* [6], shown in (b). Magenta crosses denote proposed cell centers, green dots are ground truth locations. While Arteta *et al.* need a separate classifier to post-process these hypotheses, a simple threshold on the detection confidence is sufficient to achieve the reported improved results for our method.

A qualitative illustration of the detector hypotheses on a BM image is depicted in Fig. 4. The state-of-the-art method [6] proposes many cell center hypotheses in a clear background region, where our regression method did not produce any proximity scores at all. Final localization is determined by post-processing and hence reliable hypotheses are beneficial for high accuracy.

We also compared the computation times on a standard Intel Core i7-4470 3.4GHz workstation. [6], the best performing method after ours, needs 3.6 hours for training on ten images of the BM dataset. Testing on a single BM image lasts around 60 seconds. In contrast, our regression method takes only 1.5 hours of training, and only 15 seconds for testing on $1,200 \times 1,200$ pixel images.

4 Conclusion

We showed that using a simple regression forest to predict a well-chosen function over the input images outperforms state-of-the-art methods for cell detection in histopathological images: Our approach is easy to implement and $4\times$ faster than the method of [6], while being more reliable and accurate.

References

1. Al-Adhadh, A.N., Cavill, I.: Assessment of cellularity in bone marrow fragments. J. Clin. Pathol. 36, 176–179 (1983)
2. Gurcan, M.N., Boucheron, L.E., Can, A., Madabhushi, A., Rajpoot, N.M., Yener, B.: Histopathological image analysis: a review. IEEE Rev. Biomed. Eng. 2, 147–171 (2009)
3. Bernardis, E., Yu, S.X.: Pop out many small structures from a very large microscopic image. Med. Image Anal. 15(5), 690–707 (2011)
4. Kuse, M., Wang, Y.F., Kalasannavar, V., Khan, M., Rajpoot, N.: Local isotropic phase symmetry measure for detection of beta cells and lymphocytes. J. Pathol. Inform. 2(2) (2011)
5. Wienert, S., Heim, D., Saeger, K., Stenzinger, A., Beil, M., Hufnagl, P., Dietel, M., Denkert, C., Klauschen, F.: Detection and Segmentation of Cell Nuclei in Virtual Microscopy Images: A Minimum-Model Approach. Sci. Rep. 2, 1–7 (2012)
6. Arteta, C., Lempitsky, V., Noble, J.A., Zisserman, A.: Learning to Detect Cells Using Non-overlapping Extremal Regions. In: Ayache, N., Delingette, H., Golland, P., Mori, K. (eds.) MICCAI 2012, Part I. LNCS, vol. 7510, pp. 348–356. Springer, Heidelberg (2012)
7. Nosrati, M.S., Hamarneh, G.: Segmentation of cells with partial occlusion and part configuration constraint using evolutionary computation. In: Mori, K., Sakuma, I., Sato, Y., Barillot, C., Navab, N. (eds.) MICCAI 2013, Part I. LNCS, vol. 8149, pp. 461–468. Springer, Heidelberg (2013)
8. Mualla, F., Schöll, S., Sommerfeldt, B., Maier, A., Steidl, S., Buchholz, R., Hornegger, J.: Unsupervised Unstained Cell Detection by SIFT Keypoint Clustering and Self-labeling Algorithm. In: Golland, P., Hata, N., Barillot, C., Hornegger, J., Howe, R. (eds.) MICCAI 2014, Part III. LNCS, vol. 8675, pp. 377–384. Springer, Heidelberg (2014)
9. Gurcan, M.N., Madabhushi, A., Rajpoot, N.: Pattern recognition in histopathological images: An ICPR 2010 contest. In: Ünay, D., Çataltepe, Z., Aksoy, S. (eds.) ICPR 2010. LNCS, vol. 6388, pp. 226–234. Springer, Heidelberg (2010)
10. Matas, J., Chum, O., Urban, M., Pajdla, T.: Robust Wide Baseline Stereo From Maximally Stable Extremal Regions. In: BMVC, pp. 384–393 (2002)
11. Quelhas, P., Marcuzzo, M., Mendonça, A.M., Campilho, A.: Cell nuclei and cytoplasm joint segmentation using the sliding band filter. IEEE Trans. Med. Imaging 29(8), 1463–1473 (2010)
12. Lowe, D.G.: Distinctive Image Features from Scale-Invariant Keypoints. Int. J. Comput. Vis. 60(2), 91–110 (2004)
13. Lempitsky, V., Zisserman, A.: Learning to Count Objects in Images. In: NIPS, pp. 1324–1332 (2010)
14. Fiaschi, L., Nair, R., Koethe, U., Hamprecht, F.: Learning to Count with Regression Forest and Structured Labels. In: ICPR, pp. 2685–2688 (2012)
15. Sironi, A., Lepetit, V., Fua, P.: Multiscale Centerline Detection by Learning a Scale-Space Distance Transform. In: CVPR (2014)
16. Zhou, Z.H., Jiang, Y., Yang, Y.B., Chen, S.F.: Lung cancer cell identification based on artificial neural network ensembles. Artif. Intell. Med. 24, 25–36 (2002)
17. Yin, Z., Bise, R., Chen, M., Kanade, T.: Cell segmentation in microsopy imagery using a bag of local Bayesian classifiers. In: ISBI, pp. 125–128 (2010)
18. Breiman, L.: Random Forests. Mach. Learn. 45, 5–32 (2001)

A Hybrid Approach for Segmentation and Tracking of *Myxococcus Xanthus* Swarms*

Jianxu Chen[1], Shant Mahserejian[2], Mark Alber[2,1], and Danny Z. Chen[1]

[1] Department of Computer Science and Engineering, University of Notre Dame, USA
[2] Department of Appl. and Comput. Math and Stat., University of Notre Dame, USA

Abstract. Segmentation and tracking of moving cells in time-lapse images is an important problem in biomedical image analysis. For *Myxococcus xanthus*, rod-like cells with highly coordinated motion, their segmentation and tracking are challenging because cells may touch tightly and form dense swarms that are difficult to identify accurately. Common methods fall under two frameworks: detection association and model evolution. Each framework has its own advantages and disadvantages. In this paper, we propose a new hybrid framework combining these two frameworks into one and leveraging their complementary advantages. Also, we propose an active contour model based on the Ribbon Snake and Chan-Vese model, which is seamlessly integrated with our hybrid framework. Our approach outperforms the state-of-the-art cell tracking algorithms on identifying completed cell trajectories, and achieves higher segmentation accuracy than some best known cell segmentation algorithms.

1 Introduction

Characterizing the dynamics of cell morphology and cell motility in time-lapse experiments is crucial in various biomedical studies. For example, *Myxococcus xanthus*, a type of Gram-negative bacteria showing distinguished collective motion, was considered a model organism for studying swarming behaviors for decades [2]. Because manual segmentation and tracking are tedious processes with poor reproducibility, there is an increasing need for (semi-)automated methods. In addition, *M. xanthus* poses specific challenges. The obscure boundaries of tightly touching cells, head-to-head touching, and touching in large clusters with high cell density all make cell segmentation difficult (e.g., Fig. 2(a)). The physical distances between cell boundaries may even fall below the imaging resolution. The difficulty in tracking is mainly due to three aspects: the proximity of cell positions; the similarity of nontrivial cell shapes; the diversity of cell behaviors.

Algorithms in the literature for cell segmentation and tracking in time-lapse images can be broadly classified into two categories: detection association (DA) and model evolution (ME). In the DA framework [2,7,8], segmentation is first performed in each image frame, and cell correspondences are built across all

* This work was partly supported by NSF under Grant CCF-1217906 and by NIH under Grants 1R01-GM095959 and 1R01-GM100470.

N. Navab et al. (Eds.): MICCAI 2015, Part III, LNCS 9351, pp. 284–291, 2015.
DOI: 10.1007/978-3-319-24574-4_34

frames of the image sequence into cell trajectories. One advantage of the DA framework is the flexibility in handling various cell behaviors. But, because segmentation is performed separately on each frame, the temporal context is not fully leveraged for segmentation. In some situations, like tightly touching *M. xanthus*, the segmentation may suffer from severe errors for this reason. To some extent, poor segmentation can degrade the tracking accuracy considerably. On the other hand, morphological properties, such as the dynamic changes of cell shapes, cannot be fully extracted from error prone segmentation results.

In the ME framework [3], segmentation and tracking are performed simultaneously by evolving cells in the form of contours from frame to frame, i.e., using the segmentation of one frame to initialize the evolution in the next frame. By propagating information from frame to frame, temporal context is exploited for segmentation and the results could be better than those of the DA framework, especially on images of low quality or when cells have obscure boundaries. But, due to the nature of propagation, such methods may not handle all cell behaviors very well, and may perform poorly when cell displacements are large between consecutive frames. Attempts were made to combine the DA/ME frameworks (e.g., [4]), but such methods can still face troubles when cells are tightly packed.

In this paper, we propose a new hybrid framework for segmenting and tracking cells, which combines the DA and ME frameworks and demonstrates its applicability using *M. xanthus*. In our framework, we first produce a pre-segmentation for each individual frame (the first frame is checked and corrected manually). For each frame K ($K \geq 2$), we develop a *Context Builder* module to work on frames $K-1$ to $K+t$ ($t > 1$ is constant) to build cell correspondence (similar to the DA framework), and confirm cells newly entering frame K and assign trajectory identities to cells with *reliable pre-segmentation* in frame K. Next, we apply a *Cell Tracker* module to perform an active contour evolution to segment and track the remaining cells in frame K (similar to the ME framework). The spatial-temporal context extracted from *Context Builder* is utilized to guide this contour evolution. To handle *M. xanthus* specifically, we propose an open active contour model based on Ribbon Snake [6] and the Chan-Vese model [1].

Our hybrid framework takes advantage of the complimentary strengths of the DA and ME frameworks. Our *Context Builder* extracts and analyzes the temporal context to provide information for *Cell Tracker* to guide cell evolution. The *Cell Tracker* tackles the segmentation and tracking of those cells where pre-segmentation and association fail; it refines the pre-segmentation so that *Context Builder* can build more accurate correspondence for the next frame. Consequently, our method obtains better tracking results than the state-of-the-art cell tracking algorithms, and achieves higher segmentation accuracy than some best known cell segmentation algorithms. Table 1 summarizes our results.

2 Methodology

The main steps of our framework are shown in Fig. 1. On the input image sequence, pre-segmentation is produced for each frame. The segmentation algorithm used can be application-dependent; the one we use for *M. xanthus* is

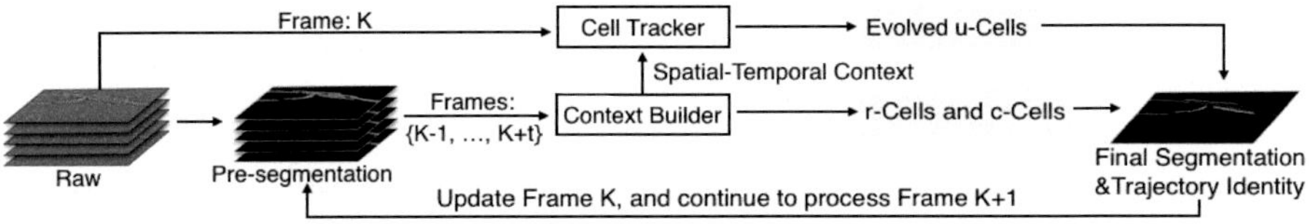

Fig. 1. An outline of our proposed framework: Pre-segmentation is first obtained. For each frame K, *Context Builder* extracts the spatial-temporal context. In frame K, reliable cells (r-Cells) are associated with existing trajectories, and entering/re-appearing cells are confirmed (c-Cells). Cells in frame $K-1$ with uncertain correspondence (u-Cells), together with the spatial-temporal context, are fed to *Cell Tracker* to find their positions in frame K. The c-Cells, r-Cells, and evolved u-Cells are merged to produce the final segmentation and trajectory identity of each cell in frame K.

described in Section 3. The first frame is manually examined and corrected. Note that it is easy to make our method fully automated. Namely, the first appearance of each cell can be confirmed by temporal context (called c-Cells, as discussed in Section 2.1). Manual correction is especially useful in low quality images, so that additional prior knowledge can be exploited to tackle extremely difficult cases.

For each frame $K \geq 2$, our method works in two steps. In step 1, the *Context Builder* employs a matching model based on the Earth Mover's Distance (EMD) [2] on frames $\{K-1, \ldots, K+t\}$, where $t \geq 1$ is a constant indicating the depth of the temporal context (we use $t = 3$). The objectives of *Context Builder* are: (1) detect and confirm the newly entering cells to frame K; (2) confirm cells in frame K that have good pre-segmentation and associate them with some existing trajectories; (3) prepare the spatial-temporal context information for *uncertain cells* (called u-Cells). Intuitively, u-Cells are cells in frame $K-1$ whose corresponding cells in frame K are hard to segment or associate with. In step 2, the *Cell Tracker* segments and tracks u-Cells by active contours controlled by three external forces: the image force, shape-prior force, and repelling force. For *M. xanthus* specifically, we propose an open active contour model based on Ribbon Snake [6] and the Chan-Vese model [1]. At the end, the final segmentation of frame K is obtained; each segmented cell in frame K either is associated with an existing trajectory or starts a new trajectory. Note that *M. xanthus* cannot merge. Yet, our framework is easy to adjust for cell fusion in other problems, by allowing some contours to merge in Cell Tracker.

2.1 Context Builder

Our *Context Builder* module works on consecutive frames $K-1$ to $K+t$ to build the temporal context by performing a hierarchical matching based on the Earth Mover's Distance (EMD) matching model [2]. The major advantages of the EMD matching model are the capability of handling cells moving in/out frames and cell divisions, and the robustness to various segmentation errors [2]. Suppose frame $K \geq 2$ is being processed and trajectories have been constructed in frames 1 to $K-1$. The matching model is applied to establish cell correspondence in frames $K-1$ to $K+t$. Frame $K-1$ is included in order to associate cells in frame K with some existing trajectories. By analyzing the cell correspondence in the temporal context, three types of objects will be extracted: confirmed cells (c-Cell), reliable cells (r-Cells), and uncertain cells (u-Cell).

C-Cells are cells in frame K that have no correspondence in frame $K-1$ but have corresponding cells with consistent shapes in frames $K+1,\ldots,K+t$. Confirmed by the temporal context, c-Cells could be entering cells with high likelihood of not being false alarm. So, manual correction is not needed for entering cells. A cell P in frame K is an r-Cell if P has a one-to-one correspondence in frame $K-1$ with consistent body shape. The pre-segmentation of P can be finalized, due to the reliable correspondence and the high shape similarity. U-Cells are cells in frame $K-1$ with no correspondence in frame K or whose corresponding cells in frame K are not r-Cells. Intuitively, u-Cells are cells at the ends of some existing trajectories, whose correspondence in frame K cannot be confidently determined. If a u-Cell is touching the image border and has no correspondence in succeeding frames, its trajectory will be terminated (i.e., considered as leaving cells). The remaining u-Cells are propagated to frame K and fed to *Cell Tracker*. The final segmentation of frame K contains all successfully evolved u-Cells, all r-Cells, and c-Cells not overlapping with any evolved contours.

The *Context Builder* also prepares the spatial-temporal context for the *Cell Tracker*. It forms a *Barrier Map* for all r-Cells, which will be used to define the repelling force in *Cell Tracker* (see Section 2.2). Moreover, it uses a *Contour Initializer* that acts on all propagated u-Cells to initialize their evolution for *Cell Tracker*. For a u-Cell Q, an initial contour in frame K is obtained by Earth Mover's Morphing (EMM) [5]. If Q has at least one corresponding cell in frame K, then EMM is applied to Q and all its corresponding cells in frame K. If Q has no corresponding cell in frame K, but at least one corresponding cell in frames $K+1$ to $K+t$, then EMM is applied to Q and the corresponding cell with the highest reliability (computed by the EMD matching model). Then, the position of Q in frame K can be extracted from the morphing result. Note that multiple u-Cells sharing common corresponding cells will be analyzed together to ensure consistent results. If no cell is associated with Q and Q is away from the image border, then Q is directly copied to frame K as the initial contour.

2.2 Cell Tracker

The *Cell Tracker* module employs an open active contour model to segment and track cells simultaneously. The initial positions of the contours are obtained from u-Cells by *Contour Initializer*. The evolution of each contour ϕ is governed by the following equation (we use $\omega_1=\omega_2=\omega_4=1$ and $\omega_3=0.25$):

$$\frac{\partial\phi}{\partial t}=\mathbf{F}\|\nabla\phi\|,\text{ where }\mathbf{F}=\omega_1\mathbf{F}_{image}+\omega_2\mathbf{F}_{internal}+\omega_3\mathbf{F}_{repel}+\omega_4\mathbf{F}_{shape}\quad(1)$$

For *M. xanthus*, the contours are represented by Ribbon Snake [6]. Each cell contour has the parametric form $\phi(s)=(x(s),y(s),w)$, where $(x(s),y(s))$ is a

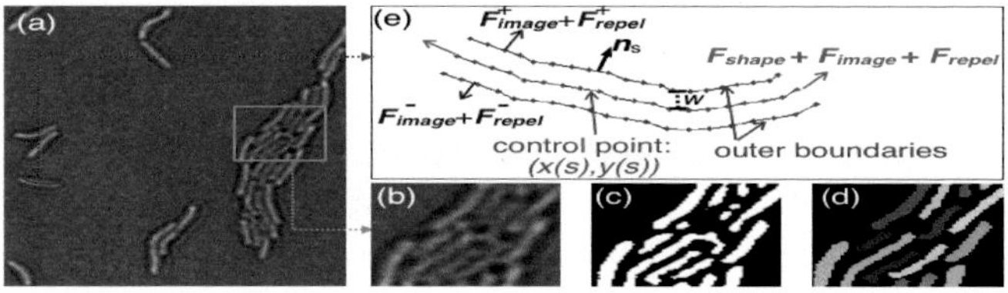

Fig. 2. (a) An input image of *M. xanthus* cells; (b) zoom-in of a clustered region; (c) segmentation of [9]; (d) segmentation of our method; (e) illustrating Ribbon Snake.

parametric curve, called the *centerline*, and w is the half width of the contour, which is computed from its segmentation result in the preceding frame. The concept is illustrated in Fig. 2(e). For each control point $(x(s), y(s))$, the image force (resp., repelling force) is the sum of the image forces (resp., repelling forces) exerted on the two outer boundaries of the contour in the normal direction. Namely, $\mathbf{F}_{image} = \mathbf{F}^{+}_{image} + \mathbf{F}^{-}_{image}$, and $\mathbf{F}_{repel} = \mathbf{F}^{+}_{repel} + \mathbf{F}^{-}_{repel}$. Here, $\mathbf{F}^{+}_{*}$ (resp., $\mathbf{F}^{-}_{*}$) is the force applied to $(x(s), y(s)) + w\mathbf{n}_s$ (resp., $(x(s), y(s)) - w\mathbf{n}_s$), where $\mathbf{n}_s$ is the unit normal vector at $(x(s), y(s))$. Additionally, for the two endpoints of the centerline, extra forces are applied in the tangential direction, including $\mathbf{F}_{shape}$, $\mathbf{F}_{image}$, and $\mathbf{F}_{repel}$. For clarification, at the two tips, the tangential component of $\mathbf{F}_{image}$ and $\mathbf{F}_{repel}$ is computed at the endpoints of the centerline, while the normal component is calculated based on the forces at the corresponding points on the outer boundaries. Finally, $\mathbf{F}_{internal}$ acts on all control points to regulate the contour smoothness, with the classic form $\mathbf{F}_{internal} = \alpha\phi'' - \beta\phi''''$, where α and β are weighting parameters (we use $\alpha = 0.4$, $\beta = 0.2$). Below, we explain the calculation of $\mathbf{F}^{+}_{image}$, $\mathbf{F}^{+}_{repel}$, and $\mathbf{F}_{shape}$. The others can be obtained similarly.

The image force is computed using the Chan-Vese model [1]. Specifically, $\mathbf{F}^{+}_{image} = -((I^{+} - \mu_1)^2 - (I^{+} - \mu_2)^2)\mathbf{n}_s$, where I^{+} is the intensity at $(x(s), y(s)) + w\mathbf{n}_s$, μ_1 is the average intensity inside the cell region enclosed by the outer boundaries, μ_2 is the average intensity outside all cell regions.

A contour will suffer from the repelling force defined by the *Barrier Map* or when it moves close to other contours. Basically, the *Barrier Map* determines the magnitude of the repelling force from r-Cells to any point in the image region. Suppose $\{\phi_1, \phi_2, \ldots, \phi_n\}$ are all evolving contours. For a point on the outer boundary of ϕ_i, say $(x(s), y(s)) + w\mathbf{n}_s$, $\mathbf{F}^{+}_{repel}(s) = -[F^{+}_{bm}(s) + \sum_{j \neq i} F^{+}_{ij}(s)]\mathbf{n}_s$. The force from *Barrier Map* is $F^{+}_{bm}(s) = 1/[1 + exp(2d^{+}(s) - d_{max})]$, if $0 < d^{+}(s) \leq d_{max}$; $F^{+}_{bm}(s) = \infty$, if $d^{+}(s) = 0$; otherwise, $F^{+}_{bm}(s) = 0$. Here, $d^{+}(s)$ is the shortest distance from $(x(s), y(s)) + w\mathbf{n}_s$ to any points on the skeletons of r-Cells, and d_{max} is a constant cut-off value of the furthest distance that the repelling force will act on. As a rule of thumb, d_{max} can be set as the maximum cell thickness. Moreover, the force from contour ϕ_j $(j \neq i)$ is $F^{+}_{ij}(s) = 1/[1 + exp(2d^{+}_{j}(s) - d_{max})]$, if $0 < d^{+}_{j}(s) \leq d_{max}$; $F^{+}_{ij}(s) = \infty$, if $d^{+}_{j}(s) = 0$; otherwise, $F^{+}_{ij}(s) = 0$. Here, $d^{+}_{j}(s)$ is the distance from $(x(s), y(s)) + w\mathbf{n}_s$ to ϕ_j, and d_{max} is the same as above.

Between consecutive frames, the shape of each cell should be consistent. In terms of *M. xanthus*, certain lengths can be expected (except for cell divisions).

Inspired by [3], we take such information as the shape prior and impose into the evolution. Specifically, the initial contours are shortened by 40% in order to reduce the possibility of part of an initial contour residing outside the cell body. Then, $\mathbf{F}_{shape}$ is imposed on the two tips of the contour in the tangential direction outwards to make the cell growing into the expected length. Suppose the length of a particular cell P in frame $K-1$ is L^{K-1}. Then the target length of P in frame K, denoted by L_T^K, is set as L^{K-1}. The magnitude of $\mathbf{F}_{shape}$ is defined as $V_{shape}^{(i)} = \gamma^{(i)} * ds$, where $i \in \{1,2\}$ is the index of the two tips. Suppose the current length of the contour is L. $ds = 1$ if $L < 0.85L_T^K$; $ds = 0.5$ if $0.85L_T^K \leq L < 0.95L_T^K$; $ds = 0$ if $0.95L_T^K \leq L < 1.2L_T^K$; $ds = -1$ if $L \geq 1.2L_T^K$. The value of γ depends on the image force and repelling force. Suppose v_1 and v_2 are the magnitudes of the tangential component of $\mathbf{F}_{image} + \mathbf{F}_{repel}$ at the two tips, respectively. If $v_1 \geq 0$ and $v_2 \geq 0$, then $\gamma^{(1)} = \gamma^{(2)} = 1$. If $v_1 < 0$ and $v_2 \geq 0$, then $\gamma^{(1)} = 0$, $\gamma^{(2)} = 1$ (similar for $v_1 \geq 0$, $v_2 < 0$). If v_1 and v_2 are both negative, suppose $v_1 > v_2$, then $\gamma^{(1)} = 2$, $\gamma^{(2)} = 0$. In general, $v_i > 0$ indicates expansion, and $v_i < 0$ means the contour will be compressed on that tip. Thus, when not both v_i's are positive, the shape force will only be exerted on the tip that will not be compressed; when v_i's are both negative, the shape force will only act on the tip suffering less compression. Finally, $\mathbf{F}_{shape}^{(i)} = V_{shape}^{i}\mathbf{t}_i$, where $\mathbf{t}_i$ is the outward tangential vector at the centerline endpoints.

There are two special cases for $\mathbf{F}_{shape}$ exerted on P. (I) If P touches the image border, $\mathbf{F}_{shape}$ is voided. In this situation, the length restriction may make contours leak to the background (when part of a cell moves out of the image region), or may make a contour not grow to the actual length (when the cell is gradually moving into the image region). (II) If the length of P after the evolution in frame K is shorter than $0.9 * L_T$, and P needs to evolve again in frame $K+1$, then the target length in frame $K+1$, i.e., L_T^{K+1}, will be set as L_T^K, not L^K. In this situation, if we always take the actual length in the preceding frame as the target length, a cell may keep shrinking frame by frame.

Finally, *Cell Tracker* checks for potential cell divisions, since *M. xanthus* may split in the middle of a cell body. After the evolution of each contour, the intensity of the centerline in the grayscale image is extracted. A local regression with the second degree polynomial is performed to smooth the values. If the minimum is located near the middle of the centerline, and the ratio of the maximum to the minimum is larger than a threshold defined experimentally, the contour will be split in the middle. The contours of the daughter cells will evolve again to find the optimal positions. Meanwhile, the cell lineage can be established. There are many advanced division detection methods in the literature, such as the training-based approach in [8]. Our trial studies showed that our division checking is effective for our problem, thus adopted for the sake of simplicity.

3 Experiments and Evaluations

We conducted experiments on seven image sequences of *M. xanthus* obtained in our lab. In general, they were all acquired by a digital camera attached to a

Table 1. Tracking and segmentation results on medium (M), low (L), high (H1-H4) quality data, and special (S) data with large cell displacements in consecutive frames.

Datasets			Tracking Results					Segmentation Accuracy			
	Traj. #	Frame #	Our	[3]	[2]	[7]	[8]	Our	Otsu	[9]	[10]
M	79	71	**70**	18	64	46	61	**0.96**	0.82	0.69	0.61
L	50	69	**41**	21	31	19	19	**0.91**	0.61	0.78	0.64
S	74	47	**67**	5	59	32	21	**0.95**	0.75	0.82	0.78
H1	168	356	**148**	57	119	79	88	**0.95**	0.77	0.92	0.87
H2	104	60	**102**	80	99	78	80	**0.95**	0.73	0.93	0.88
H3	113	100	**110**	76	98	88	92	**0.97**	0.73	0.91	0.89
H4	112	90	**106**	75	96	87	80	**0.94**	0.76	0.89	0.91

microscope with 60x oil-immersion objectives. The high quality dataset (H1-H4) were acquired with a faster camera. The metric for the tracking performance is the number of *completed trajectories*. This is a harsh metric because merely a few error correspondences in tracking may result in huge loss in completed trajectories. All results were examined visually by human experts. Our method is compared against four state-of-the-art algorithms [3,2,8,7]. [3] is a representative method under the model evolution framework. The other three are different detection association approaches. [2] is a hierarchical scheme based on the EMD matching model. [8] conducts global optimization across the whole image sequence. [7] performs frame-wise optimal matching. The pre-segmentation of our method was obtained in two steps: (i) A pixel-wise classification is performed using [9]; (ii) the detected regions were cut at the intersection points of the region centerlines or at each centerline point whose curvature is larger than an experimentally determined threshold. For fair comparison, the same pre-segmentation was used for our method and for [2] and [7]. The segmentation of [8] was also obtained by [9], but an object count classifier [8] was applied instead of explicitly cutting the regions. Note that no human intervention was made in our method except manually correcting the segmentation in the first frame. However, the model evolution method [3] may need other human interventions as discussed in [3]. All results are shown in Table 1. In dataset S, the same cell in two consecutive frames may overlap less than 50%, which showed that our method is more effective than the model evolution method [3] in dealing with large cell displacements. Also, the results showed that our method has better performance than the three detection association approaches, even in low quality images (L).

Further, we compared the segmentation results with three segmentation methods to show the advantages of our hybrid framework on segmentation, especially the benefits of leveraging temporal context in segmentation. First, the Otsu thresholding is used as the baseline method. Second, ilastik [9] is one of the best open source software for cell segmentation based on pixel classification. Finally, the method in [10] is one of the most effective cell segmentation algorithms based on correlation clustering. Except ours, the other methods are all performed on individual image frames. We manually segmented 20 frames randomly selected in each dataset as the ground truth. Suppose there are N true cells in the manual segmentation, denoted by $\{G_1, G_2, \ldots, G_N\}$, and there are M segmented cells, denoted by $\{O_1, O_2, \ldots, O_M\}$. A segmented cell O_k is a true positive (TP), if $\exists i$ s.t. $\|G_i \cap O_k\| > 0.5 * \|G_i\|$ and $\|G_i \cap O_k\| > 0.5\|O_k\|$. Then, the precision is $Pr = TP/M$, and the recall is $Re = TP/N$. Finally, the segmentation accuracy is measured by F1-score, i.e., $F = 2 * Pr * Re/(Pr + Re)$. An example of segmentation in the low quality dataset (L) is shown in Fig. 2(b)-(d). The results in Table 1 showed our hybrid framework achieves much higher segmentation accuracy than the other methods without utilizing temporal context.

4 Conclusions

In this paper, we propose a new hybrid framework for segmentation and tracking of moving cells in time-lapse images. In addition, a new active contour model is proposed for *M. xanthus*, and is seamlessly integrated with our hybrid framework. The evaluation shows that the proposed method outperforms state-of-the-art cell tracking algorithms and some best known cell segmentation algorithms.

References

1. Chan, T.F., Vese, L.A.: Active contours without edges. IEEE Trans. Image Processing 10(2), 266–277 (2001)
2. Chen, J., Harvey, C.W., Alber, M.S., Chen, D.Z.: A matching model based on earth mover's distance for tracking *myxococcus xanthus*. In: Golland, P., Hata, N., Barillot, C., Hornegger, J., Howe, R. (eds.) MICCAI 2014, Part II. LNCS, vol. 8674, pp. 113–120. Springer, Heidelberg (2014)
3. Deng, Y., Coen, P., Sun, M., Shaevitz, J.W.: Efficient multiple object tracking using mutually repulsive active membranes. PloS One 8(6), e65769 (2013)
4. Li, K., Miller, E.D., Chen, M., Kanade, T., Weiss, L.E., Campbell, P.G.: Cell population tracking and lineage construction with spatiotemporal context. Medical Image Analysis 12(5), 546–566 (2008)
5. Makihara, Y., Yagi, Y.: Earth mover's morphing: Topology-free shape morphing using cluster-based EMD flows. In: Kimmel, R., Klette, R., Sugimoto, A. (eds.) ACCV 2010, Part IV. LNCS, vol. 6495, pp. 202–215. Springer, Heidelberg (2011)
6. Mayer, H., Laptev, I., Baumgartner, A.: Multi-scale and snakes for automatic road extraction. In: Burkhardt, H.-J., Neumann, B. (eds.) ECCV 1998. LNCS, vol. 1406, pp. 720–733. Springer, Heidelberg (1998)
7. Padfield, D., Rittscher, J., Roysam, B.: Coupled minimum-cost flow cell tracking for high-throughput quantitative analysis. Med. Image Anal. 15(4), 650–668 (2011)
8. Schiegg, M., Hanslovsky, P., Kausler, B.X., Hufnagel, L., Hamprecht, F.A.: Conservation tracking. In: ICCV, pp. 2928–2935 (2013)
9. Sommer, C., Straehle, C., Kothe, U., Hamprecht, F.A.: ilastik: Interactive learning and segmentation toolkit. In: ISBI, pp. 230–233 (2011)
10. Zhang, C., Yarkony, J., Hamprecht, F.A.: Cell detection and segmentation using correlation clustering. In: Golland, P., Hata, N., Barillot, C., Hornegger, J., Howe, R. (eds.) MICCAI 2014, Part I. LNCS, vol. 8673, pp. 9–16. Springer, Heidelberg (2014)

Fast Background Removal in 3D Fluorescence Microscopy Images Using One-Class Learning*

Lin Yang[1,**], Yizhe Zhang[1], Ian H. Guldner[2], Siyuan Zhang[2], and Danny Z. Chen[1]

[1] Department of Computer Science and Engineering, University of Notre Dame, Notre Dame, IN 46556, USA
[2] Department of Biological Sciences, Harper Cancer Research Institute, University of Notre Dame, Notre Dame, IN 46556, USA
lyang5@nd.edu

Abstract. With the recent advances of optical tissue clearing technology, current imaging modalities are able to image large tissue samples in 3D with single-cell resolution. However, the severe background noise remains a significant obstacle to the extraction of quantitative information from these high-resolution 3D images. Additionally, due to the potentially large sizes of 3D image data (over 10^{11} voxels), the processing speed is becoming a major bottleneck that limits the applicability of many known background correction methods. In this paper, we present a fast background removal algorithm for large volume 3D fluorescence microscopy images. By incorporating unsupervised one-class learning into the percentile filtering approach, our algorithm is able to precisely and efficiently remove background noise even when the sizes and appearances of foreground objects vary greatly. Extensive experiments on real 3D datasets show our method has superior performance and efficiency comparing with the current state-of-the-art background correction method and the rolling ball algorithm in ImageJ.

1 Introduction

With the recent advances of optical tissue clearing technology, current imaging modalities are able to image large tissue samples (e.g., the whole mouse brain) in 3D with single-cell resolution [10]. This creates new opportunities for biomedical research, ranging from studying how the brain works to developing new medicines for cancer. But, it also brings new challenges to extract information from such large volume 3D images. Due to large imaging depth and tissue auto-fluorescence, background noise in such 3D images is often strong and highly inhomogeneous [1], not only preventing effective 3D visualization (Fig. 1(a) and 1(d)) but also causing difficulties to many image processing tasks, such as segmentation (Fig. 1(c) and 1(f)), registration, and tracking. In this paper, we present a fast background removal algorithm that is capable of precisely identifying and removing background noise in such large volume 3D images.

* Source code is available at `https://github.com/linyang519522` or upon request.
** Corresponding author.

N. Navab et al. (Eds.): MICCAI 2015, Part III, LNCS 9351, pp. 292–299, 2015.
DOI: 10.1007/978-3-319-24574-4_35

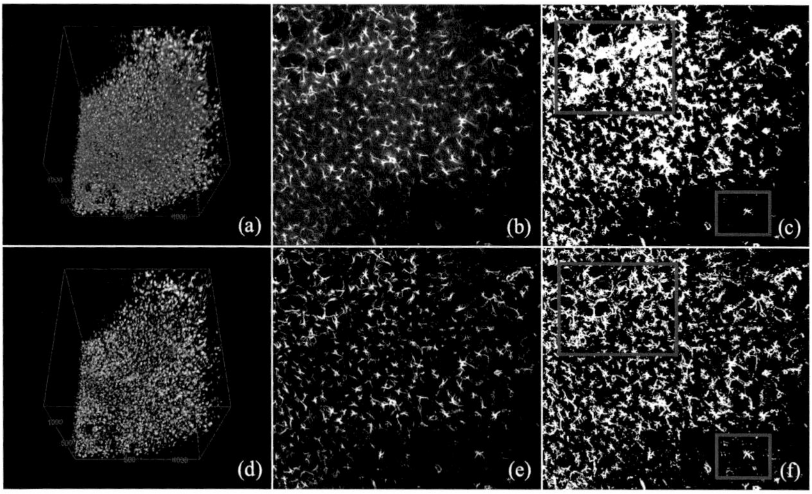

Fig. 1. (a) and (d): 3D visualization results before and after background removal by our algorithm; (b) and (e): selected 2D slices inside the sample 3D image before and after background removal; (c) and (f): segmentation results of (b) and (e) based on thresholding (more accurate segmentation is achieved in both high intensity (upper-left window) and low intensity (bottom-right window) areas after background removal).

Many methods are known for removing undesired background noise in microscopy images, such as spatial filtering [4], rolling ball algorithms [2], fitting smoothly varying function [6], entropy minimization [5], and matrix rank minimization [8]. However, due to the rapidly increasing sizes of image data, the time and space complexities of some sophisticated methods (e.g., optimization based methods and function fitting methods) are too high. With whole-body imaging at single-cell resolution [9], image sizes will continue to grow. Large 3D imaging fields yield not only large data sizes but also wide variations in the sizes of foreground objects. Although simple methods like spatial filtering and rolling ball algorithms are quite fast, significant variance of foreground objects can greatly affect their performance. For example, in some parts of our brain tumor images, cells are uniformly distributed, for which small window/ball sizes give the best performance; in other parts, tumor cells are clustered closely together and form much larger target objects, for which small window/ball sizes may include tumor cell clusters as part of the background (to be removed). We call those "small" windows that cause removal of foreground objects the *undersized windows*.

Taking advantage of the efficiency of spatial filtering methods, we develop a new spatial filtering algorithm for background removal, which is capable to overcome the "undersized window" issue. Two possible approaches may be considered for the window size issue: (1) intelligently choosing the window sizes at different parts of the images (e.g., a small window size for single cells, a big window size for large clusters); (2) first using a fixed small window size, then identifying "undersized windows", and recomputing their background accordingly. The first approach requires certain effective foreground object detection, which may not be efficient and accurate. In [6], a method in the second approach was given, which identified "undersized windows" by automatic thresholding with a kernel density estimator. However, it still fails when foreground objects are too big [6], possibly caused by a significant amount of "undersized windows". By utilizing the recently developed unsupervised one-class learning model [7], we tackle this critical window size issue even when foreground objects are $\sim$ 100 times larger than the pre-selected window size. Extensive experiments on real 3D datasets show our method has better accuracy and is $\sim$ 160 times faster than the current state-of-the-art background correction method [8]. Also, it has much better accuracy yet is only $\sim$ 1 time slower than the prevailing rolling ball algorithm in ImageJ [2]. Tables 1 and 2 show detailed comparison results.

2 Method

Our method includes three main steps: (1) estimate background noise using a fixed small window size; (2) detect "undersized windows" occurred in Step (1); (3) recompute background noise in the detected "undersized windows".

2.1 Estimating Background Noise

Common background/shading correction methods use additive models or multiplicative models to handle noise [6,8]. In our images, because multiplicative noise is significantly smaller than additive noise, we utilize an additive model $I(x,y,z) = F(x,y,z) + B(x,y,z)$, where $I(x,y,z)$ denotes the observed signal, $F(x,y,z)$ denotes the foreground signal, and $B(x,y,z)$ denotes the background noise at a voxel (x,y,z).

Our method first uses a fixed small window size w to estimate background noise in the image. Although this window size may result in a large number of "undersized windows", we will deal with them using the algorithm in Section 2.2. Because the background noise varies slowly, meaning it has low frequency in the Fourier domain, we only need to estimate the background noise for a subset of all voxels (which we call *sampled voxels*). By the Nyquist-Shannon sampling theorem, as long as our sampling frequency is more than twice as high as the frequency of the background noise, we can recover the true background noise at every voxel. Thus, we use a point grid to choose the sampled voxels. Then, centered at each sampled voxel (x_s, y_s, z_s), a $w \times w \times w$ window $W(x_s, y_s, z_s)$ is defined and p percentile of the intensities of all voxels inside $W(x_s, y_s, z_s)$ is used to estimate the background noise $B(x_s, y_s, z_s)$. In order to maximize the efficiency and quality, the interval of sampled points is chosen to be equal to the window size so that there is neither gap nor overlap between neighboring windows (Fig. 2(a)). Because the intensity of each voxel is in a small set of integers (e.g., $[0, \ldots, 255]$), this step can be computed efficiently in linear time. Since a smaller w will yield a larger sampled set and better estimation of the background (when it is not an "undersized window"), we tend to use a very small w, say 3 or 5.

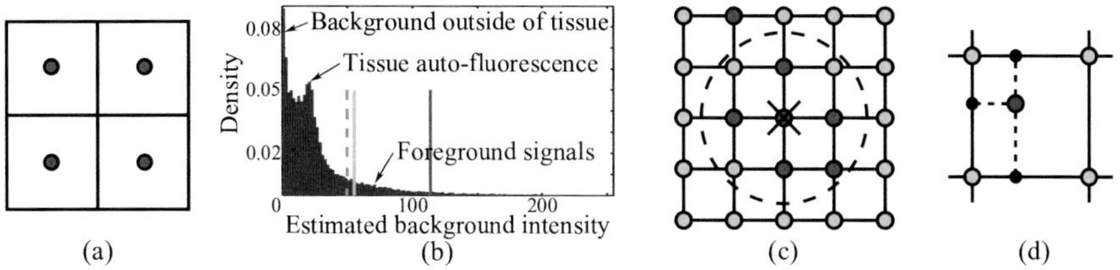

Fig. 2. (a) Each red point is a sampled voxel and the cubic window around it is used to estimate its background intensity; (b) an example histogram of estimated background noise (the green line is the threshold selected by our method, the red line is the threshold selected by median + 3 × std, and the orange dashed line is the manually selected threshold); (c) red points denote the detected "undersized windows", and green points denote the correctly estimated windows (we re-estimate the background noise of the point marked by X); (d) the blue point is a voxel amid sampled voxels, whose value is computed by linear interpolation based on its neighboring sampled voxels.

2.2 Detecting Undersized Windows

In this section, we formulate "undersized window" detection as a one-class learning problem [7], and show how to utilize the properties of our specific problem to make our one-class learning solution more accurate and efficient than in [7].

A key task to our method is to precisely detect "undersized windows". Specifically, given sampled windows $W(x_s, y_s, z_s)$, $s \in \{1, \ldots, n\}$, find all "undersized windows" $W(x_u, y_u, z_u)$ among them. A straightforward way is to use some simple histogram thresholding schemes to determine a threshold on $B(x_s, y_s, z_s)$ (e.g., using the median and standard deviation, finding the local maxima in the second derivative and the kernel density estimator [6]). However, the distribution of $B(x_s, y_s, z_s)$ could be quite complex and greatly affect the performance of such methods (Fig. 2(b)). Thus, we need to develop a more robust approach to detect these "undersized windows". Because background noise (although quite inhomogeneous to affect image processing tasks) is more homogeneous than foreground signals, correctly estimated $B(x_s, y_s, z_s)$'s are much closer to one another while $B(x_u, y_u, z_u)$'s (which are actually foreground signals) have larger variance. This property allows us to treat $B(x_u, y_u, z_u)$'s as outliers among $B(x_s, y_s, z_s)$'s. Thus, we reformulate our problem as follows: Given an unlabeled dataset $\mathcal{X} = \{x'_i = B(x_i, y_i, z_i)\}_{i=1}^n$, find a classification function $f : \mathbb{R} \to \mathbb{R}$ that is able to determine the outliers in $\mathcal{X}$. Our solution for this problem is based on the state-of-the-art unsupervised one-class learning model [7].

We first briefly review the method in [7]. Its basic idea is to use a self-guided labeling procedure to identify suspicious outliers and then train a large margin one-class classifier to separate such outliers from reliable positive samples. This procedure is achieved by minimizing the following objective function: $\min_{f \in \mathcal{H}, \{y_i\}} \sum_{i=1}^n (f(\boldsymbol{x}'_i) - y_i)^2 + \gamma_1 ||f||^2_{\mathcal{M}} - \frac{2\gamma_2}{n^+} \sum_{i, y_i > 0} f(\boldsymbol{x}'_i)$ such that $y_i \in \{c^+, c^-\}, \forall i \in [1, \ldots, n]$ and $0 < n^+ = |\{i \mid y_i > 0\}| < n$. Here, $f(\boldsymbol{x}') = \sum_{i=1}^n \kappa(\boldsymbol{x}', \boldsymbol{x}'_i)\alpha_i$ is the target classification function, where α_i is the expansion coefficient of the functional base $\kappa(\cdot, \boldsymbol{x}'_i)$. In our case, we use an RBF kernel with bandwidth $\sigma^2 = \sum_{i,j} ||\boldsymbol{x}'_i - \boldsymbol{x}'_j||^2/n^2$. y_i is the soft label assignment for each input data $\boldsymbol{x}'_i$, by choosing $(c^+, c^-) = (\sqrt{\frac{n-n^+}{n^+}}, -\sqrt{\frac{n^+}{n-n^+}})$, the model treats the positive samples and outliers in a more balanced way. The first term regularizes the target classification function to make it consistent with the label assignment. The second term $||f||^2_{\mathcal{M}}$ is the manifold regularizer that regularizes the smoothness of the intrinsic manifold structure $\mathcal{M}$. It is constructed by a neighborhood graph with affinity matrix $\mathbf{W}$. $\mathbf{W}$ is defined as follows:

$$W_{ij} = \begin{cases} \exp(-\frac{||\boldsymbol{x}'_i - \boldsymbol{x}'_j||^2}{\varepsilon^2}), & i \in \mathcal{N}_j \text{ or } j \in \mathcal{N}_i \\ 0, & \text{otherwise} \end{cases} \tag{1}$$

ε is the bandwidth parameter, and $\mathcal{N}_i$ is the set of indices of $\boldsymbol{x}'_i$'s k nearest neighbors in $\mathcal{X}$. We have $||f||^2_{\mathcal{M}} = \frac{1}{2}\sum_{i,j=1}^{n}(f(\boldsymbol{x}'_i) - f(\boldsymbol{x}'_j))^2 W_{ij}$. The last term maximizes the average margin of judged positive samples. Finally, $\gamma_1, \gamma_2 > 0$ are trade-off parameters that control the relative importance between these parts.

The above minimization problem involves a continuous function f and discrete variables $\{y_i\}$, which is very difficult to optimize. In [7], an alternative optimization algorithm was given, but it cannot guarantee finding a global minimum. Interestingly, for our specific problem, we are able to find a global minimum in a highly effective way. Note that in our setting, the data lie in a small 1D discrete space ($x'_i \in [0, \ldots, 255]$), and we seek a cut between these data points. Since there are at most 257 ways to cut our data (i.e., $C \in \{-0.5, 0.5, 1.5, \ldots, 255.5\}$), we can simply compute the optimal objective function value for each one of them and find the best cut $C_{optimal}$ that minimizes the objective function. After some transformations (see more details in [7]), the original minimization problem for any given cut point C can be put into the following matrix form:

$$\begin{aligned} &\min_{\boldsymbol{\alpha}} \; \boldsymbol{\alpha}^\top \mathbf{K}(\mathbf{I} + \gamma_1(\mathbf{D} - \mathbf{W}))\mathbf{K}\boldsymbol{\alpha} - 2\boldsymbol{\alpha}^\top \mathbf{K}\tilde{\boldsymbol{y}} \\ &s.t. \; ||\boldsymbol{\alpha}|| = 1, 0 < n^+ = |\{i \mid x'_i \leq C\}| < n \\ &\quad y_i = c^+ + \gamma_2/n^+, \forall i \in \{i \mid x'_i \leq C\}, \; y_j = c^-, \forall j \in \{j \mid x'_j > C\} \end{aligned} \tag{2}$$

where $\boldsymbol{\alpha} = [\alpha_1, \ldots, \alpha_n]^\top \in \mathbb{R}^n$, $\tilde{\boldsymbol{y}} = [y_1, \ldots, y_n]^\top$, and the kernel matrix $\mathbf{K} = [\kappa(\boldsymbol{x}'_i, \boldsymbol{x}'_j)]_{1 \leq i,j \leq n} \in \mathbb{R}^{n \times n}$. $\mathbf{D}$ is a diagonal matrix with $D_{ii} = \sum_{j=1}^{n} W_{ij}$. To take care of the constraint $0 < n^+ < n$, we add to $\mathcal{X}$ two artificial data points with values -1 and 256. Problem (2) was well studied [7], and its minimum is achieved when $\boldsymbol{\alpha} = (\mathbf{K}(\mathbf{I} + \gamma_1(\mathbf{D} - \mathbf{W}))\mathbf{K} - \lambda^* \mathbf{I})^{-1}\mathbf{K}\tilde{\boldsymbol{y}}$, where λ^* is the smallest real-valued eigenvalue of the matrix $\begin{bmatrix} \mathbf{K}(\mathbf{I} + \gamma_1(\mathbf{D} - \mathbf{W}))\mathbf{K} & -\mathbf{I} \\ -(\mathbf{K}\tilde{\boldsymbol{y}})(\mathbf{K}\tilde{\boldsymbol{y}})^\top & \mathbf{K}(\mathbf{I} + \gamma_1(\mathbf{D} - \mathbf{W}))\mathbf{K} \end{bmatrix}$.

For each cut point C, its optimal objective function value is computed using that $\boldsymbol{\alpha}$. We can then easily find $C_{optimal}$, which attains the minimum objective function value among all C's. After find $C_{optimal}$, again since $x'_i \in [0, \ldots, 255]$, we need not actually compute $f(x')$ to determine whether x' is an outlier. We only need to compare its value against $C_{optimal}$. Thus, $W(x_s, y_s, z_s)$ is classified as "undersized window" if $B(x_s, y_s, z_s) > C_{optimal}$.

Finally, we utilize a sampling strategy to make this procedure more efficient. In each 3D image, m windows are randomly sampled from all $W(x_s, y_s, z_s)$'s to calculate $\hat{C}_{optimal}$. For each class of images which are stained by the same fluorescence dye, bootstrap is used to choose a sufficiently large m [3]. More specifically, the standard error of $\hat{C}_{optimal}$, which can be computed by bootstrap, is used to decide whether m is sufficient. Initially, we set $m = 1000$, and gradually increase m until the standard error of $\hat{C}_{optimal}$ is small enough.

2.3 Recomputing Background Noise in "Undersized Windows"

After detecting all "undersized windows", we re-estimate their values based on the mean of their surrounding correctly estimated windows. Specifically, the surrounding is defined by whether the distance between the centers of the "undersized window" and the correctly estimated window is smaller than r. Initially, $r = 1$; then we gradually increase r until there are surrounding correctly estimated windows (Fig. 2(c)); finally, the background noise for each voxel is computed by linear interpolation based on the neighboring sampled voxels (Fig. 2(d)), and the estimated foreground signal is computed by $F(x, y, z) = I(x, y, z) - B(x, y, z)$.

3 Experiments and Results

To perform quantitative performance analysis, we collected four sample 3D images using two-photon microscopy on four different 3D mouse brains. Each mouse brain was made optically transparent by the method in [10]. To test the applicability of our method to different types of fluorescence dyes, Samples 1 and 3 were stained by DAPI which marks all cell nuclei in the samples. In these two samples, the background noise is moderate, but the sizes of foreground objects vary greatly (Fig. 3). Samples 2 and 4 were stained by GFAP which marks all astrocytes in the samples. In these two samples, the foreground objects are relatively sparse, but the background noise is quite severe (Fig. 3). Three representative slices were selected from each of these four 3D images for evaluation. To represent the changes across different depths, they were selected from the top, middle, and bottom of the 3D images. Human experts then labeled all the foreground objects in these representative slices. After that, the ground truth images were generated by computing the dot product between the binary human-labeled images and the original images. In this way, in the ground truth images, all the foreground objects keep their original intensities while all background intensities become 0.

Two known methods are selected for comparison with our method. The first one is a recently published shading correction method based on matrix ranking minimization [8]. The second one is the rolling ball algorithm, which is a well established method in ImageJ [2]. In the first method, for each 2D slice, its background is estimated by the neighboring d slices, where d is manually selected so that it achieves the best performance. In the second method, the ball size is selected to be equal to our window size $w = 5$. In our method, the percentile $p = 10\%$ and the parameters in the one-class learning model, $k = 7$, $\gamma_1 = 1$, $\gamma_2 = 1$, $\varepsilon = 1$, and $m = 4000$, are fixed across different samples.

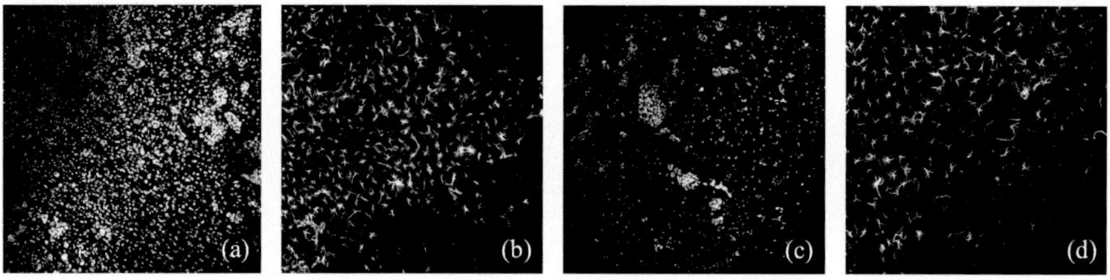

Fig. 3. (a)(b)(c)(d): Some example slices from 3D image Samples 1, 2, 3, and 4.

Table 1. Root mean squared errors (RMSE).

	Sample 1	Sample 2	Sample 3	Sample 4	Avg. Improvement
Our method	**9.21**	**8.48**	**4.26**	**7.74**	**52.53%**
Low rank [8]	18.01	9.50	5.68	7.81	34.56%
Rolling ball [2]	20.07	11.03	7.24	9.88	22.37%
Original Image	17.53	17.15	9.23	18.55	

As in [6,8], the quality of each method is measured using the root mean squared error (RMSE) between the processed slice F and the ground truth G, with RMSE $= \sqrt{\frac{1}{n}\sum_{i,j}(F_{ij} - G_{ij})^2}$. Table 1 summarizes the results. A smaller RMSE means more accurate background correction. On Table 1, one can see that when foreground objects are sparse (Samples 2 and 4), our method and [8] have comparable performance and are both much better than the rolling ball algorithm [2]. However, when foreground objects are more complicated (Samples 1 and 3), both [8] and the rolling ball algorithm are considerably worse than our method. In some cases, they can damage foreground objects (Fig. 4) and thus are even worse than the original images.

Table 2. Average processing time per voxel (in μs).

	Sample 1	Sample 2	Sample 3	Sample 4	Average
Our method	0.66μs	0.76μs	0.98μs	0.81μs	0.80μs
Low rank [8]	130.3μs	128.2μs	133.7μs	126.3μs	129.6μs
Rolling ball [2]	0.54μs	0.46μs	0.42μs	0.46μs	0.47μs

The efficiency of each method is measured by the average processing time per voxel, as shown in Table 2. Both [8] and our method were implemented in MATLAB. All these methods were tested on the same workstation. By Table 2, to process a 3D image for a whole mouse brain (with 10^{11} voxels), our method will take about 22 hours while the method in [8] will take 150 days. This shows the crucial need of efficiency for processing such large 3D images.

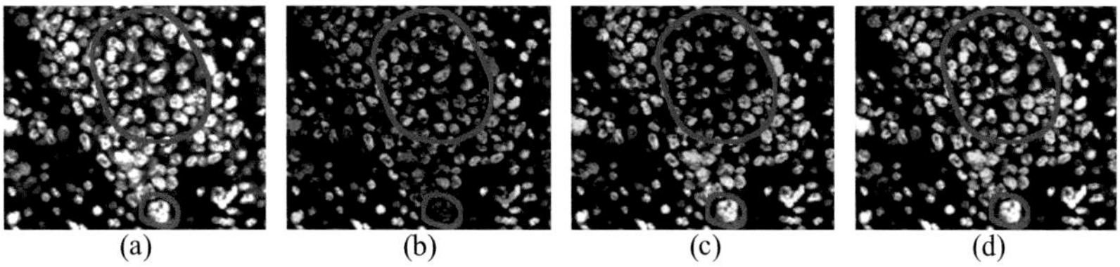

Fig. 4. A cropped window in a slice from Sample 1. (a) The labeled ground truth; (b) the result of the rolling ball algorithm; (c) the result of [8]; (d) our result. The rolling ball algorithm damages all foreground objects that are larger than its ball size. [8] is able to deal with sparse objects; but, it still damages the center of big clusters.

4 Conclusions

We present a fast background removal algorithm based on percentile filtering. The crucial "undersized window" problem in spatial filtering is tackled by unsupervised one-class learning. Extensive experiments on real 3D datasets show our method has superior performance and efficiency comparing with the current state-of-the-art background correction method and the rolling ball algorithm.

Acknowledgment. This research was supported in part by NSF under Grant CCF-1217906, and by NIH Pathway to Independence Award 5R00CA158066-04 and NIH 1R01CA194697-01.

References

1. Chen, T.W., Lin, B.J., Brunner, E., Schild, D.: In situ background estimation in quantitative fluorescence imaging. Biophysical Journal 90(7), 2534–2547 (2006)
2. Collins, T.J.: ImageJ for microscopy. Biotechniques 43(1), 25–30 (2007)
3. Efron, B., Tibshirani, R.J.: An Introduction to the Bootstrap. CRC Press (1994)
4. Gonzalez, R.C., Woods, R.E.: Digital Image Processing, 2nd edn. Addison-Wesley Longman Publishing Co., Inc., Boston (2001)
5. Likar, B., Maintz, J.A., Viergever, M.A., Pernus, F.: Retrospective shading correction based on entropy minimization. Journal of Microscopy 197(3), 285–295 (2000)
6. Lindblad, J., Bengtsson, E.: A comparison of methods for estimation of intensity non uniformities in 2D and 3D microscope images of fluorescence stained cells. In: Proc. of the Scandinavian Conf. on Image Analysis, pp. 264–271 (2001)
7. Liu, W., Hua, G., Smith, J.R.: Unsupervised one-class learning for automatic outlier removal. In: 2014 IEEE Conference on CVPR, pp. 3826–3833 (2014)
8. Peng, T., Wang, L., Bayer, C., Conjeti, S., Baust, M., Navab, N.: Shading correction for whole slide image using low rank and sparse decomposition. In: Golland, P., Hata, N., Barillot, C., Hornegger, J., Howe, R. (eds.) MICCAI 2014, Part I. LNCS, vol. 8673, pp. 33–40. Springer, Heidelberg (2014)
9. Tainaka, K., Kubota, S.I., Suyama, T.Q., Susaki, E.A., Perrin, D., Ukai-Tadenuma, M., Ukai, H., Ueda, H.R.: Whole-body imaging with single-cell resolution by tissue decolorization. Cell 159(4), 911–924 (2014)
10. Tomer, R., Ye, L., Hsueh, B., Deisseroth, K.: Advanced CLARITY for rapid and high-resolution imaging of intact tissues. Nature Protocols 9(7), 1682–1697 (2014)

Motion Representation of Ciliated Cell Images with Contour-Alignment for Automated CBF Estimation

Fan Zhang[1], Yang Song[1], Siqi Liu[1], Paul Young[2,3], Daniela Traini[2,3], Lucy Morgan[4,5], Hui-Xin Ong[2,3], Lachlan Buddle[4], Sidong Liu[1], Dagan Feng[1], and Weidong Cai[1]

[1] BMIT Research Group, School of IT, University of Sydney, Australia
[2] Woolcock Institute of Medical Research, Australia
[3] Discipline of Pharmacology, Sydney Medical School, University of Sydney, Australia
[4] Department of Respiratory Medicine,
Concord Repatriation General Hospital, Australia
[5] School of Medicine, University of Sydney, Australia

Abstract. Ciliary beating frequency (CBF) estimation is of high interest for the diagnosis and therapeutic assessment of defective mucociliary clearance diseases. Image-based methods have recently become the focus of accurate CBF measurement. The influence from the moving ciliated cell however makes the processing a challenging problem. In this work, we present a registration method for cell movement alignment, based on cell contour segmentation. We also propose a filter feature-based ciliary motion representation, which can better characterize the periodical changes of beating cilia. Experimental results on microscopic time sequence human primary ciliated cell images show the accuracy of our method for CBF computation.

1 Introduction

Mucociliary transport is a major host defense that clears mucus and inhaled debris from human airways [1]. It depends on the coordinated beating of respiratory tract cilia to generate propulsive efforts for the continuous movement of mucus. Ciliary beating frequency (CBF) is a regulated quantitative function and has been widely used for measuring ciliary beating behaviors. CBF estimation plays an important role for the diagnosis of defective mucociliary clearance diseases, e.g., primary ciliary dyskinesia (PCD) that presents cilia with stationary or slow motion (CBF $<$ 11Hz) [2]. CBF can also assist the comparisons between external stimuli on increasing ciliary motility for therapeutic assessment [3].

In the last two decades, with the more advanced digital high speed imaging (DHSI) techniques, image-based CBF estimation has demonstrated its advantages over the traditional approaches such as photomultiplier and photodiode techniques [4,5]. First of all, DHSI can visualize the actual ciliary movement, instead of detecting light changes passing through the cilia. In this way, it enables the frame-by-frame manual observation by playing the images in a slow

N. Navab et al. (Eds.): MICCAI 2015, Part III, LNCS 9351, pp. 300–307, 2015.
DOI: 10.1007/978-3-319-24574-4_36

speed, which is considered a more accurate measurement but suffers from time consumption and observer fatigue issues. There have been methods that capture the ciliary movement by extracting temporal image signals such as intensity variation and optical flow [5,6,7]. These works provide the fundamentals for automated CBF computation. However, their automaticity is restricted by the fact that regions of interest (ROIs) above the cilia should be given in advance. In addition, the accuracy of these methods can be affected by the assumption that the temporal signal variations are only caused by displacements of cilia, without considering the issues of, e.g., illumination changes. Another limitation is that the ciliated cell where the cilia are closely packed can significantly influence the CBF measurement since the cell sometimes beats simultaneously and may obscure the observation of cilia. Recent studies attempted to remove the influence by incorporating cell alignment processing [8,9]. The methods, however, conducted the rigid registration considering the cell moves only in global translation and rotation manners. This could cause inaccurate estimation if a ciliated cell presents a local shape distortion. In addition, without the overall automated processing framework, the practicability of these methods is restricted.

In this study, we present an automated CBF estimation method using the microscopic time sequence ciliary images for more accurate CBF measurement. The main contributions are: 1) we proposed a contour-alignment process consisting of a non-rigid cell registration and cell contour segmentation, which can removing the influence of more complicated cell motion; 2) we extracted a filter-based motion representation feature, which is specified to characterize periodical motion of beating cilia; 3) we designed an automated CBF estimation framework without the manual beating cycle counting or ROI annotation. We tested our method on real human ciliary image data. The experimental results compared to the photomultiplier and manual observation approaches indicate that our method provides a substantial improvement for accurate CBF computation.

2 Ciliary Beating Frequency Estimation

2.1 Data Acquisition

Ciliary images were obtained from human primary ciliated epithelial cells. We collected the sample cells via nasal brushing and dislodged them into Medium 199. The sugar alcohol (mannitol) and β-agonist (salbutamol sulfate) were used to stimulate the cells within a 24-hour period. Ciliary images were then visualized with an Olympus IX70 microscope and captured using a Nikon D7100 camera. We tested our method on a set of 32 cases/movies with moving ciliated cells of various motions such as translation, rotation and shape distortion. For each case, we used 130 consecutive images of 720×1280 pixels for CBF computation, with a recording rate at 60 frames per second.

2.2 Region Division

We first segment the image into the ciliated cell, beating cilia and background regions, by identifying an outer contour C_{out} and inner contour C_{in}. The outer

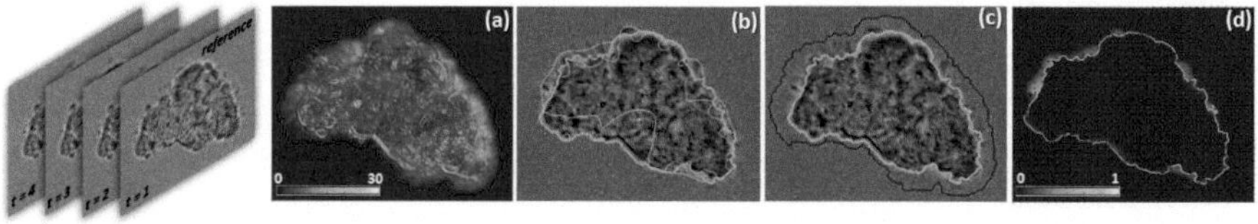

Fig. 1. Schema of cell segmentation and registration on an example image sequence: (a) C_{out} obtained given $ISDM$, (b) C_{in} computed with the DRLSE, (c) cilia region R_{cilia}, and (d) B-spline control point mesh and distance band weight.

contour C_{out} is used to separate the background. Considering that the cell and cilia can shift but background is still, we perform the segmentation on an intensity standard deviation map $ISDM$, as shown in Fig. 1(a). Given a position (x, y) in a time sequence of ciliary images $CI = \{I_t(x, y)|x \in [1, X], y \in [1, Y], t \in [1, T]\}$ with T images of size $X \times Y$, we extract its intensity curve along the time, and compute the intensity standard deviation $ISD(x, y)$. The map is then obtained as $ISDM = \{ISD(x, y)|x \in [1, X], y \in [1, Y]\}$. Due to the different moving behaviors, the cell and cilia regions present higher ISDs. We then use Sobel thresholding and extract the maximum connected component to segment the cell and cilia regions. A smoothing step is further performed to extend the contour to ensure that we include the entire cilia region.

Following that, the inner contour C_{in} is computed with a distance regularized level set evolution (DRLSE) [10] method to recognize the cell boundary. As the image sequence will be aligned to a reference $I_r \in CI$, we apply DRLSE on I_r with C_{out} as the initial segmentation. DRLSE obtains a sign matrix $\mathbf{S}$ corresponding to the level set formulation that takes negative values inside the zero level contour and positive values outside. We used the zero crossing points as C_{in}. DRLSE can also exhibit the cell contour as a signed distance band around the zero level set. The distance band can be used to weight the degree of motion of the nearby cell boundary areas. These areas normally show small beating motions, since the roots of cilia present less position displacement and become overlap with each other closer to the cell surface. This information will be incorporated into the cell registration for our contour-alignment processing.

2.3 Cell Registration

The aim of our cell registration is to ensure the observed motion of cilia only come from the ciliary beating. Hence, we do not want to over-emphasize the inside cell area nor, in particular, change the original ciliary beating behaviour, e.g., twisting the cilia based on those in the reference. The segmentation result can address these considerations by assigning higher priority to the cell boundary. Specifically, considering the cell movement mainly consists of non-rigid motions, we adopt the free-form deformation (FFD) [11] framework to get an aligned image sequence $CI' = \{I'_t|t \in [1, T]\}$ based on I_r (fixed as the first frame). FFD introduces high flexibility for local shape distortion to deform the cells while keeping the ciliary beating. It can also be naturally combined with the distance

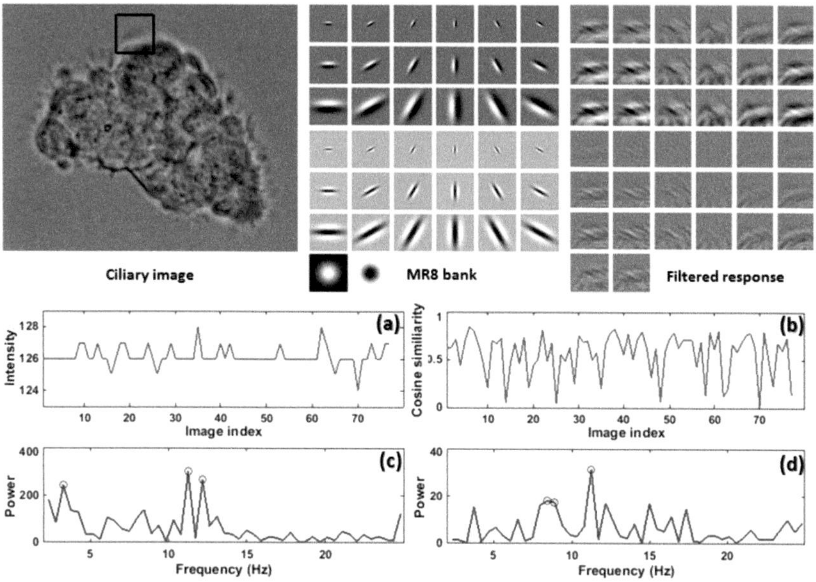

Fig. 2. Illustration of MR8-based signal extraction. The first row shows a visual representation of filtered responses given the 38 MR8 filters for a cilia ROI. The sub-figures (a) and (b) compare the original intensity and MR8 feature similarity curves for the middle position of the ROI, and (c) and (d) display the FFT frequency power distributions of the two signals, annotated with the first three dominant frequencies.

band for the contour alignment. Inspired by the work [12] that combines the structural boundary information with the textural intensity information, we incorporate the signed distance band from DRLSE for weighting the cell boundary area. The FFD with three levels of B-spline control points is implemented with the following energy function:

$$E(\mathbf{P}) = \sum((I_t(\mathbf{P}) - I_r(\mathbf{P})) \cdot w(C_{in}))^2 \tag{1}$$

$$w(x,y) = cosine(\frac{max(\mathbf{S}) - \mathbf{S}(x,y))}{max(\mathbf{S}) - min(\mathbf{S})}) \tag{2}$$

where $\mathbf{P}$ represents the B-spline control point matrix (the mesh window size is fixed at 20 for all experiments) and $\mathbf{S}$ is the sign matrix of DRLSE result. The weight $w(x,y) \in (0,1]$ gives priority to the control points in the middle of the band and gradually decreases towards the cilia and cell regions.

2.4 Ciliary Beating Signal Extraction

CBF is determined by timing a certain number of beating cycles, which is normally computed by capturing the recurrent displacement of cilia. Intensity variation is widely used in literature but can be influenced by noise, e.g., the illumination changes. In our method, after the cell registration, we apply a maximum response 8 (MR8) filtering [13], which has proved effectively for image denoising, to highlight the periodical displacement of beating cilia. MR8 bank consists of 6 oriented edge and bar filters at 3 scales, and 2 isotropic filters ($6 \times 2 \times 3 + 2$, as shown in Fig. 2). The oriented filters that correspond to the directions of cilia can reinforce the ciliary motion description, and the isotropic filters can help illumination adaption. For each I'_t, we compute a 38-dimension MR8 feature vector $f_t(x, y)$ at position (x, y), and calculate a *cosine* similarity with $f_r(x, y)$ of I_r. Concatenating the similarities along the time, we obtain a signal curve $SC(x, y) = \{cosine(f_t(x, y), f_r(x, y))|t \in [1, T]\}$ to represent the periodical motion changes. A visual example after MR8 filtering is shown in Fig. 2. The cosine similarity curve (b) can better represent the periodical variations and thus result in a frequency power distribution with the more distinct dominant component (d), when compared to the original intensity curve (a and c).

2.5 Frequency Computation

Given the beating signal, we calculate the frequency with the FFT method for each position to obtain a whole field frequency map as processed by Sisson et al [5]. The frequencies from the region R_{cilia} between C_{in} and C_{out} are considered as our CBF estimation result. Post-processing to filter noise in the frequency spectrum [6] is also applied.

3 Experimental Results

Fig. 3 shows the visual results of region division and cell registration for a case in which the cell has non-rigid movement[1]. The outer and inner contours are annotated in red and green on the reference image in Fig. 3(a). It is worth noting that the segmentations need not be very accurate if we can find the approximate cell boundary that can keep all beating cilia out of the contour (please see the last paragraph of this section for details). For this reason, we manually adjusted the coefficient α for weighting the area term of DRLSE and fixed it as $\alpha = 1$[2] that generated a better overall performance.

Figs. 3(b) and (c) display the *ISDM*s given the original CI and aligned CI'. The *ISD*s from cell region of CI' were much lower, indicating the benefit of registration on removing the cell movement. For the target image in Fig. 3(d), Figs. 3(e) and (f) compare the FFD registration results without/with the distance band, given the same parameter settings. While both of them can properly align the target, our method resulted in smaller changes in the cilia region and hence could better keep the original ciliary beating behaviour. A quantitative comparison of mean *ISD* (MISD) across different registration approaches are listed

[1] Readers are recommended to refer to the supplementary examples for better visualization, if applicable.

[2] $\alpha = 1$ generated the optimal region division results for most cases but relatively shrinked the contours for the others. For other parameters involved in DRLSE, we followed the suggestions from the reference paper [10].

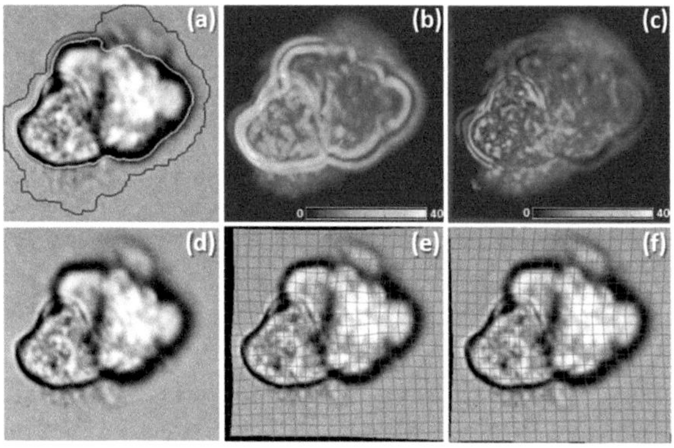

Fig. 3. Visual comparisons of the regions division and cell alignment results.

Table 1. Comparisons of MISDs across different registration methods.

	Original	Rigid	FFD	Proposed
Cell (inside C_{in})	9.67 ± 3.02	14.11 ± 6.67	**4.33 ± 2.01**	4.72 ± 2.26
Cilia (inside R_{cilia})	5.83 ± 1.91	17.42 ± 9.53	**4.16 ± 1.71**	4.23 ± 1.80
Distance band ($w > 0.5$)[3]	11.8 ± 3.76	12.38 ± 7.51	6.16 ± 3.39	**5.62 ± 3.71**

in Table 1, including a rigid intensity-based registration with gradient descent optimization, the original FFD and our method. The rigid registration obtained higher MISDs than the non-rigid registrations. Compared to the original FFD method, we obtained higher MISDs for the cell and cilia regions but smaller values in the distance band area. These results are due to that our method incorporated the weighting scheme in Eq. (2), which assigned higher priority to the control points located nearby the cell boundary. A better registration of this region could remove the influence of moving cell and keep the original ciliary beating behaviour to a large extent, and hence is more desirable even at some expense of the registration performance for the cell and cilia.

Fig. 4 illustrates the CBF estimation results given different signals. For the intensity variations, although the cell registration was incorporated in CI', the difference from CI was small. The more observable changes can be found with the MR8 feature-based signals. Firstly, the beating frequencies from the cell region were largely reduced. The higher frequencies that are usually considered originating from the beating cilia are thus more distinguishable. This can explain why a smaller cell contour has relatively negligible influence on our CBF computation. In addition, with the combination of registration and filtering, we can provide a more accurate CBF estimation. For example of the first case, given the area circled in white that contains a cluster of immotile cilia, the first two approaches failed to recognize them. The third method obtained a lower frequency spectrum that however was from the movement of ciliated cell. Our method gave the best estimation result.

[3] $w > 0.5$ gave a more suitable range of cell boundary and was thus selected. For other parameters of FFD, we followed the suggestions from the reference paper [11].

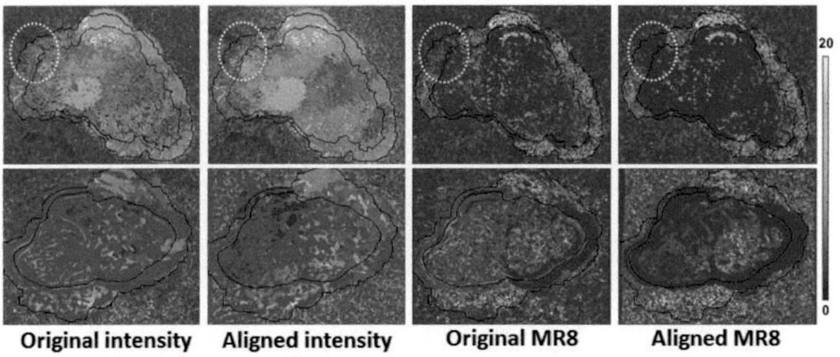

Fig. 4. Comparisons of the whole field frequency maps given different signals.

Table 2. Comparisons of MSE and MD with MO and PM estimations.

		Original intensity	Aligned intensity	Original MR8	Aligned MR8
MSE	Cell	6.216	6.135	4.217	**2.311**
	Back	4.650	5.517	**2.928**	3.701
	Cilia	7.575	7.188	5.999	**5.356**
MD	Avg	0.131	0.130	0.156	**0.551**
	SD	0.670	1.101	2.413	**2.771**
	Max	4.700	5.938	8.739	**9.609**

We conducted the manual observation (MO) estimation for quantitative performance comparison. For each case, we randomly sampled 10 points from each cell, cilia and background regions. For the cell and background points, the frequencies were set as 0Hz; for the cilia points, we conducted frame-by-frame observation to time 10 beating cycles, in terms of the relative position displacement between the cilia and nearby cell boundary. The mean square errors (MSEs) of the frequencies of these points between the MO and the various methods are listed in Table 2. With our method (Aligned MR8), the smallest difference can be observed in the cell region, showing the benefits of our contour-alignment process. Our method also obtained the best correlation with the MO estimation for the cilia region. To further validate the CBF measurement, we also compared our result with the photomultiplier (PM) approach. The PM method captured the electronic signals from the photometer through an oscilloscope and documented the signals with Mac-Lab recording system. Given the average (Avg), standard deviation (SD) and maximum (Max) of frequencies in the cilia region from the PM estimation, we report the mean difference (MD) of the statistics of our method in Table 2. The results using the original intensity method were the most similar to PM, since they shared the same signal source from the moving cell. The MR8-based approaches obtained larger MDs, but corresponded to the smaller MSEs from the MO estimation. This observation indicates that the periodical changes of beating cilia, which were essential for CBF estimation, were better characterized by the MR8 features compared to PM and the original intensity. We also suggest that the cell alignment is more important if we focus on a certain cilia region, e.g., recognizing the immotile cilia as shown in Fig. 4.

4 Conclusions

We present an image-based method for CBF estimation, based on the region division, ciliated cell registration and the signal extraction. Our method can provide a more accurate ciliary motion representation by removing the influence from the moving cell. With the MR8 feature we can better represent the periodical motion of beating cilia from the non-cilia objects. Our estimation results are expected to be more suitable for diagnosing the defective mucociliary clearance and observing the therapeutic effects of different drugs. The method also provides an alternative for the conventional CBF measures in an automated way, which avoids the time-consuming and high-cost processing.

References

1. Wanner, A., Salathé, M., et al.: Mucociliary clearance in the airways. American Journal of Respiratory and Critical Care Medicine 154(6), 1868–1902 (1996)
2. Stannard, W.A., Chilvers, M.A., et al.: Diagnostic testing of patients suspected of primary ciliary dyskinesia. American Journal of Respiratory and Critical Care Medicine 181(4), 307–314 (2010)
3. Salathe, M.: Effects of β-agonists on airway epithelial cells. Journal of Allergy and Clinical Immunology 110(6), S275–S281 (2002)
4. Chilvers, M.A., O'Callaghan, C.: Analysis of ciliary beat pattern and beat frequency using digital high speed imaging: comparison with the photomultiplier and photodiode methods. Thorax 55(4), 314–317 (2000)
5. Sisson, J.H., Stoner, J.A., et al.: All-digital image capture and whole-field analysis of ciliary beat frequency. Journal of Microscopy 211(2), 103–111 (2003)
6. Smith, C.M., Djakow, J., et al.: ciliaFA: a research tool for automated, high-throughput measurement of ciliary beat frequency using freely available software. Cilia 1(14), 1–7 (2012)
7. Kim, W., Han, T.H., et al.: An automated measurement of ciliary beating frequency using a combined optical flow and peak detection. Healthcare Informatics Research 17(2), 111–119 (2011)
8. Parrilla, E., Armengot, M., et al.: Optical flow method in phase-contrast microscopy images for the diagnosis of primary ciliary dyskinesia through measurement of ciliary beat frequency. Preliminary results. In: ISBI, pp. 1655–1658 (2012)
9. Zhang, F., et al.: Image-based ciliary beating frequency estimation for therapeutic assessment on defective mucociliary clearance diseases. In: ISBI, pp. 193–196 (2014)
10. Li, C., Xu, C., et al.: Distance regularized level set evolution and its application to image segmentation. IEEE Trans. Imag. Process. 19(12), 3243–3254 (2010)
11. Rueckert, D., Sonoda, et al.: Nonrigid registration using free-form deformations: application to breast MR images. IEEE Trans. Med. Imag. 18(8), 712–721 (1999)
12. Myronenko, A., Song, X., Sahn, D.J.: LV motion tracking from 3D echocardiography using textural and structural information. In: Ayache, N., Ourselin, S., Maeder, A. (eds.) MICCAI 2007, Part II. LNCS, vol. 4792, pp. 428–435. Springer, Heidelberg (2007)
13. Varma, M., Zisserman, A.: Classifying images of materials: achieving viewpoint and illumination independence. In: Heyden, A., Sparr, G., Nielsen, M., Johansen, P. (eds.) ECCV 2002, Part III. LNCS, vol. 2352, pp. 255–271. Springer, Heidelberg (2002)

Multimodal Dictionary Learning and Joint Sparse Representation for HEp-2 Cell Classification

Ali Taalimi[1], Shahab Ensafi[2,3], Hairong Qi[1], Shijian Lu[2], Ashraf A. Kassim[3], and Chew Lim Tan[4]

[1] University of Tennessee-Knoxville
[2] Institute for Infocomm Research, A*STAR, Singapore
[3] Department of Electrical and Computer Engineering, National University of Singapore, Singapore
[4] School of Computing, National University of Singapore, Singapore

Abstract. Use of automatic classification for Indirect Immunofluorescence (IIF) images of HEp-2 cells is increasingly gaining interest in Antinuclear Autoantibodies (ANAs) detection. In order to improve the classification accuracy, we propose a multi-modal joint dictionary learning method, to obtain a discriminative and reconstructive dictionary while training a classifier simultaneously. Here, the term 'multi-modal' refers to features extracted using different algorithms from the same data set. To utilize information fusion between feature modalities the algorithm is designed so that sparse codes of all modalities of each sample share the same sparsity pattern. The contribution of this paper is two-fold. First, we propose a new framework for multi-modal fusion at the feature level. Second, we impose an additional constraint on consistency of sparse coefficients among different modalities of the same class. Extensive experiments are conducted on the ICPR2012 and ICIP2013 HEp-2 data sets. All results confirm the higher level of accuracy of the proposed method compared with state-of-the-art.

1 Introduction

Application of automated Computer Aided Diagnosis (CAD) system to support clinicians in the field of Indirect Immunofluorescence (IIF) has been increased in recent years. Use of CAD system enables test repeatability, lowers costs and results in more accurate diagnosis. IIF imaging technique is applied to Human Epithelial Cells type 2 (HEp-2 cells), where antibodies are first stained in a tissue and then bound to a fluorescent chemical compound. In case of Antinuclear Antibodies (ANAs), the antibodies bound to the nucleus demonstrate different visual patterns which can be captured and visualized within microscope images [5]. These patterns can be used for cell classification and for assisting diagnosis. Image quality variations makes interpretation of fluorescence patterns, very challenging. To make the pattern interpretation more consistent, automated methods for classifying the cells are essential.

N. Navab et al. (Eds.): MICCAI 2015, Part III, LNCS 9351, pp. 308–315, 2015.
DOI: 10.1007/978-3-319-24574-4_37

Recently, there has been an increasing interest in sparse coding in computer vision and image processing research for reconstructive and discriminative tasks [9,7,1]. In sparse coding the input signal is approximated by a linear combination of a few atoms of the dictionary. The state-of-the-art method in HEp-2 cell classification problem is proposed in [2], where the SIFT and SURF features are extracted as the input features to learn a dictionary followed by Spatial Pyramid Matching (SPM) [8] to provide the sparse representation of the input cell images. Then a Support Vector Machine (SVM) is learned to classify the test images.

All above mentioned approaches use unsupervised dictionary learning where the dictionary is obtained purely based on minimizing the reconstruction error. However, in supervised scheme, minimization of misclassification and reconstruction errors results in a dictionary which is adapted to a task and data set [9,10] and leads to a more accurate classification compared with unsupervised formulation. In some supervised approaches the sparse codes obtained in training are not used for classifier training and test signal is classified only based on reconstruction error [10]. Although [13,1] exploit sparse codes to train classifier; it is done independent of dictionary learning. We intend to estimate the dictionary and classifier, jointly so that generated sparse codes by dictionary are more discriminative, leading to better classification result.

The majority of existing dictionary learning methods, supervised or unsupervised, can handle only single source of data [7]. Fusion of information from different sensor modalities can be more robust to single sensor failure. The information fusion happens in feature level or classifier level [14]. In feature fusion different types of features are combined to make one representation to train a classifier while in classifier fusion, for each modality one classifier is trained independent of others and their decisions would be fused. In Bag-of-Words, feature fusion is imposed by concatenating all of features in one vector. The dimension of this vector is high and suffers from curse-of-dimensionality while it does not even contain the valuable information of correlation between feature types.

We propose a supervised algorithm similar to [7] to learn a compact and discriminative dictionary in all-vs-all fashion for each modality. This method can combine information from different feature types and force them to have common sparsity patterns for each class, which is presented in Fig. 1.

2 Method

Notation. Let C represent the number of classes, $\mathcal{M} \triangleq \{1 \cdots M\}$ be a set of M different feature modalities, $\{\mathcal{Y}_{i,c}\}_{i=1}^{N}$, $c \in \{1, \cdots, C\}$ as N training samples where each sample belong to c-th class and has M feature modalities as $\mathcal{Y}_{i,c} = \{Y_i^m \in R^{n^m \times S} | m \in \mathcal{M}\}$ where n^m is the dimension of the m-th feature modality and S is the number of interest points in the image which is the same for all modalities. The binary matrix $H_i \in \mathcal{R}^{C \times S}$ is an identifier for the label of $\mathcal{Y}_{i,c}$. Given $\mathcal{Y}_{i,c}$ from c-th class, the c-th row of H_i is one and all other rows are zero. Also, consider Y^m as set of m-th feature modality of all training samples $Y^m \in \mathcal{R}^{n^m \times K} = [Y_1^m \cdots Y_N^m]$ where $K = N \times S$ is the total number of samples in m-th

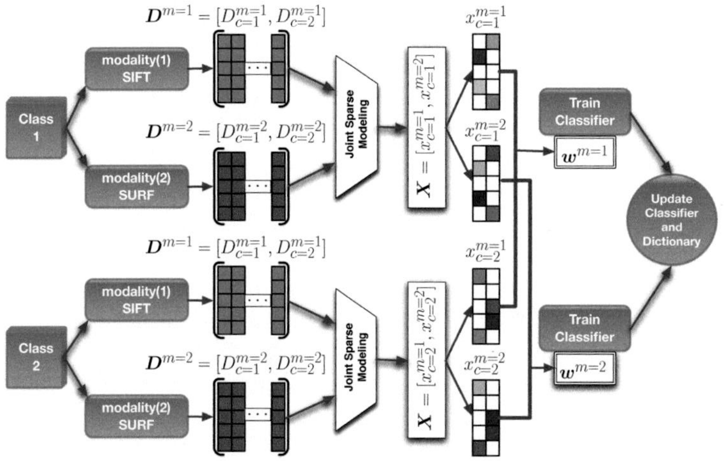

Fig. 1. Multi-modal supervised dictionary learning where two classes and two modalities for each class are assumed. We expect $X_{c=1}^{m=1}$ and $X_{c=1}^{m=2}$ have same sparsity pattern.

modality. The label matrix of Y^m is $H{=}[H_1 \cdots H_N]$. Corresponding dictionary of m-th modality $D^m \in \mathbb{R}^{n^m \times p}$ has p atoms. D^m is composed of class-specific sub-dictionaries D_c^m as $D^m{=}[D_1^m \cdots D_C^m]$. Also, assuming w^m as parameters of m-th modality classifier, W is set of all classifiers, $W = \{w^m | m \in \mathcal{M}\}$.

2.1 Supervised Dictionary Learning

Supervised dictionary learning can be done in one-vs-all scheme by training an independent dictionary for each class or in all-vs-all setting where the dictionary is shared between classes. We adopt all-vs-all scheme which allows feature sharing among the classes to obtain modality-based dictionary D^m.

Assuming sample $\mathcal{Y}_{i,c}$ from c-th class, we define binary matrix $Q_i \in \mathcal{R}^{p \times S} = [q_1 \cdots q_S]$. Each column q_i is zero everywhere except for indices of atoms which belong to the c-th class. The relation between labels of Y^m and labels of atoms in D^m is determined by matrix $Q = [Q_1 \cdots Q_N]$. The so called label consistency constraint is applied using Q so that each sample is reconstructed from atoms that belong to the same class as the sample.

The dictionary D^m can be estimated by minimizing $\mathcal{L}_u(X^m, D^m)$ using elastic-net formulation [16] as $\mathcal{L}_u(.) \triangleq \min \|Y^m - D^m X^m\|_2^2 + \lambda_1 \|X^m\|_1 + \lambda_2 \|X^m\|_F^2$ where λ_1 and λ_2 are regularization parameters. $\mathcal{L}_u$ is an *unsupervised* reconstruction loss function and is small if D^m is successful in finding sparse representation of Y^m. Given X^m obtained by elastic-net, *supervised* loss function $\mathcal{L}_{su}^m$, for dictionary learning and classifier training for modality m is formulated as [7]:

$$\underset{w^m, A^m}{\operatorname{argmin}} \mathcal{L}_{su}^m(D^m, Y^m, w^m, H, A^m, Q) + \frac{\nu_1}{2}\|w^m\|_F^2 + \frac{\nu_2}{2}\|A^m\|_F^2 \quad (1)$$

where ν_1, ν_2 are regularization parameters. The supervised loss function of m-th modality is defined as $\mathcal{L}_{su}^m \triangleq \mu\|Q - A^m X^m\|_2^2 + (1-\mu)\|H - w^m X^m\|_2^2$ with μ as a regularization and A^m as a linear transformation matrix. The so called label consistency prior $\|Q - A^m X^m\|_F^2$ allows sparse code X^m to be different from Q up to a linear transformation A^m; hence it forces sparse representation of different classes to be discriminative. The classification error in $\mathcal{L}_{su}^m$, $\|H - w^m X^m\|_F^2$ shows that how well H can be predicted by the linear classifier with parameter w^m.

We want that multi-modal sparse representation $X_c^1, \cdots, X_c^M$ of data of c-th class, $\mathcal{Y}_{i,c}$, share same sparsity pattern. We propose multi-modal supervised dictionary learning and joint sparse modeling as:

$$X_c = \underset{X_c=[X_c^1,\cdots,X_c^M]}{\operatorname{argmin}} \sum_{m=1}^{M} \mathcal{L}_{su}^m(D^m, w^m, A^m, X^m) + \eta \|X_c\|_{1,2} \tag{2}$$

each sub-matrix X_c^m is sparse representation for data reconstruction of m-th modality and c-th class. Collaboration between $X_c^1, \cdots, X_c^M$ is imposed by $\|X_c\|_{1,2}$ in (2) and is defined as $\|X\|_{1,2} = \sum_{r=1}^{p} \|x_r\|_2$; where x_r are rows of X_c. The $l_{1,2}$ regularization $\|X\|_{1,2}$ promotes solution with sparse non-zero rows x_r; hence, sparse representations share the consistent pattern across all the modalities of the same class.

Optimization. As suggested in [9], the modality-based dictionary D^m is trained over Y^m using elastic-net [16]. This is done for each modality, independently to obtain multi-modal dictionaries $D = \{D^m | m \in \mathcal{M}\}$. We expect the data of c-th class to be reconstructed by atoms that belong to the c-th class. Given multi-modal dictionaries D, the joint sparse representation of $\mathcal{Y}_i$) is calculated using (2) and solved by proximal algorithm [12]. Then, we make modality-based sparse codes of m-th modality as $X^m = [X_1^m, \cdots, X_C^m]$. Assuming $\tilde{X} = (X^m)^T$, multivariate ridge regression model with quadratic loss and l_2 norm regularization are adopted to estimate initial values of w^m and A^m:

$$A^m = Q\tilde{X}(\tilde{X}^T\tilde{X} + I)^{-1}, \quad w^m = H\tilde{X}(\tilde{X}^T\tilde{X} + I)^{-1} \tag{3}$$

where I is identity matrix. The final values of D^m and w^m is obtained using stochastic gradient descent scheme proposed in [9,7]. The proposed algorithm is summarized in Algorithm (1).

3 Experiments and Results

We evaluate proposed method on two publicly available HEp-2 image datasets, referred to as ICPR2012[1] and ICIP2013[2]. Fig. 2 shows the ICPR2012 that contains 1445 cells in six categories and divided to train and test sets by the organizers. Fig. 3 shows the ICIP2013 that has 13650 cells in six categories for the training set but the test set is not publicly available. Also, each cell image is

[1] http://mivia.unisa.it/datasets/biomedical-image-datasets/hep2-image-dataset/

[2] http://mivia.unisa.it/icip-2013-contest-on-hep-2-cells-classification/

Algorithm 1. Multi-modal Dictionary and Classifier Learning

Input: $Y^m\ \forall m \in \{1 \cdots M\}, Q, H, \mu, \eta$ and T =number of iterations
Output: $D^m, w^m\ \ \forall m \in \{1 \ldots M\}$

begin
  foreach *modality* $m \in \{1, \cdots, M\}$ **do**
    foreach *class* $c \in \{1, \cdots, C\}$ **do**
      Obtain D_c^m from $\mathcal{Y}_{i,c}$ using elastic-net;
    Find initial value of modality-based dictionary $D_0^m = [D_1^m, \cdots, D_C^m]$;
    Estimate D^m by applying elastic-net on Y^m given D_0^m
  Solve joint sparse coding problem (2) to find X_c using proximal method [12];
  Initialize w^m and A^m using (3)
  foreach *modality* $m \in \{1, \cdots, M\}$ **do**
    for *iter* $= 1 \cdots T$ **do**
      foreach *mini-batch samples of* Y^m **do**
        Update learning rate, D^m, A^m and w^m by a projected gradient step following [9];

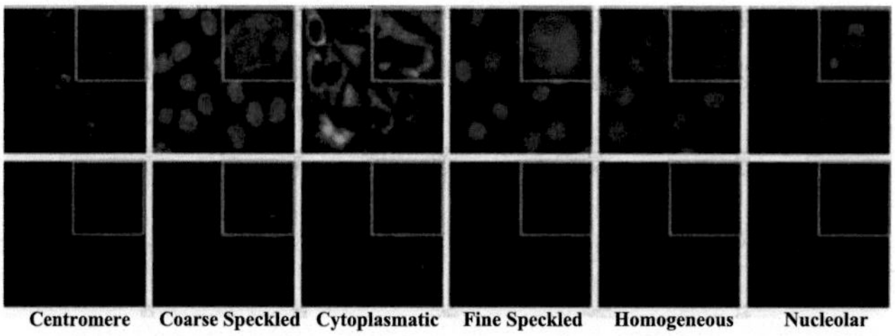

Fig. 2. ICPR2012 dataset. Positive (Top) and Intermediate (Bottom) images.

assigned to one of the two types of intensity patterns: positive or intermediate, which can be used as a prior information.

To prove the effectiveness of the proposed joint sparse representation we report our performance for four scenarios: sift (OnlySIFT), surf (OnlySURF), concatenation of sift and surf features (SIFTSURF) and joint sift and surf (Joint).

3.1 Implementation Details

Choosing the Parameters. To reduce the burden of required cross validation to set regularization parameters λ_1, λ_2 (elastic-net parameters), ν_1, ν_2 in (1), η in (2) and p (number of atoms in dictionary), we follow generally accepted heuristics proposed in [9]. To promote sparsity similar to [9,7] we set λ_2=0 and choose λ_1 by cross-validation in the set $\lambda_1 = 0.15 + 0.025k$ with $k \in \{-3, \cdots, 3\}$ and set it to $\lambda_1 = 0.5$. We observed that increasing number of atoms, p, usually leads to a better performance at the cost of higher computational complexity. We try the values p from $\{30, 60, 100, 150\}$. Our experiments on ν_1, ν_2 confirms observations in [9,7] that when p is smaller than number of normalized training patches, ν_1 and

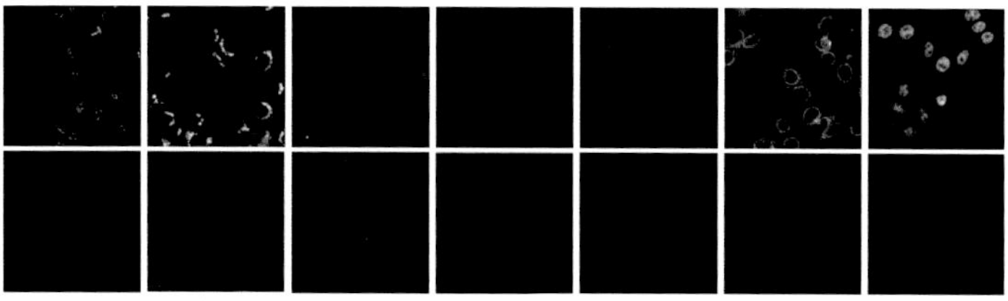

Fig. 3. ICIP2013 dataset. Positive (Top) and Intermediate (Bottom) images.

ν_2 can be arbitrarily set to small value. We try ν_1 and ν_2 from $\{10^{-1}, \cdots, 10^{-8}\}$ and choose $\nu = \nu_1 = \nu_2$ for both data sets. The regularization parameter η is selected by cross-validation in the set $\{0.001, 0.01, 0.05, 0.1, 0.2, 0.3\}$.

We extract 2-modalities of SIFT and SURF from each cell image. Each of these modalities are extracted from patches of 16×16 that are densely sampled using a grid with step size of 6 pixels. Then, spatial pyramid represents each feature-type using three grids size 1×1, 2×2 and 4×4 and codebook with $k = 900$ atoms [8]. The vector quantization codes of all spatial subregion of the spatial pyramid are pooled together to construct a pooled feature. The final spatial pyramid feature of each cell image is obtained by concatenating and l_2 normalization of the pooled features originated from subregions.

We train D_c^m from $\mathcal{Y}_{i,c}^m$ using elastic-net. Then, the initial value for dictionary of m-th modality, D_0^m is obtained by concatenating $D_c^m|_{c\in\{1\cdots C\}}$. This way we know the class label of each atom in D^m. The D^m is tuned by running elastic-net once more on training data of m-th modality Y^m given initial value D_0^m. Unlike all other methods of HEp-2 classification an explicit corresponding is made between labels of atoms in D^m and labels of data in Y^m; hence the estimated sparse codes are more distinctive. This leads to high accuracy classification result while D^m has a few atoms. We consider $p = 100$ and $p = 150$ atoms for dictionary of each cell class; hence modality-based dictionary D^m has 600 and 900 atoms for all six cell classes for ICIP2012 and ICIP2013, respectively.

The evaluation for the ICPR2012 is performed on the provided test set. Since the test set is not publicly available for ICIP2013 dataset, we follow [6] to design train and test. Training set includes 600 samples from each class except Golgi which has 300 cell samples. The remaining samples belong to the test data. In both datasets, we report performance of our method on each intensity level separately and final result is the average of classification results. As suggested by the competition organiser we evaluate our method based on Mean Class Accuracy (MCA): $MCA = \frac{1}{C}\sum_{c=1}^{C} CCR_c$; where CCR_c is correct classification rate of c-th class.

We report the performance of the proposed method for different values of ν and μ when η is changed from 0.1 to 0.7 for ICPR2012 in Fig. 4. For each ν we report the accuracy once with considering label consistency constraint as dotted line (μ=0) and once with the label consistency involved ($\mu = 0.3$). The performance is always better with label consistency constraint. Fig.4 agrees the observations made by [9,7] that ν should be set to small value when the number

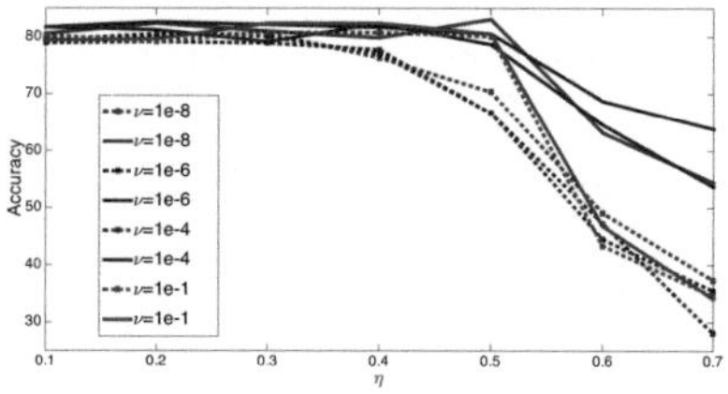

Fig. 4. The effect of changing parameters on ICIP2012 positive samples. $\mu = 0.3$ and $\mu = 0$ for the straight and dotted lines, respectively for different η values.

Table 1. The MCA accuracy on test set of ICPR2012 dataset and Comparison with state-of-the-art on ICIP2013.

ICPR2012	**OnlySIFT**	**OnlySURF**	**SIFTSURF**	**Joint**	[1]	[4]	[3]	[11]	[15]	[6]
Positive	74	72	76	**82**	81	62	63	74	69	78
Intermediate	67	66	69	**79**	62	41	60	35	48	48
Average Accuracy	70	69	73	**80**	72	52	62	55	59	63

ICPR2013	**OnlySIFT**	**OnlySURF**	**SIFTSURF**	**Joint**	[1]	[6]
Positive	88.4	90.3	90.7	**98.2**	95.8	95.5
Intermediate	76.2	72.5	81.2	**92.1**	87.9	80.9
Average Accuracy	82.3	81.4	85.9	**95.1**	91.9	88.2

of training patches is a lot more than number of atoms. We set $\eta = 0.2, \mu = 0.3$ and $\nu = 1e - 4$ in our experiments.

We compare performance of our method with state-of-the-art on ICPR2012 in Table 1. Our supervised method has 82% and 79% accuracy on positive and intermediate classification. It increases accuracy of OnlySIFT, OnlySURF more than 10% and enhances SIFTSURF around 7%. It also, outperforms other methods on average accuracy by at least 8%.

In the cell level classification on ICIP2013, Table 1 shows that applying SIFT and SURF jointly using our method enhances accuracy of OnlySIFT and Only-SURF around 13% while getting better result than simple concatenation of SIFTSURF at least 8% on average accuracy. It also outperforms other methods more than 3% on average accuracy. The proposed joint method shows superior results than concatenation of feature modalities in one vector in both datasets.

4 Conclusion

The problem of HEp-2 cell classification using sparsity scheme was studied and a supervised method was proposed to learn the reconstructive and discriminative dictionary and classifier simultaneously. Having label consistency constraint within each modality and applying joint sparse coding between modality-based sparse representations leads to discriminative dictionary with few atoms. The imposed joint sparse prior enable algorithm to fuse information in feature-level by forcing their sparse codes to collaborate and in decision-level by augmenting the classifier decisions. The result of HEp-2 cell classification experiments demonstrates that our proposed method outperforms state-of-the-art while using common features. It is trivial that our approach will further improve by adding complex and well-designed features [6].

References

1. Ensafi, S., Lu, S., Kassim, A.A., Tan, C.L.: Automatic cad system for hep-2 cell image classification. In: 2014 22nd International Conference on Pattern Recognition (ICPR), pp. 3321–3326. IEEE (2014)
2. Ensafi, S., Lu, S., Kassim, A.A., Tan, C.L.: A bag of words based approach for classification of hep-2 cell images. In: 2014 1st Workshop on Pattern Recognition Techniques for Indirect Immunofluorescence Images (I3A), pp. 29–32. IEEE (2014)
3. Ensafi, S., Lu, S., Kassim, A.A., Tan, C.L.: Sparse non-parametric bayesian model for hep-2 cell image classification. In: IEEE International Symposium on Biomedical Imaging: From Nano to Macro, ISBI 2015. IEEE (April 2015)
4. Foggia, P., Percannella, G., Soda, P., Vento, M.: Benchmarking hep-2 cells classification methods. IEEE Transactions on Medical Imaging 32(10), 1878–1889 (2013)
5. González-Buitrago, J.M., González, C.: Present and future of the autoimmunity laboratory. Clinica Chimica Acta 365(1), 50–57 (2006)
6. Han, X.H., Wang, J., Xu, G., Chen, Y.W.: High-order statistics of microtexton for hep-2 staining pattern classification. IEEE Transactions on Biomedical Engineering 61(8), 2223–2234 (2014)
7. Jiang, Z., Lin, Z., Davis, L.S.: Label consistent k-svd: learning a discriminative dictionary for recognition. IEEE Transactions on Pattern Analysis and Machine Intelligence 35(11), 2651–2664 (2013)
8. Lazebnik, S., Schmid, C., Ponce, J.: Beyond bags of features: Spatial pyramid matching for recognizing natural scene categories. In: IEEE Conference on Computer Vision and Pattern Recognition (CVPR), vol. 2, pp. 2169–2178. IEEE (2006)
9. Mairal, J., Bach, F., Ponce, J.: Task-driven dictionary learning. IEEE Transactions on Pattern Analysis and Machine Intelligence 34(4), 791–804 (2012)
10. Mairal, J., Bach, F., Ponce, J., Sapiro, G., Zisserman, A.: Discriminative learned dictionaries for local image analysis. In: IEEE Conference on Computer Vision and Pattern Recognition (CVPR), pp. 1–8. IEEE (2008)
11. Nosaka, R., Fukui, K.: Hep-2 cell classification using rotation invariant co-occurrence among local binary patterns. Pattern Recognition 47(7), 2428–2436 (2014)
12. Parikh, N., Boyd, S.: Proximal algorithms. Foundations and Trends in Optimization 1(3), 123–231 (2013)
13. Ramirez, I., Sprechmann, P., Sapiro, G.: Classification and clustering via dictionary learning with structured incoherence and shared features. In: IEEE Conference on Computer Vision and Pattern Recognition (CVPR), pp. 3501–3508. IEEE (2010)
14. Ruta, D., Gabrys, B.: An overview of classifier fusion methods. Computing and Information Systems 7(1), 1–10 (2000)
15. Wiliem, A., Sanderson, C., Wong, Y., Hobson, P., Minchin, R.F., Lovell, B.C.: Automatic classification of human epithelial type 2 cell indirect immunofluorescence images using cell pyramid matching. Pattern Recognition 47(7), 2315–2324 (2014)
16. Zou, H., Hastie, T.: Regularization and variable selection via the elastic net. J. Royal Statistical Society: Series B (Statistical Methodology) 67(2), 301–320 (2005)

Cell Event Detection in Phase-Contrast Microscopy Sequences from Few Annotations

Melih Kandemir[1], Christian Wojek[2], and Fred A. Hamprecht[1]

[1] Heidelberg University, HCI/IWR, Germany
[2] Carl Zeiss AG, Oberkochen, Germany

Abstract. We study detecting cell events in phase-contrast microscopy sequences from few annotations. We first detect event candidates from the intensity difference of consecutive frames, and then train an unsupervised novelty detector on these candidates. The novelty detector assigns each candidate a degree of surprise. We annotate a tiny number of candidates chosen according to the novelty detector's output, and finally train a sparse Gaussian process (GP) classifier. We show that the steepest learning curve is achieved when a collaborative multi-output Gaussian process is used as novelty detector, and its predictive mean and variance are used together to measure the degree of surprise. Following this scheme, we closely approximate the fully-supervised event detection accuracy by annotating only 3% of all candidates. The novelty detector based annotation used here clearly outperforms the studied active learning based approaches.

1 Introduction

Modern cell biology thrives on time lapse imaging where the fate of cells can be studied over time and in response to various stimuli. Phase-contrast microscopy is an important experimental technique in this area because it is non-invasive and allows the detection of events such as mitosis (cell division) or apoptosis (cell death). A fundamental challenge in phase-contrast microscopy images is the hardness of segmenting the cell boundaries accurately. Even though there have been attempts for segmenting cells in this type of images [5], the accuracy and the tolerance to imaging artifacts provided by the state-of-the-art are significantly below the reliability level. The suggested methods for automated analysis of phase-contrast sequences by-pass the segmentation step and jump directly to detecting events of interest from a heuristically generated set of candidate regions. Huh et al. [3] extract a candidate mitotic region from each large enough bright spot in a frame. Each candidate is represented by a Histogram of Oriented Gradients (HoG) feature set, passed through a binary classifier, and the classifier decisions are smoothed by a Conditional Random Field (CRF). In [4], apoptotic events of stem cells are detected by extracting candidate regions exploiting the image acquisition principles of phase-contrast microscopy, a rule-based filtering using application-specific heuristics, and a support vector classifier.

All the above methods require a fully-supervised training sequence. A time-lapse sequence consists of hundreds of events, which often occur simultaneously, making their annotation a tedious task. Hence, a way of reducing the annotation labor would save the biologist's precious time. This problem has first been investigated by Kandemir

N. Navab et al. (Eds.): MICCAI 2015, Part III, LNCS 9351, pp. 316–323, 2015.
DOI: 10.1007/978-3-319-24574-4_38

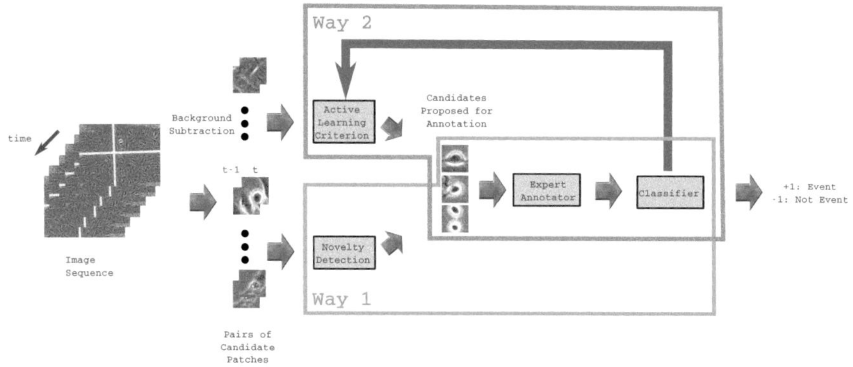

Fig. 1. Two proposed pipelines for interactive cell event detection. **Way 1:** Unsupervised event detection followed by supervised learning. **Way 2:** Active learning. The novelty detector we introduce in Way 1 gives a steeper learning curve than Way 2.

et al. [6], where a multioutput GP (MOGP) is used as an autoregressor to predict the features of a patch at time t from its features at time $t-1$. This autoregressor is trained on the first few (five) frames of the sequence where there occur no events of interest. The prediction error made by the autoregressor is used as the degree of surprise, and an event is fired if this surprise is above a preset threshold.

In this paper, we study ways of reaching high cell event detection accuracy using a supervised classifier as opposed to [6], but using only a small amount of annotations as opposed to [2,3,4]. For this, we introduce a new pipeline, and a new candidate generation scheme, which does not use labels as [2]. We then extract a set of generic features from each of these candidates, and train a novelty detector on the resulting data set. We assign a probability to each candidate proportional to its degree of surprise, and choose the candidates to be annotated by sampling from the resultant probability distribution. The annotated candidates are then fed into a binary classifier. The proposed pipeline is illustrated in Figure 1 as Way 1.

We test our pipeline and the proposed feature unpredictability based novelty detector on eight separately acquired sequences of human liver cell cultures, and three sequences of stem cell cultures. We have several interesting outcomes:

- Cell events can be detected almost as accurately as the fully-supervised case, and much more accurately than [6], by annotating less than 3% of the training data following the order suggested by the novelty detectors.
- The steepest learning curve is reached when a state-of-the-art collaborative multi-output GP regressor is used as the novelty detector, which is trained for predicting the feature vector of a candidate at frame t from its feature vector at the previous frame $t-1$, and the prediction error is calculated using the predictive mean and variance together, differently from [6] which uses only the predictive mean.
- Even though active learning (AL) looks like an intuitive solution to this problem (Figure 1 , Way 2), annotating the sequences using our unsupervised novelty detection (Way 1) performs clearly better than the studied algorithms.

2 Background Subtraction

As the common property of any event is an abrupt change in time, we propose taking the intensity difference of every consecutive frame, and fire a candidate event for each large enough connected component in the difference image. We threshold the intensity difference image from 25% of its brightest pixel value, filter out the components of the resultant binary image having an area smaller than 20 pixels, apply image opening with a 2-pixel disk, and finally fill the holes. Each connected component in the resultant image is treated as an event candidate. We represent a candidate by a 26-bin intensity histogram calculated on the intensity difference of that frame and its predecessor, 58 LBP features of the current frame, another 58 Local Binary Pattern (LBP) features for the difference from the predecessor, and 128 Scale Invariant Feature Transform (SIFT) features, similarly to earlier work on the same application [6].

3 Sparse Gaussian Processes

Let $\mathbf{X} = \{\mathbf{x}_1, \cdots, \mathbf{x}_N\}$ be a data set containing N instances $\mathbf{x}_n \in \mathbb{R}^D$, and $\mathbf{y} = \{y_1, \cdots, y_N\}$ be the corresponding real-valued outputs. The main drawback of the standard GP is the inversion of the $N \times N$ kernel matrix, which undermines the scalability of the standard GP. There exist several sparse approximations in the GP literature to overcome this problem. Here, we choose the FITC approximation [13]

$$\begin{aligned} p(\mathbf{u}|\mathbf{Z}, \boldsymbol{\theta}) &= \mathcal{N}(\mathbf{u}|\mathbf{0}, \mathbf{K}_{ZZ}), \\ p(\mathbf{f}|\mathbf{X}, \mathbf{u}, \mathbf{Z}, \boldsymbol{\theta}) &= \mathcal{N}(\mathbf{f}|\mathbf{K}_{ZX}^T \mathbf{K}_{ZZ}^{-1} \mathbf{u}, diag(\mathbf{K}_{XX} - \mathbf{K}_{ZX}^T \mathbf{K}_{ZZ}^{-1} \mathbf{K}_{ZX})), \\ p(\mathbf{y}|\mathbf{f}) &= \mathcal{N}(\mathbf{y}|\mathbf{f}, \sigma^2 \mathbf{I}), \end{aligned} \tag{1}$$

where $\mathcal{N}(\mathbf{x}|\boldsymbol{\mu}, \boldsymbol{\Sigma})$ is a multivariate normal distribution with mean $\boldsymbol{\mu}$ and covariance $\boldsymbol{\Sigma}$, is the vector of noise-free latent outputs, $\mathbf{Z}$ is the pseudo input data set, $\mathbf{u}$ is the vector of its pseudo targets, $\mathbf{K}_{ZX}$ is the kernel responses between $\mathbf{Z}$ and $\mathbf{X}$, the vector $\boldsymbol{\theta}$ has the kernel hyperparameters, and σ^2 is the variance of the white noise on the outputs. The sparse GP, denoted as $\mathcal{SGP}(\mathbf{f}, \mathbf{u}|\mathbf{Z}, \mathbf{X})$, is a parametric approximation to the non-parametric full GP. For regression, $\mathbf{u}$ is available in closed form as $p(\mathbf{u}|\mathbf{Z}, \mathbf{X}, \mathbf{y}, \boldsymbol{\theta}) = \mathcal{N}(\mathbf{u}|\mathbf{K}_{ZZ}\mathbf{Q}^{-1}\mathbf{K}_{ZX}(\boldsymbol{\Lambda} + \sigma^2\mathbf{I})^{-1}\mathbf{y}, \mathbf{K}_{ZZ}\mathbf{Q}^{-1}\mathbf{K}_{ZZ})$ where $\mathbf{Q} = \mathbf{K}_{ZZ} + \mathbf{K}_{ZX}(\boldsymbol{\Lambda} + \sigma^2\mathbf{I})^{-1}\mathbf{K}_{ZX}^T$ and $\boldsymbol{\Lambda} = \text{diag}(\boldsymbol{\lambda})$ with $\lambda_n = k_{xx} - \mathbf{k}_{Zx}^T \mathbf{K}_{ZZ}^{-1} \mathbf{k}_{Zx}$. Here, $\mathbf{k}_{Zx}$ is the kernel responses between $\mathbf{Z}$ and a single instance $\mathbf{x}$. The marginal likelihood is $p(\mathbf{y}|\mathbf{X}, \mathbf{Z}, \boldsymbol{\theta}) = \mathcal{N}(\mathbf{y}|\mathbf{0}, \mathbf{K}_{ZX}^T \mathbf{K}_{ZZ}^{-1} \mathbf{K}_{ZX} + \boldsymbol{\Lambda} + \sigma^2 \mathbf{I})$. The remaining parameters $\mathbf{Z}$ and $\boldsymbol{\theta}$ are learned by gradient descent.

For binary classification, it suffices to replace the likelihood in Equation 1 with $p(\mathbf{t}|\mathbf{f}) = \prod_{n=1}^N \Phi(f_n)^{t_n}(1 - \Phi(f_n))^{1-t_n}$, where $\Phi(s) = \dfrac{1}{\sqrt{2\pi}} \int_{-\infty}^{s} e^{-\frac{1}{2}s^2} ds$ is the probit link function and $\mathbf{t}$ is the vector of output classes $t_n \in \{-1, +1\}$. Since this likelihood is not conjugate with the normal distribution, the posterior $p(\mathbf{u}|\mathbf{Z}, \mathbf{X}, \mathbf{y}, \boldsymbol{\theta})$ is no longer available in closed form, hence has to be approximated. We choose the Laplace approximation due to its computational efficiency and yet reasonable performance [9].

Given the approximate posterior $q(\mathbf{u}|\mathbf{X}, \mathbf{Z}, \boldsymbol{\theta})$, and a newly seen instance $(\mathbf{x}_n, t_n)$, the predictive distribution is $p(t_n|\mathbf{t}) = \int \int p(t_n|f_n) p(f_n|\mathbf{X}, \mathbf{u}, \mathbf{Z}) q(\mathbf{u}|\mathbf{X}, \mathbf{Z}, \mathbf{t}) d\mathbf{u} df_n$.

We follow the common practice and take only the first integral with respect to $\mathbf{u}$, use the mean $\mu(\mathbf{x}_n)$ and variance $\sigma(\mathbf{x}_n)^2$ of the resultant normal distribution as the approximate predictive mean and variance, and replace the integral with respect to f_n with its point estimate. See [9] for further details.

4 Collaborative Multi-output Gaussian Processes for Novelty Detection

As the novelty detector, we follow the paradigm of Kandemir et al. [6] and propose the recent collaborative multi-output Gaussian process (CGP) regression model [8] as the feature predictor. The CGP is defined as

$$p(\mathbf{G},\mathbf{U}|\mathbf{Z},\mathbf{X}) = \prod_{j=1}^{Q} \mathcal{SGP}(\mathbf{g}_j,\mathbf{u}_j|\mathbf{Z}_j,\mathbf{X}), \;\; p(\mathbf{H},\mathbf{V}|\mathbf{W},\mathbf{X}) = \prod_{i=1}^{P} \mathcal{SGP}(\mathbf{h}_i,\mathbf{v}_i|\mathbf{W}_i,\mathbf{X}),$$

$$p(\mathbf{Y}|\mathbf{G},\mathbf{H}) = \prod_{i=1}^{P}\prod_{n=1}^{N} \mathcal{N}\Big(y_{in}\Big|\sum_{j=1}^{Q} w_{ij}g_j + h_i, \beta^{-1}\Big), \quad (2)$$

where $\mathbf{X}$ is a $N \times D$ matrix having D dimensional N instances in its rows, and $\mathbf{Y}$ is a $N \times P$ matrix having the corresponding P dimensional targets in its rows. Here, $\mathbf{g}_j$'s are sparse GPs shared across all output dimensions, and $\mathbf{h}_i$'s are sparse GPs specific to each output dimension. The likelihood in Equation 2 combines all these GPs linearly by the weights w_{ij}. The intractable posterior of this model is inferred by the efficient stochastic variational inference method. See [8] for further details. We use the source code provided by the authors [1].

Given the feature vector of a candidate at the previous frame $\mathbf{x}_n$, we plug its top 50 principal components into the CGP as input, and predict the top 5 principal components $\mathbf{y}_n$ of its features at the current frame as the output. As the degree of surprise, or Training Utility Value (TUV) in other terms, Kandemir et al. [6] propose using the squared distance between the mean of the predicted outputs $\boldsymbol{\mu}(\mathbf{x}_n) = [\mu_1(\mathbf{x}_n), \cdots, \mu_P(\mathbf{x}_n)]$ and the true observations $TUV(\mathbf{x}_n)_{MSE} = \|\boldsymbol{\mu}(\mathbf{x}_n) - \mathbf{y}_n\|_2^2$. We here propose to extend this measure by taking into account also the predictive variance which is shown to be useful in certain recognition tasks [11]. A principled way for this is to define a true distribution for the observed features $p_{true} = \mathcal{N}(\hat{\mathbf{y}_n}|\mathbf{y}_n, \epsilon\mathbf{I})$, with a very small ϵ, constructing spikes at the observed locations of the feature space, and use the Kullback-Leibler divergence between p_{true} and the predictive distribution $p_{pred} = \mathcal{N}(\hat{\mathbf{y}_n}|\boldsymbol{\mu}(\mathbf{x}_n), \boldsymbol{\Sigma}_n)$ as the degree of surprise, where $[\boldsymbol{\Sigma}_n]_{ii} = \sigma_i^2(\mathbf{x}_n)$ is the predictive variance for output dimension i, and $\hat{\mathbf{y}_n}$ is the predicted feature vector. The resultant training utility function becomes

$$TUV(\mathbf{x}_n)_{KL} = \frac{1}{2}\left(tr(\boldsymbol{\Sigma}_n^{-1}\epsilon\mathbf{I}) + (\boldsymbol{\mu}(\mathbf{x}_n) - \mathbf{y}_n)^T \boldsymbol{\Sigma}_n^{-1}(\boldsymbol{\mu}(\mathbf{x}_n) - \mathbf{y}_n) - \log\frac{|\epsilon\mathbf{I}|}{|\boldsymbol{\Sigma}_n|}\right).$$

Note that when $\boldsymbol{\Sigma}_n$ is equal for all instances, $TUV(\mathbf{x}_n)_{MSE}$ and $TUV(\mathbf{x}_n)_{KL}$ give identical orderings.

[1] `https://github.com/trungngv/multiplegp`

4.1 Proposal Generation by Sampling

Given the TUVs assigned to each instance, the question of how to use these values to choose the order for annotating the instances follows. We propose defining an N category multinomial distribution by assigning each instance a probability of being chosen $P(C = \mathbf{x}_n) = \frac{TUV(\mathbf{x}_n)}{\sum_{j=1}^{N} TUV(\mathbf{x}_j)}$. We determine the next instance to be annotated by taking a draw from this distribution. In multi-armed bandit formulation, each choice $C = \mathbf{x}_n$ can be viewed as an arm (a potential action), and $P(C = \mathbf{x}_n)$ the reward distribution. The most intuitive way of choosing the instances with the highest reward probability (i.e. largest TUV) corresponds to the *greedy* algorithm (exploitation), which is known to have linear regret. We have also observed it to give poor performance. Since almost all highest ranking instances are true events, choosing instances only from the top of the list causes class imbalance. Our approach, sampling from the reward distribution, corresponds to *probability matching*, which is a well-known technique for balancing exploration and exploitation.

5 Workflows

Way 1: Novelty detection plus supervised learning. As novelty detector we compare the following models: i) **CGP-KL**: CGP followed by $TUV(\mathbf{x}_n)_{KL}$, ii) **CGP-MSE**: CGP followed by $TUV(\mathbf{x}_n)_{MSE}$, iii) **OC-SVM**: The standard One-Class Support Vector Machine [10], iv) **150fps**: Sparse-coding based real-time novelty detection proposed by Lu et al. [7], as a representative of the dictionary learning based novelty detection methods.

The difference of **CGP-MSE** from [6] is that the former samples the instances to be annotated as in Section 4.1, and then trains a supervised classifier on the annotated instances, while the latter classifies the events directly by thresholding the TUVs.

Way 2: Active learning. We consider the following two active learning methods:

- **MES:** Maximum entropy sampling [12] annotates the instances in decreasing order with respect to: $TUV(\mathbf{x}_n) = \Big|p(y_n|\mathbf{X}_u, \mathbf{y}_u) - 0.5\Big|$, where $\mathbf{X}_u$ is the set of instances for which the labels $\mathbf{y}_u$ are known, $p(y_n|\mathbf{X}_u, \mathbf{y}_u)$ the predictive distribution of any probabilistic classifier, and $\mathbf{x}_n$ is an instance in the unlabeled set. In the well-known *exploration-exploitation* trade-off, this technique relies only on exploitation and ignores exploring the feature space.
- **BALD:** Bayesian Active Learning by Disagreement [1] follows a principled Bayesian approach and quantifies the importance of an instance by the change it is expected to make in the entropy of the model posterior

$$TUV(\mathbf{x}_n) = \mathbb{H}[\boldsymbol{\theta}|\mathbf{X}_u, \mathbf{y}_u] - \mathbb{E}_{p(y_n|\theta,\mathbf{x}_n)}\Big[\mathbb{H}[\boldsymbol{\theta}|\mathbf{X}_u, \mathbf{y}_u, \mathbf{x}_n, y_n]\Big],$$

  where $\mathbb{H}[\cdot] = \mathbb{E}_{p}(\cdot)[-\log p(\cdot)]$ stands for the entropy function and $p(\boldsymbol{\theta}|\mathbf{X}_u, \mathbf{y}_u)$ is the posterior of a model. BALD has been shown to handle the exploration-exploitation trade-off in a balanced way, since the first term always favors the most uncertain instance (i.e. equals to MES), hence, performs exploitation, and the second term performs exploration by penalizing the terms with high intrinsic noise. The BALD for the standard GP classifier follows as

$$TUV(\mathbf{x}_n) = \Phi\left(\frac{\mu(\mathbf{x}_n)}{\sqrt{\sigma(\mathbf{x}_n)^2+1}}\right) - \frac{\sqrt{\frac{\pi \log 2}{2}}}{\sqrt{\sigma(\mathbf{x}_n)^2+\frac{\pi \log 2}{2}}} \exp\left(\frac{\mu(\mathbf{x}_n)^2}{2\sigma(\mathbf{x}_n)^2+\pi \log 2}\right).$$

6 Experiments

We detect mitosis and apoptosis events in phase-contrast microscopy sequences independently acquired from two different live cell tissues: i) a human osteosarcoma cell line that consists of eight sequences of 134 frames each, and ii) the public stem cell line data set of Huh et al. [4] that consists of three sequences of 540 frames each. For the stem cell data set, only apoptotic events were publicly available. We also annotated the mitotic events to make the two applications comparable. In all experiments, a model is trained on one sequence and tested on another. All results are averaged over all possible training-test combinations of the sequences of a given tissue type.

We used the standard Gaussian process classifier with a probit link likelihood as the supervised event predictor (the *Classifier* box in Figure 1) and with a squared exponential kernel function with isotropic covariance $k(\mathbf{x}, \mathbf{x}') = \gamma_0 \exp(-\gamma_1 \|\mathbf{x} - \mathbf{x}'\|_2^2)$. The kernel hyperparameters γ_0 and γ_1 are learned by Type II Maximum Likelihood. Since MES and BALD cannot perform an absolute cold-start (an empty labeled set), we started these models from a randomly chosen 10 labeled instances.

6.1 Event Detection from Few Annotations

The main goal of our workflow is to direct the annotator to the relevant instances in the sequence. We achieve this without any supervision, differently from Kandemir et al.'s MOGP [6], which requires a small number of frames without any events to be provided. Figure 2 shows highest ranking five cell event candidates found by the four novelty detectors. CGP-KL, CGP-MSE, and OC-SVM all retrieve comparably relevant candidates. However, as seen in Figure 3, the TUVs found by CGP-KL lead to the steepest learning curve with respect to F1 score (harmonic mean of precision and recall), when a GP classifier is trained with an increasing number of annotated instances. For the novelty detectors, new training instances are chosen in each round using the sampling method described in Section 4.1. For the AL models, the unlabeled instances with largest TUV are chosen, following the theoretically grounded and commonly adopted way. While for the AL models the choice of new instances at a round is dependent on the choices and the trained classifiers of the previous rounds, the novelty detectors are trained once on an unsupervised sequence, and then provide a labeling order on a target sequence independently of the classifier. Despite not using any labeled data for proposal generation, the novelty detectors have a more stable learning curve. In both cell types, the two AL algorithms either saturate immaturely as for osteosarcoma, or overfit and harm the classifier in the later rounds as for the stem cell. For osteosarcoma, the fully supervised learning performance is exactly reached, and even slightly exceeded after only

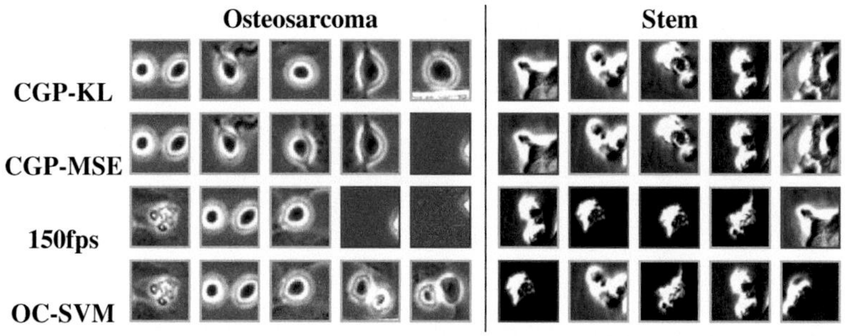

Fig. 2. Highest ranking cell event candidates are sorted from left to right in decreasing TUV. Green frame around a patch indicates that the candidate corresponds to an event, and red frame indicates that it is a false positive.

$10(initial) + 15(rounds) \times 5(questions) = 85$ annotations (2.4% of the candidates), and for the stem cell, 95% of the fully supervised learning performance is covered after $10(initial) + 30(rounds) \times 10(questions)$ annotations (1.9% of the candidates).

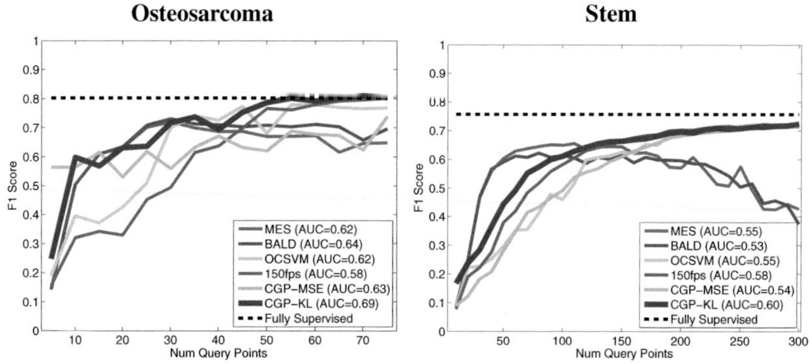

Fig. 3. Learning curves of the sparse GP classifier when it is trained with instances chosen by the novelty detectors and the AL algorithms. A higher Area Under Learning Curve (AUC) indicates faster learning, which is desired. CGP-KL provides highest AUC in both tissue types.

In both tissue types, CGP-KL outperforms Kandemir et al. [6] with $F1 = 0.81$ vs. $F1 = 0.77$ for Osteosarcoma, and $F1 = 0.74$ vs. $F1 = 0.65$ for Stem from comparably few annotator effort ($< 3\%$ of candidates from both classes for CGP-KL versus five frames from the negative class for [6]). We observed that linear combination of the TUV's of CGP-KL and any of the AL algorithms never improves on CGP-KL alone.

Failure cases of our entire framework include floating dead cells, events taking place at the image boundaries or behind the white grid in osteosarcoma sequences, and events taking place more slowly than usual.

7 Discussion

The suboptimal performance of the AL models in the problem we studied is due to the severe class imbalance coming from the nature of the event detection problem, which makes the positive instances look overly valuable for the AL models. Hence, these models focus only on refining the decision boundary, ending up overfitting. This could also be seen from the fact that MES and BALD follow very similar learning patterns for both applications. In other words, BALD reduces to MES under class imbalance. Another reason for their suboptimal performance is the cold-start problem. AL algorithms require a labeled starting subset (warm start) that includes instances from both classes, which raises yet another novelty detection problem. On the contrary, the novelty detectors benefit from the class imbalance by using it as a modeling assumption.

The fact that clearly higher accuracies can be reached with a small annotation effort could be noteworthy for further studies in the image-based cell behavior analysis field. Our pipeline can be integrated into an annotation software used by biologists, and could provide them an importance ordering of the locations to be looked in large sequences. This would bring a remarkable effort gain given that expert annotator time is very costly.

References

1. Houlsby, N., Huszar, F., Ghahramani, Z., Hernández-Lobato, J.M.: Collaborative Gaussian processes for preference learning. In: NIPS (2012)
2. Huh, S., Chen, M.: Detection of mitosis within a stem cell population of high cell confluence in phase-contrast microscopy images. In: CVPR (2011)
3. Huh, S., Ker, D.-F.E., Bise, R., Chen, M., Kanade, T.: Automated mitosis detection of stem cell populations in phase-contrast microscopy images. Trans. Medical Imaging 30(3), 586–596 (2011)
4. Huh, S., Ker, D.F.E., Su, H., Kanade, T.: Apoptosis detection for adherent cell populations in time-lapse phase-contrast microscopy images. In: Ayache, N., Delingette, H., Golland, P., Mori, K. (eds.) MICCAI 2012, Part I. LNCS, vol. 7510, pp. 331–339. Springer, Heidelberg (2012)
5. Kaakinen, M., Huttinen, S., Paavolainen, L., Marjomaki, V., Heikkila, J., Eklund, L.: Automatic detection and analysis of cell motility in phase-contrast time-lapse images using a combination of maximally stable extremal regions and kalman filter approaches. Journal of Microscopy 253(1), 65–78 (2014)
6. Kandemir, M., Rubio, J.C., Schmidt, U., Wojek, C., Welbl, J., Ommer, B., Hamprecht, F.A.: Event Detection by Feature Unpredictability in Phase-Contrast Videos of Cell Cultures. In: Golland, P., Hata, N., Barillot, C., Hornegger, J., Howe, R. (eds.) MICCAI 2014, Part II. LNCS, vol. 8674, pp. 154–161. Springer, Heidelberg (2014)
7. Lu, C., Shi, J., Jia, J.: Abnormal event detection at 150 fps in MATLAB. In: ICCV, pp. 2720–2727 (2013)
8. Nguyen, V.T., Bonilla, E.: Collaborative multi-output Gaussian processes. In: UAI (2014)
9. Rasmussen, C.E., Williams, C.I.: Gaussian processes for machine learning (2006)
10. Schölkopf, B., Platt, J.C., Shawe-Taylor, J., Smola, A.J., Williamson, R.C.: Estimating the support of a high-dimensional distribution. Neural Computation 13(7), 1443–1471 (2001)
11. Seeger, M.: Bayesian Gaussian process models: PAC-Bayesian generalisation error bounds and sparse approximations. PhD Thesis (2003)
12. Shewry, M.C., Wynn, H.P.: Maximum entropy sampling. Journal of Applied Statistics 14(2), 165–170 (1987)
13. Snelson, E., Ghahramani, Z.: Sparse Gaussian processes using pseudo-inputs. In: NIPS (2006)

Robust Muscle Cell Quantification Using Structured Edge Detection and Hierarchical Segmentation

Fujun Liu[1], Fuyong Xing[1], Zizhao Zhang[2], Mason Mcgough[3], and Lin Yang[1,3]

[1] Department of Electrical and Computer Engineering
[2] Department of Computer and Information Science and Engineering
[3] J. Crayton Pruitt Family Department of Biomedical Engineering, University of Florida, USA

Abstract. Morphological characteristics of muscle cells, such as cross-sectional areas (CSAs), are critical factors to determine the muscle health. Automatic muscle cell segmentation is often the first prerequisite for quantitative analysis. In this paper, we have proposed a novel muscle cell segmentation algorithm that contains two steps: 1) A structured edge detection algorithm that can capture the inherent edge patterns of muscle images, and 2) a hierarchical segmentation algorithm. A set of nested partitions are first constructed, and a best subset selection algorithm is then designed to choose a maximum weighted subset of non-overlapping partitions as the final segmentation result. We have experimentally demonstrated that the proposed structured edge detection based hierarchical segmentation algorithm outperforms other state of the arts for muscle image segmentation.

1 Introduction

The ability to accurately and efficiently quantify the morphological characteristics of muscle cells, such as cross-sectional areas (CSAs), is essential to determine the health conditions of muscles. Automatic muscle cell segmentation plays a significant role in calculating the morphological parameters. There are two major challenges for muscle cell segmentation: 1) Because muscle cells always touch with one another, it is critical to design an efficient and effective muscle cell edge detection algorithm, and 2) because the strength of the muscle cell boundary varies significantly, segmentation algorithms using a fixed parameter often fail to produce satisfactory results for all the regions in one digitized muscle specimens.

In this paper, we propose a structured edge detection based hierarchical segmentation algorithm for muscle image segmentation. The structured edge detection, which can better capture inherent muscle image edge structures, is achieved by extending a random decision forest framework. It is noted in [1,2] that, by storing structure information at the leaf nodes of the random decision tree other than class probabilities, random decision forest can be conveniently used for

N. Navab et al. (Eds.): MICCAI 2015, Part III, LNCS 9351, pp. 324–331, 2015.
DOI: 10.1007/978-3-319-24574-4_39

structured learning. Different from the traditional edge detection method [3], edge masks instead of edge probability values will be stored at the leaf nodes in our proposed structured edge detection algorithm. In order to accurately segment each muscle cell exhibiting both strong and weak boundaries, a hierarchical segmentation method is proposed, which takes a set of partitions produced by applying a segmentation algorithm with varying parameters as inputs, and selects a best subset of non-overlapping partition regions as the final result.

An overview of our proposed muscle image segmentation algorithm is shown in Fig. 1. Given an image patch, 1) an edge map is generated by the proposed structured edge detection algorithm; 2) an Ultrametric Contour Map (UCM) [3] is constructed and a set of segmentation candidates is generated by adjusting the thresholds of UCM; and 3) an efficient dynamic programming based subset selection algorithm is then used to choose the best regions for muscle image segmentation based on a constructed tree graph.

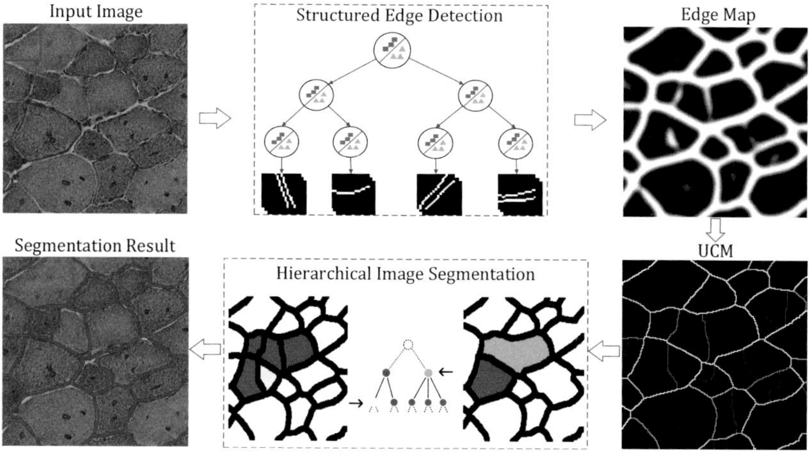

Fig. 1. An overview of the proposed muscle image segmentation algorithm.

2 Structured Edge Detection

Random Decision Forest. We start with a brief review of the random decision forest. A decision forest $\mathcal{F} = \{T_t\}$ is an ensemble of decision trees T_t, which are trained independently on randomly selected samples $S = \{s_i = (x_i \in \mathcal{X}, y_i \in \mathcal{Y})\}$, where $\mathcal{X}$ and $\mathcal{Y}$ denote the input features and output labels, respectively. A decision tree $T_t(x)$ produces the prediction results by recursively branching a feature sample $x \in \mathcal{X}$ left or right down the tree until a leaf node is reached. For a decision forest, the predictions $T_t(x)$ from individual trees are combined together using an ensemble model. Majority voting and averaging are common ensemble choices for classification and regression problems, respectively.

During the training of a decision tree, at each node n, a split function $h(x, \theta_n)$ is chosen to split the samples S_n into left S_n^L or right S_n^R. For multiclass classification, the split function $h(x, \theta_n)$ is optimized by maximizing the information gain

$$\mathcal{I}(S_n) = H(S_n) - \Big(\frac{|S_n^L|}{|S_n|}H(S_n^L) + \frac{|S_n^R|}{|S_n|}H(S_n^R)\Big), \tag{1}$$

where $H(\cdot)$ is the class entropy function. The split function $h(x, \theta_n)$ can be an arbitrary classifier. A common choice is a stump function that is found to be computationally efficient and effective in practice [2]. The training procedure continues to split the samples until either a maximum depth is reached, or too few samples are left, or information gain falls below a certain threshold.

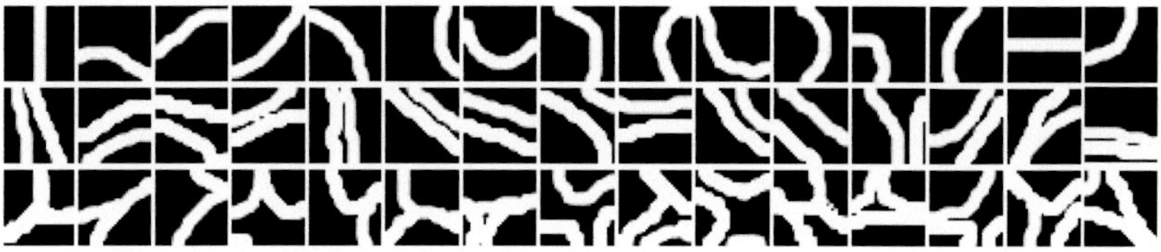

Fig. 2. Some sample edge masks learned and stored at the leaf nodes of the random decision trees.

Structured Edge Detection. Since a decision tree classifier generates the actual prediction at the leaf nodes, more information can be stored at the leaf nodes than class likelihoods. For example, in [1], structured class label information is stored at leaf nodes for semantic image segmentation. Inspired by [2,4], we propose to store edge structure information at the leaf nodes for structured muscle image edge detection. Different from traditional edge detection algorithms [3], which take an image patch x as an input and compute the probability of the edge existence at the center pixel p, the output of our proposed structured edge detection algorithm is an edge mask around the central pixel p instead of the likelihood value. As shown in Fig. 1, after learning the decision tree, the median of the edge masks sent to the leaf node will be stored as the leaf node output.

The information gain criteria in Equation (1) is effective in practice for decision tree training. In order to follow this criteria, the edge masks must be explicitly assigned proper class labels at each internal node of the tree during the training stage. One straightforward idea is to group the edge masks at a node into several clusters by an unsupervised clustering algorithm such as k-means or mean-shift, and then treat each cluster *id* as the class label for the sample belonging to that cluster. However, the edge masks $\mathcal{Y}$ do not reside in the Euclidean space and directly grouping them may not generate desired results. In addition, clustering in high dimension space ($y \in \mathbb{R}^{256 \times 1}$ for an 16×16 edge mask) is computationally expensive. In this paper, we proposed to reduce the high dimension edge masks $\mathcal{Y} \in \mathbb{R}^n$ to a lower dimensional subspace $\mathcal{Z} \in \mathbb{R}^m$ ($m << n$) using an autoencoder [5] before clustering the edge masks. In this paper, we use the matrix form and vector form of edge mask space $\mathcal{Y}$ interchangeably.

Autoencoder is one of the state-of-the-art unsupervised nonlinear dimension reduction methods. The training of an autoencoder consists of both the pretraining step, which consists of learning a stack of restricted Boltzmann machines

(RBMs) layer by layer, and the fine-tuning step that seeks to minimize the discrepancy between the original data and its reconstruction. For an autoencoder with L layers,

$$y^l = \sigma(W^l y^{l-1} + b^l), \tag{2}$$

where $\sigma(t) = 1/(1+e^{-t})$, $y^0 = y \in \mathcal{Y}, y^L = z \in \mathcal{Z}$, and W^l, b^l, $l = [1 \cdots L]$ are parameters to be learned in training the autoencoder.

Please note that although the transformed data z is used to choose split function $h(x, \theta_n)$ in training the decision tree, only the original edge mask y is stored at leaf nodes for the prediction. Some sample edge masks learned and stored at the leaf nodes are shown in Fig. 2. As one can tell that many edge structures are unique for muscle cell boundaries, which demonstrate the effectiveness of the structured edge detection procedure.

Our proposed structured edge detection algorithm takes a 32×32 image patch as input and generates a 16×16 edge mask around the input's center pixel. The image patch is represented with the same high-dimensional feature used in [2,6], which is effective and computationally efficient. In total, two million samples are randomly generated to train the structured decision random forest, which consists of 8 decision trees. The autoencoder model used in our work consists of an encoder with layers of sizes $(16 \times 16) - 512 - 256 - 30$ and a symmetric decoder. The autoencoder model is trained once offline and applied to all decision trees, and the data compression is only performed at the root node.

3 Hierarchical Image Segmentation

Hierarchical strategy has been successfully applied to image segmentation recently [7,8]. In general, the hierarchical image segmentation consists of two steps: 1) A collection of segmentation candidates is generated by running some existing segmentation algorithms with different parameters. Usually, an undirected graph is constructed from these partition candidates where an edge exists between two overlapping regions; 2) Based on some domain-specific criteria, a maximal weighted independent set (MWIS) of the constructed graph is selected as the final segmentation results. For example, Felzenszwalb's method [9] with multiple levels is used to generate the segmentation candidate pool. An optimal purity cover algorithm is used in [7] to select the most representative regions. In [8], the watershed segmentation method with different thresholds gives a collection of partitions and a conditional random field (CRF) based learning algorithm is utilized to find the best ensembles to present the final segmentation results.

However, the MWIS problem on a general graph is NP-hard and usually difficult to optimize. In this work, an Ultrametric Contour Map (UCM) [3] is first constructed on the edge map generated by the proposed structured edge detection algorithm presented in the previous section, then the pool of segmentation candidates is produced by setting different thresholds of UCM. Because of the nice property of UCM where the segmentation results using different thresholds are nested into one another, we can construct a tree graph for this pool of segmentation candidates. The final step is to solve this tree graph based MWIS problem using dynamic programming.

Given a set of segmentation candidates generated with different thresholds using UCM, an undirected and weighted tree graph, $G = (V, E, w)$, is constructed, where $V = \{v_i, i = 1, 2, ..., n\}$ represents the nodes with each v_i corresponding to a segmented region R_i. E denotes the edges of the graph. The $w(v_i)$ is learned via a general random decision forest classifier to represent the likelihood of R_i as a real muscle cell. An adjacent matrix $A = \{a_{ij}|i, j = 1, ..., n\}$ is then built with $a_{ij} = 1$ if $R_i \subset R_j$ or $R_j \subset R_i$, and otherwise 0. Denote $\mathbf{x} \in \{0,1\}^n$ the indicator vector, where its element is equal to 1 if the corresponding node is selected, otherwise 0. Finally, the constrained subset selection problem is formulated as

$$\mathbf{x}^* = \arg\max_{\mathbf{x}} w^T \mathbf{x}, \ s.\ t.\ x_i + x_j \leq 1, if\ a_{ij} = 1. \tag{3}$$

Considering the special tree graph structure, (3) can be efficiently solved via the dynamic programming approach with a bottom-to-up strategy.

Muscle Cell Likelihood Generation. In order to ensure that (3) selects the desired regions, each candidate region (node) must be assigned an appropriate muscle cell likelihood score w. In our work, each candidate region is discriminatively represented with a feature vector that consists of a descriptor to model the convexity of the shape, and two histograms to describe the gradient magnitudes of the pixels on the cell boundary and inside the cell region. These morphological features are proposed based on the following observations: 1) The shape of a muscle cell is nearly convex; 2) The cell boundaries often exhibit higher gradient magnitudes; 3) The intensities within the cell regions should be relatively homogeneous.

4 Experiments

The proposed algorithm is tested using 120 H&E-stained muscle cell images captured at 10× magnification. Each image contains around 200 muscle cells. The images are randomly split into two sets with equal size. The ground truth of each individual muscle cell is manually annotated. To quantitatively analyze the pixel-wise segmentation accuracy, we calculate the precision $P = \frac{|S \cap G|}{|S|}$, recall $R = \frac{|S \cap G|}{|G|}$, and F_1-score $F_1 = \frac{2*P*R}{P+R}$, where S denotes the segmentation result and G is the ground truth.

Both the proposed structured edge detection algorithm and the hierarchical image segmentation method are evaluated and compared with three state-of-the-art methods: 1) Isoperimetric graph partition (ISO) [10] that produces high quality segmentations as a spectral method with improved speed and stability, 2) global probability of boundary detector (gPb) [3] that is widely used in natural image segmentation, and 3) a deep convolutional neural network (DCNN) method that is widely adopted as recent state-of-the-art for detection and segmentation. The trained DCNN model consists of six learned layers including three convolutional layers with filter sizes (4 × 4, 3 × 3, and 2 × 2), and three fully connected layers with neuron numbers (500, 250, and 2). Each convolutional layer has 20 output maps and is followed by a max pooling layer with pooling size 2×2. Rectifier activation $f(x) = \max(0, x)$ is applied to all parameter layers except the last fully connected layer (output layer) where a 2-way softmax nonlinear activation is used. In total, two million image patches with size 51×51, half positive and half negative, are randomly generated from 60 images to train the DCNN model. The training of DCNN is carried out using open source tool Caffe [11].

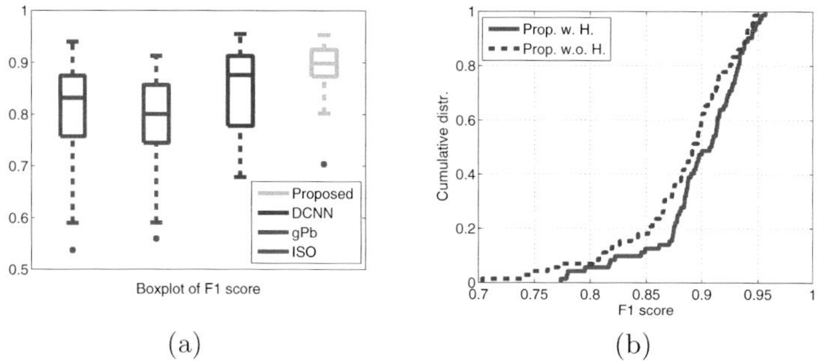

Fig. 3. The comparative segmentation results of the proposed muscle image segmentation algorithm.

Experimental Results for Structured Edge Detection. For fair comparison, UCM is first constructed for edge detection based methods including gPb [3], DCNN, and the proposed structured edge detection algorithm. The segmentation is done by changing thresholds of UCM. Different segmentation results are generated for each algorithm. Only the results with highest F_1-score are reported. Similar to ISO, multiple segmentations are produced by varying the isoperimetric parameter and the best result is reported. The comparative boxplots of F_1-scores are shown in Fig. 3 (a). We can see that our structured edge detection based segmentation algorithm outperforms other methods [10], [3] and DCNN for muscle specimens. The quantitative comparative results are shown in Table 1, where we report the average and standard variance of F_1-score, precision, and recall.

It is worth to note that the proposed structured edge detection algorithm indeed performs better than DCNN for the muscle image dataset. One reason is that we do not have sufficient training data to learn a DCNN model that is sufficient to capture all the edge variations. A larger DCNN model with more training data might be able to achieve better performance. With respect to speed, the current DCNN model takes 28 seconds to generate an edge map for segmentation on an image with size 1024×768, which is much slower than our structured edge detection (less than 1 second).

Experimental Results for Hierarchical Segmentation. In this part, five different segmentations are produced by setting thresholds $0.9, 0.8, 0.6, 0.4$, and 0.2 of UCM constructed from the proposed edge detection algorithm. The segmentation with threshold 0.6 achieves highest F_1-score. The hierarchical segmentation is achieved by solving Equation (3). In this text, we use Prop. w.o. H. to denote the proposed structured detection based segmentation algorithm

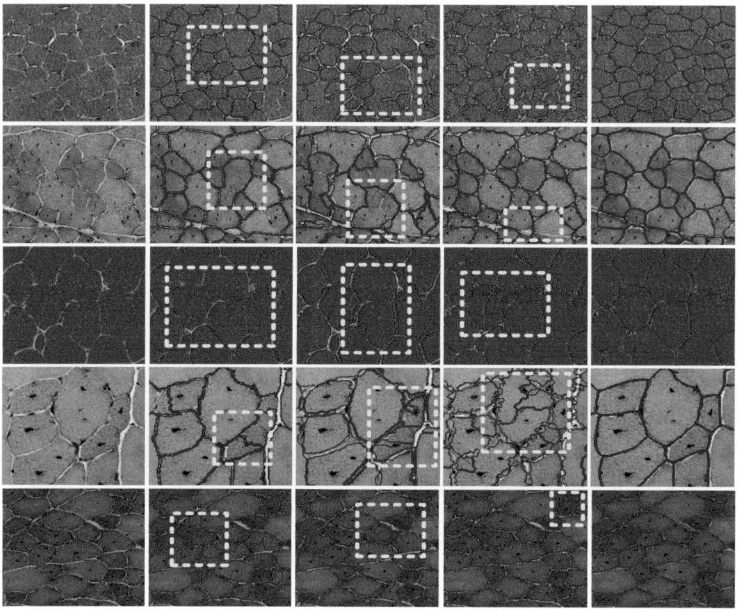

Fig. 4. Some qualitative segmentation results. From left to right, the columns denote the original image patch, the segmentation results using ISO [10], gPb [3], DCNN, and the proposed method. The yellow rectangles highlight some regions with segmentation errors.

Table 1. The pixel-wise segmentation accuracy

Method	F_1-score		Prec.		Rec.	
	mean	std	mean	std	mean	std
ISO[10]	0.8050	0.0993	0.8988	0.0589	0.7429	0.1369
gPb[3]	0.7904	0.0780	0.9123	0.0515	0.7011	0.0962
DCNN	0.8388	0.1073	**0.9464**	**0.0411**	0.7666	0.1441
Prop. w.o. H.	0.8815	0.0523	0.8861	0.0551	0.8783	0.0587
Prop. w. H.	**0.8974**	**0.0422**	0.9078	0.0433	**0.8888**	**0.0543**

without using hierarchical segmentation, and Prop. w. H. to denote the hierarchical segmentation results. The comparative results are shown in Fig. 3 (b), where the cumulative distributions $F(x) = Pr(t \leq x)$ with respect to F_1-scores are plotted. By comparing their cumulative distributions in Fig. 3, we can see that the proposed hierarchical segmentation consistently achieves better results than single segmentation with even fine-tuned parameter. In addition, as shown in Table 1, the hierarchical segmentation also gives the lowest variance with respect to F_1 score, which indicates strong robustness. The proposed hierarchical segmentation method is also more practical since it is not always possible or convenient to fine-tune the parameter at runtime for new testing images.

Based on our experimental results, we conclude that: 1) The proposed structured edge detection algorithm outperforms the state-of-the-art edge detection methods including gPb[3] and DCNN for muscle images. 2) The proposed hierarchical segmentation method consistently boosts the overall segmentation accuracy and also provides strong robustness. For better illustration, several qualitative segmentation results are presented in Fig. 4.

5 Conclusion

In this paper, we have proposed a structured edge detection based hierarchical segmentation algorithm for muscle image segmentation. Compared with traditional edge detection methods, the proposed structured edge detection algorithm can better capture the inherent muscle image edge structures such that it can accurately and efficiently detect the muscle cell boundaries. We have experimentally demonstrated that the proposed hierarchical segmentation method exceeds the performance of many state of the art segmentation methods even with fine-tuned parameters.

References

1. Kontschieder, P., Bulo, S.R., Bischof, H., Pelillo, M.: Structured class-labels in random forests for semantic image labelling. In: ICCV 2011, pp. 2190–2197. IEEE (2011)
2. Dollár, P., Zitnick, C.L.: Structured forests for fast edge detection. In: ICCV 2013, pp. 1841–1848. IEEE (2013)
3. Arbelaez, P., Maire, M., Fowlkes, C., Malik, J.: Contour detection and hierarchical image segmentation. PAMI 33(5), 898–916 (2011)
4. Chen, Y.T., Yang, J., Yang, M.H.: Extracting image regions by structured edge prediction. In: WACV 2015, pp. 1060–1067. IEEE (2015)
5. Hinton, G.E., Salakhutdinov, R.R.: Reducing the dimensionality of data with neural networks. Science 313(5786), 504–507 (2006)
6. Arbelaez, P., Pont-Tuset, J., Barron, J., Marques, F., Malik, J.: Multiscale combinatorial grouping. In: CVPR 2014, pp. 328–335. IEEE (2014)
7. Farabet, C., Couprie, C., Najman, L., LeCun, Y.: Learning hierarchical features for scene labeling. PAMI 35(8), 1915–1929 (2013)
8. Uzunbaş, M.G., Chen, C., Metaxsas, D.: Optree: A learning-based adaptive watershed algorithm for neuron segmentation. In: Golland, P., Hata, N., Barillot, C., Hornegger, J., Howe, R. (eds.) MICCAI 2014, Part I. LNCS, vol. 8673, pp. 97–105. Springer, Heidelberg (2014)
9. Felzenszwalb, P.F., Huttenlocher, D.P.: Efficient graph-based image segmentation. IJCV 59(2), 167–181 (2004)
10. Grady, L., Schwartz, E.L.: Isoperimetric graph partitioning for image segmentation. PAMI 28(3), 469–475 (2006)
11. Jia, Y., Shelhamer, E., Donahue, J., Karayev, S., Long, J., Girshick, R., Guadarrama, S., Darrell, T.: Caffe: Convolutional architecture for fast feature embedding. In: Proceedings of the ACM International Conference on Multimedia, pp. 675–678. ACM (2014)

Fast Cell Segmentation Using Scalable Sparse Manifold Learning and Affine Transform-Approximated Active Contour

Fuyong Xing[1,2] and Lin Yang[1,2]

[1] Department of Electrical and Computer Engineering
[2] J. Crayton Pruitt Family Department of Biomedical Engineering, University of Florida, Gainesville, FL 32611, USA

Abstract. Efficient and effective cell segmentation of neuroendocrine tumor (NET) in whole slide scanned images is a difficult task due to a large number of cells. The weak or misleading cell boundaries also present significant challenges. In this paper, we propose a fast, high throughput cell segmentation algorithm by combining top-down shape models and bottom-up image appearance information. A scalable sparse manifold learning method is proposed to model multiple subpopulations of different cell shape priors. Followed by a shape clustering on the manifold, a novel affine transform-approximated active contour model is derived to deform contours without solving a large amount of computationally-expensive Euler-Lagrange equations, and thus dramatically reduces the computational time. To the best of our knowledge, this is the first report of a high throughput cell segmentation algorithm for whole slide scanned pathology specimens using manifold learning to accelerate active contour models. The proposed approach is tested using 12 NET images, and the comparative experiments with the state of the arts demonstrate its superior performance in terms of both efficiency and effectiveness.

1 Introduction

Effective and efficient cell segmentation of pancreatic neuroendocrine tumor (NET) is a prerequisite for quantitative image analyses such as Ki67 counting. Many state-of-the-art approaches [11,4,16,10] have been applied to cell/nucleus segmentation on specific medical images. In order to handle partial occlusion, shape prior models have been introduced to improve touching cell separation [2,14] and liver segmentation [17].

However, it is inefficient to exploit the aforementioned shape prior models, which are not adaptive to large data sets, to fast segment thousands of cells in whole slide scanned specimens. In addition, it is necessary to learn multiple subpopulations of shape priors to handle shape variations. In this paper, we propose a high throughput and large-scale cell segmentation algorithm by combing high-level shape priors and low-level active contour models. The main contributions are: 1) A scalable sparse manifold learning algorithm to model multiple cell shape priors; 2) A novel affine transform-approximated active contour model that dramatically accelerates the shape deformation.

N. Navab et al. (Eds.): MICCAI 2015, Part III, LNCS 9351, pp. 332–339, 2015.
DOI: 10.1007/978-3-319-24574-4_40

2 Methodology

An effective cell segmentation framework combining shape prior models and image appearance information is presented in [14]; however, it requires to solve one associated partial differential equation for each contour within each iteration and therefore is not suitable to handle a large number of cells in whole slide scanned images. In this paper, we propose a novel idea by assuming that there exists an affine transformation between any two similar cell shapes, and approximate shape deformation using the affine transformation instead of solving all computationally expensive Euler-Lagrange equations. In addition, since the shapes of cells on pancreatic NET images lie on a low-dimensional manifold due to the limited number of constraints of shape control (see Figure 1), we present a scalable sparse manifold learning algorithm for cell shape modeling, which can efficiently determine the shape memberships and perform the shape inference. In our algorithm, similar shapes are effectively grouped into the same cluster by taking advantage of the manifold geometry structure to allow the affine approximation for fast shape deformation in each cluster.

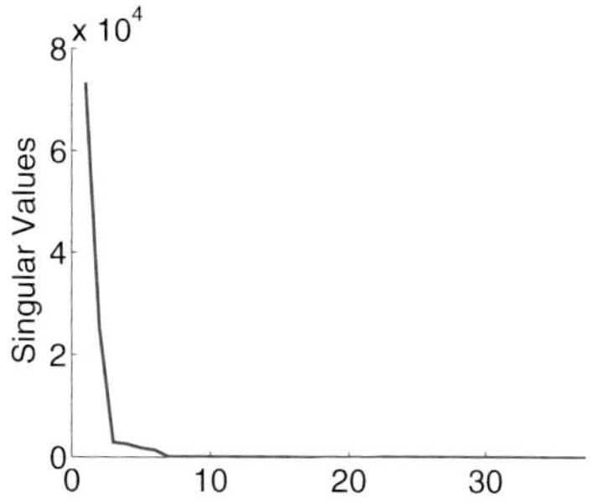

Fig. 1. The singular values of cell shapes. The first 6 singular values are nonzero and significantly larger than the rest, and thus cell shapes actually lie in a union of subspaces with dimension around 6.

In the training stage, the cell shapes aligned with Procrustes analysis [7] are utilized to learn multiple subpopulations of shape priors using sparse manifold clustering and embedding. A deep convolutional neural network (CNN) [6] is trained with small image patches for shape initialization. In the testing stage, the CNN is exploited to generate probability maps with a sliding window on images, and initial cell shapes are obtained by applying an H-minima transform [5] to the maps, one per cell. These shapes deform towards cell boundaries with the affine transform-approximated deformable model. Meanwhile, shape inference and membership update are achieved by using the scalable manifold learning based on the learned shape repositories. The proposed approach alternately performs shape deformation and inference until the active contours converge.

2.1 Scalable Sparse Manifold Learning for Shape Prior Modeling

In our model, cell shape $x \in R^{2p \times 1}$ is represented by $p = 60$ landmarks following the rules in [14]. We propose to model shape priors by clustering training shapes into multiple subpopulations considering the intrinsic dimensionality of the manifold. The sparse manifold clustering and embedding (SMCE) [8] can robustly achieve simultaneous clustering and dimensionality reduction. However, SMCE is a transductive algorithm that is not able to handle out-of-sample data, and it requires a computational complexity of $\mathcal{O}(N^3)$ to solve the optimization problem over N new testing shapes. In this paper, we efficiently extend SMCE to handle out-of-sample data and update shape clusters via sparse encoding-based shape inference. Specifically, we first apply SMCE to the limited-size training data and obtain multiple subpopulations of cell shapes, then perform sparse encoding for each new shape, and finally assign the new shapes to corresponding clusters. In this scenario, the runtime computational complexity can be reduced from $\mathcal{O}(N^3)$ to $\mathcal{O}(N \cdot M^2)$ where M is the number of training shapes with $M \ll N$.

Shape Prior Modeling via Manifold Learning: SMCE formulates an optimization problem based on sparse representation to allow simultaneous clustering and embedding of data lying in multiple manifolds. Given a set of aligned training cell shapes $\{x_i\}_{i=1}^M$, SMCE solves the following problem

$$\min_{c_i} \gamma||Q_i c_i||_1 + ||X_i c_i||_2, s.t.\ \mathbf{1}^T c_i = 1,\ \forall i, \tag{1}$$

where $Q_i \in R^{(M-1)\times(M-1)}$ represents the proximity, and it is a positive-definite diagonal matrix with the j-th diagonal element equal to $\frac{||x_j - x_i||_2}{\sum_{k\neq i}||x_k - x_i||_2}$, such that the points near x_i receive low penalties. $X_i \in R^{2p\times(M-1)}$ is the normalized shape matrix and the j-th column is $\frac{x_j - x_i}{||x_j - x_i||_2}, j \neq i$. The γ is the sparsity weight, and $\mathbf{1}^T c_i = 1$ ensures translation invariance. Based on the solution to (1), we can build a similarity graph whose nodes represent the data points [8], and the manifold clustering is achieved by applying spectral clustering to the graph.

Shape Inference and Cluster Update: After the manifold clustering, we can obtain multiple subpopulations of shape priors $\{\phi_k \in R^{2p\times M_k}\}_{k=1}^K$. The original shapes whose embedding vectors lie in the same manifold are similar to each other and form a shape repository/cluster, which is used to perform runtime shape inference for cell shapes assigned to this cluster in the testing stage. It is challenging to efficiently perform shape inference and determine the memberships of out-of-sample data considering the intrinsic dimensionality. Fortunately, any Lipschitz-smooth function defined on a smooth nonlinear manifold can be effectively approximated by a globally linear function with respect to local coordinate coding [15], and the time complexity of sparse encoding completely depends on the much lower intrinsic dimensionality. This indicates that each shape can be sufficiently represented by its coding based on its neighbors. Therefore, we propose to achieve shape inference and cluster update in a unified manner via sparse encoding. Specifically, given the learned shape repository $\Phi = [\phi_1 ... \phi_K] = [\psi_1 ... \psi_M] \in R^{2p\times M}$, we perform runtime shape inference

$$\min_{\{\alpha_i\}} \sum_{i=1}^{N} (||v_i - \Phi\alpha_i||_2 + \lambda \sum_{j=1}^{M} |\alpha_i|||\psi_j - v_i||^2), s.t.\ \mathbf{1}^T \alpha_i = 1,\ \forall i. \tag{2}$$

This local coordinate coding converts the difficult nonlinear learning into a linear problem. With the locality constraint in (2), we project each shape to its local coordinate system and solve a smaller linear system for shape inference [13]

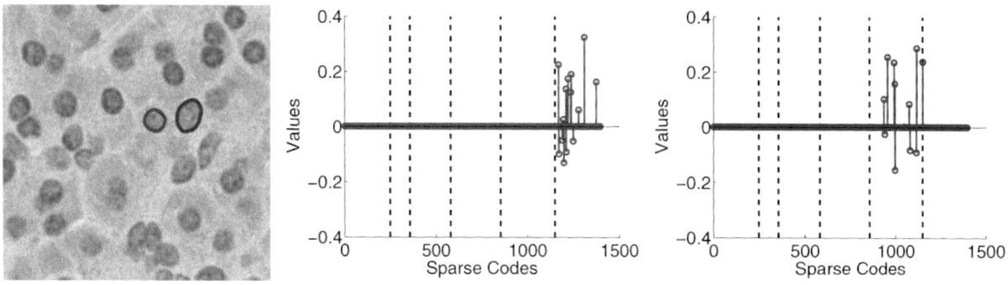

Fig. 2. Left: Two cells with different shapes in one NET image. **Middle:** The sparse codes corresponding to the red cell, where the black dash vertical lines separate different shape clusters. **Right:** The sparse codes corresponding to the blue cell.

$$\min_{\{\alpha_i\}} \sum_{i=1}^{N} ||v_i - \Phi\alpha_i||_2 + \lambda||d_i \odot \alpha_i||^2, s.t. \ \mathbf{1}^T\alpha_i = 1, \forall i, \tag{3}$$

where d_i measures the similarity between v_i and ψ_j's in Φ, and $\odot$ is the element-wise multiplication. Equation (3) has an analytical solution and it can be solved efficiently. For each shape v_i that belongs to cluster k, it selects its neighbors for sparse encoding such that only training shapes in ϕ_k are used for shape inference. Therefore, the nonzero components of the solution $\hat{\alpha}_i$ are grouped in the k-th segment of $\hat{\alpha}_i$ (see Figure 2), and we can determine the label of v_i as

$$\text{label}(v_i) = \max_k\{||\hat{\alpha}_{i1}||_0, \ ||\hat{\alpha}_{i2}||_0, \ ..., \ ||\hat{\alpha}_{ik}||_0, \ ..., \ ||\hat{\alpha}_{iK}||_0\}, \tag{4}$$

where the $\hat{\alpha}_{ik}$ corresponds to the code for cluster k, and $||\cdot||_0$ is l_0-norm.

2.2 Fast Active Contour Model

Local Repulsive Deformable Model: For shape deformation, we introduce an edge detector into the Chan-Vese model [3] to better separate cells from the background. To efficiently model the interaction among shapes, for each cell we calculate the repulsion only from its nearest neighbors [14]. Formally, for image I with N cells, the locality-constrained Chan-Vese model can be described as

$$\begin{aligned} &\min_V \lambda_1 \sum_{i=1}^{N} \int_{\Omega_i} (I(\mathbf{v}) - h_i)^2 d\mathbf{v} + \lambda_2 \int_{\Omega_b} (I(\mathbf{v}) - h_b)^2 d\mathbf{v} \\ &+\lambda_3 \sum_{i=1}^{N} \int_0^1 e(v_i(s))ds + \omega \sum_{i=1}^{N} \sum_{j\in G_i} \int_{\Omega_i \cap \Omega_j} 1 \ d\mathbf{v} + \mu \sum_{i=1}^{N} |v_i|, \end{aligned} \tag{5}$$

where Ω_i and Ω_b represent the regions inside v_i and outside all the contours, respectively, h_i (or h_b) denotes the average intensity of Ω_i (or Ω_b), $e(v_i(s))$ is the edge detector and chosen as $-||\nabla I(v_i(s))||^2$ ($s \in [0, 1]$ is the parameter for contour representation), $|v_i|$ denotes the length of v_i, and G_i represents the neighbors of v_i. The original model [3] requires to solve N associated Euler-Lagrange equations of (5) for shape deformation ($i = 1, ..., N$)

$$\frac{\partial v_i}{\partial t} = |\frac{\partial v_i}{\partial s}|\mathbf{n}_i[-\lambda_1(I-h_i)^2+\lambda_2(I-h_b)^2-\lambda_3\nabla e(v_i)-\omega\sum_{j\in G_i}o_j(v_i)+\mu\kappa(v_i)], \quad (6)$$

where $\mathbf{n}_i$ is v_i's normal unit vector, and $o_j(v_i)$ is the indicator function: $o_j(v_i) = 1$ if $v_i \in \Omega_j$, otherwise 0. $\kappa(v_i)$ is the curvature. Solving (6) for each cell in each iteration is extremely computationally expensive in whole slice scanned images.

Affine Transform Approximation: In order to avoid solving a large number of Euler-Lagrange equations, we propose to deform shapes using (6) for only a few cells and approximate all the other contour evolvements using affine transforms. Since similar cell shapes are grouped into the same clusters, we assume in each cluster there exists a certain affine transform between any two shape instances. Considering a cluster with N_k cells, $\{v_i = [x_1^i...x_p^i \ y_1^i...y_p^i]^T \in R^{2p\times 1}\}_{i=1}^{N_k}$, we assume that $v_i, i \neq 1$, is created from v_1 via affine transformation $z_i \in R^{6\times 1}$:

$$v_i = Sz_i, \ S = \begin{bmatrix} x^1 & y^1 & 0 & 0 & 1 & 0 \\ 0 & 0 & x^1 & y^1 & 0 & 1 \end{bmatrix}, \ z_i = [a_{11}^i \ a_{12}^i \ a_{21}^i \ a_{22}^i \ t_1^i \ t_2^i]^T, \ \forall i, \quad (7)$$

where $x^1 \in R^{p\times 1}$ and $y^1 \in R^{p\times 1}$ represent the first and second half of v_1. Therefore, we have $V = [v_1 \ v_2 \ ... v_{N_k}] = S[z_1 \ z_2 \ ... \ z_{N_k}]$ in each shape cluster.

For each iteration t, we randomly select only one shape in each cluster and solve its corresponding equation (6). After this selected shape deformation, we update the temporary positions of the other shapes. To preserve the cell shape information at iteration $t-1$, we apply a weight η to the update at iteration t

$$V^t = (1-\eta)V^{t-1} + \eta S^t Z^{t-1}, \quad (8)$$

where $V^t = [v_1^t \ v_2^t \ ... \ v_{N_k}^t]$ and $Z^{t-1} = [z_1^{t-1} \ z_2^{t-1} ... \ z_{N_k}^{t-1}]$. Thereafter, we perform shape inference using (3) to get the final contour positions $\hat{S}^t$ and $\hat{V}^t$ of each cluster k, and update the affine transform matrix as

$$Z^t = ((\hat{S}^t)^T\hat{S}^t)^{-1}(\hat{S}^t)^T\hat{V}^t. \quad (9)$$

In next iteration $t+1$, we repeat this procedure by alternatively performing shape deformation and inference based on results obtained at iteration t. The membership of each shape is dynamically updated to ensure that it is assigned to a correct cluster. The affine transformation approximation in (8,9), which deals with a small-size matrix inverse (6×6), is much faster than solving N Euler-Lagrange equations within each iteration. In order to finetune the final segmentation, we can deform all contours using (6) only in last iteration.

3 Experiments

The proposed approach is extensively tested on 12 pancreatic NET whole slide scanned TMA discs, which are captured at 20× magnification and contain cells

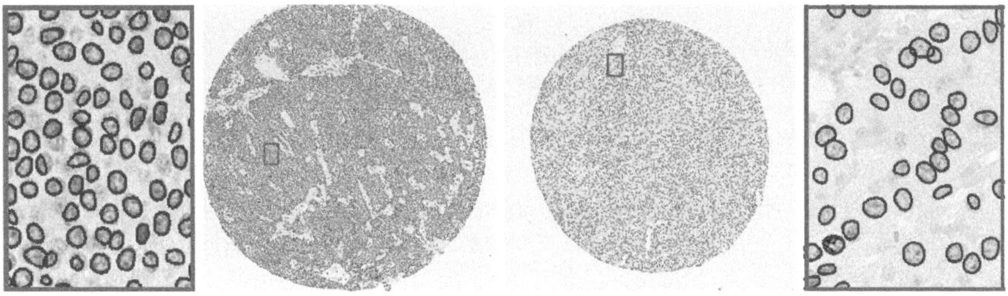

Fig. 3. Segmentation of whole slice scanned TMA discs with the proposed algorithm.

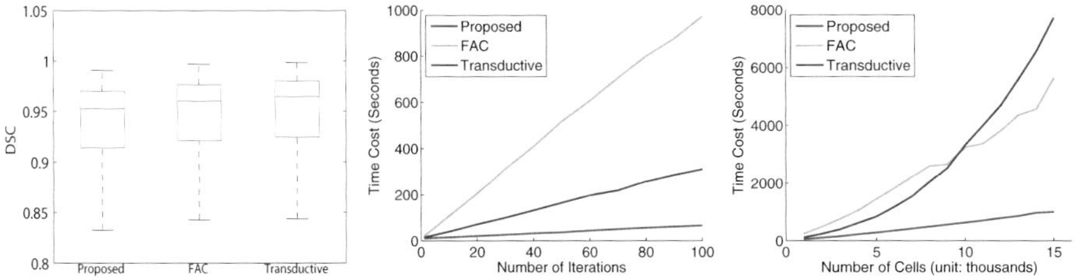

Fig. 4. Performance with the proposed method, full active contour (FAC), and transductive learning. **Left:** Dice similarity coefficient. **Middle** and **Right:** The running time with respect to the number of algorithm iterations and cells, respectively.

ranging from around 4200 to 17600. The 13-layer CNN model [6] is trained with about 1.3 million image patches with size $32 \times 32 \times 3$ (half positive and half negative). We have tested different number of training cells for shape prior modeling and observed no significant variations on the performance when the training size is larger than 1000, and thus in total 1395 cells are randomly selected. The algorithm is coded using Matlab on a PC of Intel Xeon CPU with 12 cores and 128 GB RAM. We empirically set $\gamma = 10$ in (1), $\lambda = 0.005$ in (3), $\eta = 0.2$ in (8), and $K = 6$ shape clusters. The Chan-Vese model is relatively insensitive to parameters, which are $\lambda_1 = \lambda_2 = 10, \lambda_3 = 0.2, \omega = 2.5$ and $\mu = 1$ in (6).

Figure 3 shows the segmentation results using our method on two whole slide scanned TMA discs with size of 3882×3882, where thousands of cells are accurately segmented one-by-one with shape preserving. More importantly, the average of running time for one whole slide with about 6300 cells is around 251 seconds. We randomly crop 12 image patches of size around 1300×800 from the whole slide images for quantitative analysis. The patches contain 300 to 1200 cells with large shape variations, and the ground-truth of each cell boundary is all manually annotated by pathologists for comparison. We compute the Dice similarity coefficient (DSC) [18] to measure the pixel-wise segmentation accuracy, and compare the proposed method with the *full active contour* (FAC), which does not use affine transform approximation but solves (6) for each cell within each iteration, and the transductive SMCE [8] for shape inference. Figure 4 shows that our method can produce competitive performance as the other

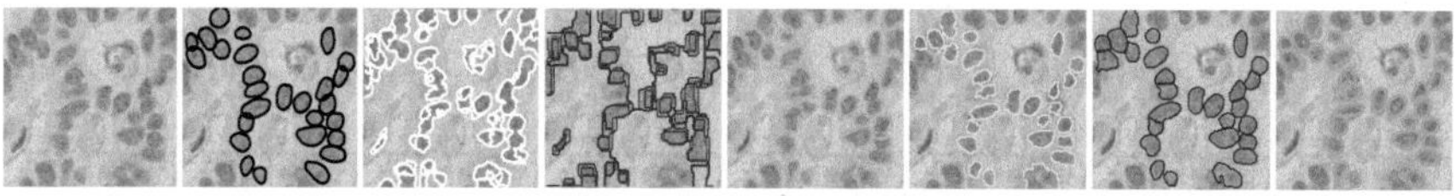

Fig. 5. Comparative segmentation using different methods. From left to right: original images, ground truth, MS, ISO [9], GCC [1], MWS, RLS [12], and the proposed. MWS, RLS, and the proposed use the same initialization, and the lymphocytes are discarded on purpose. Note that cells touching image boundaries are ignored.

Table 1. Comparative pixel-wise segmentation accuracy

	MS	ISO	GCC	MWS	RLS	Proposed
DSC	0.62 ± 0.26	0.49 ± 0.26	0.58 ± 0.26	0.81 ± 0.12	0.63 ± 0.20	0.91 ± 0.11
HD	9.59 ± 9.78	16.74 ± 19.38	7.94 ± 7.90	4.88 ± 3.39	7.83 ± 5.30	2.21 ± 3.05
MAD	5.63 ± 4.69	10.80 ± 9.84	5.55 ± 4.29	2.66 ± 1.84	5.02 ± 3.53	1.67 ± 2.04
Runtime†	10.07^{*}	139.1	32.96^{*}	3.07	317.2	36.34

†Runtime unit: seconds. *MS and GCC are coded with C++, and others with Matlab.

two in terms of the accuracy with a much lower running time (around 14(Proposed),107(FAC),39(Transductive) seconds on one patch with 465 cells). Figure 4 also shows the running time (15 iterations) with respect to the number of cells, in which the proposed method exhibits the strong scalability and is significantly faster than the other two. The more cells we need to segment, the more advantages we gain using our method.

In Figure 5, we illustrate the comparative segmentation results on one zoomed-in image patch using mean shift (MS), isoperimetric (ISO) [9], marker-based watershed (MWS), graph-cut and coloring (GCC) [1], repulsive level set (RLS) [12], and the proposed approach. It is clear that the proposed method provides best results. Table 1 summarizes the comparative performance between the proposed method and the state of the arts with multiple metrics including DSC, Hausdorff distance (HD), and mean absolute distance (MAD) [18]. As one can tell, our approach provides the best performance in terms of the mean and standard deviation of the metrics. Table 1 also lists the running time of each algorithm, which demonstrates that our method produces best performance. Except that MS and GCC are implemented in C++, all the others are coded with Matlab. Watershed (MWS), due to its simplicity, is the fastest but with poor segmentation accuracy.

4 Conclusion

We propose a fast cell segmentation approach using scalable sparse manifold learning and affine transform-approximated active contour model, which exhibits outstanding scalability and can efficiently handle large scale images (whole slide scanned specimens) for high throughput analysis using a standard PC machine without parallel computing involving complex image partitioning and stitching.

References

1. Al-Kofahi, Y., Lassoued, W., Lee, W., Roysam, B.: Improved automatic detection and segmentation of cell nuclei in histopathology images. TBME 57(4), 841–852 (2010)
2. Ali, S., Madabhushi, A.: An integrated region-, boundary-, shape-based active contour for multiple object overlap resolution in histological imagery. TMI 31(7), 1448–1460 (2012)
3. Chan, T.F., Vese, L.A.: Active contours without edges. TIP 10(2), 266–277 (2001)
4. Chang, H., Han, J., Spellman, P.T., Parvin, B.: Multireference level set for the characterization of nuclear morphology in glioblastoma multiforme. TBME 59(12), 3460–3467 (2012)
5. Cheng, J., Rajapakse, J.C.: Segmentation of clustered nuclei with shape markers and marking functions. TBME 56(3), 741–748 (2009)
6. Cireşan, D.C., Giusti, A., Gambardella, L.M., Schmidhuber, J.: Mitosis detection in breast cancer histology images with deep neural networks. In: Mori, K., Sakuma, I., Sato, Y., Barillot, C., Navab, N. (eds.) MICCAI 2013, Part II. LNCS, vol. 8150, pp. 411–418. Springer, Heidelberg (2013)
7. Cootes, T.F., Taylor, C.J., Cooper, D.H., Graham, J.: Active shape models-their training and application. CVIU 61(1), 38–59 (1995)
8. Elhamifar, E., Vidal, R.: Sparse manifold clustering and embedding. In: NIPS, pp. 55–63 (2011)
9. Grady, L., Schwartz, E.L.: Isoperimetric graph partitioning for image segmetentation. TPAMI 28(1), 469–475 (2006)
10. Irshad, H., Veillard, A., Roux, L., Racoceanu, D.: Methods for nuclei detection, segmentation, and classification in digital histopathology: A review-current status and future potential. RBME 7, 97–114 (2014)
11. Kong, H., Gurcan, M., Belkacem-Boussaid, K.: Partitioning histopathological images: an integrated framework for supervised color-texture segmentation and cell splitting. TMI 30(9), 1661–1677 (2011)
12. Qi, X., Xing, F., Foran, D.J., Yang, L.: Robust segmentation of overlapping cells in histopathology specimens using parallel seed detection and repulsive level set. TBME 59(3), 754 (2012)
13. Wang, J., Yang, J., Yu, K., Lv, F., Huang, T., Gong, Y.: Locality-constrained linear coding for image classification. In: CVPR, pp. 3360–3367 (2010)
14. Xing, F., Yang, L.: Robust selection-based sparse shape model for lung cancer image segmentation. In: Mori, K., Sakuma, I., Sato, Y., Barillot, C., Navab, N. (eds.) MICCAI 2013, Part III. LNCS, vol. 8151, pp. 404–412. Springer, Heidelberg (2013)
15. Yu, K., Zhang, T., Gong, Y.: Nonlinear learning using local coordinate coding. In: NIPS, pp. 1–9 (2009)
16. Zhang, C., Yarkony, J., Hamprecht, F.A.: Cell detection and segmentation using correlation clustering. In: Golland, P., Hata, N., Barillot, C., Hornegger, J., Howe, R. (eds.) MICCAI 2014, Part I. LNCS, vol. 8673, pp. 9–16. Springer, Heidelberg (2014)
17. Zhang, S., Zhan, Y., Dewan, M., Huang, J., Metaxas, D.N., Zhou, X.S.: Towards robust and effective shape modeling: Sparse shape composition. MedIA 16(1), 265 (2012)
18. Zhou, X., Huang, X., Duncan, J.S., Yu, W.: Active contours with group similarity. In: CVPR, pp. 2969–2976 (2013)

Restoring the Invisible Details in Differential Interference Contrast Microscopy Images*

Wenchao Jiang and Zhaozheng Yin

Department of Computer Science, Missouri University of Science and Technology
wjm84@mst.edu, yinz@mst.edu

Abstract. Automated image restoration in microscopy, especially in Differential Interference Contrast (DIC) imaging modality, has attracted increasing attention since it greatly facilitates living cell analysis. Previous work is able to restore the nuclei of living cells, but it is very challenging to reconstruct the unnoticeable cytoplasm details in DIC images. In this paper, we propose to extract the tiny movement information of living cells in DIC images and reveal the hidden details in DIC images by magnifying the cell's motion as well as attenuating the intensity variation from the background. From our restored images, we can clearly observe the previously-invisible details in DIC images. Experiments on two DIC image datasets demonstrate that the motion-based restoration method can reveal the hidden details of living cells, providing promising results on facilitating cell shape and behavior analysis.

1 Introduction

Automated image restoration, transforming an observed image that is challenging for direct analysis into a new image that can be effortless analyzed, has valuable applications in biological experiments, because it may make the segmentation and detection of specimens much easier and greatly facilitate the behavior analysis on specimens [1][2]. As predominantly phase objects, living cells are transparent and colorless under a traditional brightfield microscope, because they do not significantly alter the amplitude of the light waves passing through them, as a consequence, producing little or no contrast under a brightfield microscope. Differential Interference Contrast (DIC) microscopy technique (refer to Chapter 10 in [3]) has been widely used to observe living cells because it is noninvasive to cells. DIC microscopy converts the gradient of cells' optical path length into intensity variations which are visible to human.

Although the nucleus and some big organelles are visible in DIC microscopy images, there are many cell details which are not obvious in DIC microscopy images such as the cytoplasm and cell membrane, and they are difficult to be observed by human eyes. Fig.1(a) shows two DIC microscopy image patches and Fig.1(b) shows the ground truth cell mask obtained by combining the observation

* This research was supported by NSF CAREER award IIS-1351049, NSF EPSCoR grant IIA-1355406, ISC and CBSE centers at Missouri S&T.

N. Navab et al. (Eds.): MICCAI 2015, Part III, LNCS 9351, pp. 340–348, 2015.
DOI: 10.1007/978-3-319-24574-4_41

from corresponding phase contrast microscopy images. Fig.1(c) is the average segmentation mask by ten human annotators, from which we find that even humankind is likely to ignore the unnoticeable cytoplasm which spreads out into the background, but these hidden details can be informative to analyze cells' shape and behavior. In this paper, we focus on restoring the invisible (as well as visible) details in DIC microscopy images.

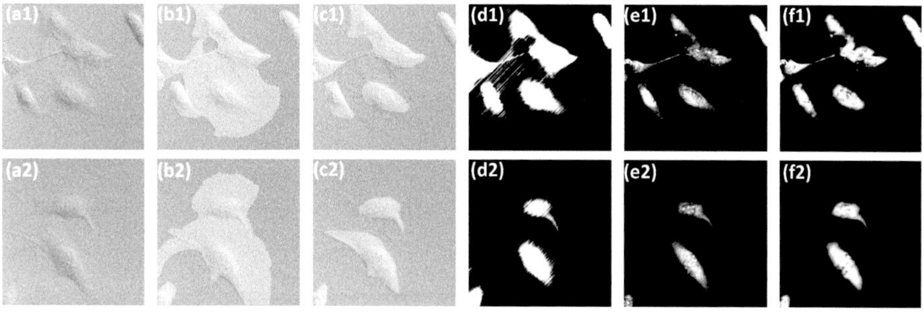

Fig. 1. Challenges in restoration of the hidden details in DIC microscopy images. (a) Two original DIC images. (b) The ground truth mask, which indicates where the cells are. (c) The mask indicates where the cells are by ten annotators merely with their naked eyes. (d) The restoration results by line integration [6]. (e) The restoration results by Wiener filter [7]. (f) The restoration results by preconditioning [8].

1.1 Related Work

The common techniques employed for microscopy image restoration include edge detection, thresholding [4], morphological operations [5]. These methods often fail when the cells are in low contrast with background. For the purpose of restoration in DIC microscopy images, lines are integrated along the shear direction inspired by the gradient interpretation property of DIC images [6], but this method introduces streaking artifacts and is sensitive to gradient noise, as shown in Fig1(d). General image processing technologies such as deconvolution by Wiener filter [7] have been investigated to restore the optical path length from DIC images. A preconditioning approach was proposed in [8] where the DIC image is reconstructed by minimizing a nonnegative-constrained convex objective function. However, neither Wiener filter nor the preconditioning method can reveal the hidden details in the DIC images and the cells are miss-segmented, as shown in Fig.1(e,f).

1.2 Our Proposal and Algorithm Overview

Although the details of living cells in a DIC image are unnoticeable by human eyes, they are likely to keep moving when we observe them in a continuous series of images, hence we are motivated to think of the following intriguing problem:

Can we extract the tiny movement information of living cells in DIC images and reveal the hidden details in DIC images by magnifying the cells' motion?

In this paper, we propose a motion-based DIC image restoration algorithm.

As shown in Fig.2, DIC image at timestamp T is to be restored. We firstly extract the spatial gradient information from every DIC image within the time sliding window $[T - \Delta t, T + \Delta t]$. The intensity values of a pixel location in the gradient images form a time-series signal and we filter it by an ideal bandpass filter to magnify small motion. The motion is further magnified in forward and backward directions independently in the temporal domain. Finally, the restoration results of two directions by motion magnification are combined to obtain the final restoration result which uncover the hidden details in the DIC image at timestamp T. Our work is different from the previous work which also considers motion information [9][10], because we do not rely on cell detection and tracking. Instead, we extract tiny motion on individual pixels and magnify it.

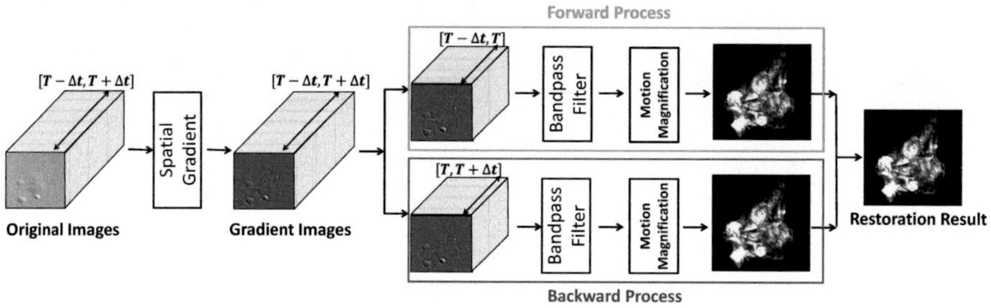

Fig. 2. Overview of our algorithm.

2 Methodology

For simplicity, we denote the original DIC image at timestamp t as $f(t)$, the pixel value of which at position (m, n) is $f(m, n, t)$. $f(T)$ is the target image to be restored at timestamp T. Let $v_m(t)$ and $v_n(t)$ denote the motion components at position (m, n) regarding to horizontal and vertical coordinates, respectively. If $f(m, n, 0) = I(m, n)$, the pixel intensity at $(m + v_m(t), n + v_n(t))$, $I(m + v_m(t), n + v_n(t))$, can be represented by image function f equivalently:

$$f(m, n, t) = I(m + v_m(t), n + v_n(t)) \tag{1}$$

By the first-order Tylor expansion, we have

$$I(m + v_m(t), n + v_n(t)) = I(m, n) + v_m(t)\frac{\partial I}{\partial m} + v_n(t)\frac{\partial I}{\partial n} \tag{2}$$

Therefore, the contrast between neighboring pixels in an image sequence (i.e., $I(m + v_m(t), n + v_n(t)) - I(m, n)$) is determined by both motion information $(v_m(t), v_n(t))$ and spatial gradient information $(\frac{\partial I}{\partial m}, \frac{\partial I}{\partial n})$. Thus we can magnify the motion by either increasing $(\frac{\partial I}{\partial m}, \frac{\partial I}{\partial n})$ or increasing $(v_m(t), v_n(t))$. This motivates us to build a Laplacian pyramid to accumulate the spatial gradient information (Subsection 2.1), design bandpass filter (Subsection 2.2) and accumulate motion information in the temporal sliding window (Subsection 2.3 and 2.4) to magnify the tiny motion caused by fine cell structures.

2.1 Gradient Images

Fig.3 illustrates the process to extract spatial gradient information from DIC microscopy images. Given a DIC image $f(t)$ (Fig.3(a)), we decompose it to several levels by the Laplacian pyramid and then reconstruct them by ignoring the last level. Fig.3(c) is the final result. Compared with the single level gradient image, such as the first level of the Laplacian pyramid in Fig.3(b), the gradient image combining several levels (Fig.3(c)) reveals more and clearer gradient information about the cells. We denote the gradient image corresponding to $f(t)$ as $g(t)$ and $g(t)$ is the input of the following motion magnification process.

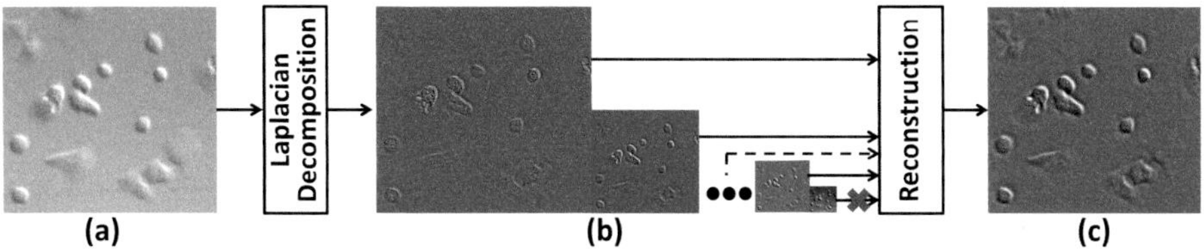

Fig. 3. Computing the gradient image $g(t)$. (a). The original image $f(t)$. (b). The Laplacian pyramid. (c). The gradient image $g(t)$.

2.2 Bandpass Filter

The original image $f(t)$ may have low signal-to-noise ratio. For example, for each image from $f(T - \Delta t)$ to $f(T + \Delta t)$, the pixel value of background is spatially stable (i.e., $(\frac{\partial I}{\partial m}, \frac{\partial I}{\partial n})$ is small on background pixels), but it can temporally change because of illumination variations, thus resulting in unwanted temporally motion in the background. Motion information $(v_m(t), v_n(t))$ can be easily extracted by the image difference of $g(t)$, but it is likely to amplify noise which is unrelated to cells' movement. We need to retain the tiny motion information of cells, meanwhile inhibiting the unwanted movement information of background pixels.

In this subsection, $g(t)$ is filtered by an ideal bandpass filter and the signal-to-noise ratio of each pixel in the temporal domain is increased. The flowchart of our bandpass filtering is shown in Fig.4 where Fig.4(a) is $g(t)$ with $t \in [T - \Delta t, T]$[1]. For each pixel (m, n), we can build a vector $g(m, n, T - \Delta t : T)$ which indicates the pixel value change at (m, n) during the time period of $[T - \Delta t : T]$. Discrete Fourier Transform (DFT) is then applied to $g(m, n, T - \Delta t : T)$ and Fig.4(b) shows examples of frequency vs. magnitude on two typical pixel locations. The principle frequency is defined as the frequency with the largest magnitude. As shown in Fig4(c), we build a principle frequency map whose pixel value at location (m, n) is the principle frequency of $g(m, n, T - \Delta t : T)$. We observe that in the cells' regions, the principle frequency is lower than that in

[1] As shown in Fig.2, the motion magnification processes towards forward and backward directions in the temporal domain are similar, thus we mainly describe the forward process in this subsection without loss of generality.

the background (presented by black regions in Fig4(c)). This is because noise variation in the background has higher frequency (fast changes) but with smaller range of variation, so people may not notice it. However, the intensity change of a pixel location caused by cell movement has lower frequency (slow changes) but with larger variation range, thus people are possible to observe cell details in continuous DIC images.

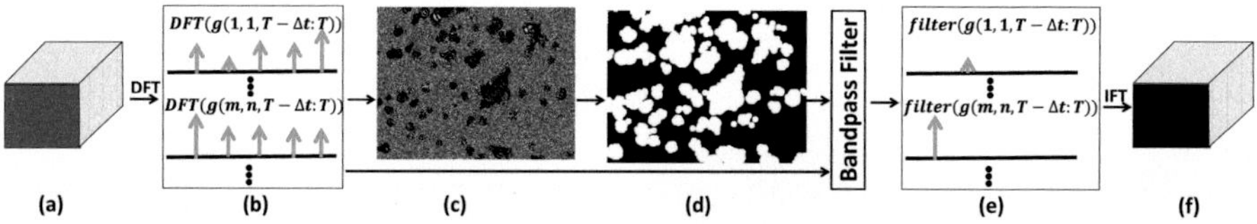

Fig. 4. Flowchart of bandpass filtering. (a) $g(t)$ with $t \in [T - \Delta t : T]$. (b) The DFT of $g(m, n, T - \Delta t : T)$. (c) Principle frequency image. (d) The bitmask by thresholding the principle frequency image, from which we can know the tentative cell and background regions. (e) Bandpass filtering result. (f) The motion image $h(t)$, which indicates the motion of each pixel.

The principle frequency map shown in Fig.4(c) inspires us to tentatively determine the cells' regions and background. We set all pixel values in the principle frequency image which are larger than the minimum of the principle frequency map as zero, yielding a bitmask that indicates the cells' regions and background as shown in Fig.4(d). The bitmask can roughly tell where the living cells are, offering us the hint on where to retain cells' tiny movement while inhibiting the motion from background noise.

For each pixel (m, n) in $g(t)$, its movement pattern may not be exactly the same during the time interval $[T - \Delta t : T]$, thus we design an ideal bandpass filter with the aid of the bitmask to keep the most salient movement of cells as well as the smallest movement in the background. The bandpass filtering increases the contrast between cell motion and background intensity variation, therefore facilitating the observation on fine details of cells.

For the tentative background regions obtained from Fig.4(d), the frequency range to be passed in the bandpass filter is set as the frequency corresponding to the *smallest* magnitude, thus all frequency components which are larger are attenuated (rejected). Note that we do not directly set all frequency components of the tentative background pixel as zero, because the tentative foreground and background segmentation in Fig.4(d) may not be accurate. For the tentative foreground regions obtained from Fig.4(d), the frequency range to be passed in the bandpass filter is set as the frequency corresponding to the *largest* magnitude, thus only the dominant frequency component related to cell motion is kept. Fig.4(e) shows the two filtering results corresponding to Fig.4(b) with the top being regarded as background and the bottom being foreground. After bandpass filtering, we apply the inverse DFT to obtain the motion images $h(t)$.

2.3 Motion Magnification

After the aforementioned processes, we obtain the motion images $h(t)$ which includes the movement information of each pixel. In this section, we further magnify the motion in a temporal sliding window to reveal cell details. This is implemented by the temporally weighted accumulation of motion. The magnification formula for forward process ($[T - \Delta t, T]$) is defined as

$$r_{fw}(T) = \sum_{t=T-\Delta t}^{T} e^{-\frac{T-t}{\Delta t}} |h(t)| \tag{3}$$

The magnification formula for backward process ($[T, T + \Delta t]$) is similarly defined as

$$r_{bw}(T) = \sum_{t=T}^{T+\Delta t} e^{-\frac{t-T}{\Delta t}} |h(t)| \tag{4}$$

where $r_{fw}(T)$ and $r_{bw}(T)$ are the motion magnified images for $f(t)$ by the forward and backward process, respectively. $e^{-\frac{T-t}{\Delta t}}$ and $e^{-\frac{t-T}{\Delta t}}$ ensure that the closer the image $h(t)$ is to the target image $h(T)$, the more contribution $h(t)$ makes to $r_{fw}(T)$ or $r_{bw}(T)$.

2.4 Combine Forward and Backward Motion Images

The final restoration image $r(T)$ for the original target image $f(T)$ can be directly defined as the elementwise min-operation on $r_{fw}(T)$ and $r_{bw}(T)$:

$$r(T) = min(r_{fw}(T), r_{bw}(T)) \tag{5}$$

As shown in Fig5(a,b,c), a cell moves from the center towards the top-right. Fig5(d,e,f) show the forward, backward and combined restoration results, respectively. In Fig5, we observe that if only one direction of motion information is used, there will be artifacts unrelated to the motion in $f(T)$. The artifacts are from the accumulated motion in the past or future DIC images. If we compute the minimum of $r_{fw}(T)$ and $r_{bw}(T)$, the artifacts are removed, leaving the cell details in the current frame only.

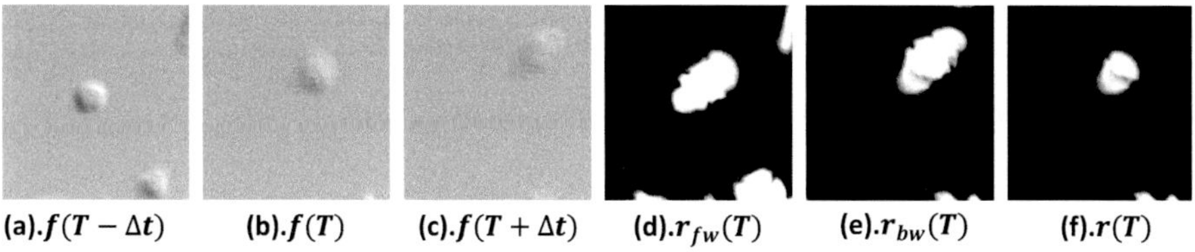

Fig. 5. Illustration of the combination of forward and backward processes.

3 Experimental Results

The proposed image restoration algorithm is tested in two different sets of Differential Interference Contrast images of 1388×1040 pixels, which were captured every 5 minutes to continuously monitor live cells. The first dataset includes 445 DIC images with each image containing about 70 cells. The second dataset includes 500 DIC images and has a wider visual field, thus each image in this dataset contains about 150 living cells. When labeling the ground truth of cell masks, we found it was likely to make mistake only with DIC images. To minimize the human errors, we took the phase contrast microscopy images on the same cell dish simultaneously when we took DIC images. Thus the ground truth was labeled by combining DIC images and corresponding phase contrast images. Δt is determined by a training dataset different from the two above-mentioned testing datasets and the following comparison on testing datasets are conducted when $\Delta t = 20$ which had the best restoration performance on the training dataset.

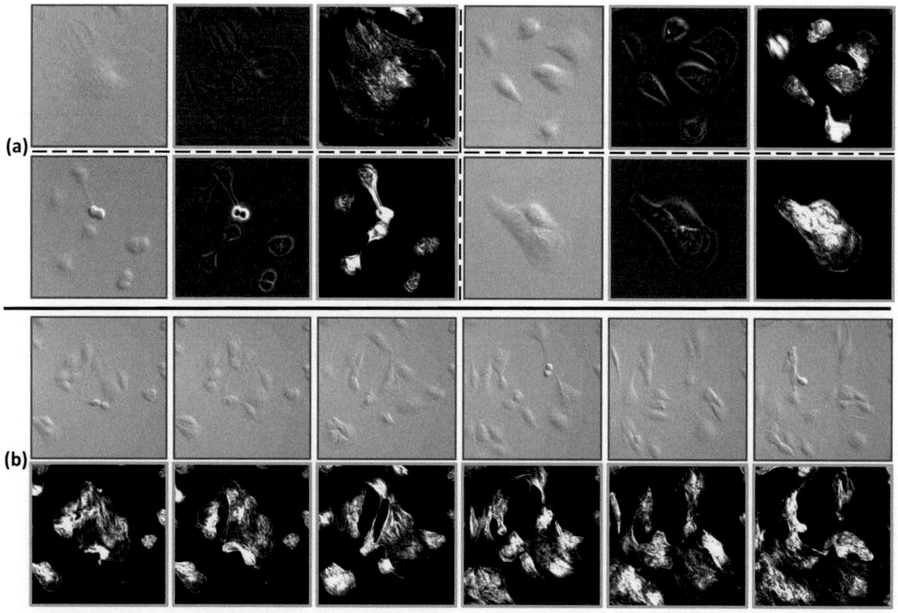

Fig. 6. The qualitative performance. (a).The images in red, blue and green boxes are the original DIC images, the corresponding phase contrast images and the restoration images obtained by the proposed algorithm, respectively. (b). The upper row shows sample DIC images during a period of 100 minutes. The bottom row is the restoration images, from which we can analyse the shape change of a cluster of cells.

3.1 Qualitative Evaluation

Fig.6 shows the qualitative performance of the proposed restoration algorithm. In Fig.6(a), the images in red or blue boxes are the original DIC images and the corresponding phase contrast images, respectively. Phase contrast images are displayed here to observe the ground truth. Unlike the previous work [6][7][8] which only reveals the nucleus of living cells (an example is in Fig.1), our approach can display the details such as the cytoplasm of living cells, even though the cytoplasm is spread out and fuses with the background (images in green boxes in Fig.6(a)). The upper row of Fig.6(b) shows some DIC images on a cluster of cells within a time interval of 100 minutes. It is clearly to observe cells' shape change and their movement, which provides more information for future cell shape and behavior analysis.

3.2 Quantitative Evaluation

The restored image enables us to achieve the cell segmentation simply using a global thresholding. Fig.7 shows the recall vs. precision curves by trying all possible thresholds for four methods: our proposed approach, line integration [6], Wiener filter [7] and preconditioning [8]. For each threshold, TP is the number of true positive pixels. FP is the number of false positive pixels. FN is the number of false negative pixels. Thus precision is defined as Precision=TP/(TP+FP) and recall is defined as Recall=TP/(TP+FN). Fig.7 shows that our proposed algorithm greatly outperforms other approaches since we can restore cell's fine details in addition to the nucleus.

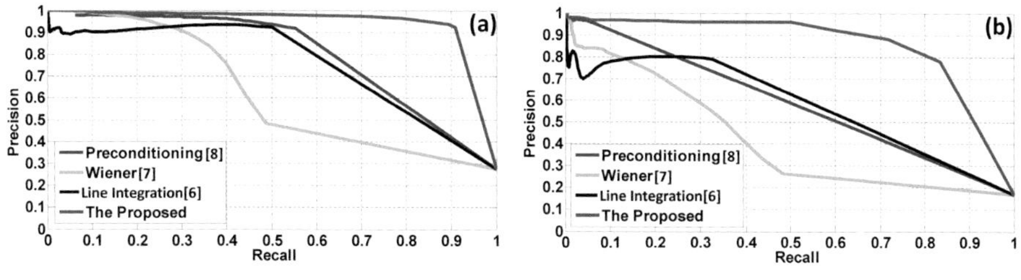

Fig. 7. The recall vs. precision comparison with other approaches. (a). Comparison in Dataset 1. (b).Comparison in Dataset 2.

4 Conclusion

In this paper, we propose a novel motion-based DIC image restoration algorithm. The tiny motion of each cell pixel is magnified by filtering a time-series of gradient signals on the pixel location using an ideal bandpass filter, while the intensity variation on the background pixels is attenuated. The motion information of a target image is further magnified by a weighted sum of a series of motion images from time-lapse image sequences. From our restored images, we can clearly observe the previously-invisible details in DIC images. The restored images facilitate the cell segmentation greatly compared to three other image restoration methods. In the future, we will further explore cell image analysis tasks based on our restoration algorithm such as the cell proliferation event detection.

References

1. Yin, Z., Ker, D.F.E., Kanade, T.: Restoring DIC Microscopy Images from Multiple Shear Directions. In: Székely, G., Hahn, H.K. (eds.) IPMI 2011. LNCS, vol. 6801, pp. 384–397. Springer, Heidelberg (2011)
2. Kaakinen, M., et al.: Automatic Detection and Analysis of Cell Motility in Phase contrast Time lapse Images Using a Combination of Maximally Stable Extremal Regions and Kalman Filter Approaches. Journal of Microscopy (2014)
3. Murphy, D.B.: Fundamentals of Light Microscopy and Electronic Imaging. John Wiley & Sons (2001)
4. Neumann, B., et al.: High-throughput RNAi Screening by Time-lapse Imaging of Live Human Cells. Nature Methods (2006)
5. Li, K., et al.: Cell Population Tracking and Lineage Construction with Spatiotemporal Context. Medical Image Analysis (2008)
6. Kam, Z.: Microscopic Differential Interference Contrast Image Processing by Line Integration (LID) and Deconvolution. Bioimaging (1998)
7. Heise, B., Sonnleitner, A., Klement, E.P.: DIC image Reconstruction on Large Cell Scans. Microscopy Research and Technique (2005)
8. Li, K., Kanade, T.: Nonnegative mixed-norm preconditioning for microscopy image segmentation. In: Prince, J.L., Pham, D.L., Myers, K.J. (eds.) IPMI 2009. LNCS, vol. 5636, pp. 362–373. Springer, Heidelberg (2009)
9. Liu, K., et al.: Optical Flow Guided Cell Segmentation and Tracking in Developing Tissue. In: International Symposium on Biomedical Imaging (2014)
10. Hennies, J., et al.: Cell Segmentation and Cell Splitting Based on Gradient Flow Tracking in Microscopic Images. Springer, Heidelberg (2014)

A Novel Cell Detection Method Using Deep Convolutional Neural Network and Maximum-Weight Independent Set

Fujun Liu[1] and Lin Yang[1]

[1] Department of Electrical & Computer Engineering, University of Florida, USA
[2] Crayton Pruitt Family Department of Biomedical Engineering, University of Florida, USA

Abstract. Cell detection is an important topic in biomedical image analysis and it is often the prerequisite for the following segmentation or classification procedures. In this paper, we propose a novel algorithm for general cell detection problem: Firstly, a set of cell detection candidates is generated using different algorithms with varying parameters. Secondly, each candidate is assigned a score by a trained deep convolutional neural network (DCNN). Finally, a subset of best detection results are selected from all candidates to compose the final cell detection results. The subset selection task is formalized as a maximum-weight independent set problem, which is designed to find the heaviest subset of mutually non-adjacent nodes in a graph. Experiments show that the proposed general cell detection algorithm provides detection results that are dramatically better than any individual cell detection algorithm.

1 Introduction

Cell detection is an important topic in biomedical image analysis because it is often the first step for the following tasks, including cell counting, segmentation, and morphological analysis. Many automatic cell detection algorithms are proposed in recent literatures [1,2,3]. Parvin *et al.* proposed an iterative voting algorithm based on oriented kernels to localize cell centers, in which the voting direction and areas were dynamically updated within each iteration. In [2], a simple and reliable cell detector was designed based on a Laplacian of Gaussian filter. A learning based cell detection algorithm was proposed in [3]. It used an efficient maximally stable extremal regions (MSER) detector [4] to find a set of nested candidate regions that will form a tree graph. Then a non-overlapping subset of those regions was selected for cell detection via dynamic programming.

All the methods reviewed above give good detection results under certain circumstances. However, in general, they all have some limitations. For example, both [1] and [2] are sensitive to the selection of proper cell diameter parameters. However, finding an appropriate parameter that works under all conditions is extremely difficult when the cells exhibit large size variations. In [3], the algorithm heavily depends on the quality of MSER detector that does not take advantage

N. Navab et al. (Eds.): MICCAI 2015, Part III, LNCS 9351, pp. 349–357, 2015.
DOI: 10.1007/978-3-319-24574-4_42

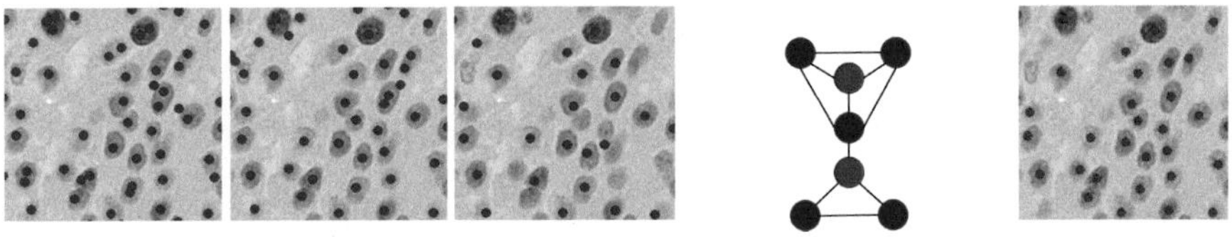

(a) (b) (c)

Fig. 1. An overview of the proposed general cell detection algorithm. (a) A set of detections candidates generated using multiple detection algorithms. Each candidate is marked with blue dot. (b) An undirected weighted graph was constructed from all detection candidates. The red color indicates the selected nodes. (c) The final cell detection results using the proposed method.

the prior cell shape information and the performance will deteriorate when the cells overlap with one another.

In this paper, we propose a novel algorithm for general cell detection that does not require the fine tuning of parameters. First, a set of cell detection candidates is produced from different algorithms with varying parameters. Second, each candidate will be assigned a score using a trained deep convolutional neural network (DCNN) [5,6]. Third, we will construct a weighted graph that has the detection candidates as nodes and the detection scores (DCNN outputs) as weights (an edge exists between two nodes if their corresponding detection results lie in the same cell). Finally, a subset of mutually non-adjacent graph nodes is chosen to maximize the sum of the weights of the selected nodes. An overview of the algorithm is shown in Fig. 1. The selection of the best subset is formulated as a maximum-weight independent set problem (MWIS). MWIS is a combinatorial optimization problem that has been successfully applied in clustering [7], segmentation [8], and tracking [9], etc.

To the best of our knowledge, this is the first work that formulates the general cell detection problem as a MWIS problem, and this is also the first work to introduce DCNN to provide weights to a graph for future combinational optimization.

2 Methodology

2.1 Cell Detection Using MWIS

A set of cell detection candidates (points), $P = \{p_1, ..., p_n\}$, are first generated based on different cell detection algorithms with various parameters. An undirected and weighted graph, $G = (V, E, w)$, is constructed, where the node v_i corresponds to the i-th cell detection candidate p_i, E denotes undirected edges between nodes, and w_i denotes weight for the i-th node v_i. Two nodes v_i and v_j are adjacent, $(v_i, v_j) \in E$, if the Euclidean distance between their respective detection results p_i and p_j is smaller than a threshold λ. A node v_i will be assigned a larger weight value w_i if its corresponding detection result p_i is close to the real cell center, otherwise smaller weight will be assigned. After graph G is constructed, an optimal subset of V will be selected with the constraint that two nodes adjacent to each other will not be selected simultaneously. A subset is represented by an indicator vector $\mathbf{x} = \{x_1, .., x_i, ...x_n\}$, where $x_i \in \{0, 1\}$. $x_i = 1$ indicates that node v_i is in the subset, and $x_i = 0$ represents that v_i is not in the subset. This best subset selection is then formulated as finding the maximum weight independent set (MWIS) $\mathbf{x}^*$.

$$\mathbf{x}^* = \arg\max_{\mathbf{x}} w^T \mathbf{x},\ s.\ t.\ \ \mathbf{x}^T A \mathbf{x} = 0,\ x_i \in \{0, 1\}, \tag{1}$$

where $A = (a_{ij})_{n \times n}$ is the adjacent matrix, $a_{ij} = 1$ if $(v_i, v_j) \in E$ and $a_{ij} = 0$ otherwise. The diagonal elements of A are zeros. The quadric constraints can be integrated into the object function to reformulate the optimization as

$$\mathbf{x}^* = \arg\max_{\mathbf{x}} \left(w^T \mathbf{x} - \frac{1}{2} \alpha \mathbf{x}^T A \mathbf{x} \right),\ s.\ t.\ x_i \in \{0, 1\}, \tag{2}$$

where α is a positive regularization parameter to encode the non-adjacent constraints in (1).

The MWIS optimization can be solved by some numerical approximation algorithms [10,8]. In [10], the integer constraints in (2) are relaxed, and a graduated assignment algorithm iteratively maximizes a Taylor series expansion of the object function in (2) around the previous solution in the continuous domain. The relaxed continuous solution will then be binarized to obtain the discrete solution. This binarization procedure might lead to errors. In order to avoid this type of error, [8] directly seeks a discrete solution in each iteration in maximizing the Taylor series approximation. However, in this case the solution of (2) might not satisfy the non-adjacent constraints in (1). In our algorithm, unlike all the previous procedures, we propose to find the optimal results iteratively only in the solution space of (1).

Denote $f(\mathbf{x})$ as the objective function in (2), let $x^{(t)} \in \{0, 1\}^n$ denotes the current solution in the t-th iteration, each iteration consists of the following two steps in our algorithm.

Step 1: For any point $x \in \{0, 1\}^n$ in the neighborhood of $x^{(t)}$, we first find the first-order Taylor series approximation of $f(x)$ as

$$f(\mathbf{x}) \approx T(\mathbf{x}) = f(x^{(t)}) + (x - x^{(t)})^T (w - \alpha A x^{(t)}) = x^T (w - \alpha A x^{(t)}) + const, \tag{3}$$

where *const* represents an item that does not depends on x. Define $y^{(t)}$ as the intermediate solution to (3), it can be computed by maximizing the approximation $T(x)$ as $y^{(t)} = \mathbb{1}(w - \alpha A x^{(t)} \geq 0)$, where $\mathbb{1}(\cdot)$ is an indicator function.

Step 2: The solution of (3) might not satisfy the non-adjacent constraints listed in (1). If this is the case, we need to find a valid solution of (1) based on $y^{(t)}$. This is achieved by the following steps: 1) We first sort all the nodes based on their weights with an decreasing order. The nodes with $y^{(t)} = 1$ will be placed in front of the nodes that have $y^{(t)} = 0$. 2) The nodes are then selected from the

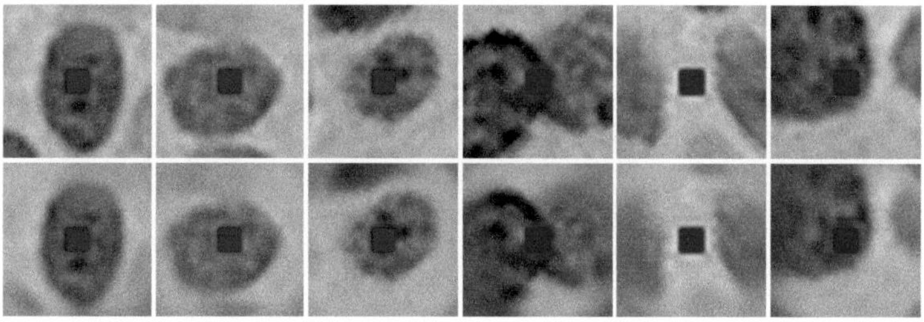

Fig. 2. Some training samples for DCNN and their foveation versions. The first row denote original training samples. Positive samples are marked with red rectangles and negatives are marked with blue. The second row denote the samples after foveation.

front of the queue sequentially with a constraint that the picked node will not be adjacent to those that are already chosen.

After we find the valid solution, the $x^{(t+1)}$ in the solution space of (1) based on $y^{(t)}$ is computed using a local search method by first randomly removing k selected nodes and the probability to remove each node is inversely proportional to its weight, then choosing the maximum weighted node in the queue that are not adjacent to those selected until all nodes are considered. This procedure continues until convergence or maximum iterations reached and the best solution is selected as $x^{(t+1)}$. The reason that we randomly remove k selected nodes is to help the optimization escape from potential local maxima.

2.2 Deep Convolutional Neural Network

In this section, we need to calculate the weight w_i for each detection candidate $v_i \in V$ from section 2.1. A deep convolutional neural network (DCNN) is trained for this purpose to assign each node a proper score as its weight. In our algorithm, a detection candidate is described by a small rectangle region centering around the detected position. Some training samples are shown in the first row in Fig. 2. The patches whose centers are close to the true cell centers are annotated as positive (+1) samples, marked with red rectangles in Fig. 2. Patches that have centers far away from true cell centers will be annotated as negative (-1) samples, marked with blue rectangles in Fig. 2.

DCNN Architecture: In our algorithm, the input features are the raw intensities of 31 $\times$ 31 image patches around the detected position. Considering the staining variations and the generality of the detection framework, color information is disregarded since they may change dramatically with respect to different staining protocols. The DCNN consists of seven layers: three convolutional (C) layers, two pooling layers, and two fully connected (FC) layers. In our implementation, max pooling (MP) is applied. The MP layers select the maximal activations over non-overlapping patches of the input layers. Except the output layer, where the two-way *softmax* function is used as activation function, the rectifier nonlinear activation functions are used in the convolutional layers and

Table 1. The configuration of the proposed DCNN architecture in our algorithm.

Layer	Type	Maps (M) and neurons (N)	Filter size	Nonlinearity	Weights
0	I	1M × 31N × 31N	–	–	–
1	C	6M × 28N × 28N	4 × 4	rectifier	102
2	MP	6M × 14N × 14N	2 × 2	–	–
3	C	12M × 12N × 12N	3 × 3	rectifier	660
4	MP	12M × 6N × 6N	2 × 2	–	–
5	C	12M × 4N × 4N	3 × 3	rectifier	1308
6	FC	100N	1 × 1	rectifier	19300
7	FC	2N	1 × 1	softmax	202

the fully connected layer prior to the output layer. A detailed configuration of the DCNN used in our algorithm is shown in Table 1.

Foveation: The task of DCNN is to classify the center pixel of each rectangle patch, so it will be ideal if we can keep the focus on the central region (fovea) and also retain the general structure of the image. Foveation, inspired by the structure of human photoreceptor topography, has been shown to be effective in imposing a spatially-variant blur on images [11]. In our algorithm, a Gaussian pyramid is first built for each input image, then all the pyramid layers are resized to the input image scale. In the foveated image, pixels closer to the image center are assigned intensity values in higher resolution layers at the same coordinate, pixels far away from the centers will be assigned values from lower resolution layers. Some foveation examples are shown in the second row of Fig. 2.

DCNN Training: Several cell detection algorithms [1,2] with varying parameters are chosen to generate training samples for the DCNN. All the true cell centers are manually annotated in training images. The detected results within a certain distance τ_1 to the annotated cell centers are marked as positive training samples, others that locate far away from the centers (measured by τ_2) are marked as negative training samples, where $\tau_2 \geq \tau_1$. Each training sample is further rotated by seven angles. In our implementation, a mini-batch of size 10, which is a compromise between the standard and stochastic gradient descent forms, is used to train the DCNN. The learning rate is initiated as 0.01, and decreases as the number of epoches increases.

3 Experiments

The proposed algorithm is tested with two datasets: 1) 24 neuroendocrine (NET) tissue microarray (TMA) images, and 2) 16 lung cancer images. Each image contains roughly 150 cells. For each dataset, two fold cross-validation is used to evaluate the accuracy. All the true cell centers are manually labeled by doctors. An automatic detection is considered as true positive (TP) if the detected result is within a circle centered at the ground-truth annotation with a radius r. The detected results that do not fall into the circle will be labeled as false positive (FP). All missed true cell centers are counted as false negative (FN). The results are reported in terms of precision ($P = \frac{TP}{TP+FP}$) and recall ($R = \frac{TP}{TP+FN}$). Both the maximum-weight independent set (MWIS) and the deep convolutional neural network (DCNN) are evaluated in the following sections.

Firstly, in order to justify the proposed two-step iterative algorithm to solve the MWIS problem stated in Equation (1), we have compared it with a commonly used greedy non-maximum suppression (NMS) method [6], which keeps selecting an available node with the highest score and then removing the node and its neighbors until all the nodes are checked. As defined before, two nodes are considered as neighbors if their Euclidean distance is smaller than a threshold parameter λ. Taking detection results obtained from [1], [2], and [3] as inputs, we generate a set of detection results for both the proposed algorithm and NMS by changing the parameter λ. The comparison of the converged object function values of Equation (1) achieved by the proposed algorithm (Ours) and NMS are shown in Fig. 3 (a) and (d). The comparative results of detection accuracy (F_1 score) are shown in Fig. 3 (b) and (e) for Net and Lung dataset, respectively. We can observe that: 1) Both the proposed algorithm and NMS method are insensitive to parameter λ, and 2) the proposed algorithm consistently produces solutions of better qualities in terms of maximizing the object function in Equation (1) and outperforms the NMS method in most cases in terms of detection accuracy, F_1 score. For both methods, the detect candidates with scores below than 0 (1 denotes positive and -1 denotes negative while training) will not be considered.

Secondly, the proposed cell detection algorithm is compared with three detection algorithms: 1) Iterative radial voting (IRV) [1] with different cell diameter parameter {19, 22, 25, 28, 31} for NET and {17, 20, 23, 26, 29} for Lung dataset; 2) Image-based tool for counting nuclei (ITCN) [2] with diameter parameter set as {20, 23, 26, 29, 32} for NET and {17, 20, 23, 26, 29} for Lung dataset; 3) A learning based cell detection algorithm (Arteta *et al.* [3]) that does not require the parameter selection once a structured supported vector machine is learned on the training images. Both algorithms (1) and (2) will generate a pool of detection candidates, and we will evaluate whether the proposed algorithm is capable of finding the best subset that outperforms each individual algorithm. Please note that we use IRV+OURS and ITCN+OURS to denote the proposed algorithm using the detection results of IRV and ITCN as candidates for best subset selection, respectively. The experimental results are shown in Fig. 3. The first row denotes the testing results using the NET dataset, and the second row presents the testing results using the lung cancer dataset. The detailed comparative results are explained below.

The comparative results of IRV, IRV+OURS, ITCN, ITCN+OURS with respect to different parameters are shown in Fig. 3 (c) and (f). As one can tell, whether or not IRV and ITCN can provide satisfactory results heavily depend on proper parameter selections, which is not always feasible or convenient during runtime. When the parameter is not selected correctly, the performance will deteriorate significantly as illustrated in (c) and (f) (red and blue dotted lines). However, our proposed algorithm does not require careful selection of parameters

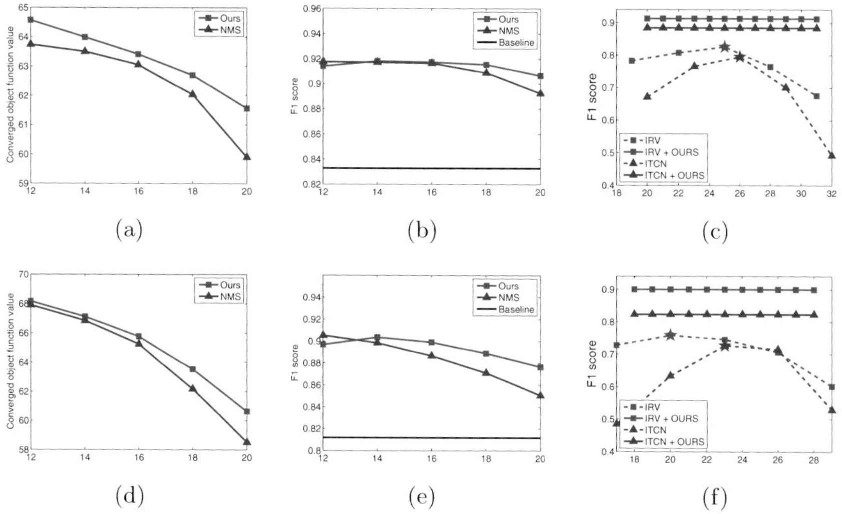

Fig. 3. The evaluation of the proposed general cell detection algorithm using two different datasets. The first and second row denotes results of the NET and Lung datasets, respectively. (a) and (d): The comparison of the object values of Equation (1) achieved by the proposed algorithm (Ours) and NMS with different parameter λ. (b) and (e): The comparison of the proposed algorithm (Ours) and NMS by changing the parameter λ. The baseline method is the algorithm presented by Arteta *et al.* [3]. (c) and (f): The comparison of detection accuracies among IRV, ITCN (different parameters), and our algorithm. The best results of IRV and ITCN are marked with stars.

Table 2. Comparison of cell detection accuracy

Method	NET			Lung		
	F_1-score	Prec.	Rec.	F_1-score	Prec.	Rec.
IRV [1]	0.8260	0.7999	0.8539	0.7584	0.6657	0.8812
ITCN [2]	0.7950	0.8277	0.7647	0.7264	0.6183	0.8804
Arteta *et al.* [3]	0.8328	0.8806	0.7899	0.8118	0.8820	0.7520
[1]+[2]+[3]+OURS	**0.9182**	**0.9003**	**0.9369**	**0.9036**	**0.8843**	**0.9237**

as shown in Fig . 3 (b) and (e). In addition, it consistently outperforms any best individual detection result using IRV and ITCN (red and blue lines).

In order to justify the accuracy of the assigned weights w using DCNN in Equ. (1), we have compared DCNN with a random forest (RF) classifier using different features: 1) Global scene descriptor (GIST) and 2) raw pixel values following by a principle component analysis (PCA) for the dimension reduction. The comparison results can be seen in Fig. 5. It is obvious that DCNN consistently provides better results than other methods on both Net and Lung datasets.

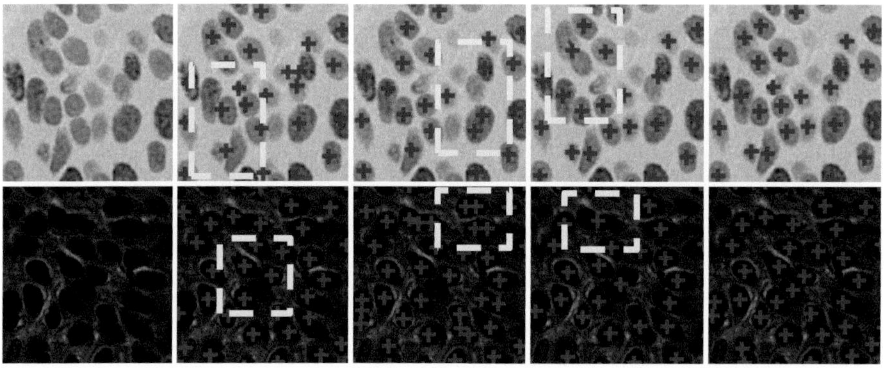

Fig. 4. Qualitative cell detection results using different algorithms. The first row denotes the cell detection results using NET and the second row denotes the cell detection results using the Lung cancer dataset. From left to right, the columns denote: cropped image patch, cell detection results of [1], [2], [3], and the proposed algorithm. The detection errors are labeled with dotted yellow rectangles.

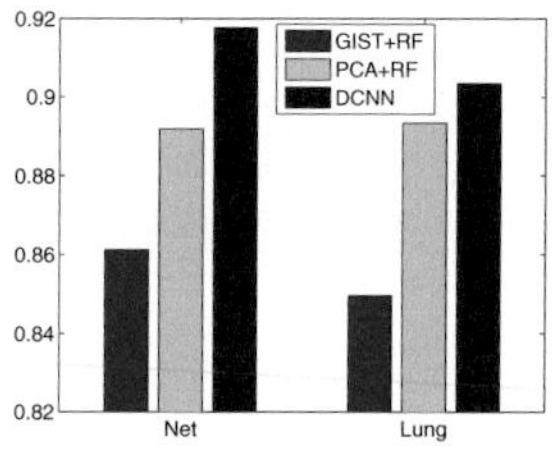

Fig. 5. Comparisons of methods to compute w in Equ. (1)

The quantitative detection results are summarized in Table 2. We can see that the proposed algorithm consistently performs better than both the parameter sensitive methods (IRV and ITCN) and the parameter non-sensitive method [3]. Please note that in Table 2, we report the best detection results of [1] and [2] using the optimal parameters. Some qualitative automatic cell detection results are shown in Fig. 4 using both NET and lung cancer data.

4 Conclusion

In this paper, we have proposed a novel cell detection algorithm based on maximum weight independent set selection that will choose the heavies subset from a pool of cell detection candidates generated from different algorithms using various parameters. The weights of the graph are computed using a deep convolutional neural network. Our experiments show that this novel algorithm provide ensemble detection results that can boost the accuracy of any individual cell detection algorithm.

References

1. Parvin, B., Yang, Q., Han, J., Chang, H., Rydberg, B., Barcellos-Hoff, M.H.: Iterative voting for inference of structural saliency and characterization of subcellular events. TIP 16(3), 615–623 (2007)

2. Byun, J., Verardo, M.R., Sumengen, B., Lewis, G.P., Manjunath, B., Fisher, S.K.: Automated tool for the detection of cell nuclei in digital microscopic images: application to retinal images. Mol. Vis. 12, 949–960 (2006)
3. Arteta, C., Lempitsky, V., Noble, J.A., Zisserman, A.: Learning to detect cells using non-overlapping extremal regions. In: Ayache, N., Delingette, H., Golland, P., Mori, K. (eds.) MICCAI 2012, Part I. LNCS, vol. 7510, pp. 348–356. Springer, Heidelberg (2012)
4. Matas, J., Chum, O., Urban, M., Pajdla, T.: Robust wide-baseline stereo from maximally stable extremal regions. Image and Vision Computing 22(10), 761–767 (2004)
5. LeCun, Y., Bottou, L., Bengio, Y., Haffner, P.: Gradient-based learning applied to document recognition. Proceedings of the IEEE 86(11), 2278–2324 (1998)
6. Cireşan, D.C., Giusti, A., Gambardella, L.M., Schmidhuber, J.: Mitosis detection in breast cancer histology images with deep neural networks. In: Mori, K., Sakuma, I., Sato, Y., Barillot, C., Navab, N. (eds.) MICCAI 2013, Part II. LNCS, vol. 8150, pp. 411–418. Springer, Heidelberg (2013)
7. Li, N., Latecki, L.J.: Clustering aggregation as maximum-weight independent set. In: NIPS, pp. 791–799 (2012)
8. Brendel, W., Todorovic, S.: Segmentation as maximum-weight independent set. In: NIPS, pp. 307–315 (2010)
9. Brendel, W., Amer, M., Todorovic, S.: Multiobject tracking as maximum weight independent set. In: CVPR, pp. 1273–1280. IEEE (2011)
10. Gold, S., Rangarajan, A.: A graduated assignment algorithm for graph matching. PAMI 18(4), 377–388 (1996)
11. Ciresan, D., Giusti, A., Schmidhuber, J., et al.: Deep neural networks segment neuronal membranes in electron microscopy images. In: NIPS, pp. 2852–2860 (2012)

Beyond Classification: Structured Regression for Robust Cell Detection Using Convolutional Neural Network

Yuanpu Xie[1], Fuyong Xing[2], Xiangfei Kong[1], Hai Su[1], and Lin Yang[1]

[1] J. Crayton Pruitt Family Department of Biomedical Engineering, University of Florida, FL 32611, USA
[2] Department of Electrical and Computer Engineering, University of Florida, FL 32611, USA

Abstract. Robust cell detection serves as a critical prerequisite for many biomedical image analysis applications. In this paper, we present a novel convolutional neural network (CNN) based structured regression model, which is shown to be able to handle touching cells, inhomogeneous background noises, and large variations in sizes and shapes. The proposed method only requires a few training images with weak annotations (just one click near the center of the object). Given an input image patch, instead of providing a single class label like many traditional methods, our algorithm will generate the structured outputs (referred to as proximity patches). These proximity patches, which exhibit higher values for pixels near cell centers, will then be gathered from all testing image patches and fused to obtain the final proximity map, where the maximum positions indicate the cell centroids. The algorithm is tested using three data sets representing different image stains and modalities. The comparative experiments demonstrate the superior performance of this novel method over existing state-of-the-art.

1 Introduction

In microscopic image analysis, robust cell detection is a crucial prerequisite for biomedical image analysis tasks, such as cell segmentation and morphological measurements. Unfortunately, the success of cell detection is hindered by the nature of microscopic images such as touching cells, background clutters, large variations in the shape and the size of cells, and the use of different image acquisition techniques.

To alleviate these problems, a non-overlapping extremal regions selection method is presented in [2] and achieves state-of-the-art performance on their data sets. However, this work heavily relies on a robust region detector and thus the application is limited. Recently, deep learning based methods, which exploit the deep architecture to learn the hierarchical discriminative features, have shown great developments and achieved significant success in biomedical image analysis [11,10]. Convolutional neural network (CNN) attracts particular attentions among those works because of its outstanding performance. Ciresan *et al.*

N. Navab et al. (Eds.): MICCAI 2015, Part III, LNCS 9351, pp. 358–365, 2015.
DOI: 10.1007/978-3-319-24574-4_43

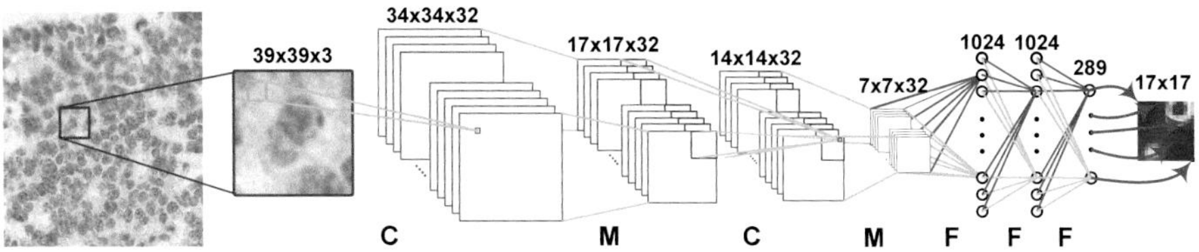

Fig. 1. The CNN architecture used in the proposed structured regression model. C, M and F represents the convolutional layer, max pooling layer, and fully connected layer, respectively. The purple arrows from the last layer illustrate the mapping between the final layer's outputs to the final proximity patch.

adopt CNN for mitosis detection [4] in breast cancer histology images and membrane neuronal segmentation [5] in microscopy images. Typically, CNN is used as a pixel-wise classifier. In the training stage, local image patches are fed into the CNN with their labels determined by the membership of the central pixel. However, this type of widely used approach ignores the fact the labeled regions are coherent and often exhibit certain topological structures. Failing to take this topological information into consideration will lead to implausible class label transition problem [7].

In this paper, we propose a novel CNN based structured regression model for cell detection. Our contributions are summarized as two parts: 1) We modify the conventional CNN by replacing the last layer (classifier) with a structured regression layer to encode topological information. 2) Instead of working on the label space, regression on the proposed structured proximity space for patches is performed so that centers of image patches are explicitly forced to get higher value than their neighbors. The proximity map produced with our novel fusion scheme contains much more robust local maxima for cell centers. To the best of our knowledge, this is the first study to report the application of structured regression model using CNN for cell detection.

2 Methodology

We formulate the cell detection task as a structured learning problem. We replace the last (classifier) layer that is typically used in conventional CNN with a structured regression layer. Our proposed model encodes the topological structured information in the training data. In the testing stage, instead of assigning hard class labels to pixels, our model generates a proximity patch which provides much more precise cues to locate cell centers. To obtain the final proximity map for an entire testing image, we propose to fuse all the generated proximity patches together.

CNN-Based Structured Regression. Let $\mathcal{X}$ denote the patch space, which consists of $d \times d \times c$ local image patches extracted from c-channel color images. An image patch $x \in \mathcal{X}$ centered at the location (u, v) of image I is represented by a quintuple $\{u, v, d, c, I\}$. We define $\mathcal{M}$ as the proximity mask corresponding to image I, and compute the value of the ij-th entry in $\mathcal{M}$ as

$$\mathcal{M}_{ij} = \begin{cases} \frac{1}{1+\alpha D(i,j)} & \text{if } D(i,j) \leq r, \\ 0 & \text{otherwise}, \end{cases} \tag{1}$$

where $D(i, j)$ represents the Euclidean distance from pixel (i, j) to the nearest human annotated cell center. r is a distance threshold and is set to be 5 pixels. α is the decay ration and is set to be 0.8.

The $\mathcal{M}_{ij}$ can have values belongs to the interval $\mathcal{V} = [0, 1]$. An image patch x has a corresponding proximity patch on the proximity mask (shown in Fig.1). We define $s \in \mathcal{V}^{d' \times d'}$ as the corresponding proximity patch for patch x, where $d' \times d'$ denotes the proximity patch size. Note that d' is not necessarily equal to d. We further denote the proximity patch s of patch x as $s = \{u, v, d', \mathcal{M}\}$. It can be viewed as the *structured label* of patch $x = \{u, v, d, c, I\}$.

We define the training data as $\{(\boldsymbol{x}^i, \boldsymbol{y}^i) \in (\mathcal{X}, \mathcal{Y})\}_{i=1}^{\mathcal{N}}$, whose elements are pairs of inputs and outputs: $\boldsymbol{x}^i \in \mathcal{X}$, $\boldsymbol{y}^i = \Gamma(\boldsymbol{s}^i)$, $\mathcal{N}$ is the number of training samples, and $\Gamma : \mathcal{V}^{d' \times d'} \rightarrow \mathcal{Y}$ is a mapping function to represent the vectorization operation in column-wise order for an proximity patch. $\mathcal{Y} \subset \mathcal{V}^{p \times 1}$ represents the output space of the structured regression model, where $p = d' \times d'$ denotes the number of units in the last layer. Define functions $\{f_l\}_{l=1}^{L}$ and $\{\boldsymbol{\theta}_l\}_{l=1}^{L}$ as the operations and parameters corresponding to each of the L layers, the training process of the structured regression model can be formulated as learning a mapping function ψ composed with $\{f_1, ..., f_L\}$, which will map the image space $\mathcal{X}$ to the output space $\mathcal{Y}$.

Given a set of training data $\{(\boldsymbol{x}^i, \boldsymbol{y}^i) \in (\mathcal{X}, \mathcal{Y})\}_{i=1}^{\mathcal{N}}$, $\{\boldsymbol{\theta}_l\}_{l=1}^{L}$ will be learned by solving the following optimization problem

$$\underset{\boldsymbol{\theta}_1, \ldots, \boldsymbol{\theta}_L}{\arg\min} \frac{1}{\mathcal{N}} \sum_{i=1}^{\mathcal{N}} \mathcal{L}(\psi(\boldsymbol{x}^i; \boldsymbol{\theta}_1, ..., \boldsymbol{\theta}_L), \boldsymbol{y}^i), \tag{2}$$

where $\mathcal{L}$ is the loss function that is defined in the following.

Equation (2) can be solved using the classical back propagation algorithm. In order to back propagate the gradients from the last layer (structured regression layer) to the lower layers, we need to differentiate the loss function defined on one training sample with respect to the inputs to the last layer. Let $\boldsymbol{a}^i$ and $\boldsymbol{o}^i$ represent the inputs and the outputs of the last layer. For one training example $(\boldsymbol{x}^i, \boldsymbol{y}^i)$, we can have $\boldsymbol{o}^i = \psi(\boldsymbol{x}^i; \boldsymbol{\theta}_1, ..., \boldsymbol{\theta}_L)$. Denote y_j^i, a_j^i and o_j^i as the j-th element of $\boldsymbol{y}^i$, $\boldsymbol{a}^i$ and $\boldsymbol{o}^i$, respectively. The loss function $\mathcal{L}$ for $(\boldsymbol{x}^i, \boldsymbol{y}^i)$ is given by

$$\begin{aligned} \mathcal{L}(\psi(\boldsymbol{x}^i; \boldsymbol{\theta}_1, ..., \boldsymbol{\theta}_L), \boldsymbol{y}^i) = \mathcal{L}(\boldsymbol{o}^i, \boldsymbol{y}^i) &= \frac{1}{2} \sum_{j=1}^{p} (y_j^i + \lambda)(y_j^i - o_j^i)^2 \\ &= \frac{1}{2} \left\| (Diag(\boldsymbol{y}^i) + \lambda \mathbf{I})^{1/2} (\boldsymbol{y}^i - \boldsymbol{o}^i) \right\|_2^2, \end{aligned} \tag{3}$$

where $\mathbf{I}$ is an identity matrix of size $p \times p$, and $Diag(\boldsymbol{y}^i)$ is a diagonal matrix with the j-th diagonal element equal to y_j^i. Since the non-zero region in the proximity patch is relatively small, our model might return a trivial solution. To alleviate this problem, we adopt a weighting strategy [13] to give the loss coming from the network's outputs corresponding to the non-zero area in the proximity patch more weights. A small λ indicates strong penalization that is applied to errors coming from the outputs with low proximity values in the training data. Our model is different from [13] which applies a bounding box mask regression approach on the entire image.

We choose the sigmoid activation function in the last layer, i.e., $o_j^i = sigm(a_j^i)$. The partial derivative of (3) with respect to the input of the j-th unit in the last layer is given by

$$\frac{\partial \mathcal{L}(\boldsymbol{o}^i, \boldsymbol{y}^i)}{\partial a_j^i} = \frac{\partial \mathcal{L}(\boldsymbol{o}^i, \boldsymbol{y}^i)}{\partial o_j^i} \frac{\partial o_j^i}{\partial a_j^i} = (y_j^i + \lambda)(o_j^i - y_j^i) a_j^i (1 - a_j^i). \tag{4}$$

Based on (4), we can evaluate the gradients of (2) with respect to the model's parameters in the same way as [9]. The optimization procedure is based on mini-batch stochastic gradient descent.

CNN Architecture. The proposed structured regression model contains several convolutional layers (C), max-pooling layers (M), and fully-connected layers (F). Figure 1 illustrates one of the architectures and mapped proximity patches in the proposed model. The detailed model configuration is: Input($49 \times 49 \times 3$) – C($44 \times 44 \times 32$) – M($22 \times 22 \times 32$) – C($20 \times 20 \times 32$) – M($10 \times 10 \times 32$)– C($8 \times 8 \times 32$) – F(1024) – F(1024) – F(289). The activation function of last F (regression) layer is chosen as the sigmoid function, and ReLu function is used for all the other F and C layers. The sizes of C and M layers are defined as $width \times height \times depth$, where $width \times height$ determines the dimensionality of each feature map and $depth$ represents the number of feature maps. The filter size is chosen as 6×6 for the first convolutional layer and 3×3 for the remaining two. The max pooling layer uses a window of size 2×2 with a stride of 2.

Structured Prediction Fusion and Cell Localization. Given a testing image patch $x = (u, v, d, c, I)$, it is easy to get the corresponding proximity mask as $s = \Gamma^{-1}(y)$, where $y \in \mathcal{Y}$ represent the model's output corresponding to x. In the fusion process, s will cast a proximity value for every pixel that lies in the $d' \times d'$ neighborhood area of (u, v), for example, pixel $(u + i, v + j)$ in image I will get a prediction s_{ij} from pixel (u, v). In other words, as we show in Fig.2(B), each pixel actually receives $p' \times p'$ predictions from its neighboring pixels. To get the fused proximity map, we average all the predictions for each pixel from its neighbors to calculate it's final proximity prediction. After this step, the cell localization can be easily obtained by finding the local maximum positions in the average proximity map.

Speed Up. Traditional sliding window method is time consuming. However, we have implemented two strategies to speed up. The first one comes from the property that our model generates a $d' \times d'$ proximity patch for each testing patch. This makes it feasible to skip a lot of pixels and only test the image

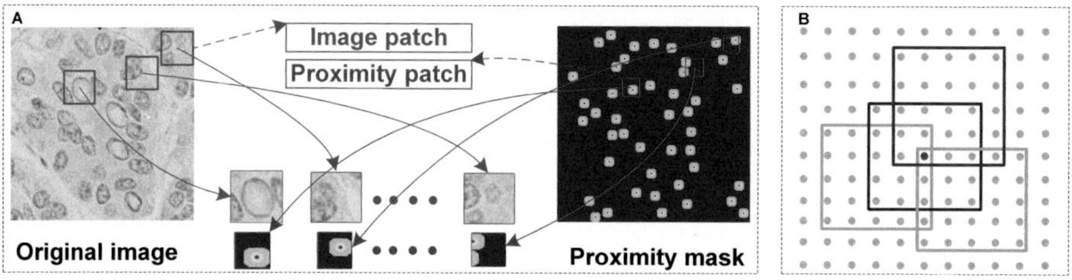

Fig. 2. (A): The training data generation process. Each original image has a proximity mask of the same size and each local image patch has an proximity patch used as the structured *label.* (B) The fusion process. Each pixel receives predictions from it's neighborhoods. For example, the red dot collects all the predictions from its 25 neighboring pixels and an average value will be assigned as final result. In this figure, we only display 4 out of 25 proximity patches.

patches at a certain stride ss ($1 \leq ss \leq d'$) without significantly sacrificing the accuracy. The second strategy, called *fast scanning* [6], is based on the fact that there exists a lot of redundant convolution operations among adjacent patches when computing the sliding-windows.

3 Experimental Results

Data Set and Implementation Details. Our model is implemented in C++ and CUDA based on the fast CNN kernels [8], and *fast scanning* [6] is implemented in MATLAB. The proposed algorithm is trained and tested on a PC with an Intel Xeon E5 CPU and a NVIDIA Tesla k40C GPU. The learning rate is set as 0.0005 and a dropout rate of 0.2 is used for the fully connected layers. The λ is set as 0.3 in (3).

Three data sets are used to evaluate the proposed method. First, The Cancer Genome Atlas (TCGA) dataset, from which we cropped and annotated 32 400×400 H&E-stained microscopy images of breast cancer cells, the magnification is 40×. The detection task in this data set is challenging due to highly inhomogeneous background noises, a large variability of the size of cells, and background similarities. The second dataset is obtained from [2] that contains 22 phase contrast images of HeLa cervical cancer cell. These images exhibit large variations in sizes and shapes. The third dataset contains 60 400×400 Ki67-stained neuroendocrine tumor (NET) images of size 400×400, the magnification is 40×. Many touching cells, weak staining, and fuzzy cell boundaries are presented in this dataset. All of the data are randomly split into halves for training and testing.

Model Evaluation. Figure 3 shows the qualitative detection results on three datasets. For quantitative analysis, we define the ground-truth areas as circular regions within 5 pixels of every annotated cell center. A detected cell centroid

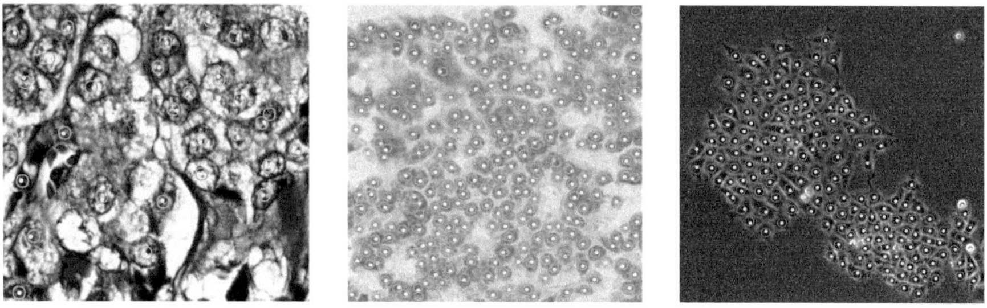

(a) H&E breast cancer (b) Ki-67 stained NET (c) Phase-contrast HeLa

Fig. 3. Cell detection results on three sample images from the three data sets. Yellow dots represent the detected cell centers. The ground truth annotations are represented by green circles for better illustrations.

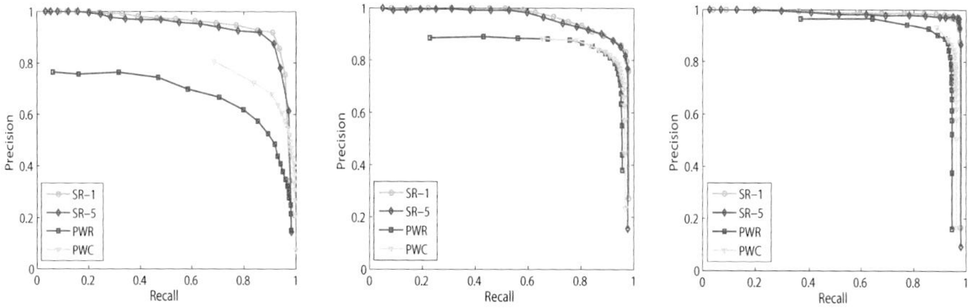

(a) H&E breast cancer (b) Ki-67 stained NET (c) Phase-contrast HeLa

Fig. 4. Precision-recall curves of the four variations of the proposed algorithm on three data sets. SR-5 achieves almost the same results as SR-1. The proposed SR-1 significantly outperforms the other two pixel-wise methods using CNN.

is considered to be a true positive (TP) only if it lies within the ground-truth areas; otherwise, it is considered as a false positive (FP). Each TP is matched with the nearest ground-truth annotated cell center. The ground-truth cell centers that are not matched by any detected results are considered to be false negatives (FN). Based on the above definitions, we can compute the precision (P), recall(R), and F_1 score as $P = \frac{TP}{TP+FP}$, $R = \frac{TP}{TP+FN}$ and $F_1 = \frac{2PR}{P+R}$, respectively.

We evaluated four variations of the proposed methods. (1, 2) *Structured Regression + testing with a stride ss* (SR-ss), ss is chosen to be 1 for (1) and 5 for (2). (3) *CNN based Pixel-Wise Classification* (PWC), which shares the similar architecture with the proposed method except that it utilizes the softmax classifier in the last layer. (4) *CNN based Pixel-Wise Regression* (PWR), which is similar to SR-1 but only predicts the proximity value for the central pixel of each patch.

Figure 4 shows the precision-recall curves of the four variations of the proposed method on each data set. These curves are generated by changing the threshold ζ

Table 1. The comparative cell detection results on three data sets. μ_d, σ_d represent the mean and standard deviation of $\mathbf{E_d}$, and μ_n, σ_n represent the mean and standard deviation of $\mathbf{E_n}$.

Data Set	Methods	P	R	F_1	$\mu_d \pm \sigma_d$	$\mu_n \pm \sigma_n$
H&E breast cancer	SR-1	**0.919**	0.909	**0.913**	$\mathbf{3.151 \pm 2.049}$	4.8750 ± 2.553
	NERS [2]	–	–	–	–	–
	IRV [12]	0.488	0.827	0.591	5.817 ± 3.509	9.625 ± 4.47
	LoG [1]	0.264	**0.95**	0.398	7.288 ± 3.428	$\mathbf{2.75 \pm 2.236}$
	ITCN [3]	0.519	0.528	0.505	7.569 ± 4.277	26.188 ± 8.256
NET	SR-1	0.864	**0.958**	**0.906**	$\mathbf{1.885 \pm 1.275}$	$\mathbf{8.033 \pm 10.956}$
	NERS [2]	**0.927**	0.648	0.748	2.689 ± 2.329	32.367 ± 49.697
	IRV [12]	0.872	0.704	0.759	2.108 ± 3.071	15.4 ± 14.483
	LoG [1]	0.83	0.866	0.842	3.165 ± 2.029	11.533 ± 21.782
	ITCN [3]	0.797	0.649	0.701	3.643 ± 2.084	24.433 ± 40.82
Phase Contrast	SR-1	**0.942**	**0.972**	**0.957**	$\mathbf{2.069 \pm 1.222}$	$\mathbf{3.455 \pm 4.547}$
	NERS [2]	0.934	0.901	0.916	2.174 ± 1.299	11.273 ± 11.706
	IRV [12]	0.753	0.438	0.541	2.705 ± 1.416	58.818 ± 40.865
	LoG [1]	0.615	0.689	0.649	3.257 ± 1.436	29.818 ± 16.497
	ITCN [3]	0.625	0.277	0.371	2.565 ± 1.428	73.727 ± 41.867

on the final proximity maps before finding the local maximum. We can see that SR-5 achieves almost the same performance as SR-1, and both PWC and PWR don't work as well as the proposed structured regression model, especially for the H&E breast cancer data set that exhibits high background similarity and large variations in cell size. This demonstrates that the introduction of the structured regression increases the overall performance. The computational cost for SR-1, SR-5 and *fast scanning* are 14.5, 5 and 19 seconds for testing a 400 $\times$ 400 RGB image. In the training stage, our model takes about 5 hours to converge in our machine.

Comparison with Other Works: We also compare our structured regression model (SR) with four state-of-the-art, including Non-overlapping Extremal Regions Selection (NERS) [2], Iterative Radial Voting (IRV) [12], Laplacian-of-Gaussian filtering (LoG) [1], and Image-based Tool for Counting Nuclei (ITCN) [3]. In addition to Precision, Recall, and F_1 score, we also compute the mean and standard deviation of two terms: 1) The absolute difference $\mathbf{E_n}$ between the number of true positive and the ground-truth annotations, and 2) the Euclidean distance $\mathbf{E_d}$ between the true positive and the corresponding annotations. The quantitative experiment results are reported in Table 1. It is obvious that our method provides better performance than others in all three data sets, especially in terms of F_1 score. Our method also exhibits strong reliability with the lowest mean and standard deviations in $\mathbf{E_n}$ and $\mathbf{E_d}$ on NET and phase contrast data sets.

3.1 Conclusion

In this paper, we propose a structured regression model for robust cell detection. The proposed method differs from the conventional CNN classifiers by introducing a new structured regressor to capture the topological information exhibiting in the training data. Spatial coherence is maintained across the image at the same time. In addition, our proposed algorithm can be implemented with several fast implementation options. We have experimentally demonstrate the superior performance of the proposed method compared with several state-of-the-art. We also show that the proposed method can handle different types of microscopy images with outstanding performance. In future work, we will validate the generality of the proposed model on other image modalities.

References

1. Al-Kofahi, Y., Lassoued, W., Lee, W., Roysam, B.: Improved automatic detection and segmentation of cell nuclei in histopathology images. TBME 57(4), 841–852 (2010)
2. Arteta, C., Lempitsky, V., Noble, J.A., Zisserman, A.: Learning to detect cells using non-overlapping extremal regions. In: Ayache, N., Delingette, H., Golland, P., Mori, K. (eds.) MICCAI 2012, Part I. LNCS, vol. 7510, pp. 348–356. Springer, Heidelberg (2012)
3. Byun, J., Verardo, M.R., Sumengen, B., Lewis, G.P., Manjunath, B.S., Fisher, S.K.: Automated tool for the detection of cell nuclei in digital microscopic images: application to retinal images. Mol. Vis. 12, 949–960 (2006)
4. Cireşan, D.C., Giusti, A., Gambardella, L.M., Schmidhuber, J.: Mitosis detection in breast cancer histology images with deep neural networks. In: Mori, K., Sakuma, I., Sato, Y., Barillot, C., Navab, N. (eds.) MICCAI 2013, Part II. LNCS, vol. 8150, pp. 411–418. Springer, Heidelberg (2013)
5. Ciresan, D., Giusti, A., Gambardella, L.: Schmidhuber: Deep neural networks segment neuronal membranes in electron microscopy images. In: NIPS, pp. 2852–2860 (2012)
6. Giusti, A., Ciresan, D.C., Masci, J., Gambardella, L.M., Schmidhuber, J.: Fast image scanning with deep max-pooling convolutional neural networks. In: ICIP, pp. 4034–4038 (2013)
7. Kontschieder, P., Bul, S., Bischof, H., Pelillo, M.: Structured class-labels in random forests for semantic image labelling. In: ICCV, pp. 2190–2197 (2012)
8. Krizhevsky, A., Sutskever, I., Hinton, G.E.: Imagenet classification with deep convolutional neural networks. In: NIPS, pp. 1106–1114 (2012)
9. Lecun, Y., Bottou, L., Bengio, Y., Haffner, P.: Gradient-based learning applied to document recognition, vol. 86, pp. 2278–2324 (1998)
10. Li, R., Zhang, W., Suk, H.-I., Wang, L., Li, J., Shen, D., Ji, S.: Deep learning based imaging data completion for improved brain disease diagnosis. In: Golland, P., Hata, N., Barillot, C., Hornegger, J., Howe, R. (eds.) MICCAI 2014, Part III. LNCS, vol. 8675, pp. 305–312. Springer, Heidelberg (2014)
11. Liao, S., Gao, Y., Oto, A., Shen, D.: Representation learning: A unified deep learning framework for automatic prostate mr segmentation. In: Mori, K., Sakuma, I., Sato, Y., Barillot, C., Navab, N. (eds.) MICCAI 2013, Part II. LNCS, vol. 8150, pp. 254–261. Springer, Heidelberg (2013)
12. Parvin, B., Yang, Q., Han, J., Chang, H., Rydberg, B., Barcellos-Hoff, M.H.: Iterative voting for inference of structural saliency and characterization of subcellular events. TIP 16, 615–623 (2007)
13. Szegedy, C., Toshev, A., Erhan, D.: Deep neural networks for object detection. In: NIPS, pp. 2553–2561 (2013)

Joint Kernel-Based Supervised Hashing for Scalable Histopathological Image Analysis

Menglin Jiang[1], Shaoting Zhang[2,*], Junzhou Huang[3], Lin Yang[4], and Dimitris N. Metaxas[1]

[1] Department of Computer Science, Rutgers University, Piscataway, NJ, USA
[2] Department of Computer Science, UNC Charlotte, Charlotte, NC, USA
[3] Department of Computer Science and Engineering, UT Arlington, Arlington, TX, USA
[4] Department of Biomedical Engineering, University of Florida, Gainesville, FL, USA

Abstract. Histopathology is crucial to diagnosis of cancer, yet its interpretation is tedious and challenging. To facilitate this procedure, content-based image retrieval methods have been developed as case-based reasoning tools. Recently, with the rapid growth of histopathological images, hashing-based retrieval approaches are gaining popularity due to their exceptional scalability. In this paper, we exploit a joint kernel-based supervised hashing (JKSH) framework for fusion of complementary features. Specifically, hashing functions are designed based on linearly combined kernel functions associated with individual features, and supervised information is incorporated to bridge the semantic gap between low-level features and high-level diagnosis. An alternating optimization method is utilized to learn the kernel combination and hashing functions. The obtained hashing functions compress high-dimensional features into tens of binary bits, enabling fast retrieval from a large database. Our approach is extensively validated on thousands of breast-tissue histopathological images by distinguishing between actionable and benign cases. It achieves 88.1% retrieval precision and 91.2% classification accuracy within 14.0 ms query time, comparing favorably with traditional methods.

1 Introduction

For years, histopathology has played a key role in the early diagnosis of breast cancer, which is the second leading cause of cancer-related death among women. Unfortunately, examination of histopathological images is very tedious and error-prone due to their large size, inter- and intra-observer variability among pathologists, and several other factors [11]. To facilitate this procedure, many content-based image retrieval (CBIR) methods have been proposed as computer-aided diagnosis (CAD) tools [1, 3, 13, 14]. These approaches compare a query histopathological image with previously diagnosed cases stored in a database, and return the most similar cases along with the likelihood of abnormality of the query. Compared with classifier-based CAD methods [2, 5], CBIR approaches could provide more clinical evidence to assist the diagnosis. In addition, they can also contribute to digital slide archiving, pathologist training, and various

* Corresponding author.

N. Navab et al. (Eds.): MICCAI 2015, Part III, LNCS 9351, pp. 366–373, 2015.
DOI: 10.1007/978-3-319-24574-4_44

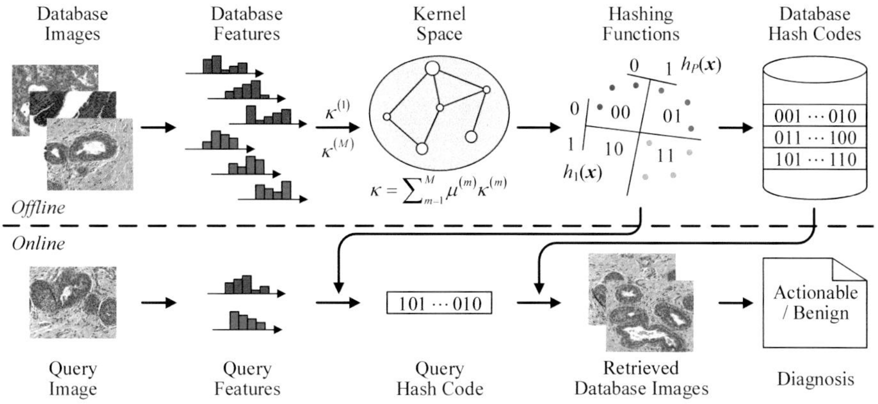

Fig. 1. Overview of the proposed approach.

other applications. Especially, along with the dramatic increase in digital histopathology, hashing-based retrieval methods are drawing more and more attention because of their remarkable computational efficiency and excellent scalability [13, 14].

In the image retrieval community, it is a common practice to employ multiple features to improve performance. Nevertheless, few hashing-based methods have put this principle into practice. A pioneer work [14] adopts the strategy of affinity aggregation. In particular, several affinity matrices calculated using individual features are averaged, and traditional hashing methods are applied to the combined matrix. However, this approach is not suitable for those features that need different kernel functions during the hashing process. Besides, it introduces extra parameters (i.e. the weights of all the matrices) which need to be elaborately tuned. Other widely used feature fusion methods in medical image retrieval include feature concatenation [1] and result-level fusion [12]. The former approach simply concatenates several features to form a new one. Similar to affinity aggregation, it is not appropriate for intrinsically different features even with feature normalization, because various features may need different similarity measures during subsequent feature matching. The latter method first conducts similarity search using individual features, and then integrates their results. Obviously, this approach compromises the computational efficiency, since its processing time will be at least the sum of time required by each feature.

To overcome the above drawbacks, we employ joint kernel-based supervised hashing (JKSH) [6,8,9] to incorporate feature fusion into the supervised hashing framework, and apply it to scalable analysis of histopathological images [13, 14]. The overview of our approach is shown in Fig. 1. Specifically, a joint kernel function is defined as a linear combination of the kernels for individual features, and a series of hashing functions are constructed based on this kernel. Diagnostic information of histopathological images in the database is utilized to learn the weights of individual kernels and the hash functions, which bridges the semantic gap between low-level features and high-level diagnosis. With the learned hashing functions, high-dimensional features are compressed into tens of binary hash bits, enabling efficient search from a large-scale database. At last, a query image is classified (as actionable or benign) according to a weighted majority vote of its retrieved database images [7].

Our approach has many advantages over current methods. First, it could adopt multiple kernel functions as similarity measures for various features, rather than employ the same kernel. Second, the parameter tuning issue is solved, as all the important parameters are automatically learned. Finally, utilizing the kernel representation, compressing multiple features into hash code has little computational overhead than using a single feature.

2 Methodology

In this section, we first formulate the multiple-feature hashing problem as a linear combination of individual kernels, and then explain how to simultaneously learn the kernel weights and hashing functions. After obtaining the hashing functions, features extracted from the database histopathological images can be mapped to compact hash codes and stored in a hash table. Given a query histopathological image, its hash code is computed using the same hashing functions and searched from the hash table to find the most similar database images, which then vote to determine its diagnosis [7].

Joint Kernel-Based Hashing: Suppose we extract M features from N histopathological images. Denote $\boldsymbol{x}_n^{(m)} \in \mathbb{R}^{d^{(m)}}$ as the m-th feature of the n-th image, which is a $d^{(m)}$-dimensional column vector. Then $\boldsymbol{x}_n = \left[\left(\boldsymbol{x}_n^{(1)}\right)^T, \cdots, \left(\boldsymbol{x}_n^{(M)}\right)^T\right]^T \in \mathbb{R}^d$ is the concatenation of all features extracted from the n-th image, where $d = \sum_{m=1}^{M} d^{(m)}$. A hashing method aims at finding P hashing functions $\{h_1, \cdots, h_P\}$, where P is the desired number of hash bits. Each hashing function, $h_p : \mathbb{R}^d \mapsto \{-1, 1\}$, maps a concatenated feature vector into a binary bit. The n-th image is represented as $\boldsymbol{y}_n = [h_1(\boldsymbol{x}_n), \cdots, h_P(\boldsymbol{x}_n)]^T$.

When designing hashing functions, a classic idea is to preserve "local sensitivity", i.e., similar feature vectors are compressed into similar hash codes. Unfortunately, sometimes it is difficult to distinguish between the original features. To solve this problem, kernel functions are introduced to operate the data in an *implicit* higher-dimensional feature space [6]. Given M features, we can choose M kernel functions $\{\kappa^{(1)}, \cdots, \kappa^{(M)}\}$, where each kernel $\kappa^{(m)}$ is associated with an implicit feature mapping function $\varphi^{(m)}$, i.e. $\kappa^{(m)}\left(\boldsymbol{x}_i^{(m)}, \boldsymbol{x}_j^{(m)}\right) = \varphi^{(m)}\left(\boldsymbol{x}_i^{(m)}\right)^T \varphi^{(m)}\left(\boldsymbol{x}_j^{(m)}\right)$. Without ever computing the mapped features $\varphi^{(m)}\left(\boldsymbol{x}_i^{(m)}\right)$ and $\varphi^{(m)}\left(\boldsymbol{x}_j^{(m)}\right)$, $\kappa^{(m)}$ directly calculates their inner product. Such "kernel trick" improves computational efficiency dramatically. Following [3], the joint mapping function φ and corresponding kernel κ are defined as:

$$\varphi(\boldsymbol{x}_n) = \left[\sqrt{\mu^{(1)}}\varphi^{(1)}\left(\boldsymbol{x}_n^{(1)}\right)^T, \cdots, \sqrt{\mu^{(M)}}\varphi^{(M)}\left(\boldsymbol{x}_n^{(M)}\right)^T\right]^T, \tag{1}$$

$$\kappa(\boldsymbol{x}_i, \boldsymbol{x}_j) = \varphi(\boldsymbol{x}_i)^T \varphi(\boldsymbol{x}_j) = \sum_{m=1}^{M} \mu^{(m)} \kappa^{(m)}\left(\boldsymbol{x}_i^{(m)}, \boldsymbol{x}_j^{(m)}\right), \tag{2}$$

where $\mu^{(m)}$ is the weight for the m-th feature. Later we will show how to automatically learn the weight vector $\boldsymbol{\mu} = \left[\mu^{(1)}, \cdots, \mu^{(M)}\right]^T$. Eq. (2) demonstrates that $\kappa = \sum_{m=1}^{M} \mu^{(m)} \kappa^{(m)}$ is actually a linear combination of individual kernels for each feature.

To reduce computational complexity, R $(R \ll N)$ landmark points, denoted as $\{\boldsymbol{z}_1, \cdots, \boldsymbol{z}_R\}$, are randomly selected from all the database feature vectors $\{\boldsymbol{x}_1, \cdots, \boldsymbol{x}_N\}$. Then, for the p-th hashing function h_p, its hyperplane vector $\boldsymbol{v}_p$ in the kernel space is represented as a linear combination of projections of landmarks in that space:

$$\boldsymbol{v}_p = \sum_{r=1}^{R} W(r, p)\, \varphi(\boldsymbol{z}_r),\ p = 1, \cdots, P, \tag{3}$$

where W is a $R \times P$-dimensional matrix, its element $W(r, p)$ denotes the weight of $\boldsymbol{z}_r$ for $\boldsymbol{v}_p$. $h_p(\boldsymbol{x}_n)$ is defined based on the projection of $\varphi(\boldsymbol{x}_n)$ on $\boldsymbol{v}_p$:

$$h_p(\boldsymbol{x}_n) = \operatorname{sgn}\left(\boldsymbol{v}_p^T \varphi(\boldsymbol{x}_n) + b_p\right),\ p = 1, \cdots, P, \tag{4}$$

where b_p is the threshold parameter. Denote $\boldsymbol{b} = [b_1, \cdots, b_P]^T$ as the threshold vector, $K_{R\times N} = [\kappa(\boldsymbol{z}_r, \boldsymbol{x}_n)]_{R\times N}$ as the kernel matrix between R landmarks and N database features, and $K_{R\times N}(:, n)$ as the n-th column of K. Utilizing the fact $\kappa = \sum_{m=1}^{M} \mu^{(m)} \kappa^{(m)}$, we can represent the hash code of the n-th image in a kernel form:

$$\boldsymbol{y}_n = \operatorname{sgn}\left(W^T K_{R\times N}(:, n) + \boldsymbol{b}\right),\ n = 1, \cdots, N. \tag{5}$$

W and $\boldsymbol{b}$ determine the hashing functions, and they are learned using supervised information along with $\boldsymbol{\mu}$.

Supervised Optimization: In the image retrieval field, "semantic gap", which refers to the difference between low-level features and high-level concepts, is a long-standing problem. Supervised methods, such as kernel-based supervised hashing (KSH) [8], offer a promise to address this issue. Developed from the idea of "local sensitivity", supervised hashing approaches map semantically similar images to similar hash codes. To this end, we incorporate diagnostic information into affinity matrix S. $S(i, j)$, representing the similarity score between the i-th and the j-th images, is defined as:

$$S(i, j) = \begin{cases} \exp\left(-\frac{\|\boldsymbol{x}_i - \boldsymbol{x}_j\|^2}{\sigma^2}\right), & \text{if } \boldsymbol{x}_j \text{ is among the } k \text{ nearest neighbors} \\ & \text{of } \boldsymbol{x}_i \text{ with the same label} \\ 0, & \text{otherwise} \end{cases}, \tag{6}$$

where σ is a scaling parameter estimated from the data. Note that S is a sparse matrix, i.e., most of its elements are 0.

The objective function of the proposed JKSH is formulated as:

$$\begin{aligned} &\min_{W, \boldsymbol{b}, \boldsymbol{\mu}} \ \tfrac{1}{2} \sum_{i,j=1}^{N} S(i, j) \|\boldsymbol{y}_i - \boldsymbol{y}_j\|^2 + \lambda \|V\|_F^2 = \operatorname{Tr}\left(YLY^T\right) + \lambda \|V\|_F^2 \\ &\text{s.t.} \ \sum_{n=1}^{N} \boldsymbol{y}_n = \boldsymbol{0},\ \tfrac{1}{N} \sum_{n=1}^{N} \boldsymbol{y}_n \boldsymbol{y}_n^T = I,\ \boldsymbol{1}^T \boldsymbol{\mu} = 1,\ \boldsymbol{\mu} \succcurlyeq \boldsymbol{0}. \end{aligned} \tag{7}$$

Here $\sum_{i,j=1}^{N} S(i, j) \|\boldsymbol{y}_i - \boldsymbol{y}_j\|^2$ guarantees that histopathological images with the same label and similar features are compressed into similar hash codes, $V = [\boldsymbol{v}_1, \cdots, \boldsymbol{v}_P]$

is the hyperplane matrix, $\|V\|_F^2$ is a regularized term used to control the smoothness of hashing functions, $Y = [\boldsymbol{y}_1, \cdots, \boldsymbol{y}_N]$ includes all the database hash codes, $L = \text{diag}(S\mathbf{1}) - S$ is the graph Laplacian matrix, the constraints ensure that the generated hash codes are balanced and uncorrelated. To solve this NP-hard problem, we employ spectral relaxation, which ignores the discrete constraint for $\boldsymbol{y}_n$ in Eq. (5) and allows $\boldsymbol{y}_n = W^T K_{R\times N}(:, n) + \boldsymbol{b} \in \mathbb{R}^P$.

The above problem, when either $(W, \boldsymbol{b})$ or $\boldsymbol{\mu}$ is fixed, is convex with respect to the other. Therefore we perform an alternating optimization algorithm, which mainly consists of the following two steps.

Step 1. Optimize $(W, \boldsymbol{b})$ ***for given*** $\boldsymbol{\mu}$. Similar to [6], we can find the optimal W by solving the following problem using eigen-decomposition:

$$\min_W \text{Tr}\left(W^T C W\right) \text{ s.t. } W^T G W = I, \tag{8}$$

where $C = K_{R\times N} L K_{R\times N}^T + \lambda K_{R\times R}$, $K_{R\times R} = [\kappa(\boldsymbol{z}_i, \boldsymbol{z}_j)]_{R\times R}$ is the kernel matrix between R landmarks, and $G = (1/N) K_{R\times N}\left(I - (1/N)\mathbf{1}\mathbf{1}^T\right) K_{R\times N}^T$. $\boldsymbol{b}$ has a close-form solution depending on W:

$$\boldsymbol{b} = -\frac{1}{N} W^T K_{R\times N}\mathbf{1}. \tag{9}$$

Step 2. Optimize $\boldsymbol{\mu}$ ***for given*** $(W, \boldsymbol{b})$. The optimal $\boldsymbol{\mu}$ can be obtained by solving the following quadratic programming problem:

$$\min_{\boldsymbol{\mu}} \frac{1}{2}\boldsymbol{\mu}^T E \boldsymbol{\mu} + \boldsymbol{f}^T \boldsymbol{\mu} \text{ s.t. } \mathbf{1}^T \boldsymbol{\mu} = 1,\ \boldsymbol{\mu} \succcurlyeq \mathbf{0}, \tag{10}$$

where E is defined as $E(i,j) = 2\,\text{Tr}\left(W^T K_{R\times N}^{(i)} L \left(K_{R\times N}^{(j)}\right)^T W\right)$ $(i, j = 1, \cdots, M)$, $\boldsymbol{f} = \left[f^{(1)}, \cdots, f^{(M)}\right]^T$, $f^{(m)} = \lambda\,\text{Tr}\left(W^T K_{R\times R}^{(m)} W\right)$, $K_{R\times N}^{(m)} = \left[\kappa^{(m)}\left(\boldsymbol{z}_r^{(m)}, \boldsymbol{x}_n^{(m)}\right)\right]_{R\times N}$ is the kernel matrix for the m-th feature between R landmarks and N database images, and $K_{R\times R}^{(m)} = \left[\kappa^{(m)}\left(\boldsymbol{z}_i^{(m)}, \boldsymbol{z}_j^{(m)}\right)\right]_{R\times R}$ is the kernel matrix for the m-th feature between R landmarks $(m = 1, \cdots, M)$.

In summary, the optimization approach works as follows. First, it initializes $\boldsymbol{\mu} = [1/M, \cdots, 1/M]^T$. Then, it iteratively updates $(W, \boldsymbol{b})$ according to step 1 and updates $\boldsymbol{\mu}$ according to step 2 until they converge. In practice, our method usually finds the optimal $(W, \boldsymbol{b})$ and $\boldsymbol{\mu}$ within a few iterations.

3 Experiments

Experimental Settings: Our experiments are carried out on the breast-tissue microscopic image dataset built in [5,13]. Briefly speaking, this dataset comprises 20 actionable (atypical ductal hyperplasia, ADH, and ductal carcinoma in situ, DCIS) cases and 20 benign (usual ductal hyperplasia, UDH) cases. 654 and 1723 images, each of which

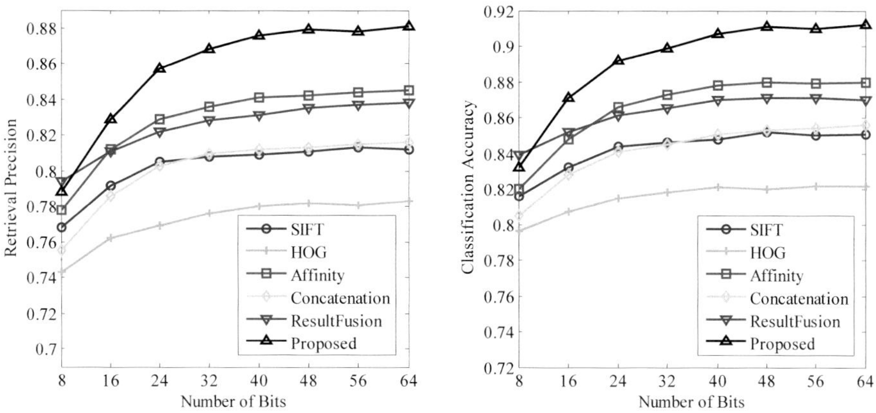

Fig. 2. Retrieval precision (left) and classification accuracy (right) at different hash code lengths.

has about 2.25M pixels, are sampled from the slides of these two categories. Four-fold cross-validation is performed for reliable results. That is, both actionable and benign cases are divided into four parts, and the proposed approach is evaluated four times. During each time, images in three parts form a database, and images in the other part are used as queries. Note that the query and database images are selected from different cases to avoid positive bias. The average performance from four runs is reported.

The proposed approach employs two texture-related features, namely scale-invariant feature transform (SIFT) [10] and histogram of oriented gradient (HOG) [4], which have demonstrated good performance in medical image retrieval and analysis [2, 3, 7, 13, 14]. In particular, scale-invariant keypoints are first detected by finding local extrema in difference-of-Gaussian (DoG) space, then SIFT and HOG features are calculated around these keypoints. Both features are quantized using bag-of-words (BoW) method [2, 3] and represented as 2000-dimensional histograms. As for kernel function, the proposed approach adopts Gaussian radial basis function (RBF) for both SIFT and HOG. Gaussian RBF is very popular in kernelized learning methods, and has been successfully applied to medical image analysis [2].

Five baseline methods are implemented for comparison. The first two methods, following [13], apply traditional KSH [8] on SIFT and HOG BoW respectively. The other three methods exploit KSH on both features, which are unified through affinity aggregation [14], feature catenation [1], and result-level fusion [12], respectively. These feature fusion methods have been widely used in medical image retrieval and demonstrated good performance.

Results and Analysis: We first evaluate the *retrieval precision* of all the methods, which is defined as the percentage of retrieved database images that are relevant to query image. The top 20 retrieved images are considered for this purpose. To demonstrate parameter sensitivity, each method uses a series of hash code lengths, ranging from 8 to 64 bits. The results are summarized in Fig. 2. For all the methods, as the hash code length increases to 64 bits, the precision scores first improve and then converge. This observation indicates that hashing-based methods can transform high-dimensional

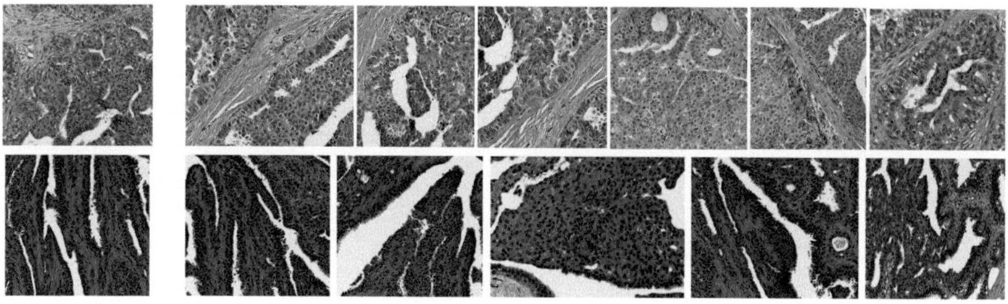

Fig. 3. Two query images (left) and their retrieved database images obtained by our approach (right). Images in the top row are all actionable, and images in the bottom row are all benign.

Table 1. Query time with 64-bit hash code

Method	SIFT	HOG	Affinity	Concatenation	ResultFusion	Proposed
Time (millisecond)	13.2	13.1	14.1	13.8	26.4	14.0

image features to compact yet descriptive image "signatures". Among all the six approaches, the two methods utilizing single feature perform worst. As for the fusion methods, feature concatenation gains marginal improvement over "SIFT + KSH", while affinity aggregation and result-level fusion obtain considerable improvement. The proposed approach substantially outperforms all compared methods, and achieves a precision score of 88.1% when using 64-bit hash code. Two retrieval examples are provided in Fig. 3 for visual evaluation, which demonstrate that our approach could find visually and semantically similar database images for queries.

Then, *classification accuracy* is measured, which refers to the percentage of query images that are correctly classified. Remember that a query image is classified as actionable or benign tissue according to a weighted majority vote of its retrieved database images [7]. The accuracy scores are reported in Fig. 2. Apparently, these scores exhibit similar intra- and inter-method trends to those of the precision scores. Furthermore, the accuracy scores are systematically higher than the precision scores, since irrelevant retrieved images would not cause a misclassification as long as they remain a minority of the retrieval set. Once again, our approach considerably surpasses all the baseline methods. Especially, it achieves a satisfactory classification accuracy of 91.2% at 64-bit hash code length.

Finally, *query time*, i.e. the time needed to retrieve and classify a query image, is investigated when using 64-bit hash code. Here, the time cost of SIFT and HOG BoW calculation is not taken into account, since it remains fixed as the database expands and therefore is not the bottleneck for large-scale image analysis. As shown in Table 1, these hashing-based methods exhibit outstanding computational efficiency. This is attributed to the compactness of hash codes, as well as adoption of hash table and "kernel trick". It is noteworthy that our approach, along with affinity aggregation and feature concatenation, has only a small computational overhead compared with methods using a single feature. As expected, the time cost for result-level fusion is the sum of those for "SIFT + KSH" and "HOG + KSH".

4 Conclusion

In this paper, we adopt joint kernel-based supervised hashing (JKSH) for fusion of complementary features. Multiple-feature hashing is transformed to a similarity preserving problem with linearly combined kernel functions, which are corresponding to the similarity measures for individual features. An alternating optimization algorithm is performed to learn both the kernel combination and hashing functions efficiently. Superior to traditional fusion methods, the proposed approach is suitable for heterogeneous features and doesn't introduce new parameters. Extensive experiments on breast cancer histopathological images demonstrate the efficacy of our approach. Future endeavors will be devoted to improve the performance by choosing better image features and kernel functions. In addition, we plan to extend our approach with online learning so that it could efficiently update hashing functions as new images are added into the database.

References

1. Akakin, H.C., Gurcan, M.N.: Content-based microscopic image retrieval system for multi-image queries. IEEE TITB 16(4), 758–769 (2012)
2. Caicedo, J.C., Cruz, A., González, F.A.: Histopathology image classification using bag of features and kernel functions. In: Combi, C., Shahar, Y., Abu-Hanna, A. (eds.) AIME 2009. LNCS, vol. 5651, pp. 126–135. Springer, Heidelberg (2009)
3. Caicedo, J.C., González, F.A., Romero, E.: Content-based histopathology image retrieval using a kernel-based semantic annotation framework. JBI 44(4), 519–528 (2011)
4. Dalal, N., Triggs, B.: Histograms of oriented gradients for human detection. In: Proc. IEEE CVPR, pp. 886–893 (2005)
5. Dundar, M.M., Badve, S., Bilgin, G., Raykar, V.C., Jain, R.K., Sertel, O., Gurcan, M.N.: Computerized classification of intraductal breast lesions using histopathological images. IEEE TBME 58(7), 1977–1984 (2011)
6. He, J., Liu, W., Chang, S.: Scalable similarity search with optimized kernel hashing. In: Proc. ACM SIGKDD, pp. 1129–1138 (2010)
7. Jiang, M., Zhang, S., Li, H., Metaxas, D.N.: Computer-aided diagnosis of mammographic masses using scalable image retrieval. IEEE TBME 62(2), 783–792 (2015)
8. Liu, W., Wang, J., Ji, R., Jiang, Y., Chang, S.: Supervised hashing with kernels. In: Proc. IEEE CVPR, pp. 2074–2081 (2012)
9. Liu, X., He, J., Lang, B.: Multiple feature kernel hashing for large-scale visual search. PR 47(2), 748–757 (2014)
10. Lowe, D.G.: Distinctive image features from scale-invariant keypoints. IJCV 60(2), 91–110 (2004)
11. Veta, M., Pluim, J.P.W., van Diest, P.J., Viergever, M.A.: Breast cancer histopathology image analysis: A review. IEEE TBME 61(5), 1400–1411 (2014)
12. Wei, C.H., Li, Y., Huang, P.J.: Mammogram retrieval through machine learning within BI-RADS standards. JBI 44(4), 607–614 (2011)
13. Zhang, X., Liu, W., Dundar, M., Badve, S., Zhang, S.: Towards large-scale histopathological image analysis: Hashing-based image retrieval. IEEE TMI 34(2), 496–506 (2015)
14. Zhang, X., Yang, L., Liu, W., Su, H., Zhang, S.: Mining histopathological images via composite hashing and online learning. In: Golland, P., Hata, N., Barillot, C., Hornegger, J., Howe, R. (eds.) MICCAI 2014, Part II. LNCS, vol. 8674, pp. 479–486. Springer, Heidelberg (2014)

Deep Voting: A Robust Approach Toward Nucleus Localization in Microscopy Images

Yuanpu Xie[1], Xiangfei Kong[1], Fuyong Xing[2], Fujun Liu[2], Hai Su[1], and Lin Yang[1]

[1] J. Crayton Pruitt Family Department of Biomedical Engineering, University of Florida, FL 32611, USA
[2] Department of Electrical and Computer Engineering, University of Florida, FL 32611, USA

Abstract. Robust and accurate nuclei localization in microscopy image can provide crucial clues for accurate computer-aid diag In this paper, we propose a convolutional neural network (CNN) based hough voting method to localize nucleus centroids with heavy cluttering and morphologic variations in microscopy images. Our method, which we name as deep voting, mainly consists of two steps. (1) Given an input image, our method assigns each local patch several pairs of voting *offset* vectors which indicate the positions it votes to, and the corresponding voting *confidence* (used to weight each votes), our model can be viewed as an implicit hough-voting codebook. (2) We collect the weighted votes from all the testing patches and compute the final voting density map in a way similar to Parzen-window estimation. The final nucleus positions are identified by searching the local maxima of the density map. Our method only requires a few annotation efforts (just one click near the nucleus center). Experiment results on Neuroendocrine Tumor (NET) microscopy images proves the proposed method to be state-of-the-art.

1 Introduction

Nuclei localization in microscopy image is the foundation of many subsequent biomedical image analysis tasks (e.g., cell segmentation, counting and tracking, etc). However, robust and accurate nucleus localization, especially for microscopy images that exhibit dense nucleus clutters and large variations in both nucleus sizes and shapes, has been a challenging task for a long time. In the past few years, a large number of methods have been proposed, including kernel based radial voting [10], spatial filtering [1] and graph partition based methods [3]. However, because of the large variations in microscopy modality, nucleus morphology, and the inhomogeneous background, it remains to be a challenging topic for these non-learning approaches.

Supervised learning based methods have also attracted a lot of interests due to their promising performance. For example, a general and efficient maximally stable extremal region (MSER) section method is presented in [2]. However this

N. Navab et al. (Eds.): MICCAI 2015, Part III, LNCS 9351, pp. 374–382, 2015.
DOI: 10.1007/978-3-319-24574-4_45

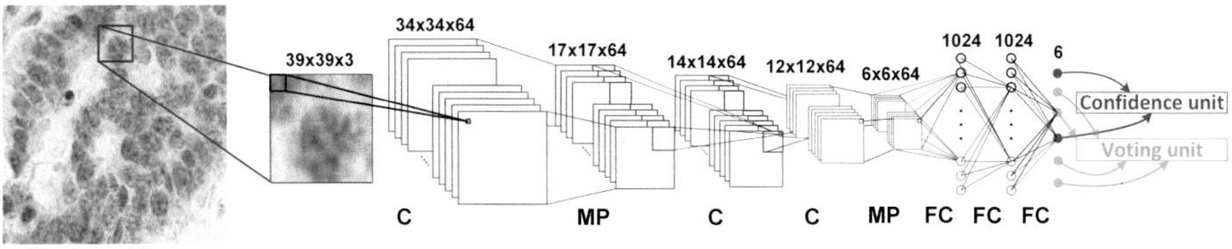

Fig. 1. The architecture of the proposed deep voting model. The C, MP and FC represent the convolutional layer, max-pooling layer, and fully connected layer, respectively. The two different types of units (voting units and weight units) in the last layer are marked with different color. Please note that in this model, the number of votes for each patch (k) is 2.

method requires a robust MSER detector and thus the usage is limited. Codebook based hough transformation has also been widely studied and shown to be able to produce promising performance. In [6], a class specific random forest method is applied to learn a discriminative codebook. However, it only associates one voting *offset* vector to a patch during the training process, and in the testing stage, one patch can only vote along the directions that have already appeared in the training data.

Recently, deep learning has been revived and achieved outstanding performance in both natural and biomedical image analysis tasks [12,11,5]. In this work, we extend the traditional CNN model to learn the voting *offset* vectors and voting *confidence* jointly. Different from [6,11], our method assigns more than one pairs of prediction for each image patch, which together with our specific loss function render our method more robust and capable of handling touching cases. As shown in Fig.1, our deep voting model can be viewed as an implicit hough-voting codebook, via which, each testing patch can vote towards several directions with specific voting *confidence*. We then collect all the weighted votes from all the image patches in an additive way, and estimate the voting density map in a way similar to Parzen-window estimation. Comparative experimental results using several datasets show superiority of the proposed deep voting method.

2 Methodology

2.1 Learning The Deep Voting Model

Preprocessing: In our method, each patch votes to several possible nucleus positions (the coordinates for the nucleus center specified by voting *offsets*) with voting *confidence*. We propose to learn an implicit codebook for these voting *offsets* and corresponding voting *confidence*. During the training stage, we denote the input image patch space as $\mathcal{P}$, composed of a set of image patches with size $d \times d$; and the target space as $\mathcal{T}$, defining the space of the proposed *target* *information.* We define the *target information* as the coalescence of voting *offsets* and voting *confidence.*

For each training patch, we first get its k nearest nucleus positions from a group of human annotated nucleus centers (ground-truth) on training images. Then, corresponding *target information* is computed. Let $\{\mathcal{D}^i = (\mathcal{P}^i, \mathcal{T}^i)\}$ represent the training set where $\mathcal{P}^i \in \mathcal{P}$ is the i-th input image patch and $\mathcal{T}^i \in \mathcal{T}$ is the corresponding *target informationc.* $\mathcal{T}^i$ is further defined as $\{\alpha^i_j, \mathbf{v}^i_j\}^k_{j=1}$, where k denotes the number of total votes from each image patch and $\mathbf{v}^i_j$ is the 2D *offset* vector equals to the displacement from the $j-$th nearest ground-truth nucleus aligned to the center of patch $\mathcal{P}^i$. α^i_j represents the voting *confidence* corresponding to $\mathbf{v}^i_j$. We define it based on the length of the voting *offset* $|\mathbf{v}^i_j|$:

$$\alpha^i_j = \begin{cases} 1, & \text{if } |\mathbf{v}^i_j| \leq r_1, \\ \frac{1}{1+\beta|\mathbf{v}^i_j|}, & \text{if } r_1 < |\mathbf{v}^i_j| \leq r_2, \\ 0, & \text{otherwise}, \end{cases} \tag{1}$$

where β represents the *confidence* decay ratio. r_1, r_2 are used to tune the voting range and are chosen as d and $1.5d$, respectively. Please note that α^i_j is given the flexibility to associate with many properties of the training patches such as foreground area ratio, class membership, distance to the voting position, etc.

Hybrid Non-linear Transformation: We categorize the units of the output layer in our CNN as *voting units* and *confidence units* as shown in Fig.1. Thus, voting *offset* vectors and voting *confidence* are jointly learned. *Voting units* can take any values and are used to specify the positions that each patch will vote to. The values for *confidence units* are confined to $[0, 1]$ and are used as weights for each vote. Existing activation functions (sigmoid, linear, or ReLu) associated to the output layer do not satisfy our needs. We therefore introduce a **hybrid non-linear transformation** *Hy* as our new activation function. Units of the output layer are treated differently based on their category:

$$Hy(x) = \begin{cases} sigm(x), & \text{if } x \text{ is the input to the } \textit{confidence units}, \\ x, & \text{otherwise}, \end{cases} \tag{2}$$

where *sigm* denotes the sigmoid function, Hy takes a vector as it's input and computed the value in element-wise. For example, for a vector $\boldsymbol{a} = \{a_i\}^m_{i=1}$, $Hy(\boldsymbol{a})$ equals to $\{Hy(a_i)\}^m_{i=1}$.

Inference In Deep Voting Model: Denote L as the number of layers, let functions $f_1, ..., f_L$ represent each layer's computations (e.g., linear transformations and convolution, etc.), and denote $\boldsymbol{\theta}_1, ..., \boldsymbol{\theta}_L$ as the parameters of those layers, our model can be viewed as a mapping function: ψ, which maps input image patches to *target information.* Denote $\circ$ as the composition of functions, ψ can be further defined as $f_L \circ f_{L-1}, ..., \circ f_1$ with parameters $\boldsymbol{\Theta} = \{\boldsymbol{\theta}_1, ..., \boldsymbol{\theta}_L\}$.

Given a set of training data $\{\mathcal{D}^i = (\mathcal{P}^i, \mathcal{T}^i)\}_{i=1}^N$, where N is the number of training samples. We evaluate the proposed model's parameters by solving

$$\arg\min_{\boldsymbol{\Theta}} \frac{1}{N} \sum_{i=1}^{N} l(\psi(\mathcal{P}^i; \boldsymbol{\Theta}), T^i), \tag{3}$$

where l is a proper loss function defined in the following sections. Let $\psi(\mathcal{P}^i; \boldsymbol{\Theta}) = \{w_j^i, \boldsymbol{d}_j^i\}_{j=1}^k$ denote the model's output corresponding to the input $\mathcal{P}^i$, where w_j^i and $\boldsymbol{d}_j^i$ are predicted voting *confidence* and *offsets*, respectively. Recall that $\mathcal{T}^i = \{\alpha_j^i, \mathbf{v}_j^i\}_{j=1}^k$ is the *target information* of $\mathcal{P}^i$ and k represents the number of votes from each training image patch. The loss function defined on one training example $(\mathcal{P}^i, \mathcal{T}^i)$ is given by

$$l(\psi(\mathcal{P}^i; \boldsymbol{\Theta}), \mathcal{T}^i) = \sum_{j=1}^{k} \frac{1}{2}(\alpha_j^i w_j^i \|\boldsymbol{d}_j^i - \boldsymbol{v}_j^i\|^2 + \lambda(w_j^i - \alpha_j^i)^2), \tag{4}$$

where λ is a regularization factor. There are two benefits of the proposed loss function: (1) The first term punishes uninformative votes that have either low predicted voting *confidence* or low voting *confidence* in the *target information.* (2) The second term acts as a regularization term to prevent the network producing trivial solutions (setting all voting *confidence* to zero).

The optimization problem defined in (3) is highly non-convex. We use the back propagation algorithm [9] to solve it. In order to calculate the gradient of (3) with respect to the model's parameters $\boldsymbol{\Theta}$, we need to calculate the partial derivatives of the loss function defined on one single example with respect to the inputs of the nodes in the last layer. As shown in Fig.1, the outputs of the proposed model are organized as k pairs of $\{confidence\ units, offset\ units\}$. Let $\{Iw_j^i, \boldsymbol{Iv}_j^i\}_{j=1}^k$ represent the inputs to the units in the last layer for one training sample $(\mathcal{P}^i, \mathcal{T}^i)$, we can easily get $w_j^i = Hy(Iw_j^i)$ and $\boldsymbol{v}_j^i = Hy(\boldsymbol{Iv}_j^i)$. The partial differentiations of (4) with respect to Iw_j^i and $\boldsymbol{Iv}_j^i$ are then given as

$$\begin{aligned}\frac{\partial l(\psi(\mathcal{P}^i; \boldsymbol{\Theta}), \mathcal{T}^i)}{\partial Iw_j^i} &= \frac{\partial l(\psi(\mathcal{P}^i; \boldsymbol{\Theta}), \mathcal{T}^i)}{\partial w_j^i} \frac{\partial w_j^i}{\partial Iw_j^i} \\ &= (\frac{1}{2}\alpha_j^i \|\boldsymbol{d}_j^i - \boldsymbol{v}_j^i\|^2 + \lambda(w_j^i - \alpha_j^i)) Iw_j^i(1 - Iw_j^i), \\ \frac{\partial l(\psi(\mathcal{P}^i; \boldsymbol{\Theta}), \mathcal{T}^i)}{\partial \boldsymbol{Id}_j^i} &= \frac{\partial \boldsymbol{d}_j^i}{\partial \boldsymbol{Id}_j^i} \frac{\partial l(\psi(\mathcal{P}^i; \boldsymbol{\Theta}), \mathcal{T}^i)}{\partial \boldsymbol{d}_j^i} = \alpha_j^i w_j^i(\boldsymbol{d}_j^i - \boldsymbol{v}_j^i),\end{aligned} \tag{5}$$

where $\boldsymbol{Id}_j^i$, $\boldsymbol{d}_j^i$ and $\frac{\partial l(\psi(\mathcal{P}^i;\boldsymbol{\Theta}),\mathcal{T}^i)}{\partial \boldsymbol{Id}_j^i}$ are 2D vectors. After getting the above partial derivatives, the following inferences used to obtain the gradients of (3) with respect to the model's parameters are exactly the same to the classical back propagation algorithm used in conventional CNN [9].

2.2 Weighted Voting Density Estimation

Given a testing image, denote $\mathcal{P}(\boldsymbol{y})$ as a testing patch centered at position $\boldsymbol{y}$ on the testing image, and let $\{w_j(\boldsymbol{y}), \boldsymbol{d}_j(\boldsymbol{y})\}_{j=1}^{k}$ represent our model's output for $\mathcal{P}(\boldsymbol{y})$, where $w_j(\boldsymbol{y})$ and $\boldsymbol{d}_j(\boldsymbol{y})$ represents the $j-$th voting *confidence* and voting *offset* vector for patch $\mathcal{P}(\boldsymbol{y})$, respectively. Furthermore, denote $V(\boldsymbol{x}|\mathcal{P}(\boldsymbol{y}))$ as the accumulated voting score of position $\boldsymbol{x}$ coming from patch $\mathcal{P}(\boldsymbol{y})$. Similar to the kernel density estimation using Parzen-window, we write $V(\boldsymbol{x}|\mathcal{P}(\boldsymbol{y}))$ as

$$V(\boldsymbol{x}|\mathcal{P}(\boldsymbol{y})) = \sum_{j=1}^{k} w_j(\boldsymbol{y}) \frac{1}{2\pi\sigma^2} exp(-\frac{\|(\boldsymbol{y} - \boldsymbol{d}_j(\boldsymbol{y})) - \boldsymbol{x}\|^2}{2\sigma^2}). \quad (6)$$

In this paper, we restrict the votes to a location $\boldsymbol{x}$ to be calculated from a limited area $B(\boldsymbol{x})$, which can be a circle or a bounding box centered at position $\boldsymbol{x}$. To compute the final weighted voting density map $V(\boldsymbol{x})$, we accumulate the weighted votes:

$$V(\boldsymbol{x}) = \sum_{\boldsymbol{y} \in B(\boldsymbol{x})} V(\boldsymbol{x}|\mathcal{P}(\boldsymbol{y})). \quad (7)$$

After obtaining the voting density map $V(\boldsymbol{x})$, a small threshold $\xi \in [0, 1]$ is applied to remove the values smaller than $\xi \cdot \max(V)$. The following procedure for Nucleus localization is to find all the local maxima in V.

2.3 Efficient Nuclei Localization

Traditional localization methods with sliding window are computationally expensive. However, there are two methods to boost the testing speed of the proposed algorithm. The first strategy, which is called fast scanning [7], achieves three orders of magnitude speedup compared to standard sliding window. The basic idea is to remove the redundant convolution operations appeared in adjacent testing patches by doing the convolutional operations on the entire image. The second strategy is straight-forward: instead of performing the testing on the entire image for every sliding window, we can perform the computation in an s stride manner. Both of the methods are evaluated in the experiment part and are proven to be efficient.

In order to reduce the complexity for computing the voting density map in (7), we provide a fast implementation: Given a testing image, instead of following the computation order of (6) and (7), we go through every possible patch $\mathcal{P}(\mathbf{y})$ centered at position $\mathbf{y}$, and add weighted votes $\{w_j(\boldsymbol{y})\}_{j=1}^{k}$ to pixel $\{\boldsymbol{y} - \boldsymbol{d}_j(\boldsymbol{y})\}_{j=1}^{k}$ in a cumulative way. The accumulated vote map are then filtered by a Gaussian kernel to get the final voting density map $V(\boldsymbol{x})$.

3 Experiments

Data and Implementation Details: The proposed method has been extensively evaluated using 44 Ki67-stained NET microscopy images (400$\times$400 pixels).

Testing images are carefully chosen to cover challenging cases like touching cells, inhomogeneous intensity, blurred cell boundaries, and weak staining.

The architecture of our model is summarized in Fig.1. The patch size is set as 39×39. The convolutional kernel sizes are set as 6×6, 4×4, and 3×3 for the three convolutional layers, respectively. All the max pooling layers have a window size of 2×2, and a stride of 2. A dropout ratio 0.25 is used at the training stage to prevent over fitting and the learning rate is set as 0.0001. β and λ are set to be 0.5 and 384 in (1) and (4), respectively. The threshold ξ is set to be 0.2. The Parzen-window size is 5×5 and σ is 1 in (6). These parameters are set either by following conventions from the existing works or by empirical selection. In fact, out method is robust not sensitive to parameters. Our implementation is based on the fast CUDA kernel provided by Krizhevsky [8]. The proposed model is trained and tested using a PC with NVIDIA Tesla K40C GPU and a Intel Xeon E5 CPU.

Evaluate the Deep Voting Model: For quantitative evaluation, we define the ground-truth region as the circular regions of radius r centered at every human annotated nucleus centers. In our case, r is roughly chosen to be half of the average radius of all nucleus. True positive (TP) detections are defined as detected results that lie in the ground-truth region. False positive (FP) detections refer to detection results that lie outside of the ground-truth region. The human annotated nucleus centers that do not match with any detection results are considered to be false negative (FN). Based on TP, FP, and FN, we can calculate the recall (R), precision (P), and F_1 scores, which are given by $R = \frac{TP}{TP+FN}$, $P = \frac{TP}{TP+FP}$ and $F_1 = \frac{2PR}{P+R}$. In addition to P, R, and F_1 score, we also compute the mean μ and standard deviation σ of the Euclidean distance (defined as $\mathbf{E_d}$) between the human annotated nucleus centers and the true positive detections, and also of the absolute difference (defined as $\mathbf{E_n}$) between the number of human annotation and the true positive nucleus centers.

We compare our deep voting with no stride (referred as **DV-1**), deep voting with stride 3 (referred as **DV-3**), and standard patch wise classification using CNN (referred as **CNN+PC**). **CNN+PC** has the same network architecture to the proposed model, except that its last layer is a softmax classifier and produce a probability map for every testing image. Please note that the fast scanning strategy produces the same detection result as **DV-1**.

We also compare our algorithm with three state of the arts, including kernel based Iterative Radial Voting method (**IRV**) [10], structured SVM based Non-overlapping Extremal Regions Selection method (**NERS**) [2], and Image based Tool for Counting Nuclei method (**ITCN**) [4]. For fair comparison, we carefully preprocess the testing image for ITCN and IRV. We do not compare the proposed deep voting model with other methods, such as SVM and boosting using handcrafted features, because CNN is widely proven in recent literatures to produce superior performance in classification tasks.

Experimental Results: Figure 2 shows some qualitative results using three randomly selected image patches. Hundreds of nuclei are correctly detected

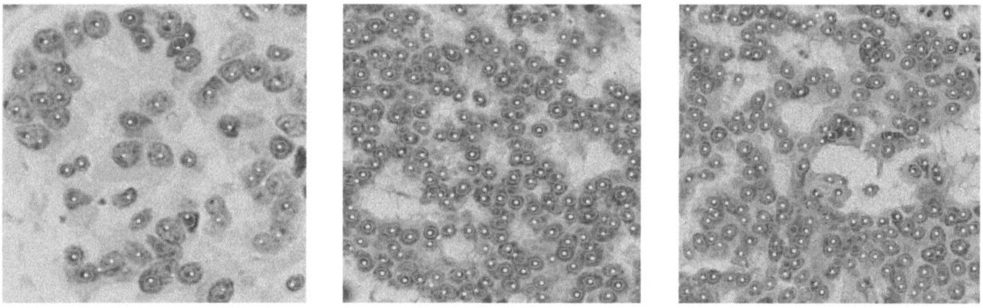

Fig. 2. The Nucleus detection results using deep voting on several randomly selected example images from Ki-67 stained NET dataset. The detected cell centers are marked with yellow dots. The ground-truth is represented with small green circles.

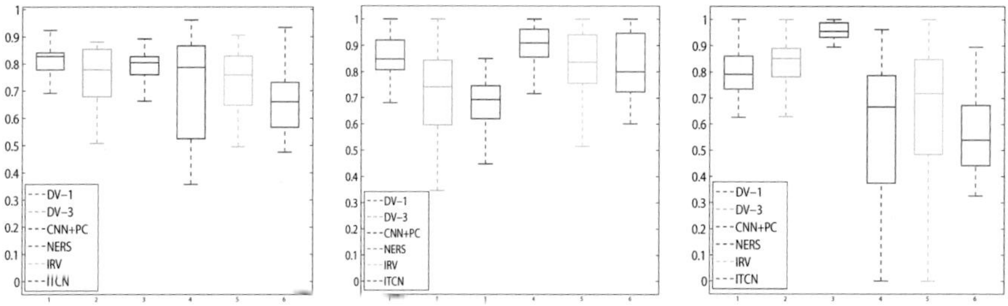

(a) F_1 (b) Precision (c) Recall

Fig. 3. The boxplot of F_1 score, precision, and recall on the NET data set.

using our method. Deep voting is able to handle the touching objects, weak staining, and inhomogeneous intensity variations. Detailed quantitative results are summarized in Table 1. Fast scanning produces exactly the same result as **DV-1** and thus is omitted in the table. It can be observed that deep voting consistently outperforms other methods, especially in terms of F_1 score. Although NERS [2] achieves comparable P score, it does not produce good F_1 score because Ki-67 stained NET images contain a lot of nucleus exhibiting weak staining and similar intensity values between nucleus and background, leading to a large number of FP. Due to the relatively noisy probability map, both **DV-3** and **CNN-PC** provide higher R score but with a large sacrifice of precision. On the other hand, our method, which encodes the geometric information exhibited between the nucleus centroids and patch centers, produces much better overall performance than others. The **DV-3** also gives reasonable results with faster computational time. The boxplot in Fig.3 provides detailed comparisons in terms of precision, recall, and F_1 score.

The computation time for testing a 400×400 RGB image is 22, 5.5 and 31 seconds for our three deep voting implementations: **DV-1**, **DV-3**, and fast scanning, respectively. In our work, both **DV-1** and **DV-3** are implemented using GPU, and deep voting using fast scanning is implemented with MATLAB.

Table 1. The nucleus localization evaluation on the three data sets. μ_d, μ_n and σ_d, σ_n represent the mean and standard deviation of the two criteria $\mathbf{E_d}$ and $\mathbf{E_n}$, respectively

Methods	P	R	F_1	$\mu_d \pm \sigma_d$	$\mu_n \pm \sigma_n$
DV-1	0.852	0.794	**0.8152**	$2.98 \pm \mathbf{1.939}$	$\mathbf{9.667} \pm \mathbf{10.302}$
DV-3	0.727	0.837	0.763	3.217 ± 2.069	17.238 ± 18.294
CNN+PC	0.673	0.9573	0.784	2.51 ± 1.715	37.714 ± 39.397
NERS [2]	0.859	0.602	0.692	2.936 ± 2.447	41.857 ± 57.088
IRV [10]	0.806	0.682	0.718	3.207 ± 2.173	17.714 ± 16.399
ITCN [4]	0.778	0.565	0.641	3.429 ± 2.019	33.047 ± 46.425

3.1 Conclusion

In this paper, we propose a novel deep voting model for accurate and robust nucleus localization. We extend the conventional CNN model to jointly learn the voting *confidence* and voting *offset* by introducing a **hybrid non-linear activation function**. We formulate our problem as a minimization problem with incorporating a novel loss function. In addition, we also demonstrate that our method can be accelerated significantly using simple strategies without sacrificing the overall detection accuracy. Both qualitative and quantitative experimental results demonstrate the superior performance of the proposed deep voting algorithm compared with several state of the arts. We will carry out more experiments and test our method on other image modalities in the future work.

References

1. Al-Kofahi, Y., Lassoued, W., Lee, W., Roysam, B.: Improved automatic detection and segmentation of cell nuclei in histopathology images. TBME 57(4), 841–852 (2010)
2. Arteta, C., Lempitsky, V., Noble, J.A., Zisserman, A.: Learning to detect cells using non-overlapping extremal regions. In: Ayache, N., Delingette, H., Golland, P., Mori, K. (eds.) MICCAI 2012, Part I. LNCS, vol. 7510, pp. 348–356. Springer, Heidelberg (2012)
3. Bernardis, E., Yu, S.X.: Finding dots: segmentation as popping out regions from boundaries. In: CVPR, pp. 199–206 (2010)
4. Byun, J., Verardo, M.R., Sumengen, B., Lewis, G.P., Manjunath, B.S., Fisher, S.K.: Automated tool for the detection of cell nuclei in digital microscopic images: application to retinal images. Mol. Vis. 12, 949–960 (2006)
5. Cireşan, D.C., Giusti, A., Gambardella, L.M., Schmidhuber, J.: Mitosis detection in breast cancer histology images with deep neural networks. In: Mori, K., Sakuma, I., Sato, Y., Barillot, C., Navab, N. (eds.) MICCAI 2013, Part II. LNCS, vol. 8150, pp. 411–418. Springer, Heidelberg (2013)
6. Gall, J., Lempitsky, V.: Class-specific hough forests for object detection. In: CVPR, pp. 1022–1029 (2009)
7. Giusti, A., Ciresan, D.C., Masci, J., Gambardella, L.M., Schmidhuber, J.: Fast image scanning with deep max-pooling convolutional neural networks. In: ICIP, pp. 4034–4038 (2013)

8. Krizhevsky, A., Sutskever, I., Hinton, G.E.: Imagenet classification with deep convolutional neural networks. In: NIPS, pp. 1106–1114 (2012)
9. Lecun, Y., Bottou, L., Bengio, Y., Haffner, P.: Gradient-based learning applied to document recognition, vol. 86, pp. 2278–2324 (1998)
10. Parvin, B., Yang, Q., Han, J., Chang, H., Rydberg, B., Barcellos-Hoff, M.H.: Iterative voting for inference of structural saliency and characterization of subcellular events. TIP 16, 615–623 (2007)
11. Riegler, G., Ferstl, D., Rüther, M., Bischof, H.: Hough networks for head pose estimation and facial feature localization. In: BMVC (2014)
12. Toshev, A., Szegedy, C.: Deeppose: Human pose estimation via deep neural networks, pp. 1653–1660 (2014)

Robust Cell Detection and Segmentation in Histopathological Images Using Sparse Reconstruction and Stacked Denoising Autoencoders

Hai Su[1], Fuyong Xing[2], Xiangfei Kong[1], Yuanpu Xie[1], Shaoting Zhang[3], and Lin Yang[1,2]

[1] J. Crayton Pruitt Family Dept. of Biomedical Engineering, University of Florida, FL 32611
[2] Department of Electrical and Computer Engineering, University of Florida, FL 32611
[3] Department of Computer Science, University of North Carolina at Charlotte, NC 28223

Abstract. Computer-aided diagnosis (CAD) is a promising tool for accurate and consistent diagnosis and prognosis. Cell detection and segmentation are essential steps for CAD. These tasks are challenging due to variations in cell shapes, touching cells, and cluttered background. In this paper, we present a cell detection and segmentation algorithm using the sparse reconstruction with trivial templates and a stacked denoising autoencoder (sDAE). The sparse reconstruction handles the shape variations by representing a testing patch as a linear combination of shapes in the learned dictionary. Trivial templates are used to model the touching parts. The sDAE, trained with the original data and their structured labels, is used for cell segmentation. To the best of our knowledge, this is the first study to apply sparse reconstruction and sDAE with structured labels for cell detection and segmentation. The proposed method is extensively tested on two data sets containing more than 3000 cells obtained from brain tumor and lung cancer images. Our algorithm achieves the best performance compared with other state of the arts.

1 Introduction

Reproducible and accurate analysis of digitized histopathological specimens plays a critical role in successful diagnosis and prognosis, treatment outcome prediction, and therapy planning. Manual analysis of histopathological slides is not only laborious, but also subject to inter-observer variability. Computer-aided diagnosis (CAD) is a promising solution. In CAD, cell detection and segmentation are often prerequisite steps for critical morphological analysis [10,16].

The major challenges in cell detection and segmentation are: 1) large variations of cell shapes and inhomogeneous intensity, 2) touching cells, and 3) background clutters. In order to handle touching cells, radial voting based detection

N. Navab et al. (Eds.): MICCAI 2015, Part III, LNCS 9351, pp. 383–390, 2015.
DOI: 10.1007/978-3-319-24574-4_46

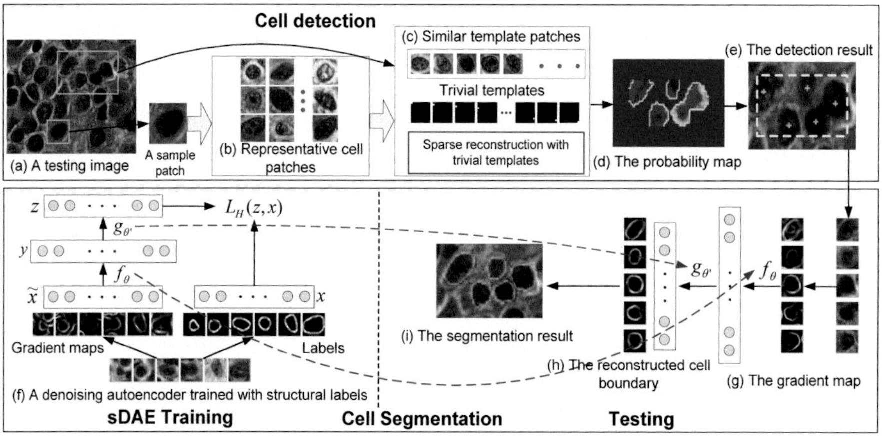

Fig. 1. An overview of the proposed algorithm.

method achieves robust performance with an assumption that most of the cells have round shapes [7]. In [14], an active contour algorithm is applied for cell segmentation. Recently, shape prior model is proposed to improve the performance in the presence of weak edges [2,15].

In this paper, we propose a novel cell detection and segmentation algorithm. To handle the shape variations, inhomogeneous intensity, and cell overlapping, the sparse reconstruction using an adaptive dictionary and trivial templates is proposed to detect cells. In the segmentation stage, a stacked denoising autoencoder (sDAE) trained with structural labels is used for cell segmentation.

2 Methodology

An overview of the proposed method is shown in Figure 1. During the training for cell detection, a compact cell dictionary (Figure 1(b)) is learned by applying K-selection [6] to a cell patch repository containing single centered cells. In the testing (Figure 1(a)-(e)), a sample patch from the testing image is first used as a query to retrieve similar patches in the learned dictionary. Since the appearance variation within one particular image is small, any sample patch containing a centered cell can be used. Next, sparse reconstruction using *trivial templates* [13] is utilized to generate a probability map to indicate the potential locations of the cells. Finally, weight-guided mean-shift clustering is used to compute the seed detection. Different from [13], our algorithm removes the sparsity constraints for the trivial templates. Therefore, the proposed method is more robust to the variations of the cell size and background. During the segmentation stage (Figure 1(f)-(i)), the sDAE is trained using the gradient maps of the training patches and their corresponding human annotated edges (Figure 1(f)). Our proposed segmentation algorithm is designed to handle touching cells and inhomogeneous cell intensities. As shown in (Figure 1(h)), the false edges are removed, the broken edges are connected, and the weak edges are recovered.

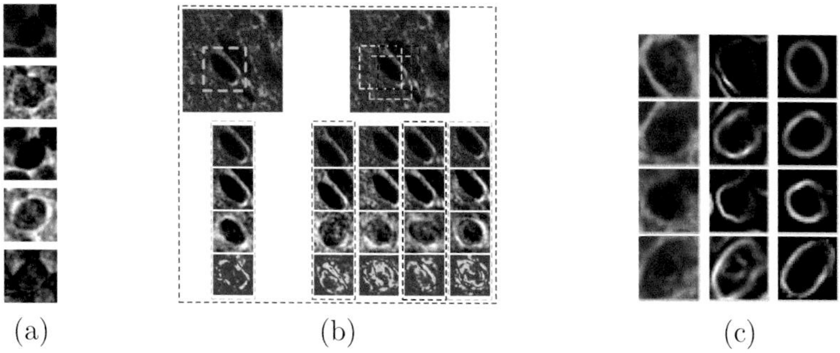

Fig. 2. (a) A demonstration of sparse reconstruction with/without trivial templates. From row 1 to 3: a testing patch, the sparse reconstruction without trivial templates, the sparse reconstruction with trivial templates. Row 4 and 5 are the first term and the second term in equation $\mathbf{p}_{ij} \approx \mathbf{Bc} + \mathbf{e}$, respectively. (b) A demonstration of reconstruction errors obtained from a testing patch aligned to the center of the cell and from those misaligned patches. Row 1 displays a small testing image. The green box shows a testing patch aligned to the cell. Boxes in other colors show misaligned testing patches. From row 2 to row 5: A testing image patch with occlusion from a neighboring cell, the reconstruction of the testing patch, the reconstructed patches with the occlusion part removed, and the visualization of the reconstruction errors. Note that the aligned testing patch has the smallest error. (c) From left to right: the original testing patches, the gradient magnitude maps, and the recovered cell boundaries using sDAE.

2.1 Detection via Sparse Reconstruction with Trivial Templates

Adaptive Dictionary Learning. During cell dictionary learning, a set of relevant cell patches are first retrieved based on their similarities compared with the sample patch. Considering the fact that pathological images commonly exhibit staining variations, the similarities are measured by normalized *local steering kernel* (nLSK) feature and *cosine similarity*. nLSK is more robustness to contrast change [9]. An image patch is represented by the densely computed nLSK features. Principal component analysis (PCA) is used for dimensionality reduction. Cosine distance: $D_{cos} = (\mathbf{v}_i^T \mathbf{v}_j)/(\|\mathbf{v}_i\| \|\mathbf{v}_j\|)$, where $\mathbf{v}_i$ denotes the nLSK feature of patch i, is proven to be the optimal similarity measurement under maximum likelihood decision rule [9]. Therefore, it is used to measure the similarities. The dictionary patches are selected by a nearest neighbor search.

Probability Map Generation via Sparse Reconstruction with Trivial Templates: Given a testing image, we propose to utilize sparse reconstruction to generate the probability map by comparing the reconstructed image to the original patch via a sliding window approach. Because the testing image patch may contain part of other neighboring cells, trivial templates are utilized to model these noise parts. When the testing image patch is aligned to the center of a cell, it can be linearly represented by the cell dictionary with small reconstruction errors. The touching part can be modeled with trivial templates. Let $\mathbf{p}_{ij} \in \mathbb{R}^{\sqrt{m} \times \sqrt{m}}$ denote a testing patch located at (i, j), and $\mathbf{B}$

represent the learned cell dictionary, this patch can be sparsely reconstructed by: $\mathbf{p}_{ij} \approx \mathbf{B}\mathbf{c} + \mathbf{e} = [\mathbf{B}\ \mathbf{I}][\mathbf{c}\ \mathbf{e}]^T$, where $\mathbf{e}$ is the error term to model the touching part, and $\mathbf{I}_{m \times m}$ is an identity matrix containing the trivial templates. The optimal sparse reconstruction can be found by:

$$\min_{\tilde{\mathbf{c}}} \|\mathbf{p}_{ij} - \tilde{\mathbf{B}}\tilde{\mathbf{c}}\|^2 + \lambda \|\mathbf{d} \odot \mathbf{c}\|^2 + \gamma \|\mathbf{e}\|^2, \ s.t.\ \mathbf{1}^T\mathbf{c} = 1, \tag{1}$$

where $\tilde{\mathbf{B}} = [\mathbf{B}\ \mathbf{I}], \tilde{\mathbf{c}} = [\mathbf{c}\ \mathbf{e}]^T$, and $\mathbf{d}$ represents the distance between the testing patch and the dictionary atoms, $\odot$ denotes element-wise multiplication, and λ controls the importance of the locality constraints, and γ controls the contribution of the trivial templates. The first term incorporates trivial templates to model the touching cells, and the second term enforces that only local neighbors in the dictionary are used for the sparse reconstruction. The locality constraint enforces sparsity [12]. In order to solve the locality-constrained sparse optimization, we first perform a KNN search in the dictionary excluding the trivial templates. The selected nearest neighbor bases together with the trivial templates form a smaller local coordinate system. Next, we solve the sparse reconstruction problem with least square minimization [12].

The reconstruction error is defined as $\epsilon_{rec} = \|(\mathbf{p}_{ij} - \tilde{\mathbf{B}}\tilde{\mathbf{c}}) \odot k(u, v)\|$, where $k(u, v)$ is a "bell-shape" spatial kernel that penalizes the errors in the central region. A probability map is obtained by $P_{ij} = \frac{|\epsilon_{rec} - \max(E)|}{\max(E) - \min(E)}$, where P_{ij} denotes the probability at location (i, j), and E represents the reconstruction error map. We demonstrate the reconstruction results of touching cells with and without trivial templates in Figure 2(a)-(b). The final cell detection is obtained by running a weight-guided mean-shift clustering on the probability map.

2.2 Cell Segmentation via Stacked Denoising Autoencoders

In this section, we propose to train a stacked denoising autoencoder (sDAE) [11] with structural labels to remove the fake edges while preserving the true edges. An overview of the training and testing procedure is shown in Figure 1 (f)-(i). Traditionally, denoising autoencoders (DAE) are trained with corrupted versions of the original samples, which requires the clean image as a premise. In our proposed method, we use the gradient images of the original image patches as the noisy inputs and the human annotated boundaries as the clean images. The DAE is trained to map a noisy input to a clean (recovered) image patch that can be used for segmentation.

We first focus on training a single layer of the DAE. Let $\tilde{\mathbf{X}} \in \mathbb{R}^m$ denote the noisy gradient magnitude map of the original image patch centered on a detected center of the cell (seed). The DAE learns a parametric encoder function $f_\theta(\tilde{\mathbf{x}}) = s(\mathbf{W}\tilde{\mathbf{x}} + \mathbf{b})$, where $s(\cdot)$ denotes the sigmoid function to transform the input from the original feature space into the hidden layer representation $\mathbf{y} \in \mathbb{R}^h$, where $\theta = \{\mathbf{W}, \mathbf{b}\}$ and $\mathbf{W} \in \mathbb{R}^{h,m}$. A parametric decoder function $g_{\theta'}(\mathbf{y}) = s(\mathbf{W}'\mathbf{y} + \mathbf{b}'), \theta' = \{\mathbf{W}', \mathbf{b}'\}$ is learned to transform the hidden layer representation back to a reconstructed version $\mathbf{Z} \in \mathbb{R}^m$ of the input $\tilde{\mathbf{X}}$.

Since it is a reconstruction problem based on real-valued variables, a square error loss function of the reconstruction $\mathbf{z}$ and the manually annotated structural label $\mathbf{x}$ is chosen, and the sigmoid function in $g_{\theta'}$ is omitted. The parameters $\{\theta, \theta'\}$ are obtained by:

$$\min_{\mathbf{W},\mathbf{b},\mathbf{W}',\mathbf{b}'} \|\mathbf{x} - g_{\theta'} \circ f_\theta(\tilde{\mathbf{x}})\|^2. \quad (2)$$

We choose *tied weights* by setting $\mathbf{W}' = \mathbf{W}^T$ [11]. The fake edges are suppressed in the reconstructed patches (Figure 2(c)). The final results are obtained by applying five iterations of an active contour model to the convex hull computed from the reconstructed image.

3 Experimental Results

Data set: The proposed algorithm is extensively tested on two data sets including about 2000 lung tumor cells and 1500 brain tumor cells, respectively. For the detection part, 2000 patches of size 45×45 with a centralized single cell are manually cropped from both data sets. $K = 1400$ patches are selected by K-selection. The parameter γ in equation (1) is set to 10^{-4}. In the segmentation part, contours of more than 4900 cells are annotated. Training sample augmentation is conducted via rotation and random translation. In total more than 14×10^4 training patches are used and each of them is resized to 28×28. A two-layer sDAE with 1000 maps in the first layer and 1200 maps in the second layer is trained on the data set. An active contour model [4] is applied to obtain the final segmentation result. All the experiments are implemented with MATLAB on a workstation with Intel Xeon E5-1650 CPU and 128 GB memory.

Detection Performance Analysis: We evaluate the proposed detection method through both qualitative and quantitative comparison with four state of the arts, including Laplacian-of-Gaussian (LoG) [1], iterative radial voting (IRV) [7], and image-based tool for counting nuclei (ITCN) [3], and single-pass voting (SPV) [8]. The qualitative comparison of two patches is shown in Figure 3.

To evaluate our algorithm quantitatively, we adopt a set of metrics defined in [14], including false negative rate (FN), false positive rate (FP), over-detection rate (OR), and effective rate (ER). Furthermore, precision (P), recall (R), and F_1 score are also computed. In our experiment, a true positive is defined as a detected seed that is within the circular neighborhood with 8-pixel distance to a ground truth and there is no other seeds within the 12-pixel distance neighborhood. The comparison results are shown in Table 1. It can be observed that the proposed method outperforms other methods in terms of most of the metrics on the two data sets. We also observed that in solving equation (1), increase of the number of nearest neighbors can help the detection performance. Such effect vanishes when more than 100 nearest neighbors are selected. Friedman test is performed on the F_1 scores obtained by the methods under comparison. $P-$values< 0.05 are observed. The proposed detection algorithm is based on

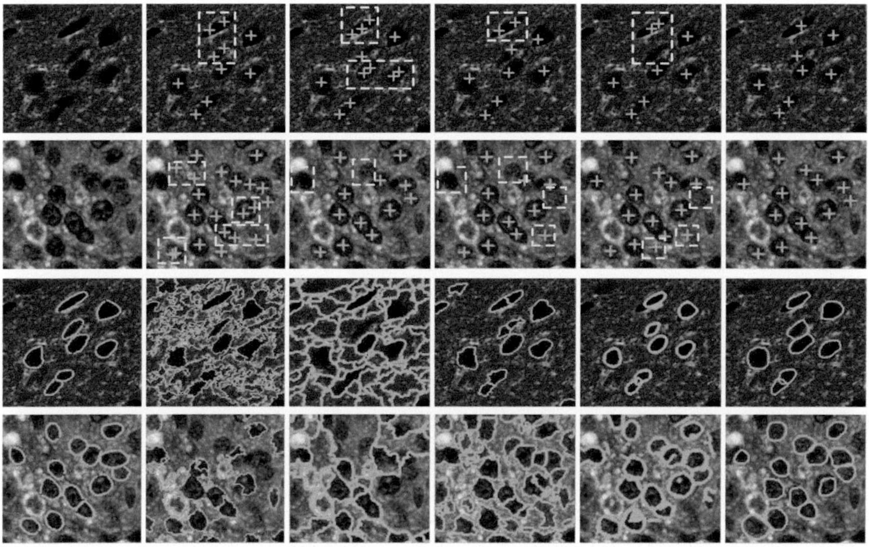

Fig. 3. Detection and segmentation results of two testing images randomly selected from the two data sets. Row 1 and row 2 show the comparison of the detection results: (a) is the original image patches. (b)-(f) are the corresponding results obtained by LoG [1], IRV [7], ITCN [3], SPV [8], and the proposed method. Row 3 and row 4 show the comparison of the segmentation results: (a) is the ground truth. (b)-(f) are the corresponding results obtained by MS, ISO [5], GCC [1], RLS [8], and the proposed method.

Table 1. The comparison of the detection performance.

	Brain tumor data							Lung cancer data						
Methods	FN	FP	OR	ER	P	R	F_1	FN	FP	OR	ER	P	R	F_1
LoG [1]	0.15	0.004	0.3	0.8	0.94	0.84	0.89	0.19	0.003	0.13	0.78	0.96	0.80	0.88
IRV [7]	0.15	0.04	0.07	0.76	0.95	0.83	0.88	0.33	0.014	0.21	0.64	0.98	0.66	0.79
ITCN [3]	0.22	0.0005	**0.01**	0.77	0.99	0.77	0.87	0.31	0.002	0.05	0.68	0.98	0.69	0.81
SPV [8]	0.1	0.02	0.06	0.86	0.98	0.89	0.93	0.18	0.008	0.006	0.79	0.98	0.81	0.89
Ours	**0.07**	0.0007	0.04	**0.92**	0.99	**0.93**	**0.96**	**0.15**	0.01	0.06	0.81	0.96	**0.85**	**0.90**

MATLAB and is not yet optimized with respect to efficiency. It takes about 10 minutes to scan an image of size 1072×952.

Segmentation Performance Analysis: A qualitative comparison of performance between the sDAE and the other four methods, including mean-shift (MS), isoperimetric graph partitioning (ISO) [5], graph-cut and coloring (GCC) [1], and repulsive level set (RLS) [8], is shown in Figure 3. It is clear that the

Table 2. The comparison of the segmentation performance.

	Brain tumor data						Lung cancer data					
Methods	P.M.	P.V.	R.M.	R.V.	F_1 M.	F_1. V.	P.M.	P.V.	R.M.	R.V.	F_1 M.	F_1. V.
MS	**0.92**	0.02	0.59	0.08	0.66	0.05	**0.88**	**0.01**	0.73	0.04	0.77	0.02
ISO [5]	0.71	0.04	0.81	0.03	0.71	0.03	0.75	0.03	0.82	0.025	0.75	0.02
GCC [1]	0.87	0.03	0.77	0.044	0.78	0.024	0.87	0.03	0.73	0.04	0.77	0.02
RLS [8]	0.84	**0.01**	0.75	0.09	0.74	0.05	0.85	0.013	0.82	0.04	0.81	0.02
Ours	0.86	0.018	**0.87**	**0.01**	**0.85**	**0.009**	0.86	0.023	**0.85**	**0.012**	**0.84**	**0.01**

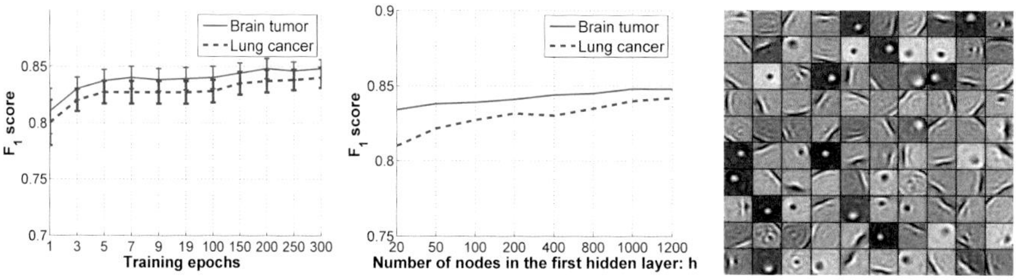

(a) (b) (c)

Fig. 4. (a) F_1 score as a function of the number of training epochs. (b) F_1 score as a function of the model complexity. (c) A set of learned feature maps in the first hidden layer.

proposed method learns to capture the structure of the cell boundaries. Therefore, the true boundaries can be recovered in the presence of inhomogeneous intensity, and a better segmentation performance is achieved. The quantitative comparison based on the mean and variance of precision (P), recall (R), and F_1 score is shown in Table 2. In addition, Friedman test followed by Bonferroni-Dunn test is conducted on the F_1 scores. $P-$values are all significantly smaller than 0.05. The Bonferroni-Dunn test shows there does exist significant difference between our methods and the other state of the arts.

We also explored the interaction between the segmentation performance and the number of training epochs. The result is shown in Figure 4(a). As one can tell that the performance increases as the number of training epochs increases, and it converges after 200 epochs. The number of training samples needed for a reasonable performance depends on the variation of the data. In our setting, it is observed that around 5000 samples are sufficient. The interaction between the performance and the model complexity is shown in Figure 4(b), where the dimension of the second layer is fixed to 200. The proposed segmentation algorithm is very efficient. It takes only 286 seconds for segmenting 2000 cells. This is because it takes only four vector-matrix multiplications using the two-layer sDAE to compute the outputs for one cell. Finally, a set of learned feature maps are shown in Figure 4(c).

4 Conclusion

In this paper we have proposed an automatic cell detection and segmentation algorithm for pathological images. The detection step exploits sparse reconstruction with trivial templates to handle shape variations and touching cells. The segmentation step applies a sDAE trained with structural labels to remove the non-boundary edges. The proposed algorithm is a general approach that can be adapted to many pathological applications.

References

1. Al-Kofahi, Y., Lassoued, W., Lee, W., Roysam, B.: Improved automatic detection and segmentation of cell nuclei in histopathology images. TBME 57(4), 841–852 (2010)
2. Ali, S., Madabhushi, A.: An integrated region-, boundary-, shape-based active contour for multiple object overlap resolution in histological imagery. IEEE Transactions on Medical Imaging 31(7), 1448–1460 (2012)
3. Byun, J., Verardo, M.R., Sumengen, B., Lewis, G.P., Manjunath, B., Fisher, S.K.: Automated tool for the detection of cell nuclei in digital microscopic images: Application to retinal images. Mol. Vis. 12, 949–960 (2006)
4. Chan, T.F., Vese, L.A.: Active contours without edges. TIP 10(2), 266–277 (2001)
5. Grady, L., Schwartz, E.L.: Isoperimetric graph partitioning for image segmentation. PAMI 28(3), 469–475 (2006)
6. Liu, B., Huang, J., Yang, L., Kulikowsk, C.: Robust tracking using local sparse appearance model and k-selection. In: CVPR, pp. 1313–1320 (2011)
7. Parvin, B., Yang, Q., Han, J., Chang, H., Rydberg, B., Barcellos-Hoff, M.H.: Iterative voting for inference of structural saliency and characterization of subcellular events. TIP 16(3), 615–623 (2007)
8. Qi, X., Xing, F., Foran, D., Yang, L.: Robust segmentation of overlapping cells in histopathology specimens using parallel seed detection and repulsive level set. TBME 59(3), 754–765 (2012)
9. Seo, H.J., Milanfar, P.: Training-free, generic object detection using locally adaptive regression kernels. PAMI 32(9), 1688–1704 (2010)
10. Veta, M., Pluim, J.P., van Diest, P.J., Viergever, M.A.: Breast cancer histopathology image analysis: A review. TBME 61(5), 1400–1411 (2014)
11. Vincent, P., Larochelle, H., Lajoie, I., Bengio, Y., Manzagol, P.A.: Stacked denoising autoencoders: Learning useful representations in a deep network with a local denoising criterion. JMLR 11, 3371–3408 (2010)
12. Wang, J., Yang, J., Yu, K., Lv, F., Huang, T., Gong, Y.: Locality-constrained linear coding for image classification. In: CVPR, pp. 3360 –3367 (2010)
13. Wright, J., Yang, A.Y., Ganesh, A., Sastry, S.S., Ma, Y.: Robust face recognition via sparse representation. PAMI 31(2), 210–227 (2009)
14. Xing, F., Su, H., Neltner, J., Yang, L.: Automatic ki-67 counting using robust cell detection and online dictionary learning. TBME 61(3), 859–870 (2014)
15. Xing, F., Yang, L.: Robust selection-based sparse shape model for lung cancer image segmentation. In: Mori, K., Sakuma, I., Sato, Y., Barillot, C., Navab, N. (eds.) MICCAI 2013, Part III. LNCS, vol. 8151, pp. 404–412. Springer, Heidelberg (2013)
16. Zhang, X., Liu, W., Dundar, M., Badve, S., Zhang, S.: Towards large-scale histopathological image analysis: Hashing-based image retrieval. IEEE Transactions on Medical Imaging 34(2), 496–506 (2015)

Automatic in Vivo Cell Detection in MRI

Muhammad Jamal Afridi[1], Xiaoming Liu[1], Erik Shapiro[2], and Arun Ross[1]

[1] Department of Computer Science and Engineering, Michigan State University
[2] Department of Radiology, Michigan State University
{afridimu,liuxm,shapir86,rossarun}@msu.edu

Abstract. Due to recent advances in cell-based therapies, non-invasive monitoring of *in vivo* cells in MRI is gaining enormous interest. However, to date, the monitoring and analysis process is conducted manually and is extremely tedious, especially in the clinical arena. Therefore, this paper proposes a novel computer vision-based learning approach that creates superpixel-based 3D models for candidate spots in MRI, extracts a novel set of superfern features, and utilizes a partition-based Bayesian classifier ensemble to distinguish spots from non-spots. Unlike traditional ferns that utilize pixel-based differences, superferns exploit superpixel averages in computing difference-based features despite the absence of any order in superpixel arrangement. To evaluate the proposed approach, we develop the first labeled database with a total of more than 16 thousand labels on five *in vivo* and four *in vitro* MRI scans. Experimental results show the superiority of our approach in comparison to the two most relevant baselines. To the best of our knowledge, this is the first study to utilize a learning-based methodology for *in vivo* cell detection in MRI.

1 Introduction

As a promising alternative to organ transplants in humans, cell transplant-based therapies have recently gained enormous interest in medical research. However, its long term success in humans has not been proven, where one key obstacle is the ability to non-invasively monitor the transplanted cells via MRI, and measure both transplant efficiency and long-term cell repopulation. Overcoming this obstacle is equivalent to achieving two goals: (i) display the transplanted cells in MRI scans under *in vivo* conditions, and (ii) perform comprehensive quantitative analysis on the behavior of transplanted cells. To display transplanted cells in MRI scans, cells are injected with an MRI contrast agent prior to or during imaging [8]. This has been demonstrated in many *in vivo* studies, e.g., [7,2].

While such cell studies use efficient magnetic particles and high-resolution MRI, they stopped short of quantification and hence cannot accomplish the second goal. For comprehensive quantitative analysis, *manual* enumeration of cells in MRI is *laborious*, *subjective*, and *limited* in capturing all patterns of cell behaviors. Further, current commercial tools can only assist humans in conducting

N. Navab et al. (Eds.): MICCAI 2015, Part III, LNCS 9351, pp. 391–399, 2015.
DOI: 10.1007/978-3-319-24574-4_47

manual analysis. Therefore, there is a need to automatically and accurately perform such quantitative analysis of cells or spots. Note that we use *cell* or *spot* interchangeably since a cell visually appears as a spot in MRI scans.

Recognizing this need, a recent study utilized a simple threshold-based strategy to automatically detect cell spots in 2D MRI images of a rat's brain [4]. However, they did not quantitatively report the spot detection accuracy against any ground truth. In contrast, supervised machine learning-based solutions are more robust and have recently shown enormous success in a wide range of medical applications. Unfortunately, there is no prior work that utilizes learning-based approaches for automatically detecting *in vivo* spots in MRI. In a related area of 2D microscopic image analysis, authors in [9] conducted a comparative study of various machine learning approaches in detecting spots. The study concluded that a Haar-based Adaboost approach performs the best on their data. Nevertheless, *in vivo* 3D MRI scans present more challenging in nature than florescence based microscopic images of [9]. E.g., MRI scans also contain spot-like tissue's structural entities in the image background that are absent in microscopic images. Secondly, based on the size and shape of the spots in [9], HAAR-like features are extracted from a fixed sized mask that slides on a 2D image, which may not work for our 3D spots due to the large size and shape variations of spots.

Moving towards accomplishing the second goal, this paper presents the first comprehensive study on learning-based detection of cell spots in MRI scans. Our cell detection framework has novelty in terms of spot modelling, feature representation, and classification. Our approach considers spots as 3D entities and represents its general structural model using superpixels. We then extract a novel set of "superferns" features and finally classify it using a partition-based ensemble of Bayesian networks. Experimental results show that our proposed approach performs significantly better than previously related approaches.

In summary, this paper makes the following contributions: (i) It proposes a novel superpixel-based 3D model to characterize cellular spots and that can potentially be used in other medical problems. (ii) It introduces the *superferns* feature that exploits superpixel-based representations and is more discriminative than traditional fern features. (iii) It demonstrates *how* a partition-based ensemble learning can be effectively utilized for MRI spot detection. (iv) It presents a labeled publicly available database of five *in vivo* and four *in vitro* MRI scans, and a total of 16,298 spot labels for quantitative evaluation.

2 Proposed Approach

The cell/spot detection problem in MRI scans has unique challenges, where a number of questions should be carefully considered prior to algorithm design. First, since a spot is essentially a 3D entity in an MRI cube, *how* can we model

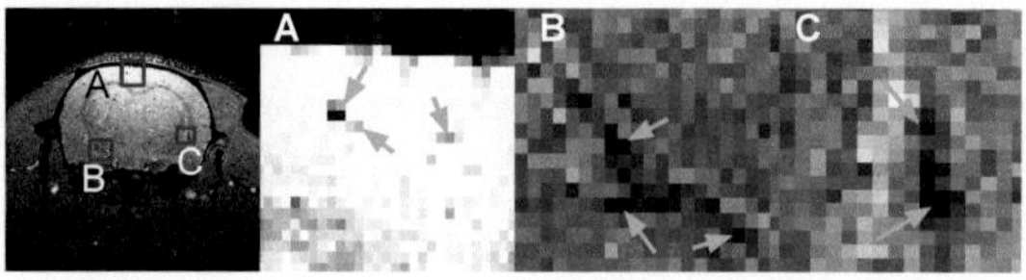

Fig. 1. Spot variations in diverse region contexts.

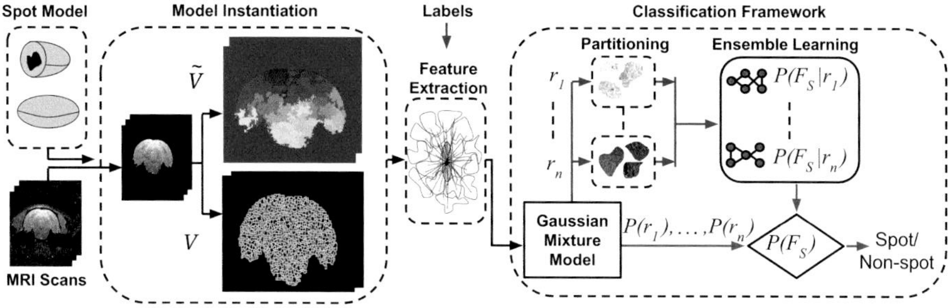

Fig. 2. Our approach has four main modules. Blue, red, and black arrows are the processing flow during the training stage, testing stage and both stages, respectively.

its three dimensional characteristics? Second, a spot is also a small group of dark pixels with varying shapes and sizes. *What* is the basic *unit* within an MRI cube (e.g., one, two, or N pixels) for which the two-class classification decision can be made? Third, there is a huge number of candidate locations. So, *how* to construct discriminative and efficient feature representation for spots? Fourth, the appearance of a spot varies relative to its local and regional neighborhood (Fig. 1). *How* to make learning robust to these variations should be addressed. Considering these challenges, we design our technical approach as in Fig. 2.

2.1 Spot Modeling

Visually, a cellular spot $\mathbf{S}$ appears as a cluster of dark 3D pixels with high variations in its 3D shape and intensity, wrapped inside a cover of background pixels as conceptually illustrated in Fig. 3. In this work, we call the small group of dark pixels as a spot's interior I, and their local neighboring pixels in the background as the exterior E of a 3D spot. This model is consistent with the manual labeling of spots by domain experts, who inspect the cross-sections of spots in consecutive 2D MRI slices, and look for a small region (interior) that is darker than its neighboring pixels (exterior). Furthermore, the human visual system can also adjust for the amount of relative darkness based on the characteristics of the *specific brain region* containing that spot. E.g., Fig. 1 shows that the way to classify spots in region A and B might be different, and one spot in C is comparatively larger. Thus, in addition to modeling a spot with its interior/exterior, we also model the specific region it belongs to, termed *region context* R.

2.2 Model Instantiation via Superpixel

Given the conceptual spot model $\mathbf{S} = \{I, E, R\}$, we now describe how to define I, E, and R for a spot, by three steps. Since no spot should be outside the brain region, the first step is to perform brain segmenation in every 2D MRI slice with basic image processing techniques. The second step is to define I and E by applying 2D superpixel extraction [3] to the segmented brain

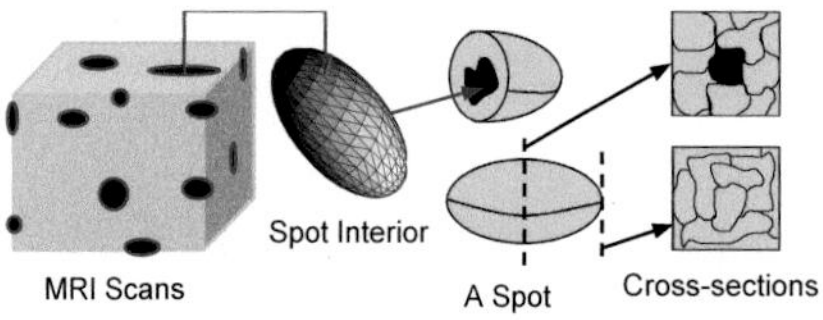

Fig. 3. Conceptual Spot Model

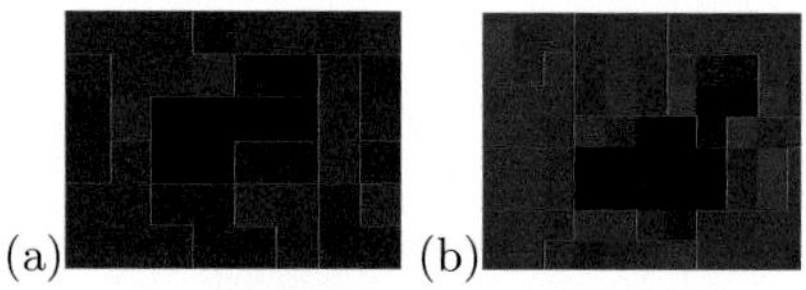

Fig. 4. Superpixels capture a tight (a) or loose (b) boundary of a spot's interior.

region of each slice. A superpixel is a group of N neighboring pixels with similar intensities, i.e., $V_{z,u} = \{x_i, y_i, z\}_{i=1}^N$ where u is the superpixel ID in slice z. In general superpixels can tightly capture the boundary of a spot's interior; however, some imprecise localization is also expected in practice (Fig. 4). After extraction, we denote $\mathbb{M} = \{V_{z,u}\}_{z=u=1}^{L,U}$ as the set of all superpixels in the 3D brain region, where L is the number of slices and U is the number of superpixels per slice. Due to the exclusiveness of the interior and exterior of spots, we have $\mathbb{M} = \mathbb{I} \cup \mathbb{E}$ where $\mathbb{I}$ and $\mathbb{E}$ are the set of all interior and exterior superpixels, respectively. With that, for a spot $\mathbf{S}$ with length l in z-axis, we formally define its interior as $I = \{V_{z,u}, \cdots, V_{z+l-1,u} \mid V \subset \mathbb{I}\}$ and the exterior as $E = \{V_{z-1,.}, V_{z,\bar{u}}, \ldots, V_{z+l-1,\bar{u}}, V_{z+l,.} \mid ||(m(I) - m(V)|| \leq \tau, V \subset \mathbb{E}\}$, where $m()$ is the mean of a set, τ is the maximum L^2 distance between the centers of a spot and an exterior superpixel, and $V_{z-1,.}$ and $V_{z+l,.}$ are superpixels in two adjacent neighboring slices. To define the region context R, in the third step we extract very large superpixels $\{\tilde{V}_{z,u}\}_{z=u=1}^{L,\tilde{U}}$, where the number of superpixels $\tilde{U} \ll U$, by assuming that large superpixels are representative of the regional appearance. Thus, we define the region context of a spot as $R = \{\tilde{V}_{z,u} \mid m(I) \subset \tilde{V}_{z,u}\}$, which is the large superpixel enclosing the spot center $m(I)$. Consequently, this process allows each superpixel to act an an interior of a potential spot and therefore naturally generates a large number of candidates.

The superpixel-based 3D spot model has a few advantages. First, it addresses the issue of *unit*, by going beyond pixels and using superpixel-based feature extraction and classification. Second, it substantially limits the total candidate spots to be tested, since the candidates are nominated via superpixels rather than pixels. Note that we may extend our 3D spot model by directly using 3D supervoxels instead of joining 2D superpixels. We choose the latter in this work due to its superior reliability than well-known 3D supervoxel methods.

2.3 Superferns Feature Extraction

With an instantiated spot model $\mathbf{S} = \{I, E, R\}$, the next step is to extract a discriminative and efficient feature representation. Since a spot generally has darker interior than its exterior, it makes sense to define features based on the computationally efficient intensity differences between pixels in the interior and exterior. Difference-based fern features have shown great success in computer vision [5]. Ferns compute the intensity difference between a *subject pixel* and another pixel with a certain offset w.r.t. the subject pixel. Using the same offset in different images leads to feature correspondence among these images.

For our problem, the spot center $m(I)$ can be regarded as the subject pixel, and its intensity is the average intensity of all interior pixels $m(\mathbf{G}(I))$. We then randomly generate h 3D offsets $O = \{\mathbf{o}_i\}_{i=1}^h$ with a uniform distribution, whose center is the spot center and radius is τ. Finally, the feature set is computed as $F = \{f_i\}_{i=1}^h$, where $f_i = \mathbf{G}(m(I) + \mathbf{o}_i) - m(\mathbf{G}(I))$. While f_i is efficient to compute, $\mathbf{G}(m(I) + \mathbf{o}_i)$ is the intensity of a single pixel, which can be noisy, specially in *in vivo* MRI and lead to low discriminability of f_i. Thus, it is desirable to replace it with the average intensity of all pixels within an exterior superpixel. However, the exterior superpixels around different spots have no correspondence, and, as a result, f_i for different spots also have the correspondence issue.

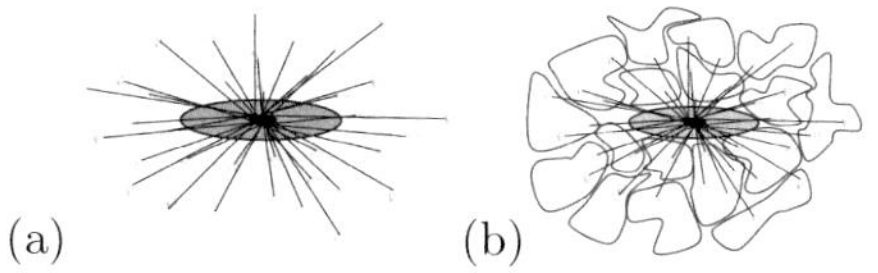

Fig. 5. The ferns (a) and superferns (b).

To address this issue, we present an approach to exploit the average intensity without losing correspondence information. The new feature, termed as "superferns", is similar to F except it replaces the single pixel-based intensity with the average intensity of the superpixel (Fig. 5 (b)), i.e., $F' = \{f_i'\}_{i=1}^h$, where $f_i' = m(\mathbf{G}(V)) - m(\mathbf{G}(I))$, $\forall\, m(I) + \mathbf{o}_i \in V$. Note that it is possible to have the same feature at two different offsets due to them being in the same superpixel, i.e., $f_i' = f_j'$. This is not an issue because this equality may not be true for other spots, hence the feature distributions of f_i' and f_j' are not the same, and they contribute differently to the classification.

Features are also needed for the region context R. Given its role of supporting region-dependent classifiers, we find that simple features work well for R, e.g., the mean and standard deviation of pixel intensities in R, $F_r = (m(\mathbf{G}(R)), \sigma(\mathbf{G}(R)))$.

2.4 Partition-Based Bayesian Classification

Having computed the feature $F_s = (F', F_r)$ for a set of spots and non-spots, we now present our approach to learn an accurate two-class classifier. Since different local regions have different appearance as shown in Fig. 1, we parition the brain region into N_0 partitions, learn a set of N_0 classifiers each for one partition, and fuse them via a probabilistic Bayesian formulation. Specifically, for any spot candidate $\mathbf{S}$, its probability of being a spot is

$$P(F_s) = \sum_{i=1}^{N_0} P(F_s, r_i) = \sum_{i=1}^{N_0} P(F_s|r_i)P(r_i), \tag{1}$$

where r_i represents the ith partition, $P(r_i)$ is the probability of $\mathbf{S}$ belonging to r_i, and $P(F_s|r_i)$ is the conditional probability of being a spot at partition r_i.

We learn $P(r_i)$ using Gaussian Mixture Models (GMM) with random initialization. By collecting the F_r for all training samples, we perform GMM to estimate N_0 component Gaussian densities (using Aikake Information Criterion), each considered as one partition. During the testing, $\{P(r_i)\}_{i=1}^{N_O}$ is obtained by evaluating F_r of the testing sample w.r.t. each component densities.

In order to learn $P(F_s|r_i)$, we group all training samples into N_O groups based on their respective maximum $\{P(r_i)\}$, and train the $P(F_s|r_i)$ using the standard implementation of Bayesian Networks in [1], where the maximum number of parent nodes is set to 4. During the test, for a testing candidate spot, GMM enables a soft partition assignment, and its final probability of being a spot is the weighted average from the classifier ensemble.

3 MRI Database for Cell Detection

Since there is no public database for cell detection in MRI, we collect a database in both *in vivo* and *in vitro* settings, and manually label the ground truth spots.

***In vitro* MRI:** A phantom was constructed consisting of a known number of 4.5 micron diameter, magnetic microparticles with 10 pg iron per particle, suspended in 1% agarose. T2*-weighted gradient echo MRI was performed on this sample at a resolution of 100 micron isotropic voxels ($128 \times 80 \times 80$ pixels). Using a field strength of 7T, a total of four MRI *in vitro* scans of different tubes were developed. One of these tubes was naïve whereas the rest contained spots.

***In vivo* MRI:** At a field strength of 11.7T, five rat brains are scaned to obtain MRI cubes of $256 \times 256 \times 256$ pixels. Three rats were injected intracardiac with MPIO-labeled MSCs, delivering cells to the brain, and two rats were naïve.

Labeling: For quantitative evaluation, for every MRI scan with spots, a domain expert manually clicked on a set of 2D dark pixels on every slice, using our GUI labeling tool that allows zooming in locally. The superpixel of one clicked pixel, or the concatenation of multiple nearby pixels, forms the interior of one ground truth 3D spot. This leads to a set of ground truth spots $S = \{\mathbf{s}_i\}_{i=1}^{K}$, $\mathbf{s}_i = (x_i, y_i, z_i)^\intercal$, where x_i, y_i, z_i are the 3D spot center. There are 841 and 15,457 ground truth spots on three *in vitro* scans and three *in vivo* scans, respectively. Labeling such data is not only time consuming but also *subjective*. Therefore, to learn the inter-rater variability, we compute $Dv = 1 - \frac{1}{3}\sum_{i=1}^{3} |J1 \cap J2|/|J1 \cup J2|$ to be $\sim$36% on three *in vitro* scans, where $J1$ and $J2$ are labels of two experts.

4 Experimental Results

In this section we design experiments to investigate answers to the following questions: (i) how does our approach perform and compare with the previous approaches using both *in vivo* and *in vitro* data? (ii) how does the discriminating potential of superferns quantitatively compare with the fern features? (iii) how diverse is the classifier ensemble created by our proposed approach?

Experimental Setup: For each detected spots $\hat{\mathbf{s}}$, we claim a true detection if there is a ground truth spot within a small distance, i.e., $||\hat{\mathbf{s}} - \mathbf{s}_i|| < 0.5$ pixel. The ROC, and Area Under the Curve (AUC) are the evaluation metrics. For the

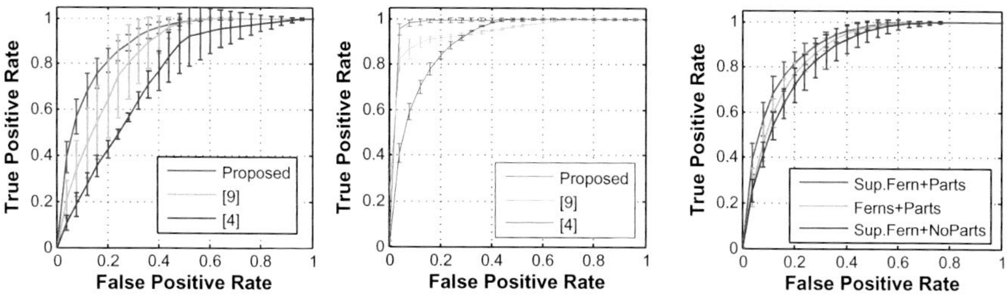

(a) *In vivo* data (b) *In vitro* data (c) No superferns or partition

Fig. 6. Detection performance comparisons and with various components.

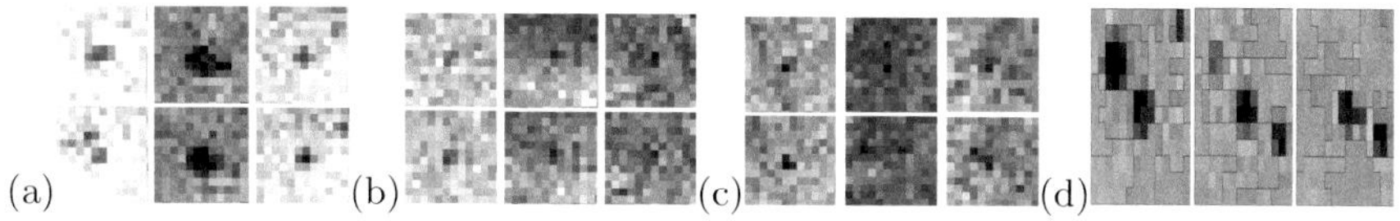

Fig. 7. Spot detection examples: (a) true detection, (b) false negative, and (c) false positive of *in vivo* data. Each column shows two consecutive slices of a spot. Note the amount of appearance variations in *in vivo* data. (d) visualization for a 3 sliced spot.

5-scans *in vivo* data, we adopt a leave-two-out scheme such that our testing set contains one labeled and one spotless scan. This creates six pairs of training and testing sets, which allows us to compute the error bar of ROC. For the 4-scans *in vitro* data, three pairs of training and testing sets are formed such that the naïve scan remains in the testing set accompanied by every other scan once. Since [4] and [9] are the most relevant examples of MRI cell detection using learning-based and rule-based methods, we implement them as the baselines. We experimentally determine $\tau = 9$, $h = 215$, $N_0 \in [6, 9]$ for *in vivo* data, and $U \in [200, 2000]$ and $\tilde{U} \in [20, 60]$ depending on the size of brain regions.

Performance and Comparison: As shown in Fig. 6 (a,b), the proposed method outperforms two baselines with an average AUC of 98.9% (*in vitro*) and 89.1% (*in vivo*). The improvement margin is especially larger at lower FPRs, which are the main operation points in practice. Fig. 6 (c) shows that with *in vivo* data, by using ferns instead of superferns or by making no partitions of the brain region, we observe a decrease in AUC to 87.1% and 85.3%, respectively. We also applied the standard implementation of C4.5 decision tree to our data, since decision trees naturally splits data based on features, however, the obtained results were significantly inferior to our approach. Fig. 7 shows three types of spot detection results with our method. The appearance and shape variations among the spots clearly show the challenge of this problem.

Superferns vs. Ferns: To further illustrate the strength of the novel superferns feature, we compare the discriminating potential of superferns with ferns, *regardless* of the classifier design. Information gain (IG) is a standard tool to measure the worth of a feature, where a higher IG indicates its higher discrimi-

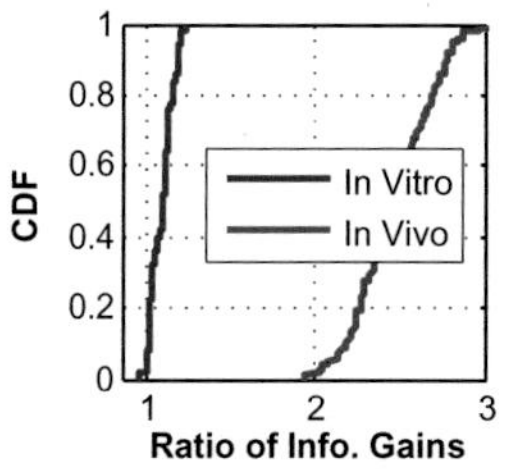

Fig. 8. The ratio of IGs.

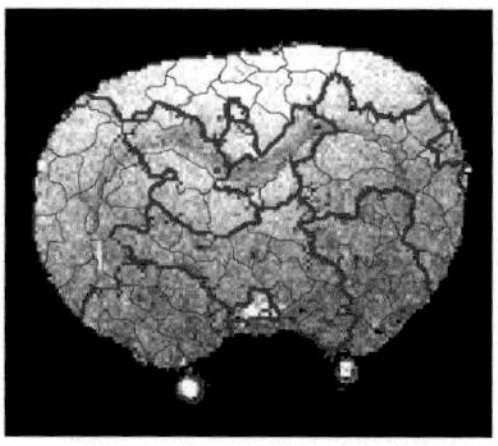

Fig. 9. $\tilde{V}_{z,\cdot}$ & 8 partitions.

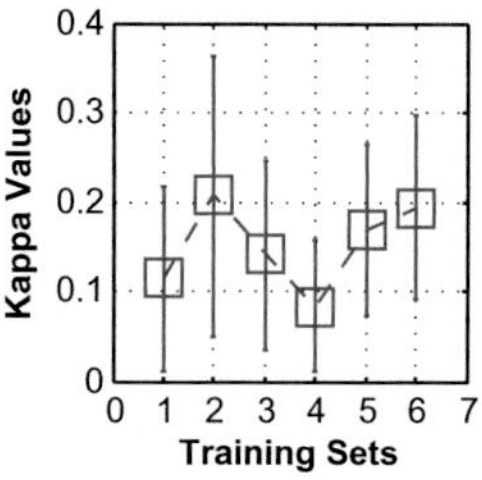

Fig. 10. Classifier diversity.

nating potential. Given a set of 50 randomly generated offsets $\{\mathbf{o}_i\}$, we calculate their superferns features on the *in vitro* data including both spots and non-spots, which allows us to compute A_s containing the IG of each superfern. The *same* offsets are applied to the fern features and then their corresponding set of IGs A_f is computed. Finally we compute the ratio of both IGs, $\frac{A_s(i)}{A_f(i)}$, for each offset $\mathbf{o}_i$, and show the Cumulative Density Function (CDF) of 50 ratios in Fig. 8. Using 100 random offsets, the same experiment is repeated for the *in vivo* data. The fact that almost all ratios are larger than 1 shows the superiority of superferns.

Diversity Analysis: Our classification framework includes an ensemble of classifiers, one for each partition. Fig. 9 shows for one slice the $N_0(=8)$ partitions and the enclosured large superpixels $\tilde{V}_{z,\cdot}$. Since diverse discriminative features are likely to be utilized in different partitions, learning on disjoint partitions should favor high diversities among classifiers – an indicator for effective classification. To evaluate the diversity of our classifier ensemble, we use the standard Cohen's kappa value [6], which ranges from 0 to 1, with a lower value indicating a higher diversity. For each of six *in vivo* training sets, we compute $\frac{N_0(N_0-1)}{2}$ kappa values, each between a pair of classifiers learned on different partitions. Fig. 10 shows their mean and standard deviation for each training set. According to [6], our kappa values is very low, indicating the high diversity of learned ensemble.

5 Conclusions and Future Work

This paper presents the first comprehensive study on learning-based cell/spot detection in MRI. We propose a novel framework that employs a superpixel-based 3D spot model, extracts *superferns* features, and utilizes a partition-based classifier ensemble. We collected a total of nine MRI scans with more than 16 thousand labels for evaluation. Experimental results demonstrate the superiority of our approach. In future, we intend to investigate two directions: (i) further improving the detection accuracy by learning more contextual information of the brain; (ii) extend the spot detection from brain to other organs, such as liver.

References

1. Bouckaert, R., Frank, E., Hall, M., Kirkby, R., Reutemann, P., Seewald, A., Scuse, D.: Weka manual for version 3-7-8 (2013)
2. Heyn, C., Ronald, J.A., Mackenzie, L.T., MacDonald, I.C., Chambers, A.F., Rutt, B.K., Foster, P.J.: In vivo magnetic resonance imaging of single cells in mouse brain with optical validation. Magnetic Resonance in Medicine 55(1), 23–29 (2006)
3. Liu, M., Tuzel, O., Ramalingam, S., Chellappa, R.: Entropy rate superpixel segmentation. In: IEEE CVPR, pp. 2097–2104 (2011)
4. Mori, Y., Chen, T., Fujisawa, T., Kobashi, S., Ohno, K., Yoshida, S., Tago, Y., Komai, Y., Hata, Y., Yoshioka, Y.: From cartoon to real time MRI: in vivo monitoring of phagocyte migration in mouse brain. Scientific Reports 4 (2014)
5. Ozuysal, M., Calonder, M., Lepetit, V., Fua, P.: Fast keypoint recognition using random ferns. IEEE T-PAMI 32(3), 448–461 (2010)
6. Rodriguez, J.J., Kuncheva, L.I., Alonso, C.J.: Rotation forest: A new classifier ensemble method. IEEE T-PAMI 28(10), 1619–1630 (2006)
7. Shapiro, E.M., Sharer, K., Skrtic, S., Koretsky, A.P.: In vivo detection of single cells by MRI. Magnetic Resonance in Medicine 55(2), 242–249 (2006)
8. Slotkin, J.R., Cahill, K.S., Tharin, S.A., Shapiro, E.M.: Cellular magnetic resonance imaging: nanometer and micrometer size particles for noninvasive cell localization. Neurotherapeutics 4(3), 428–433 (2007)
9. Smal, I., Loog, M., Niessen, W., Meijering, E.: Quantitative comparison of spot detection methods in fluorescence microscopy. IEEE T-MI 29(2), 282–301 (2010)

Quantitative Image Analysis III: Motion, Deformation, Development and Degeneration

Automatic Vessel Segmentation from Pulsatile Radial Distension

Alborz Amir-Khalili[1], Ghassan Hamarneh[2], and Rafeef Abugharbieh[1]

[1] BiSICL, University of British Columbia, Vancouver, Canada
[2] Medical Image Analysis Lab, Simon Fraser University, Burnaby, Canada

Abstract. Identification of vascular structures from medical images is integral to many clinical procedures. Most vessel segmentation techniques ignore the characteristic pulsatile motion of vessels in that formulation. In a recent effort to automatically segment vessels that are hidden under fat, we motivated the use of the magnitude of local pulsatile motion extracted from surgical endoscopic video. In this paper we propose a new approach that leverages the local orientation, in addition to magnitude of motion, and demonstrate that the extended computation of motion vectors can improve the segmentation of vascular structures. We implement our approach using two alternatives to magnitude-only motion estimation by using traditional optical flow and by exploiting the monogenic signal for fast flow estimation. Our evaluations are conducted on both synthetic phantoms as well as real ultrasound data showing improved segmentation results (0.36 increase in DSC and 0.11 increase in AUC) with negligible change in computational performance.

1 Introduction

Identification of blood vessels from medical images is important to many clinical procedures. Extraction of vascular structures are of such importance that many acquisition techniques and imaging modalities have been developed to image vasculature. Such techniques include contrast enhanced computed tomography (CT) or magnetic resonance (MR) angiography, laser speckle imaging [1], color Doppler ultrasound (US) and optical coherence tomography (OCT) [2].

Attempts have been made to automatically extract, or segment, these structures by applying advanced image analysis techniques to the intensity information acquired from the aforementioned modalities. Such attempts include the exploitation of ridge-like features in the image [3], a combination of wavelet-based features and machine learning [4], Hessian-based vesselness features [5,6], model/physics based approaches [7,6], active contours [8], and supervised machine learning techniques [9]. With the exception of Doppler US and OCT, the listed techniques focus on extracting features from static information, ignoring the most characteristic feature of a pulsating vessel, i.e. its temporal behavior.

US and OCT are capable of measuring the directionality and relative velocity of structures (usually blood) by leveraging the Doppler effect. The flow of blood,

N. Navab et al. (Eds.): MICCAI 2015, Part III, LNCS 9351, pp. 403–410, 2015.
DOI: 10.1007/978-3-319-24574-4_48

however, is not the only temporal characteristic of vascular structures. The pulsatile radial distension of the vascular walls (from the lumen to tunica externa) is another characteristic that can be observed and measured using almost any imaging modality so long as the temporal and spatial resolutions are adequate.

Recently, we demonstrated in [10] that phased-based (PB) Eulerian techniques can be used to detect the motion of renal vessels at a sub-pixel level by analyzing the temporal change in phase. Our early work did not explicitly compute the deformation vectors (magnitude and orientation) of structures in the image through time. The estimation of said vectors is computationally expensive and thus not appropriate in the context of robotic surgery. In this contribution, we propose that 1) a more detailed computation of motion characteristics (i.e. an estimation of the *local orientation* of motion) can increase the accuracy of motion based vessel segmentation, and 2) by reconstructing the monogenic signal (MON) [11], the local orientation of motion may be estimated concurrently while increasing the computational performance of the method.

We propose a robust vessel segmentation technique that models local motion of vessels subject to pulsatile radial distension. We estimate all components of motion using traditional optical flow (OF) and faster MON based flow estimation [12]. This complete representation of motion allows us to analyze the local orientation of motion to remove outliers on objects that are undergoing more translational motion while amplifying the response of structures that behave like a truly pulsating vessel, i.e., periodically expand and contract in time. Using computational phantoms, we evaluate the performance of our motion estimation methods while comparing it to our old PB method [10]. Finally. we validate our segmentations on US images acquired from human volunteers.

2 Methods

Our method relies on a complete estimation of motion. Optical flow methods, such as the one proposed by Sun et al. [13], compute apparent local motions of objects in a sequence of images by imposing the brightness consistency assumption. Similarly, the MON signal may be used to estimate this local motion more efficiently. The MON signal is a 2D extension of the analytic signal and it provides a framework for extracting the local orientation θ and the local phase ϕ features from an image. By measuring the temporal change in θ and ϕ in a sequence of images, we can estimate motion [12]. In this paper, each jth frame of such sequence is defined as a scalar valued (grayscale) function $f_j : \mathbf{x} \subset \mathbb{R}^2 \to \mathbb{R}$ mapping a pixel $\mathbf{x} = (x_1, x_2)^\intercal$ in the spatial domain to an intensity value. The MON signal is constructed from a trio of bandpass filters with finite spatial support. This trio is called a spherical quadrature filter (SQF) [11]. To estimate the motion of both small and large structures in each frame, we generate different SQFs by tuning the spatial passband of the filters to varying scales. We first provide a brief summary of the SQFs used and how we estimate local motion vectors from the MON signal of a sequence of frames. Lastly, we explain how local motion extracted using MON or OF is used to identify pulsating structures.

The Monogenic Framework: Each SQF is comprised of an even (symmetric) radial bandpass filter and two odd (antisymmetric) filters. The odd filters are computed from the Riesz transform, a 2D generalization of the Hilbert transform, of the radial bandpass filter [11]. We employ Log-Gabor bandpass filters as they suit the natural statistics of an image [4,14] and maintain zero DC gain at lower spatial scales. For every scale s, the even component of the SQF is expressed as

$$B_e(\mathbf{u}; s) = \exp\left(\frac{-\left[\log\left(|\mathbf{u}|/\omega_s\right)\right]^2}{2\left[\log k\right]^2}\right), \tag{1}$$

in the frequency domain $\mathbf{u} = (u_1, u_2)^\intercal$, where k and ω_s are parameters of the filter. The parameter $k = \sigma/\omega_s$ is a fixed constant representing the ratio of the standard deviation σ of the Gaussian describing the Log-Gabor filter's transfer function in the frequency domain to the filter's center frequency ω_s. At each scale s, the center frequency is defined as $\omega_s = (\lambda_0 2^{(s-1)})^{-1}$, where λ_0 is an initial minimum wavelength. Note that B_e is symmetric as it is only a function of the magnitude of the frequency $\mathbf{u}$. Using the Riesz transform, we compute the two odd components (B_{o1} and B_{o2}) associated to this SQF as

$$B_{o1}(\mathbf{u}; s) = i\frac{u_1}{|\mathbf{u}|}B_e; \quad B_{o2}(\mathbf{u}; s) = i\frac{u_2}{|\mathbf{u}|}B_e. \tag{2}$$

In the spatial domain, the components of the MON signal $(h_{j,e}, \mathbf{h}_{j,o})$ are obtained by convolving the SQF with a given frame of the sequence such that

$$\begin{aligned} h_{j,e}(\mathbf{x}; s) &= \mathcal{F}^{-1}\left[B_e(\mathbf{u}; s)F_j(\mathbf{u})\right] \\ h_{j,o1}(\mathbf{x}; s) &= \mathcal{F}^{-1}\left[B_{o1}(\mathbf{u}; s)F_j(\mathbf{u})\right] \\ h_{j,o2}(\mathbf{x}; s) &= \mathcal{F}^{-1}\left[B_{o2}(\mathbf{u}; s)F_j(\mathbf{u})\right] \\ \mathbf{h}_{j,o}(\mathbf{x}, s) &= (h_{j,o1}(\mathbf{x}; s), h_{j,o2}(\mathbf{x}; s))^\intercal, \end{aligned} \tag{3}$$

where $F_j(\mathbf{u}) = \mathcal{F}[f_j(\mathbf{x})]$ is the frequency domain representation of the frame.

Extraction of Local Motion from the Local Phase Vector: Let $\mathbf{r}$ be the phase vector, the continuous representation of local orientation θ and local phase information ϕ, which can be computed from (3) such that

$$\mathbf{r}_j(\mathbf{x}; s) = \phi(\cos\theta, \sin\theta)^\intercal = \frac{\mathbf{h}_{j,o}}{|\mathbf{h}_{j,o}|}\arg\left(h_{j,e} + i|\mathbf{h}_{j,o}|\right). \tag{4}$$

Local motion may then be calculated by first computing the components of a 3D rotation that relates the response of two adjacent frames in the video

$$\begin{aligned} h_{\text{diff},e} &= h_{j,e}h_{j+1,e} + \mathbf{h}_{j,o}^\intercal\mathbf{h}_{j+1,o} \\ \mathbf{h}_{\text{diff},o} &= h_{j,e}\mathbf{h}_{j+1,o} - h_{j+1,e}\mathbf{h}_{j,o} \end{aligned} \tag{5}$$

and then computing the phase differences $\mathbf{r}_{\text{diff}}$ by solving (4) using (5). Given a local neighborhood $\mathcal{N}$, the local displacement $\mathbf{d}_{\mathcal{N}}$ is calculated from

$$\sum_{\mathbf{x}\in\mathcal{N}}\left[\nabla^\intercal\mathbf{r}_j(\mathbf{x}; s)\right]\mathbf{d}_{\mathcal{N},j} = \sum_{\mathbf{x}\in\mathcal{N}}\mathbf{r}_{\text{diff}}(\mathbf{x}; s) \tag{6}$$

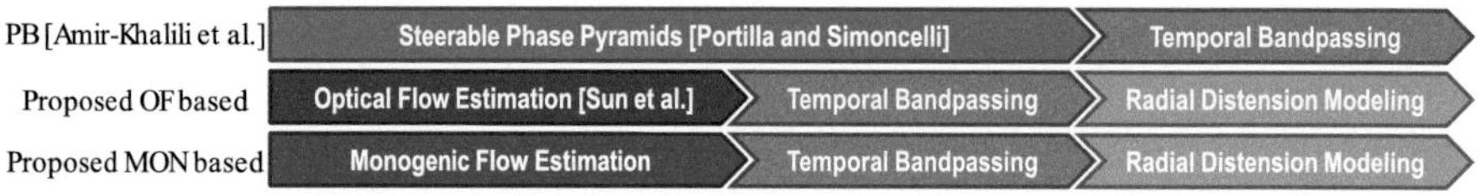

Fig. 1. Overview of the motion based vessel segmentation pipelines.

where ∇^{T} is the divergence operator. The derivation of (4), (5), and (6) from the response to the SQF is outside the scope of this paper and can be found in [12]. To improve the estimate for the displacement vector $\mathbf{d}_{\mathcal{N},j}$, we compute the mean of this value across all scales s. The computed $\mathbf{d}_{\mathcal{N},j}$ is an estimate of the true motion vectors $\mathbf{d}_j(\mathbf{x})$ that relates two frames in a sequence $f_{j+1}(\mathbf{x}) = f_j(\mathbf{x} - \mathbf{d}_j(\mathbf{x}))$. This is the same motion vector that is computed by traditional OF techniques.

Modeling of Radial Distension: Let $\mathbf{d}(\mathbf{x}, j)$ define motion field containing the motion vectors estimated for all adjacent fames inside a given sequence. We first isolate the motions that are in sync with the heart rate by applying the same ideal temporal bandpass filter (Fig. 1) used in [10] to each location in $\mathbf{x}$ of the motion vector $\mathbf{d}(\mathbf{x}, j)$ independently. Let h be the temporal filter defined as

$$h(\mathbf{x}, j) = 2b_H \mathtt{sinc}(2b_H j) - 2b_L \mathtt{sinc}(2b_L j), \tag{7}$$

where b_L is the low frequency cutoff and b_H is the high frequency cutoff. We define the temporally bandpassed motion vectors as $\hat{\mathbf{d}}(\mathbf{x}, j) = \mathbf{d}(\mathbf{x}, j) * h(\mathbf{x}, j)$.

Temporal filtering alone does not distinguish between structures that distend radially and tissues that translate at pulsatile frequency. Pulsating vessels are subject to periodic expansion and contraction, which implies that the orientation of the motion vectors are opposing each other along the centerline of the vessel. Such vector fields thus exhibit high *divergence* along the centerline.

Due of the tubular geometry of vessels, the radial motion along the centerline of the vessels are weaker compared to the regions that are along the walls. We account for this by computing the divergence across multiple spatial scales; the motion field at each scale denoted $\hat{\mathbf{d}}(\mathbf{x}, j; s)$. At each scale, we downsample the vector field by a factor of two using bilinear interpolation. Our resulting vessel labels are computed to be

$$I(\mathbf{x}) = \frac{1}{M} \sum_{\forall j} \sum_{\forall s} |\nabla^{\mathsf{T}} \hat{\mathbf{d}}(\mathbf{x}, j; s)|, \tag{8}$$

where M is a normalizing factor to fix the range of I to [0 1].

3 Results and Discussion

In this section we present two experiments to evaluate the performance of our method against the state-of-the-art. In the experiments, we compare our proposed MON and OF pipelines with the PB method (Fig. 1).

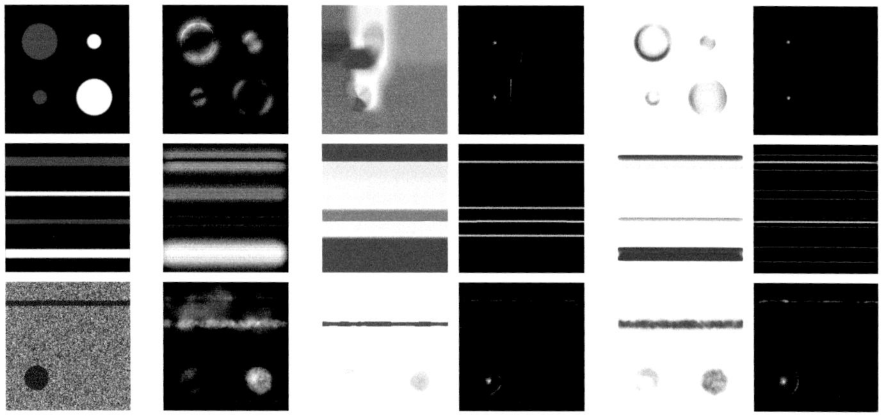

(a) Phantom (b) PB Seg. (c) OF (d) OF Seg. (e) MON (f) MON Seg.

Fig. 2. Qualitative phantom experiments showing segmentation results of PB and our vessel extraction applied to OF and MON. All resulting segmentations were thresholded at 0.3 for visibility. Fuzzy segmentations of our method depict high (white) response at the center of the pulsating structures. Top row: phantom with circular shapes of varying sizes. Middle row: tubular shapes of varying sizes. Bottom row: A randomly generated texture subjected to local deformations that include a combination of translating/pulsating circular/tubular structures. Column (a): the first image of the phantom with red overlay indicating structures that distend radially, the other structures are subject to translation only. Column (c & e): the color encoding of the motion vectors extracted using OF and MON respectively.

Materials and Experimental Setup: For the real data experiments, we use eight US sequences of the common carotid artery (CCA) acquired from three volunteers. Although our methods are applicable to other imaging modalities, US is ideal for validation as it can image vessels in the transverse and longitudinal axes, it has high temporal resolution, and the vessels can be manually delineated with accuracy for evaluation against ground truth. The first frame of each sequence was segmented manually for quantitative analysis. All of the computational phantoms and the methods described were implemented in MATLAB 2011b running on a workstation with two Intel 3GHz Xeon x5472 processors and 8GB of RAM. We use the MATLAB code and default parameters of PB [10] and the `classic+nl-fast` setting of OF [13]. For the MON method, the minimum wavelength λ_0 is set to 2, ratio k was set to 0.05, and a 7×7 square filter was used to average the displacements over the neighborhood of $\mathcal{N}$. The number of scales are set such that $s = \lfloor \log_2(L) \rfloor - 1$ where L is the smallest image dimension.

Phantom Experiment: We use three computational phantoms, in a two-frame matching experiment, to compare the effectiveness of our proposed MON and OF based segmentation techniques to the PB method. Temporal filtering was not used in this experiment. We constructed three computational phantoms containing: Pulsating and translating circles (top row in Fig. 2), pulsating and

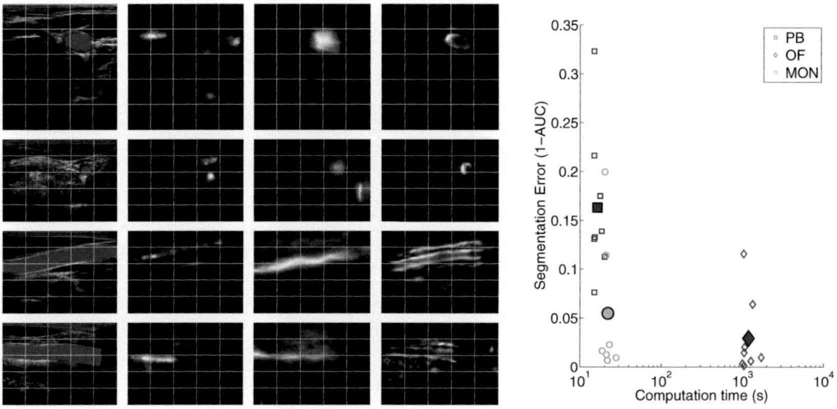

(a) US **(b)** PB Seg. **(c)** OF Seg. **(d)** MON Seg. **(e)**

Fig. 3. Experiment with real data. Exemplar US image of CCA in axial and longitudinal axes. The corresponding US ground truth for the vessel is shown in red. Yellow gridlines are superimpsoed to enhance correspondence. All resulting segmentations were thresholded at 0.3 for visibility. (e) Performance of each segmentation method, corresponding averages illustrated with filled markers and black outline.

translating tubular structures (middle row in Fig. 2), and a noise pattern that undergoes a combination of pulsating and translating motions in the shapes of circles and tubes (bottom row in Fig. 2). The OF flow estimation code used relies heavily on regularization in regions that do not contain salient textures (Fig. 2c). We thus used the third phantom to perform further quantitative comparison between the OF and MON flow estimation modules. We computed the error in flow endpoint to the ground truth $\mathbf{d}_{GT}$ defined as $\|\mathbf{d} - \mathbf{d}_{GT}\|_2$ and observed only a small increase in the mean error from 0.21 pixels (OF) to 0.28 (MON).

Real Data Experiment: Real data evaluation was done on eight US sequences of the CCA along the transverse and longitudinal axes, where the vessel appears as a pulsating ellipsoid and tube respectively. The passband of the temporal filter was tuned depending on the patient's approximate heart rate, denoted b_r. The filter parameters were set such that $b_L = b_r/2$ and $b_H = 2b_r$. Four exemplar cases of our fuzzy segmentation labels are shown in Fig. 3. To clarify the advantages to each approach as a trade-off between accuracy and computation time, we present quantitative analysis (Fig 3e) using the ground truth segmentations of the US sequences. We report the area under the receiver operating characteristics curve (AUC) for each case (thresholding the fuzzy segmentations from 0 to 1) as a measure of segmentation accuracy, in which the value of 1 indicates perfect segmentation and 0.5 is the noise threshold.

Discussions: From our analysis, we conclude that the MON approach is the best candidate for segmenting vasculature from pulsatile motion. Fig. 3e shows that the MON method can, on average, achieve comparable accuracy with OF method while maintaining similar performance as the PB method. The comparable performance of MON vs OF flow estimation is further confirmed by the analysis of the endpoint errors. Compared to PB (Fig 3b), with the addition of our proposed orientation based vessel segmentation, our MON (Fig 3d) and OF (Fig 3c) pipelines are more specific to motion of the CCA. In Fig. 3b, the false positives that occur on the surrounding soft tissues have been reduced.

Quantitatively, the average AUC was increased from 0.84 (PB) to 0.97 (OF) and 0.95 (MON). Binarizing the segmentations at 0.5 yields a significant increase in average Dice similarity coefficient (DSC) from 0.16 (PB) to 0.55 (OF) and 0.52 (MON). The average run times for the 40 frame US sequences (without distension modeling) are: 16 s for PB, 19.6 min for OF, and 15 s for the MON method; the modeling step costs an additional 7 s for OF and MON. Our unoptimized MATLAB implementation of MON is drastically faster than OF and slightly faster than the PB method. We predict that the MON method has the potential to further outperform the PB method, as our SQF is composed of three filters per scale whereas the PB method uses a total of eight filters per scale.

In the domain of US image processing, SQFs have been shown to improve the extraction of structures, during radio frequency (RF) signal to B-mode conversion, by demodulating the RF in a 2D context [15]. This implies that our method may be used to extract local motion information from raw RF data, allowing for direct implementation in a native representation of acquired data.

Our Eulerian approach is not yet able to cope with gross out-of-plane motion, common during 2D US acquisitions, because our current implementation of the MON framework is in two spatial dimensions. As noted in [16], the steerable approach of Portilla and Simoncelli [17] that was used in the PB method is hard to transpose into 3D due to its invertibility. The MON formulation can however be extended to 3D [16]. This will allow our proposed method to be extended to volumetric images such as 3D CT fluoroscopy, Cine MRI, and 3D US.

4 Conclusions

We presented evidence that more robust automatic segmentation of vasculature is achievable by analyzing the characteristic pulsatile radial distension of vascular structures. Specifically we have shown that 1) the local orientation of motion extracted from a sequence can be used to highlight the center of a pulsating vessel where the *divergence* of the motion vector field is high, and 2) the MON framework is capable of estimating the amplitude *and* orientation of local motion faster than the PB method. Using US sequences acquired from the CCA, we have shown that the performance of the PB method can be increased from an average AUC of 0.84 to 0.95 while slightly increasing the computation time from 15 to 22 seconds. The proposed MON method can be optimized further through the precomputation of the SQFs, may be applied to native RF data, and can be extended to process volumetric (3D+time) data.

References

1. Murari, K., Li, N., Rege, A., Jia, X., et al.: Contrast-enhanced imaging of cerebral vasculature with laser speckle. Applied Optics 46(22), 5340–5346 (2007)
2. Izatt, J.A., Kulkarni, M.D., Yazdanfar, S., Barton, J.K., Welch, A.J.: In vivo bidirectional color doppler flow imaging of picoliter blood volumes using optical coherence tomography. Optics Letters 22(18), 1439–1441 (1997)
3. Staal, J., Abràmoff, M.D., Niemeijer, M., Viergever, M.A., van Ginneken, B.: Ridge-based vessel segmentation in color images of the retina. Transactions on Medical Imaging 23(4), 501–509 (2004)
4. Soares, J.V., Leandro, J.J., Cesar, R.M., Jelinek, H.F., Cree, M.J.: Retinal vessel segmentation using the 2-D Gabor wavelet and supervised classification. Transactions on Medical Imaging 25(9), 1214–1222 (2006)
5. Frangi, A.F., Niessen, W.J., Vincken, K.L., Viergever, M.A.: Multiscale vessel enhancement filtering. In: Wells, W.M., Colchester, A.C.F., Delp, S.L. (eds.) MICCAI 1998. LNCS, vol. 1496, pp. 130–137. Springer, Heidelberg (1998)
6. Hennersperger, C., Baust, M., Waelkens, P., Karamalis, A., Ahmadi, S., Navab, N.: Multiscale tubular structure detection in ultrasound imaging. Transactions on Medical Imaging 34(1), 13–26 (2015)
7. Vermeer, K.A., Vos, F.M., Lemij, H., Vossepoel, A.M.: A model based method for retinal blood vessel detection. Computers in Biology and Medicine 34(3), 209–219 (2004)
8. Lorigo, L.M., Faugeras, O.D., Grimson, W.E.L., Keriven, R., Kikinis, R., Nabavi, A., Westin, C.-F.: Curves: Curve evolution for vessel segmentation. Medical Image Analysis 5(3), 195–206 (2001)
9. Becker, C., Rigamonti, R., Lepetit, V., Fua, P.: Supervised feature learning for curvilinear structure segmentation. In: Mori, K., Sakuma, I., Sato, Y., Barillot, C., Navab, N. (eds.) MICCAI 2013, Part I. LNCS, vol. 8149, pp. 526–533. Springer, Heidelberg (2013)
10. Amir-Khalili, A., Hamarneh, G., Peyrat, J.M., Abinahed, J., Al-Alao, O., Al-Ansari, A., Abugharbieh, R.: Automatic segmentation of occluded vasculature via pulsatile motion analysis in endoscopic robot-assisted partial nephrectomy video. Medical Image Analysis (2015)
11. Felsberg, M., Sommer, G.: The monogenic signal. Transactions on Signal Processing 49(12), 3136–3144 (2001)
12. Felsberg, M.: Optical flow estimation from monogenic phase. In: Complex Motion, pp. 1–13 (2007)
13. Sun, D., Roth, S., Black, M.J.: Secrets of optical flow estimation and their principles. In: IEEE Computer Vision and Pattern Recognition, pp. 2432–2439 (2010)
14. Field, D.J.: Relations between the statistics of natural images and the response properties of cortical cells. JOSA A 4(12), 2379–2394 (1987)
15. Wachinger, C., Klein, T., Navab, N.: The 2D analytic signal on RF and B-mode ultrasound images. In: Information Processing in Medical Imaging, pp. 359–370 (2011)
16. Chenouard, N., Unser, M.: 3D steerable wavelets and monogenic analysis for bioimaging. In: IEEE International Symposium on Biomedical Imaging, pp. 2132–2135 (2011)
17. Portilla, J., Simoncelli, E.P.: A parametric texture model based on joint statistics of complex wavelet coefficients. IJCV 40(1), 49–70 (2000)

A Sparse Bayesian Learning Algorithm for Longitudinal Image Data

Mert R. Sabuncu*

A.A. Martinos Center for Biomedical Imaging, Massachusetts General Hospital, Harvard Medical School, Charlestown, MA, USA

Abstract. Longitudinal imaging studies, where serial (multiple) scans are collected on each individual, are becoming increasingly widespread. The field of machine learning has in general neglected the longitudinal design, since many algorithms are built on the assumption that each datapoint is an independent sample. Thus, the application of general purpose machine learning tools to longitudinal image data can be sub-optimal. Here, we present a novel machine learning algorithm designed to handle longitudinal image datasets. Our approach builds on a sparse Bayesian image-based prediction algorithm. Our empirical results demonstrate that the proposed method can offer a significant boost in prediction performance with longitudinal clinical data.

Keywords: Machine learning, Image-based prediction, Longitudinal data.

1 Introduction

Machine learning algorithms are increasingly applied to biomedical image data for a range of clinical applications, including computer aided detection/diagnosis (CAD) and studying group differences, e.g. [1,2,3] . In early biomedical applications, off-the-shelf algorithms such as Support Vector Machines were employed on image intensity data. However, there has been a recent proliferation of customized methods that derive optimal image features and incorporate domain knowledge about the clinical context and imaging data, e.g. [4,5,6,7,8]. Such customized methods can offer a significant increase in prediction accuracy.

Machine learning in general, and its application to population-level biomedical image analysis in particular, has largely been concerned with the cross-sectional design, where each sample is treated as independent. Yet, as data acquisition costs continue to fall and data collection efforts become more collaborative and standardized, longitudinal designs have become increasingly widespread. Longitudinal studies, where serial data are collected on each individual, can offer increased sensitivity and specificity in detecting associations, and provide insights into the temporal dynamics of underlying biological processes.

Real-life longitudinal data suffer from several technical issues, which make their analysis challenging. Subject drop-outs, missing visits, variable number of

* Supported by NIH NIBIB 1K25EB013649-01 and a BrightFocus grant (AHAF-A2012333). Data used were obtained from ADNI: http://tinyurl.com/ADNI-main.

N. Navab et al. (Eds.): MICCAI 2015, Part III, LNCS 9351, pp. 411–418, 2015.
DOI: 10.1007/978-3-319-24574-4_49

Table 1. Data from annual ADNI MRI visits analyzed in this study. Note some subjects had MRI visits at 6, 18, 30, 42, 54, and 66 months too.

Planned visit time (months)	Baseline	12	24	36	48	60	72
Mean± Std. time (months)	0	$13.1 \pm .8$	25.5 ± 1.2	37.7 ± 1.2	50.7 ± 2.2	62.4 ± 1.7	74.2 ± 2.0
Number of imaging sessions	791	649	518	336	216	159	131

visits, and heterogeneity in the timing of visits are commonplace. For example, Table 1 illustrates these challenges with longitudinal data from the Alzheimer's disease neuroimaging initiative (ADNI) [9]. The number of subjects completing each planned longitudinal visit diminishes gradually as subjects drop out, and scan timings are highly variable. Recently, several methods have been proposed to appropriately examine this type of data in a (mass-)univariate fashion and using classical statistical techniques suitable for longitudinal designs, e.g., linear mixed effects (LME) models [10] and generalized estimating equations (GEE) [11].

To our knowledge, however, there exists no purpose-built machine learning method that would offer the ability to optimally handle serial data, particularly from real-life longitudinal designs. We note that the scenario we consider is different from time-series data, which also deals with temporal dynamics. Yet in time-series analysis (e.g., of financial data), which has received considerable attention in machine learning, e.g. [12], temporal processes are typically sampled densely and at uniform intervals. A common goal is to fully characterize a single process in order to make forecasts. Instead, the longitudinal scenario we consider here assumes that each subject has a separate temporal process, which has been sampled a small number of times, possibly at non-uniform intervals.

We adopt the framework of the recently proposed Relevance Voxel Machine (RVoxM) [5], which offers state-of-the-art image-based prediction for a range of clinical applications and has a publicly available implementation. RVoxM builds on the Relevance Vector Machine (RVM) [13], a sparse Bayesian learning technique, and adapts it to model the spatial smoothness in images. Like virtually all machine learning algorithms, both RVM and RVoxM treat each datapoint as an independent sample, likely making their use sub-optimal for longitudinal data analysis. Inspired by LME models [10], we propose to introduce subject-specific random effects into the RVoxM model in order to capture the within-subject correlation structure in longitudinal data. Section 2 introduces the theoretical concepts of the proposed method. Section 3 presents empirical results and Section 4 provides a conclusion and discussion.

2 Theory

We aim to predict a target variable, $t \in \mathbb{R}$, from an image scan, $\boldsymbol{x}$, which denotes vectorized voxel values. We append 1 to $\boldsymbol{x}$ to account for the bias. Thus $\boldsymbol{x}$ is $V+1$ dimensional, where V is the number of voxels. As in RVoxM [5], we assume:

$$t = y(\boldsymbol{x}, \boldsymbol{w}) + \epsilon, \tag{1}$$

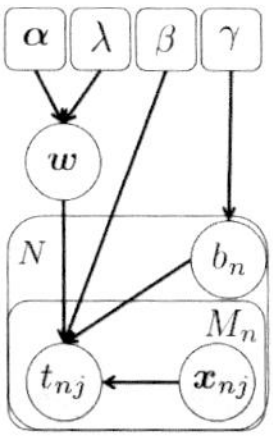

Fig. 1. Graphical model depicting the dependency structure between model variables. Circles represent random variables and model parameters are in squares. Plates indicate replication. Shaded variables are observed (during training), whereas remaining variables are unknown (latent). For variable names and further details, refer to text.

where the error is zero-mean Gaussian, $\epsilon \sim \mathcal{N}(0, \beta^{-1})$, with variance $\beta^{-1} > 0$.

Similar to RVoxM we adopt a linear model for y. Unlike RVoxM, however, we utilize subject-specific random variables to account for the within-subject correlation structure in longitudinal data. Thus, we assume:

$$y_{nj} = \boldsymbol{x}_{nj}^{\mathrm{T}} \boldsymbol{w} + b_n, \tag{2}$$

where the subscripts n and j denote the subject and subject-specific time-point indices, respectively; $\boldsymbol{w}$ is the vector of latent model coefficients shared across subjects (one for each voxel and a bias term); and b_n is the latent, subject-specific bias term. As in RVoxM [5], the coefficients are assumed to be drawn from a sparsity-inducing, spatial-smoothness-encouraging prior:

$$\boldsymbol{w} \sim N(\mathbf{0}, \mathbf{P}^{-1}), \tag{3}$$

where $\mathbf{P} = \mathrm{diag}(\boldsymbol{\alpha}) + \lambda L$, $\boldsymbol{\alpha} = [\alpha_1, \cdots, \alpha_{V+1}] > 0$, and $\lambda \geq 0$ are hyperparameters; and L is a Laplacian matrix defined as:

$$L(u, v) = \begin{cases} -1 & \text{, if } u \text{ and } v \text{ are indices of neighboring voxels} \\ \text{Number of neighbors} & \text{, if } u = v \\ 0 & \text{, otherwise.} \end{cases} \tag{4}$$

The critical component of Eq. 2 is the subject-specific bias term b_n, which we assume to be drawn from a zero-mean Gaussian, $b_n \sim N(0, \gamma^{-1})$, with variance $\gamma^{-1} > 0$. Fig. 1 shows the graphical model illustrating the relationship between model variables. Similar to LME models, b_n captures the positive correlation between serial datapoints on the same individual. That is, we expect the error of the core prediction algorithm (e.g., RVoxM with $b_n = 0$) to be positively correlated for longitudinal data. So, for example, if the prediction is smaller than the ground truth (i.e., negative error) for the first time-point of a subject, we expect the error to be negative for a second time-point of the same individual too. The subject-specific bias term is intended to correct for this error. Empirical evidence presented in Fig. 2 supports our theoretical expectation of positive correlation between the prediction errors made on serial scans. The details of these data, which come from our empirical analysis, can be found in Section 3.

2.1 Training Phase

Let us assume we are given N training subjects, each with $M_n \geq 1$ time-points, where n denotes the subject index. Thus, we have $M = \sum_n M_n$ samples and

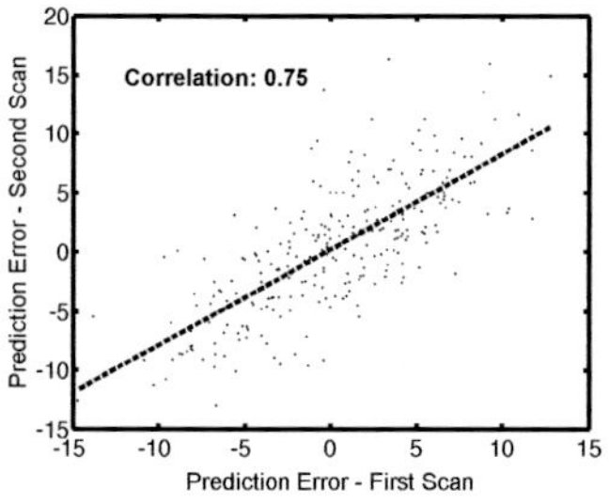

Fig. 2. Scatter plot of prediction error (predicted minus true value) of mini-mental state exam score (MMSE, a cognitive test that is associated with dementia). Prediction computed with RVoxM on brain MRI-derived cortical thickness data from ADNI. "First scan" was acquired at baseline and "Second scant" at the month 12 visit. Each point represents an individual. See experiment section for further details.

each sample consists of an image scan $\boldsymbol{x}$ and corresponding target variable value t. Let $\mathbf{X} \in \mathbb{R}^{M\times(V+1)}$ and $\boldsymbol{t} \in \mathbb{R}^M$ denote the stacked up training data. The goal of training is to learn the hyper-parameters $\boldsymbol{\alpha}$, λ, β and γ from the training data, e.g., via maximizing the type II likelihood:

$$\begin{aligned}(\boldsymbol{\alpha}^*, \lambda^*, \beta^*, \gamma^*) &= \underset{\boldsymbol{\alpha},\lambda,\beta,\gamma}{\operatorname{argmax}}\, p(\boldsymbol{t}|\mathbf{X}; \boldsymbol{\alpha}, \lambda, \beta, \gamma) \\ &= \underset{\boldsymbol{\alpha},\lambda,\beta,\gamma}{\operatorname{argmax}} \int p(\boldsymbol{w}; \boldsymbol{\alpha}, \lambda) \prod_n p(\boldsymbol{t}_n|\mathbf{X}_n, \boldsymbol{w}; \beta, \gamma) d\boldsymbol{w}, \end{aligned} \tag{5}$$

where $\boldsymbol{t}_n \in \mathbb{R}^{M_n}$ and $\mathbf{X}_n \in \mathbb{R}^{M_n\times(V+1)}$ are the stacked up data (target variables and images) for the n'th training subject. The likelihood term for the n'th subject can be derived by marginalizing over the unknown subject-specific bias:

$$p(\boldsymbol{t}_n|\mathbf{X}_n, \boldsymbol{w}; \beta, \gamma) = \int p(\boldsymbol{t}_n|\mathbf{X}_n, \boldsymbol{w}; \beta, b_n) p(b_n; \gamma) db_n = \mathcal{N}(\mathbf{X}_n^{\mathrm{T}}\boldsymbol{w}, \boldsymbol{\Lambda}_n), \tag{6}$$

where

$$\boldsymbol{\Lambda}_n = \left(\beta(\mathbf{I}_{M_n} - \frac{\beta}{\beta M_n + \gamma}\mathbf{1}_{M_n}\mathbf{1}_{M_n}^{\mathrm{T}})\right)^{-1} = \beta^{-1}\mathbf{I}_{M_n} + \gamma^{-1}\mathbf{1}_{M_n}\mathbf{1}_{M_n}^{\mathrm{T}}. \tag{7}$$

$\mathbf{I}_{M_n}$ denotes the $M_n \times M_n$ identity matrix and $\mathbf{1}_{M_n}$ denotes a length M_n column vector of 1's. Note $\boldsymbol{\Lambda}_n$ is in general not a diagonal matrix, thus modeling correlation structure between serial data. Inserting Eq. 6 into Eq. 5 and working out the integral yields $p(\boldsymbol{t}|\mathbf{X}; \boldsymbol{\alpha}, \lambda, \beta, \gamma) = \mathcal{N}(\mathbf{0}, \mathbf{C})$, where $\mathbf{C} = \boldsymbol{\Lambda} + \mathbf{X}^{\mathrm{T}}\mathbf{P}^{-1}\mathbf{X}$, $\boldsymbol{\Lambda} = \mathbf{I}_N \otimes \boldsymbol{\Lambda}_n$ and $\otimes$ is the Kronecker product. Note $\mathbf{C}$ depends on all hyper-parameters $(\boldsymbol{\alpha}, \lambda, \beta, \gamma)$ and the optimization (learning) problem of Eq. 5 can be re-written as:

$$\underset{\boldsymbol{\alpha},\lambda,\beta,\gamma}{\operatorname{argmin}}\, \boldsymbol{t}^{\mathrm{T}}\mathbf{C}^{-1}\boldsymbol{t} + \log|\mathbf{C}|, \tag{8}$$

where $|\cdot|$ denotes matrix determinant. Let's define:

$$\boldsymbol{\Sigma} = (\mathbf{P} + \mathbf{X}^{\mathrm{T}}\boldsymbol{\Lambda}^{-1}\mathbf{X})^{-1}, \text{ and } \boldsymbol{\mu} = \boldsymbol{\Sigma}\mathbf{X}^{\mathrm{T}}\boldsymbol{\Lambda}^{-1}\boldsymbol{t}. \tag{9}$$

Following the algebraic manipulations of [5,13], we arrive at the following update equation for the elements of the hyper-parameter vector $\boldsymbol{\alpha}$:

$$\alpha_i \leftarrow \frac{1 - \alpha_i\boldsymbol{\Sigma}_{ii} - \lambda\left(\mathbf{P}^{-1}\mathbf{L}\right)_{ii}}{\mu_i^2}, \tag{10}$$

which satisfies the non-negativity constraints and optimizes Eq. 8. As originally observed by Tipping [13], this optimization procedure tends to yield many α_i's that diverge to ∞ in practice, effectively turning off the contribution of the corresponding voxel (see next subsection) and producing a sparse model. We estimate the three scalar hyper-parameters, (β, λ, γ), by solving Eq. 8 via gradient-descent.

2.2 Testing Phase

The training phase provides a set of learned hyper-parameters $(\boldsymbol{\alpha}^*, \lambda^*, \beta^*, \gamma^*)$. The testing phase involves computing the posterior distribution of the target variable given longitudinal image data from a novel test subject, $\mathbf{X}_{N+1} \in \mathbb{R}^{M_{N+1}\times(V+1)}$, with $M_{N+1} \geq 1$ time-points. It can be shown that this posterior is a Gaussian:

$$p(\boldsymbol{t}_{N+1}|\mathbf{X}_{N+1};\boldsymbol{\alpha}^*, \lambda^*, \beta^*, \gamma^*) = \mathcal{N}(\mathbf{X}_{N+1}\boldsymbol{\mu}^*, \tilde{\boldsymbol{\Sigma}}_{N+1}), \tag{11}$$

where

$$\tilde{\boldsymbol{\Sigma}}_{N+1} = \boldsymbol{\Lambda}^*_{N+1} + \mathbf{X}_{N+1}\boldsymbol{\Sigma}^*\mathbf{X}^{\mathrm{T}}_{N+1}, \tag{12}$$

$\boldsymbol{\Lambda}^*_{N+1} = (\beta^*)^{-1}\mathbf{I}_{M_{N+1}} + (\gamma^*)^{-1}\mathbf{1}_{M_{N+1}}\mathbf{1}^{\mathrm{T}}_{M_{N+1}}$, and $\boldsymbol{\mu}^*$ and $\boldsymbol{\Sigma}^*$ are computed based on Eq. 9 with learned hyper-parameters. From Eq. 11, the maximum a posteriori probability (MAP) estimate of the target variable is:

$$\hat{\boldsymbol{t}}_{N+1} = \mathbf{X}_{N+1}\boldsymbol{\mu}^*. \tag{13}$$

Using Eq 9 it can be shown that if $\alpha_i \to \infty$, then $\mu_i = 0$. Thus, the corresponding voxel has no influence on the MAP prediction.

In certain scenarios with $M_{N+1} > 1$, target variable values might be available for some time-points of the test subject. Without loss of generality, let us decompose $\boldsymbol{t}_{N+1} = [\boldsymbol{t}^{\text{known}}_{N+1}; \boldsymbol{t}^{\text{unknown}}_{N+1}]$, where the superscript indicates whether the target variable is known or not. Using well-known formulae for conditional multivariate Gaussians, the MAP estimate for $\boldsymbol{t}^{\text{unknown}}_{N+1}$ can be written as:

$$\hat{\boldsymbol{t}}^{\text{unknown}}_{N+1} = \mathbf{X}^{\text{unknown}}_{N+1}\boldsymbol{\mu}^* + [\tilde{\boldsymbol{\Sigma}}^{\text{unknown, known}}_{N+1}][\tilde{\boldsymbol{\Sigma}}^{\text{known, known}}_{N+1}]^{-1}(\boldsymbol{t}^{\text{known}}_{N+1} - \mathbf{X}^{\text{known}}_{N+1}\boldsymbol{\mu}^*), \tag{14}$$

where we have used: $\tilde{\boldsymbol{\Sigma}}_{N+1} = \left[\begin{array}{c|c} \tilde{\boldsymbol{\Sigma}}^{\text{known, known}}_{N+1} & \tilde{\boldsymbol{\Sigma}}^{\text{known, unknown}}_{N+1} \\ \hline \tilde{\boldsymbol{\Sigma}}^{\text{unknown, known}}_{N+1} & \tilde{\boldsymbol{\Sigma}}^{\text{unknown, unknown}}_{N+1} \end{array}\right]$.

2.3 Implementation

The learning algorithm is initialized with: $\boldsymbol{\mu}^{\text{init}} = \mathbf{X}^{\mathrm{T}}(\mathbf{X}\mathbf{X}^{\mathrm{T}})^{-1}\boldsymbol{t}$, $\alpha_i^{\text{init}} = \frac{1}{(\mu_i^{\text{init}})^2}$, $\lambda^{\text{init}} = 1$, $\beta^{\text{init}} = \frac{5}{\text{var}(\boldsymbol{t})}$, $\gamma^{\text{init}} = \frac{50}{\text{var}(\boldsymbol{t})}$. The objective function of Eq. 8 is monitored at each iteration and the optimization terminates once the change in the value is below a preset tolerance threshold. As RVoxM and RVM, the computational demands of the proposed algorithm are significant. A naive implementation, for example, can require $\mathcal{O}(V^3)$ time, and V, the number of voxels, can reach hundreds of thousands. Instead, we use a greedy algorithm, originally proposed for RVM [13], that permanently "turns off" voxels when their corresponding α_i exceeds a threshold (e.g., 10^{12}). Finally, all update equations can be expressed only using effective voxels (that haven't been turned off) and we can exploit the sparsity of $\mathbf{P}$ to speed up some matrix operations, as described in [5].

Our implementation is based on publicly available RVoxM code in Matlab. We call the proposed algorithm LRVoxM, for longitudinal RVoxM. We implemented a surface-based version designed to handle FreeSurfer-derived cortical surface data. FreeSurfer [14] is a freely available toolkit for automatically processing brain MRI scans. For example, given a structural brain MRI scan, FreeSurfer can compute a cortical thickness map sampled onto a common template surface mesh that represents a population average.

3 Empirical Results

In our experiment, we considered the problem of predicting the mini-mental state exam score (MMSE ranges between 0-30 and a lower score is associated with heightened dementia risk) from a 1.5T structural brain MRI scan. We analyzed longitudinal data from ADNI [9]. We generated two groups that consisted of pairs of matched subjects with three or more longitudinal scans at $>$ 6 month intervals. The matching was done based on baseline characteristics (age, sex, and diagnosis), yielding two groups of $N = 273$ with the following composition: 77 ± 7.1 years, %40 female, 76 healthy controls, 135 subjects with mild cognitive impairment (MCI, a clinical stage associated with high dementia risk), and 62 Alzheimer's disease (AD) patients. Total number of scans across both groups was 3069, i.e., an average of 5.62 MRI scans per subject. We assigned an MMSE score to each scan based on the clinical assessment closest to the MRI date.

Each matched pair of subjects were randomly split into a test subject and a training subject. We repeated this random split 10 times to obtained 10 random matched train/test datasets. Note that, since each subject contained a variable number of ($\geq$ 3) longitudinal time-points, the sizes of the train/test datasets were in general different.

The input to the prediction algorithm was FreeSurfer-derived cortical thickness data sampled on a common template surface (*fsaverage6* with $>$ 70k vertices) and smoothed with a Gaussian of FWHM = 5mm. As the baseline method, we considered the public implementation of RVoxM, which corresponded to setting $\gamma = \infty$ in the proposed LRVoxM algorithm. For LRVoxM, we examined three test phase scenarios: (**S0**) target variable was unknown for all test subject scans (LRVoxM-0), (**S1**) target variable was given for first scan (LRVoxM-1), and (**S2**) first two scans (LRVoxM-2) of each test subject. For **S1** and **S2**, LRVoxM used Eq. 14 to compute predictions. In assessing testing accuracy, we only used the scans for which none of the algorithms had access to the target variable (i.e., we excluded first two scans of each subject). Note that testing accuracy metrics for LRVoxM-0 and RVoxM remained virtually unchanged when we included the first two scans of each subject.

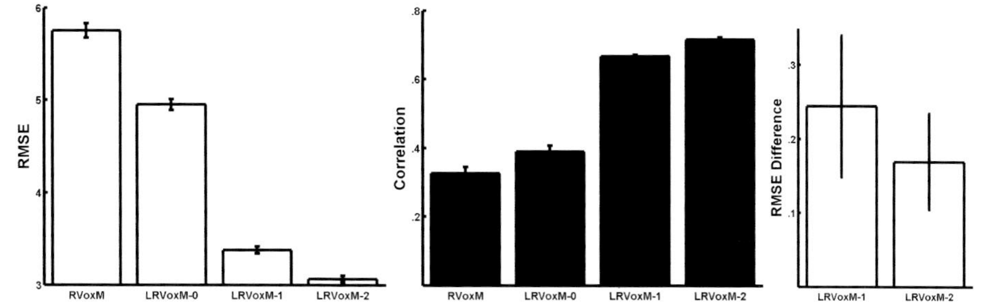

Fig. 3. Average testing accuracy (left: RMSE, middle: Correlation) in predicting MMSE from MRI scan. RVoxM: baseline method. LRVoxM: proposed longitudinal RVoxM algorithm. Right: Avg. RMSE improvement over MRI-blind predictions in scenarios **S1** and **S2** (see text). The bar charts show the mean values over the 10 test phase sessions. Errorbars indicate standard error of the mean.

Fig. 2 shows a scatter plot of the prediction error (predicted minus true MMSE value) of RVoxM, the benchmark algorithm, on the baseline and year 1 scans of a test dataset. This plot reveals the strong positive correlation of the prediction error in longitudinal data, which was the core motivation of our approach. The main empirical results are presented in Fig. 3, which shows the root mean squared error (RMSE) and correlation between the predictions and ground truth values. LRVoxM-0 clearly outperforms RVoxM on both metrics (avg. RMSE: 4.95 v. 5.75, avg. correlation: 0.39 v. 0.33, paired t-test across 10 sessions, $p < 10^{-7}$), which demonstrates the accuracy boost achieved by appropriately accounting for longitudinal data in a prediction algorithm.

Moreover, LRVoxM-1 and LRVoxM-2 offer progressively better prediction performance. For example, providing the target variable value for only a single timepoint reduces RMSE by about 32% to an average of 3.38, whereas LRVoxM-2 achieves a further improved average RMSE of 3.07. These results demonstrate that LRVoxM exploits subject-specific information to compute improved predictions (via the use of Eq. 14). We conducted an additional comparison of the LRVoxM results with "MRI-blind" predictions, which were computed based on the available MMSE values for each test subject (scenarios **S1** and **S2**, see Fig. 3-right). LRVoxM-1's RMSE was significantly lower than a prediction that assigned the first time point's MMSE value to all remaining time-points of the same subject (paired t-test $p < 0.02$). For **S2**, the MRI-blind prediction was computed by fitting a line to the given MMSE values of the first two timepoints. The predictions were then computed from this line at subsequent visits. LRVoxM-2's RMSE was also significantly lower than this MRI-blind prediction ($p < 0.04$).

4 Discussion and Conclusion

We presented a novel, sparse Bayesian learning algorithm suitable for longitudinal image data. Our experiments demonstrated a significant boost in performance achieved by the proposed method in comparison with the conventional strategy that ignores the longitudinal structure. Although we utilized the RVoxM framework, our approach is general and can be adopted within alternative probabilistic models, e.g., Gaussian processes, or for other data types. Future work will include extending LRVoxM to handle discrete target variables (classification), compute predictions about future outcome (prognosis), and examine alternative priors that might be more appropriate for handling discrete jumps in spatial data. We further plan to explore the use of additional subject-specific terms (such as those depending on time) to capture more complex correlation patterns, e.g, that depend on the time interval between visits.

References

1. Davatzikos, C., et al.: Individual patient diagnosis of AD and FTD via high-dimensional pattern classification of MRI. Neuroimage 41(4), 1220–1227 (2008)
2. Gaonkar, B., Davatzikos, C.: Deriving statistical significance maps for svm based image classification and group comparisons. In: Ayache, N., Delingette, H., Golland, P., Mori, K. (eds.) MICCAI 2012, Part I. LNCS, vol. 7510, pp. 723–730. Springer, Heidelberg (2012)
3. Sabuncu, M.R., et al.: Clinical prediction from structural brain MRI scans: A large-scale empirical study. Neuroinformatics, 1–16 (2014)
4. Cuingnet, R., et al.: Spatial regularization of SVM for the detection of diffusion alterations associated with stroke outcome. Medical Image Analysis, 15 (2011)
5. Sabuncu, M.R., Van Leemput, K.: The Relevance Voxel Machine (RVoxM): A self-tuning bayesian model for informative image-based prediction. IEEE Transactions on Medical Imaging (2012)
6. Suk, H.-I., Shen, D.: Deep learning-based feature representation for AD/MCI classification. In: Mori, K., Sakuma, I., Sato, Y., Barillot, C., Navab, N. (eds.) MICCAI 2013, Part II. LNCS, vol. 8150, pp. 583–590. Springer, Heidelberg (2013)
7. Liu, M., et al.: Identifying informative imaging biomarkers via tree structured sparse learning for AD diagnosis. Neuroinformatics 12(3) (2014)
8. Jie, B., et al.: Manifold regularized multitask feature learning for multimodality disease classification. Human Brain Mapping 36(2) (2015)
9. Jack, C.R., et al.: The Alzheimer's disease neuroimaging initiative (ADNI): MRI methods. Journal of Magnetic Resonance Imaging 27(4) (2008)
10. Bernal-Rusiel, J., et al.: Statistical analysis of longitudinal neuroimage data with linear mixed effects models. Neuroimage 66 (2013)
11. Li, Y., et al.: Multiscale adaptive generalized estimating equations for longitudinal neuroimaging data. Neuroimage 72 (2013)
12. Cao, L.-J., Tay, F.E.H.: Support vector machine with adaptive parameters in financial time series forecasting. IEEE T. on Neural Networks (2003)
13. Tipping, M.E.: Sparse Bayesian learning and the relevance vector machine. Journal of Machine Learning Research 1, 211–244 (2001)
14. Fischl, B.: FreeSurfer. Neuroimage 62(2), 774–781 (2012)

Descriptive and Intuitive Population-Based Cardiac Motion Analysis via Sparsity Constrained Tensor Decomposition

K. McLeod[1,2,3], M. Sermesant[3], P. Beerbaum[4], and X. Pennec[3]

[1] Simula Research Laboratory, Cardiac Modelling Project, Oslo, Norway
[2] Centre for Cardiological Innovation, Norway
[3] INRIA Méditerranée, Asclepios Project, Sophia Antipolis, France
[4] Hanover Medical University, Germany

Abstract. Analysing and understanding population-specific cardiac function is a challenging task due to the complex dynamics observed in both healthy and diseased subjects and the difficulty in quantitatively comparing the motion in different subjects. Affine parameters extracted from a Polyaffine motion model for a group of subjects can be used to represent the 3D motion regionally over time for a group of subjects. We propose to construct from these parameters a 4-way tensor of the rotation, stretch, shear, and translation components of each affine matrix defined in an intuitive coordinate system, stacked per region, for each affine component, over time, and for all subjects. From this tensor, Tucker decomposition can be applied with a constraint of sparsity on the core tensor in order to extract a few key, easily interpretable modes for each subject. Using this construction of a data tensor, the tensors of multiple groups can be stacked and collectively decomposed in order to compare and discriminate the motion by analysing the different loadings of each combination of modes for each group. The proposed method was applied to study and compare left ventricular dynamics for a group of healthy adult subjects and a group of adults with repaired Tetralogy of Fallot.

1 Introduction

Given the challenges in quantitatively measuring cardiac function, beyond simple 1D measures such as volume, strain, and so on, a number of cardiac motion tracking methods have been proposed. Cardiac motion tracking provides a non-invasive means to quantify cardiac motion and can be used to assess global and regional functional abnormalities such as akinesia or dyskinesia, to classify subjects as healthy/diseased or according to the severity of motion abnormalities, as well as to aid with diagnosis and therapy planning by providing quantitative measures of function.

While single-subject motion tracking can provide useful insight into the motion dynamics for a given subject, population-based (i.e. atlas-based) motion analysis can give further understanding on how the motion dynamics are typically affected by a pathology. The key challenge with analysing population-wide

N. Navab et al. (Eds.): MICCAI 2015, Part III, LNCS 9351, pp. 419–426, 2015.
DOI: 10.1007/978-3-319-24574-4_50

motion dynamics is in finding a method to be able to compare the motion from one subject to another in a consistent manner. Recent work to address this has been focused on comparing either the regional strain values directly, or the aligned displacements computed from subject-specific motion tracking. Comparing the strain values can provide useful insight to aid with classification, such as in [1], however, 1D strain measures are not sufficient for fully characterising abnormalities. The displacement fields from a set of subjects can provide further characterisation of motion abnormalities, though this requires spatio-temporal alignment of either the images prior to motion tracking ([2]), or the displacements themselves ([3]). In either case, spatio-temporal alignment of 3D data is not straightforward and subsequent analysis of the motion from 3D displacements remains difficult to interpret and analyse. In order to address these issues, a method was recently proposed to describe the full motion of a group of subjects in a consistent and low-dimensional manner as the tensor of Polyaffine parameters for a set of regions in the heart over the cardiac cycle [4].

Given that a set of motion parameters is typically high dimensional (due to the need to account for the spatial and temporal factors), model reduction can be useful to reduce the dimensionality of the data while retaining a small number of variables that describe the data. Tensor decomposition is one such technique that has been widely studied in the last years for a wide range of applications (see [5] for a review of tensor decomposition methods). PCA of displacement field has already been proposed for population-based cardiac motion analysis in [3], and Tucker tensor decomposition of Polyaffine motion parameters was proposed in [4]. A difficulty with these methods is in interpreting the results since both PCA and Tucker are unconstrained and can thus result in factor matrices with a large number of mode combinations required for each subject.

Inspired by the method developed in [4], we propose a method for population-wide cardiac motion analysis with intelligible and easy to interpret mode combinations. In contrast to this previous work, we study the motion of different population subgroups using descriptive anatomical motion parameters (namely the circumferential twisting, radial thickening, and longitudinal shrinking). Furthermore, we identify much fewer, and thus more easily interpretable, factors discriminating between the motion patterns of healthy and unhealthy subjects thanks to a Tucker decomposition on Polyaffine motion parameters with a constraint on the sparsity of the core tensor (which essentially defines the loadings of each mode combination). Sparsity of the discriminating factors and their individual intelligibility is important for clear and intuitive interpretation of differences between populations. The key contributions of the present work are summarised in the following:

- Re-orientation of the polyaffine matrices to a prolate spheroidal coordinate system
- Analysis of the rotation, stretch, shear, and translation components
- Combined basis computation of multiple groups
- 4-way tensor decomposition, decoupling the spatial components
- Tucker decomposition performed with sparsity constraints on the core tensor

2 Methods

A method for performing population-based cardiac motion analysis methods by considering spatio-temporally aligned Polyaffine motion parameters and performing decomposition of these for a group of subjects was recently proposed in [4]. The method involves a cardiac motion tracking step that takes a dense displacement field computed using the LogDemons algorithm and projects this to a Polyaffine space [6], subject to some cardiac-specific constraints (namely incompressibility and regional smoothing). The obtained Polyaffine parameters are then spatially and temporally aligned to a common reference frame, and the parameters for all subjects are grouped to a data tensor of [space $\times$ time $\times$ subject]. Non-constrained Tucker decomposition is applied to the data tensor to extract the dominant spatial and temporal patterns.

In order to obtain more meaningful parameters and interpretations, we propose in this work to first re-orient the affine parameters from a Cartesian frame to a prolate-spheroidal coordinate system, as described in Sec. 2.1. The rotation, stretch, shear, and translation components can be extracted, as described in Sec. 2.2. A 4-way tensor can be extracted by decoupling the spatial components into the affine and regional parts (Sec 2.3), from which Tucker decomposition with a constraint on the sparsity of the core tensor can be applied, as described in Sec. 2.4. Finally, the analysis can be performed by stacking together multiple groups as a single tensor to compute a combined basis, as described in Sec 2.5.

2.1. Re-orientation of Affine Matrices to Local Coordinates: Analysing the affine parameters directly when they are described in Cartesian coordinates creates a difficulty in interpreting differences (or similarities) between groups. In contrast, the parameters can be more easily interpreted once they are in a prolate spheroidal system (which can be computed using the methods described in [7]), given that the parameters will then directly represent motion along the circumferential (c), radial (r), and longitudinal (l) directions. The Jacobian matrices defined at the barycentre of each region in prolate spheroidal coordinates ($J_{i(PSS)}$) were computed as in [4]: $M_{i(PSS)} = J_{i(PSS)} * M_i$, where M_i is the log-affine matrix at region i in Cartesian coordinates, and $M_{i(PSS)}$ is the transformation of M_i to prolate spheroidal coordinates.

2.2. Extraction of Rotation, Stretch, Shear, and Translation: Rather than performing the decomposition on the affine matrices M_w^u:

$$M_w^u = \begin{bmatrix} a_{1,1} & a_{2,1} & a_{3,1} & t_1 \\ a_{1,2} & a_{2,2} & a_{3,2} & t_2 \\ a_{1,3} & a_{2,3} & a_{3,3} & t_3 \end{bmatrix}$$

the analysis can be performed on vectors $P_{u,v,w}$ made up of the rotation, stretch, shearing and translation components for subject u at time v in region w. The components are given by:

$$Rotation: \begin{bmatrix} R_c \\ R_r \\ R_l \end{bmatrix} = \begin{bmatrix} 1/2(a_{2,3} - a_{3,2}) \\ 1/2(a_{1,3} - a_{3,1}) \\ 1/2(a_{1,2} - a_{2,1}) \end{bmatrix} \qquad Stretch: \begin{bmatrix} S_c \\ S_r \\ S_l \end{bmatrix} = \begin{bmatrix} a_{1,1} \\ a_{2,2} \\ a_{3,3} \end{bmatrix}$$

$$Shear: \begin{bmatrix} S_{cr} \\ S_{cl} \\ S_{rl} \end{bmatrix} = \begin{bmatrix} 1/2(a_{1,2} + a_{2,1}) \\ 1/2(a_{1,3} + a_{3,1}) \\ 1/2(a_{2,3} + a_{3,2}) \end{bmatrix} \qquad Translation: \begin{bmatrix} T_c \\ T_r \\ T_l \end{bmatrix} = \begin{bmatrix} t_1 \\ t_2 \\ t_3 \end{bmatrix}$$

Combining the re-scaled affine parameters to a new [12 × 1] vector, we obtain $P_{u,v,w} = [R_c\ R_r\ R_l\ S_c\ S_r\ S_l\ S_{cr}\ S_{cl}\ S_{rl}\ T_c\ T_r\ T_l]^T$. The elements of $P_{u,v,w}$ can then be scaled by the variance of each element described by: $\sigma = [\sigma_{R_c}, \sigma_{R_r} \cdots \sigma_{t_l}]$. Scaling by the variance ensures that all parameters are equally weighted in the decomposition. Tensor analysis can then be performed on the final vectors $\mathcal{T}_{u,v,w} = [P_{u,v,w}]_{[i]}/\sigma_{[i]}$.

2.3. 4-Way Tensor Decomposition: In order to analyse the spatial motion features independently (in terms of regional and affine components), Tucker Decomposition can be performed on a 4-way tensor $\mathcal{T}$ stacked by [motion parameters × region × time × subject]. Given the complex nature of cardiac motion with several key components, trying to analyze these independently is difficult. Performing decomposition on the full tensor directly has the advantage of describing how all the components interact.

The Tucker tensor decomposition method [8] is a higher-order extension of PCA which computes orthonormal subspaces associated with each axis of $\mathcal{T}$. The Tucker decomposition of a 4-way tensor $\mathcal{T}$ is expressed as an n-mode product:

$$\begin{aligned} \mathcal{T} &\approx \mathcal{G} \times_1 A_1 \times_2 A_2 \times_3 A_3 \times_4 A_4 \\ &= \sum_{m_1=1}^{M_1} \sum_{m_2=1}^{M_2} \sum_{m_3=1}^{M_3} \sum_{m_4=1}^{M_4} g_{m_1 m_2 m_3 m_4} a_{1m_1} \otimes a_{2m_2} \otimes a_{3m_3} \otimes a_{4m_4} \\ &= [[\mathcal{G}; A_1, A_2, A_3, A_4]], \end{aligned} \tag{1}$$

where $\times_n$ denotes the mode-n tensor-matrix product, and ⊗ denotes the vector outer product. A_i are factor matrices in the ith direction ($i = 1 \ldots 4$) that can be thought of as the tensor equivalent of principal components for each axis. The core tensor $\mathcal{G}$ gives the relationship between the modes in each direction and describes how to re-combine the modes to obtain the original tensor $\mathcal{T}$. We propose to perform 4-way Tucker decomposition with A_1: the extracted re-oriented affine parameters, A_2: the regions, A_3: time, and A_4: the subject axis.

2.4. Tucker Decomposition with Sparsity Constraints: In order to improve the interpretability of the solution, a sparsity constraint on the core tensor can be incorporated into the Tucker decomposition. In [9], an alternating proximal gradient method is used to solve the sparse non-negative Tucker decomposition (NTD) problem:

$$\min \frac{1}{2} \parallel \mathcal{T} - \mathcal{G} \times_1 A_1 \times_2 A_2 \times_3 A_3 \times_4 A_4 \parallel_F^2 + \lambda_{\mathcal{G}} \parallel \mathcal{G} \parallel_1 + \sum_{n=1}^{N} \lambda_n \parallel A_n \parallel_1$$

$$s.t \;\; \mathcal{G} \in \mathbb{R}_+^{J_1 \times J_2 \times J_3 \times J_4}, A_n \in \mathbb{R}_+^{I_n \times J_n} \forall n,$$

where J_n is the dimension of the core tensor for axis n and $\lambda_{\mathcal{G}}, \lambda_n$ are parameters controlling the balance of the data fitting and sparsity level. The core tensor $\mathcal{G}$ and factor matrices A_n are alternately updated in the order: $\mathcal{G}, A_1, \mathcal{G}, A_2, \mathcal{G}, A_3, \mathcal{G}, A_4$ (see [9] for details on the λ parameters).

In this work, the tensor $\mathcal{T}$ represents the log-affine parameters and are typically not non-negative. In order to satisfy the non-negativity constraint of the NTD algorithm, the exponential of each element of $\mathcal{T}$ can be analysed rather than $\mathcal{T}$ directly.

2.5. Combined Basis Computation of Multiple Groups: In order to compare the two populations with the same basis, a combined model can be generated by forming a 4-way tensor of all subjects grouped together, yielding an observation tensor M of size $[12 \times 17 \times 29 \times N]$ for the affine, regional, temporal, and the N patient-specific components respectively. 4-way tensor decomposition can then be applied to this data tensor (as described in the previous sections). By performing the decomposition jointly to obtain a combined basis for multiple groups, the modes relevant to a given population can be extracted by studying the loadings of each patient of a chosen mode to identify mutual and distinct motion patterns.

3 Experiments and Results

The proposed methodology was applied to the STACOM 2011 cardiac motion tracking challenge dataset [10]: an openly available data-set of 15 healthy subjects (3 female, mean age $\pm$ SD $= 28 \pm 5$), as well as a data-set of 10 Tetralogy of Fallot patients (5 female, mean age $\pm$ SD $= 21 \pm 7$). For all subjects, short axis cine MRI sequences were acquired with 12 - 16 slices, isotropic in-plane resolution ranging from 1.15×1.15mm^2 to 1.36×1.36mm^2, slice thickness of $8mm$, and 15 - 30 image frames.

The sparse NTD algorithm described in Sec. 2 was applied to the stacked parameters for the combined tensor of healthy controls and the Tetralogy of Fallot subjects with the size of the core tensor chosen as $[5 \times 5 \times 5]$ (to retain only the first 5 dominant modes in each axis). The choice of the number of modes is a trade-off between maintaining a sufficient level of accuracy (in terms of the percentage of variance explained), while minimizing the number of output parameters. In this work, 5 modes were considered to be a reasonable trade-off. The core tensor loadings for each subject were averaged for the different groups, in order to visualise the dominant mode combinations in each group. These are plotted in Fig. 1 and indicate that the two groups share some common dominant loadings, though the Tetralogy of Fallot group have some additional dominant loadings, which is expected since additional modes may be required to represent the abnormal motion patterns in these patients.

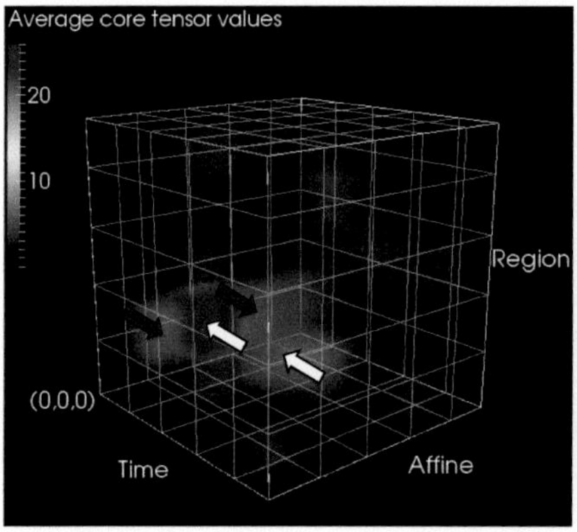

(a) Healthy control group

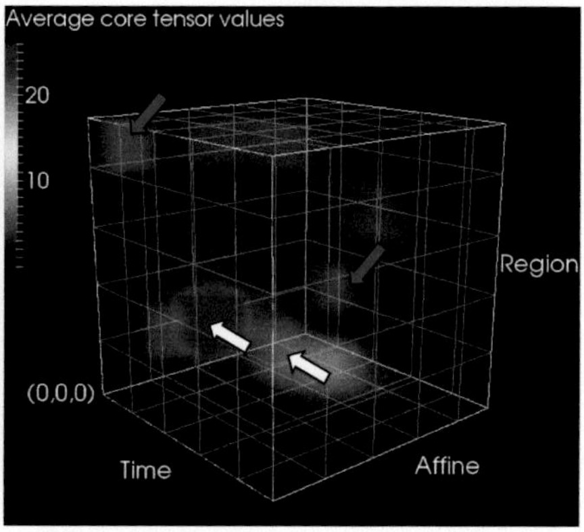

(b) Tetralogy of Fallot group

Fig. 1. Average core tensor loadings for the healthy control group (a) and the Tetralogy of Fallot group (b). The groups share some common dominant loadings (white arrows), however, the control group have some distinct mode combinations (purple arrows). The Tetralogy of Fallot group have some additional extreme values (blue arrows), which indicates that additional modes are needed to represent the abnormal motion patterns in these patients.

The dominant modes unique to the control group (indicated by purple arrows in Fig. 1) have the same regional component as the dominant mode in Fig. 2 and the same temporal component (mode 2: black line in Fig. 2 b), along with affine mode 1,3 (see Fig. 2 for description of each matrix element):

$$Aff_1 = \begin{bmatrix} 0 & 0.053 & 0.002 & 0 \\ 0.015 & \mathbf{0.697} & 0.009 & 0 \\ 0.328 & 0 & 0 & 0.009 \end{bmatrix} \qquad Aff_3 = \begin{bmatrix} 0 & 0.144 & 0.126 & 0 \\ 0.099 & 0.101 & 0.076 & 0.083 \\ 0 & \mathbf{0.847} & 0 & 0.007 \end{bmatrix}$$

The affine modes suggest dominance in the radial stretch (thickening) and longitudinal rotation (twisting) for mode 1, and dominance in the longitudinal stretch for mode 3, which are the expected motion dynamics in healthy subjects. The temporal mode (2) accounts for differences around peak systole and diastole (given that the temporal resampling used in this work was linear).

The common dominant mode combinations are plotted in Fig. 2 (top row). The affine mode for the dominant mode combinations (Fig. 2, a) shows predominant stretching in the circumferential direction, which may be related to the twisting motion in the left ventricle. The temporal modes (Fig. 2, b) show a dominant pattern around the end- and mid-diastolic phases for mode 2, which may be due to the end of relaxation and end of filling. The dominant regions for these mode combinations are anterior (Fig. 2, c).

The dominant mode combinations for the Tetralogy of Fallot group are plotted in Fig. 2. The affine mode for the first dominant combination (Fig. 2, d) indicates little longitudinal motion. The corresponding temporal mode (Fig. 2, e) represents a peak at the end systolic frame (around one third of the length

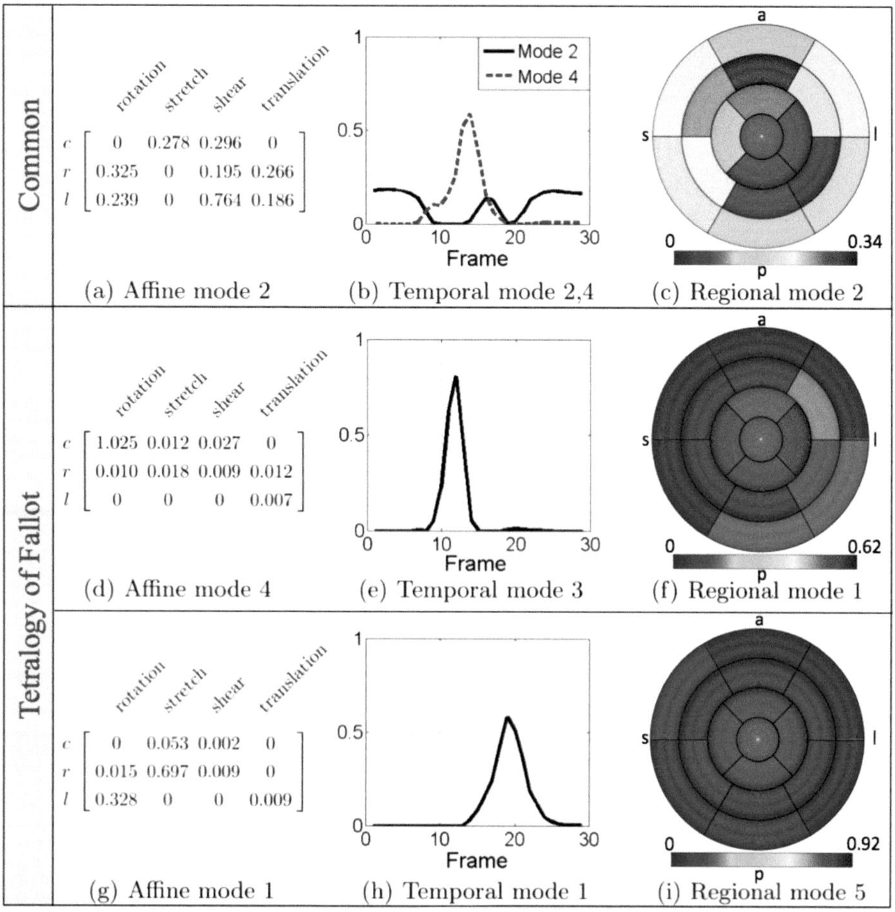

Fig. 2. Dominant mode combinations common to both cohorts: affine mode 2 (a), temporal modes 2 and 4 (b), and regional mode 2 (c). Key - a: anterior, p: posterior, s: septal, l: lateral.

of the cardiac cycle). The corresponding regional mode (Fig. 2, f) indicates that there is a dominance in the motion in the lateral wall. This is an area with known motion abnormalities in these patients given that the motion in the free wall of the left ventricle is dragged towards the septum. The temporal mode for the second dominant mode (Fig. 2, h) has instead a peak around mid-systole, with corresponding regional mode (Fig. 2, i), indicating dominance around the apex, which may be due to poor resolution at the apex.

4 Conclusion

A method for descriptive and intuitive analysis of cardiac motion in different populations is described. The proposed method makes use of a Polyaffine motion model that represents the motion with reasonable accuracy (i.e. on a par with state-of-the-art methods) while requiring only few, consistently defined parameters for motion tracking of different subjects. The parameters are described in terms of intuitive physiological parameters and the key affine descriptors of the motion (namely the rotation, stretch, shear, and translation) are analysed collectively for multiple populations in order to determine common and distinct motion patterns between different groups. By performing sparse tensor decomposition of the combined parameters, dominant loadings can be extracted in order to make the analysis and comparison more straightforward, and we believe that obtaining a very small number of expressive and intelligible parameters is crucial for the future automatic discovery of key motion features in different cardiac diseases. The proposed method shows promise for analysing pathology-specific motion patterns in terms of the affine, temporal, and regional factors.

Acknowledgements. This project was partially funded by the Centre for Cardiological Innovation (CCI), Norway funded by the Norwegian Research Council, and the MD Paedigree European project ICT-2011.5.2 grant no. 600932. These tools are largely based on the Tensor Toolbox from Sandia National Laboratories. The NTD method used in the work was provided by the authors of [9].

References

1. Qian, Z., Liu, Q., Metaxas, D.N., Axel, L.: Identifying regional cardiac abnormalities from myocardial strains using nontracking-based strain estimation and spatio-temporal tensor analysis. IEEE Trans. Med. Imaging 30(12) (2011)
2. Perperidis, D., Rao, A., Lorenzo-Valdés, M., Mohiaddin, R., Rueckert, D.: Spatio-temporal alignment of 4D cardiac MR images. In: Magnin, I.E., Montagnat, J., Clarysse, P., Nenonen, J., Katila, T. (eds.) FIMH 2003. LNCS, vol. 2674, pp. 205–214. Springer, Heidelberg (2003)
3. Rougon, N.F., Petitjean, C., Preteux, F.J.: Building and using a statistical 3D motion atlas for analyzing myocardial contraction in MRI. In: Med. Imaging, International Society for Optics and Photonics (2004)
4. McLeod, K., Sermesant, M., Beerbaum, P., Pennec, X.: Spatio-temporal tensor decomposition of a polyaffine motion model for a better analysis of pathological left ventricular dynamics. IEEE Trans. Med. Imaging (2015)
5. Kolda, T.G., Bader, B.W.: Tensor decompositions and applications. SIAM Review 51(3) (2009)
6. Seiler, C., Pennec, X., Reyes, M.: Capturing the multiscale anatomical shape variability with polyaffine transformation trees. Med. Image Anal. (2012)
7. Toussaint, N., Stoeck, C.T., Sermesant, M., Schaeffter, T., Kozerke, S., Batchelor, P.G.: In vivo human cardiac fibre architecture estimation using shape-based diffusion tensor processing. Med. Image Anal. (2013)
8. Tucker, L.R.: Implications of factor analysis of three-way matrices for measurement of change. Problems in Measuring Change (1963)
9. Xu, Y.: Alternating proximal gradient method for sparse nonnegative tucker decomposition. Mathematical Programming Computation (2014)
10. Tobon-Gomez, C., De-Craene, M., et al.: Benchmarking framework for myocardial tracking and deformation algorithms: An open access database. Med. Image Anal. (2013)

Liver Motion Estimation via Locally Adaptive Over-Segmentation Regularization

Bartłomiej W. Papież[1], Jamie Franklin[2], Mattias P. Heinrich[4], Fergus V. Gleeson[3], and Julia A. Schnabel[1]

[1] Institute of Biomedical Engineering, Department of Engineering Science, University of Oxford, UK
bartlomiej.papiez@eng.ox.ac.uk
[2] Department of Oncology, University of Oxford, UK
[3] Department of Radiology, Churchill Hospital, Oxford University Hospitals NHS Trust, Oxford, UK
[4] Institute of Medical Informatics, University of Lübeck, Germany

Abstract. Despite significant advances in the development of deformable registration methods, motion correction of deformable organs such as the liver remain a challenging task. This is due to not only low contrast in liver imaging, but also due to the particularly complex motion between scans primarily owing to patient breathing. In this paper, we address abdominal motion estimation using a novel regularization model that is advancing the state-of-the-art in liver registration in terms of accuracy. We propose a novel regularization of the deformation field based on spatially adaptive over-segmentation, to better model the physiological motion of the abdomen. Our quantitative analysis of abdominal Computed Tomography and dynamic contrast-enhanced Magnetic Resonance Imaging scans show a significant improvement over the state-of-the-art Demons approaches. This work also demonstrates the feasibility of segmentation-free registration between clinical scans that can inherently preserve sliding motion at the lung and liver boundary interfaces.

1 Introduction

Analysis of functional abdominal imaging (e.g. dynamic magnetic resonance imaging (DCE-MRI)) and structural imaging (such as CT or MRI) is an emerging research area that can potentially lead to improved strategies for differential diagnosis and planning of personalized treatment (e.g. patient stratification) of abdominal cancer. In this work, we present a generic approach for intra-subject motion correction of time sequences, applied to both standard 4D CT acquisition, and relatively new quantitative imaging techniques such as DCE-MRI. This will ultimately provide new opportunities for tumor heterogeneity assessment for patients, with the potential of extending our understanding of human liver tumor complexity [10]. Deformable registration of time scans acquired using modalities with contrast agent is challenging due to: 1) significant amount of motion between consecutive scans including sliding motion at the lung and liver

N. Navab et al. (Eds.): MICCAI 2015, Part III, LNCS 9351, pp. 427–434, 2015.
DOI: 10.1007/978-3-319-24574-4_51

interface; 2) low contrast of liver tissue; and 3) local volume intensity changes due to either contrast uptake in DCE-MRI. Thus, robust image registration is an inevitable post-acquisition step to enable quantitative pharmacokinetic analysis of motion-free DCE-MRI data.

Conventional motion correction algorithms use generic similarity measures such as sum-of-squared differences with a statistical prior to find an optimal transformation [5]. Alternatively, registration can be performed using a physiological image formation model [3]. However in both cases, the estimated transformation is highly influenced by the chosen regularization model. In the classic Demons framework, the diffusion regularization is performed by Gaussian smoothing of the estimated deformation field [14] that generates a smooth displacement field. However, the complex physiology of abdominal motion during breathing involves modeling of the liver sliding at the thoracic cage, which has been addressed by only a few registration algorithms [15,16,11]. Limitations of the aforementioned motion correction methods include the need for segmenting the liver surface [15,16,11]. Moreover, hepatic deformations [4] that is secondary to breathing has not been analyzed in motion models proposed so far.

In this paper, we propose a novel registration approach, referred to as SLIC Demons, owing to the use of the Simple Linear Iterative Clustering algorithm [1] for a liver motion estimation model. This model is used then for an accurate deformable registration of DCE-MRI data to enforce the plausibility of the estimated deformation field, e.g. preservation of sliding motion at the thoracic cage and at the lung boundaries whilst not requiring any prior liver segmentation. The contributions of this work are as follows. First, we introduce an accurate model for the regularization of the deformation field, which incorporates additional (anatomical) information from so-called *guidance* images in a computationally efficient manner. This regularization is embedded in a classic non-rigid Demons registration framework using the local correlation coefficient [9] as a similarity measure to handle local intensity changes due to contrast uptake. The improved performance on a publicly available liver CT data [11] is demonstrated. Finally, the robustness of the method on a challenging clinical application of DCE-MRI liver motion compensation is quantitatively assessed.

2 Methodology

Deformable Image Registration. In the classic formulation [8], deformable image registration is defined as a global energy minimization problem with respect to the geometrical transformation describing the correspondences between input images I_F and I_M:

$$\hat{\boldsymbol{u}} = \arg\min_{\boldsymbol{u}} \left(Sim(I_F, I_M(\boldsymbol{u})) + \alpha Reg(\boldsymbol{u}) \right) \tag{1}$$

where $\hat{\boldsymbol{u}}$ is the optimal displacement field, Sim is a similarity measure, Reg is a regularization term, and $\alpha > 0$ is a weighting parameter. The Demons framework [14], due to its simplicity and efficiency, is a common choice to solve Eq. (1)

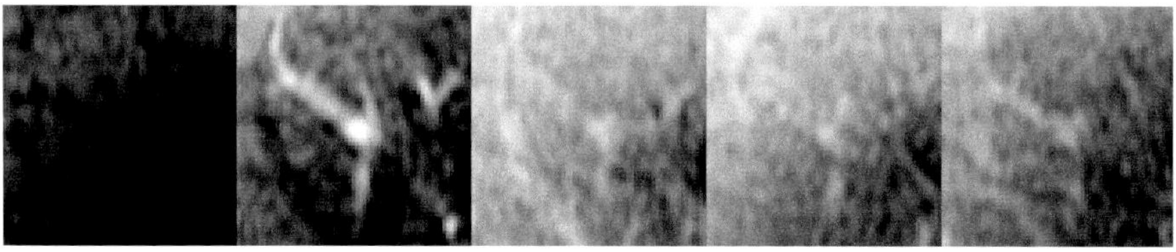

Fig. 1. Corresponding region of interest (axial view of the segmental branch of hepatic artery) selected by the expert from consecutive volumes of DCE-MRI sequence. Besides intensity changes caused by the contrast agent, local structures are visibly correlated, which is also confirmed by quantitative evaluation of LCC Demons.

when sum-of-squared differences (or any other point-wise difference metric) is used as a similarity measure, and a diffusion model is used for regularization. For the Demons framework, the optimization procedure alternates between minimizing the energy related to the similarity Sim and the regularization Reg in an iterative manner. In this work, due to the low contrast of the liver in CT, and change of intensity values owing to the contrast uptake between consecutive DCE-MRI volumes (see an example in Fig. 1), we propose to use the local correlation coefficient (LCC) as a similarity measure. This is further motivated by recent work that used LCC-Demons for brain MRI registration due to their independence of any additive and multiplicative bias in the data [9].

Filtering of the Deformation Field. Accurate alignment of intra-subject dynamic imaging data is challenging not only because of intensity changes due to contrast uptake, but also due to the complexity of motion to be estimated. In the Demons framework, diffusion regularization is performed by Gaussian smoothing of the estimated deformation field. However, the complex physiology of respiratory motion involves more than just modeling of the liver sliding at the thoracic wall [11,12]. The human liver is non-uniform in composition as it is built of vascular structures and filamentous tissue. Hence it is not adequate to model hepatic motion by performing segmentation of the whole liver prior to registration [15,16]. Thus, inspired by a previous approach of spatially adaptive filtering of the deformation field [13,12], and the guided image filtering technique developed for computer vision applications [6], we present a generic approach for regularization. In our approach, the estimated deformation field is spatially filtered by considering the context of the guidance information coming either from one of the input images itself or another auxiliary image (e.g. from a segmentation mask). The output deformation field $\boldsymbol{u}_{out}$ of the guided image filtering technique of the input deformation field $\boldsymbol{u}_{in}$ is based on a linear model of the guidance image I_G in the local neighborhood $\mathcal{N}$ centered at the spatial position $\boldsymbol{x}$, and is defined as follows [6]:

$$\boldsymbol{u}_{out}(\boldsymbol{x}) = \sum_{\boldsymbol{y} \in \mathcal{N}} W_{\boldsymbol{y}}(I_G)\boldsymbol{u}_{in}(\boldsymbol{y}) \tag{2}$$

where $W_{\boldsymbol{y}}$ is a filter kernel derived from the guidance image I_G. An example of such local filter kernel weights $W_{\boldsymbol{y}}$ are the bilateral filtering kernels proposed by [12].

Note that a guided image filter can be implemented using a sequence of box filters making the computing time independent of the filter size [6].

Guidance for Accurate Modeling of Complex Liver Motion. An additional motivation for using the guided filter technique is that it allows incorporation of prior knowledge for deformation field regularization. For example, the output deformation field can be filtered with respect to the registered image (*self-guidance*), or labels obtained from segmentation of the entire thoracic cage. While the use of masks in [15,16] is limited to just a few objects, multi-object segmentation can be easily added to the presented approach by using a multi-channel guidance image (e.g. similarly to the channels in an RGB image) without a significant increase of computational complexity [6]. Therefore, we consider an alternative guidance image, which is built based on the concept of sparse image representation based on supervoxel clustering. Following [7], we adapt Simple Linear Iterative Clustering (SLIC) [1] for supervoxel clustering. SLIC performs an image segmentation that corresponds to spatial proximity (spatial compactness) and image boundaries (color similarity). SLIC is designed to generate K approximately equally-sized supervoxels. The Euclidean distance between voxel $\boldsymbol{x}$ and a cluster center $\boldsymbol{y}$ is calculated as $d_{\boldsymbol{xy}} = \|\boldsymbol{x} - \boldsymbol{y}\|$ and the distance measuring the gray-color proximity is given by: $d_I = \sqrt{(I(\boldsymbol{x}) - I(\boldsymbol{y}))^2}$. The combination of the two normalized distances $d_{\boldsymbol{xy}}$ and d_I is defined in the following way: $D = \sqrt{(d_{\boldsymbol{xy}}/S)^2 + (d_I/m)^2}$ where m is a parameter determining the relative importance between color and spatial proximity. A larger value of m results in supervoxels with more compact shapes, whereas for small m the resulting clusters have less regular shapes and sizes, but they are more adapted to image details and intensity edges. The parameter $S = \sqrt[3]{N/K}$ corresponds to the sampling interval of the initial spacing of the cluster centers. The algorithm starts from a set of equally spaced cluster centers. After each iteration the cluster centers are recomputed, and the algorithm is iterated until the convergence.

Because SLIC performs an image segmentation that corresponds to spatial and intensity proximity, it removes the redundant intensity information of voxels in the homogeneous regions. However, such clustering becomes also very inconsistent in such regions. In the context of filtering the deformation field during registration, this is a major drawback, because filtering with respect to the clustered image would introduce artificial discontinuities. This is called over-segmentation, and it is a common problem for simple image-driven regularization models. In [7] the authors proposed to use multiple channel (layers) of supervoxels to obtain a piecewise smooth deformation model. To generate such different channels of supervoxels, the SLIC algorithm was run several times with randomly perturbed initial cluster centers. Image clustering in homogeneous regions will result in different clusters for each channel. However, image regions with sufficient structural content will not be affected by random perturbation of SLIC cluster centers. Furthermore, the displacement fields obtained for each channel separately can be averaged to construct the final displacement field, and therefore avoid discontinuities in homogeneous regions [7]. In our case, we can use each channel of supervoxels S as a separate channel of our guidance image $I_G = [S_1, S_2, \cdots, S_N]$ and then perform an efficient filtering of the deformation field with respect to such multichannel guidance image.

For a given I_G, the weights W_{GIF} of the guided filter at the position $\boldsymbol{x}$ are explicitly expressed in the following way:

$$W_{GIF}(I_G) = 1 + (I_G - \mu_{I_G})^T (\boldsymbol{\Sigma}_{I_G} + \varepsilon \mathbf{U})^{-1} (I_G - \mu_{I_G}) \tag{3}$$

where μ_{I_G} and $\boldsymbol{\Sigma}_{I_G}$ are the mean and covariance of the guidance image I_G in the local neighborhood $\mathcal{N}$, and $\mathbf{U}$ denotes the identity matrix. It has been shown [6] that in the case of the guidance image I_G being a multichannel image, the weights of the guided filter (defined in Eq. (3)) can be computed without a significant increase of computational complexity compared to single-channel image guidance (however for N numbers of channels, inversion of an $N \times N$ matrix is required for each voxel). The SLIC [1] algorithm is reported to have a linear complexity with respect to the number of image voxels and therefore is easily applicable to large medical data sets. It is also important to note that the SLIC algorithm is memory efficient when dealing with large volumes (see more details [1]). Our implementation of SLIC is based on jSLIC[1].

Physiological Plausibility. The estimated sliding motion should have three properties: 1) Motion normal to the organ boundary should be smooth both across organ boundaries and within organs, 2) Motion tangential to the organ boundary should be smooth in the tangential direction within each individual organ, and 3) Motion tangential to the organ boundary is not required to be smooth across organ boundaries [11]. The presented regularization model addresses explicitly 2) and 3), while diffeomorphic formulation of the overall registration [9] prevents folding between organs. Furthermore, filtering the deformation field using a guided filter, which is derived from a locally linear model, provides an invertibility constraint (due to the log-Euclidean parameterization [2]).

3 Evaluation and Results

We performed deformable registration using diffeomorphic logDemons with a symmetric local correlation coefficient (LCC) as a similarity criterion [9]. We use the following parameter settings for the optimization: three multi-resolution levels, and a maximum number of iterations of 50. For liver CT data, we empirically determined the LCC smoothing parameter σ_{LCC}=2 the regularization parameter $\sigma = 3$ for LCC-Demons, a filter radius r=5 and a regularization parameter α=0.1 was found to give the best results for the SLIC Demons. For registration of DCE-MRI, we employ a larger patch σ_{LCC}=5 to calculate the local correlation coefficient, while the other parameters remain the same. It is worth noting that the parameters for the SLIC Demons have a low sensitivity, causing an increase of Target Registration Error (TRE) of only 0.1mm when changing r between 4

[1] jSLIC: superpixels in ImageJ, `http://fiji.sc/CMP-BIA_tools`

and 6, and α between 0.2 and 0.01. For SLIC, the weighting parameter m=20 was selected empirically (for intensity range between 0 - 255). We found that three channels of the SLIC guidance image provides satisfactory results, and further increasing the number of channels does not improve the overall TRE significantly.

Results on 4DCT. For the quantitative evaluation of liver motion, the SLIC Demons are tested on volumes of abdominal 4D-CT data sets that are publicly available. Four inhale and exhale abdominal CT image pairs were obtained from the Children's National Medical Center/Stanford[2] that were previously used for validation purposes in [11]. Following preprocessing steps performed in [11], the volumes were cropped, thresholded, intensity-normalized, and finally linearly resampled to isotropic spacing of 2mm^3. To quantify the registration accuracy, the TRE was calculated for the well-distributed set of landmarks, which are provided with this data set ($\approx$50 landmarks per case for lungs, and $\approx$20 landmarks per case for the abdomen including liver). For all cases in this data set, the end-of-inspiration volume was chosen as a reference, and the end-of-expiration volume as a moving image. The initial average TRE is 7.04$\pm$4.3mm for lung landmarks, and 6.44$\pm$3.4mm for abdominal landmarks. A significantly lower TRE (p-value$<$0.05 using a two-sample Wilcoxon rank sum test) is obtained by deformation fields estimated using the framework based on the guided filtering of deformation fields (TRE=2.08mm for lungs and TRE=2.19mm for abdomen) when compared to the classic Demons (TRE=3.24mm for lungs and =2.5mm for abdomen). All resulting deformation fields are invertible within the region of interest (indicated by the positive value of the Jacobian). Moreover, the TRE yielded by the proposed method is lower than the best results reported so far in the literature (2.15mm for lungs and 2.56mm for abdomen [11]). Employing registration with guidance for regularization of the deformation field preserves discontinuities at the pleural boundaries whilst satisfying smoothness requirements inside the lungs and liver (e.g. the difference between the estimated deformation fields close to the lung boundaries shown in Fig. 2).

Results on DCE-MRI. The presented registration approach was additionally applied for two abdominal DCE-MRI sequences acquired at the Churchill Hospital in Oxford as a part of an ongoing clinical trial exploring the feasibility of novel imaging techniques to assess how tumors are responding to treatment. The DCE-MRI data were acquired with a variable time, yielding 25 volumes with the volume resolution of 0.78$\times$0.78$\times$2.5mm. The initial average TRE is 15.82mm$\pm$8.5 for the landmarks annotated within the liver region. Similarly as for the previous experiment on the 4D liver CT, a significantly lower TRE (p-value$<$0.05 using a two-sample Wilcoxon rank sum test) was obtained using the framework based on the guided filtering of deformation fields (TRE=2.3mm$\pm$0.9 for the liver) when compared to the classic Demons (TRE=2.7mm$\pm$1.7 for the liver). The results of this evaluation indicate that the proposed spatially adaptive

[2] MIDAS Community: 4D CT Liver with segmentations

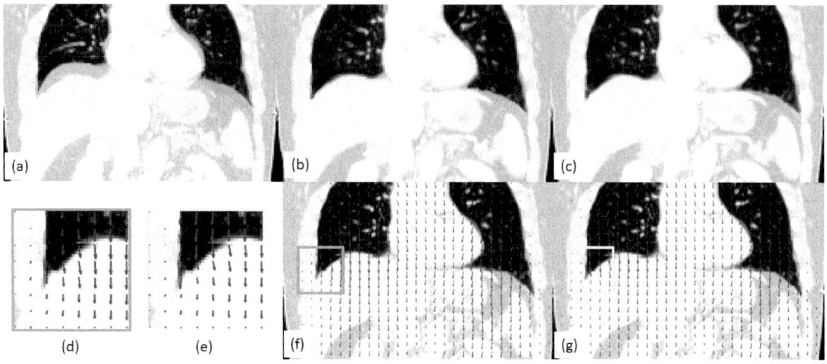

Fig. 2. Coronal view of 3D deformable CT/CT registration results. Color-coded intensity differences between image pair: (a) before registration, using (b) Demons, and (c) SLIC Demons. The estimated deformation field depicted: using (f) Demons, and (g) SLIC Demons with the corresponding zoomed images of the region of interest (labeled by box in the bottom row). Registration with SLIC yields a smooth deformation field inside the liver, while capturing the sliding motion across the pleural cavity boundaries.

regularization is capable of handling complex hepatic motion that is naturally present during DCE-MRI acquisition of the liver.

4 Discussion and Conclusions

We have presented an automated regularization approach for deformable registration that enables estimation of physiologically plausible hepatic deformations. For this purpose, the classic diffusion regularization using Gaussian smoothing was replaced by a fast image guidance technique that filters the estimated deformation field with respect to the anatomical tissue properties directly derived from the guidance image. The presented approach forms a spatially adaptive regularization that is capable of accurately preserving discontinuities that naturally occur between the lungs, liver and the pleura. We verified the robustness of our method on a publicly available data set [11], for which the results clearly demonstrated its advantages in terms of accuracy and computational efficiency when compared to the state-of-the-art methods. The computation time per registration using the presented framework is $\approx$5 mins per 3D pair (a standard CPU, with a non-optimized C++ code), and is several times faster compared to the bilateral filtering procedure proposed in [12]. We also applied our proposed method to an on-going clinical trial, where patients are scanned with DCE-MRI, and for which we obtained a good visual alignment of the data. The presented technique has the potential to generalize to other modalities and clinical applications in which compensation of the complex motion is essential.

Acknowledgments. We would like to acknowledge funding from the CRUK/ EPSRC Oxford Cancer Imaging Centre. BWP would like to thank D.F. Pace for providing the additional 4D liver CT patient annotations.

References

1. Achanta, R., Shaji, A., Smith, K., Lucchi, A., Fua, P., Süsstrunk, S.: SLIC Superpixels compared to state-of-the-art superpixel methods. IEEE Trans. Pattern Anal. Mach. Intell. 34(11), 2274–2282 (2012)
2. Arsigny, V., Commowick, O., Pennec, X., Ayache, N.: A log-Euclidean framework for statistics on diffeomorphisms. In: Larsen, R., Nielsen, M., Sporring, J. (eds.) MICCAI 2006. LNCS, vol. 4190, pp. 924–931. Springer, Heidelberg (2006)
3. Bhushan, M., Schnabel, J.A., Risser, L., Heinrich, M.P., Brady, J.M., Jenkinson, M.: Motion correction and parameter estimation in dceMRI sequences: application to colorectal cancer. In: Fichtinger, G., Martel, A., Peters, T. (eds.) MICCAI 2011, Part I. LNCS, vol. 6891, pp. 476–483. Springer, Heidelberg (2011)
4. Clifford, M.A., Banovac, F., Levy, E., Cleary, K.: Assessment of hepatic motion secondary to respiration for computer assisted interventions. Comput. Aided Surg. 7(5), 291–299 (2002)
5. Hamy, V., Dikaios, N., Punwani, S., Melbourne, A., Latifoltojar, A., et al.: Respiratory motion correction in dynamic MRI using robust data decomposition registration–Application to dce-MRI. Med. Image Anal. 18(2), 301–313 (2014)
6. He, K., Sun, J., Tang, X.: Guided image filtering. IEEE Trans. Pattern Anal. Mach. Intell. 35(6), 1397–1409 (2013)
7. Heinrich, M.P., Jenkinson, M., Papiez, B.W., Glesson, F.V., Brady, M., Schnabel, J.A.: Edge- and detail-preserving sparse image representations for deformable registration of chest MRI and CT volumes. In: Gee, J.C., Joshi, S., Pohl, K.M., Wells, W.M., Zöllei, L. (eds.) IPMI 2013. LNCS, vol. 7917, pp. 463–474. Springer, Heidelberg (2013)
8. Hermosillo, G., Chefd'Hotel, C., Faugeras, O.D.: Variational methods for multimodal image matching. Int. J. Comput. Vision 50, 329–343 (2002)
9. Lorenzi, M., Ayache, N., Frisoni, G., Pennec, X.: LCC-Demons: a robust and accurate symmetric diffeomorphic registration algorithm. Neuroimage 81, 470 (2013)
10. Mescam, M., Kretowski, M., Bezy-Wendling, J.: Multiscale model of liver dce-MRI towards a better understanding of tumor complexity. IEEE Trans. Med. Imag. 29(3), 699–707 (2010)
11. Pace, D.F., Aylward, S.R., Niethammer, M.: A locally adaptive regularization based on anisotropic diffusion for deformable image registration of sliding organs. IEEE Trans. Med. Imag. 32(11), 2114–2126 (2013)
12. Papież, B.W., Heinrich, M.P., Fehrenbach, J., Risser, L., Schnabel, J.A.: An implicit sliding-motion preserving regularisation via bilateral filtering for deformable image registration. Med. Image Anal. 18(8), 1299–1311 (2014)
13. Staring, M., Klein, S., Pluim, J.P.W.: Nonrigid registration with tissue-dependent filtering of the deformation field. Phys. Med. Biol. 52, 6879–6892 (2007)
14. Vercauteren, T., Pennec, X., Perchant, A., Ayache, N.: Diffeomorphic Demons: Efficient non-parametric image registration. NeuroImage 45, S61–S72 (2009)
15. Wu, Z., Rietzel, E., Boldea, V., Sarrut, D., Sharp, G.C.: Evaluation of deformable registration of patient lung 4DCT with subanatomical region segmentations. Med. Phys. 35(2), 775–781 (2008)
16. Xie, Y., Chao, M., Xiong, G.: Deformable image registration of liver with consideration of lung sliding motion. Med. Phys. 38(10), 5351–5361 (2011)

Motion-Corrected, Super-Resolution Reconstruction for High-Resolution 3D Cardiac Cine MRI

Freddy Odille[1,2,3], Aurélien Bustin[4,5], Bailiang Chen[1,2,3], Pierre-André Vuissoz[1,2], and Jacques Felblinger[1,2,3]

[1] U947, Inserm, Nancy, France
[2] IADI, Université de Lorraine, Nancy, France
[3] CIC-IT 1433, Inserm, Nancy, France
[4] Computer Science, Technische Universitat Munchen, Munich, Germany
[5] GE Global Research Center, Garching, Germany

Abstract. Cardiac cine MRI with 3D isotropic resolution is challenging as it requires efficient data acquisition and motion management. It is proposed to use a 2D balanced SSFP (steady-state free precession) sequence rather than its 3D version as it provides better contrast between blood and tissue. In order to obtain 3D isotropic images, 2D multi-slice datasets are acquired in different orientations (short axis, horizontal long axis and vertical long axis) while the patient is breathing freely. Image reconstruction is performed in two steps: (i) a motion-compensated reconstruction of each image stack corrects for nonrigid cardiac and respiratory motion; (ii) a super-resolution (SR) algorithm combines the three motion-corrected volumes (with low resolution in the slice direction) into a single volume with isotropic resolution. The SR reconstruction was implemented with two regularization schemes including a conventional one (Tikhonov) and a feature-preserving one (Beltrami). The method was validated in 8 volunteers and 10 patients with breathing difficulties. Image sharpness, as assessed by intensity profiles and by objective metrics based on the structure tensor, was improved with both SR techniques. The Beltrami constraint provided efficient denoising without altering the effective resolution.

Keywords: Magnetic resonance imaging, super-resolution, motion-compensated reconstruction.

1 Introduction

High-resolution, 3D isotropic cine imaging of the heart is challenging because it requires lengthy acquisitions, even with efficient imaging sequences, and therefore advanced patient motion management. Such an imaging technique would be useful for understanding complex anatomy and function in congenital heart diseases or for imaging small cardiac structures such as the atrium or the valves. It might also help reducing the variability of ventricular volumetric assessment in cardiovascular diseases (stroke volume, ejection fraction…) which is generally high with the conventional 2D cine image stacks due to the difficulty of segmenting the myocardium near the base of the ventricles.

N. Navab et al. (Eds.): MICCAI 2015, Part III, LNCS 9351, pp. 435–442, 2015.
DOI: 10.1007/978-3-319-24574-4_52

The b-SSFP (balanced steady-state free precession) sequence is one of the most widely used imaging techniques for cardiac cine imaging. This is because it provides the highest signal-to-noise ratio per unit time among all known sequence, with good T_2/T_1 contrast [1]. Moreover when the slice thickness is not too small (5 to 10 mm) the 2D b-SSFP does not suffer from severe motion-induced signal dropouts thanks to its fully balanced gradients. Unlike its 3D version, the 2D b-SSFP provides excellent contrast between tissues and blood/vessels due to the inflow effect (fresh spins moving in/out of the slice) [1]. A multi-slice 2D b-SSFP acquisition is therefore a good candidate but it suffers from poor resolution in the slice direction. One possible way to overcome this limitation is to combine multiple 2D stacks acquired in different orientations using a super-resolution (SR) reconstruction [2–4]. Applying SR techniques to chest or abdominal imaging is difficult because the image stacks to be combined need to be perfectly aligned. Rigid motion correction techniques have been combined with SR algorithms [5] but nonrigid motion is even more challenging and has not been addressed yet.

In this paper we propose a method for high-resolution, 3D isotropic cine imaging of the heart. The acquisition strategy consists of multiple 2D image stacks with different orientations obtained by a 2D multi-slice b-SSFP sequence during free breathing. The image reconstruction consists of two steps: (i) a motion-compensated 3D cine reconstruction of each stack; (ii) a super-resolution reconstruction combining the multiple cine volume stacks into an isotropic cine volume. The objective of this paper is to show the feasibility of the method in actual volunteer and patient experiments.

2 Image Reconstruction

2.1 Motion-Compensated 3D Cine Reconstructions

In the first step each stack of 2D slices (from one particular volume orientation) is reconstructed with a nonrigid motion compensation approach named cine-GRICS (generalized reconstruction by inversion of coupled systems) [6, 7]. Here the method reconstructs $N_{ph} = 32$ volumes corresponding to 32 phases of the cardiac cycle. In order to reconstruct a given cardiac phase, k-space data within a cardiac acceptance window (here $W_{card} = 120\,ms$) are selected. As described hereafter the motion-compensated reconstruction for this cardiac phase is formulated as the joint reconstruction of a 3D image ρ_i ($i = 1,2,3$ for SA, HLA, VLA) and a motion model α accounting for respiratory motion and for cardiac motion within the acceptance window.

The motion model approximates 3D time-varying nonrigid displacement fields $u(x,y,z,t)$ in the imaged volume such that $u(x,y,z,t) \simeq \sum_{k=1}^{N_s} \alpha_k(x,y,z) s_k(t)$ as described in Ref. [7], with some motion signals $s_k(t)$ acquired simultaneously with the k-space data m. Here we use $N_s = 5$ motion signals: $[s_1(t)\ s_2(t)]$ are the signals from two pneumatic belts (chest and abdomen); $[s_3(t)\ s_4(t)]$ are their first-order time derivatives; and $s_5(t)$ is the cardiac phase signal derived from the ECG recordings ($s_5(t)$ has values between 0 and the mean cardiac cycle length in ms).

For each cardiac phase the joint reconstruction is achieved by solving:

$$\min_{(\rho_i,\alpha)} \|E(\alpha,s)\rho_i - m\|^2 + \lambda\|\rho_i\|^2 + \mu \|\nabla\alpha\|^2. \tag{1}$$

Here $E(\alpha,s)$ denotes the forward acquisition model, i.e. the motion-corrupted 2D multi-slice acquisition. It includes a 3D nonrigid transformation operator for each motion state, followed by a slice selection, receiver coil sensitivity weightings, 2D Fourier transforms and k-space sampling operators similar to the description in Ref. [7]. The respiratory signals $s_1(t) \dots s_4(t)$ are centered on their most likely value (i.e. end-expiratory plateaus) so that all image stacks are reconstructed in a consistent motion state. Problem (1) is solved by a multi-resolution Gauss-Newton scheme, alternating between optimization with respect to ρ and α as described in [7].

2.2 Super-Resolution Reconstruction

In a second step the N motion-compensated 3D cine volumes (obtained from different orientations, $N = 3$ in this study) are combined using SR reconstruction. For a given cardiac phase if $\rho_1 \dots \rho_N$ denote the N motion-compensated 3D images, the SR image is found by solving:

$$\min_x \sum_{i=1}^{N} \|D_i B_i T_i x - \rho_i\|^2 + \lambda R(x). \tag{2}$$

Here T_i is a rigid image transformation that takes the SR image from the desired reconstructed orientation to the orientation of the ith acquisition (i.e. it is an interpolation operator that can describe an arbitrary orientation); $D_i B_i$ is a slice selection operator including a blurring operator B_i (i.e. a sum in the slice direction in the range of the slice thickness) and a downsampling operator D_i (in the slice direction).

Two regularizers were tested in this study: Tikhonov regularization, i.e. $R(x) = \|x\|^2$ and Beltrami regularization [8], i.e. $R(x) = (1 + \beta^2|\nabla x|^2)^{1/2}$. The Beltrami regularizer is a modified version of the well-known total variation and has better feature-preserving properties. In the case of Tikhonov regularization the SR reconstruction is a linear least-squares problem and is solved by a conjugate gradient solver. For the Beltrami regularization a primal-dual projected gradient scheme is used [8].

3 MRI Experiments

8 healthy volunteers and 10 patients with major breathing difficulties (Duchenne muscular dystrophy) underwent a cardiac functional MRI. Experiments were conducted on either a 1.5 T Signa HDxt (10 patients and 5 volunteers) or a 3 T Signa HDxt scanner (3 volunteers) (General Electric Healthcare, USA). For both the volunteers and the patients written informed consent was obtained and both studies were approved by an ethical committee. A 2D multi-slice b-SSFP sequence was used to cover the left ventricle in three different orientations: short-axis (SA), horizontal long-axis (HLA) and vertical long axis (VLA). The orientations were those planned by the

MR technologist (they were chosen to be independent but not strictly orthogonal). All acquisitions were performed during free breathing and were ungated (retrospective gating was included in the cine-GRICS reconstruction step). Typical parameters were: 224x224 acquisition matrix, 20 frames (i.e. 20 k-spaces acquired per slice), native in-plane resolution 1.6 x 1.6 mm^2, 8 mm slice thickness, TE/TR=1.8/4.1ms.

The cine-GRICS motion correction step provided three cine volumes (with 32 cardiac phases) of resolution 1.6 x 1.6 x 8 mm^3 (by solving Eq. (1)) which were combined by the SR reconstruction to form an isotropic volume of resolution 1.6 x 1.6 x 1.6 mm^3 (by solving Eq. (2)). The SR reconstruction was performed on the smallest cube encompassing the intersection volume of the three image stacks.

4 Validation

In order to validate the method we compared the SR reconstructed images (with Tikhonov and Beltrami regularization) against the native images. We first analyzed the images visually with cine-loop movies. We also drew intensity profiles across the ventricle to highlight differences in effective resolution in various oblique directions.

We then proposed a quantitative assessment. Isotropic images are expected to provide good depiction of features/edges in all three dimensions unlike the images with native resolution which are blurred in the slice direction. It is proposed to assess the presence of features in specific directions using the structure tensor [9]. The structure tensor S of a 3D image I characterizes, for each voxel p in the image, the local orientation of the anatomical structure based on the gradients in a small neighborhood of p:

$$S[p] = \begin{bmatrix} S_{xx}[p] & S_{xy}[p] & S_{xz}[p] \\ S_{xy}[p] & S_{yy}[p] & S_{yz}[p] \\ S_{xz}[p] & S_{yz}[p] & S_{zz}[p] \end{bmatrix}, \quad (3)$$

$$with\ S_{ij}[p] = \left(W * (\partial I/\partial i \times \partial I/\partial j)\right)[p]\ \ for\ (i,j) \in \{x,y,z\}^2.$$

Here W is a Gaussian convolution kernel defining the size of the neighborhood. Before computing the structure tensor, the SA images (native resolution of 1.6 x 1.6 x 8 mm^3) were interpolated to the same isotropic resolution as the SR images (i.e. 1.6 x 1.6 x 1.6 mm^3) using a windowed *sinc* interpolation (Lanczos window).

We compared the following metrics based on the structure tensor in the different reconstructions: $< S_{xx} >$, $< S_{yy} >$ and $< S_{zz} >$ (i.e. the average of S_{xx}, S_{yy} and S_{zz} respectively over the reconstructed volume). $< S_{xx} >$ and $< S_{yy} >$ can be viewed as the amount of details (edges, features…) present in the SA plane while $< S_{zz} >$ relates to the direction orthogonal to SA. It is expected that the SR images can preserve directional information from the native in-plane resolution and that they can retrieve additional information in the orthogonal direction (z) from the VLA and HLA images (increased $< S_{zz} >$). Statistical differences between the native and SR images were assessed by Wilcoxon signed rank tests. A significance level of 5% was used.

5 Results

The time needed to acquire the three cine stacks was approximately 10 min (4 min for SA, 3 min for HLA and 3 min for VLA). The cine-GRICS reconstruction time was 180 min (SA+HLA+VLA) using a parallel C++ code running on a cluster of 16 workstations; the SR step for a full cine dataset took 14/16 min (Tikhonov/Beltrami) using Matlab (single-thread, sequential reconstruction of the 32 cardiac phases).

Example reconstructed images are shown in Fig. 1. Images are shown both in end-diastole and in end-systole position. The visual comparison between the native SA images and the SR images shows preserved image quality in the short-axis plane with a slight noise amplification for the Tikhonov regularization. Important differences are observed in the through-plane direction, i.e. in the VLA and HLA orientations. Several anatomical structures and vessels were not visible in the native SA images but were recovered by both SR reconstruction techniques. Differences are mostly noticed near the base and near the apex of the left ventricle where the structures are orthogonal to the slice direction (see arrows in Fig. 1).

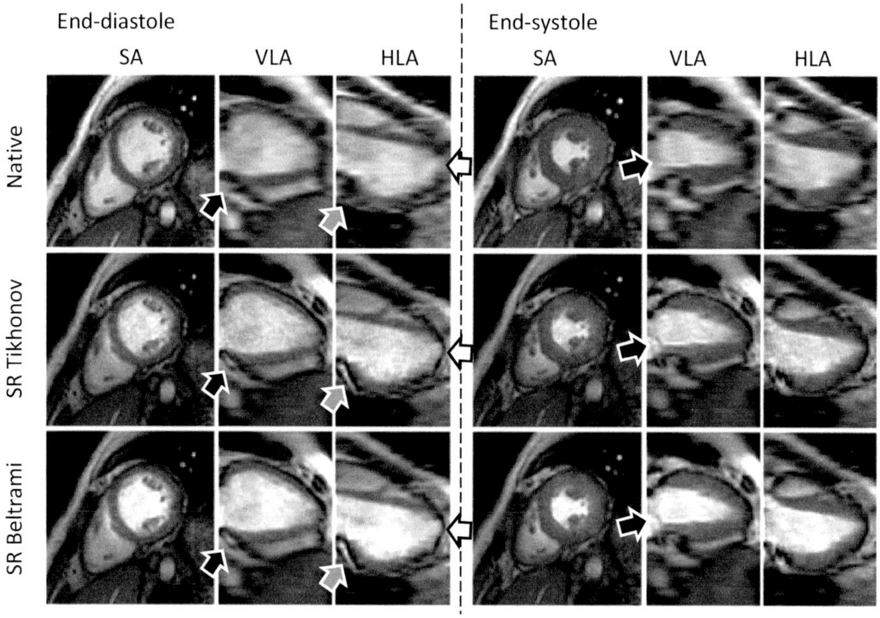

Fig. 1. Example 3D cine datasets from a patient: native short-axis images (top row), super-resolution with Tikhonov (middle row) and with Beltrami regularization (bottom row). The arrows point out noticeable anatomical details which were not visible in the native images but were recovered by both SR techniques, especially near the base and apex of the left ventricle.

Example intensity profiles drawn across the left ventricle are shown in Fig. 2. Again the resolution improvement compared to the native images can be observed, especially near the mitral plane and at the apex. Structures like the myocardial wall and papillary muscles appear much sharper in SR images. Beltrami regularized images appear less noisy than Tikhonov images.

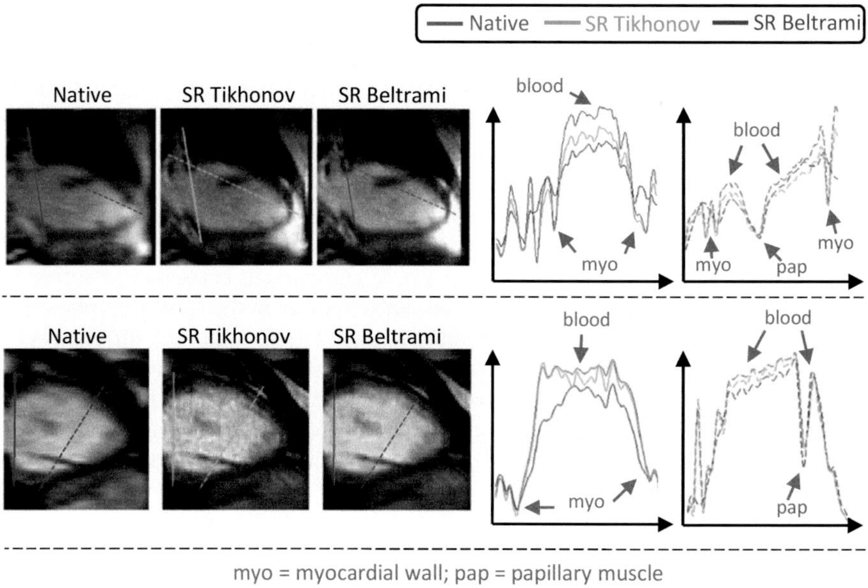

Fig. 2. Example intensity profiles from two volunteers (top and bottom row). Two line profiles were drawn on the images (left side: native and SR images) with various oblique orientations and the corresponding intensity profiles are shown on the right. Finer details better observed in the SR images and Beltrami regularized images appear less noisy than Tikhonov ones.

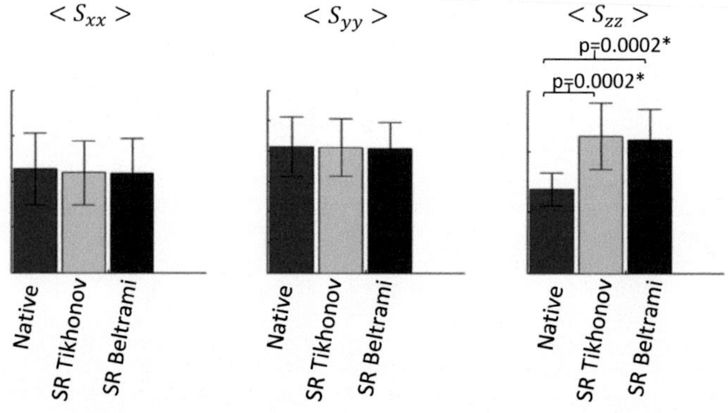

Fig. 3. Directional information (derived from the structure tensor S) contained in the native short-axis images and in the SR images (with Tikhonov and Beltrami regularization) in the short-axis plane ($< S_{xx} >$ and $< S_{yy} >$) and in the orthogonal direction ($< S_{zz} >$). Differences between native and SR images were not significant for x and y directions and were significant for z direction.

Measures of directional information, as measured by the structure tensor metrics in the 18 subjects (volunteers and patients), are summarized in Fig 3. In-plane information (SA plane) was preserved between native SA images and SR images, as differences in

$< S_{xx} >$ (p>0.1) and $< S_{yy} >$ (p>0.6) were not statistically significant. Information in the orthogonal direction was improved with SR reconstruction compared to the native images since $< S_{zz} >$ was significantly different (p=0.0002). Beltrami denoising did not seem to affect this resolution enhancement as differences in all three metrics between Tikhonov and Beltrami regularized images were not significant (p>0.5).

6 Discussion and Conclusion

The proposed reconstruction combines nonrigid motion-correction and super-resolution. Our hypothesis was that SR reconstruction can be guaranteed if two conditions are met: (i) images with good quality and good motion-consistency can be provided as inputs of the SR algorithm, i.e. the input volumes need to have high in-plane resolution, minimal blurring/ghosting artifacts, and the misalignments from one volume to another should be minimal; (ii) an efficient SR solver can be implemented, i.e. efficient regularization schemes can be implemented in order to solve this under-determined inverse problem. For these reasons the joint reconstruction of image and motion (GRICS approach) and the feature-preserving Beltrami regularization were key technical choices. Our results in healthy volunteers and patients with breathing difficulties show the feasibility of the technique.

Alternative methods for SR cine reconstruction include dictionary learning approaches [10, 11] which do not explicitly require motion correction. Our cine-GRICS approach has the advantage of using a motion model that inherently compensates intra-image motion (ghosting/blurring), intra-stack motion (slice-to-slice consistency) and inter-stack motion (stack-to-stack consistency). Compared to other total variation schemes [12] our Beltrami scheme yields similar results with faster convergence [8].

The proposed approach still has limitations that should be mentioned. Despite its high efficiency the b-SSFP sequence is sensitive to B_0 field inhomogeneity that may result in dark banding artifacts. Although the requirement in terms of B_0 homogeneity is less for the 2D b-SSFP than it is for its 3D version, it does rely on efficient shimming in the volume to be scanned. It should also be noted that both the in-flow effect and the location of the dark-band artifacts depend on the slice orientation and may result in outliers in the native images. This might be overcome with robust SR algorithms [13]. Another limitation is that the motion correction and the SR steps were applied sequentially. The final reconstruction might still be improved by merging the two steps into a single optimization problem. Such an approach would consist of searching for the isotropic SR image directly from the motion-corrupted k-space data.

In conclusion we have proposed a strategy for 3D isotropic cine MRI. The data acquisition consists of multiple stacks of 2D b-SSFP datasets with different orientations. Efficient SR reconstruction of an isotropic 3D cine dataset was rendered possible by (i) advanced nonrigid motion correction (using 3D cine GRICS) providing artifact-free and motion consistent images for each stack; (ii) regularized inversion of the SR model (with either Tikhonov or feature-preserving Beltrami regularization). The feasibility has been demonstrated in healthy volunteers and patients with breathing difficulties. The approach might be adapted to other imaging sequences or applications such as 3D late gadolinium enhancement.

Acknowledgement. The authors would like to thank AFM (French association against myopathy) for funding the patient study (ID C13-04). This publication was supported by the European Commission, through Grant Number 605162. The content is solely the responsibility of the authors and does not necessarily represent the official views of the EU.

References

1. Scheffler, K., Lehnhardt, S.: Principles and applications of balanced SSFP techniques. European Radiology 13(11), 2409–2418 (2003)
2. Greenspan, H., Oz, G., Kiryati, N., Peled, S.: MRI inter-slice reconstruction using super-resolution. Magnetic Resonance in Medicine 20(5), 2409–2418 (2003)
3. Gholipour, A., Estroff, J., Warfield, S.: Robust super-resolution volume reconstruction from slice acquisitions: application to fetal brain MRI. IEEE Transactions on Medical Imaging 29(10), 1739–1758 (2010)
4. Plenge, E., Poot, D., Bernsen, M., Kotek, G., Houston, G., Wielopolski, P., van der Weerd, L., Niessen, W., Meijering, E.: Super-resolution methods in MRI: Can they improve the trade-off between resolution, signal-to-noise ratio, and acquisition time? Magnetic Resonance in Medicine 68(6), 1522–2594 (2012)
5. Rousseau, F., Glenn, O., Iordanova, B., Rodriguez-Carranza, C., Vigneron, D., Barkovich, J., Studholme, C.: Registration-based approach for reconstruction of high-resolution in utero fetal MR brain images. Academic Radiology 13(9), 1072–1081 (2006)
6. Vuissoz, P., Odille, F., Fernandez, B., Lohezic, M., Benhadid, A., Mandry, D., Felblinger, J.: Free-breathing imaging of the heart using 2D cine-GRICS (generalized reconstruction by inversion of coupled systems) with assessment of ventricular volumes and function. Journal of Magnetic Resonance Imaging 35(2), 340–351 (2012)
7. Odille, F., Vuissoz, P., Marie, P., Felblinger, J.: Generalized reconstruction by inversion of coupled systems (GRICS) applied to free-breathing MRI. Magnetic Resonance in Medicine 60(1), 146–157 (2008)
8. Zosso, D., Bustin, A.: A primal-dual projected gradient algorithm for efficient Beltrami regularization. UCLA CAM Report, 14-52 (2014)
9. Bigun, J., Granlund, G., Wiklund, J.: Multidimensional orientation estimation with applications to texture analysis and optical-flow. IEEE Trans. Pattern Anal. Mach. Intell. 13(8), 775–790 (1991)
10. Caballero, J., Price, A., Rueckert, D., Hajnal, J.: Dictionary learning and time sparsity for dynamic MR data reconstruction. IEEE Trans. Med. Imaging 33(4), 979–994 (2014)
11. Bhatia, K., Price, A., Shi, W., Hajnal, J., Rueckert, D.: Super-resolution reconstruction of cardiac MRI using coupled dictionary learning. In: Proc. of ISBI, pp. 947–950 (2014)
12. Tourbier, S., Bresson, X., Hagmann, P., Thiran, J.-P., Meuli, R., Cuadra, M.B.: Efficient total variation algorithm for fetal brain MRI reconstruction. In: Golland, P., Hata, N., Barillot, C., Hornegger, J., Howe, R. (eds.) MICCAI 2014, Part II. LNCS, vol. 8674, pp. 252–259. Springer, Heidelberg (2014)
13. Kuklisova-Murgasova, M., Quaghebeur, G., Rutherford, M., Hajnal, J., Schnabel, J.: Reconstruction of fetal brain MRI with intensity matching and complete outlier removal. Med. Image Anal. 16(8), 1550–1564 (2012)

Motion Estimation of Common Carotid Artery Wall Using a H_∞ Filter Based Block Matching Method

Zhifan Gao[1,2,3], Huahua Xiong[4], Heye Zhang[1,3], Dan Wu[1,2,3], Minhua Lu[5], Wanqing Wu[1,3], Kelvin K.L. Wong[6], and Yuan-Ting Zhang[1,3,7]

[1] Shenzhen Institutes of Advanced Technology, Chinese Academy of Sciences, China
[2] Shenzhen College of Advanced Technology, University of Chinese Academy of Sciences, China
[3] Key Lab for Health Informatics of Chinese Academy of Sciences, China
[4] Department of Ultrasound, The Second People's Hospital of Shenzhen, China
[5] Department of Biomedical Engineering, School of Medicine, Shenzhen University, China
[6] School of Computer Science and Software Engineering, University of Western Australia, Australia
[7] The Joint Research Centre for Biomedical Engineering, Department of Electronic Engineering, Chinese University of Hong Kong, China

Abstract. The movement of the common carotid artery (CCA) vessel wall has been well accepted as one important indicator of atherosclerosis, but it is still one challenge to estimate the motion of vessel wall from ultrasound images. In this paper, a robust H_∞ filter was incorporated with block matching (BM) method to estimate the motion of carotid arterial wall. The performance of our method was compared with the standard BM method, Kalman filter, and manual traced method respectively on carotid artery ultrasound images from 50 subjects. Our results showed that the proposed method has a small estimation error (96 μm for the longitudinal motion and 46 μm for the radial motion), and good agreement (94.03% results fall within 95% confidence interval for the longitudinal motion and 95.53% for the radial motion) with the manual traced method. These results demonstrated the effectiveness of our method in the motion estimation of carotid wall in ultrasound images.

Keywords: vessel wall motion, carotid ultrasound, H_∞ filter, block matching.

1 Introduction

Stiffness of carotid artery has been considered as an important risk marker of severe atherosclerosis [1], which is the main cause of morbidity and mortality related to cardiovascular diseases. A number of studies have attempted to characterize the arterial stiffness from the motion of carotid artery [2]. In particular, the longitudinal motion of carotid wall have recently been recognized in an Editorial

N. Navab et al. (Eds.): MICCAI 2015, Part III, LNCS 9351, pp. 443–450, 2015.
DOI: 10.1007/978-3-319-24574-4_53

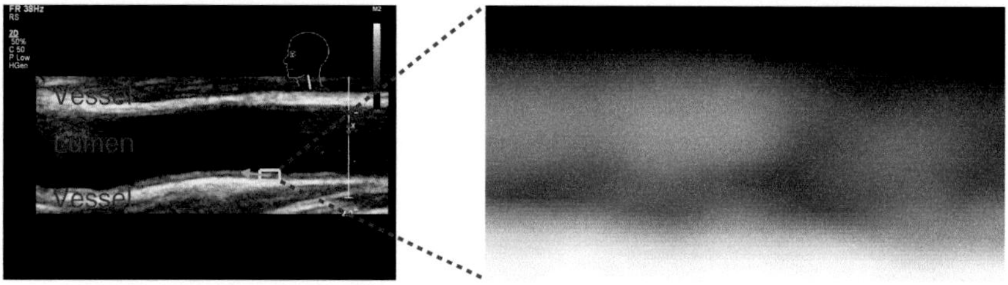

Fig. 1. Example of the ultrasound image of the CCA. The enlarged region (right), corresponding to the yellow rectangle (left), represents the ROI for tracking the motion of carotid vessel. The green arrow is the displacement vector of ROI.

in American Journal of Physiology for its potential importance for the development process of atherosclerosis and recognized at the Royal Swedish Academy of Engineering Sciences annual meeting 2012 [3,4]. Most of these attempts utilized the block matching (BM) method to estimate radial and longitudinal tissue motion of carotid artery from ultrasound image sequences [5]. There are four important issues in the BM method: 1) the size of reference block, 2) the searching range, 3) the distortion function, and 4) the estimation strategy.

The size of reference block always plays an important role in BM method [6]. The influence from the size of reference block on the motion estimation of carotid artery was investigated in [5] by comparing longitudinal and radial displacements generated by different reference blocks. The searching range is another factor to determine the accuracy of BM method. However, the large search range would lead to high computation cost. The tradeoff between the computational cost and the accuracy has been carefully evaluated in the motion estimation from the ultrasound image of carotid artery [7]. The distortion function is used to measure the similarity between the reference block and the candidate block [8], and the cross correlation is one frequently used distortion function in the motion tracking of carotid artery [9]. However, the cross correlation can be easily influenced by the time-variant speckle noise in the ultrasound images. Therefore, normalized cross correlation was proposed to compress the speckle noise in the motion estimation in carotid artery ultrasound images [5]. The estimation strategy is to determine the location of the block from frame to frame in the ultrasound image sequences. Most recent works adopted the adaptive schemes, such as the Kalman filter [2] and the Hilbert transform [10], for estimating the motion of carotid artery. The main problem of Kalman filter is under the Gaussian statistics assumptions. However, uncertainties, such as image noise, sparse image data, and model uncertainty often encountered in practical cases might not be Gaussian statistics. Furthermore, the Kalman filter always performs well only if the filter parameters are reasonably set. In practice, it is very difficult to obtain proper filter parameters because of complexity of the problem. Thus, the issue of robust estimation becomes paramountly important.

In this paper, we introduce a modified BM method using the H_∞ filter to estimate longitudinal and radial motion of CCA. This algorithm differs from the

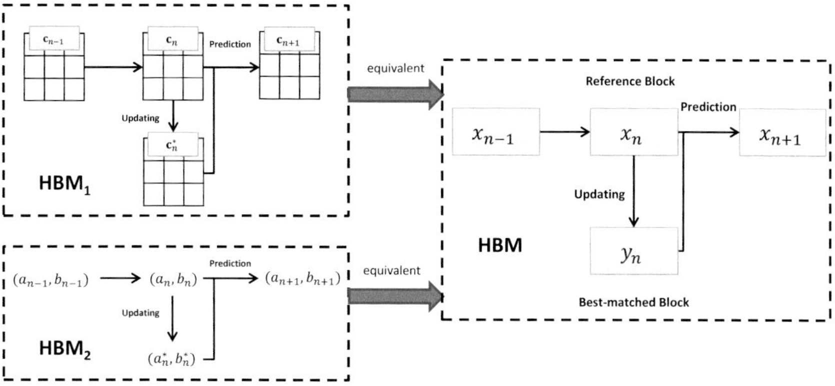

Fig. 2. The flowcharts of HBM_1 and HBM_2, that can be generalized to the same flowcharts HBM.

previous Kalman approach mainly in the following two aspects: 1) no a priori knowledge of noise statistics is required; and 2) the worst possible effects of the image noises can be minimized because H_∞ filter is a minimax estimator [11], which will ensure that if the disturbances are small, the estimation errors will be as small as possible [12,13]. The performance of our method is evaluated using a set of 50 ultrasound image sequences from 50 subjects by comparing to the manual traced results by one ultrasound physician and three other methods: standard BM method (BM), Kalman-based BM (KBM), update of BM's estimation applying Kalman filter during tracking (KDBM).

2 Methodology

The proposed H_∞-based Block Matching (HBM) for motion estimation of carotid vessel from frame to frame can be divided into two steps: 1) prediction step and 2) updating step. In the prediction step, the best-matched block $\mathcal{B}_{best}$ is estimated from the reference block $\mathcal{B}_{ref}$ in the same frame. In the updating step, the reference block $\mathcal{B}'_{ref}$ in the next frame is estimated from $\mathcal{B}_{best}$ in the current frame. Before HBM, the ultrasound sequence should be preprocessed as follows: 1) inhomogeneity of intensity distributions across frames can influence the subsequent block matching method. It leads to the different dynamic ranges in frames, and moreover makes the same tissues in frames have different range of the pixel value. Thus, every frame in the ultrasound sequence should be normalized into [0, 255] [14]. It can also improve the image quality by changing image contrast; 2) considering the tradeoff between the tracking accuracy and the computational cost, the ultrasound sequence is spatially interpolated using the bilinear method for tracking the sub-pixel motion of carotid artery, which magnifies the image by 3 times and 3) an user-defined reference block (ROI) on the carotid arterial wall in the first frame of the ultrasound sequence is selected with size 0.36 mm × 0.18 mm. And then the search range can be located, which

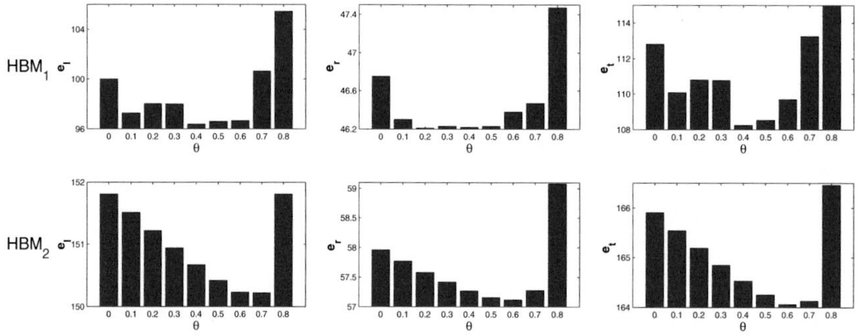

Fig. 3. The mean error of the longitudinal (e_l), radial (e_r) and total displacement (e_t) in μm of the proposed method (HBM$_1$ in the top row and HBM$_2$ in the bottom row).

is a rectangle region with size 1.08 mm $\times$ 0.36 mm, and its center is same with its corresponding ROI. Figure 1 shows the example of ROI.

Prediction Step. In the prediction step, the reference block $\mathcal{B}'_{ref}$ in the next frame is estimated from the reference block $\mathcal{B}_{ref}$ and the best-matched block $\mathcal{B}_{best}$ in the current frame by H$_\infty$ filter. H$_\infty$ filter can generate the best estimate of the state of a dynamic system by minimizing the worst-case estimation error, and the variation of the reference block $\mathcal{B}_{ref}$ can be modeled as a time-invariant discrete dynamic system:

$$\begin{aligned} \mathbf{x}_{n+1} &= \mathbf{x}_n + \mathbf{w}_n, \\ \mathbf{y}_n &= \mathbf{x}_n + \mathbf{v}_n, \\ \mathbf{z}_n &= \mathbf{x}_n, \end{aligned} \tag{1}$$

where n is the frame index, $\mathbf{w}_n$ and $\mathbf{v}_n$ are noise terms, $\mathbf{x}_n$ and $\mathbf{y}_n$ are matrices corresponding to the reference block $\mathcal{B}_{ref}$ and the best-matched block $\mathcal{B}_{best}$. $\mathbf{x}_{n+1}$ corresponds to the reference block $\mathcal{B}'_{ref}$ in the next frame.

In order to find an optimal estimate $\hat{\mathbf{z}}_n$ of $\mathbf{z}_n$, we need to minimize the cost function J [11], Because the direct minimization of J is not tractable, a strategy for generating the best estimation of $\hat{\mathbf{x}}_{n+1}$ is developed by making the cost function J satisfying an upper bound. Let θ be the reciprocal of the upper bound. This strategy can be formulated as follows [11]:

$$\begin{aligned} \mathbf{K}_n &= \mathbf{P}_n[\mathbf{I} - \theta \mathbf{S}_n \mathbf{P}_n + \mathbf{R}_n^{-1} \mathbf{P}_n]^{-1} \mathbf{R}_n^{-1}, \\ \mathbf{P}_{n+1} &= \mathbf{P}_n[\mathbf{I} - \theta \mathbf{S}_n \mathbf{P}_n + \mathbf{R}_n^{-1} \mathbf{P}_n]^{-1} + \mathbf{Q}_n, \\ \hat{\mathbf{x}}_{n+1} &= \hat{\mathbf{x}}_n + \mathbf{K}_n(\mathbf{y}_n - \hat{\mathbf{x}}_n), \end{aligned} \tag{2}$$

where $\mathbf{Q}_n$ and $\mathbf{R}_n$ are the covariance matrices of the noise terms $\mathbf{w}_n$ and $\mathbf{v}_n$ respectively, $\mathbf{S}_n$ is the user-specified symmetric positive definite matrix, $\mathbf{P}_n$ is the covariance of the estimation error in the frame index n, and $\mathbf{I}$ is the identity matrix. In our method, we set $\mathbf{Q}_n = \mathbf{R}_n = \mathbf{S}_n = \mathbf{I}$, and $\mathbf{x}_1$ corresponds to the ROI selected in the first frame. In addition, in order to obtain the steady-state solution of Equation (2), we set $\mathbf{P}_{n+1} = \mathbf{P}_n$ and $\mathbf{K}_{n+1} = \mathbf{K}_n$.

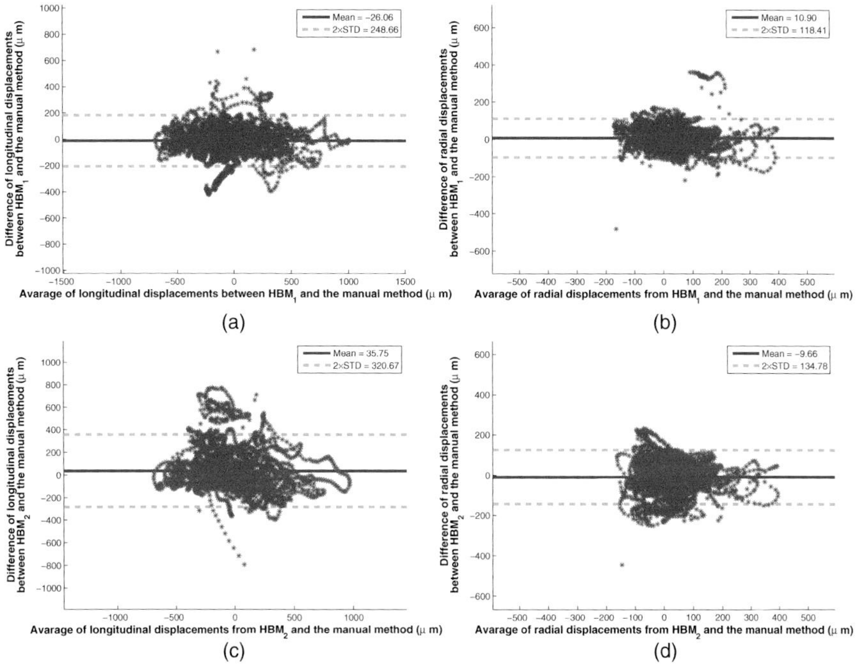

Fig. 4. The Bland-Altman analysis between HBM and manual method. (a) and (b) represent the longitudinal displacements and radial displacements for HBM1 respectively. (c) and (d) represent the longitudinal displacements and radial displacements for HBM2 respectively.

Updating Step. In the updating step, the best-matched block $\mathcal{B}_{best}$ is estimated from the reference block $\mathcal{B}_{ref}$ by the block matching method with normalized cross correlation [5].

Two Implementations. We execute the HBM through two indenpendent implementations: HBM_1 and HBM_2. In HBM_1, $\mathbf{x}_n$ is the vector of the pixel intensity $\mathbf{c}_n$ in the reference block $\mathcal{B}_{ref}$, that is for $\forall i \in \{1, 2, ..., M\}$, the value of the ith element in $\mathbf{x}_n$ equals to the gray value of the ith pixel in the reference block, and M is number of elements in $\mathbf{x}_n$. Similarly, $\mathbf{y}_n$ is the vector of pixel intensity $\mathbf{c}_n^*$ in the best-matched block $\mathcal{B}_{best}$, computed from $\mathcal{B}_{ref}$ by the block matching algorithm. Then, the pixel intensity $\mathbf{c}_{n+1}$ of the reference block $\mathcal{B}'_{ref}$ in the next frame is estimated by $\mathbf{x}_n$ and $\mathbf{y}_n$ using Equation (2). In HBM_2, $\mathbf{x}_n$ is the center location of the reference block $\mathcal{B}_{ref}$, that is $\mathbf{x}_n = (a_n, b_n)$, where a_n and b_n are x-coordinate value and y-coordinate value, respectively. Similarly, $\mathbf{y}_n$ is the center location (a_n^*, b_n^*) of the best-matched block $\mathcal{B}_{best}$, computed from $\mathcal{B}_{ref}$ by the block matching algorithm. Then the center location (a_{n+1}, b_{n+1}) of the reference block $\mathcal{B}'_{ref}$ in the next frame is estimated by $\mathbf{x}_n$ and $\mathbf{y}_n$ using Equation (2). Figure 2 illustrates the flowcharts of HBM1 and HBM2 and shows that the two flowcharts are equivalent.

Table 1. The comparison between BM, KBM, KDBM, $HBM_1(\theta=0.4)$ and $HBM_2(\theta=0.6)$ in μm.

Error	BM	KBM	KDBM	HBM_1	HBM_2
e_l	150.42±148.24	100.00±100.37	151.81±147.18	96.37±85.93	150.22±148.86
e_r	57.16±39.83	50.76±41.52	57.96±39.46	46.22±38.26	57.12±39.92
e_t	164.25±149.83	112.81±106.08	165.91±148.57	109.25±91.24	164.06±150.13

3 Results

One ultrasound physician with more than 10-year experiences collected all the ultrasound data on CCA using a high-resolution ultrasound system (iU22, Philips Ultrasound, Bothell, WA, USA) and a 7.5MHz liner array transducer. All the imaging data then were saved as DICOM format into CDs for off-line analysis. During the collection, the subjects were supine in the bed, with the head turned 45° away from the examined side. In the end, a total of 50 ultrasound image sequences from 50 subjects are used in this study. The study protocol was designed according to the principles of the Declaration of Helsinki and then approved by the Ethics Committee of the Second People's Hospital of Shenzhen in China. Each participant was informed of the purpose and procedure of this study. Informed consent was obtained from each participant. We implement all the codes using Matlab R2012a on a desktop computer with Intel(R) Xeon(R) CPU E5-2650(2.00 GHz) and 32GB DDR2 memory. In the experiments, the motion of carotid artery estimated by our method were compared to the manual traced results by the same ultrasound physician, which is considered as the ground truth.

In order to evaluate the performance of our method quantitatively, we calculated the radial displacement D_r and the longitudinal displacement D_l with respect to the first frame in the ultrasound image sequence. Then the longitudinal error e_l and the radial error e_r of the displacement were computed to analyze the difference between our method and manual traced results,

$$e_l = \sqrt{\frac{1}{N}\sum_{n=1}^{N}(D_l^m(n) - D_l^h(n))^2}, \quad e_r = \sqrt{\frac{1}{N}\sum_{n=1}^{N}(D_r^m(n) - D_r^h(n))^2}, \quad (3)$$

where $D_l^m(n)$ and $D_r^m(n)$ are measured by manual, $D_l^h(n)$ and $D_r^h(n)$ are estimated by our method. Then the total error can be computed by $e_t = \sqrt{e_l^2 + e_r^2}$. Through e_l, e_r and e_t, we can determine the value of θ. In Figure 3, we can see that the $\theta = 0.4$ is better than other values of θ in HBM_1. Similarly, $\theta = 0.6$ in HBM_2 is better than other values. Moreover, HBM_1 is better than HBM_2 because all the minimum errors in HBM_1 are less than those in HBM_2. Additionally, we used the Bland-Altman method to analyze the agreement between our method and the manual method. As seen in Figure 4. For the longitudinal displacement and the radial displacement in HBM_1, 94.03% and 95.53% of points fall within the 95% confidence interval in the Student t-test, respectively.

In HBM_2, the results are 93.47% and 92.38%. At last, our method was compared with three other methods using manual traced results as ground truth: the standard BM method [5], Kalman-based BM (KBM) [7], update of BM's estimation applying Kalman filter during tracking (KDBM) [7]. Table 1 shows the comparative results of these methods.

4 Discussion and Conclusion

We developed a H_∞ filter based BM method to estimate the motion of carotid artery wall from the ultrasound image sequences. In each imaging frame, we compute the best-matched block by the reference block using the block matching method. Then, the reference block in the next frame can be estimated by the reference block and the best-matched block in the current frame using a H_∞ filter. Additionally, we used two independent strategies (HBM_1 and HBM_2) to implement the proposed method. And the two implementations are based on the pixel intensity and center location of the reference block, respectively. In the experiments, the results generated by our H_∞ filter based BM method with different values of θ were evaluated using 50 ultrasound image sequences and compared to manual traced results by one experienced ultrasound physician. Based on these experiments, the optimal values of θ for HBM_1 (= 0.4) and HBM_2 (= 0.6) can be obtained according to minimum error shown in Table 1. In addition, we can see that the proposed H_∞ filter with $\theta \geqslant 0.9$ is unstable as the error is significantly in Figure 3. Moreover, our method were also compared to three recent methods using manual traced results as the ground truth: BM, KBM and KDBM. Table 1 shows that the motion trajectory computed by our H_∞ filter based BM method (HBM_1 with $\theta = 0.4$ and HBM_2 with $\theta = 0.6$) are more accurate than three other methods. These experiments can demonstrate the effectiveness of our method in the motion estimation of carotid artery wall from ultrasound image sequences. Using the motion tracking of carotid vessel, we will focus on the investigation of the properties of vessel wall (especially the longitudinal motion) and its relationship with physiological parameters related to cardiovascular disease (such as wall shear strain and pulse wave velocity) in the future.

Acknowledgements. We thank support from the Guang-dong Innovation Research Team Fund for Low-cost Health-care Technologies in China, the Key Lab for Health Informatics of the Chinese Academy of Sciences, the External Cooperation Program of the Chinese Academy of Sciences (GJHZ1212), National Natural Science Foundation of China (No. 61471243) and Shenzhen Innovation Funding (JCYJ20140414170821190).

References

1. Yli-Ollila, H., Laitinen, T., Weckström, M., Laitinen, T.M.: Axial and radial waveforms in common carotid artery: An advanced method for studying arterial elastic

properties in ultrasound imaging. Ultrasound in Medicine & Biology 39(7), 1168–1177 (2013)
2. Zahnd, G., Orkisz, M., Srusclat, A., Moulin, P., Vray, D.: Evaluation of a kalman-based block matching method to assess the bi-dimensional motion of the carotid artery wall in b-mode ultrasound sequences. Medical Image Analysis 17(5) (2013)
3. Cinthio, M., Ahlgren, R., Bergkvist, J., Jansson, T., Persson, W., Lindström, K.: Longitudinal movements and resulting shear strain of the arterial wall. American Journal of Physiology-Heart and Circulatory Physiology 291(1) (2006)
4. Ahlgren, R., Cinthio, M., Steen, S., Nilsson, T., Sjöberg, T., Persson, W., Lindström, K.: Longitudinal displacement and intramural shear strain of the porcine carotid artery undergo profound changes in response to catecholamines. American Journal of Physiology-Heart and Circulatory Physiology 302(5) (2012)
5. Golemati, S., Sassano, A., Lever, M.J., Bharath, A.A., Dhanjil, S., Nicolaides, A.N.: Carotid artery wall motion estimated from b-mode ultrasound using region tracking and block matching. Ultrasound in Medicine & Biology 29, 387–399 (2003)
6. Ramirez, B.: Performance evaluation and recent advances of fast block-matching motion estimation methods for video coding. In: Kropatsch, W.G., Kampel, M., Hanbury, A. (eds.) CAIP 2007. LNCS, vol. 4673, pp. 801–808. Springer, Heidelberg (2007)
7. Gastounioti, A., Golemati, S., Stoitsis, J.S., Nikita, K.S.: Carotid artery wall motion analysis from b-mode ultrasound using adaptive block matching: in silico evaluation and in vivo application. Physics in Medicine and Biology 58(24), 8647–8661 (2013)
8. Metkar, S., Talbar, S.: Motion Estimation Techinques for Digital Video Coding. Springer (2013)
9. Lewis, J.P.: Fast template matching. In: Proceeding of Vision Interface, pp. 120–123 (1995)
10. Zahnd, G., Orkisz, M., Balocco, S., Sérusclat, A., Moulin, P., Vray, D.: A fast 2d tissue motion estimator based on the phase of the intensity enables visualization of the propagation of the longitudinal movement in the carotid artery wall. In: IEEE International Ultrasonics Symposium (IUS), pp. 1761–1764. IEEE (2013)
11. Simon, D.: Optimal State Estimation: Kalman, H_∞ and Nonlinear Approaches. Wiley-Interscience (2006)
12. Hassibi, B., Sayed, A.H., Kailath, T.: H_∞ Optimality of the LMS Algorithm. IEEE Transactions on Signal Processing 44(2) (1996)
13. Liu, H., Wang, S., Fei, G., Tian, Y., Chen, W., Hu, Z., Shi, P.: Robust Framework for PET Image Reconstruction Incorporating System and Measurement Uncertainties. PLOS One 7(3) (2012)
14. Gonzalez, R., Woods, R., Digital Image Processing. Pearson Education (2009)

Gated-tracking: Estimation of Respiratory Motion with Confidence

Valeria De Luca*, Gábor Székely, and Christine Tanner

Computer Vision Laboratory, ETH Zürich, 8092 Zürich, Switzerland
vdeluca@vision.ee.ethz.ch

Abstract. Image-guided radiation therapy during free-breathing requires estimation of the target position and compensation for its motion. Estimation of the observed motion during therapy needs to be reliable and accurate. In this paper we propose a novel, image sequence-specific confidence measure to predict the reliability of the tracking results. The sequence-specific statistical relationship between the image similarities and the feature displacements is learned from the first breathing cycles. A confidence measure is then assigned to the tracking results during the real-time application phase based on the relative closeness to the expected values. The proposed confidence was tested on the results of a learning-based tracking algorithm. The method was assessed on 9 2D B-mode ultrasound sequences of healthy volunteers under free-breathing. Results were evaluated on a total of 15 selected vessel centers in the liver, achieving a mean tracking accuracy of 0.9 mm. When considering only highly-confident results, the mean (95th percentile) tracking error on the test data was reduced by 12% (16%) while duty cycle remained sufficient (60%), achieving a 95% accuracy below 3 mm, which is clinically acceptable. A similar performance was obtained on 10 2D liver MR sequences, showing the applicability of the method to a different image modality.

Keywords: confidence, tracking, learning, respiratory motion, image guidance, ultrasound.

1 Introduction

Image-guided radiation therapy of abdominal organs during free-breathing requires estimation of the target position and compensation for its motion over the duration of the entire treatment session [9]. Examples of imaging techniques available for observing the internal motion are ultrasound (US) and magnetic resonance imaging (MRI). US is increasingly used, as it can image soft tissues in real time, and with higher temporal and spatial resolution than other modalities, is non-ionizing and inexpensive [4]. MRI is a popular choice for guidance of focused ultrasound surgery as it provides thermometry images, also used for tracking [15], yet the temporal resolution is about 5 times lower than US.

* We thank the European Union's 7th Framework Program (FP7/2007-2013) under grant agreement no. 611889 (TRANS-FUSIMO) for funding.

N. Navab et al. (Eds.): MICCAI 2015, Part III, LNCS 9351, pp. 451–458, 2015.
DOI: 10.1007/978-3-319-24574-4_54

The intrafraction motion estimation needs to be reliable and accurate, to reduce the size of the safety margins due to expected residual tumor motion in the planned dose delivery [19]. Gating is commonly used to reduce motion uncertainties. Yet it generally leads to relatively low duty cycles (20-50%) for maintaining acceptable accuracy [9,16]. Following the tumor motion by tracking keeps duty cycle at 100%, but can have high errors. Here we propose gated-tracking, where gating (i.e. accepting motion predictions) is based on the estimated accuracy (confidence) of the current tracking result and tracking is used to follow the tumor.

Confidence measures for motion estimation from images can generally be based on image appearance, motion field properties, or both. Estimates are likely more accurate for strong image features, high image similarity and realistic motion patterns. Usually maximization of these criteria has been incorporated in the tracking approach to increase accuracy. For example, methods based on optical flow [10,2,11] and probabilistic approaches [18,13] include already confidence values in their tracking formulation. Yet they are tailored for the specific tracking strategy. Learning-based methods have been employed for detecting the areas of the images which can be most reliably tracked [1,6,8]. A probabilistic confidence measure, based on the local image similarity, was provided for a block matching method [13]. Consistency of motion estimates across groups of image has been used in image registration to detect errors and improve accuracy [5]. However such a strategy is too time-consuming for real-time applications.

We propose a different approach for assigning confidence measures, which is independent from the motion estimation strategy and image modality, and is based on the relationship between image similarity and estimated displacement vectors. This method exploits the recurring similarities of both motion and image appearance in pseudo-repetitive scenarios, like breathing. The aim is to keep the tracking errors below 5 mm, to fulfill the clinical requirements for target margins in radiation therapies [9]. Further reductions will facilitate to keep the overall system error within this limit, when also having to incorporate spatio-temporal motion prediction [12]. A strategy was devised to automatically determine the required thresholds of the confidence values to stay within these limits.

2 Materials

We collected nine 2D US sequences of the liver of healthy volunteers under free-breathing, from the same spatial location. In details, second harmonic B-mode US sequences were acquired over 3-10 min, using a Siemens Antares scanner (CH4-1 transducer, center frequency 1.82 - 2.22 MHz) [14]. These images (longitudinal or intercostal planes) are characterized by spatial and temporal resolution ranging in $[0.28, 0.71]$ mm and $[14, 25]$ Hz, and size in $[82632, 279300]$ pixels. To explore the validity of the method independently of the image modality, we gathered 2D MR sequences from 10 healthy volunteers under free-breathing. These consisted of sagittal navigator slices, acquired at 2.6-3.4 Hz for 4D-MRI [17]. The MRIs were captured using a balanced Steady State Free Precession sequence (flip angle 70°, TR=3.1 ms) on a 1.5T Philips Achieva MR system. Image resolution and size ranged in $[1.29, 1.37]$ mm and $[50176, 65536]$ pixels.

Given a sequence of T 2D images $I(t)$, with $t \in [0, T-1]$, the tracking objective is to compute the position of anatomical landmarks inside the liver (vessel centers) $P_j(t) \in \mathbb{R}^2$ in each image. $ROI_{j,\tilde{t}}(t)$ and $\mathbf{d}_j(t) = P_j(t) - P_j(0)$ denote a rectangular region of interest from $I(\tilde{t})$ centered in $P_j(t)$ and the displacement of the landmark with respect to the initial frame, respectively.

3 Method

We propose a novel, sequence-specific confidence measure to predict the reliability of tracking results. The sequence-specific statistical relationship between the image similarities and the feature displacements is learned from the first breathing cycles. A confidence measure is then assigned to the tracking results during the real-time application phase based on the relative closeness to the expected values. The proposed measure was tested on the results of two tracking methods and two image modalities: an automatic learning-based tracking algorithm for US images; and a deformable registration for MRIs.

3.1 Tracking Algorithm

For US, we used the learning-based block matching algorithm (LB-BMA) proposed in [3], which exploits the pseudo-repetitive nature of respiration. During an initial training phase of 10 breathing cycles the images are registered and the relationship between the image appearance and the displacements is learned. Image registration is performed non-iteratively by optimizing a local affine transformation with respect to normalized cross-correlation (NCC). The transformation is defined for $ROI_{j,0}(0)$, which is automatically extracted by finding the blob-like feature centered at $P_j(0)$ [3] and expanding it by 3 times its size. The ROI_j image appearance for the training set is efficiently stored by dimensionality reduction via principal component analysis (PCA). For each landmark in the real-time application phase, the most similar ROI from the training set is selected based on the distance in the PCA space and used for temporal alignment of the BMA. For previously unseen image variations (outliers), affine registration is performed to stay adaptive to non-periodic motions. For tracking the MR slices we used the deeds registration method [7], which can cope with sliding boundaries, is relatively fast ($\approx$0.5 s per slice) for a deformable registration and publicly available.

3.2 Confidence Measure

Independently from the tracking algorithm, the confidence measure is learned from an initial set of T_{in} images $I(t')$ in a sequence, with $t' \in [0, T_{in} - 1]$, where we extract the tracked position of J landmarks $P_j(t')$. For each landmark, we compute the magnitude of the Euclidean distances to the initial frame $d_j(t') = ||\mathbf{d}_j(t')||$ and normalize it to the range of the distances from the T_{in} frames, $\bar{d}_j(t')$.

We also compute NCC between the initial $ROI_{j,0}(0)$ and the same sized and positioned, non-transformed ROI at t', i.e. $NCC_j(t') = NCC(ROI_{j,0}(0), ROI_{j,0}(t'))$.

We collect all 2D data points $N_j(t') = [\bar{d}_j(t'), NCC_j(t')]$ for the training data and fit a polynomial curve $F(\mathbf{c}) = \sum_{i=0}^{n} \alpha_i \mathbf{c}^i$ of degree $n \in \{1, 2, 3\}$ to the 5%-95% of this distribution, with α_i the estimated parameters and $\mathbf{c}$ the vector of $\mathbf{c}(t') = \bar{d}_j(t')$. Degree n is selected to minimize the sum of squared errors and maximize the coefficient of determination of the fit, while avoiding zero-crossing of the α_i confidence bounds and hence overfitting. We also extract the 99% confidence bounds ($F^{99}(\mathbf{c})$) of the fit via the Matlab `fit` function. An example of $F(\mathbf{c})$ is shown in Fig. 1.

For each $P_j(\tau)$ during the application phase ($\tau \in [T_{in}, T-1]$), we calculated $N_j(\tau) = [\bar{d}_j(\tau), NCC_j(\tau)]$ and find its projection to $F(\mathbf{c})$ with minimum distance $p_j(\tau) = ||N_j(\tau) - F(c^*)||$, where $c^* = argmin_c ||p_j(\tau, \mathbf{c})||$. If the distance $p_j(\tau)$ of the data point $N_j(\tau)$ to $F(\mathbf{c})$ is within the 99% confidence bounds and $\bar{d}_j(\tau)$ does not exceed the observed $\bar{d}_j(t')$ (to avoid extrapolation), the confidence measure $C_j(\tau) \in [0, 1]$ is assigned according to the local 99% confidence as follows:

If $p_j(\tau) < F^{99}(c^*)$ **and** $\bar{\mathbf{d}}_j(\tau) \leq max_{t'} \bar{\mathbf{d}}_j(t')$ **do** $C_j(\tau) = 1 - 2p_j(\tau)/F^{99}(c^*)$
else do $C_j(\tau) = 0$

3.3 Evaluation

Quantitative evaluation of the tracking and the gated-tracking method was performed on a total of 15 selected vessel centers inside the liver from the US data and 20 from the MRIs. We randomly selected 10% of the application images in each sequence and annotated the landmark position $\hat{P}_j(\hat{t})$ corresponding to $P_j(0)$, and computed the tracking error $TE_j(\hat{t}) = ||P_j(\hat{t}) - \hat{P}_j(\hat{t})||$. Results were summarized by the mean (MTE), standard deviation (SD) and the 95th percentile (TE^{95}) of the single distribution including all $TE_j(\hat{t})$ belonging to the data subset. We also determined the motion magnitude $M_j(\hat{t}) = ||P_j(0) - \hat{P}_j(\hat{t})||$.

The confidence values $C_j(t) \in [0, 1]$ were divided into $S = 20$ intervals $CI_s = [s, 1]$, with $s \in \{0, 0.05, 0.10, \ldots, 0.95\}$. We computed S tracking errors based on accepting results with confidence $C_j(t) \in CI_s$. For each CI_s we define its duty cycle (DC) as the the ratio between the number of accepted tracking results ($T_{j,s}$) and the total number of frames in the application phase: $DC_j = T_{j,s}/(T - T_{in})$.

In order to select one confidence interval to apply during the application phase to all sequences, we split the US data into two similar sized subsets for training and testing. Subset Set_1^{US} included 7 landmarks from 5 sequences and subset Set_2^{US} consisted of the remaining 8 points from 4 sequences. Similarly, we annotated 2 vessel landmarks per MR sequence and selected alternately the sequences in order of acquisition for the training and test set, e.g. training on volunteers $\{1, 3, \ldots, 9\}$ (Set_1^{MR}), testing on volunteers $\{2, 4, \ldots, 10\}$ (Set_2^{MR}).

For the training data we selected s^*, which minimized the 95th percentile error (TE_{j,s^*}^{95}) while keeping $DC_{j,s^*} > 60\%$. During gated-tracking we considered only the frames whose confidence values are within the selected interval CI_{s^*}.

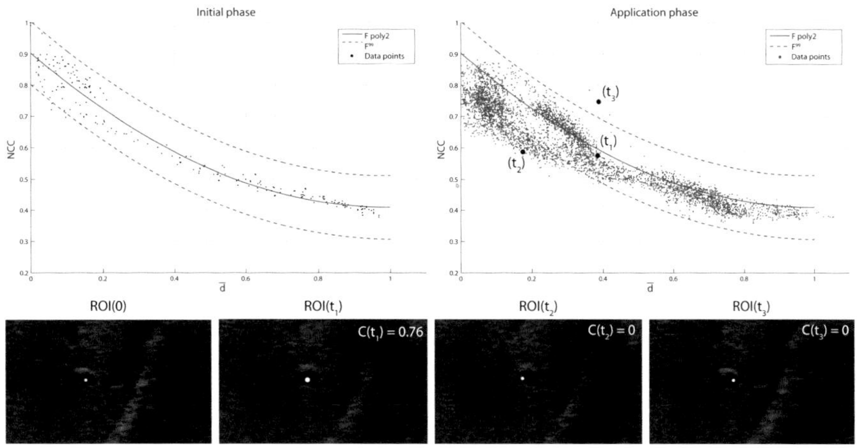

Fig. 1. (Top) example of confidence curve $F(\mathbf{c})$ and 99% bounds $F^{99}(\mathbf{c})$ obtained from training data points (in black) for a representative sequence. (Bottom) example of tracking results in $ROI_{j,0}$ for 3 points with different confidence values, showing $P(t_1)$ with similar NCC as $P(t_2)$, and $P(t_1)$ with similar distance $\bar{d}$ as $P(t_3)$. The initial image $ROI_{j,0}(0)$, with point-landmark $P(0)$ in yellow, is shown as a reference.

Two experiments were conducted, where the role of the subsets as training and test set was swapped to assess the sensitivity of the results to the data selection.

Finally, we compared the gated-tracking results to the ones of gating, where we accepted tracking results with small displacement, i.e. $d_j(\tau) < 3$ mm.

4 Results

For US, we used 5 breathing cycles (260-453 frames) for T_{in}. The number of application frames ranged in [2233, 14211]. The MTE±SD (TE^{95}) for all landmarks was 0.90±0.77 (2.04) mm. MTE ranged in [0.38, 2.34] mm, while the TE_j^{95} was in [0.90, 6.57] mm. For these landmarks the motion magnitude M was 5.17±3.21 mm, and the 95th percentile was 10.59 mm. Fig. 1 shows the relationship between motion and image similarity for (left) the initial phase and (right) the application phase. It can be observed that some of the application phase data falls outside the confidence region and will be discarded first. The example images illustrate outliers with respect to motion and image similarity.

The overall 95th percentile errors in comparison to duty cycle values can be seen for the training set on the left graphs in Fig. 2. The lowest TE^{95} in the objective region was 1.91 mm (-24%) and 1.50 mm (-11%) for Set$_1^{US}$ and Set$_2^{US}$ respectively, see Table 1. Using the resulting s^* for gated-tracking on the test set provided the same TE^{95} reduction, while keeping overall duty cycle at 59% and 68%. Gating results showed similar or worse TE^{95}, but DC<47%.

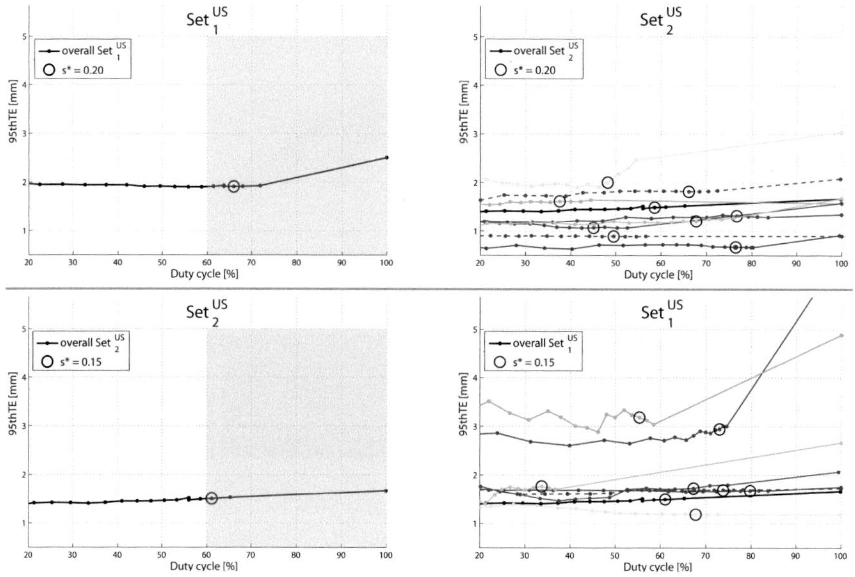

Fig. 2. 95th percentile of TE vs. duty cycle for (left) training set with determined optimum confidence interval $CI_{s^*} = [s^*, 1]$ and (right) test set with sequence-specific curves (in colors) and indicated result for CI_{s^*} (circles).

Table 1. Summary of the results for the two **US** subsets (Set_1^{US} and Set_2^{US}) used interchanged as test and training set. Results of the TE are in mm, while DC is in %.

		Tracking	**Gated-tracking trained on Set_1^{US} CI = [0.20, 1]**	**Gated-tracking trained on Set_2^{US} CI = [0.15, 1]**	**Gating**
Set_1^{US}	**MTE±SD**	1.10±0.93	0.97±0.56	0.97±0.57	1.23±1.20
	TE^{95}	2.51	1.91	1.91	3.64
	range MTE_j	[0.65, 2.34]	[0.70, 1.55]	[0.69, 1.58]	[0.58, 3.14]
	range TE_j^{95}	[1.18, 6.57]	[1.19, 3.24]	[1.18, 3.18]	[1.07, 6.89]
	DC	100	65.90	67.96	46.15
	range DC_j	[100, 100]	[31.82, 77.61]	[33.66, 79.75]	[15.30, 68.38]
Set_2^{US}	**MTE±SD**	0.73±0.54	0.62±0.44	0.63±0.45	0.62±0.47
	TE^{95}	1.68	1.49	1.50	1.52
	range MTE_j	[0.38, 1.06]	[0.33, 1.02]	[0.33, 1.02]	[0.35, 1.03]
	range TE_j^{95}	[0.90, 3.04]	[0.67, 2.00]	[0.67, 2.18]	[0.88, 2.28]
	DC	100	58.57	61.06	38.02
	range DC_j	[100, 100]	[37.53, 76.66]	[39.98, 79.21]	[16.12, 53.72]

Due to the lower temporal resolution of the MRIs, we considered 25 breathing cycles ($T_{in} \in [141, 519]$ frames). The following 1160 frames (7 min) were used for testing. For a mean motion amplitude of 5.63±5.12 mm, tracking results

Table 2. Summary of **MR** results as in Table 1.

		Tracking	Gated-tracking trained on Set_1^{MR} CI = [0.35, 1]	Gated-tracking trained on Set_2^{MR} CI = [0.55, 1]	Gating
Set_1^{MR}	MTE±SD	1.14±1.75	1.03±1.40	1.05±1.42	1.66±0.95
	TE^{95}	2.99	2.31	2.38	3.24
	DC	100	81.12	64.56	41.24
Set_2^{MR}	MTE±SD	0.96±0.91	0.90±0.74	0.88±0.70	1.63±0.87
	TE^{95}	2.21	2.07	1.95	3.17
	DC	100	83.21	67.79	39.28

achieved an overall accuracy of 1.05±1.38 mm (TE^{95}=15.69 mm). Similarly to US, gated-tracking trained on the same subset resulted in an improvement of the TE^{95} by 23% and 12% for Set_1^{MR} and Set_2^{MR} respectively, see Table 2. On the test set, the 95th percentile error reduction was 20% and 6%, with overall DC of 65% and 83%. Gating resulted in higher errors and lower DCs (≈ 40%).

The mean run-time of the confidence estimation is 0.2 ms/frame, with Matlab implementation on a single PC with Intel®Core™i7 CPU (2.66 GHz, 8 GB).

5 Conclusion

We proposed a method for estimating the confidence of tracking results for pseudo-repetitive motion scenarios. It is based on learning the sequence-specific relationship between image similarity and motion vectors, based on the assumption that during the initial learning phase the tracking errors are low. The confidence prediction is independent from the tracking method and image modality. The actually applied confidence interval is decided based on training data. Tested on US sequences, the method reduced 95th percentile errors by between 11% and 24% (to below 1.7 mm on average) while keeping duty cycle at 59% and 68%. Similar results were obtained for the MR sequences, with a reduction of the 95th percentile errors between 6% and 20% while keeping duty cycle at 65% and 83%. For both scenarios, performance was improved by gated-tracking over gating.

In future work we will verify the method's general applicability to other tracking algorithms and larger datasets. For slow varying drift of the target, we envision to update the learning phase. Integration of the estimated confidence values in an overall motion prediction system is the long term plan to facilitate robust and reliable therapy guidance.

References

1. Avidan, S.: Ensemble tracking. IEEE Trans. Pattern Anal. Mach. Intell. 29(2), 261 (2007)

2. Brox, T., Bregler, C., Malik, J.: Large displacement optical flow. In: Proc. IEEE Int. Conf. Comp. Vis. Pattern Recognit., p. 41 (2009)
3. De Luca, V., Tschannen, M., Székely, G., Tanner, C.: Learning-based approach for fast and robust vessel tracking in long ultrasound sequences. In: Mori, K., Sakuma, I., Sato, Y., Barillot, C., Navab, N. (eds.) MICCAI 2013, Part I. LNCS, vol. 8149, pp. 518–525. Springer, Heidelberg (2013)
4. Fontanarosa, D., van der Meer, S., Bamber, J., Harris, E., O'Shea, T., Verhaegen, F.: Review of ultrasound image guidance in external beam radiotherapy. Phys. Med. Biol. 60, R77 (2015)
5. Gass, T., Szekely, G., Goksel, O.: Detection and correction of inconsistency-based errors in non-rigid registration. In: SPIE Medical Imaging, p. 90341B (2014)
6. Grabner, H., Leistner, C., Bischof, H.: Semi-supervised on-line boosting for robust tracking. In: Forsyth, D., Torr, P., Zisserman, A. (eds.) ECCV 2008, Part I. LNCS, vol. 5302, pp. 234–247. Springer, Heidelberg (2008)
7. Heinrich, M., Jenkinson, M., Brady, M., Schnabel, J.: MRF-based deformable registration and ventilation estimation of lung CT. IEEE Trans. Med. Imag. 32, 1239 (2013)
8. Kalal, Z., Mikolajczyk, K., Matas, J.: Tracking-learning-detection. IEEE Trans. Pattern Anal. Mach. Intell. 34(7), 1409 (2012)
9. Keall, P.J., Mageras, G.S., Balter, J.M., Emery, R.S., Forster, K.M., Jiang, S.B., Kapatoes, J.M., Low, D.A., Murphy, M.J., Murray, B.R., Ramsey, C.R., Van Herk, M.B., Vedam, S.S., Wong, J.W., Yorke, E.: The management of respiratory motion in radiation oncology report of AAPM Task Group 76. Med. Phys. 33, 3874 (2006)
10. Kondermann, C., Mester, R., Garbe, C.S.: A statistical confidence measure for optical flows. In: Forsyth, D., Torr, P., Zisserman, A. (eds.) ECCV 2008, Part III. LNCS, vol. 5304, pp. 290–301. Springer, Heidelberg (2008)
11. Kybic, J., Nieuwenhuis, C.: Bootstrap optical flow confidence and uncertainty measure. Comput. Vis. Image. Und. 115, 1449 (2011)
12. McClelland, J., Hawkes, D.J., Schaeffter, T., King, A.P.: Respiratory motion models: a review. Med. Image Anal. 17, 19 (2013)
13. Patras, I., Hendriks, E.A., Lagendijk, R.L.: Probabilistic confidence measures for block matching motion estimation. IEEE Trans. Circuits Syst. Video Technol. 17(8), 988 (2007)
14. Petrusca, L., Cattin, P., De Luca, V., Preiswerk, F., Celicanin, Z., Auboiroux, V., Viallon, M., Arnold, P., Santini, F., Terraz, S., Scheffler, K., Becker, C.D., Salomir, R.: Hybrid Ultrasound/Magnetic Resonance Simultaneous Acquisition and Image Fusion for Motion Monitoring in the Upper Abdomen. Invest. Radiol. 48, 333 (2013)
15. Roujol, S., Moonen, C., De Senneville, B.D.: Motion correction techniques for MR-guided HIFU ablation of abdominal organs. Frontiers of Medical Imaging, 355 (2014)
16. Shirato, H., Shimizu, S., Kitamura, K., Onimaru, R.: Organ motion in image-guided radiotherapy: lessons from real-time tumor-tracking radiotherapy. Int. J. Clin. Oncol. 12, 8 (2007)
17. von Siebenthal, M., Szekely, G., Gamper, U., Boesiger, P., Lomax, A., Cattin, P.: 4D MR imaging of respiratory organ motion and its variability. Phys. Med. Biol. 52, 1547 (2007)
18. Simoncelli, E.P., Adelson, E.H., Heeger, D.J.: Probability distributions of optical flow. In: Proc. IEEE Int. Conf. Comp. Vis Pattern Recognit., p. 310 (1991)
19. Van Herk, M.: Errors and margins in radiotherapy. Seminars in Radiation Oncology 14, 52 (2004)

Solving Logistic Regression with Group Cardinality Constraints for Time Series Analysis

Yong Zhang[1] and Kilian M. Pohl[1,2]

[1] Department of Psychiatry and Behavioral Sciences, Stanford University, USA
[2] Center for Health Sciences, SRI International, USA

Abstract. We propose an algorithm to distinguish 3D+t images of healthy from diseased subjects by solving logistic regression based on cardinality constrained, group sparsity. This method reduces the risk of overfitting by providing an elegant solution to identifying anatomical regions most impacted by disease. It also ensures that consistent identification across the time series by grouping each image feature across time and counting the number of non-zero groupings. While popular in medical imaging, group cardinality constrained problems are generally solved by relaxing counting with summing over the groupings. We instead solve the original problem by generalizing a penalty decomposition algorithm, which alternates between minimizing a logistic regression function with a regularizer based on the Frobenius norm and enforcing sparsity. Applied to 86 cine MRIs of healthy cases and subjects with Tetralogy of Fallot (TOF), our method correctly identifies regions impacted by TOF and obtains a statistically significant higher classification accuracy than logistic regression without and relaxed grouped sparsity constraint.

1 Introduction

Identifying image phenotypes by automatically classifying 3D+t MRIs is popular in medical image analysis, such as for cardiac motion [1,2] and brain development [3,4]. Automatic classification is difficult due to the complex information captured by MRIs coupled with small sample sizes of most MRI studies. Besides avoiding overfitting, the image phenotypes extracted by the classifiers need to be meaningful to clinicians. To address both issues, group sparsity constrained logistic regression models [5,6] first reduce the dense image information to a small number of features by grouping image features via the l_2-norm and counting the number of non-zero groupings (l_0 "norm"). The identified groupings then often can be directly linked to specific anatomy or function. Motivated by [5,7], these methods generally find a solution by relaxing the l_0 "norm" to the sum over the l_2-norm values. However, this solution relates to the original sparse problem only in specific conditions, e.g. compressed sensing [8], which generally do not hold for medical image applications. We now propose an algorithm for solving the logistic regression problem with the group cardinality constraint and show on a data set of cine MRIs that it produces statistically significant better results than the corresponding approach based on the relaxed norm .

N. Navab et al. (Eds.): MICCAI 2015, Part III, LNCS 9351, pp. 459–466, 2015.
DOI: 10.1007/978-3-319-24574-4_55

Specifically, we model consistency constraints of disease patterns across the series of images via group sparsity, i.e. we group the weights associated with each image feature across time and then apply the l_0 "norm" to those groupings. We find a solution within this model by generalizing Penalty Decomposition (PD) [9] from solving sparse logistic regression problem with group size one to more than one. In detail, we decouple the logistic regression function from enforcing the group sparsity constraint by introducing a penalty term based on the Forbenius norm. We minimize the smooth and convex logistic regression with the penalty term via gradient descent and derive a closed form solution for the modified group sparsity problem. We then find a local minimum of the original problem by iteratively solving the two subproblems via block coordinate descent.

We apply our method to cine MRI of 40 patients with reconstructive surgery of Tetralogy of Fallot (TOF) and 46 healthy volunteers, whose diagnosis we view as ground truth. As the residual effects of TOF mostly impact the shape of the RV [10], the regions impacted by TOF should not change across time, i.e. an ideal test bed for our logistic regression approach. We encode each cine MRI by first non-rigidly registering the image series to a 3D+t template, which divides the left and right ventricle into subregions. For each of those regions, we then record the average of the Jacobian determinant of the deformation map.

We measure the accuracy of our model via five-fold cross-validation. During training, we automatically set all important parameters of our approach by first creating a separate classifier for each setting of the parameter space. We then reduce the risk of overfitting by combining those classifiers into a single *ensemble of classifiers* [11], i.e. we compute a weighted average across the outputs of the individual classifiers. As we will show later, the ensemble of classifiers correctly favors subregions of the ventricles most likely impacted by TOF. Furthermore, the accuracy of the ensemble of classifiers is statistically significant higher than the outcomes obtained by relaxing and omitting group cardinality constraint, i.e. the classical logistic regression model that keeps all regions for disease detection.

2 Solving Sparse Group Logistic Regression

Our aim is to train a classifier to correctly assign subjects to cohorts based on their corresponding image data. To do so, we first describe the logistic regression model with group cardinality constraint. We then find a solution within that model by generalizing the PD approach.

Model: We assume that our training set consists of N subjects that are represented by their corresponding diagnosis $\{b_1, \ldots, b_N\}$ and the encoding of 3D+t medical images $\{Z^1, \ldots, Z^N\}$ with T time points. The value of $b_s \in \{-1, +1\}$ depends on the subject 's' being healthy (+1) or diseased (−1). The corresponding feature matrix $Z^s := [z_1^s \; z_2^s \ldots z_T^s] \in \mathbb{R}^{M \times T}$ of that subject is composed of vectors $z_t^s \in \mathbb{R}^M$ encoding the tth frame with M features.

Next, we train the classifier on that data by solving the *logistic regression* problem confined by group sparsity. To define the problem, we introduce the variable $A^s := b_s \cdot Z^s$ for $s = 1, \ldots, N$, the weight matrix $W \in \mathbb{R}^{M \times T}$ defining the importance of each feature in correctly classifying 3D+t images, the trace of a matrix $\text{Tr}(\cdot)$, the logistic function $\theta(y) := \log(1 + \exp(-y))$, and the *average logistic loss* function with respect to the label weight $v \in \mathbb{R}$

$$l_{\text{avg}}(v, W) := \frac{1}{N} \sum_{s=1}^{N} \theta\left(\text{Tr}(W^\top A^s) + v \cdot b_s\right). \tag{1}$$

Ignoring the time point associated with each feature, we now assume that the disease is characterized by $r \in \mathbb{N}$ features, i.e. 'r' rows of the feature matrix Z^s subject to (s.t.) $r \leq M$. Then the logistic regression problem with group sparsity constraint is defined as

$$(\hat{v}, \widehat{W}) := \underset{v \in \mathbb{R}, W \in \mathbb{R}^{M \times T}}{\arg\min} \; l_{\text{avg}}(v, W) \;\text{ s.t. }\; \|\widetilde{W}\|_0 \leq r, \tag{2}$$

where $\widetilde{W} := (\|W^1\|_2, \ldots, \|W^M\|_2)^\top$ groups the weight vectors over time as $W^i := (W_1^i, \ldots, W_T^i)$ is the ith row of matrix W. Note, $\|\widetilde{W}\|_0$ equals the number of nonzero components of $\widetilde{W}$, i.e. the model accounts for the relationship of the same features across all the time points. Intuitively, if the model chooses a feature in one frame, the corresponding features in other frames should also be chosen since the importance of a feature should be similar across time. Replacing $\|\widetilde{W}\|_0$ with $\|W\|_0$ (or in the case of $T = 1$) results in the more common *sparse logistic regression* problem, which, in contrast, chooses individual features of W ignoring any temporal dependency, which is not desired for our application.

Algorithm: We find a local minimum to Eq. (2) by decoupling the minimization of $l_{\text{avg}}(\cdot, \cdot)$ from the sparsity constraint

$$\mathcal{X} := \{W \in \mathbb{R}^{M \times T} : \widetilde{W} := (\|W^1\|_2, \ldots, \|W^M\|_2)^\top \text{ and } \|\widetilde{W}\|_0 \leq r\}.$$

Specifically, we approximate the sparse weights $W \in \mathcal{X}$ via the unconstrained variable $Y \in \mathbb{R}^{M \times T}$ so that Eq. (2) changes to

$$(\hat{v}, \widehat{Y}, \widehat{W}) := \underset{v \in \mathbb{R}, Y \in \mathbb{R}^{M \times T}, W \in \mathcal{X}}{\arg\min} \; l_{\text{avg}}(v, Y) \;\text{ s.t. }\; W - Y = 0. \tag{3}$$

Denoting with $\varrho > 0$ a penalty parameter and the matrix Frobenius norm with $\|\cdot\|_F$, we solve Eq. (3) by generalizing PD proposed in [9] from enforcing the cardinality constraint for group size $T = 1$ to $T \geq 1$, i.e. we obtain a local solution $(\hat{v}, \widehat{Y}, \widehat{W})$ of the following nonconvex problem

$$\min_{v \in \mathbb{R}, Y \in \mathbb{R}^{M \times T}, W \in \mathcal{X}} f(v, Y, W) = l_{\text{avg}}(v, Y) + \frac{\varrho}{2}\|W - Y\|_F^2. \tag{4}$$

Ascending ϱ at each iteration, we use Block Coordinate Descent (BCD) to determine the solution by alternating between minimizing Eq. (4) with fixed W and by fixing v and Y. When W is set to W', finding the minimum with respect to v and Y turns into a smooth and convex problem

$$(v', Y') \leftarrow \underset{v \in \mathbb{R}, Y \in \mathbb{R}^{M \times T}}{\arg\min} \left\{ l_{\text{avg}}(v, Y) + \frac{\varrho}{2}\|W' - Y\|_F^2 \right\}, \tag{5}$$

which can be solved via a gradient descent. In turn, minimizing the objective function just with respect to W, i.e.

$$W' \leftarrow \arg\min_{W \in \mathcal{X}} \|W - Y'\|_F^2, \tag{6}$$

can now be solved in closed form. We derive the closed form solution by assuming (without loss of generality) that the rows of Y' are nonzero and listed in descending order according to their l_2-norm, i.e. let $(Y')^i$ be the ith row of Y' for $i = 1, \ldots, M$ then $\|(Y')^1\|_2 \geq \|(Y')^2\|_2 \geq \ldots \geq \|(Y')^M\|_2 > 0$. It can then be easily shown (see [1]) that W' is defined by the first 'r' rows of Y', i.e.

$$(W')^i = \begin{cases} (Y')^i, & \text{if } i \leq r; \\ 0, & \text{otherwise,} \end{cases} \quad \text{for } i = 1, \ldots, M. \tag{7}$$

In theory, the global solution derived above is not unique for Eq. (6), which we have not experienced in practice. One can also prove (similar to [9]) that the method converges with respect to $\varrho \rightarrow +\infty$ to a local minimum of Eq. (2).

3 Characterizing TOF Based on Cine MRIs

We apply our approach to cine MRIs of 40 TOF cases and 46 healthy controls. We choose this dataset due to the ground-truth diagnosis, i.e. each subject received reconstructive surgery for TOF during infancy or not. Furthermore, refining the quantitative analysis of these scans could lead to improved timing for follow-up surgeries in TOF patients. Finally, the assumption of our group sparsity model, i.e. the features extracted from each time point of the image series are sample descriptions of the same phenomena, fits well to this dataset. As we describe next, the features of this experiment are deformation-based shape encodings of the heart. As the residual effects of TOF reconstructive surgery mostly impact the shape of the right ventricle [10], our encoding should capture differences between the two groups in the same heart regions across time. We not only show that this is the case but our approach defined by Eq. (2) achieves significantly higher accuracy than logistic regression with relaxed sparsity constraints, i.e. given the sparse regularizing parameter λ solving

$$\min_{v \in \mathbb{R}, W \in \mathbb{R}^{M \times T}} l_{\text{avg}}(v, W) + \lambda \sum_{i=1}^{M} \|W^i\|_2, \tag{8}$$

and without sparsity constraints, *i.e.*, $\lambda = 0$. Note we omit comparison to implementations replacing the l_2-norm in Eq. (8) with the l_1-norm since the resulting regularizor ignores consistency of the features across time. In other words, the regions identified by those approaches most likely have no relevance with respect to TOF, whose residual effects should be consistent across time.

Extract Image Feature: All 86 cine MR scans are defined by 30 time points. Each time point of a cine MRI is represented by a 3D image and a semi-automatically segmented label map of the right ventricular blood pool (RV)

[1] `http://www.stanford.edu/~yzhang83/MICCAI2015_supplement.pdf`

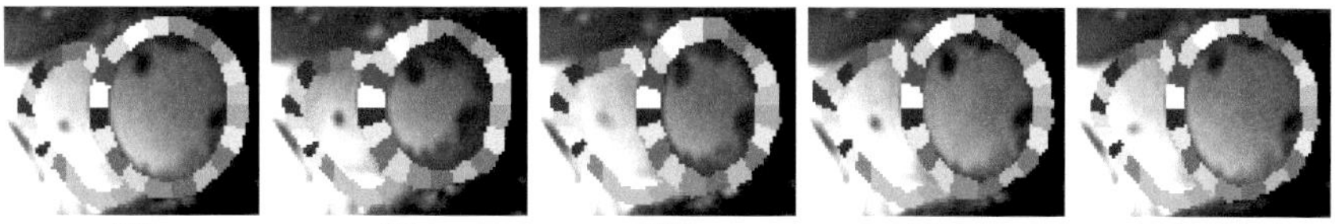

Fig. 1. Example of partitioning the template at different time points (T1 to T25) of the heart cycle. Each section of the RV is subtended by 9° and by 18° for the LV.

and the myocardium of the left ventricle (LV). Based on those segmentations, we omitted non cardiac structures from the scans and corrected each scan for image inhomogeneity and slice motion [12]. Next, we randomly choose the first time point of a healthy subject as a template and rigidly registered each case to the template. We encode the shape of the RV and LV by non-rigidly registering (via Demon's approach [13]) each time point of the remaining 85 scans to the template. We then compute the Jacobian determinant of the deformation maps [14]. We confine the determinant maps to the LV segmentations and for the RV reduce the maps to a 7mm band along its boundary, which is similar to the width of the LV myocardium. We also parcellate the RV and LV into smaller regions by first computing its corresponding mass center and then sectoring it into region of interests by the subtended angles as shown in Fig. (1). We finalize our shape descriptor by mapping the refined Jacobians into the template space and computing their average value with respect to individual sections. The size of the sections are defined with respect to degrees.

Measure Accuracy: We measure the accuracy of our approach via five-fold cross validation. We define the parameter space of the smoothness parameter $p = \{0, 0.5, \ldots, 5.0\}$ of the Demon's algorithm, the subtended angle $d = \{45°, 36°, 30°, 24°, 20°, 18°, 15°, 12°, 10°, 8°, 6°, 5°, 4°\}$ of each section of the LV and RV, and the sparsity constraint $r \in \{5, 10, \ldots, 50\}$, i.e. the number of average regional values chosen by our approach. Note, that we choose such a broad parameter space to allow for a fair comparison with other logistic regression models. For each parameter setting, we specify a regressor by computing the optimal weights $\widehat{W}$ with respect to training data. We do so by initializing the penalty parameter ρ at 0.1 and increase ρ by a factor of $\sqrt{10}$ at each PD iteration until convergence, *i.e.*, $\|\widehat{W} - \widehat{Y}\|_F^2 \leq 10^{-3} \cdot f(v, \widehat{Y}, \widehat{W})$. We also compute its training accuracy with respect to correctly assigning cine MRIs to each patient group. We account for the imbalance in cohort size by computing the normalized accuracy (nAcc), i.e. we separately compute the accuracy for each cohort and then average their values. On our dataset, parameter exploration on the training set resulted in multiple settings with 100% training accuracy. We therefore cross-validate a classifier based on training a single ensemble of classifiers [11]. We do so by treating the training nAcc score of a regressor as its weight in the decision of the ensemble of classifiers. In other words, the final label is then determined by the weighted average across the set of regressors, all of whom have different parameter settings. We also refer to this ensemble of classifier as $\boldsymbol{l_0}$**-Grp**. Fig. (2) shows the weight of each region according to the l_0-Grp across time. We notice

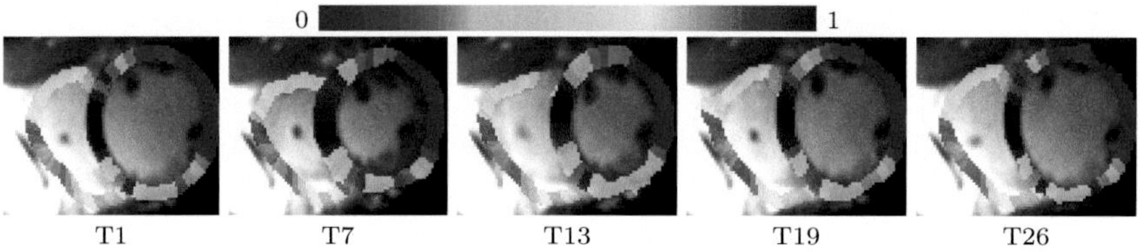

Fig. 2. Regions weighted by importance according to the proposed l_0-Grp approach. The sparsity constraints correctly identified the RV (left side) and specifically the right ventricular outflow tract (the regions where RV and LV meet) as important markers for identifying the residual TOF effects.

that the weights are fairly consistent across time due to the group sparsity term. In addition, the maps correctly point out (in red and yellow) the importance of the RV (left side) and more specifically the right ventricular outflow tract (the area where RV meets the LV) in identifying TOF.

Alternative Models: For comparison, we also generated an ensemble of logistic regression classifiers omitting the sparsity constraint (called **No-Grp**) and one by relaxing the group cardinality constraint (called **Rlx-Grp**) as defined by Eq. (8) [15]. These ensembles of classifiers used the same parameter space for the smoothness parameter p and the subtended angle d of each section. For Rlx-Grp, the sparsity parameter λ of Eq. (8) was automatically set so that the number of chosen group features were similar to the group cardinality, i.e. $\{5, 10, \ldots, 50\}$. We applied each ensemble implementation to the dataset of just the LV, RV, and both ventricles.

Classification Results: The accuracy scores in % of all three ensembles are listed in Table 1 with respect to the encoding of the LV, RV, and both ventricles (LV&RV). Scores in bold represent results, which are significantly better (p-value < 0.05) than those of the other two methods. We compute the p-value based on the DeLongs Test [16] of the methods' ROC curves.

All three methods have similar accuracy scores for the LV (around 74.5%). As expected, the accuracy scores of all methods improve (by at least 9.9%) when the classification is based on the RV. The scores further improve for No-Grp and l_0-Grp by including both ventricles in the analysis. The increase in the score of l_0-Grp is explained by looking at the weight map of LV&RV in Fig. (3) (a), which, compared to the map of RV only in Fig. (3) (b), also highlights part of the LV. The impact of TOF on the LV was also recently echoed by [10].

Not only does the proposed l_0-Grp achieve the overall best score with 94% but the scores involving the RV are significantly better than those of the other two methods (p-values ≤ 0.036). While these results further validate the proposed group cardinality constraint model for logistic regression, the relatively poor accuracy scores by Rlx-Grp is somewhat surprising (84.7%). Comparing the regional weight maps of the two approaches (see Fig. (3) (a) + (d)), the map of Rlx-Grp mostly ignores the RV failing to identify regions impacted by TOF. It not only explains the relatively low score but further highlights the superiority of the group cardinality over the l_2-norm relaxation with respect to this experiment.

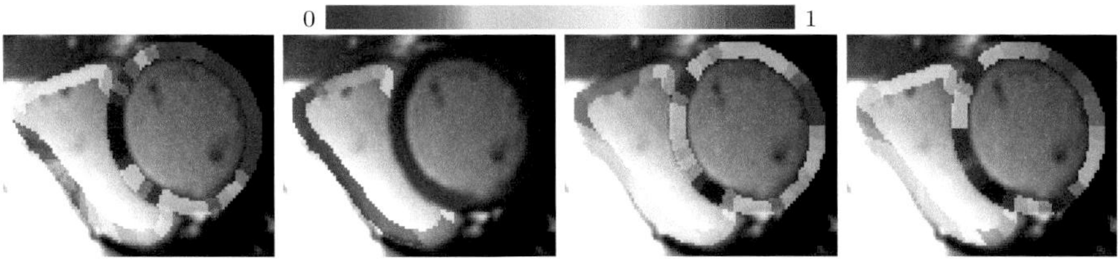

(a) l_0-Grp RV&LV (b) l_0-Grp RV only (c) l_0-Grp 1st TP only (d) Rlx-Grp RV&LV

Fig. 3. Regions of the first time point weighted by importance according to different implementations: l_0-Grp based on RV&LV (a), just based on the RV (b), based only on the first time point (c), and l_0-Grp based on RV&LV (d). Note, implementations putting more emphasis on the RV (a+b) are those with the higher accuracy scores.

Table 1. Accuracy scores (nAcc) in % of No-Grp, Rlx-Grp, and our proposed model (l_0-Grp). As expected, all methods achieve higher accuracy scores based on RV encoding vs. LV encoding. Including both ventricles in the analysis, leads to higher accuracy scores for No-Grp and the proposed l_0-Grp. The bold accuracy scores of l_0-Grp are significantly higher ($p\text{-value} < 0.05$) than the other two implementations, which was the case for the two experiments including the RV.

	LV	RV	LV&RV
No-Grp	74.5	85.1	86.2
Rlx-Grp	74.8	84.7	83.8
l_0-Grp	74.1	**91.8**	**94.0**

To study the importance of the group-sparsity over just sparsity, we confined l_0-Grp to the first time point, i.e. reducing the sparsity term to the cardinality constraint without group constraint. The accuracy of l_0-Grp dropped for all three experiments by a minimum of 4.5%. The weight map in Fig. (3) (c) reveals the reason for the drop in accuracy as it puts less emphasis on the RV. Furthermore, its scores are now similar to those of No-Grp (less than 2.5% difference). We therefore conclude that the l_0 group sparsity takes proper advantage of the repeat samples of the same disease patterns provided by the image time series.

4 Conclusion

We proposed an algorithm for solving logistic regression based on the group cardinality constraint. Unlike existing approaches, our algorithm did not relax the l_0-norm regularizer but instead used penalty decomposition to solve the original problem. Applied to 86 cine MRIs of healthy cases and subjects with TOF, our method not only correctly identified regions impacted by TOF but also obtains statistically significant higher classification accuracy than logistic regression without and with relaxed group sparsity constraints.

Acknowledgement. We would like to thank DongHye Ye for his help on generating the cardiac 515 dataset. This project was supported in part by the NIH grant R01HL127661. It was also supported by the Creative and Novel Ideas in HIV Research Program through a supplement to NIH P30 AI027763. This funding was made possible by collaborative efforts of the Office of AIDS Research, the National Institutes of Allergies and Infectious Diseases, and the International AIDS Society.

References

1. Yu, Y., Zhang, S., Li, K., Metaxas, D., Axel, L.: Deformable models with sparsity constraints for cardiac motion analysis. Med. Image Anal. 18(6), 927–937 (2014)
2. van Assen, H.C., Danilouchkine, M.G., Frangi, A.F., Ordás, S., Westenberg, J.J.M., Reiber, J.H.C., Lelieveldt, B.: SPASM: Segmentation of sparse and arbitrarily oriented cardiac MRI data using a 3D-ASM. In: Frangi, A.F., Radeva, P., Santos, A., Hernandez, M. (eds.) FIMH 2005. LNCS, vol. 3504, pp. 33–43. Springer, Heidelberg (2005)
3. Serag, A., Gousias, I.S., Makropoulos, A., Aljabar, P., Hajnal, J.V., Boardman, J.P., Counsell, S.J., Rueckert, D.: Unsupervised learning of shape complexity: Application to brain development. In: Durrleman, S., Fletcher, T., Gerig, G., Niethammer, M. (eds.) STIA 2012. LNCS, vol. 7570, pp. 88–99. Springer, Heidelberg (2012)
4. Bernal-Rusiel, J.L., Reuter, M., Greve, D.N., Fischl, B., Sabuncu, M.R.: Spatiotemporal linear mixed effects modeling for the mass-univariate analysis of longitudinal neuroimage data. NeuroImage 81, 358–370 (2013)
5. Meier, L., Van De Geer, S., Bühlmann, P.: The group lasso for logistic regression. J. Roy. Soc. Ser. B 70(1), 53–71 (2008)
6. Wu, F., Yuan, Y., Zhuang, Y.: Heterogeneous feature selection by group lasso with logistic regression. In: ACM-MM, pp. 983–986 (2010)
7. Friedman, J., Hastie, T., Tibshirani, R.: A note on the group lasso and a sparse group lasso. arXiv preprint arXiv:1001.0736 (2010)
8. Candès, E.J., Romberg, J., Tao, T.: Robust uncertainty principles: Exact signal reconstruction from highly incomplete frequency information. IEEE Trans. Inf. Theory 52(2), 489–509 (2006)
9. Lu, Z., Zhang, Y.: Sparse approximation via penalty decomposition methods. SIAM J. Optim. 23(4), 2448–2478 (2013)
10. Atrey, P.K., Hossain, M.A., El Saddik, A., Kankanhalli, M.S.: Multimodal fusion for multimedia analysis: a survey. Multimedia Syst. 16(6), 345–379 (2010)
11. Rokach, L.: Ensemble-based classifiers. Artif. Intell. Rev. 33(1-2), 1–39 (2010)
12. Ye, D., Desjardins, B., Hamm, J., Litt, H., Pohl, K.: Regional manifold learning for disease classification. IEEE T. Med. Imaging 33(6), 1236–1247 (2014)
13. Vercauteren, T., Pennec, X., Perchant, A., Ayache, N.: Diffeomorphic demons: Efficient non-parametric image registration. NeuroImage 45(1), S61–S72 (2009)
14. Shen, D., Davatzikos, C.: Very high-resolution morphometry using mass-preserving deformations and hammer elastic registration. NeuroImage 18(1), 28–41 (2003)
15. Liu, J., Ji, S., Ye, J.: SLEP: Sparse Learning with Efficient Projections. Arizona State University (2009)
16. DeLong, E., DeLong, D., Clarke-Pearson, D.: Comparing the areas under two or more correlated receiver operating characteristic curves: a nonparametric approach. Biometrics 44(3), 837–845 (1988)

Spatiotemporal Parsing of Motor Kinematics for Assessing Stroke Recovery

Borislav Antic[1,⋆], Uta Büchler[1,⋆], Anna-Sophia Wahl[2], Martin E. Schwab[2], and Björn Ommer[1]

[1] HCI/IWR, Heidelberg University, Germany
[2] Department of HST, ETH Zurich, Switzerland

Abstract. Stroke is a major cause of adult disability and rehabilitative training is the prevailing approach to enhance motor recovery. However, the way rehabilitation helps to restore lost motor functions by continuous reshaping of kinematics is still an open research question. We follow the established setup of a rat model before/after stroke in the motor cortex to analyze the subtle changes in hand motor function solely based on video. Since nuances of paw articulation are crucial, mere tracking and trajectory analysis is insufficient. Thus, we propose an automatic spatiotemporal parsing of grasping kinematics based on a max-projection of randomized exemplar classifiers. A large ensemble of these discriminative predictors of hand posture is automatically learned and yields a measure of grasping similarity. This non-parametric distributed representation effectively captures the nuances of hand posture and its deformation over time. A max-margin projection then not only quantifies functional deficiencies, but also back-projects them accurately to specific defects in the grasping sequence to provide neuroscience with a better understanding of the precise effects of rehabilitation. Moreover, evaluation shows that our fully automatic approach is reliable and more efficient than the prevalent manual analysis of the day.

1 Introduction

Generation and control of movements are fundamental requirements to interact and respond to the environment. Complex hand functions such as grasping depend on well-orchestrated and precisely coordinated sequences of motor actions. When a stroke occurs, they are often impaired and the subject suffers from lost skilled motor functions. Studying motor impairment and establishing new therapeutic strategies, is a key challenge of neuroscience typically conducted in rodents to provide, as demonstrated in [1,2], information about the human model too. Often a tedious visual inspection of the grasping function is the only means to determine outcome levels after stroke. To tackle this challenge, we propose a fully automatic approach for analyzing the kinematics of grasping. These characteristic patterns of hand deformation are significantly more intricate than mere trajectories shown in Fig. 1. Our goal is not only to identify *if* motor function is impaired, but also *how* exactly the limb paresis affects grasping.

⋆ Indicates equal contribution.

N. Navab et al. (Eds.): MICCAI 2015, Part III, LNCS 9351, pp. 467–475, 2015.
DOI: 10.1007/978-3-319-24574-4_56

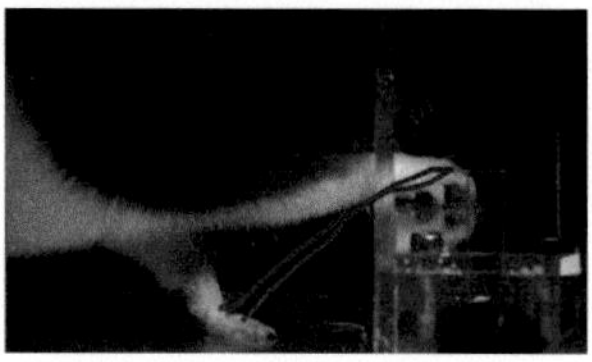

Fig. 1. Side view (cutout) of a rat performing single pellet grasping in a Plexiglas box with opening at the side. The paw trajectory of a successful grasp is superimposed (time running from blue to red).

To accurately represent and detect paws we extend the powerful exemplar-based paradigm by max-projection of randomized versions of an exemplar classifier. A large set of these paw classifiers is then aggregated to define similarities between hand postures and group them. Grasping is characterized by the deformation of the paw over time. Since we also need to represent the vastly different abnormal grasps of impaired animals, neither priors on the smoothness of kinematics, nor explicit models for a grasp are appropriate. Therefore, we propose a non-parametric representation that is based on robust matching of grasp sequences. Using this compact model, max-margin multiple-instance learning yields a classifier that not only recognizes impaired grasping but also identifies fragments of a grasp that are characteristically altered due to the injury.

This study analyzes the recovery of motor function in Long-Evans rats performing single pellet grasping [3] before and after a photothrombotic stroke destroys the corresponding sensorimotor cortex of the grasping paw. We compare recovery under *i)* a rehabilitative therapy (*Anti-Nogo* neuronal growth promoting immunotherapy followed by rehabilitation [4], denoted green group), *ii)* for a cohort without treatment (red), *iii)* and a control of sham operated rats (black).

Due to its importance for understanding and analyzing motor function, there has been considerable effort on analyzing grasping behavior. A main focus has been on studying hand trajectories [5,4], thus ignoring the crucial, intricate kinematics of hand motion [1], which involve the temporal deformation of fingers and the overall shape of the hand. Representing, detecting, and distinguishing the fine articulation of small, hairy, fast moving fingers of a rat paw under self-occlusion, noise, and variations between animals pose tremendous challenges for evaluation. Consequently, previous studies mainly rely on tedious manual identification of hand posture in individual video frames [5,1,2]. In large evaluations, motion analysis is often simplified by applying reflective motion capture markers [6] or even electromagnetic tracking gloves [7]. However, these techniques are typically used on human or primate subjects but are not applicable to rats, due to the small size of their paws and distraction that attached devises impose. In [8] human hand is tracked by relying on depth from structured light, which is too coarse and slow for the fast moving, small rat paws. Moreover, [8] discard appearance and solely depend on weak contour information and articulation models of normal hands, which are not appropriate for abnormal locomotion after stroke.

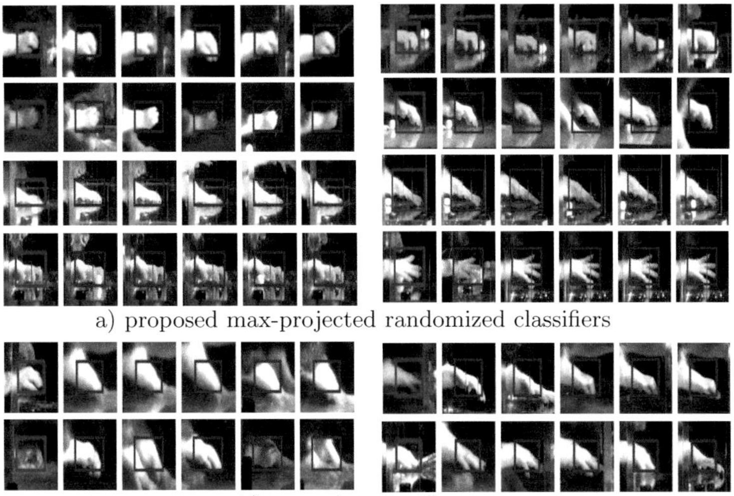

a) proposed max-projected randomized classifiers

b) exemplar classifiers

Fig. 2. a) Subset of our pooled classifiers proposed in Sect. 2.2. For each classifier (blue) we show the five best detections on query videos (magenta). Note the subtle difference that the model captures, such as pronation (1st row left), supination (2nd row left), or the different stages of hand closure (1st, 2nd row right). b) Baseline: Subset of classifiers trained by exemplar Support Vector Machine (SVM) [9] without our pooling. The matches are significantly less specific than the proposed approach.

2 Approach

2.1 Creating Candidate Foreground Regions

To focus our analysis on hand motor function we first extract a large set of candidate foreground regions. Following [10] we decompose frames of video into a low-rank background model and a sparse vector corresponding to foreground pixels. Candidate regions $x_i \in \mathcal{X}$ are then randomly sampled from the estimated foreground of a set of sample videos to initialize the subsequent learning of classifiers and compute their HOG features (size 10×10). K-Nearest Neighbors density estimation then reveals rare outliers, which are then removed from $\mathcal{X}$.

2.2 Robust Exemplar Classification

We seek a representation of rat paws that i) facilitates detection and tracking of hands in novel videos and ii) exposes the subtle differences in hand posture, while being robust to noise, illumination differences, and intra-class variability.

Max-projected Randomized Exemplar Classifiers: To measure the similarity to a sampled region x_i, we train a discriminative exemplar classifier w_i, using x_i as positive example. Since $\mathcal{X}$ likely contains other samples similar to x_i, we cannot use all remaining samples in $\mathcal{X}$ as negatives for training or perform hard negative mining [9]—too much overlap with the single positive makes

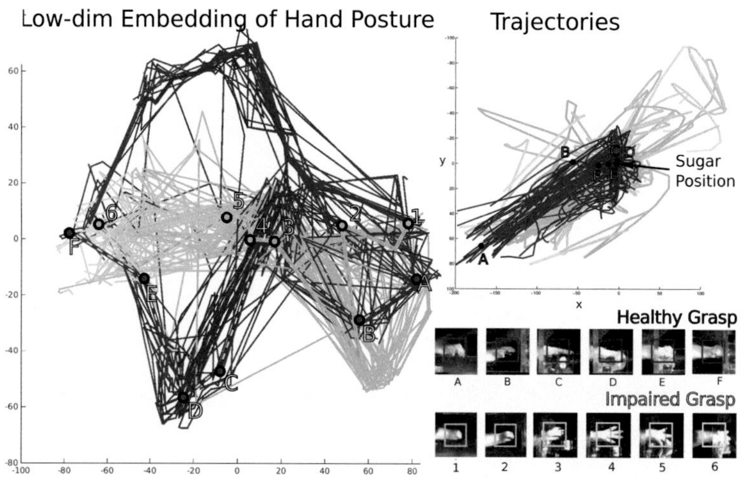

Fig. 3. *Left:* Paws are represented using the proposed non-parametric representation of hand posture. A distance preserving embedding then maps all detected hands onto 2D and straight lines connect successive frames within a single grasp. Time is encoded as blue to red for healthy animals and cyan to yellow for impaired 2 days post stroke. For one healthy and one impaired grasping sequence selected frames (marked as 1,2,.. and A,B,.. along the sequence) are shown *bottom right.* On *top right* the grasping trajectories of all grasps are depicted relative to the position of the sugar pellet at the origin. The non-parametric representation of postures helps to accurately distinguish impaired grasping patterns from healthy ones and emphasizes characteristic abnormal postures within individual grasps, such as D vs. 4.

learning unreliable. Thus we train in Eq. 1 an ensemble of K exemplar classifiers w_i^k with their offsets b_i^k, $k \in \{1, \dots, K\}$, using randomly selected negative sets $\mathcal{X}_i^k \subset \mathcal{X} \backslash x_i$. The soft margin parameter $C = .01$ was chosen via cross-validation.

$$\min_{w_i^k, b_i^k} \|w_i^k\|^2 + C \max\big(0, 1 - \langle w_i^k, x_i\rangle - b_i^k\big) + \frac{C}{|X_i^k|} \sum_{j=1}^{|X_i^k|} \max\big(0, 1 + \langle w_i^k, x_j\rangle + b_i^k\big). \quad (1)$$

To compensate for the unreliability of individual classifiers, we aggregate them using a max-projection that selects for each feature dimension the most confident classifier $w_i(\bullet) := \max_k w_i^k(\bullet)$. The scores of these max-projected randomized exemplar classifiers w_i are then calibrated by a logistic regression [9].

Dictionary of Paw Classifiers: Now we reduce the large candidate set $\mathcal{X}$ (size 1000) and create a dictionary $\mathcal{D} \subseteq \mathcal{X}$ to canonically represent hand postures of previously unseen rats. The randomized exemplar classifiers provide a robust measure of pair-wise similarity $s(x_i, x_j) := \frac{1}{2}\big(\langle w_i, x_j\rangle + \langle w_j, x_i\rangle\big)$. Redundant candidates are merged by Normalized Cuts to obtain a dictionary $\mathcal{D}$ (size 100) that is sufficiently diverse and rich non-parametric representation of all viable hand-postures.[1] See Fig. 2 for examples and a comparison to standard exemplars.

[1] A coarser discretization is possible by discarding elements with small contribution.

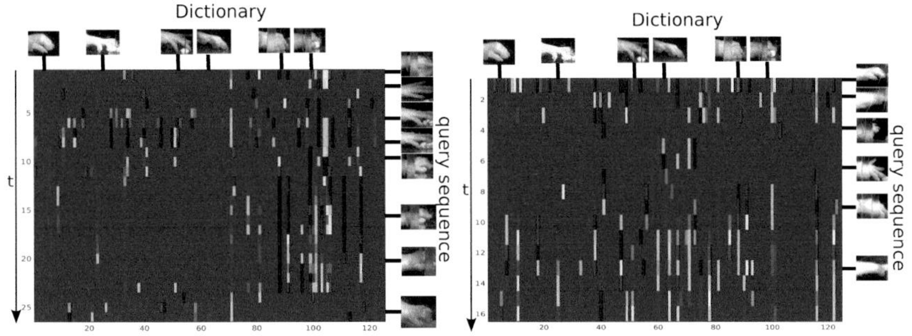

Fig. 4. Representation of hand posture for all frames of a successful (left) and a failed grasping sequence (right). On each query frame (rows) all classifiers (columns) from the dictionary of characteristic hand configurations of Sect. 2.2 are evaluated. In this representation successful grasps typically first exhibit activations of pronation, followed by a characteristic opening and closing (t=4..10, left) and retraction of the closed hand.

In a new video all classifiers w_i from dictionary $\mathcal{D}$ are applied densely. Averaging the scores of the top scoring k classifiers and taking the location with the highest score yields the final paw detection and its trajectories over time, Fig. 3.

Non-parametric Representation of Hand Posture: On a novel paw sample x the joint activation pattern of all $\{w_i\}_{i\in\mathcal{D}}$ yields an embedding $e := [\langle w_1, x\rangle, \ldots, \langle w_{|\mathcal{D}|}, x\rangle]$. Moreover, novel hand configurations can now be related by comparing their embedding vectors, since similar samples give rise to similar classifier activations. To visualize a hand posture, the high-dimensional embedding is mapped to a low-dimensional projection using the t-SNE method [11].

2.3 Spatiotemporal Parsing

While hand posture is a crucial factor, its deformation during a grasp is even more decisive. We represent an M frame long grasp j as a sequence in the embedding space $S_j := [e_1^j, \ldots, e_M^j]$. Measuring the similarity of grasps based on their embeddings requires a sequence matching since they are not temporally aligned. We thus seek a mapping $\pi : \{1,\ldots,M\} \mapsto \{0,\ldots,M'\}$ that aligns S_j of length M with $S_{j'}$ of length M' (0 denotes outliers), cf. Fig. 5. Their distance is then defined in the embedding space as $d(S_j, S_{j'}) := \sum_{i=1}^{M} \|e_i^j - e_{\pi(i)}^{j'}\|$. A matching $\pi(\bullet)$ should penalize outliers and variations in the temporal order,

$$\min_{\pi} \sum_{i=1}^{M} \|e_i^j - e_{\pi(i)}^{j'}\| + \lambda \sum_{i=1}^{M-1} \mathbf{1}\big(\pi(i) > \pi(i+1)\big), \text{ s.t. } |\pi(i) - i| \leq B, \forall i, \quad (2)$$

where $\mathbf{1}(\cdot)$ denotes the identity function. The constraint in Eq. 2 prevents matched frames to be more than B frames apart from each other. The second sum in

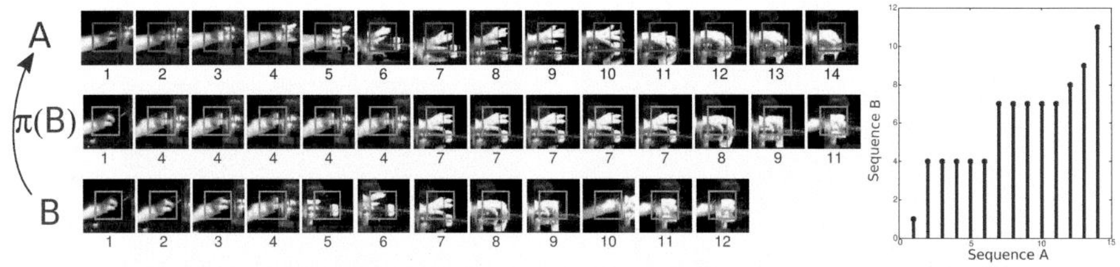

Fig. 5. Sequence matching: Sequence A is matched to B by permuting and warping this sequence into $\pi(B)$ using the approach of Sect. 2.3. Frames are numbered and the permutations $\pi(\bullet)$ are shown on the right.

Fig. 6. Novel grasps are represented by automatically explaining them with a compact set of prototypical grasping sequences (Sect. 2.3), yielding an embedding. For all animals of the black (sham control), green (therapy), and red (no treatment) cohort the mean representation of all graspings of a trial session is visualized by distance preserving projection to a 3D subspace. The mean representations of successive trial sessions are then connected to show recovery within each cohort (time runs from dark to light, from 4 weeks before stroke to 4 weeks after). Note that black and green cohort show similar final recovery, whereas red ends up close to its state 2 days post stroke, indicating only little recovery (the red loop at right is actually elevated and far away from the others).

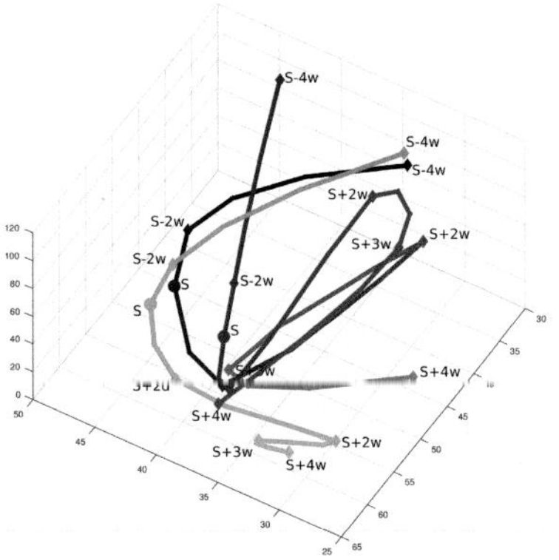

Eq. 2 allows for more flexible matching than the standard string matching or dynamic time warping. Substitution $z_{i,i'_1,i'_2} := \mathbf{1}(\pi(i) = i'_1 \wedge \pi(i+1) = i'_2)$ in Eq. 2 transforms the sequence matching problem to an integer linear program (ILP),

$$\max_{z_\bullet \in \{0,1\}} \sum_{i=1}^{M-1} \sum_{i'_1,i'_2=0}^{M'} z_{i,i'_1,i'_2} \psi_{i,i'_1,i'_2}, \text{ s.t. } \sum_{i'_1,i'_2=0}^{M'} z_{i,i'_1,i'_2} = 1 \wedge \sum_{i'_1=0}^{M'} z_{i,i'_1,i'_2} = \sum_{i'_3=0}^{M'} z_{i+1,i'_2,i'_3}, \tag{3}$$

where ψ_{i,i'_1,i'_2} is the sum of all terms in Eq. 2 that correspond to $z_{i,i'_1,i'_2} = 1$. IBM ILOG CPLEX software is applied to solve Eq. 3 (tenth of a second for sequences of 30 frames).

Due to a large number of grasping actions in our dataset, it is computationally prohibitive to match a novel sequence to all others. Thus we reduce redundancy as in Sect. 2.2 and construct a dictionary $\mathcal{D}_{seq} := \{S_1, \ldots, S_Q\}$ with canonical grasping sequences that then explain novel grasps yielding a spatiotemporal parsing. Measuring the distances of a new sequence S' to all prototypical ones in $\mathcal{D}_{seq}$ yields the sequence-level embedding $E' := [d(S', S_1), ..., d(S', S_Q)]$, after aligning grasps by our sequence matching to compute distances.

2.4 Automatic Grasping Diagnostics

Multiple instance learning (MIL) [12] is utilized to train an SVM on few successful pre-stroke grasps against failed grasps from directly after stroke using the representation from Sect. 2.3. Since even before stroke there are failed attempts, the pre-stroke grasps are randomly aggregated in bags (20 attempts per bag) and the successful positive training samples are inferred using MIL. To diagnose a novel grasping sequence S', the MIL trained linear SVM is applied before transforming the classifier scores into the probability of a grasping sequence being abnormal. To automatically discover what made a grasp fail and how impaired motor function manifests, we back-project the kernel-based sequence representation onto frames that are indicative for grasping failure, i.e., the parts of the sequence that have highest responsibility for yielding a bad SVM score, Sect. 3.

3 Experimental Results

Recording Setup: For the three cohorts of 10 rats described in Sect. 1, grasping has been filmed from the side, cf. Fig. 1, with a Panasonic HDC-SD800 camcorder at 50fps, shutter 1/3000, ~8 hours of video in total. Recording sessions were -4, -2, 2, 3, 4 weeks before/after stroke, each with 100 grasp trials per animal per session, yielding in total 15000 individual grasps for evaluation of our analysis.

Grasping Diagnostics: In an initial experiment we computed paw trajectories during grasping, Fig. 3 (top right). However, since the unilateral stroke has most impact on the fine motor skills of the hand rather than the full arm, its implications for grasping are only truly revealed by the detailed analysis of hand posture, Fig. 3 (left). From a neurophysiological view, this unsupervised analysis reveals characteristics of impaired grasping such as incorrect supination (D vs. 4), evident by the large distances between healthy and impaired kinematics especially around the moment of pellet capture (C,D). The difference in hand posture around this moment is also evident around t=4..10 in Fig. 4.

Fig. 6 visualizes the recovery of all animals within one cohort by averaging over all their grasp trials conducted at the same time pre/post stroke. This unsupervised approach highlights the positive effect of the rehabilitation during the recovery process. Based on the same sequence representation, the classifier of Sect. 2.4 predicts if grasps are healthy or impaired in Fig. 8. This analysis not only underlines the positive outcome of the therapy, but also compare our prediction of fitness of a grasp against a manual labeling provided by 5 experts. They accurately annotated sequences as 1, .5, 0 if they were successful, partially successful (correct up to final supination), or failed. Statistical hypothesis testing, Tab. 1, shows that our automatic prediction compares favorably with manual annotations (p-value between .002 and .02, two-tailed t-test capturing deviations

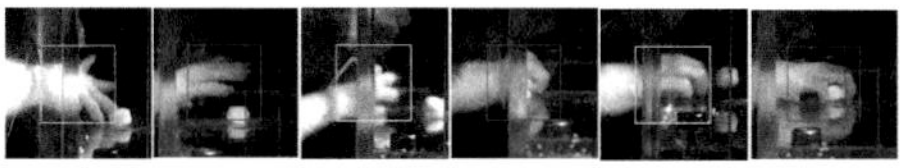

Fig. 7. Examples of hand postures that deteriorated grasping fitness (yellow) vs. those that improved it (magenta).

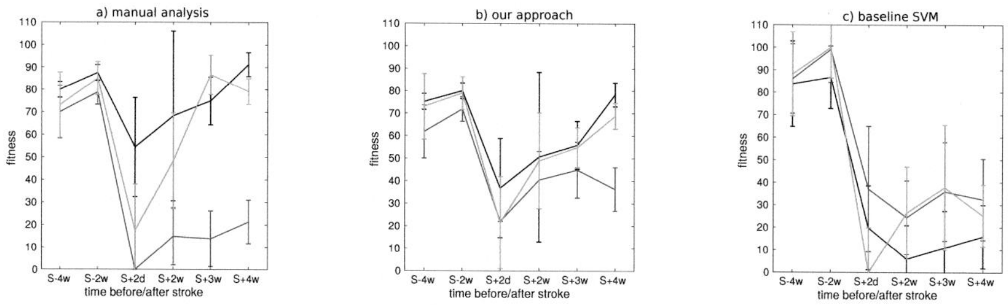

Fig. 8. Prediction of grasping fitness using a) manual analysis by neuroscientists, b) our approach, c) baseline SVM approach

Table 1. Comparing predictions of our approach Fig. 8b) and of the baseline approach (no randomized pooling and sequence matching) 8c) against the manual annotation of neuroscientists 8a). Overall our approach significantly improves upon the baseline.

	Our Approach			Baseline SVM		
Cohort	p-value	RMSE	R^2	p-value	RMSE	R^2
Sham control (black)	0.002	4.06	0.927	0.401	13.6	0.18
No treatment (red)	0.004	11.8	0.896	0.003	11.1	0.909
Therapy (green)	0.019	14.2	0.779	0.161	23	0.425

in both directions from the ground truth) and are significantly more robust than a baseline approach without the proposed randomized pooling and sequence matching. Finally we also retrieve frames of an impaired sequence that mostly deteriorated the grasp by causing bad alignments in sequence matching, Fig. 7.

4 Conclusion

To analyze grasping function and its restoration after stroke we have presented a fully automatic video-based approach. Details of hand posture are captured by a non-parametric representation based on a large set of max-projected randomized exemplar classifiers. The spatiotemporal kinematics of grasping is then explained by a robust sequence matching. With this representation an unsupervised and a supervised approach have been presented to automatically analyze the recovery after stroke and predict the impairment of individual grasps. This approach has the potential to open up new possibilities of studying motor restoration over time and evaluating the efficiency of therapeutic interventions after stroke.[2]

[2] This research has been funded in part by the Ministry for Science, Baden-Wuerttemberg and the Heidelberg Academy of Sciences, Heidelberg, Germany.

References

1. Alaverdashvili, M., Whishaw, I.Q.: A behavioral method for identifying recovery and compensation: hand use in a preclinical stroke model using the single pellet reaching task. Neurosci. Biobehav. Rev. 37, 950–967 (2013)
2. Sacrey, L.A., Alaverdashvili, M., Whishaw, I.Q.: Similar hand shaping in reaching-for-food (skilled reaching) in rats and humans provides evidence of homology in release, collection, and manipulation movements. Behav. Brain Res. (2009)
3. Metz, G.A., Whishaw, I.Q.: Skilled reaching an action pattern: stability in rat (rattus norvegicus) grasping movements as a function of changing food pellet size. Behav. Brain Res. 116(2), 111–122 (2000)
4. Wahl, A.S., Omlor, W., Rubio, J.C., Chen, J.L., Zheng, H., Schröter, A., Gullo, M., Weinmann, O., Kobayashi, K., Helmchen, F., Ommer, B., Schwab, M.E.: Asynchronous therapy restores motor control by rewiring of the rat corticospinal tract after stroke. Science 344, 1250–1255 (2014)
5. Whishaw, I., Pellis, S.: The structure of skilled forelimb reaching in rat: a proximally driven movement with single distal rotatory component. Behav. Brain Res. (1990)
6. Goebl, W., Palmer, C.: Temporal control and hand movement efficiency in skilled music performance. PLoS One 8 (2013)
7. Schaffelhofer, S., Agudelo-Toro, A., Scherberger, H.: Decoding wide range of hand configurations from macaque motor, premotor, and parietal cortices. J. N. Sci. (2015)
8. Hamer, H., Schindler, K., Koller-Meier, E., Gool, L.V.: Tracking a hand manipulating an object. In: ICCV, pp. 1475–1482 (2009)
9. Eigenstetter, A., Takami, M., Ommer, B.: Randomized max-margin compositions for visual recognition. In: CVPR, pp. 3590–3597 (2014)
10. Wright, J., Ganesh, A., Rao, S., Peng, Y., Ma, Y.: Robust principal component analysis: Exact recovery of corrupted low-rank matrices via convex optim. In: NIPS (2009)
11. Van der Maaten, L., Hinton, G.: Visualizing data using t-sne. JMLR 9 (2008)
12. Andrews, S., Tsochantaridis, I., Hofmann, T.: Support vector machines for multiple-instance learning. In: NIPS, pp. 577–584 (2003)

Longitudinal Analysis of Pre-term Neonatal Brain Ventricle in Ultrasound Images Based on Convex Optimization

Wu Qiu[1,⋆], Jing Yuan[1,⋆], Jessica Kishimoto[1], Yimin Chen[2], Martin Rajchl[3], Eranga Ukwatta[4], Sandrine de Ribaupierre[5], and Aaron Fenster[1]

[1] Robarts Research Institute, University of Western Ontario, London, ON, CA
[2] Department of Electronic Engineering, City University of Hong Kong, CN
[3] Department of Computing, Imperial College London, London, UK
[4] Sunnybrook Health Sciences Centre, Toronto, CA; Department of Biomedical Engineering, Johns Hopkins University, MD, USA
[5] Neurosurgery, Department of Clinical Neurological Sciences, University of Western Ontario, London, ON, CA

Abstract. Intraventricular hemorrhage (IVH) is a major cause of brain injury in preterm neonates and leads to dilatation of the ventricles. Measuring ventricular volume quantitatively is an important step in monitoring patients and evaluating treatment options. 3D ultrasound (US) has been developed to monitor ventricle volume as a biomarker for ventricular dilatation and deformation. Ventricle volume as a global indicator, however, does not allow for the precise analysis of local ventricular changes. In this work, we propose a 3D+t spatial-temporal nonlinear registration approach, which is used to analyze the detailed local changes of the ventricles of preterm IVH neonates from 3D US images. In particular, a novel sequential convex/dual optimization is introduced to extract the optimal 3D+t spatial-temporal deformable registration. The experiments with five patients with 4 time-point images for each patient showed that the proposed registration approach accurately and efficiently recovered the longitudinal deformation of the ventricles from 3D US images. To the best of our knowledge, this paper reports the first study on the longitudinal analysis of the ventriclar system of pre-term newborn brains from 3D US images.

Keywords: 3D ultrasound, pre-term neonatal ventricles, spatial-temporal registration, convex optimization.

1 Introduction

Ventriculomegaly (VM) is often seen in pre-term neonates born at < 32 weeks gestation or with very low birth weight (< 1500 g). Intraventricular hemorrhage (IVH) is one of the primary non-congenital causes of VM, which is caused by bleeding in the brain that occurs in 15-30% of very low birth weight pre-term neonates and is predictive of an adverse neurological outcome [9]. Preterm infants

⋆ Contributed equally.

N. Navab et al. (Eds.): MICCAI 2015, Part III, LNCS 9351, pp. 476–483, 2015.
DOI: 10.1007/978-3-319-24574-4_57

with IVH are at risk of white matter injury, and the development of post hemorrhagic ventricular dilatation (PHVD) increases the risk of an adverse neurodevelopmental outcome. It is difficult to follow the dynamic of ventricle dilatation with current techniques (2D ultrasound (US) and MR imaging) determine the level by which ventricle dilatation is progressing. While clinicians have a good sense of what VM looks like compared to normal ventricles, there is little information available on how the cerebral ventricles change locally and temporally in pre-term IVH neonates. Additionally, the PHVD patients require interventional therapies, and about 20-40% of these patients will consequently develop hydrocephalus, necessitating surgery. Currently, there is no means of accurately predicting PHVD or determining if and when ventricular dilation requires treatment [14]. 3D US has proven to be a useful tool to measure the ventricle volume size, which can be used as a global indicator of ventricle changes [8,10]. However, differential enlargement of specific parts of the ventricles occurs over time, which cannot be identified by volume measurement alone. Thus, the longitudinal analysis of ventricle changes could provide rich information explaining some specific neurological and neuropsychological deficits, and can greatly improve the diagnosis, prognosis, and treatment of VM [3]. Longitudinal analysis of brains has been extensively studied using MR images, mostly focusing on adult populations, leading to several successful methods and software packages, such as SPM [1], FreeSurfer [7], and aBEAT [6]. However repeated MRI are not feasible in the context of preterm infants, as they are too weak to leave the unit for the first few weeks of their life. There are a few studies on the development of early brains [4,5]. However, methods employed for the longitudinal analysis of MR images are not suited for the unique challenges posed by US imaging, such as US image speckle, low tissue contrast, fewer image details of structures, and dramatic inter-subject shape deformation [8,10]. In addition, 3D neonatal US images can only provide the partial view of the neonatal brain, rather than the whole brain as in 3D MR images.

Contributions: A novel 3D+t deformable image registration technique is developed for the longitudinal analysis of 3D neonatal ventricle US images, which makes use of a sequential convex optimization technique to address the resulting nonlinear and non-smooth image fidelity function. Each convex optimization sub-problem is solved under a dual optimization perspective. The developed approach allows for the registration of all the follow-up 3D ventricle US images onto the baseline image in the same spatial coordinates. To the best of our knowledge, this paper reports the first study on the longitudinal analysis of lateral ventricles of pre-mature newborn brains from the temporal sequence of 3D US images.

2 Method

Optimization Model: Given a sequence of 3D US images $I_1(x) \dots I_{n+1}(x)$, we aim at computing the temporal sequence of 3D deformation fields $u_k(x)$, $k = 1 \dots n$, within each two adjacent images $I_k(x)$ and $I_{k+1}(x)$, while imposing both spatial and temporal smoothness of the 3D+t spatial-temporal deformation fields $u_k(x) = (u_k^1(x), u_k^2(x), u_k^3(x))^{\mathrm{T}}$, $k = 1 \dots n$.

In this work, we apply the sum of absolute intensity differences (SAD) to evaluate the dissimilarities between each two adjacent images $I_k(x + u_k(x))$ and $I_{k+1}(x)$, $k = 1 \dots n$, over the deformation field $u_k(x)$. Hence, we have

$$P(I_{1\dots n+1}; u) := \sum_{k=1}^{n} \int_{\Omega} |I_k(x + u_k(x)) - I_{k+1}(x)| \, dx \tag{1}$$

to measure the 3D+t intensity-based dissimilarities within the input 3D image sequence I_k, over the sequence of 3D deformation fields $u_k(x)$, $k = 1 \dots n$.

For each 3D deformation field $u_k(x)$, $k = 1 \dots n$, we prefer a smooth deformation field, hence penalize its spatial non-smoothness; in this work, we minimize the convex quadratic function of the spatial non-smoothness of deformations, *i.e.*,

$$R(u) := \alpha \sum_{k=1}^{n} \int_{\Omega} \left(\left|\nabla u_k^1\right|^2 + \left|\nabla u_k^2\right|^2 + \left|\nabla u_k^3\right|^2 \right) dx \,, \tag{2}$$

where $\alpha > 0$ is the positive spatial regularization parameter. Actually, spatial regularization function significantly restricts the solution space of deformation fields and sets up the well-posedness of the deformable registration problem. In addition, we also employ a temporal smoothness prior which encourages the similarities between each two adjacent deformation fields $u_k(x)$ and $u_{k+1}(x)$, $k = 1 \dots n - 1$, and penalizes their total absolute differences, *i.e.*,

$$T(u) := \gamma \sum_{k=1}^{n-1} \int_{\Omega} \left(\left|u_k^1 - u_{k+1}^1\right| + \left|u_k^2 - u_{k+1}^2\right| + \left|u_k^3 - u_{k+1}^3\right| \right) dx \,, \tag{3}$$

where $\gamma > 0$ is the temporal regularization parameter. Such absolute function-based proposed temporal regularization function (3) can eliminate undesired sudden changes within each two neighbouring deformation fields, which is mainly due to the poor image quality of US including US speckle and shadows, low tissue contrast, fewer image details of structures, and improve robustness of the introduced 3D+t non-rigid registration method.

Considering (1), (2) and (3), we formulate the studied 3D+t deformable registration of the input 3D US image sequence as the following optimization problem:

$$\min_{u_{1\dots n}(x)} \; P(I_{1\dots n+1}; u) + R(u) + T(u) \,, \tag{4}$$

where the spatial and temporal regularization functions $R(u)$ and $T(u)$ allow the well-posed optimization formulation (4).

Sequential Convex and Dual Optimization: The image fidelity term $P(I_{1\dots n+1}; u)$ of (4) is highly nonlinear, which is challenging to be minimized directly. In this regard, we use an incremental Gauss-Newton optimization scheme [2], which results in a series of linearization of the nonlinear function $P(I_{1\dots n+1}; u)$ over the incremental warping steps, hence a sequence of convex optimization problems, where each convex optimization problem properly computes an optimal update $h(x)$ to the current deformation approximation $u(x)$, till convergence, *i.e.*, the updated deformation $t(x)$ is sufficiently small.

Given the current estimated deformation $u(x)$, the linearization of $P(I_{1\dots n+1}; u + h)$ over its incremental update $h(x)$ gives rise to the following approximation:

$$P(I_{1\dots n+1}; u + h) \simeq \left(\tilde{P}(h) := \sum_{k=1}^{n} \int_{\Omega} \left|\nabla \tilde{I}_k \cdot h_k + \tilde{G}_k\right| dx\right), \tag{5}$$

where $\tilde{I}_k := I_k(x + u_k(x))$, $i = 1 \dots n$, denotes the deformed image $I_k(x)$ over the current deformation field $u_k(x)$, and $\tilde{G}_k := I_k(x + u_k(x)) - I_{k+1}(x)$.

Therefore, we can compute each deformation update $h(x)$ by solving the following optimization problem

$$\min_{h_{1\dots n}(x)} \sum_{k=1}^{n} \int_{\Omega} \left|\nabla \tilde{I}_k \cdot h_k + \tilde{G}_k\right| dx \, + \, R(u + h) \, + \, T(u + h)\, dx\,, \tag{6}$$

which is convex, due to the convexity of the absolute function and the spatial-temporal regularization functions $R(\cdot)$ and $T(\cdot)$, and can be optimized globally. Note that a small number n of time point images leads to approximation errors in practice, and a large number n results in a more smooth temporal deformation field.

Dual Optimization Formulation. In this work, we solve the convex minimization problem (6) under a dual-optimization perspective, which not only avoids directly tackling the non-smooth functions of (6) but also derives a new duality-based algorithm. Moreover, the proposed dual optimization-based approach can be easily extended to minimize the energy function (6) with any other spatial and temporal regularizars, for example the non-smooth total-variation based regularization function $\sum_{i=1}^{3} \int_{\Omega} |\nabla(u)|\, dx$.

Through variational analysis, we can derive a mathematically equivalent *dual model* to the convex minimization problem (6):

Proposition 1. *The convex minimization problem* (6) *can be equally reformulated by its* dual model*:*

$$\max_{w,q,r} \sum_{k=1}^{n} \int_{\Omega} \big(w_k \tilde{G}_k \, + \sum_{i=1}^{n} u_k^i \operatorname{div} q_k^i\big)\, dx \; - \; \frac{1}{2\alpha} \sum_{k=1}^{n} \sum_{i=1}^{3} \int_{\Omega} \left(q_k^i\right)^2 dx$$
$$+ \sum_{k=1}^{n-1} \sum_{i=1}^{3} \int_{\Omega} \big(r_k^i (u_k^i - u_{k+1}^i)\big)\, dx \tag{7}$$

subject to

$$F_1^i(x) := (w_1 \cdot \partial_i \tilde{I}_1 + \operatorname{div} q_1^i + r_1^i)(x) \, = \, 0\,, \tag{8}$$
$$F_k^i(x) := (w_k \cdot \partial_i \tilde{I}_k + \operatorname{div} q_k^i + (r_k^i - r_{k-1}^i))(x) \, = \, 0\,, \quad k = 2 \dots n-1\,, \tag{9}$$
$$F_n^i(x) := (w_n \cdot \partial_i \tilde{I}_n + \operatorname{div} q_n^i - r_{n-1}^i)(x) \, = \, 0\,, \tag{10}$$

where $i = 1 \dots 3$, and

$$|w_k(x)| \, \leq \, 1\,, \; \left|r_k^1(x)\right| \, \leq \, \gamma\,, \; \left|r_k^2(x)\right| \, \leq \, \gamma\,, \; \left|r_k^3(x)\right| \, \leq \, \gamma\,; \; k = 1 \dots n\,.$$

The proof follows the facts that $\gamma\,|x| = \max_{|w|\leq\gamma} wx$, and the convex optimization problem (6) can be equally rewritten by the minimax of its associated primal-dual Lagrangian function, *i.e.*,

$$\min_h \max_{w,q,r} L(h,w,q,r) := \sum_{k=1}^{n} \int_\Omega \left(w_k \tilde{G}_k + \sum_{i=1}^{n} u_k^i \operatorname{div} q_k^i\right) dx - \frac{1}{2\alpha} \sum_{k=1}^{n} \sum_{i=1}^{3} \int_\Omega \left(q_k^i\right)^2 dx$$
$$+ \sum_{k=1}^{n-1} \sum_{i=1}^{3} \int_\Omega \left(r_k^i (u_k^i - u_{k+1}^i)\right) dx + \sum_{k=1}^{n} \sum_{i=1}^{3} \left\langle h_k^i, F_k^i \right\rangle , \quad (11)$$

subject to $|w(x)| \leq 1$ and $\left|r_k^i(x)\right| \leq \gamma$, $i = 1,2,3$; where the functions $F_k^i(x)$, $k = 1 \ldots n$ and $i = 1,2,3$, are defined in (8). We refer to [15,11,12] for the detailed primal-dual analysis. Given Prop. 1 and the Lagrangian function (11), each component of the incremental deformation $h_k(x)$ just works as the multiplier function to the respective linear equalities (8) under the primal-dual perspective. In addition, the associated primal-dual energy function of (11) is just the Lagrangian function to the *dual formulation* (7), which can be solved by an efficient duality-based Lagrangian augmented algorithm [15,11,12].

3 Experiments and Results

Image Acquistion: A motorized 3D US system developed for cranial US scanning of pre-term neonates was used for image acquisition in the neonatal intensive care unit (NICU) [8]. The 3D image sizes ranged from 300 × 300 × 300 to 450 × 450 × 450 voxels with a voxel spacing of 0.22 × 0.22 × 0.22 mm^3. Five patients were enrolled in this study. Once enrolled, patients underwent serial US exams 1-2 times per week until the discharge from NICU, or transfer to a secondary care center. Four time-point 3D images were acquired per patient. Each

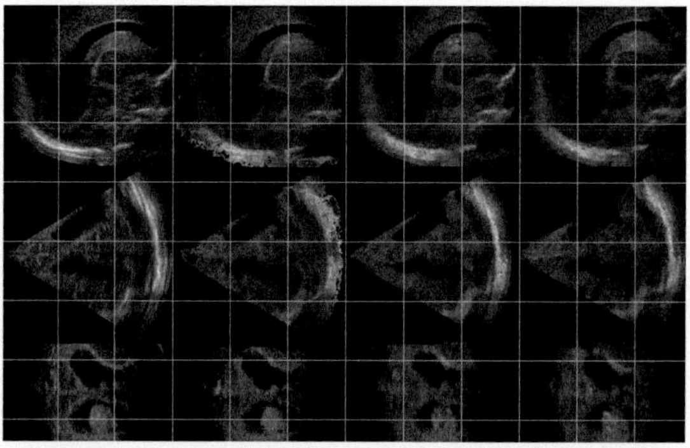

Fig. 1. Registration results of an IVH neonatal ventricles in 3D US image. 1 - 4 columns: baseline, registered images at time points 1-3. The first - third row: sagittal, coronal, and transvers view.

image was manually segmented on parallel sagittal slices by a trained observer and verified by an experienced clinician. Manual segmentations were used to evaluate the 3D+t registration results.

Evaluation Metrics: Our registration method was evaluated by comparing the registered follow-up image with the corresponding baseline image in terms of the overlap of two ventricle surfaces extracted from the two images using *volume-based metrics*: Dice similarity coefficient (DSC); and *distance-based metrics*: the mean absolute surface distance (MAD) and maximum absolute surface distance (MAXD) [11,12].

Results: Figure 1 shows an example of registered follow-up and baseline images from transverse, coronal and sagittal views. Table 1 summarizes the quantitative registration results for the initial rigid alignment, pair-wise deformable registration without the spatial-temporal constraint [13], and the proposed 3D+t non-linear registration, which shows that the proposed 3D+t deformable registration improved the target ventricle overlap in terms of DSC, MAD, and MAXD, compared to the results after rigid registration and pair-wise deformable registration without the spatial-temporal constraint. The ventricles at each time point were additionally compared to the previous time point using the generated 3D+t deformation results. The local 3D volume changes can be well represented by the divergence of deformations, *i.e.*, $\operatorname{div} u(x) := (\partial_1 u_1 + \partial_2 u_2 + \partial_3 u_3)(x)\,, \quad \forall x \in \mathcal{R}_{ventricle}$. The local volume changes within the ventricle regions over the computed deformation field $u_k(x)$ are shown in Fig. 2.

The proposed 3D+t non-rigid registration algorithm was implemented in Matlab (Natick, MA), and the experiments were conducted on a Windows desktop with an Intel i7-2600 CPU (3.4 GHz). The registration time was calculated as the mean run time of five registrations. The mean registration time of our method was 8.1 ± 1.2 minutes per patient dataset.

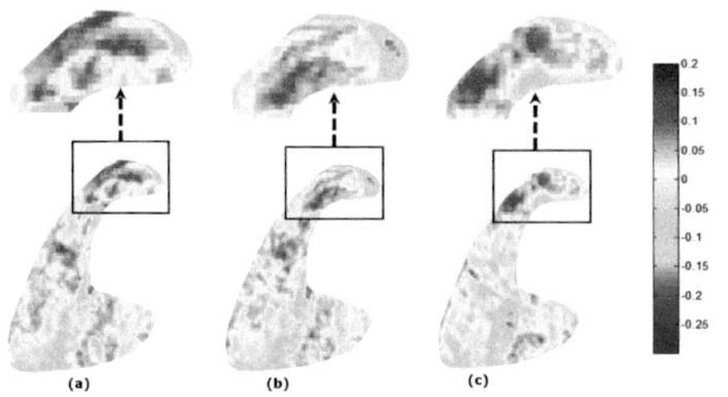

Fig. 2. Local volume changes represented by the divergence of the deformation field, *i.e.*, $\operatorname{div} u(x)$, at each time point. (a)-(c): the first-third time points. The local volume expansion is colored in red, while the local volume shrinkage is colored in blue. Magnifications of all regions of interest are depicted in the top row.

Table 1. Registration results of 5 patient images (4 time points each patient) in terms of DSC, MAD, and MAXD (p1-p5: patient ID), represented as the mean ± standard deviation.

	DSC (%)	MAD (mm)	MAXD (mm)
Rigid	66.4 ± 4.3	1.2 ± 1.3	7.0 ± 4.4
Pair-wise nonlinear registration	78.5 ± 3.3	0.7 ± 0.8	3.8 ± 3.0
3D+t nonlinear registration	$\mathbf{80.1 \pm 2.4}$	$\mathbf{0.5 \pm 0.6}$	$\mathbf{3.1 \pm 2.2}$

4 Discussion and Conclusion

Longitudinal analysis of 3D neonatal brain US images can reveal structural and anatomical changes of neonatal brains during aging or in patients with IVH disease. The analysis has the potential to be used to monitor patients and evaluate treatment options with quantitative measurements of ventricular dilatation or shrinkage in pre-term IVH neonates over time. The unique challenges provided by 3D US images of neonatal brains make most registration-based analysis methods used in MR images not useful. To cater for this clinical need, a deformable 3D+t registration approach is proposed to accurately and efficiently analyze the longitudinal pre-term neonatal brain from 3D US images. Specifically, the proposed 3D+t registration approach makes use of convex and dual optimization technique to efficiently extract the optimal 3D+t spatial-temporal deformation field and enjoys both efficiency and simplicity in numerics. In addition, the proposed dual optimization-based algorithm can be parallelized on GPUs to accelerate the computation.

The experimental results show that the proposed 3D+t registration approach can capture the longitudinal deformation of neonatal ventricles in 3D US images accurately and efficiently, suggesting that it could help physicians to locally quantify the neonatal ventricle changes over time. The proposed method was preliminarily evaluated on a small database. Additional validation on a large number of images would be required. Future work will involve mapping different subject images onto a healthy template image for classification of disease grade and progression. Moreover, based on the developed registration technique, an IVH-grade- and age-specific 3D US neonatal ventricle atlas may clinically useful for the diagnosis and treatment of developing neonatal brains with VM.

Acknowledgments. The authors are grateful for the funding support from the Canadian Institutes of Health Research (CIHR) and Academic Medical Organization of Southwestern Ontario (AMOSO).

References

1. Ashburner, J., Friston, K.J.: Unified segmentation. NeuroImage 26(3), 839–851 (2005)
2. Baust, M., Zikic, D., Navab, N.: Diffusion-based regularisation strategies for variational level set segmentation. In: BMVC, pp. 1–11 (2010)
3. Breeze, A.C., Alexander, P., Murdoch, E.M., Missfelder-Lobos, H.H., Hackett, G.A., Lees, C.C.: Obstetric and neonatal outcomes in severe fetal ventriculomegaly. Prenatal Diagnosis 27(2), 124–129 (2007)
4. Chen, Y., An, H., Zhu, H., Jewells, V., Armao, D., Shen, D., Gilmore, J.H., Lin, W.: Longitudinal regression analysis of spatial–temporal growth patterns of geometrical diffusion measures in early postnatal brain development with diffusion tensor imaging. NeuroImage 58(4), 993–1005 (2011)
5. Dai, Y., Shi, F., Wang, L., Wu, G., Shen, D.: ibeat: a toolbox for infant brain magnetic resonance image processing. Neuroinformatics 11(2), 211–225 (2013)
6. Dai, Y., Wang, Y., Wang, L., Wu, G., Shi, F., Shen, D., Initiative, A.D.N., et al.: abeat: A toolbox for consistent analysis of longitudinal adult brain mri. PloS One 8(4), e60344 (2013)
7. Fischl, B., Salat, D.H., Busa, E., Albert, M., Dieterich, M., Haselgrove, C., van der Kouwe, A., Killiany, R., Kennedy, D., Klaveness, S., et al.: Whole brain segmentation: automated labeling of neuroanatomical structures in the human brain. Neuron 33(3), 341–355 (2002)
8. Kishimoto, J., de Ribaupierre, S., Lee, D., Mehta, R., St Lawrence, K., Fenster, A.: 3D ultrasound system to investigate intraventricular hemorrhage in preterm neonates. Physics in Medicine and Biology 58(21), 7513 (2013)
9. Klebermass-Schrehof, K., Rona, Z., Waldhör, T., Czaba, C., Beke, A., Weninger, M., Olischar, M.: Can neurophysiological assessment improve timing of intervention in posthaemorrhagic ventricular dilatation? Archives of Disease in Childhood-Fetal and Neonatal Edition 98(4), F291–F297 (2013)
10. Qiu, W., Yuan, J., Kishimoto, J., McLeod, J., de Ribaupierre, S., Fenster, A.: User-guided segmentation of preterm neonate ventricular system from 3d ultrasound images using convex optimization. Ultrasound in Medicine & Biology 41(2), 542–556 (2015)
11. Qiu, W., Yuan, J., Ukwatta, E., Sun, Y., Rajchl, M., Fenster, A.: Dual optimization based prostate zonal segmentation in 3D MR images. Medical Image Analysis 18(4), 660–673 (2014)
12. Qiu, W., Yuan, J., Ukwatta, E., Sun, Y., Rajchl, M., Fenster, A.: Prostate segmentation: An efficient convex optimization approach with axial symmetry using 3D TRUS and MR images. IEEE Trans. Med. Imag. 33(4), 947–960 (2014)
13. Sun, Y., Yuan, J., Qiu, W., Rajchl, M., Romagnoli, C., Fenster, A.: Three-dimensional non-rigid mr-trus registration using dual optimization. IEEE Transactions on Medical Imaging 34(5), 1085–1094 (2015)
14. de Vries, L.S., Brouwer, A.J., Groenendaal, F.: Posthaemorrhagic ventricular dilatation: when should we intervene? Archives of Disease in Childhood-Fetal and Neonatal Edition 98(4), F284–F285 (2013)
15. Yuan, J., Bae, E., Tai, X.C.: A study on continuous max-flow and min-cut approaches. In: CVPR (2010)

Multi-GPU Reconstruction of Dynamic Compressed Sensing MRI

Tran Minh Quan, Sohyun Han, Hyungjoon Cho, and Won-Ki Jeong*

Ulsan National Institute of Science and Technology (UNIST)
{quantm,hansomain,hcho,wkjeong}@unist.ac.kr

Abstract. Magnetic resonance imaging (MRI) is a widely used in-vivo imaging technique that is essential to the diagnosis of disease, but its longer acquisition time hinders its wide adaptation in time-critical applications, such as emergency diagnosis. Recent advances in compressed sensing (CS) research have provided promising theoretical insights to accelerate the MRI acquisition process, but CS reconstruction also poses computational challenges that make MRI less practical. In this paper, we introduce a fast, scalable parallel CS-MRI reconstruction method that runs on graphics processing unit (GPU) cluster systems for dynamic contrast-enhanced (DCE) MRI. We propose a modified Split-Bregman iteration using a variable splitting method for CS-based DCE-MRI. We also propose a parallel GPU Split-Bregman solver that scales well across multiple GPUs to handle large data size. We demonstrate the validity of the proposed method on several synthetic and real DCE-MRI datasets and compare with existing methods.

1 Introduction

Magnetic resonance imaging (MRI) has been widely used as an in-vivo imaging technique due to its safety to living organisms. Because the acquisition process is the major bottleneck of MRI, many acceleration techniques have been developed using parallel imaging techniques [2]. Recently, the compressed sensing (CS) theory [3] has been successfully adopted to MRI to speed up the acquisition process [10]. However, CS-MRI introduces additional computational overhead in the reconstruction process because the ℓ_1 minimization is a time-consuming nonlinear optimization problem. Therefore, there exists a need to develop fast CS reconstruction methods to make the entire MRI reconstruction process practical for time-critical applications.

One research direction for accelerating CS reconstruction has focused on developing efficient numerical solvers for the ℓ_1 minimization problem [7,5,1]. The other direction has been leveraging the state-of-the-art parallel computing hardware, such as the graphics processing unit (GPU), to push the performance to the limit [9,13,1]. We believe that GPU acceleration is the most promising approach to make CS-MRI reconstruction clinically feasible, but multi-GPU acceleration has not been fully addressed in previously published literature.

* Corresponding author.

N. Navab et al. (Eds.): MICCAI 2015, Part III, LNCS 9351, pp. 484–492, 2015.
DOI: 10.1007/978-3-319-24574-4_58

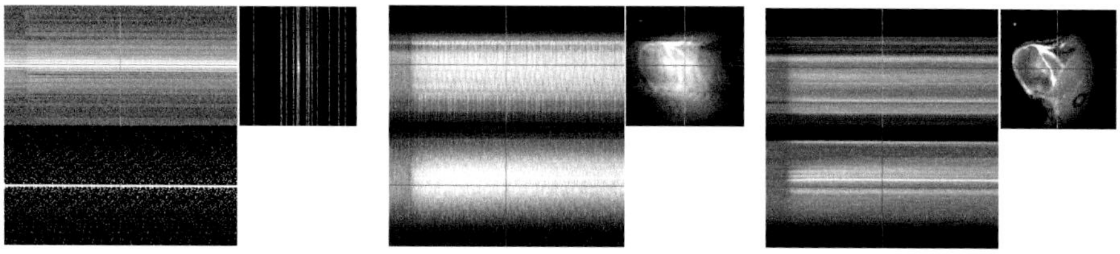

(a) ×8 subsampled k-space (b) Zero padding recon. (c) CS-DCE-MRI recon.

Fig. 1. CS-DCE-MRI examples. Red line: time axis, Blue–green lines: x–y axis

In this paper, we introduce a novel multi-GPU reconstruction method for CS-based dynamic contrast-enhanced (DCE) MRI. DCE-MRI is widely used to detect tumors, and its diagnostic accuracy highly depends on the spatio-temporal resolution of data. Fig. 1 shows an example of CS-based DCE-MRI reconstruction from a sub-sampled k-space data. CS has been successfully adopted to DCE-MRI to increase the resolution of data, but CS also imposes a high computational burden due to the increasing data size. In addition, we observed that a popular numerical method for CS reconstruction, i.e., Split-Bregman, is not directly applicable to the CS-based DCE-MRI formulation because the time and spatial domains of DCE-MRI data cannot be treated equally.

The main contributions of this paper can be summarized as follows. First, we present a modified Split-Bregman iteration to solve CS-based time-varying 2D DCE-MRI reconstruction problems. The proposed method splits time (1D) and spatial (2D) operators in the sub-optimization problem in the original Split-Bregman method, which can be efficiently solved by a single-step implicit integration method. The proposed method runs 3× faster than the conjugate gradient method and 5× faster than the fixed-point iteration method, which makes the entire reconstruction process converge up to about 7× faster than the state-of-the-art GPU DCE-MRI method [1]. Second, we introduce a scalable GPU implementation of the proposed reconstruction method and further extend to a multi-GPU system by leveraging advanced communication and latency hiding strategies. We demonstrate the performance of the proposed method on several CS-based DCE-MRI datasets with up to 12 GPUs.

2 Method

The input to our system is 2D DCE MRI data (a collection of 2D k-space data over time) defined on a 3D domain by the parameter (x, y, t), where x and y are spatial coordinates for 2D k-space data, and t denotes a temporal coordinate on the time axis. In the following, the subscript of an operator represents its dimension, e.g., F_{xy} stands for a Fourier operator applied to a 2D x-y grid.

2.1 Compressed Sensing Formulation for DCE-MRI

Let U be a collection of 2D MRI k-space data u_i, i.e., $U = \{u_1, u_2, ..., u_n\}$, acquired over time. Then the general CS formulation for DCE-MRI reconstruction problem can be described as follows:

$$\min_U \{J(U)\} \quad s.t. \quad \sum_i \|Ku_i - f_i\|_2^2 < \sigma^2 \tag{1}$$

where $J(U)$ is the ℓ_p-norm energy function to minimize (i.e., regularizer), f_i is the measurement at time i from the MRI scanner, and $K = RF$ is the sampling matrix that consists of a sampling mask R and a Fourier matrix F for 2D data. Since DCE-MRI does not change abruptly along the time axis, we enforce the temporal coherency by introducing a total variation energy along t axis and decouple the sparsifying transform on the x-y plane and temporal axis as follows:

$$J(U) = \|W_{xy}U\|_1 + \|\nabla_{xy}U\|_1 + \|\nabla_t U\|_1 \tag{2}$$

where W is the wavelet transform. Then Eq. 1 can be solved as a constrained optimization problem using a Bregman iteration [5] where each update of U^{k+1} in line 3 solves an unconstrained problem as shown in Algorithm 1. Using the

Algorithm 1. Constrained CS Optimization Algorithm

1: $k = 0, u_i^0 = f_i^0 = \mathbf{0}$ for all i
2: **while** $\sum_i \|R_i F_{xy} u_i^k - f_i\|_2^2 > \sigma^2$ **do**
3: $\quad U^{k+1} = \min_U \{J(U) + \frac{\mu}{2} \sum_i \|R_i F_{xy} u_i - f_i^k\|_2^2\}$
4: $\quad f_i^{k+1} = f_i^k + f_i - R_i F_{xy} u_i^{k+1}$ for all i
5: **end while**

Split Bregman algorithm [5], we can decouple ℓ_1 and ℓ_2 components in line 3 in Algorithm 1 and iteratively update using a two-step process (more details can be found in [5]). Note that in the original Split-Bregman algorithm, U and $J(U)$ are defined on the same dimensional grid, i.e., if U is a 3D volume then $J(U)$ is a hybrid of 3D total variation (TV) and wavelet regularizers, which allows a closed-form solution for U^{k+1}. However, because our $J(U)$ consists of 1D and 2D operators, the same closed-form solution is not applicable. To be more specific, U^{k+1} can be updated by solving the linear system defined as follows:

$$(\mu F_{xy}^{-1} R^T R F_{xy} - \lambda \Delta_{xy} - \theta \Delta_t + \omega) U^{k+1} = rhs^k \tag{3}$$

where the parameters λ, θ, ω and μ are used to control the amount of regularization energy, and refer to [5] for the definition of rhs^k. Goldstein et al. [5] proposed a closed form solution to invert the left-hand side of the given linear system using the forward and inverse 3D Fourier transforms, but we cannot apply the same method since the k-space data is 2D in our formulation.

Since the left-hand side of Eq. 3 is not directly invertible, we can use iterative methods, such as the fixed-point iteration or the conjugate gradient method, that converge slower than the explicit inversion in the original method. In order to speed up the convergence, we propose a *single iteration* method, which further reduces the iteration cost by splitting the left-hand side of Eq. 3 and solve for

U^{k+1} directly in a single step. If we separate 1D and 2D operators in the left-hand side, then Eq. 3 can be represented as follows:

$$(A_1 + A_2)U^{k+1} = rhs^k \tag{4}$$

where $A_1 = (\mu F_{xy}^{-1} R^T R F_{xy} - \lambda \Delta_{xy})$ and $A_2 = -\theta \Delta_t + \omega$. If we treat A_2 as the operator applied to U from the previous iteration, i.e., U^k at $(k+1)$-th iteration, then Eq. 4 can be expressed as follows:

$$A_1 U^{k+1} + A_2 U^k = rhs^k. \tag{5}$$

Because U^k is known, we can move it to the right-hand side to make the update rule for U^{k+1}

$$U^{k+1} = A_1^{-1}(rhs^k - A_2 U^k). \tag{6}$$

This assumption holds for a sufficiently large k because U^k and U^{k+1} will converge. Then, A_1 can be inverted by making the system circulant as shown in [5]

$$U^{k+1} = F_{xy}^{-1} \mathcal{K}^{-1} F_{xy}(rhs^k + (\theta \Delta_t - \omega)U^k) \tag{7}$$

where $\mathcal{K}$ is the diagonal operator defined as $\mathcal{K} = \mu R^T R - \lambda F_{xy} \Delta_{xy} F_{xy}^{-1}$.

We evaluated the convergence rates of three different minimization strategies for U^{k+1} – fixed-point iteration, conjugate gradient, and single iteration methods (Fig. 2). We observed that the conjugate gradient method converges about twice faster than the fixed-point iteration, and our single iteration converges about 2–3-fold faster than the conjugate gradient method to reach the same PSNR.

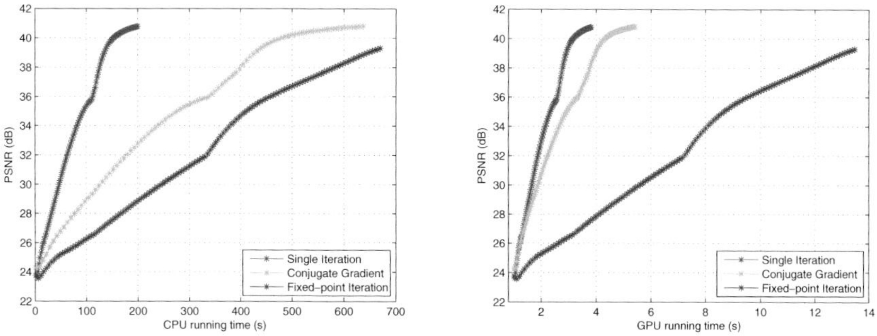

Fig. 2. PSNR vs. CPU (left) and GPU running times (right) of various methods.

2.2 Multi-GPU Implementation

As the temporal resolution of DCE-MRI increases, the entire k-space can not be mapped onto a single GPU. We decompose the domain along the t-axis into chunks where each chunk consists of three parts: *interior*, *exterior*, and *ghost*, similar to [12]. Interior and exterior regions form a computational domain for a given chunk, and ghost is the region extends to its neighbor chunk that is

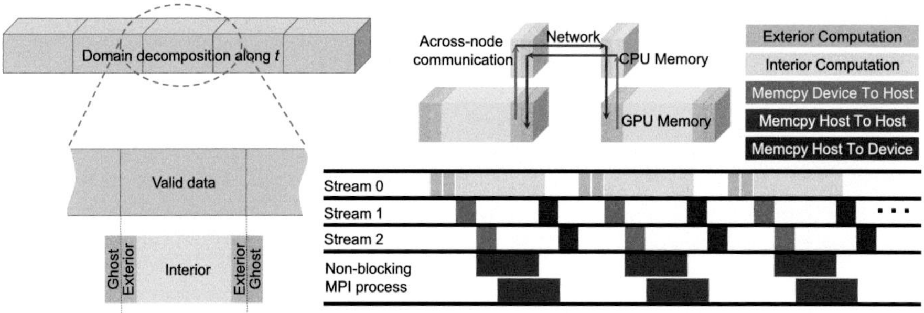

Fig. 3. Ghost region communication between neighbour GPUs

required for computation (Fig. 3 left). In our method, we increase the ghost and exterior size (up to 5 slices in our experiment) in order to run the algorithm multiple iterations without communication.

Data communication between adjacent GPUs is performed as follows (see Fig. 3 bottom right): First, we perform the computation on the exterior regions, which are the ghost regions of the neighborhood GPU, using the main stream (stream 0, Fig. 3 cyan). Note that we can run n iterations in this step for the ghost size n (one slice of ghost region is invalidated per each iteration, so we can run up to n iterations). Next, the other concurrent streams (stream 1 and 2) will perform the peer copies from GPU (device) to CPU (host) memory, one stream per an exterior region (Fig. 3 green). Because streams run in parallel, stream 0 can continue to compute on the interior region during the communication (Fig. 3 yellow). Then each exterior region data on the CPU will be transferred to the ghost region of its neighborhood CPU via MPI send and receive (Fig. 3 magenta). Because the MPI process becomes available right after invoking the GPU asynchronous calls, it can be used to perform a non-blocking transaction across the GPUs (note that stream 2 is overlapped with MPI transfer). Finally, the valid ghost data is copied from the host to device asynchronously to complete one round of ghost communication (Fig. 3 purple). By doing this, we can effectively hide the communication latency by allowing the ghost transfers occur on the different GPU streams while the main stream continues the computation on the interior region. If GPUs are in the same physical node, this communication can be implemented using asynchronous peer-to-peer device communication via PCI bus. In addition, if the system supports infiniband network, we can use NVIDIA GPUDirect for RDMA communication.

3 Result

We used an NVIDIA GeForce GTX 680 GPU with Jacket for MATLAB for the single GPU evaluation (same environment as Bilen's). We ran our scalability test on a 6-node GPU cluster system with two NVIDIA K20m per node, 12 GPUs in total. Gd-DTPA contrast agent was used for data preparation, and the CS-undersampling factor is ×8.

3.1 Image Quality and Running Time Evaluation

We compared our methods with IMPATIENT [4], kt-SPARSE [11], kt-FOCUSS [8], GPU Split-Bregman [9] and GPU ADMM [1], and our method is comparable to or outperforms those. Among them, we discuss Bilen et al. [1] in detail because it is the most recent work close to our method in the sampling strategy, energy function, numerical method, and GPU implementation. For a direct comparison with Bilen's, the wavelet term in the formulation is ignored in this experiment.

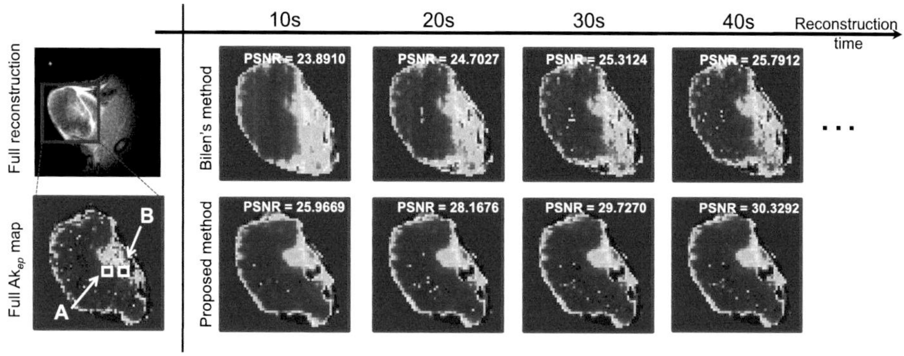

(a) Ak_{ep} maps at specific moments of reconstruction time

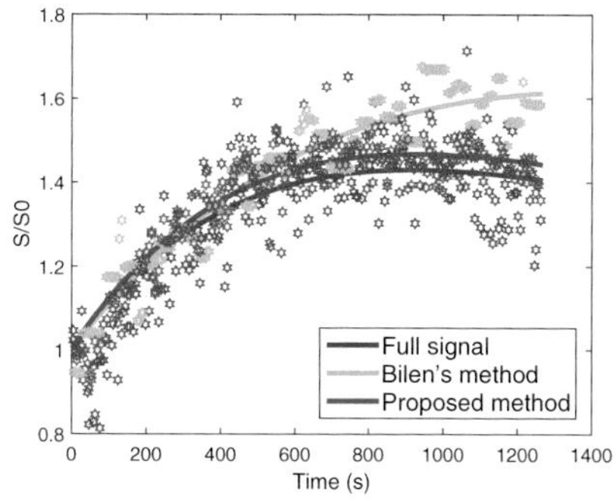

(b) Temporal profile of A

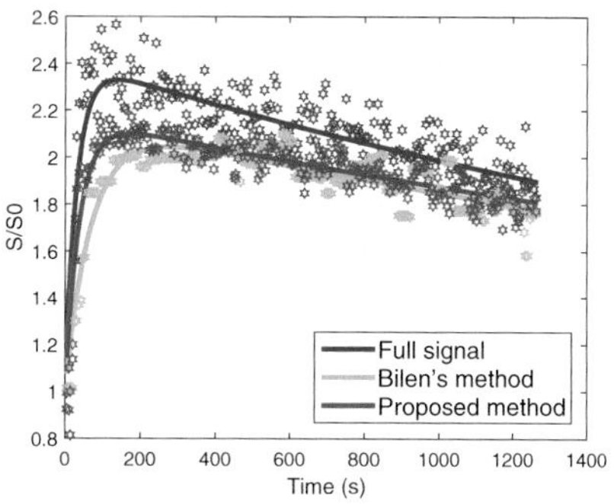

(c) Temporal profile of B

Fig. 4. Comparison between Bilen's method and the proposed solution

Fig. 4 (a) compares Ak_{ep} maps [6] of reconstructed images at different points in time. The Ak_{ep} maps in the bottom row (our method) is much closer to the ground truth (Full Akmap on the left) than those in the upper row at the same point in time, which implies our method converges faster. Fig. 4 (b) and (c) show the least-square fitting curve to the temporal profile of the region of interest in the Ak_{ep} map (A and B, high vascularity regions), which is also a commonly used quality measure to characterize the perfusion and permeability in DCE-MRI data. For this test, we ran each method until its reconstruction image reaches the same PSNR. While both methods generate the curves similar to that of the full reconstruction, our result is more accurate (i.e., close to the full reconstruction curve), which is due to the different numerical characteristics of the algorithm. Table 1 shows the running time of each method on several tumor datasets until convergence (i.e., reaching a steady state). The result also confirms that our method converges much faster than Bilen's, up to 6.9× in GPU implementation.

Table 1. Running times of Bilen's and the proposed method on various datasets of size 128 × 128 × 256.

Metrics	Tumor 1		Tumor 2		Tumor 3		Tumor 4	
	Bilen	Ours	Bilen	Ours	Bilen	Ours	Bilen	Ours
PSNR(dB)	30.598	30.636	40.169	39.931	39.678	39.479	33.559	34.174
CPU time(s)	448.451	360.689	797.056	340.143	719.187	327.868	715.004	407.461
GPU time(s)	292.341	61.637	475.155	68.002	394.241	66.125	367.759	63.276

3.2 Multi-GPU Performance Evaluation

In this evaluation, we check the scalability up to 12 GPUs on a distributed GPU cluster. We first measure the computation-only time to obtain the best possible running times, and then measure the total running times including data communication (i.e., ghost region exchange). As shown in Fig. 5, the total time including the ghost exchange is approximately close to the computation-only time, in both strong and weak scaling tests. This result confirms that our multi-GPU implementation can effectively hide the communication latency while performing the CS DCE-MRI reconstruction solver on distributed systems.

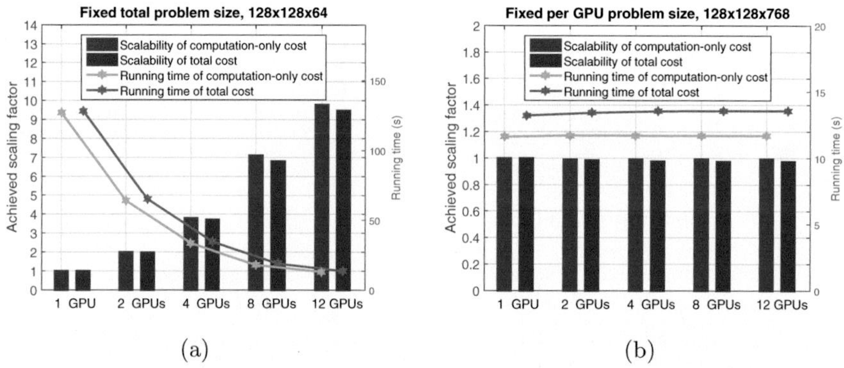

Fig. 5. Strong (a) and weak scaling (b) on a distributed GPU cluster.

4 Conclusion

In this paper, we presented our new CS-based DCE-MRI reconstruction system for the multi-GPU computing environment. The proposed method delivered a new numerical method in order to apply the Split-Bregman algorithm to

CS-based time-variant DCE-MRI problem. We also introduced a scalable implementation of the proposed CS-MRI reconstruction method on a distributed multi-GPU system. As discussed, the proposed method outperforms the existing GPU CS-reconstruction algorithm in quality and running time. For future work, we plan to extend the proposed CS-MRI method to large-scale dynamic 3D DCE-MRI reconstruction. Assessing the clinical feasibility of the proposed method would be another interesting future research.

Acknowledgements. This work was partially supported by the National Research Foundation of Korea grant NRF-2012R1A1A1039929 and NRF- 2013K2A1 A2055315.

References

1. Bilen, C., Wang, Y., Selesnick, I.: High-speed CS reconstruction in dynamic parallel MRI using augmented lagrangian and parallel processing. IEEE Journal on Emerging and Selected Topics in Circuits and Systems 2(3), 370–379 (2012)
2. Blaimer, M., Breuer, F., Mueller, M., Heidemann, R.M., Griswold, M.A., Jakob, P.M.: SMASH, SENSE, PILS, GRAPPA: How to choose the optimal method. Topics in Magnetic Resonance Imaging 15(4), 223–236 (2004)
3. Donoho, D.: Compressed sensing. IEEE Transactions on Information Theory 52(4), 1289–1306 (2006)
4. Gai, J., Obeid, N., Holtrop, J.L., Wu, X.L., Lam, F., Fu, M., Haldar, J.P., Hwu, W.M.W., Liang, Z.P., Sutton, B.P.: More IMPATIENT: a gridding-accelerated toeplitz-based strategy for non-cartesian high-resolution 3D MRI on GPUs. Journal of Parallel and Distributed Computing 73(5), 686–697 (2013)
5. Goldstein, T., Osher, S.: The split bregman method for $\ell 1$–regularized problems. SIAM Journal on Imaging Sciences 2(2), 323–343 (2009)
6. Hoffmann, U., Brix, G., Knopp, M.V., Hess, T., Lorenz, W.J.: Pharmacokinetic mapping of the breast: a new method for dynamic MR mammography. Magnetic Resonance in Medicine 33(4), 506–514 (1995). PMID: 7776881
7. Jung, H., Sung, K., Nayak, K.S., Kim, E.Y., Ye, J.C.: k–t FOCUSS: a general compressed sensing framework for high resolution dynamic MRI. Magnetic Resonance in Medicine 61(1), 103–116 (2009)
8. Jung, H., Ye, J.C., Kim, E.Y.: Improved k–t BLAST and k–t SENSE using FOCUSS. Physics in Medicine and Biology 52(11), 3201–3226 (2007)
9. Kim, D., Trzasko, J., Smelyanskiy, M., Haider, C., Dubey, P., Manduca, A.: High–performance 3D compressive sensing MRI reconstruction using many–core architectures. Journal of Biomedical Imaging, 1–11, January 2011
10. Lustig, M., Donoho, D., Santos, J., Pauly, J.: Compressed sensing MRI. IEEE Signal Processing Magazine 25(2), 72–82 (2008)
11. Lustig, M., Donoho, D., Pauly, J.M.: Sparse MRI: the application of CS for rapid MR imaging. Magnetic Resonance in Medicine 58(6), 1182–1195 (2007)

12. Micikevicius, P.: 3D finite difference computation on GPUs using CUDA. In: Proceedings of 2nd Workshop on General Purpose Processing on Graphics Processing Units, GPGPU 2009, pp. 79–84. ACM, New York (2009)
13. Murphy, M., Alley, M., Demmel, J., Keutzer, K., Vasanawala, S., Lustig, M.: Fast - SPIRiT compressed sensing parallel imaging MRI: scalable parallel implementation and clinically feasible runtime. IEEE Transactions on Medical Imaging 31(6), 1250–1262 (2012)

Prospective Identification of CRT Super Responders Using a Motion Atlas and Random Projection Ensemble Learning

Devis Peressutti[1], Wenjia Bai[2], Thomas Jackson[1], Manav Sohal[1], Aldo Rinaldi[1], Daniel Rueckert[2], and Andrew King[1]

[1] Division of Imaging Sciences & Biomedical Engineering, King's College London, UK
[2] Biomedical Image Analysis Group, Imperial College London, UK

Abstract. Cardiac Resynchronisation Therapy (CRT) treats patients with heart failure and electrical dyssynchrony. However, many patients do not respond to therapy. We propose a novel framework for the prospective characterisation of CRT 'super-responders' based on motion analysis of the Left Ventricle (LV). A spatio-temporal motion atlas for the comparison of the LV motions of different subjects is built using cardiac MR imaging. Patients likely to present a super-response to the therapy are identified using a novel ensemble learning classification method based on random projections of the motion data. Preliminary results on a cohort of 23 patients show a sensitivity and specificity of 70% and 85%.

1 Introduction

Cardiac resynchronisation therapy (CRT) has the potential to improve both morbidity and mortality in selected heart failure patients with electrical dyssynchrony. Standard selection criteria for CRT are a New York Heart Association functional class of II to IV, a QRS duration $> 120ms$, and a Left Ventricular (LV) ejection fraction (EF) $\leq 35\%$. However, when applying such criteria, a large variability in the response rate has been reported [1]. Improved characterisation of patients likely to respond to the treatment is therefore of clinical interest.

In recent years, there has been a growing interest in the characterisation of CRT *super-response*. Super-responders exhibit an enhanced level of LV Reverse Remodelling (RR) after CRT, which leads to an almost complete recovery of cardiac function [2]. Recent studies have shown strong evidence for super-response in patients with strict left bundle branch block (LBBB) [11] and a type II electrical activation pattern (also known as U-shaped activation) [8]. A strict LBBB is characterised by a longer QRS duration ($\geq 140ms$ in men and $\geq 130ms$ in women) and a mid-QRS notching, while a U-shaped activation pattern is typically characterised by a line of functional block located between the septum and the lateral wall and by a delayed trans-septal conduction time [8].

However, characterisation of the complex LV electrical activation based only on strict LBBB and a U-shaped activation pattern, although promising, is rather

N. Navab et al. (Eds.): MICCAI 2015, Part III, LNCS 9351, pp. 493–500, 2015.
DOI: 10.1007/978-3-319-24574-4_59

simplistic. As noted in [8], assessment of contraction patterns is a subjective process and it is possible that such a classification might fail to capture the complex variation in electrical and mechanical activation patterns. Assuming a coupled electrical and mechanical LV activation, we propose a more sophisticated characterisation of LV contraction for the prediction of CRT super-response. Using Cardiac Magnetic Resonance (CMR) imaging, the LV mechanical contraction of a population of CRT patients is estimated and a spatio-temporal LV motion atlas is built, allowing direct comparison of LV contractions of different patients. Random projection ensemble learning is used to prospectively identify super-responders based on the LV contraction information only. Previous related work includes [5,4], where a LV motion atlas was used to identify specific abnormal activation patterns, such as Septal Flash. However, to the authors' knowledge, this is the first work seeking to characterise CRT super-responders using machine learning on 3D motion descriptors.

2 Materials

A cohort of 23 patients[1] fulfilling the conventional criteria for CRT (see Sect. 1) was considered. The study was approved by the institutional ethics committee and all patients gave written informed consent. All patients underwent CMR imaging using a 1.5T scanner (Achieva, Philips Healthcare, Best, Netherlands) with a 32-element cardiac coil. The acquired CMR sequences are as follows:

cine MR: A multi-slice SA and three single-slice LA (2, 3 and 4-chamber view) 2D cine Steady State Free Precession (SSFP) sequences were acquired (TR/TE $= 3.0/1.5ms$, flip angle $= 60°$). Typical slice thickness is of $8mm$ for SA and $10mm$ for LA with an in-plane resolution $\approx 1.4 \times 1.4mm^2$;

T-MR: Tagged MR sequences in three orthogonal directions with reduced field-of-view enclosing the left ventricle were acquired (TR/TE $= 7.0/3.2ms$, flip angle $= 19 - 25°$, tag distance $= 7mm$). The typical spatial resolution in the plane orthogonal to the tagging direction is $\approx 1.0 \times 1.0mm^2$;

All images were ECG-gated and acquired during sequential breath-holds. Given their high in-plane spatial resolution, the cine MR images at end-diastole (ED) were employed to estimate LV geometry (see Sect. 3.1), while the cine MR images at the other cardiac phases were not used in this work. An average high resolution $3D + t$ T-MR sequence was derived from the three T-MR acquisitions with orthogonal tagging directions and was used to estimate the LV contraction (see Sect. 3.1). Prior to the estimation of LV geometry and motion, the SA and LA cine MR sequences were spatially aligned to the T-MR coordinate system. Such spatial alignment compensates for motion occurring between sequential breath-holds. The T-MR sequence is free from respiratory artefacts and therefore was chosen as the reference coordinate system.

Different super-response measures that quantify the degree of RR have been proposed [2,11]. In this work, we employ a combined measure of super-response,

[1] Data were acquired from different projects and cannot be made publicly available due to lack of ethical approval or patient consent on data sharing.

characterised by a LV end-diastolic volume reduction $\leq 20\%$, a LV end-systolic volume reduction $\leq 15\%$ and a two-fold increase in LV ejection fraction or an absolute value $\geq 40\%$. According to this classification, 10 out of 23 patients in our cohort were classified as super-responders. This binary classification was used to train the proposed ensemble learning classifier (see Sect. 3.2).

3 Methods

The main novelty of the proposed method lies in the application of a novel dimensionality reduction technique for the characterisation of CRT super-response. The proposed framework is summarised in Fig. 1.

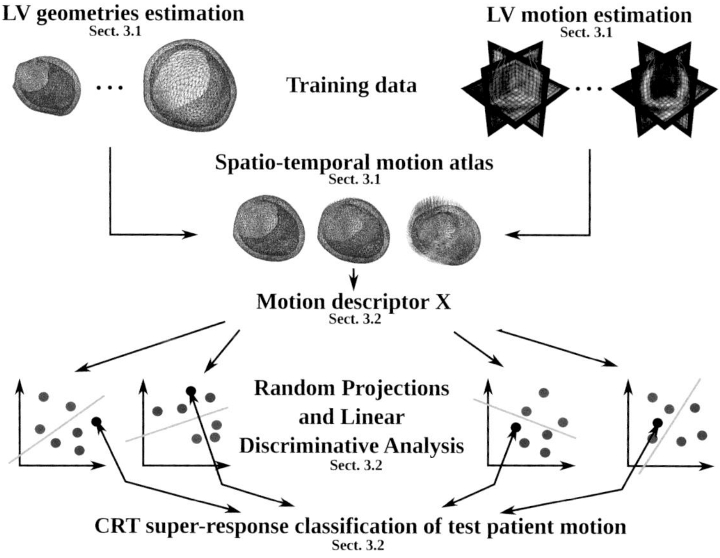

Fig. 1. Overview of the proposed framework.

Similarly to [4], a spatio-temporal motion atlas of the LV was built to allow motion comparison from different patients. The atlas removes differences in LV anatomy and cardiac cycle duration from the comparison of LV motion. Details of the atlas formation are reported in Sect. 3.1, while Sect. 3.2 describes the random projection ensemble classifier used to characterise super-responders.

3.1 Spatio-Temporal Motion Atlas

The LV spatio-temporal motion atlas formation comprises the following steps:

Estimation of LV Geometry. For each patient, the LV myocardium, excluding papillary muscles, was manually segmented from the ED frames of the multi-slice SA and three LA cine MR images and the four binary masks were fused together into an isotropic $2mm^3$ binary image. Following a further manual refinement of the binary mask to obtain a smooth LV segmentation, an open-source statistical shape model (SSM) of the LV [7] was employed to enforce point correspondence amongst all LV geometries. After an initial landmark-based rigid alignment, the SSM was optimised to fit the LV segmentation. Non-rigid registration followed the mode optimisation to refine local alignment. An example of a LV surface is shown in Fig. 2(a)-(e).

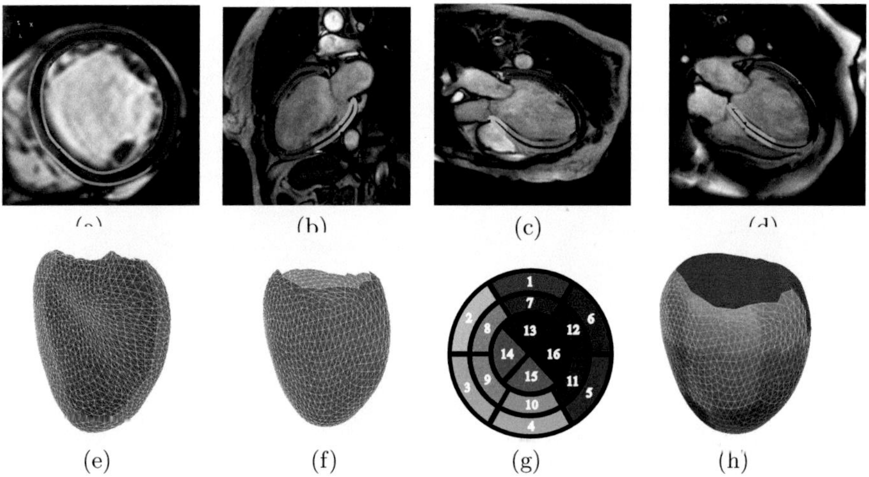

Fig. 2. Example of estimated LV geometry at end-diastole overlaid onto (a) mid SA slice, (b) 2-, (c) 3-, and (d) 4-chamber cine LA slices. Fig. (e) shows the resulting SSM epi- and endo-cardial meshes, while (f) shows the resampled medial mesh. Fig. (g) shows the AHA bull's eye plot, while (h) shows the unbiased medial shape.

In order to spatially regularise the number of vertices, a medial surface mesh with regularly sampled vertices (≈ 1500) was generated from the personalised SSM epi- and endo-cardial surfaces (Fig. 2(f)). The same resampling strategy was employed for all patients to maintain point correspondence.

Estimation of LV Motion. An average high resolution $3D+t$ T-MR sequence was derived from the $3D+t$ T-MR sequences with orthogonal tagging planes. For each T-MR volume, the trigger time t_T specified in the DICOM meta-tag was normalised with respect to the patient's average cardiac cycle, such that $t_T \in [0, 1)$, with 0 being ED. LV motion with respect to the ED cardiac phase was estimated using a $3D+t$ free-form-deformation algorithm with sparse spatial and temporal constraints [10]. This algorithm estimates a smooth and continuous $3D+t$ transformation for any $t \in [0, 1)$. This way, temporal normalisation was achieved for each patient, regardless of the number of acquired T-MR volumes and cycle length.

Spatial Normalisation. The aim of spatial normalisation is to remove bias towards patient-specific LV geometries from the motion analysis. From the previous steps, LV shapes at ED (see Fig. 2(f)) were derived from N patients.

An initial Procrustes alignment based on the point correspondences was performed on the N medial LV shapes, obtaining a set of affine transformations $\{\phi_{aff}^n\}, n = 1, \ldots, N$ with respect to a randomly chosen reference shape. An unbiased LV medial shape was computed by transforming the average shape of the aligned surfaces by the inverse of the average affine transformation $\tilde{\phi}_{aff} = \frac{1}{n}\sum_n \phi_{aff}^n$. An example of an unbiased LV shape is shown in Fig. 2(h). In order to enforce an identity average transformation, the original transformations $\{\phi_{aff}^n\}$ were similarly normalised $\hat{\phi}_{aff}^n = \phi_{aff}^n \circ (\tilde{\phi}_{aff})^{-1}$. All shapes were consequently aligned to the unbiased medial LV shape using Thin Plate Spline (TPS) transformations $\{\phi_{TPS}^n\}$. The transformation from the patient-specific coordinate system to the unbiased LV mesh is thus given by $\phi^n = \phi_{TPS}^n \circ \hat{\phi}_{aff}^n$ [4].

Motion Reorientation. In order to compare cardiac phases amongst all patients, for each patient, the reference ED medial surface was warped to $T = 24$ cardiac phases equally distributed in $[0, 0.8]$ by using the estimated $3D + t$ transformation. Only the first 80% of the cardiac cycle was considered since it represents the typical coverage of T-MR sequences, and the estimated motion for $t \in (0.8, 1]$ is due to interpolation. The patient-specific LV motion was therefore fully represented by the T shapes. Under a small deformation assumption [4], $\mathbf{v}_{p,t}^n = \mathbf{u}_{p,t}^n - \mathbf{u}_{p,0}^n$ denotes the motion at location $\mathbf{u}$ of vertex $p \in 1, .., P$ at the cardiac phase $t \in 1, .., T$ with respect to the ED phase for patient $n \in 1, .., N$. The patient-specific motion $\mathbf{v}_{p,t}^n, \forall n, t, p$ is transported to the coordinate system of the unbiased average shape by computing $\mathbf{v}_{n,p,t}^{atlas} = J^{-1}(\phi^n(\mathbf{u}_p)) \cdot \mathbf{v}_{p,t}^n$, where $J(\phi^n)$ denotes the Jacobian of the transformation ϕ^n [4].

AHA Segmentation. For a more intuitive understanding of the LV motion, the atlas was segmented into the standard 16 AHA segments [3] (see Fig. 2(g) and 2(h)) and the LV motion $\mathbf{v}_{n,p,t}^{atlas}$ was decomposed into longitudinal, radial and circumferential cylindrical coordinates ($\mathbf{v}_{n,p,t}^{atlas} = [l_{n,p,t}, r_{n,p,t}, c_{n,p,t}]^T$) with respect to the long axis of the LV ED medial surface.

3.2 Random Projection Ensemble Learning

The spatio-temporal atlas permits representation of the LV motion in a common coordinate system $\mathbf{v}_{n,p,t}^{atlas}, \forall n, p, t$. For each patient n, a LV motion descriptor was derived by concatenating $\mathbf{v}_{p,t}^{atlas}, \forall p, t$ into a single column vector $\mathbf{v}_n \in \mathbb{R}^F$, where F denotes the number of features of the motion descriptor. After normalisation, $\tilde{\mathbf{v}}_n = \frac{\mathbf{v}_n}{\|\mathbf{v}_n\|}$, the training data set was given by $\mathbf{X} = [\tilde{\mathbf{v}}_1 \cdots \tilde{\mathbf{v}}_N] \in \mathbb{R}^{F \times N}$. The aim of the proposed technique is to find a set of low-dimensional representations of the high dimensional motion matrix $\mathbf{X}$ that maximises super response classification.

Typical limitations in the analysis of high dimensional data are the presence of noisy features and the curse of dimensionality (i.e. data is very sparse in a high dimensional space). These factors can hinder the identification of the underlying structure of the data. To overcome these limitations, linear and non-linear dimensionality reduction techniques have been proposed to transform the original high dimensional data onto lower dimensional subspaces, where the underlying data structure is described according to some criteria. For instance, Principal Component Analysis (PCA) projects the original data onto a linear subspace that preserves the variance of the data. However, the resulting subspace might not be optimal for the classification task at hand.

A novel ensemble learning classifier employing Random Projections (RPs) has been recently proposed in [6]. In our work, we extend [6] by using RPs and Linear Discrimant Analysis (LDA) to identify an optimal set of subspaces that best performs on the given classification. Let $\mathbf{Y} \in \mathbb{R}^N$, $y_n \in \{0, 1\}$ be the CRT super-response labels (0-no super-response, 1-super-response, see Sect. 2 for the classification criteria), L the number of classifiers in the ensemble and D the number of dimensions of the random subspace ($D \ll F$). In the training phase, for each classifier C_l, $l = 1, .., L$, the motion matrix $\mathbf{X}$ was projected onto a random subspace defined by a sparse random matrix $\mathbf{R}_l \in \mathbb{R}^{D \times F}$, in which the elements of each column vector $\{r_i\}_{i=1}^F$ are drawn from a Bernoulli $\{+1, -1\}$ distribution with $\|r_i\| = 1$. As a result of the random projection, a new set of low-dimensional descriptors $\mathbf{Z} = \mathbf{R} \cdot \mathbf{X}$, $\mathbf{Z} \in \mathbb{R}^{D \times N}$ was generated and a LDA classifier was trained on the descriptors $\mathbf{Z}$ and the class labels $\mathbf{Y}$.

In this work we extend [6] to improve the robustness of the random subspace generation, as follows. The performance of each classifier was evaluated on the same training data and the number of misclassified patients M was computed. If the misclassification was larger than a predefined percentage $M > k \cdot N$, $\mathbf{R}$ was discarded and a new random projection was generated. This process was repeated for each classifier C_l until an acceptable projection $\mathbf{R}_l$ was found. As a consequence, the random subspace selection is more robust, even with a low number of classifiers. The value of k defines the accuracy of the selected subspace. Low values of k generate very discriminative subspaces at the cost of a higher computational time (a maximum number of iterations can also be introduced).

The result was a set of linear classifiers trained on RPs of the motion matrix $\mathbf{X}$ which are highly discriminative with respect to CRT super-response. In the testing phase, the motion vector of a test patient $\mathbf{x}_{test} \in \mathbf{R}^F$ was projected onto the selected random subspaces $\{\mathbf{R}_l\}_{l=1}^L$ and the CRT super-response class was predicted by the L trained LDA classifiers. The final super-response class y_{test} was derived by a weighted average of the L predicted classes $\{y_{test_l}\}_{l=1}^L$, where the weight for each classifier C_l is given by the residual misclassification error M (the higher the residual misclassification error M, the lower the weight) [9]. The super-response class with highest cumulative weights was assigned to y_{test}.

4 Experiments and Results

To evaluate the proposed technique, a leave-one-out cross-validation was employed. Each patient was left-out in turn and the motion descriptor $\mathbf{X}$ was built using the remaining $N = 22$ patients. The LV motion of the left-out patient constituted the test motion descriptor $\mathbf{x}_{test}$.

Since both strict LBBB and U-shaped activation are related to localised activation patterns [8], we investigated the influence of different LV regions on the super-response classification. Three different motion descriptors $\mathbf{X}_{16}$, $\mathbf{X}_6$ and

$\mathbf{X}_3$ were built considering a different number of AHA segments as follows. $\mathbf{X}_{16}$ was built considering all the vertices in the atlas ($F \approx 110,000$), $\mathbf{X}_6$ was built considering the six AHA segments $7-12$ in the mid LV ($F \approx 38,000$) and $\mathbf{X}_3$ was built considering only the three AHA segments $7, 8, 12$ ($F \approx 17,000$) located in proximity to the conduction block line [8] (see Fig. 2(g)).

The proposed technique ($RLDA_{wr}$) was compared to: a LDA classification applied to the high dimensional motion matrices (LDA), a LDA classification applied to a low-dimensional subspace given by PCA ($PLDA$), and to the RPs ensemble classifier with no subspace rejection ($RLDA$) [6]. For the $PLDA$ technique, a dual formulation was employed since $N \ll F$, and the modes retaining 95% of the original variance were considered. A super-response classification based on the presence of strict LBBB only is also reported for comparison. The set of parameters used for $RLDA_{wr}$ was determined from an initial pilot study using the same training data (see Table 1). The same parameters L, D were employed for $RLDA$, while the value of k was fixed $k = 0.1$.

Results of the leave-one-out cross-validation are reported in Table 1.

Table 1. Cross-validation results for sensitivity, specificity, positive (PPV) and negative predictive value (NPV). The subspace dimensionality D and, where applicable, the number of classifiers L is also reported. Best classification results are shown in bold.

	$\mathbf{X}_{16}$				$\mathbf{X}_6$				$\mathbf{X}_3$				LBBB
	LDA	$PLDA$	$RLDA$	$RLDA_{wr}$	LDA	$PLDA$	$RLDA$	$RLDA_{wr}$	LDA	$PLDA$	$RLDA$	$RLDA_{wr}$	
Sens	.40	.70	.50	.60	.40	.50	.40	.50	.50	.60	.60	**.70**	.80
Spec	.62	.62	.62	.69	.62	.69	.77	.85	.77	.61	.77	**.85**	.62
PPV	.44	.58	.50	.60	.44	.55	.57	.71	.63	.55	.66	**.78**	.62
NPV	.57	.72	.62	.69	.57	.64	.63	.69	.67	.67	.71	**.79**	.80
D	F	17	20	20	F	15	30	30	F	13	200	200	NA
L	NA	NA	61	61	NA	NA	61	61	NA	NA	61	61	NA

5 Discussion

We have presented a method for the automatic prospective identification of CRT super-responders based purely on motion information estimated from CMR imaging. The novelty of this paper lies in the application and extension of a recently proposed dimensionality reduction algorithm to a clinically important, but previously untackled problem in medical image processing. Our extension to the random projections ensemble learning technique [6] consists of a more robust selection of the random subspace with respect to the classification accuracy.

Results on a cohort of 23 CRT patients show the proposed technique $RLDA_{wr}$ to outperform $PLDA$ and $RLDA$ in the selection of an optimal subspace for classification of CRT super-responders. The best classification results were achieved considering only three AHA segments localised around the conduction block line, which supports the findings in [8] on the correlation between the presence of a U-shaped contraction and super-response. Compared to a LBBB-based classification [11] (last column in Table 1), better specificity and PPV were achieved.

In the future, we plan to expand our patient cohort to enable our algorithm to learn a wider range of motion-based biomarkers that are correlated with CRT super-response. Much work remains to be done to better understand CRT response and super-response. At the moment, relatively simple indicators are used to select patients for CRT and many that undergo the invasive therapy do not respond. Furthermore, there is currently no consensus on the definition of a super-responder. It may be that a better characterisation of LV mechanical activation patterns could lead to a more functional definition of super-response. Our method offers the possibility of providing insights into these motion patterns, which could lead to a more refined characterisation of LV function than is currently possible. We have demonstrated our technique on the problem of identifying super-responders, but we believe that it could one day complement or even replace conventional indicators for predicting CRT response in general.

Acknowledgements. This work was funded by EPSRC Grants EP/K030310/1 and EP/K030523/1. We acknowledge financial support from the Department of Health via the NIHR comprehensive Biomedical Research Centre award to Guy's & St Thomas' NHS Foundation Trust with KCL and King's College Hospital NHS Foundation Trust.

References

1. Abraham, W.T., et al.: Cardiac resynchronization in chronic heart failure. The New England Journal of Medicine 346(24), 1845–1853 (2002)
2. António, N., et al.: Identification of 'super-responders' to cardiac resynchronization therapy: the importance of symptom duration and left ventricular geometry. Europace 11(3), 343–349 (2009)
3. Cerqueira, M.D., et al.: Standardized Myocardial Segmentation and Nomenclature for Tomographic Imaging of the Heart. Circulation 105(4), 539–542 (2002)
4. De Craene, M., et al.: SPM to the heart: Mapping of 4D continuous velocities for motion abnormality quantification. In: 2012 IEEE ISBI, pp. 454–457 (2012)
5. Duchateau, N., et al.: A spatiotemporal statistical atlas of motion for the quantification of abnormal myocardial tissue velocities. Medical Image Analysis 15(3), 316–328 (2011)
6. Durrant, R., et al.: Random projections as regularizers: learning a linear discriminant from fewer observations than dimensions. Machine Learning, 1–16 (2014)
7. Hoogendoorn, C., et al.: A High-Resolution Atlas and Statistical Model of the Human Heart From Multislice CT. IEEE Transactions on Medical Imaging 32(1), 28–44 (2013)
8. Jackson, T., et al.: A U-shaped type II contraction pattern in patients with strict left bundle branch block predicts super-response to cardiac resynchronization therapy. Heart Rhythm 11(10), 1790–1797 (2014)
9. Kim, H., et al.: A weight-adjusted voting algorithm for ensembles of classifiers. Journal of the Korean Statistical Society 40(4), 437–449 (2011)
10. Shi, W., et al.: Temporal sparse free-form deformations. Medical Image Analysis 17(7), 779–789 (2013)
11. Tian, Y., et al.: True complete left bundle branch block morphology strongly predicts good response to cardiac resynchronization therapy. Europace 15(10), 1499–1506 (2013)

Motion Compensated Abdominal Diffusion Weighted MRI by Simultaneous Image Registration and Model Estimation (SIR-ME)

Sila Kurugol[1], Moti Freiman[1], Onur Afacan[1], Liran Domachevsky[2], Jeannette M. Perez-Rossello[1], Michael J. Callahan[1], and Simon K. Warfield[1,⋆]

[1] Radiology, Boston Children's Hospital, Harvard Medical School, Boston, USA
[2] Nuclear Medicine, Rabin Medical Center, Petah-Tikva, Israel

Abstract. Non-invasive characterization of water molecule's mobility variations by quantitative analysis of diffusion-weighted MRI (DW-MRI) signal decay in the abdomen has the potential to serve as a biomarker in gastrointestinal and oncological applications. Accurate and reproducible estimation of the signal decay model parameters is challenging due to the presence of respiratory, cardiac, and peristalsis motion. Independent registration of each b-value image to the b-value=0 s/mm^2 image prior to parameter estimation might be sub-optimal because of the low SNR and contrast difference between images of varying b-value. In this work, we introduce a motion-compensated parameter estimation framework that simultaneously solves image registration and model estimation (SIR-ME) problems by utilizing the interdependence of acquired volumes along the diffusion weighting dimension. We evaluated the improvement in model parameters estimation accuracy using 16 in-vivo DW-MRI data sets of Crohn's disease patients by comparing parameter estimates obtained using the SIR-ME model to the parameter estimates obtained by fitting the signal decay model to the acquired DW-MRI images. The proposed SIR-ME model reduced the average root-mean-square error between the observed signal and the fitted model by more than 50%. Moreover, the SIR-ME model estimates discriminate between normal and abnormal bowel loops better than the standard parameter estimates.

Keywords: Diffusion-weighted imaging, abdomen, motion compensation, Crohn's disease, block matching registration.

1 Introduction

DW-MRI enables characterization of the tissue microenvironment by measuring variations in the mobility of water molecules due to cellularity, cell membrane

⋆ This work is supported by the National Institute of Diabetes & Digestive & Kidney Diseases of the NIH under award R01DK100404 and by the Translational Research Program at Boston Childrens Hospital. The content is solely the responsibility of the authors and does not necessarily represent the official views of the NIH.

N. Navab et al. (Eds.): MICCAI 2015, Part III, LNCS 9351, pp. 501–509, 2015.
DOI: 10.1007/978-3-319-24574-4_60

integrity, and the compartment in which water molecules are located (intravascular, extracellular, or intracellular spaces) [1]. The water molecule mobility leads to attenuation in the diffusion signal, which is measured at multiple b-values. The signal decay at high b-values associated with the slow-diffusion component reflects water molecules' mobility in the tissue and the decay at low b-values associated with the fast-diffusion component reflects micro-capillaries' blood flow. Combined with an appropriate model, the variations in both fast and slow diffusion between normal tissue and regions with pathology can be quantified.

Quantitative DW-MRI has been increasingly used for various diseases of abdominal organs including spleen, liver and bowel [1,2,3]. Recently, a more accurate probabilistic model with a spatial homogeneity prior have been proposed [4] to increase the robustness and reproducibility of parameter estimation in low signal-to-noise ratio (SNR) DW-MRI images. However, respiratory, cardiac and peristalsis motion still pose a challenge to robust and reproducible parameter estimation and reduces enthusiasm for using abdominal DW-MRI for diagnostic purposes. A possible solution is to acquire images using breath-holding, gating, respiratory or cardiac triggering. These techniques have disadvantages, and they do not entirely correct for motion. For example, breath holding only allows for a short scan time window at each breath hold, which is not enough to acquire all b-value images at once. It also requires the cooperation of the imaged subject, which is not practical for pediatric patients. Triggering and gating increase scan duration and do not always perform well due to varying breathing pattern.

Another possible solution is to use post-processing techniques based on image-registration algorithms to bring the volumes acquired at different b-values into the same physical coordinate space before fitting a signal decay model [5]. However, each b-value image has different contrast and therefore independent registration of different b-value images to a b=0 image may not be very accurate, especially for high b-value images where the signal is significantly attenuated. Incorporating additional information may improve the registration performance.

A unique feature in DW-MRI in particular, and in parametric imaging techniques in general, is the interdependence of acquired volumes along the fourth parametric dimension, which is the diffusion weighting dimension in the case of DW-MRI. The images at each b-value are related to each other through a signal decay function which models the signal as a function of the b-value used to acquire the image. This interdependence can be exploited as an additional source of information that can be utilized for improved image alignment.

In this work, we introduce a motion-compensated parameter estimation framework that simultaneously solves image registration and model estimation (SIR-ME) problems by utilizing the interdependence of acquired data along the diffusion weighting dimension. The proposed SIR-ME solver jointly estimates transformations between images for alignment, reconstructs high SNR registered diffusion images and estimates the signal decay model parameters from these images.

We evaluated the improvement in parameter estimation accuracy obtained with the SIR-ME model on DW-MR datasets of 16 patients with Crohn's disease. We compared the root-mean-square error (RMSE) of the SIR-ME parameter estimates to the RMSE of the parameter estimates obtained with fitting to: 1) the original non-registered DW-MRI data, and; 2) the independently registered DW-MRI data. The proposed method reduced parameter estimation error by more than 50% compared to parameters estimated without using registration. We also demonstrated potential clinical impact by assessing group differences between normal and inflamed bowel loops of the same patient cohort. The SIR-ME parameter estimates were more precise with smaller in-group standard deviation and a better discrimination power between inflamed and normal bowel loops.

2 Methods

2.1 Simultaneous Image Registration and Model Estimation (SIR-ME) for Motion Compensated DW-MRI Parameter Estimation

In abdominal DW-MRI, we acquire images at multiple ($i = 1..N$) b-values. We then select a signal decay model to estimate the decay rate parameters by fitting that model to the measured signal. The signal decay model proposed by Le Bihan et al. [6] called the intra-voxel incoherent motion (IVIM) model assumes a bi-exponential signal decay function ($g(\Theta, i)$) of the form:

$$g(\Theta, i) = S_0 \left(f \exp\left(-b_i(D + D^*)\right) + (1 - f)(\exp(-b_i D))\right), \tag{1}$$

where $g(\Theta, i)$ is the expected signal at b-value b_i, $\Theta = \{s_0, f, D^*, D\}$ are the IVIM model parameters describing the baseline signal (S_0); the fast diffusion fraction coefficient (f); the fast diffusion coefficient (D^*), characterizing the fast diffusion component related to blood flow in micro-capillaries; and the slow diffusion coefficient (D) associated with extravascular water.

We estimate the parameters by solving a maximum-likelihood estimation problem. The measured signal DW-MRI (S_i) is a sum of the signal component and the noise component. When the non-central χ-distributed parallel imaging acquisition noise is approximated by a Gaussian in the maximum likelihood estimator, the following least-squares minimization problem is obtained:

$$\hat{\Theta} = \arg\min_{\Theta} \sum_{i=1}^{N} \left(S_i - g(\Theta, i)\right)^2, \tag{2}$$

where $g(\Theta, i)$ is given by Eqn. 1.

However, the inherent low SNR of each b-value image may introduce error to the parameter estimates. To improve the SNR before model fitting, multiple DW-MRI signals ($S^{'}_{i,j}$) are acquired at different gradient directions ($j = 1..M$) at the same b-value (b_i). An improved SNR image (S_i) is then estimated from these multiple acquisitions at each b-value. Formally, we obtain a maximum-likelihood estimate of the underlying DW-MRI signal (S_i) by assuming a normal distribution of $S^{'}_{i,j}$'s around S_i, and minimizing the following least-squares problem:

$$\hat{S}_i = \operatorname*{argmin}_{S_i} \sum_{j=1}^{M} (S_i - S^{'}_{i,j})^2 \tag{3}$$

We find the underlying signal ($\hat{S}_i$) by simply averaging the multiple gradient directions ($\hat{S}_i = \frac{1}{M}\sum_{j=1}^{M} S'_{i,j}$) at each b-value i assuming isotropic diffusion.

However, in the presence of motion, measured images ($S'_{i,j}$) are not spatially aligned and therefore cannot be directly averaged. One solution is independently registering each low SNR image ($S'_{i,j}$) to a reference image, which is usually chosen to be the high SNR b=0 s/mm^2 image (S_0) before averaging the low SNR images and then estimating the model parameters by fitting the model to the average of the registered images at each b-value. However, registration of high b-value images to a b=0 s/mm^2 image is challenging due to contrast differences between these images and the even lower SNR of high b-value images.

Instead, we introduce a motion compensated parameter estimation framework that simultaneously solves image registration and model estimation (SIR-ME) problems by utilizing the interdependence of volumes in the acquired data along the fourth parametric dimension, i.e. diffusion weighting dimension as an additional term in the cost function. Our joint formulation is then given by:

$$[\hat{S}, \hat{\Theta}, \hat{T}', \hat{T}] = \underset{S,\Theta,T,T'}{\operatorname{argmin}} \sum_{i=1}^{N}\sum_{j=1}^{M}(S_i - T'_{i,j} \circ S'_{i,j})^2 + \sum_{i=1}^{N}(T_i \circ S_i - g(\Theta, i))^2 \quad (4)$$

where ($S'_{i,j}$) is the low SNR measured image, S_i is the noisy high SNR image template and $g(\Theta, i)$ is the expected signal at b-value b_i given the signal decay model parameters Θ, $T'_{i,j}$ is the transformation between the observed image $S'_{i,j}$ and the high SNR image at b_i, and T_i is the transformation between S_i and S_0.

The first term in this cost function is used to reconstruct the high SNR images from registered low SNR images and the second term is the signal decay model fitting prior. When solving this equation, the expected signal, $g(\Theta, i)$), is dependent on the parameters of the signal decay model (i.e. Θ) and transformations $\hat{T}', \hat{T}$ which are unknown. Therefore, we cannot optimize this equation directly. Instead, we solve it as a simultaneous optimization problem, where registration, reconstruction of the high SNR DW-MRI images and estimation of the signal decay model parameters are iteratively performed.

2.2 Optimization Scheme

We solve Eq. 4 by iteratively estimating the signal decay model parameters Θ and transformation T' given the current estimate of the signal S and T, and estimating the signal S and transformation T, given the current estimate of the model parameters Θ and T'. We describe these steps in detail next.

Signal Decay Model (Θ) Estimation: We use the spatially constrained probability distribution model of slow and fast diffusion (SPIM) [4] to robustly estimate the fast and slow diffusion parameters of the signal decay model Θ. Given the current estimate of the DW-MRI signal S^t and transformation T^t at iteration t, the model parameter Θ^{t+1} is obtained by minimizing:

$$\hat{\Theta}^{t+1} = \underset{\Theta}{\operatorname{argmin}} \sum_{i=1}^{N} (T_i^t \circ S_i^t - g(\Theta, i))^2 + \sum_{v_p \sim v_q} \psi(\Theta_{v_p}, \Theta_{v_q}) \tag{5}$$

where $\psi(\cdot, \cdot)$ is the spatial constraint given by:

$$\psi(\Theta_{v_p}, \Theta_{v_q}) = \alpha W |\Theta_{v_p} - \Theta_{v_q}| \tag{6}$$

and $\alpha \geq 0$ is the spatial coupling factor, W is a diagonal weighting matrix which accounts for the different scales of the parameters in Θ and v_p, v_q are the neighboring voxels according to the employed neighborhood system.

We estimated the model parameters Θ by minimizing Eq. 5 using the "fusion bootstrap moves" combinatorial solver introduced by Freiman et al. [7] and applied in Kurugol et al. [4] to solve the SPIM model.

Estimation of Transformation $T'_{i,j}$: Given the current estimate of expected signal from the signal decay model $g(\Theta, i)$, we solve the registration problem and compute the transformation $T'^{t+1}_{i,j}$ that aligns each low SNR acquired image $S'_{i,j}$ to $g(\Theta, i)$ at each b-value i. We apply the block matching based non-rigid registration algorithm proposed by Commowick et al. [8], using cross-correlation as a measure of intra b-value image similarity.

Reconstruction of High SNR DW-MRI Signal S_i: In this step we update S_i given the current estimate of $T'^{t+1}_{i,j}$ from the registration step. We minimize Eq. 4 to get the next estimate of the signal S^{t+1}.

Estimation of Transformation T_i: We finally estimate transformation T_i^{t+1} to align each reconstructed high SNR template image (S_i) to b=0 s/mm^2 image (S_1) to correct for the remaining misalignments between multiple b-value images. Inter b-value alignment is more accurate at this stage since S_i images have higher SNR than $S'_{i,j}$ images even for high b-values. We use the same block-matching registration algorithm for inter b-value registration but replace the similarity measure with squared cross correlation.

We initialize the algorithm with the acquired DW-MRI data as the current estimate of the signal after application of an initial registration algorithm. We then iteratively alternate between estimating the model parameters, estimation of transformations for registration and estimating the high SNR DW-MRI signal until the change in the model parameter estimations is negligible. The steps of the optimization algorithm are summarized in Table 1.

3 Results

We have tested the performance of the proposed model in DW-MRI data of 16 Crohn's Disease patients. The images were acquired using a 1.5-T scanner (Magnetom Avanto, Siemens Medical Solutions) with free-breathing single-shot echo-planar imaging using the following parameters: repetition/echo time (TR/TE)= 7500/77ms; matrix size=192x156; field of view=300x260 mm; slice thickness/gap = 5mm/0mm; 40 axial slices; 7 b-values = 0,50,100,200,400,600,800 s/mm^2 with 1 excitation, 6 gradient directions; acquisition time = 5.5 min.

Table 1. SIR-ME optimization algorithm

Input:	$S'_{i,j}$: measured signal at b-value i and gradient j.
Output:	$\Theta \leftarrow \Theta^{t+1}$: final parameter values after t^{th} iteration
Initialize:	An initial registration to estimate $T'^{1}_{i,j}$ and T^1_i is applied.
Step 1.	**Estimate signal decay model parameters Θ:**
	Given the current estimate of the high SNR signal S^t and transformation T^t, estimate model parameters Θ^{t+1} by minimizing Eq. 5.
Step 2.	**Estimate transformation $T'_{i,j}$:**
	Given the current estimate of expected signal $g(\Theta, i)$, solve the registration problem and compute the transformation $T'^{t+1}_{i,j}$ that aligns each $S'_{i,j}$ to $g(\Theta, i)$ at each b-value i using the block matching non-rigid registration algorithm [8].
Step 3.	**Estimate high SNR template image at b-value i, S_i, $i = 1..N$**
	Given the current estimate of parameters $T'^{t+1}_{i,j}$, compute the high SNR template signal S^{t+1}_i by minimizing Eq. 4.
Step 4.	**Estimate transformation T_i**
	Estimate transformation T^{t+1}_i to align each b-value high SNR image (S^{t+1}_i) to b=0 s/mm^2 image using the same block-matching registration algorithm. Go back to **Step 1** until convergence.

A region of normal bowel wall and a region of inflamed bowel wall with active Crohn's disease identified in Gd-DTPA contrast enhanced images were delineated on DW-MRI images of each subject by an expert radiologist.

We computed the average RMSE between the measured signal (S_i) and the signal of fitted model ($g(\Theta, i)$) in both normal and inflamed bowel regions to evaluate the effect of motion-compensation on parameter estimation accuracy. Fig. 1 a) and b) compares the RMSE using no registration, independent registration and SIR-ME. The mean error computed over inflamed bowel regions of all subjects reduced from 12.39 ± 8.01 to 6.66 ± 2.91 with registration, and further reduced to 5.63 ± 2.57 with SIR-ME. The error in normal-looking bowel walls reduced from 12.23 ± 5.54 to 7.77 ± 3.17 with registration and further reduced to 6.27 ± 2.42 with SIR-ME. While the independent registration decreased the RMSE in average, it increased the RMSE for some cases. SIR-ME model was consistent and performed either equally well or better in all of the cases. A representative signal decay curve plotted in Fig. 1 c) shows the reduction in error using the SIR-ME model. Fig. 2 b) shows an image region plotted for b-values from 0 to $800 s/mm^2$. The image intensity decays smoothly with increasing b-values when SIR-ME model is used, compared to original signal w/o registration.

We also compared the performance of estimated parameters in differentiating normal and inflamed bowel regions. In Table 3, the mean values of the parameters for normal and inflamed bowel regions, computed using no registration, independent registration, and SIR-ME model, are listed. These results demonstrated that the proposed SIR-ME model estimated f and D parameters with greater precision and lower intra-group standard deviation compared to the other two models. Moreover, we observed an increased statistically significant difference between the two groups using the SIR-ME model compared to other two models, which indicates a better discrimination power. We also trained Naive Bayes classifiers for D and f parameters independently, and obtained the classification errors of 0.41 w/o registration, 0.28 with registration and 0.15 with

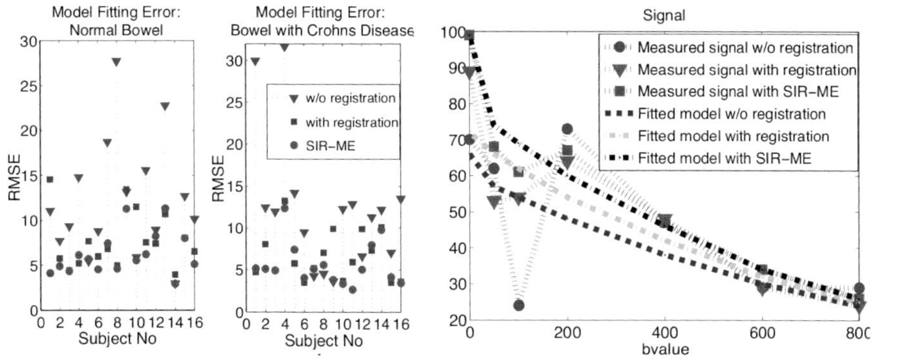

Fig. 1. Average RMSE between DW-MRI signal and signal of fitted model compared for 1) without registration, 2) with registration, and 3) with simultaneous image registration and motion estimation (SIR-ME) are plotted for a) normal and b) inflamed bowel regions in 16 patients. c) Signal decay plot for one voxel from an inflamed region.

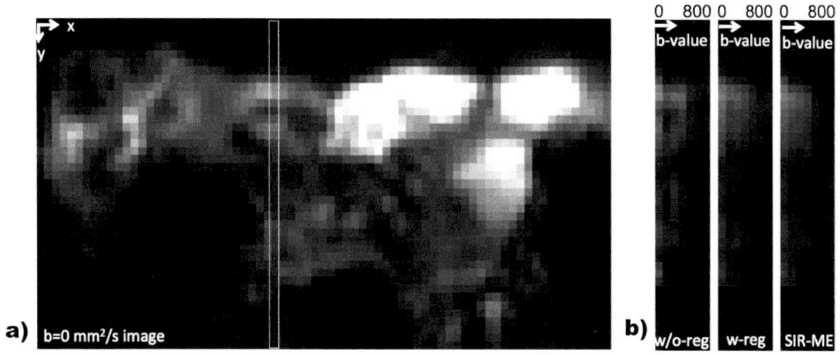

Fig. 2. a) shows a sample b=$0mm^2/s$ image region. The white rectangle shows a selected image column that is plotted for increasing b-values in b) for w/o-registration, with registration and with SIR-ME images. SIR-ME method successfully compensates for motion and results in smoothly decaying intensities in b-value direction.

SIR-ME using D parameter; 0.28 w/o registration, 0.28 with registration and 0.15 with SIRME using f parameter. These results showed that SIR-ME model achieved the best classification accuracy for both f and D parameters.

4 Conclusions

Abdominal DW-MRI enables characterization of tissue microstructure of pathological regions such as inflamed bowel in Crohn's disease. The presence of motion and low SNR reduces the accuracy and reproducibility of parameter estimates and prevents more extensive clinical utility. In this work, we introduced a motion-compensated parameter estimation framework that simultaneously solves image registration and model estimation (SIR-ME) problems by utilizing the interdependence of acquired volumes along the diffusion weighting dimension. Our

Table 2. Comparison of parameters estimated without registration, with independent registration and with SIR-ME models for normal and Crohn's disease bowel regions

		Normal bowel regions	Inflamed bowel regions	
	parameter	mean ± sd	mean ± sd	p-value
D	w/o reg	1.56 ± 0.92	0.98 ± 0.62	0.04
	with reg	1.99 ± 0.59	1.25 ± 0.47	**5x10^{-4}**
	SIR-ME	2.15 ± 0.33	1.45 ± 0.26	**3x10^{-7}**
f	w/o reg	0.65 ± 0.23	0.47 ± 0.23	0.03
	with reg	0.57 ± 0.18	0.35 ± 0.20	**0.003**
	SIR-ME	0.56 ± 0.16	0.28 ± 0.11	**2x10^{-6}**
D*	w/o reg	24.51 ± 16.60	32.75 ± 50.97	0.54
	with reg	31.34 ± 19.31	64.88 ± 62.98	0.05
	SIR-ME	38.03 ± 21.17	57.55 ± 59.99	0.23

experiments on 16 Crohn's disease patients showed that the SIR-ME method reduced the model fitting error by more than 50% compared to the errors obtained from non-registered original DW-MRI images. We demonstrated potential clinical impact by evaluating group differences between normal and inflamed bowel loops. The parameters obtained with the SIR-ME model had lower intra-group standard deviation and a better discrimination power compared to parameter estimates obtained without any registration and with independent registration.

References

1. Chavhan, G.B., AlSabban, Z., Babyn, P.S.: Diffusion-weighted imaging in pediatric body MR imaging: Principles, technique, and emerging applications. RadioGraphics 34(3), E73–E88 (2014)
2. Jang, K.M., Kim, S.H., Hwang, J., Lee, S.J., Kang, T.W., Lee, M.W., Choi, D.: Differentiation of malignant from benign focal splenic lesions: Added value of diffusion-weighted MRI. American Journal of Roentgenology 203(4), 803–812 (2014)
3. Yoon, J.H., et al.: Evaluation of hepatic focal lesions using diffusion-weighted MRI: Comparison of apparent diffusion coefficient and intravoxel incoherent motion-derived parameters. J. of Magnetic Resonance Imaging 39(2), 276–285 (2014)
4. Kurugol, S., Freiman, M., Afacan, O., Perez-Rossello, J.M., Callahan, M.J., Warfield, S.K.: Spatially-constrained probability distribution model of incoherent motion (SPIM) in diffusion weighted MRI signals of crohn's disease. In: Yoshida, H., Näppi, J.J., Saini, S. (eds.) ABDI 2014. LNCS, vol. 8676, pp. 117–127. Springer, Heidelberg (2014)
5. Guyader, J.M., Bernardin, L., Douglas, N.H., Poot, D.H., Niessen, W.J., Klein, S.: Influence of image registration on apparent diffusion coefficient images computed from free-breathing diffusion MRI of the abdomen. JMRI (2014)
6. Le Bihan, D., Breton, E., Lallemand, D., Aubin, M.L., Vignaud, J., Laval-Jeantet, M.: Separation of diffusion and perfusion in intravoxel incoherent motion MR imaging. Radiology 168(2), 497–505 (1988)

7. Freiman, M., Perez-Rossello, J.M., Callahan, M.J., Voss, S.D., Ecklund, K., Mulkern, R.V., Warfield, S.K.: Reliable estimation of incoherent motion parametric maps from diffusion-weighted MRI using fusion bootstrap moves. MEDIA 17(3), 325–336 (2013)
8. Commowick, O., Wiest-Daesslé, N., Prima, S.: Automated diffeomorphic registration of anatomical structures with rigid parts: Application to dynamic cervical MRI. In: Ayache, N., Delingette, H., Golland, P., Mori, K. (eds.) MICCAI 2012, Part II. LNCS, vol. 7511, pp. 163–170. Springer, Heidelberg (2012)

Fast Reconstruction of Accelerated Dynamic MRI Using Manifold Kernel Regression

Kanwal K. Bhatia[1], Jose Caballero[1], Anthony N. Price[2], Ying Sun[3], Jo V. Hajnal[2], and Daniel Rueckert[1]

[1] Biomedical Image Analysis Group, Imperial College London, UK
[2] Division of Imaging Sciences and Biomedical Engineering, King's College London, UK
[3] Department of Electrical and Computer Engineering, National University of Singapore, Singapore

Abstract. We present a novel method for fast reconstruction of dynamic MRI from undersampled k-space data, thus enabling highly accelerated acquisition. The method is based on kernel regression along the manifold structure of the sequence derived directly from k-space data. Unlike compressed sensing techniques which require solving a complex optimisation problem, our reconstruction is fast, taking under 5 seconds for a 30 frame sequence on conventional hardware. We demonstrate our method on 10 retrospectively undersampled cardiac cine MR sequences, showing improved performance over state-of-the-art compressed sensing.

1 Introduction

Dynamic Magnetic Resonance imaging (MRI), for example, cardiac imaging, functional MRI, angiography or contrast agent uptake studies, is constrained by motion or intensity changes that occur over the duration of the image acquisition. Due to physical limits on the speed of acquisition in MRI, a compromise between the proportion of k-space and the frequency of time points acquired needs to be determined, resulting in a trade-off between spatial and temporal resolution. Accelerating the acquisition of each frame of a dynamic sequence is therefore a popular approach used to improve spatial or temporal resolution, or to enhance patient comfort by reducing scanning time [1]. One method of acceleration is through the undersampling of k-space, for example, by acquiring only a subset of phase-encode lines. The resultant missing lines of k-space, can then be completed through interpolation [8][11] or compressed sensing [7][5][9] techniques, which are active areas of current research.

While MRI acquisition of dynamic sequences is difficult to obtain at high-resolution ordinarily, the additional temporal structure of the images can be utilised to aid reconstruction. Compressed sensing methods such as [9][5][10][14] have been developed which incorporate temporal information, allowing for high rates of k-space undersampling. These methods require the reconstructed images to adhere to a specified model (such as sparsity in some domain), typically resulting in complex optimisation problems that can be slow to solve.

N. Navab et al. (Eds.): MICCAI 2015, Part III, LNCS 9351, pp. 510–518, 2015.
DOI: 10.1007/978-3-319-24574-4_61

Interpolation techniques have also previously been used in the reconstruction of undersampled k-space [8][11]. These generally require regular sampling in the k-t domain, and interpolate from neighbouring sampled locations in space and time. However, while these methods are fast, they typically have not been able to obtain the same levels of acquisition acceleration with comparable image quality as compressed sensing methods.

In this paper, we propose an alternative method of completing the missing lines of k-space, based on learning the underlying temporal manifold structure of k-space directly from the acquired data. Recent work [4][12] has shown that the inter-frame changes involved in dynamic MRI sequences, such as free-breathing cardiac or lung motion MRI, can be well-parameterised by non-linear dimensionality reduction techniques such as manifold learning. Motivated by developments in compressive manifold learning [2], we propose to exploit this to build a temporal manifold directly from undersampled k-space data. We then reconstruct the unknown lines of k-space through kernel regression in manifold space.

We demonstrate the performance of our proposed algorithm on ten retrospectively undersampled cardiac cine sequences, comparing to state-of-the-art compressed sensing techniques [9][5]. As our algorithm requires computation solely in k-space, our method is significantly faster than compressed sensing algorithms, while achieving comparable rates of acceleration and improved accuracy. Furthermore, the algorithm does not require strict conditions on the sampling pattern used.

2 Methods

Dynamic MRI involves acquisition of raw data in k-t space, that is, acquiring a time series of k-space frames (often 2D) at varying time points t. Cartesian undersampling in MRI is a common method used to accelerate acquisition of a frame by sampling a subset of k-space locations in the phase-encode direction (and fully in the frequency-encode direction). In this paper, we aim to use manifold learning to extract the temporal structure of a sequence directly from the common locations of k-space that are sampled in all frames.

2.1 Manifold Learning

Manifold learning has been applied to dynamic MR images in a number of recent applications [4][12]. While most medical imaging applications have so far involved manifold learning in image space, recent work [12], in which the learnt structure of a temporal sequence was used for respiratory gating, has shown that manifold learning can also be performed directly on k-space data.

In this paper, we use Laplacian Eigenmaps, which has been successfully applied in dynamic MRI applications [13][4][12]. The aim is to find an embedding which preserves the structure of the dataset by ensuring that data points (k-space samples of each frame of the sequence) which are “close” in the high-dimensional space remain "close" in the low-dimensional embedding. This is done by minimising the following cost function:

$$C(\mathbf{x}) = \sum_{ij} (\mathbf{x}_i - \mathbf{x}_j)^T (\mathbf{x}_i - \mathbf{x}_j) W_{ij} \tag{1}$$

which minimises the weighted Euclidean distance between the embedding coordinates $\mathbf{x}_i$ and $\mathbf{x}_j$ of data points i and j, respectively, in the low-dimensional embedding. The measure of closeness between points i and j is defined by the weight, W_{ij}, which indicates their similarity. The solution to (1) is obtained using properties of the graph of the data. We define a diagonal matrix as the column (or row) sum of the weights for each vertex $D_{ii} = \sum_j W_{ij}$, and the graph Laplacian as an operator on the graph vertices $\mathbf{L} = \mathbf{D} - \mathbf{W}$. Using these, we can rewrite the cost function as [3]:

$$C(\mathbf{x}) = \sum_{ij} (\mathbf{x}_i - \mathbf{x}_j)^T (\mathbf{x}_i - \mathbf{x}_j) W_{ij} = 2\mathbf{x}^T \mathbf{L}\mathbf{x} \tag{2}$$

After adding the constraint $\mathbf{x}^T \mathbf{D}\mathbf{x} = 1$ to eliminate arbitrary scale factors in the solution, the m-dimensional solution to (2) is given by the eigenvectors $\mathbf{x}$ of the generalised eigenvalue problem:

$$\mathbf{L}\mathbf{x} = \lambda \mathbf{D}\mathbf{x} \tag{3}$$

corresponding to the m smallest non-zero eigenvalues (λ).

In order to maintain the local structure of the data, the graph edge weights $\mathbf{W}$ are set to correspond to the neighbourhood (defined using k-nearest neighbours in the space of the original data) similarities between data points. One commonly-used metric is based on the ℓ_2 (Euclidean) norm distance $d_{st} = \|\mathbf{y}_s - \mathbf{y}_t\|_2^2$ between the sampled k-space lines at times s and t. Here $\mathbf{y}_.$ represents all the k-space values at a given time point which have been commonly sampled in all time frames. The final weights are then obtained using a Gaussian kernel function:

$$W_{st} = \begin{cases} e^{-\frac{\|\mathbf{y}_s - \mathbf{y}_t\|^2}{2\sigma^2}} & \text{if } s, t \text{ are neighbours in distance;} \\ 0 & \text{otherwise.} \end{cases}$$

where σ indicates the variance of the Gaussian.

2.2 Manifold Learning of Under-Sampled k-space

We require a time-varying sampling mask with a number of lines of k-space which are sampled in all frames of the sequence in order to construct the manifold. Recent work [2][12] has introduced the theory of *compressive manifold learning*, showing that for data that lies on a low-dimensional manifold, only a random subsample of the data is needed to retrieve that manifold. However, the data distribution of k-space is such that the majority of energy lies in the centre of k-space; we therefore require the central line of k-space to be fully-sampled in all frames. We show in Section 3.1 how the manifold created varies with number of lines of k-space used and that good approximations can be obtained even when using a single line. The left panel of Fig. 3b shows an example of a temporal mask with a sixth of the k-space phase-encoding lines sampled.

2.3 k-space Interpolation Using Manifold Kernel Regression

We assume, for the purposes of interpolation, that the manifold co-ordinates obtained as above would be common to all lines of k-space. Empirically, we have found this to give a good approximation when interpolating k-space. Each missing phase-encoding line of k-space is interpolated individually using manifold kernel regression along the manifold. This has previously been used to estimate the appearance of brain images of particular populations at unsampled locations [6]. For each frame, each unknown line in k-space is interpolated from the filled frames of the same line using weights based on the manifold co-ordinates as found in the previous section. The values $\mathbf{y}_f$ of each line of k-space in frame f are calculated using:

$$\mathbf{y}_f = \frac{\sum_i \kappa(\mathbf{x}_f, \mathbf{x}_i)\mathbf{y}_i}{\sum_j \kappa(\mathbf{x}_f, \mathbf{x}_j)} \tag{4}$$

Here $\mathbf{y}_i$ are the values of the sampled k-space line in frame i and $\kappa(\mathbf{x}_f, \cdot)$ is a kernel determining the distance between the manifold co-ordinates $\mathbf{x}_f$ of frame f and all other filled frames. As with the construction of the manifold, we use a Gaussian kernel given by:

$$\kappa(\mathbf{x}_f, \mathbf{x}_i) = \frac{1}{\sqrt{2\pi}\phi} e^{-\frac{\|\mathbf{x}_f - \mathbf{x}_i\|_2}{2\phi^2}} \tag{5}$$

where ϕ is chosen to be half the standard deviation of the manifold embedding co-ordinates. This means that data which are very far away in manifold co-ordinates are given less weight than those close together.

2.4 Algorithm Summary

Given time-varying sampling mask with at least the central line of k-space sampled in all frames, the missing lines of k-space are interpolated as follows:

1. Calculate manifold co-ordinates from the common line(s) of k-space sampled in all frames using Equation 3.
2. Interpolate each remaining line of k-space from the sampled frames of the same line using Equation 4.

3 Experiments and Results

Fully-sampled, short-axis cardiac cine scans were acquired from 10 subjects on a Siemens 1.5T scanner using retrospective gating. All datasets contain 30 temporal frames of size 256 × 256 with a 320 × 320 mm field of view and 10 mm slice thickness. These were generated using a combination of 32-channel data. Coil sensitivity maps were normalised to a body coil image to produce a single complex-valued image set that could either be back-transformed to regenerate complex k-space samples or further processed to form magnitude images. These images were then retrospectively undersampled for analysis.

3.1 Manifold Creation

We first show that even a subsample of the k-space lines can approximate the low-dimensional manifold of a full acquisition if the central line of k-space is included. Fig. 3.1 shows the 1-dimensional manifold created from the commonly-sampled lines of k-space of an example subject, using varying numbers of k-space lines. It can be seen that this manifold approximates the changes occurring during the cardiac cycle, even when only a single central line is used.

3.2 Comparison to State-of-the-Art Compressed Sensing Algorithms

We compare the results of our proposed reconstruction with those from two state-of-the-art dynamic MRI acceleration schemes: Dictionary Learning Temporal Gradient (DLTG) compressed sensing [5] and a Low Rank plus Sparse (LRS) reconstruction [9]. In both cases, we use the implementations and sampling masks provided by the toolboxes of the authors to ensure no bias in performance is caused by sub-optimal sampling for their method. All reconstructions were implemented in MATLAB and run on a 3.4GHz Intel Core i7-2600 CPU.

Fig. 3.2 shows the mask and example frames using the proposed method compared to DLTG. The mask in this case uses an 8 times undersampling scheme with the central nine lines of k-space used to build a 1-D manifold. The DLTG framework uses a patch size of 4×4×4 and 600 dictionary atoms for all subjects.

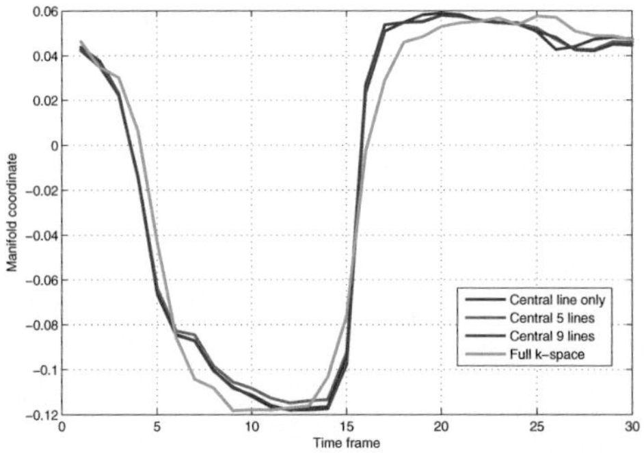

Fig. 1. 1-D Manifold created from cardiac cine sequence of example subject using varying number of lines of k-space.

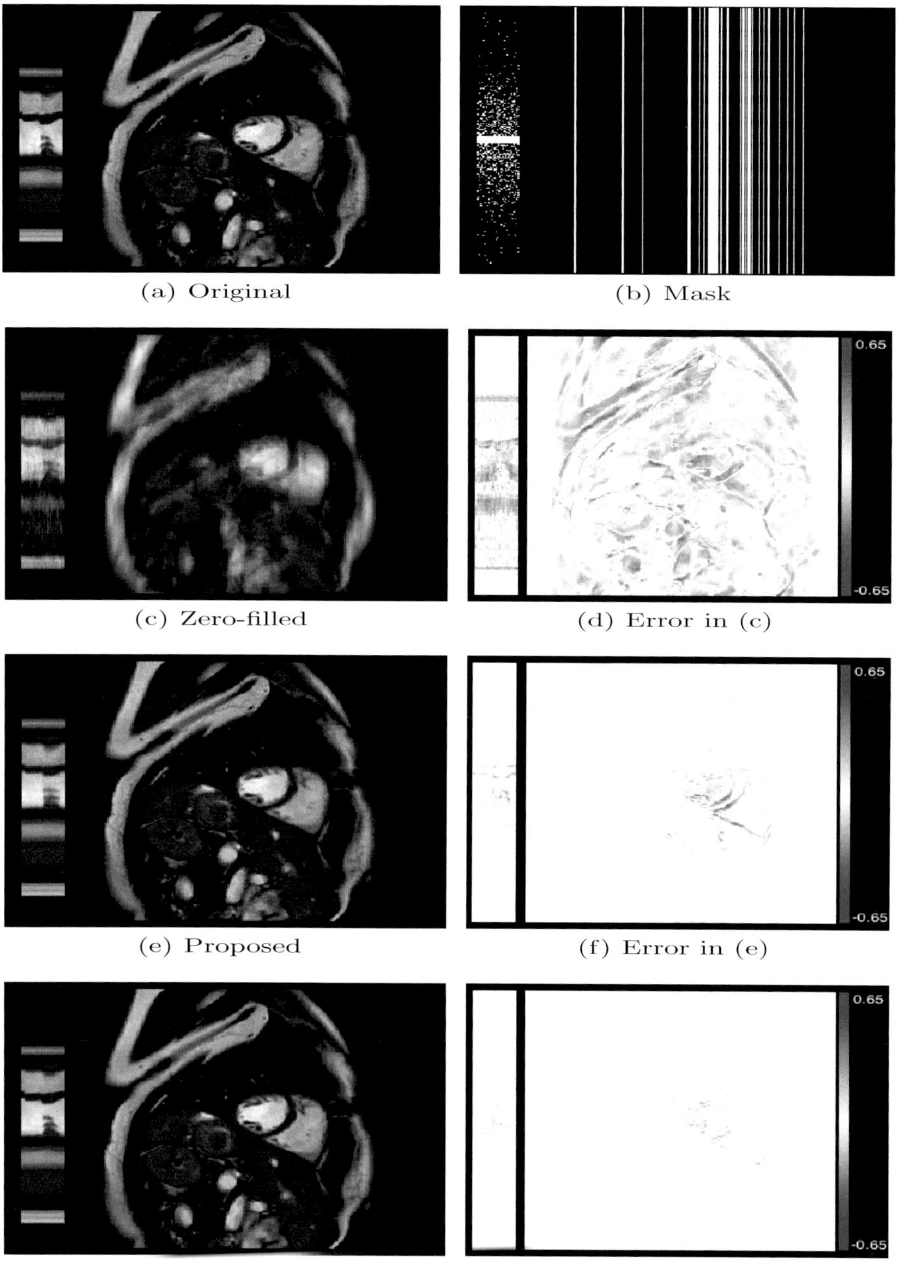

(a) Original (b) Mask

(c) Zero-filled (d) Error in (c)

(e) Proposed (f) Error in (e)

(g) DLTG (h) Error in (g)

Fig. 2. Example reconstruction of retrospectively undersampled (x8) cardiac cine images comparing proposed reconstructions with DLTG [5]. The temporal profile of the sequence and errors are shown on the left of each sub-figure.

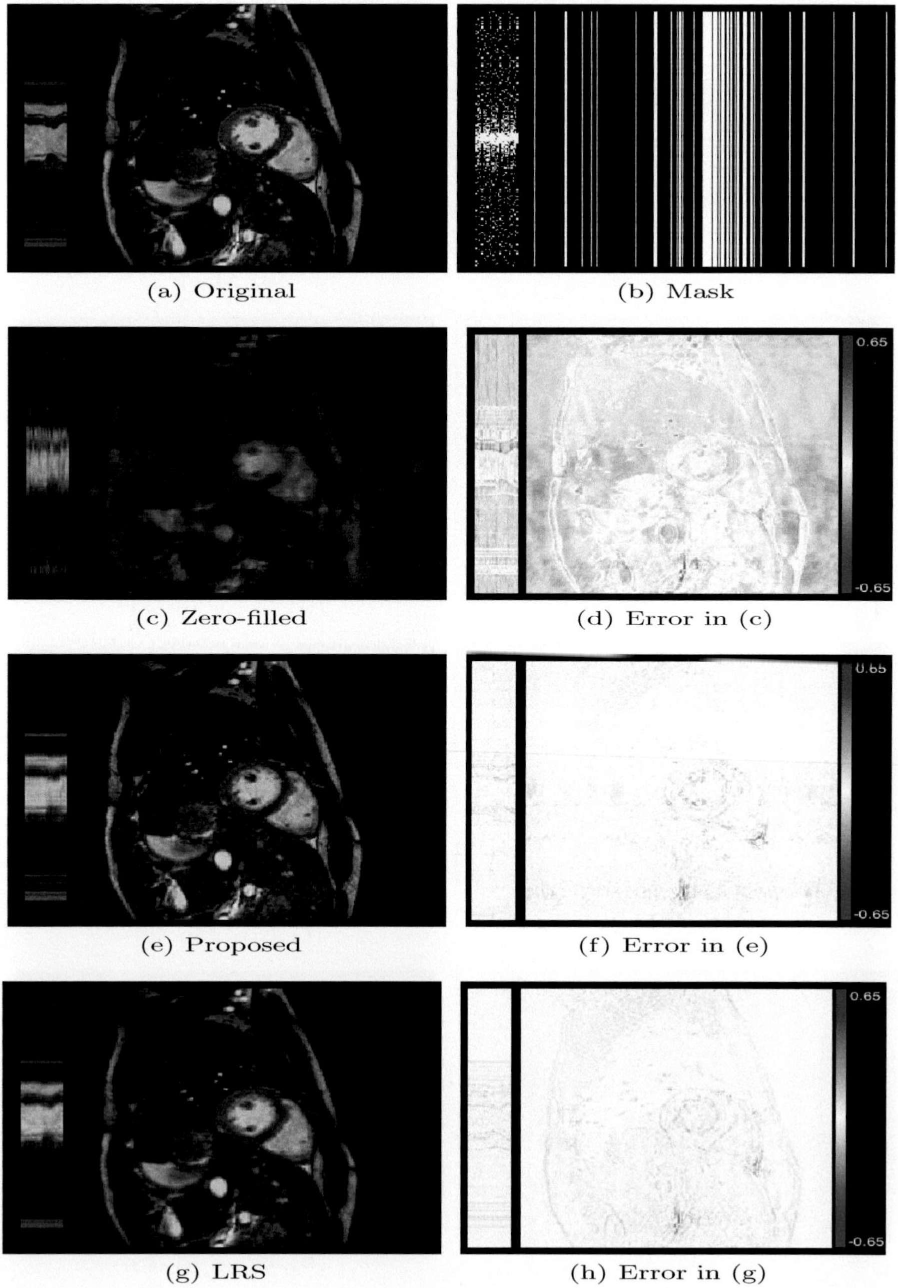

Fig. 3. Example reconstruction of retrospectively undersampled (x6) cardiac cine images comparing proposed reconstruction and LRS [9]. The temporal profile of the sequence and errors are shown on the left of each sub-figure.

The initial mean PSNR, taken over the all frames of all sequences, of the zero-filled reconstruction is 21.7dB. The mean PSNR of the DLTG reconstruction was 32.8±2.2dB while that of our proposed method was 31.6±1.7dB. However the gain in reconstruction time is significant - our method taking under 5 seconds for every sequence while the mean reconstruction time for DLTG being 53 hours.

We also compare our method to LRS using the mask provided by the authors for cardiac cine sequences, providing a 6 times undersampling. Default LRS parameters are used for all sequences. Example sequence, mask and reconstructions are shown in Fig. 3.2. The 1-D manifold here is constructed from the central line of k-space only. The mean PSNR over all sequences of the zero-filled reconstructions is 21.2dB. Our proposed method improves the PSNR to 33.1±1.4dB compared to 30.7±1.9dB for LRS, while taking 3 seconds for each subject compared to the 46 seconds of LRS on average.

4 Discussion

We have presented a method for fast reconstruction of undersampled k-space for accelerated dynamic MRI acquisition. Compared to state-of-the-art compressed sensing, our method achieves good reconstruction quality at significantly faster speeds. In this paper, we have not optimised sampling for our method, instead showing how it can be used with existing strategies for comparison. Optimising the sampling mask is the subject of ongoing work.

References

1. Axel, L., Sodickson, D.K.: The need for speed: Accelerating CMR imaging assessment of cardiac function. JACC Cardiovasc. Imaging 7(9), 893–895 (2014)
2. Baraniuk, R.G., Wakin, M.B.: Random projections of smooth manifolds. Foundations of Computational Mathematics 9, 51–77 (2009)
3. Belkin, M., Niyogi, P.: Laplacian eigenmaps for dimensionality reduction and data representation. Neural Computation 15(6), 1373–1396 (2003)
4. Bhatia, K.K., Rao, A., Price, A.N., Wolz, R., Hajnal, J., Rueckert, D.: Hierarchical manifold learning for regional image analysis. IEEE T. Med. Im. 33, 444–461 (2014)
5. Caballero, J., Price, A.N., Rueckert, D., Hajnal, J.: Dictionary learning and time sparsity for dynamic mr data reconstruction. IEEE T. Med. Im. 33, 979–994 (2014)
6. Davis, B.C., Fletcher, P.T., Bullitt, E., Joshi, S.: Population shape regression from random design data. International Journal of Computer Vision 90, 255–266 (2010)
7. Lustig, M., Donoho, D., Pauly, J.M.: Sparse mri: The application of compressed sensing for rapid MR imaging. Medical Image Analysis 58(6), 1182–1195 (2007)
8. Madore, B., Hoge, W., Chao, T.: Retrospectively gated cardiac cine imaging with temporal and spatial acceleration. Mag. Resonance in Medicine 29, 457–469 (2011)
9. Otazo, R., Candes, E., Sodickson, D.K.: Low-rank plus sparse matrix decomposition for accelerated dynamic MRI with separation of background and dynamic components. Magnetic Resonance in Medicine 73(3), 1125–1136 (2015)
10. Poddar, S., Lingala, S.G., Jacob, M.: Real-time cardiac MRI using manifold sensing. In: International Society of Magnetic Resonance in Medicine, p. 5309 (2014)

11. Tsao, J., Boesiger, P., Pruessmann, K.P.: k-t blast and k-t sense: Dynamic mri with high frame rate exploiting spatiotemporal correlations. MRM 50, 1031–1042 (2003)
12. Usman, M., Vaillant, G., Schaefter, T., Prieto, C.: Compressive manifold learning: estimating one-dimensional respiratory motion directly from undersampled k-space data. Magnetic Resonance in Medicine 72, 1130–1140 (2014)
13. Wachinger, C., Yigitsoy, M., Navab, N.: Manifold learning for image-based breathing gating with application to 4D ultrasound. In: Jiang, T., Navab, N., Pluim, J.P.W., Viergever, M.A. (eds.) MICCAI 2010, Part II. LNCS, vol. 6362, pp. 26–33. Springer, Heidelberg (2010)
14. Zhao, B., Haldar, J.P., Christodoulou, A.G., Liang, Z.P.: Image reconstruction from highly undersampled (k-t)-space data with joint partial separability and sparsity constraints. IEEE T. Med. Im. 31, 1809–1820 (2012)

Predictive Modeling of Anatomy with Genetic and Clinical Data

Adrian V. Dalca[1], Ramesh Sridharan[1], Mert R. Sabuncu[1,2], and Polina Golland[1,⋆]

[1] Computer Science and Artificial Intelligence Lab, EECS, MIT
[2] Martinos Center for Biomedical Imaging, Harvard Medical School

Abstract. We present a semi-parametric generative model for predicting anatomy of a patient in subsequent scans following a single baseline image. Such predictive modeling promises to facilitate novel analyses in both voxel-level studies and longitudinal biomarker evaluation. We capture anatomical change through a combination of population-wide regression and a non-parametric model of the subject's health based on individual genetic and clinical indicators. In contrast to classical correlation and longitudinal analysis, we focus on predicting new observations from a single subject observation. We demonstrate prediction of follow-up anatomical scans in the ADNI cohort, and illustrate a novel analysis approach that compares a patient's scans to the predicted subject-specific healthy anatomical trajectory.

1 Introduction

We present a method for predicting anatomy based on external information, including genetic and clinical indicators. Specifically, given only a single baseline scan of a new subject in a longitudinal study, our model predicts anatomical changes and generates a subsequent image by leveraging subject-specific genetic and clinical information. Such voxel-wise prediction opens up several new areas of analysis, enabling novel investigations both at the voxel level and at the level of derivative biomarker measures. For example, voxel level differences between the true progression of a patient with dementia and their predicted healthy anatomy highlight spatial patterns of disease. We validate our method by comparing measurements of volumes of anatomical structures based on predicted images to those extracted from the acquired scans.

Our model describes the change from a single (or *baseline*) medical scan in terms of population trends and subject-specific external information. We model how anatomical appearance changes with age on average in a population, as well as deviations from the population average using a person's *health profile*. We characterize such profiles non-parametrically based on the genotype, clinical information, and the baseline image. Subject-specific change is constructed

⋆ A listing of ADNI investigators is available at `http://tinyurl.com/ADNI-main`. Data used via AD DREAM Challenge: `https://www.synapse.org/#!Synapse:syn2290704`

N. Navab et al. (Eds.): MICCAI 2015, Part III, LNCS 9351, pp. 519–526, 2015.
DOI: 10.1007/978-3-319-24574-4_62

from the similarity of health profiles in the cohort, using a Gaussian process parametrized by a population health covariance. Given the predicted change, we synthesize new images through an appearance model.

Statistical population analysis is one of the central topics in medical image computing. The classical correlation-based analysis has yielded important characterization of relationships within imaging data and with independent clinical variables [2,11,12,14]. Regression models of object appearance have been previously used for atlas construction and population analysis [2,14]. These methods characterize population trends with respect to external variables, such as age or gender, and construct clinically relevant population averages. Longitudinal analyses also characterize subject-specific temporal effects, usually in terms of changes in the biomarkers of interest. Longitudinal cohorts and studies promise to provide crucial insights into aging and disease [11,12]. Mixed effects models have been shown to improve estimation of subject-specific longitudinal trends by using inter-population similarity [3,15]. While these approaches offer a powerful basis for analysis of biomarkers or images in a population, they require multiple observations for any subject, and do not aim to provide subject-specific predictions given a single observation. The parameters of the models are examined for potential scientific insight, but they are not tested for predictive power. In contrast, we define the problem of population analysis as predicting anatomical changes for individual subjects. Our generative model incorporates a population trend and uses subject-specific genetic and clinical information, along with the baseline image, to generate subsequent anatomical images. This prediction-oriented approach provides avenues for novel analysis, as illustrated by our experimental results.

2 Prediction Model

Given a dataset of patients with longitudinal data, and a single baseline image for a new patient, we predict follow-up anatomical states for the patient. We model anatomy as a phenotype y that captures the underlying structure of interest. For example, y can be a low-dimensional descriptor of the anatomy at each voxel. We assume we only have a measurement of our phenotype at baseline y_b for a new subject. Our goal is to predict the phenotype y_t at a later time t. We let x_t be the subject age at time t, and define $\Delta x_t = x_t - x_b$ and $\Delta y_t = y_t - y_b$. We model the change in phenotype y_t using linear regression:

$$\Delta y_t = \Delta x_t \beta + \epsilon, \tag{1}$$

where β is the subject-specific regression coefficient, and noise $\epsilon \sim \mathcal{N}(0, \sigma^2)$ is sampled from zero-mean Gaussian distribution with variance σ^2.

2.1 Subject-Specific Longitudinal Change

To model subject-specific effects, we define $\beta = \bar{\beta} + H(g, c, f_b)$, where $\bar{\beta}$ is a global regression coefficient shared by the entire population, and H captures a deviation from this coefficient based on the subject's genetic variants g, clinical information c, and baseline image features f_b.

We assume that patients' genetic variants and clinical indicators affect their anatomical appearance, and that subjects with similar health profiles exhibit similar patterns of anatomical change. We let $h_G(\cdot)$, $h_C(\cdot)$, $h_I(\cdot)$ be functions that capture genetic, clinical and imaging effects on the regression coefficients:

$$H(g, c, I_b) = h_G(g) + h_C(c) + h_I(f_b). \tag{2}$$

Combining with (1), we arrive at the full model

$$\Delta y_t = \Delta x_t \bar{\beta} + \Delta x_t \big(h_G(g) + h_C(c) + h_I(f_b)\big) + \epsilon, \tag{3}$$

which captures the population trend $\bar{\beta}$, as well as the subject-specific deviations $[h_G(\cdot), h_C(\cdot), h_I(\cdot)]$.

For a longitudinal cohort of N subjects, we group all T_i observations for subject i to form $\boldsymbol{\Delta y}_i = [y_{i_1}, y_{i_2}, ...y_{i_{T_i}}]$. We then form the global vector $\boldsymbol{\Delta y} = [\boldsymbol{\Delta y}_1, \boldsymbol{\Delta y}_2, ..., \boldsymbol{\Delta y}_N]$. We similarly form vectors $\boldsymbol{\Delta x}$, $\boldsymbol{h}_G$, $\boldsymbol{h}_C$, $\boldsymbol{h}_I$, $\boldsymbol{g}$, $\boldsymbol{c}$, $\boldsymbol{f_b}$ and $\boldsymbol{\epsilon}$, to build the full regression model:

$$\boldsymbol{\Delta y} = \boldsymbol{\Delta x}\bar{\beta} + \boldsymbol{\Delta x} \odot (\boldsymbol{h}_G(\boldsymbol{g}) + \boldsymbol{h}_C(\boldsymbol{c}) + \boldsymbol{h}_I(\boldsymbol{f}_b)) + \boldsymbol{\epsilon}, \tag{4}$$

where $\odot$ is the Hadamard, or element-wise product. This formulation is mathematically equivalent to a General Linear Model (GLM) [9] in terms of the health profile predictors $[\boldsymbol{h}_G, \boldsymbol{h}_C, \boldsymbol{h}_I]$.

We employ Gaussian process priors to model the health functions:

$$h_D(\cdot) \sim GP(\mathbf{0}, \tau_D^2 K_D(\cdot, \cdot)), \tag{5}$$

where covariance kernel function $\tau_D^2 K_D(z_i, z_j)$ captures the similarity between subjects i and j using feature vectors $\boldsymbol{z}_i$ and $\boldsymbol{z}_j$ for $D \in \{G, C, I\}$. We discuss the particular form of $K(\cdot, \cdot)$ used in the experiments later in the paper.

2.2 Learning

The Bayesian formulation in (4) and (5) can be interpreted as a linear mixed effects model (LMM) [10] or a least squares kernel machine (LSKM) regression model [5,8]. We use the LMM interpretation to learn the parameters of our model, and the LSKM interpretation to perform final phenotype predictions.

Specifically, we treat $\bar{\beta}$ as the coefficient vector of fixed effects and $\boldsymbol{h}_G, \boldsymbol{h}_C$, and $\boldsymbol{h}_I$ as independent random effects. We seek the maximum likelihood estimates of parameters $\bar{\beta}$ and $\boldsymbol{\theta} = (\tau_G^2, \tau_C^2, \tau_I^2, \sigma^2)$ by adapting standard procedures for LMMs [5,8]. As standard LMM solutions become computationally expensive for thousands of observations, we take advantage of the fact that while the entire genetic and the image phenotype data is large, the use of kernels on baseline data reduces the model size substantially. We obtain intuitive iterative updates that project the residuals at each step onto the expected rate of change in likelihood, and update $\bar{\beta}$ using the best linear unbiased predictor.

2.3 Prediction

Under the LSKM interpretation, the terms $h(\cdot)$ are estimated by minimizing a penalized squared-error loss function, which leads to the following solution [5,7,8,16]:

$$h(z_i) = \sum_{j=1}^{N} \alpha_j K(\boldsymbol{z}_i, \boldsymbol{z}_j) \quad \text{or} \quad \boldsymbol{h} = \boldsymbol{\alpha}^T \boldsymbol{K} \tag{6}$$

for some vector $\boldsymbol{\alpha}$. Combining with the definitions of the LMM, we estimate coefficients vectors $\boldsymbol{\alpha}_G, \boldsymbol{\alpha}_C$ and $\boldsymbol{\alpha}_I$ from a linear system of equations that involves our estimates of $\hat{\beta}$ and θ. We can then re-write (4) as

$$\Delta \boldsymbol{y} = \Delta \boldsymbol{x} \bar{\beta} + \Delta \boldsymbol{x} \left(\boldsymbol{\alpha}_G^T \boldsymbol{K}_G + \boldsymbol{\alpha}_C^T \boldsymbol{K}_C + \boldsymbol{\alpha}_I^T \boldsymbol{K}_I \right) \tag{7}$$

and predict a phenotype at time t for a new subject i:

$$y_t = y_b + \Delta x_t \left[\bar{\beta} + \sum_{j=1}^{N} \alpha_{G,j} K_G(g_i, g_j) + \alpha_{C,j} K_C(c_i, c_j) + \alpha_{I,j} K_I(f_i, f_j) \right]. \tag{8}$$

3 Model Instantiation for Anatomical Predictions

The full model (3) can be used with many reasonable phenotype definitions. Here, we describe the phenotype model we use for anatomical predictions and specify the similarity kernels of the health profile.

3.1 Anatomical Phenotype

We define a voxel-wise phenotype that enables us to predict entire anatomical images. Let Ω be the set of all spatial locations v (voxels) in an image, and $I_b = \{I_b(v)\}_{v \in \Omega}$ be the acquired baseline image. We similarly define $A = \{A(v)\}_{v \in \Omega}$, to be the population atlas template. We assume each image I is generated through a deformation field Φ_{AI}^{-1} parametrized by the corresponding displacements $\{\boldsymbol{u}(v)\}_{v \in \Omega}$ from the common atlas to the subject-specific coordinate frame [14], such that $I(v) = A(v + \boldsymbol{u}(v))$. We further define a follow-up image I_t as a deformation Φ_{Bt} from the baseline image I_b, which can be composed to yield an overall deformation from the atlas to the follow-up scan via $\Phi_{At}^{-1} = \Phi_{AB}^{-1} \circ \Phi_{Bt}^{-1} = \{\boldsymbol{u}'(v)\}_{v \in \Omega}$:

$$I_t(v) = A(v + \boldsymbol{u}'(v)). \tag{9}$$

Using displacements $\boldsymbol{u}'(v)$ as the phenotype of interest in (1) captures the necessary information for predicting new images, but leads to very high dimensional descriptors. To regularize the transformation and to improve efficiency, we define a low-dimensional embedding of $\boldsymbol{u}'(v)$. Specifically, we assume that the atlas provides a parcellation of the space into L anatomical labels $\mathcal{L} = \{\Psi\}_{l=1}^{L}$.

We build a low-dimensional embedding of the transformation vectors $\boldsymbol{u}(v)$ within each label using PCA. We define the relevant phenotypes $\{y_{l,c}\}$ as the coefficients associated with the first C principal components of the model that capture 95% of the variance in each label, for $l = 1 \dots L$.

We predict the phenotypes using (8). To construct a follow-up image I_t given phenotype y_t, we first form a deformation field $\widehat{\Phi}_{At}^{-1}$ by reconstruction from the estimated phenotype y_t, and use $\widehat{\Phi}_{At}$ assuming an invertible transformation. Using the baseline image, we predict a subsequent image via $\Phi_{Bt} = \widehat{\Phi}_{At} \circ \Phi_{AB}^{-1}$. Note that we do not directly model changes in image intensity. While population models necessitate capturing such changes, we predict changes from a baseline image. We also assume that affine transformations are not part of the deformations of interest, and thus all images are affinely registered to the atlas.

3.2 Health Similarities

To fully define the health similarity term $H(\cdot, \cdot, \cdot)$, we need to specify the forms of the kernel functions $K_G(\cdot, \cdot)$, $K_C(\cdot, \cdot)$, and $K_I(\cdot, \cdot)$.

For genetic data, we employ the identical by state (IBS) kernel often used in genetic analysis [13]. Given a vector of genetic variants g of length S, each genetic locus is encoded as $g(s) \in \{0, 1, 2\}$, and

$$K_G(g_i, g_j) = \frac{1}{2S} \sum_{s=1}^{S} (2 - |g_i(s) - g_j(s)|). \tag{10}$$

To capture similarity of clinical indicators c, we form the kernel function

$$K_C(c_i, c_j) = \exp\left(-\frac{1}{\sigma_C^2} (c_i - c_j)^T \boldsymbol{W} (c_i - c_j) \right), \tag{11}$$

where diagonal weight matrix $\boldsymbol{W}$ captures the effect size of each clinical indicator on the phenotype, and σ_C^2 is the variance of the clinical factors.

We define the image feature vectors f_b as the set of all PCA coefficients defined above for the baseline image. We define the image kernel matrix as

$$K_I(f_{b,i}, f_{b,j}) = \exp\left(-\frac{1}{\sigma_I^2} ||f_{b,i} - f_{b,j}||_2^2 \right), \tag{12}$$

where σ_I^2 is the variance of the image features.

4 Experiments

We illustrate our approach by predicting image-based phenotypes based on genetic, clinical and imaging data in the ADNI longitudinal study [6] that includes two to ten follow-up scans acquired $0.5 - 7$ years after the baseline scan. We use affine registration to align all subjects to a template constructed from 145 randomly chosen subjects, and compute non-linear registration warps Φ_{AI} for

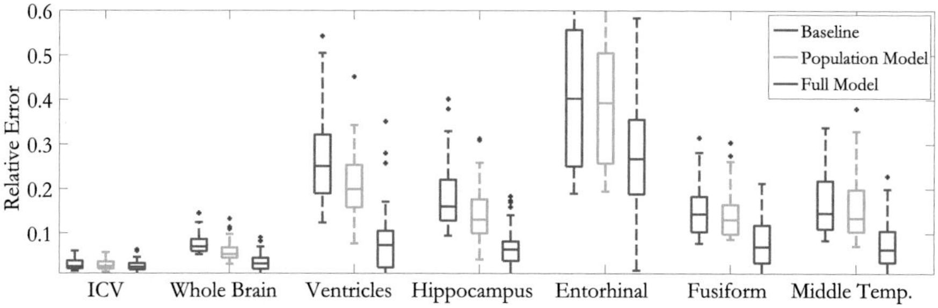

Fig. 1. Relative error (lower is better) of volume prediction for seven structures for subjects in the top decile of volume change. We report relative change between the baseline and the follow-up measurement (red), relative error in prediction using a population model (green), and the complete model (blue).

each image using ANTs [1]. We utilize a list of 21 genetic loci associated with Alzheimer's disease (AD) as the genetic vector g, and the standard clinical factors including age, gender, marital status, education, disease diagnostic, and cognitive tests, as the clinical indicator vector c. We learn the model parameters from 341 randomly chosen subjects and predict follow-up volumes on a separate set of 100 subjects. To evaluate the advantages of the proposed predictive model, we compare its performance to a population-wide linear regression model that ignores the subject-specific health profiles (i.e., $H = 0$).

4.1 Volumetric Predictions

In the first simplified experiment, we define phenotype y to be a vector of several scalar volume measurements obtained using FreeSurfer [4]. In addition to the population-wide linear regression model, we include a simple approach of using the baseline volume measurements as a predictor of the phenotype trajectory, effectively assuming no volume change with time. Since in many subjects, the volume differences are small, all three methods perform comparably when evaluated on the whole test set. To evaluate the differences between the methods, we focus on the subset of subjects with substantial volume changes, reported in Fig. 1. Our method consistently achieves smaller relative errors than the two baseline approaches.

4.2 Anatomical Prediction

We also evaluate the model for full anatomical scan prediction. To quantify prediction accuracy, we propagate segmentation labels of relevant anatomical structures from the baseline scan to the predicted scan using the predicted warps. We compare the predicted segmentation label maps with the actual segmentations of the follow-up scans. The warps computed based on the actual follow-up scans through the atlas provide an indication of the best accuracy the predictive

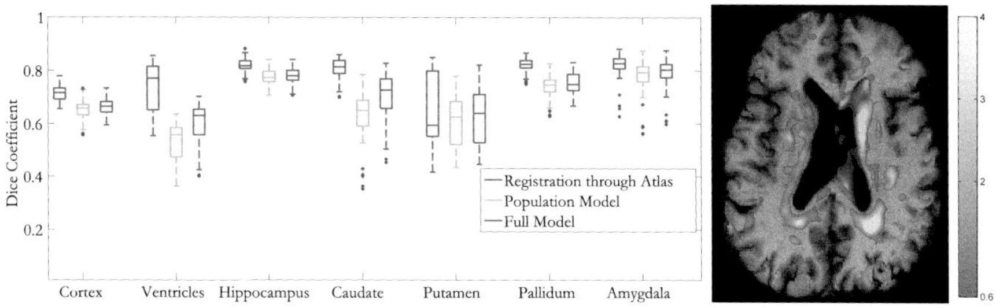

Fig. 2. Prediction results. Left: Dice scores of labels propagated through three methods for several structures implicated in AD in subjects with the most volume change for each structure. We report the prediction based on the registration of the actual follow-up scan to the atlas as an upper bound for warp-based prediction accuracy (red), predictions based on the population-wide linear regression model (green), and the full model (blue). Right: A predicted anatomical image for a patient diagnosed with AD using a healthy model. The color overlay shows the squared magnitude of the difference in predicted versus observed deformations, indicating a significantly different expansion trajectory of the ventricles.

model could achieve when using warps to represent images. Similar to the volumetric predictions, the full model offers modest improvements when evaluated on the entire test set, and substantial improvements in segmentation accuracy when evaluated in the subjects who exhibit large volume changes between the baseline scan and the follow-up scan, as reported in Fig. 2. In both experiments, all components h_g, h_c and h_I contributed significantly to the improved predictions.

Our experimental results suggest that the anatomical model depends on registration accuracy. In particular, we observe that directly registering the follow-up scan to the baseline scan leads to better alignment of segmentation labels than when transferring the labels through a composition of the transformations from the scans to the atlas space. This suggests that a different choice of appearance model may improve prediction accuracy, a promising direction for future work.

To demonstrate the potential of the anatomical prediction, we predict the follow-up scan of a patient diagnosed with dementia as if the patient were healthy. Specifically, we train our model using healthy subjects, and predict follow-up scans for AD patients. In Fig. 2 we illustrate an example result, comparing the areas of brain anatomy that differ from the observed follow-up in the predicted *healthy* brain of this AD patient. Our prediction indicates that ventricle expansion would be different if this patient had a healthy trajectory.

5 Conclusions

We present a model to predict the anatomy in patient follow-up images given just a baseline image using population trends and subject-specific genetic and clinical information. We validate our prediction method on scalar volumes and anatomical images, and show that it can be used as a powerful tool to illustrate how a subject-specific brain might differ if it were healthy. Through this and other new applications, our prediction method presents a novel opportunity for the study of disease and anatomical development.

Acknowledgements. We acknowledge the following funding sources: NIH NIBIB 1K25EB013649-01, BrightFocus AHAF-A2012333, NIH NIBIB NAC P41EB015902, NIH DA022759, and Wistron Corporation.

References

1. Avants, B.B., Tustison, N.J., Song, G., Cook, P.A., Klein, A., Gee, J.C.: A reproducible evaluation of ants similarity metric performance in brain image registration. Neuroimage 54(3), 2033–2044 (2011)
2. Davis, B.C., Fletcher, P.T., Bullitt, E., Joshi, S.: Population shape regression from random design data. Int. J. Comp. Vis. 90(2), 255–266 (2010)
3. Durrleman, S., Pennec, X., Trouvé, A., Braga, J., Gerig, G., Ayache, N.: Toward a comprehensive framework for the spatiotemporal statistical analysis of longitudinal shape data. International Journal of Computer Vision 103(1), 22–59 (2013)
4. Fischl, B.: Freesurfer. Neuroimage 62(2), 774–781 (2012)
5. Ge, T., Nichols, T.E., Ghosh, D., Mormino, E.C., Smoller, J.W., Sabuncu, M.R., et al.: A kernel machine method for detecting effects of interaction between multidimensional variable sets: An imaging genetics application. NeuroImage (2015)
6. Jack, C.R., Bernstein, M.A., Fox, N.C., Thompson, P., Alexander, G., Harvey, D., Borowski, B., Britson, P.J., L Whitwell, J., Ward, C., et al.: The alzheimer's disease neuroimaging initiative (adni): Mri methods. Journal of Magnetic Resonance Imaging 27(4), 685–691 (2008)
7. Kimeldorf, G., Wahba, G.: Some results on tchebycheffian spline functions. Journal of Mathematical Analysis and Applications 33(1), 82–95 (1971)
8. Liu, D., Lin, X., Ghosh, D.: Semiparametric regression of multidimensional genetic pathway data: Least-squares kernel machines and linear mixed models. Biometrics 63(4), 1079–1088 (2007)
9. McCullagh, P.: Generalized linear models. European Journal of Operational Research 16(3), 285–292 (1984)
10. McCulloch, C.E., Neuhaus, J.M.: Generalized linear mixed models. Wiley Online Library (2001)
11. Misra, C., Fan, Y., Davatzikos, C.: Baseline and longitudinal patterns of brain atrophy in mci patients, and their use in prediction of short-term conversion to ad: results from adni. Neuroimage 44(4), 1415–1422 (2009)
12. Pfefferbaum, A., Rohlfing, T., Rosenbloom, M.J., Chu, W., Colrain, I.M., Sullivan, E.V.: Variation in longitudinal trajectories of regional brain volumes of healthy men and women (ages 10 to 85years) measured with atlas-based parcellation of mri. Neuroimage 65, 176–193 (2013)
13. Queller, D.C., Goodnight, K.F.: Estimating relatedness using genetic markers. Evolution, 258–275 (1989)
14. Rohlfing, T., Sullivan, E.V., Pfefferbaum, A.: Regression models of atlas appearance. In: Prince, J.L., Pham, D.L., Myers, K.J. (eds.) IPMI 2009. LNCS, vol. 5636, pp. 151–162. Springer, Heidelberg (2009)
15. Sadeghi, N., Prastawa, M., Fletcher, P.T., Vachet, C., Wang, B.: et al.: Multivariate modeling of longitudinal mri in early brain development with confidence measures. In: 2013 IEEE Inter. Symp. Biomed. Imag., pp. 1400–1403. IEEE (2013)
16. Wahba, G.: Spline models for observational data, vol. 59. SIAM (1990)

Joint Diagnosis and Conversion Time Prediction of Progressive Mild Cognitive Impairment (pMCI) Using Low-Rank Subspace Clustering and Matrix Completion

Kim-Han Thung, Pew-Thian Yap, Ehsan Adeli-M., and Dinggang Shen

Department of Radiology and BRIC,
University of North Carolina at Chapel Hill, USA
dgshen@med.unc.edu

Abstract. Identifying progressive mild cognitive impairment (pMCI) patients and predicting when they will convert to Alzheimer's disease (AD) are important for early medical intervention. Multi-modality and longitudinal data provide a great amount of information for improving diagnosis and prognosis. But these data are often incomplete and noisy. To improve the utility of these data for prediction purposes, we propose an approach to denoise the data, impute missing values, and cluster the data into low-dimensional subspaces for pMCI prediction. We assume that the data reside in a space formed by a union of several low-dimensional subspaces and that similar MCI conditions reside in similar subspaces. Therefore, we first use incomplete low-rank representation (ILRR) and spectral clustering to cluster the data according to their representative low-rank subspaces. At the same time, we denoise the data and impute missing values. Then we utilize a low-rank matrix completion (LRMC) framework to identify pMCI patients and their time of conversion. Evaluations using the ADNI dataset indicate that our method outperforms conventional LRMC method.

1 Introduction

Alzheimer's disease (AD) is the most prevalent dementia that is commonly associated with progressive memory loss and cognitive decline. It is incurable and requires attentive care, thus imposing significant socio-economic burden on many nations. It is thus vital to detect AD at its earliest stage or even before its onset, for possible therapeutic treatment. AD could be traced starting from its prodromal stage, called mild cognitive impairment (MCI), where there is mild but measurable memory and cognitive decline. Studies show that some MCI patients will recover over time, but more than half will progress to dementia within five years [2]. In this paper, we focus on distinguishing progressive MCI (pMCI) patients who will progress to AD from stable MCI (sMCI) patients who will not. We will at the same time predict when the conversion to AD will occur.

Biomarkers based on different modalities, such as magnetic resonance imaging (MRI), positron emission topography (PET), and cerebrospinal fluid (CSF), have been proposed to predict AD progression [15,4,12,14]. The Alzheimer's disease neuroimaging initiative (ADNI) collects these data longitudinally from subjects ranging from

N. Navab et al. (Eds.): MICCAI 2015, Part III, LNCS 9351, pp. 527–534, 2015.
DOI: 10.1007/978-3-319-24574-4_63

cognitively normal elders to AD patients in an effort to use all these information to accurately predict AD progression. However, these data are incomplete because of dropouts and unavailability of a certain modality. The easiest and most popular way to deal with missing data is by discarding the samples with missing values [15]. But this will decrease the number of samples as well as the statistical power of analyses. One alternative is to impute the missing data, via methods like k-nearest neighbour (KNN), expectation maximization (EM), or low-rank matrix completion (LRMC) [10,16,1]. But these imputation methods do not often perform well on datasets with a large amount of values missing in blocks [9,13]. To avoid the need for imputation, Yuan *et al.* [13] divides the data into subsets of complete data, and then jointly learn the sparse classifiers for these subsets. Through joint feature learning, [13] enforces each subset classifier to use the same set of features for each modality. However, this will restrain samples with certain modality missing to use more features in available modality for prediction. Goldberg *et al.* [3], on the other hand, imputes the missing features and unknown targets simultaneously using a low-rank assumption. Thus, all the features are involved in the prediction of the target through rank minimization, while the propagation of the missing feature's imputation errors to the target outputs is largely averted, as the target outputs are predicted directly and simultaneously. Thung *et al.* [9] improves the efficiency and effectiveness of [3] by performing feature and sample selection before matrix completion. However, by applying matrix completion on all the samples, the authors implicitly assumes that the data are from a single low-dimensional subspace. This assumption hardly holds for real and complex data.

To capture the complexity and heterogeneity of the pathology of AD progression, we assume that the longitudinal multi-modality data reside in a space that is formed by a union of several low-dimensional subspaces. Assuming that the data is low-rank as a whole is too optimistic, and missing values might not be imputed correctly. A better approach is to first cluster the data and then perform matrix completion on each cluster. In this paper, we propose a method, called low-rank subspace clustering and matrix completion (LRSC-MC), which will cluster the data into subspaces for improving prediction performance. More specifically, we first use incomplete low rank representation (ILRR) [5,8] to simultaneously determine a low-rank affinity matrix, which gives us an indication of the similarity between any pair of samples, estimate the noise, and obtain the denoised data. We then use spectral clustering [6] to split the data into several clusters and impute the output targets (status labels and conversion times) using low-rank matrix completion (LRMC) algorithm for each cluster. We tested our framework using longitudinal MRI data (and cross-sectional multi-modality data) for both pMCI identification and conversion time prediction, and found that the LRSC-MC outperforms LRMC. In addition, we also found that using denoised data will improve the performance of LRMC.

2 Materials and Preprocessing

2.1 Materials

We used both longitudinal and cross-sectional data from ADNI[1] for our study. We used MRI data of MCI subjects that were scanned at baseline, 6th, 12th and 18th months

[1] http://adni.loni.ucla.edu

Table 1. Demographic information of subjects involved in this study. (Edu.: Education; std.: Standard Deviation)

	No. of subjects	Gender (M/F)	Age (years)	Edu. (years)
pMCI	65	49/16	75.3 ± 6.7	15.6 ± 3.0
sMCI	53	37/16	76.0 ± 7.9	15.5 ± 3.0
Total	118	86/32	-	-

to predict who progressed to AD in the monitoring period from 18th to 60th month. MCI subjects that progressed to AD within this monitoring period were retrospectively labeled as pMCI, whereas those that remained stable were labeled as sMCI. MCI subjects that progressed to AD on and before 18th month were not used in this study. There are two target outputs in this study – class label and conversion month. For estimating these outputs, we used the MRI data, PET data, and clinical scores (e.g., Mini-Mental State Exam (MMSE), Clinical Dementia Rating (CDR), and Alzheimer's Disease Assessment Scale (ADAS)). Table 1 shows the demographic information of the subjects used in this study.

2.2 Preprocessing and Feature Extraction

We use region-of-interest (ROI)-based features from the MRI and PET images in this study. The processing steps involved, for each MRI image, are described as follows. Each MRI image was AC-PC corrected using MIPAV[2], corrected for intensity inhomogeneity using the N3 algorithm, skull stripped, tissue segmented, and registered to a common space [11,7]. Gray matter (GM) volumes, normalized by the total intracranial volume, were extracted as features from 93 ROIs [11]. We also linearly aligned each PET image to its corresponding MRI image, and used the mean intensity value at each ROI as feature.

3 Method

Figure 1 shows an overview of the proposed low-dimensional subspace clustering and matrix completion framework. The three main components in this framework are 1) incomplete low-rank representation, which computes the low-rank affinity matrix, 2) spectral clustering, which clusters data using the affinity matrix acquired from the previous step, and 3) low-rank matrix completion, which predicts the target outputs using the clustered data. In the following subsections, each of these steps will be explained in detail.

3.1 Notation

We use $\mathbf{X} \in \mathbb{R}^{n \times m}$ to denote the feature matrix with n samples of m features. n depends on the number of time points and the number of modalities used. Each sample

[2] http://mipav.cit.nih.gov

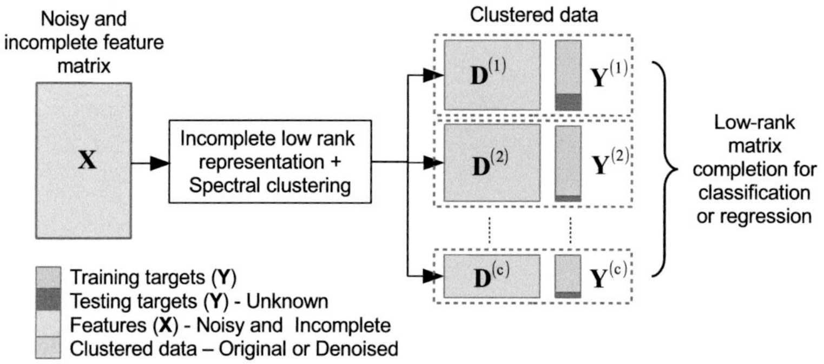

Fig. 1. Low-rank subspace clustering and matrix completion for pMCI diagnosis and prognosis.

(i.e., row) in $\mathbf{X}$ is a concatenation of features from different time points and different modalities (MRI, PET and clinical scores). Note that $\mathbf{X}$ can be incomplete due to missing data. The corresponding target matrix is denoted as $\mathbf{Y} \in \mathbb{R}^{n \times 2}$, where the first column is a vector of labels (1 for pMCI, -1 for sMCI), and the second column is a vector of conversion times (e.g., the number of months to AD conversion). The conversion times associated with the sMCI samples should ideally be set to infinity. But to make the problem feasible, we set the conversion times to a large value computed as 12 months in addition to the maximum time of conversion computed for all pMCI samples. For any matrix $\mathbf{M}$, $M_{j,k}$ denotes its element indexed by (j,k), whereas $M_{j,:}$ and $M_{:,k}$ denote its j-th row and k-th column, respectively. We denote $\|\mathbf{M}\|_* = \sum \sigma_i(\mathbf{M})$ as the nuclear norm (i.e., sum of the singular values $\{\sigma_i\}$ of $\mathbf{M}$), $\|\mathbf{M}\|_1 = \sum |M_{j,k}|$ as l_1 norm, and $\mathbf{M}'$ as transpose of $\mathbf{M}$. $\mathbf{I}$ is the identity matrix.

3.2 Low-Rank Matrix Completion (LRMC)

Assuming linear relationship between $\mathbf{X}$ and $\mathbf{Y}$, we let for the k-th target $Y_{:,k} = \mathbf{X}\mathbf{a}_k + b_k = [\mathbf{X}\ \mathbf{1}] \times [\mathbf{a}_k; b_k]$, where $\mathbf{1}$ is a column vector of 1's, $\mathbf{a}_k$ is the weight vector, and b_k is the offset. Assuming a low rank $\mathbf{X}$, then the concatenated matrix $\mathbf{M} = [\mathbf{X}\ \mathbf{1}\ \mathbf{Y}]$ is also low-rank [3], i.e., each column of $\mathbf{M}$ can be linearly represented by other columns, or each row of $\mathbf{M}$ can be linearly represented by other rows. Based on this assumption, low-rank matrix completion (LRMC) can be applied on $\mathbf{M}$ to impute the missing feature values and the output target simultaneously by solving $\min_{\mathbf{Z}}\{\|\mathbf{Z}\|_* \mid \mathbf{M}_\Omega = \mathbf{Z}_\Omega\}$, where Ω is the index set of known values in $\mathbf{M}$. In the presence of noise, the problem can be relaxed as [3]

$$\min_{\mathbf{Z}} \mu\|\mathbf{Z}\|_* + \frac{\lambda}{|\Omega_l|} L_l(\mathbf{Z}_{\Omega_l}, \mathbf{M}_{\Omega_l}) + \frac{1}{|\Omega_s|} L_s(\mathbf{Z}_{\Omega_s}, \mathbf{M}_{\Omega_s}), \tag{1}$$

where $L_l(\cdot,\cdot)$ and $L_s(\cdot,\cdot)$ are the logistic loss function and mean square loss function, respectively. Ω_l and Ω_s are the index sets of the known target labels and conversion times, respectively. The nuclear norm $\|\cdot\|_*$ in Eq. (1) is used as a convex surrogate for matrix rank. Parameters μ and λ are the tuning parameters that control the effect of each term.

If the samples come from different low-dimensional subspaces instead of one single subspace, applying (1) to the whole dataset is inappropriate and might cause inaccurate imputation of missing data. We thus propose instead to apply LRMC to the subspaces, where samples are more similar and hence the low-rank constraint is more reasonable. The problem now becomes

$$\min_{\mathbf{Z}} \sum_{c=1}^{C} \mu \|\mathbf{Q}_c\mathbf{Z}\|_* + \frac{\lambda}{|\Omega_l|} L_l(\mathbf{Z}_{\Omega_l}, \mathbf{M}_{\Omega_l}) + \frac{1}{|\Omega_s|} L_s(\mathbf{Z}_{\Omega_s}, \mathbf{M}_{\Omega_s}), \tag{2}$$

where $\mathbf{Q}_c \in \mathbb{R}^{n\times n}$ is a diagonal matrix with values $\{0, 1\}$, C is the number of clusters, and $\sum_{c=1}^{C} \mathbf{Q}_c = \mathbf{I}$. The effect of $\mathbf{Q}_c\mathbf{Z}$ is to select from the rows of $\mathbf{Z}$ the samples that are associated with each cluster. For example, if the value of $\mathbf{Q}(i, i)$ is one, the i-th sample (i.e., the i-th row) in $\mathbf{Z}$ will be selected. $\mathbf{Q}_c$ is estimated from the feature matrix $\mathbf{X}$ by performing low-rank representation subspace clustering [5] and spectral clustering [6], which will be discussed next.

3.3 Incomplete Low-Rank Representation (ILRR)

Low-rank representation (LRR) [5] is widely used for subspace clustering. LRR assumes that data samples are approximately (i.e., the data are noisy) drawn from a union of multiple subspaces and aims to cluster the samples into their respective subspaces and at the same time remove possible outliers. However, LRR cannot be applied directly to our data because they are incomplete. We therefore apply instead the method reported in [8], which is called incomplete low-rank representation (ILRR). For an incomplete matrix $\mathbf{X}$, the ILRR problem is given by

$$\min_{\mathbf{A},\mathbf{E},\boldsymbol{\mathcal{X}}} \|\mathbf{A}\|_* + \alpha\|\mathbf{E}\|_1 \text{ s.t. } \boldsymbol{\mathcal{X}} = \mathbf{A}\boldsymbol{\mathcal{X}} + \mathbf{E}, \boldsymbol{\mathcal{X}}_{\Omega} = \mathbf{X}_{\Omega} \tag{3}$$

where $\boldsymbol{\mathcal{X}}$ is the completed version of $\mathbf{X}$, which is self-represented by $\mathbf{A}\boldsymbol{\mathcal{X}}$, $\mathbf{A} \in \mathbb{R}^{n\times n}$ is the low-rank affinity matrix, $\mathbf{E}$ is the error matrix, and α is the regularizing parameter. Each element of $\mathbf{A}$ indexed by (i, j) is an indicator of the similarity between the i-th sample and the j-th sample. Eq. (3) is solved using inexact augmented Lagragrian multiplier (ALM), as described in [8]. ILRR 1) denoises the data through prediction of $\mathbf{E}$, providing us with clean data $\mathbf{D} = \mathbf{A}\boldsymbol{\mathcal{X}}$, and 2) predicts the affinity matrix $\mathbf{A}$, which is used next to cluster the data.

3.4 Spectral Clustering

After acquiring the affinity matrix $\mathbf{A}$ between all the subjects, we perform spectral clustering [6] on $\mathbf{X}$ (or $\mathbf{D}$). The clustering procedures are:

1. Symmetrize the affinity matrix, $\mathbf{A} \leftarrow \mathbf{A} + \mathbf{A}'$ and set $\texttt{diag}(\mathbf{A}) = \mathbf{0}$.
2. Compute Laplacian matrix, $\mathbf{L} = \mathbf{S}^{-1/2}\mathbf{A}\mathbf{S}^{-1/2}$, where $\mathbf{S}$ is a diagonal matrix consisting of the row sums of $\mathbf{A}$.
3. Find k largest eigenvectors of $\mathbf{L}$ and stack them as columns of matrix $\mathbf{V} \in \mathbb{R}^{n\times k}$.
4. Renormalize each row of $\mathbf{V}$ to have unit length.

5. Treat each row of $\mathbf{V}$ as a point in $\mathbb{R}^k$ and cluster them into k clusters using the k-means algorithm.

Based on the clustering indices, we now have clustered data $\mathbf{X}^{(c)}$ (or $\mathbf{D}^{(c)}$), which together with the corresponding target $\mathbf{Y}^{(c)}$, can be used for classification. As can be seen in Fig. 1, we now have multiple classification problems, one for each subspace. Thus, in practice, we implement (2) by completing concatenated matrix $[\mathbf{X}^{(c)} \mathbf{1} \mathbf{Y}^{(c)}]$ (or $[\mathbf{D}^{(c)} \mathbf{1} \mathbf{Y}^{(c)}]$) using LRMC, and combine the outputs predicted in all subspaces to obtain a single classification or regression outcome.

4 Results and Discussions

We evaluated the proposed method, LRSC-MC, using both longitudinal and multi-modality data. In both Fig. 3 and Fig. 2, the baseline method – LRMC using original data, is denoted by light blue bar, while the rests either using part(s) or full version of the proposed method – LRMC using the denoised data, and LRSC-MC using the original and the denoised data. Two clusters ($C = 2$) were used for LRSC-MC. Parameter $\alpha = 0.005$ is used for LRSC, and parameters μ and λ of LRMC are searched through the range $\{10^{-n}, n = 6, \ldots, 3\}$ and $\{10^{-3} - 0.5\}$, respectively. All reported results are the average of the 10 repetitions of a 10-fold cross validation.

Fig. 2 shows the comparison result between the conventional LRMC and LRSC-MC, using different combinations of MRI, PET, and clinical scores, at first time point. The result shows that LRSC-MC always outperforms the conventional LRMC, using either original or denoised data, both in terms of pMCI identification and conversion time prediction (i.e., red bar is higher than light blue bar). This confirms the effectiveness of our method for heterogeneous data that exhibit multiple low dimensional subspaces. In addition, we also found that LRMC is improved using the denoised data from the first component of our method (ILRR) (i.e., dark blue bar is higher than light blue bar). This is probably because denoising the data using ILRR is similar to smoothing the data to a low-dimensional subspace, (when affinity matrix $\mathbf{A}$ is low rank, $\mathbf{A}\mathcal{X}$ is also low rank), which fulfills the assumption of LRMC. Sometimes, the improvement due to the use of denoised data is more than the use of clustering. Thus, there are 2 ways to improve LRMC on data that consists of multiple subspaces, i.e., by first denoise/smooth the data, or by clustering the data. Nevertheless, the best pMCI classification is still achieved by LRSC-MC using modality combination of MRI+Cli, at around 81%, using the original data.

In Fig. 3, we show the results of using only MRI data at 1 to 4 time points for pMCI identification and conversion time prediction. The results indicate that LRSC-MC outperforms LRMC using either data from 1, 2 and 3 time points. The improvement of the LRSC-MC is more significant for the case of 1 time point (at 18th month), where the pMCI identification is close to 80% of accuracy using the denoised data, while LRMC on the original data is only about 72%. In general, when using the original data, LRSC-MC outperforms LRMC, while when using the denoised data, LRSC-MC is either better or on par with LRMC. This is probably because the denoised data is closer to the assumption of single low-dimensional subspace, opposing the assumption made by the LRSC-MC – the data is a union of several low-dimensional subspaces.

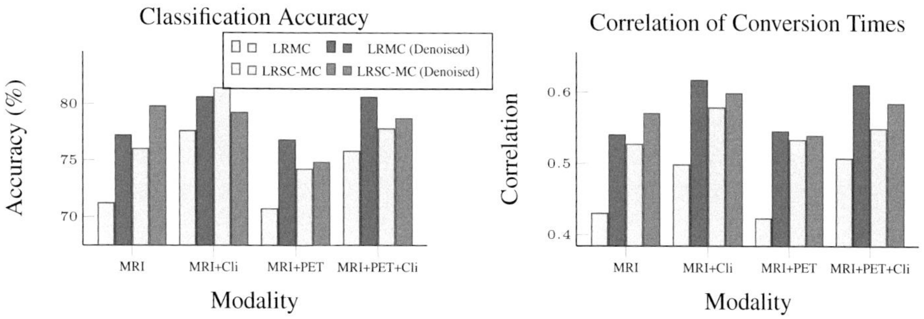

Fig. 2. Average pMCI/sMCI classification accuracy and the correlation of conversion month predictions using multi-modality data.

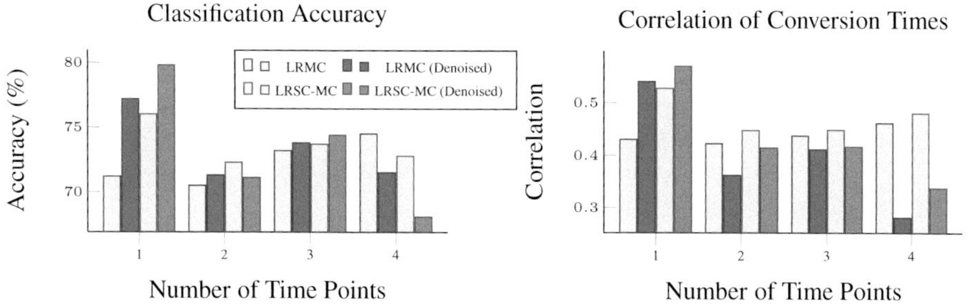

Fig. 3. Average pMCI/sMCI classification accuracy and the correlation of conversion month predictions, using data from different number of time points.

Table 2. Comparison with other methods.

1TP Data	[13]	[9]	LRSC-MC
MRI	70.0	72.8	76.0
MRIPET	71.0	74.8	74.2
MRICli	81.6	-	81.4

MRI data	[13]	[9]	LRSC-MC
2TPs	57.0	55.0	72.3
3TPs	-	63.2	73.7
4TPs	-	72.0	72.8

The only case where LRSC-MC performs worse than LRMC is when data from 4 time points are used. This is probably because when 2 or more TPs are used, the earlier data (e.g., 12th, 6th month) are added. These added data is farther away from the conversion time and could be noisier and less reliable for prediction. Since in our current model, we assume equal reliability of features, when the noisy features started to dominate the feature matrix using 4 TPs, LRSC is unable to give us a good affinity matrix and thus poorer performance.

In addition, we also compare our method with [9,13] in Table 2. However, since both methods rely on the subset of complete data for feature selection and learning, they fail in cases when the subset contains too little samples for training (those cases are left blank in the table). The results show that the proposed method outperforms or on par with these state-of-the-art methods.

5 Conclusion

We have demonstrated that the proposed method, LRSC-MC, outperforms conventional LRMC using longitudinal and multi-modality data in many situations. This is in line with our hypothesis that, for data that reside in a union of low-dimensional subspaces, subspace low-rank imputation is better than whole-space low-rank imputation.

Acknowledgment. This work was supported in part by NIH grants EB009634, AG041721, and AG042599.

References

1. Candès, E.J., et al.: Exact matrix completion via convex optimization. Foundations of Computational Mathematics 9(6), 717–772 (2009)
2. Gauthier, S., et al.: Mild cognitive impairment. The Lancet 367(9518), 1262–1270 (2006)
3. Goldberg, A., et al.: Transduction with matrix completion: three birds with one stone. Advances in Neural Information Processing Systems 23, 757–765 (2010)
4. Li, F., et al.: A robust deep model for improved classification of AD/MCI patients. IEEE Journal of Biomedical and Health Informatics 99 (2015)
5. Liu, G., et al.: Robust recovery of subspace structures by low-rank representation. IEEE Transactions on Pattern Analysis and Machine Intelligence 35(1), 171–184 (2013)
6. Ng, A.Y., et al.: On spectral clustering: Analysis and an algorithm. Advances in Neural Information Processing Systems 2, 849–856 (2002)
7. Shen, D., et al.: HAMMER: hierarchical attribute matching mechanism for elastic registration. IEEE Transactions on Medical Imaging 21(11), 1421–1439 (2002)
8. Shi, J., et al.: Low-rank representation for incomplete data. Mathematical Problems in Engineering 2014 (2014)
9. Thung, K.H., et al.: Neurodegenerative disease diagnosis using incomplete multi-modality data via matrix shrinkage and completion. Neuroimage 91, 386–400 (2014)
10. Troyanskaya, O., et al.: Missing value estimation methods for DNA microarrays. Bioinformatics 17(6), 520–525 (2001)
11. Wang, Y., Nie, J., Yap, P.-T., Shi, F., Guo, L., Shen, D.: Robust deformable-surface-based skull-stripping for large-scale studies. In: Fichtinger, G., Martel, A., Peters, T. (eds.) MICCAI 2011, Part III. LNCS, vol. 6893, pp. 635–642. Springer, Heidelberg (2011)
12. Weiner, M.W., et al.: The Alzheimer's disease neuroimaging initiative: A review of papers published since its inception. Alzheimer's & Dementia 9(5), e111–e194 (2013)
13. Yuan, L., et al.: Multi-source feature learning for joint analysis of incomplete multiple heterogeneous neuroimaging data. NeuroImage 61(3), 622–632 (2012)
14. Zhan, L., et al.: Comparison of nine tractography algorithms for detecting abnormal structural brain networks in Alzheimers disease. Frontiers in Aging Neuroscience 7 (2015)
15. Zhang, D., et al.: Multi-modal multi-task learning for joint prediction of multiple regression and classification variables in Alzheimer's disease. Neuroimage 59(2), 895–907 (2012)
16. Zhu, X., et al.: Missing value estimation for mixed-attribute data sets. IEEE Transactions on Knowledge and Data Engineering 23(1), 110–121 (2011)

Learning with Heterogeneous Data for Longitudinal Studies

Letizia Squarcina[1], Cinzia Perlini[1], Marcella Bellani[1], Antonio Lasalvia[1], Mirella Ruggeri[1], Paolo Brambilla[3], and Umberto Castellani[2,⋆]

[1] University of Verona, Department of Psychiatry, Verona, Italy
[2] University of Verona, Department of Computer Science, Verona, Italy
[3] Department of Neurosciences and Mental Health, Psychiatric Clinic, Fondazione IRCCS Ca Granda Ospedale Maggiore Policlinico, University of Milan, Milan, Italy

Abstract. Longitudinal studies are very important to understand cerebral structural changes especially during the course of pathologies. For instance, in the context of mental health research, it is interesting to evaluate how a certain disease degenerates over time in order to discriminate between pathological and normal time dependent brain deformations. However longitudinal data are not easily available, and very often they are characterized by a large variability in both the age of subjects and time between acquisitions (follow up time). This leads to heterogeneous data that may affect the overall study. In this paper we propose a learning method to deal with this kind of heterogeneous data by exploiting covariate measures in a Multiple Kernel Learning (MKL) framework. Cortical thickness and white matter volume of the left middle temporal region are collected from each subject. Then, a subject-dependent kernel weighting procedure is introduced in order to obtain the correction of covariate effect simultaneously with classification. Experiments are reported for First Episode Psychosis detection by showing very promising results.

Keywords: Support Vector Machines, Multiple Kernel Learning, Longitudinal study, First Episode Psychosis.

1 Introduction

The analysis of anatomical variability over time is a relevant topic in neuroimaging research to characterize the progression of a certain disease [8]. The overall aim is to detect structural changes in spatial and time domains that are able to differentiate between patients and healthy controls. To this end, longitudinal studies are considered where the same subject is observed repeatedly at several time points [4]. In the simplest scenarios only two time points are defined, namely *baseline* and *follow up*. In this fashion a classification method, like Support Vector Machine (SVM) [18], can be designed for each time point and, more interestingly, for the differential degeneracy measurements to evaluate how

⋆ Corresponding author.

N. Navab et al. (Eds.): MICCAI 2015, Part III, LNCS 9351, pp. 535–542, 2015.
DOI: 10.1007/978-3-319-24574-4_64

the dynamics of the observed features may change across the populations (i.e., patients and controls). Unfortunately, a relevant issue in longitudinal studies is the lack of reliable datasets. In many cases collected data are heterogeneous due to the large variability of the considered population. In particular, there are different factors that may contribute to brain deformations such as gender, age, follow up time, and so on. In general, these factors are considered as *nuisance* variables that cause a *dispersion* of the observed values (i.e., the main variable) by possible affecting the final analysis result [15]. For instance, in brain classification if the volume reduction is dependent on both the analysed disease and the age of subject, it may be difficult to discriminate between a young patient and an elderly control. A common approach to deal with this problem consists of introducing some correction procedure based on statistical regression. As an example the *Generalized Linear Model* (GLM) [13] can be employed to predict and remove the effect of the confounding covariates. In general this procedure is carried out as a pre-processing before classification. In this paper our intent is to integrate the data correction into the learning phase by defining a classification model that explicitly takes into account of the nuisance covariates. We exploit Multiple Kernel Learning (MKL) as a powerful and natural approach to combine different sources of information [7] that has already been successfully applied in the neuro-imaging field [2,8]. The main idea behind MKL methods [1,7] is to learn an optimal weighted combination of several kernels while simultaneously training the classifier ([7]). In general, each kernel is associated to a specific feature and their combination is carried out aiming at exploiting interdependent information from the given features. In this work, we propose to adapt the standard MKL formulation to enable the correction of the covariate effect in the kernel space by overcoming the hypotesis of linear progression. We show that this approach leads to a subject-specific kernel weighting scheme where each weight is locally dependent on the subject covariate. A similar strategy is known in literature as *localized* kernel learning [6,7] where the idea consists of assigning different weights to a kernel in different regions of the input space. We evaluate our method to improve the classification performance of longitudinal study [4] to automatically detect First Episode Psychosis (FEP) [10,17]. Research on the first stages of psychosis is very important to understand the causes of the disease, excluding the consequence of chronicity and treatment on the study outcomes. In our study we evaluate the brain variation by analysing several cortical features, namely the *volume* and the surface *thickness* [3,5]. In our paper we focus on the *middle temporal* region since it is already known its relation with psychosis [10,17]. We considered as confounding covariate the age of subjects since in our population the span of age is quite large and heterogeneous. For each subject two MRI scans are available, i.e., baseline and follow up. Classification is carried out for the two time points, and for the differential values of volume and thickness. In the latter experiment the follow up time is considered as covariate together with the age. Experiments show promising results by reporting a clear improvement when covariates are integrated in the learning phase. Moreover our study evidences that also brain deformation over the time can be used to discriminate between patients and controls by confirming the idea that speed of structural changes is faster in mental disorders.

2 CO-MKL: Multiple Kernel Learning with Covariate

2.1 Background

The overall idea of kernel methods is to project non-linearly separable data into a higher dimensional space where the linear class separation becomes feasible [18]. Support Vector Machine (SVM) is an example of discriminative classifier belonging to this class of methods for binary classification problems. Given a training set of N samples $\{(\boldsymbol{x}_i, y_i)\}_{i=1}^N$ where $\boldsymbol{x}_i \in R^d$ is a vector of the input space and $y_i \in \{-1, +1\}$ is the sample class label, SVM finds the best discriminative hyperplane in the feature space according to the maximum margin principle [18]. Therefore, after training, the discriminative function is defined as:

$$f(\boldsymbol{x}) = \sum_{i=1}^{N} \alpha_i y_i \langle \Phi(\boldsymbol{x}_i), \Phi(\boldsymbol{x}) \rangle + b, \tag{1}$$

where Φ is the mapping function, and α_i are the dual variables. Considering the so called "kernel trick" the dot product in Equation 1 is replaced by a kernel function $k(\boldsymbol{x}_i, \boldsymbol{x}) = \langle \Phi(\boldsymbol{x}_i), \Phi(\boldsymbol{x}) \rangle$. Several kernel functions can be defined such as the linear kernel, the polynomial kernel, and the Gaussian Radial Basis Function (RBF) kernel. An interesting extension of SVMs is represented by Multiple Kernel Learning (MKL) methods[7], recently proposed in [1,11]. MKL aims at selecting or combining a set of different kernels that usually describes different data sources. The simplest combination strategy is given by the linear MKL model:

$$k_w(\boldsymbol{x}_i, \boldsymbol{x}_j) = \sum_{m=1}^{P} w_m k_m(\boldsymbol{x}_i^m, \boldsymbol{x}_j^m), \tag{2}$$

where $w_m \in \mathbb{R}$, $\boldsymbol{x}_i = \{\boldsymbol{x}_i^m\}_{m=1}^P$, $\boldsymbol{x}_i^m \in R^{d_m}$, and d_m is the size of the mth feature. In particular, MKL methods enable the estimation of the kernel weights and the coefficients of the associated predictor in a single learning framework.

2.2 Proposed Approach

In our method we address the problem of integrating the confounding covariate in a supervised fashion by including the data correction in the learning phase. We assume the knowledge of covariate for each subject. Therefore, each sample is now represented by $\{(\boldsymbol{x}_i, \boldsymbol{c}_i, y_i)\}$ where $\boldsymbol{c}_i \in R^h$ encodes the covariates associated to sample i. Rather than working on the original space, our main idea consists of correcting the effect of the covariate in the kernel space. More specifically, the decision function reported in Equation 1 is redefined as:

$$f(\boldsymbol{x}) = \sum_{i=1}^{N} \alpha_i y_i \langle w(\boldsymbol{c}_i)\Phi(\boldsymbol{x}_i), w(\boldsymbol{c})\Phi(\boldsymbol{x}) \rangle + b, \tag{3}$$

where a weighting function $w(\boldsymbol{c})\colon R^h \to R$ is introduced to take into account of the covariates. Note that in this fashion all the covariate are simultaneously considered in the correction procedure. In order to deal with multiple features the proposed correction method is extended to a MKL framework by combining Equations 3 and 2:

$$k_w^c(\boldsymbol{x}_i, \boldsymbol{x}_j) = \sum_{m=1}^{P} \langle w_m(\boldsymbol{c}_i)\Phi(\boldsymbol{x}_i^m), w_m(\boldsymbol{c}_j)\Phi(\boldsymbol{x}_j^m)\rangle = \sum_{m=1}^{P} w_m(\boldsymbol{c}_i)k_m(\boldsymbol{x}_i^m, \boldsymbol{x}_j^m)w_m(\boldsymbol{c}_j). \quad (4)$$

As an important assessment we observe that kernel definition of Equation 4 has the same form of the so called *localized kernel* [6]. The difference regards the meaning of the weighting function $w_m(.)$ that in [6] is defined on the original space rather than on the covariates. This leads to a different interpretation of the weighting effect. In [6] the weighting aims at estimating different classification criteria at different region of the input space [16]. In our approach the main contribution of the weighting function is to attenuate the conditioning of nuisance variables. Moreover, we can consider the covariate as a sort of *side* information that are included in the classification model. The weighting function $w_m(.)$ is defined as a softmax model[7]. The model parameters of the proposed MKL with covariate (CO-MKL) are computed using standard alternating optimization[7]: first, the kernel weights are fixed and standard solvers (i.e., libSVM) are used to estimate the SVM parameters, second, the SVM parameters are fixed and a gradient descent strategy is employed to compute kernels weights. The two steps are iterated until convergence.

3 Materials and Methods

The pipeline we adopted can be schematically visualized in Figure 1. After data collection, extracted features and covariates are fed to the classifier. This

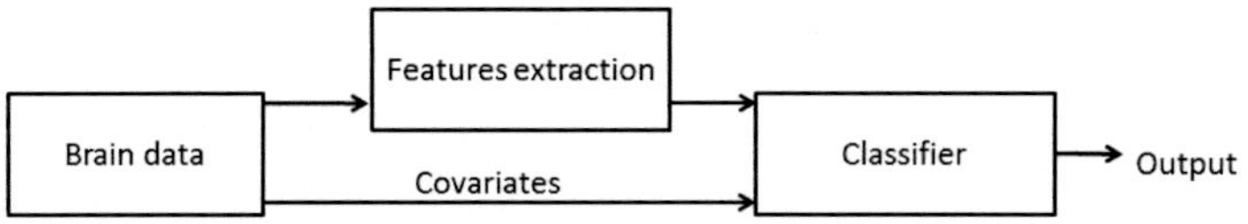

Fig. 1. Features, i.e. thickness and volume of temporal white and gray matter, were extracted from brain data, and features were used for classification together with covariates (age or months between different acquisitions).

study was conducted in the frame of Psychosis Incident Cohort Outcome Study (PICOS), a multi-site naturalistic research study, which aimed at analyzing clinical, social, cognitive, genetic and imaging features of FEP patients [12]. 22 First

Episode of Psychosis patients (FEP, 12 males, mean age 37.5 ± 7.9 y.o. at baseline, 39.4 ± 7.6 y.o. at follow up) and 22 healthy controls (HC, 12 males, 39.0 ± 11.7 y.o. at baseline, 42.0 ± 12.2 y.o. at follow up) underwent two Magnetic Resonance Imaging sessions (months between acquisitions (Δ_m) 21.1 ± 8.4 for FEP, 36.7 ± 7.8 for HC) with a 1.5 Siemens Symphony scanner. The two populations were matched for age and sex both at baseline and at follow up (t-test, $p>0.05$). The difference in months between the two scans (follow up time) was significantly higher for controls (t-test, $p<0.05$). To avoid bias in the classification we normalized the values independently in the two populations in order to obtain two vectors ranging from 0 to 1, with no statistical difference (t-test, $p>0.05$). T1-weighted images(256x256x18 voxels, 1x1x5 mm^3, TR 2160 ms, TE 47 ms, flip angle 90°) were acquired for all subjects. Data were analyzed using FreeSurfer [3] and volume and cortical thickness were computed for the left medial temporal gray and white matter. With this methodology meshes of the boundaries between white and gray matter and between gray matter and cerebrospinal fluid are built. Thickness is defined as the distance between the meshes. Volume is computed assigning a label corresponding to a brain structure to each voxel of the image based on probabilistic information [5]. Thickness and volume are computed for several regions of interest (ROIs). We chose to restrict our analyses to the medial temporal white and gray matter, because of the involvement of this area of the brain with early psychosis. Mean region volume at baseline (μ_A^V) and at follow up (μ_B^V) and mean region thickness at baseline (μ_A^T) and follow up (μ_B^T) were computed for each subject, and used as features for the classifier. We also computed the difference in mean thickness and volume for each subject and used it as features $\Delta\mu^X = \frac{\mu^X{}_A - \mu^X{}_B}{\mu^X{}_A}$, where X is T or V in the case of thickness or volume, respectively.

All experiments were conducted with radial basis functions (RBF) kernels. The optimal values for free parameters were chosen with a search in a grid as shown in [9]. Cross validation was done with a leave-one-out procedure for all classification methods. For each subject, the complete set of features is $\boldsymbol{x} = [\mu_A^T, \mu_B^T, \mu_A^V, \mu_B^V, \Delta\mu^T, \Delta\mu^V]$ and that of covariates is $\boldsymbol{c} = [\text{age}_A, \text{age}_B, \Delta_m]$ where age_A and age_B are age at baseline and at follow up.

4 Results

We evaluated classification methods using baseline, follow-up, and difference values, considering as covariate baseline age, follow-up age and baseline age in conjunction with the normalized follow up time in months (Δ_m), respectively. For comparison, we employed standard SVM on single features and simple MKL [14] on both thickness and volume, to evaluate if the introduction of covariates in the CO-MKL method overtakes the effect of considering more than one feature simultaneously. We also used the covariates as features in SVM and MKL classification of baseline and follow-up data, to ensure that these values do not discriminate between the classes when used as features. More in details, analyses were carried out as follows:

- SVM classification using either middle temporal thickness or volume as features, adjusted for age using GLM. When considering the difference in thickness of volume ($\Delta\mu^T$ and $\Delta\mu^V$ respectively) the adjustment with GLM was done also for differences in follow up months.
- MKL where features are both thickness and volume adjusted for differences using GLM.
- CO-MKL with a single feature that can be the mean volume (at baseline, or at follow up) or thickness (at baseline, or at follow up), or the difference $\Delta\mu^X$ (thus $\boldsymbol{x} = \mu^T_{AorB}$ or $\boldsymbol{x} = \mu^V_{AorB}$ or $\boldsymbol{x} = \Delta\mu^X$). The covariate is age of subjects (at baseline or at follow up) or both age at baseline and follow up time in the case of the difference ($\boldsymbol{c} = \text{age}_A$ or age_B, or $\boldsymbol{c} = [\text{age}_A, \Delta_m]$).
- CO-MKL with multiple features at baseline, or at follow up, or for differences ($\boldsymbol{x} = [\mu^T_A, \mu^V_A]$ or $\boldsymbol{x} = [\mu^T_B, \mu^V_B]$ or $\boldsymbol{x} = [\Delta\mu^T, \Delta\mu^V]$). The covariate $\boldsymbol{c}$ is age of subjects for baseline and follow up, or both age at baseline and follow up time in the case of differences ($\boldsymbol{c} = \text{age}_A$ or $\boldsymbol{c} = \text{age}_B$, or $\boldsymbol{c} = [\text{age}_A, \Delta_m]$).
- MKL where both main variables and covariates are used as features. Therefore at baseline $\boldsymbol{x} = [\mu^T_A, \mu^V_A, age_A]$, at follow up $\boldsymbol{x} = [\mu^T_B, \mu^V_B, \text{age}_B]$, and for the difference $\boldsymbol{x} = [\Delta\mu^T, \Delta\mu^V, \text{age}_A, \Delta_m]$.
- SVM with the concatenation of both main variables and covariates.

Table 1. Results from classification from data of thickness and volume of middle temporal gray and white matter.

	Baseline			Follow up			Δ		
	Acc	Sens	Spec	Acc	Sens	Spec	Acc	Sens	Spec
CO-MKL									
Thickness	70.4	54.6	86.4	**81.8**	77.3	86.4	70.5	59.1	81.8
Volume	**72.7**	54.6	89.0	68.2	59.0	77.3	**72.7**	63.6	81.8
SVM									
Thickness	65.9	50.0	81.8	61.3	63.6	59.0	56.8	59.0	54.6
Volume	72.7	50.0	95.5	65.9	54.5	77.3	56.9	72.7	42.0

All results are reported in Table 1 and 2. We observe that CO-MKL reached higher values of accuracy than SVM where data are adjusted for age or between scans (82% vs 66%), demonstrating that correcting for nuisance variables in a MKL framework is more efficient than adjusting the values with a linear model. Moreover, CO-MKL with both thickness and volume values as features did not improve the accuracy in respect with employing CO-MKL using only the thickness as feature, but reaches better results than standard simple MKL used with both features μ^V and μ^T, demonstrating that out methods improves the classification performances in merging different information. As expected, MKL using covariates as features did not reach good values of accuracy, with a maximum of 66% in the case of follow up data. Also using SVM concatenating all variables of interest did not improve classification results, demonstrating once again that age and follow up time are useful when used to correct the classification but not if considered as features.

Table 2. Results from classification from data of thickness and volume of middle temporal gray and white matter considered together.

	Baseline			**Follow up**			Δ		
	Acc	Sens	Spec	Acc	Sens	Spec	Acc	Sens	Spec
CO-MKL	**70.5**	68.2	72.7	**81.8**	86.4	77.3	**70.45**	81.8	59.1
MKL	43.2	61.4	27.3	61.3	50.0	72.7	59.1	77.3	31.8
MKL + cov.	59.1	45.5	72.7	47.7	54.5	40.9	54.5	31.8	77.2
CON - SVM	72.7	50.0	95.4	65.9	54.6	77.3	65.9	59.1	72.7

It is to be noted that the use of both thickness and volume simultaneously did not improve performances in this specific case, but could allow a more comprehensive evaluation of degeneracy processes in respect to the analysis of a single brain feature. Moreover, even if classification using $\Delta\mu^X$ did not reach very high values, an accuracy of around 70% can be considered promising, since changes in brain structure are not easily detectable in psychosis patients, and points towards possible modifications in the rate of brain changes in patients in respect to healthy.

5 Conclusions

In this work, we propose CO-MKL to exploit supervised correction of the effects of confounding variables, with the aim of compensating possible unbalanced dataset. In fact, the presence of heterogeneity in longitudinal datasets is very common in neuropsychiatry research. We showed how automatic classification improves when the spurious differences between populations are taken into account into a process of supervised correction instead of ignored or integrated in simple models, as GLM. We focused our analysis to the middle temporal region of the brain, because it is known that it is involved in psychosis. We obtained high accuracies, up to more than 80%, demonstrating that brain structure and in particular thickness and volume of definite ROIs are markers of psychosis also at early stages. Moreover, we showed that the progression of the disease by itself, which we measured computing the difference in thickness or volume over time, could be employed to distinguish healthy from patients, suggesting that there could be a change in the speed of brain deformation in psychiatric diseases. The number of subjects we considered is limited: we plan on recruiting more patients and controls, as well as extending the analysis to other confounds to use as covariates, as for example medications or clinic scales both at baseline and at follow-up.

References

1. Bach, F.R., Lanckriet, G.R.G., Jordan, M.I.: Multiple kernel learning, conic duality, and the smo algorithm. In: ICML 2004, pp. 41–48 (2004)
2. Castro, E., Martínez-Ramón, M., Pearlson, G., Sui, J., Calhoun, V.D.: Characterization of groups using composite kernels and multi-source fmri analysis data: Application to schizophrenia. Neuroimage 58, 526–536 (2011)

3. Dale, A.M., Fischl, B., Sereno, M.I.: Cortical surface-based analysis. I. Segmentation and surface reconstruction. Neuroimage 9(2), 179–194 (1999)
4. Durrleman, S., Pennec, X., Trouvé, A., Braga, J., Gerig, G., Ayache, N.: Toward a comprehensive framework for the spatiotemporal statistical analysis of longitudinal shape data. International Journal of Computer Vision 103(1), 22–59 (2013)
5. Fischl, B., Salat, D.H., Busa, E., Albert, M., Dieterich, M., Haselgrove, C.E.A.: Whole brain segmentation: automated labeling of neuroanatomical structures in the human brain. Neuron 33(3), 341–355 (2002)
6. Gönen, M., Alpaydın, E.: Localized multiple kernel learning. In: ICML 2008, pp. 352–359 (2008)
7. Gönen, M., Alpaydın, E.: Multiple kernel learning algorithms. Journal of Machine Learning Research 12, 2181–2238 (2011)
8. Hinrichs, C., Singh, V., Xu, G., Johnson, S.C., Initiative, T.A.D.N.: Predictive markers for ad in a multi-modality framework: An analysis of mci progression in the adni population. Neuroimage 55, 574–589 (2011)
9. Hsu, C.W., Chang, C.C., Lin, C.J.: A practical guide to support vector classification (2010). http://www.csie.ntu.edu.tw/~cjlin/papers/guide/guide.pdf
10. Kuroki, N., Shenton, M.E., Salisbury, D.F., Hirayasu, Y., Onitsuka, T., Ersner-Hershfield, H., Yurgelun-Todd, D., Kikinis, R., Jolesz, F.A., McCarley, R.W.: Middle and inferior temporal gyrus gray matter volume abnormalities in first-episode schizophrenia: an MRI study. Am. J. Psychiatry 163(12), 2103–2110 (2006)
11. Lanckriet, G., Cristianini, N., Bartlett, P., Ghaoui, L.E., Jordan, M.: Learning the kernel matrix with semidefinite programming. Journal of Machine Learning Research 5, 27–72 (2004)
12. Lasalvia, A., Tosato, S., Brambilla, P., Bertani, M., Bonetto, C., Cristofalo, D.E.A.: Psychosis Incident Cohort Outcome Study (PICOS). A multisite study of clinical, social and biological characteristics, patterns of care and predictors of outcome in first-episode psychosis. Background, methodology and overview of the patient sample. Epidemiol. Psychiatr. Sci. 21(3), 281–303 (2012)
13. Peter, P.M., Nelder, J.: Generalized Linear Models. Chapman and Hall (1989)
14. Rakotomamonjy, A., Bach, F., Canu, S., Grandvalet, Y.: SimpleMKL. Journal of Machine Learning Research 9, 2491–2521 (2008)
15. Sederman, R., Coyne, J.C., Ranchor, A.V.: Age: Nuisance variable to be eliminated with statistical control or important concern? Patient Education and Counseling 61(37), 315–316 (2006)
16. Segate, N., Blanzieri, E.: Fast and scalable local kernel machines. Journal of Machine Learning Research 11, 1883–1926 (2010)
17. Tang, J., Liao, Y., Zhou, B., Tan, C., Liu, W., Wang, D., Liu, T., Hao, W., Tan, L., Chen, X.: Decrease in temporal gyrus gray matter volume in first-episode, early onset schizophrenia: an MRI study. PLoS One 7(7), e40247 (2012)
18. Vapnik, V.N.: Statistical Learning Theory. John Wiley and Sons (1998)

Parcellation of Infant Surface Atlas Using Developmental Trajectories of Multidimensional Cortical Attributes

Gang Li[1], Li Wang[1], John H. Gilmore[2], Weili Lin[1], and Dinggang Shen[1]

[1] Department of Radiology and BRIC, University of North Carolina at Chapel Hill, NC, USA
{gang_li,dgshen}@med.unc.edu
[2] Department of Psychiatry, University of North Carolina at Chapel Hill, NC 27599, USA

Abstract. Cortical surface atlases, equipped with anatomically and functionally defined parcellations, are of fundamental importance in neuroimaging studies. Typically, parcellations of surface atlases are derived based on the sulcal-gyral landmarks, which are extremely variable across individuals and poorly matched with microstructural and functional boundaries. Cortical developmental trajectories in infants reflect underlying changes of microstructures, which essentially determines the molecular organization and functional principles of the cortex, thus allowing better definition of developmentally, microstructurally, and functionally distinct regions, compared to conventional sulcal-gyral landmarks. Accordingly, a parcellation of infant cortical surface atlas was proposed, based on the developmental trajectories of *cortical thickness* in infants, revealing regional patterning of cortical growth. However, cortical anatomy is jointly characterized by biologically-distinct, multidimensional cortical attributes, i.e., cortical thickness, surface area, and local gyrification, each with its distinct genetic underpinning, cellular mechanism, and developmental trajectories. To date, the parcellations based on the development of surface area and local gyrification is still missing. To bridge this critical gap, for the first time, we parcellate an infant cortical surface atlas into distinct regions based solely on developmental trajectories of surface area and local gyrification, respectively. For each cortical attribute, we first *nonlinearly fuse* the subject-specific similarity matrices of vertices' developmental trajectories of all subjects into a single matrix, which helps better capture common and complementary information of the population than the conventional method of *simple averaging* of all subjects' matrices. Then, we perform spectral clustering based on this fused matrix. We have applied our method to parcellate an infant surface atlas using the developmental trajectories of surface area and local gyrification from 35 healthy infants, each with up to 7 time points in the first two postnatal years, revealing biologically more meaningful growth patterning than the conventional method.

Keywords: Surface area, local gyrification, infant, atlas, parcellation.

1 Introduction

Magnetic resonance imaging (MRI) allows for an unparalleled *in vivo* study of early dynamic development of the human brain. In MRI studies, cortical surface atlases, encoding anatomical structures and other reference information of the cortex, play

N. Navab et al. (Eds.): MICCAI 2015, Part III, LNCS 9351, pp. 543–550, 2015.
DOI: 10.1007/978-3-319-24574-4_65

fundamental roles in normalization, analysis, visualization, and comparison of results across subjects and studies [1]. Parcellations, defined in cortical surface atlases, help localize structural and functional regions, and partition individuals into regions of interest (ROIs), for region-based and network-based analyses [2]. Typically, these parcellations are defined based on sulcal-gyral landmarks [2], which are actually extremely variable across individuals and poorly matched with microstructurally, functionally, and developmentally defined boundaries [3]. Therefore, there is increasing interest to parcellate surface atlases into distinct regions based on other sources of information, e.g., the functional connectivity derived from fMRI [4] and the genetic correlation of surface area and cortical thickness derived from twin MRI studies [5]. However, owing to the dynamic development of cortical size, shape and folding in early postnatal stages, existing surface atlases and their parcellations created for adult brains are not suitable for infant brain studies [6]. For precise charting dynamic developmental trajectories of infant brains, the infant-dedicated surface atlases with parcellations, based on cortical developmental trajectories, are more appropriate. This is because cortical developmental trajectories in infants reflect underlying changes of microstructures, which essentially determine molecular organization and functional principles of the cortex [3], thus allowing for better definition of developmentally, microstructurally, and functionally distinct regions on surface atlases, compared to conventional sulcal-gyral landmarks. Accordingly, the first infant surface atlas, equipped with a parcellation based solely on the developmental trajectories of *cortical thickness*, has been recently created, revealing intriguing and meaningful regional patterning of cortical development [6].

Although promising, the parcellation based on cortical thickness trajectories has two major limitations. *First*, cortical thickness only reflects one aspect of the multidimensional nature of the cortex. Essentially, cortical structural development is jointly characterized by biologically-distinct, multidimensional cortical attributes, i.e., cortical thickness, surface area, and local gyrification, each with its distinct genetic underpinning, cellular mechanism, and developmental trajectories [7-9]. For example, in the first postnatal year, the cortex increases 31% in cortical thickness, 76% in surface area [8], and 17% in local gyrification [9]. Moreover, these cortical attributes are differently correlated with cognitive functioning, and differentially affected in a variety of brain disorders [8]. To date, parcellations of infant cortical surface atlases based on the developmental trajectories of *surface area* and *local gyrification* are still critically missing. *Second*, the existing method simply averages the subject-specific similarity matrices of vertices' developmental trajectories of all individuals as a population-mean similarity matrix for parcellation [6]; however, it ignores remarkable individual variability in terms of growth patterns and uneven distribution of time points, thus failing to fully capture common and complementary information of individuals.

In this paper, we unprecedentedly parcellate an infant cortical surface atlas into distinct regions, based on dynamic developmental trajectories of surface area and local gyrification in infants, respectively. To address the limitations of using population-mean similarity matrix for parcellation [6], we propose to first *nonlinearly fuse* the similarity matrices of vertices' developmental trajectories of all subjects into a single matrix and then perform spectral clustering based on this fused matrix. This strategy accounts for individual variability of growth patterns and the uneven distribution of time points, thus making full use of both common and complementary information across individuals. Based on 202 longitudinal MRI of 35 typical infants, each with up to 7 time points in the first two postnatal years, we reveal hitherto unseen, biologically meaningful surface atlas parcellations that capture the distinct patterns of developmental trajectories of surface area and local gyrification, respectively.

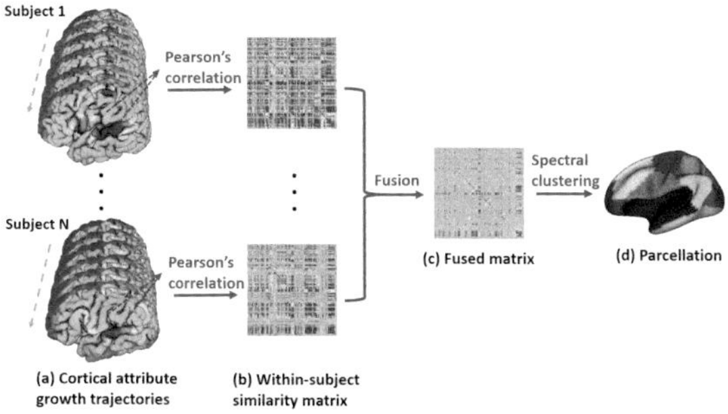

Fig. 1. Flowchart of developmental trajectories based parcellation of infant surface atlases.

2 Method

2.1 Dataset and Cortical Surface Mapping

We adopted a longitudinal infant MRI dataset, including 35 healthy infants, each with up to 7 scans in the first two postnatal years [6]. For each infant, T1-, T2-, and diffusion-weighted MRI were acquired using a Siemens 3T head-only scanner every 3 months in the first year since birth, and then every 6 months in the second year. Any scans with strong motion effects, leading to poor quality of tissue segmentation, were discarded. T1 images were acquired with the parameters: TR/TE = 1900/4.38 ms, flip angle = 7, resolution = $1 \times 1 \times 1$ mm^3. T2 images were acquired with the parameters: TR/TE = 7380/119 ms, flip angle = 150, resolution = $1.25 \times 1.25 \times 1.95$ mm^3. Diffusion-weighted images (DWI) were acquired with the parameters: TR/TE = 7680/82 ms, resolution = $2 \times 2 \times 2$ mm^3, 42 non-collinear diffusion gradients, and diffusion weighting b =1000s/mm^2. Data distribution included 8 infants each with 7 scans, 15 infants each with 6 scans, 8 infants each with 5 scans, and 4 infants each with 4 scans.

Infant cortical surfaces reconstruction and mapping were performed by an infant-dedicated computational pipeline [6]. Briefly, *first*, non-cerebral tissues were removed, and longitudinally-consistent tissue segmentation, using multimodal information of T1, T2 and FA images, were performed [10]. *Second*, each brain was divided into left and right hemispheres after filling of non-cortical structures. *Third*, inner and outer surfaces for each hemisphere were reconstructed by first tessellating the topology corrected white matter as a triangular mesh representation and then deforming the mesh using a deformable model [11]. *Fourth*, for each infant, all longitudinal inner surfaces were mapped to a standard sphere and groupwisely aligned to establish within-subject cortical correspondences and generate within-subject mean cortical folding using Spherical Demons [12]. *Fifth*, within-subject mean cortical folding maps of all subjects were groupwisely aligned to establish longitudinally-consistent inter-subject cortical correspondences, for construction of infant cortical surface atlases [6], and each surface was then resampled to a standard mesh tessellation. *Finally*, for each vertex of each resampled surface, both surface area (SA) and local gyrification index (LGI, Fig. 1(a)) were computed using an infant-specific method [9].

2.2 Atlas Parcellation Using Cortical Developmental Trajectories

To perform cortical surface atlas parcellation based on the developmental trajectories of cortical attributes, we adopted the spectral clustering method, which projects the data into the eigenspace of the similarity matrix (encoding the similarity between each pair of data points) to better capture distributions of original data points [13]. To this end, we first defined for each subject a *subject-specific* similarity matrix of the developmental trajectories for each cortical attribute (i.e., SA and LGI) between each pair of vertices in the surface atlas, using Pearson's correlation (Fig. 1(b)). Of note, as each subject had a different number and different temporal distribution of time points owing to missing scans, the subject-specific similarity matrix naturally solved this issue. For each cortical attribute of each subject, we computed its subject-specific similarity matrix $\boldsymbol{A}^s$ as: $\boldsymbol{A}^s(i,j) = (1 + r^s(i,j))/2$, where $r^s(i,j)$ is Pearson's correlation coefficient between the developmental trajectories of a cortical attribute between each pair of vertices i and j. One intuitive method to perform surface atlas parcellation is to first *simply average* similarity matrices of all subjects as a population-mean matrix and then perform spectral clustering based on this mean matrix [6]. This, however, ignores the remarkable individual variability in terms of growth patterns and scan distributions, thus failing to fully capitalize on both common and complementary information across individuals, leading to less meaningful parcellations.

To fully integrate both common and complementary information of individuals, we propose to first *nonlinearly fuse* their similarity matrices into a single matrix (Fig. 1(c)) and then perform spectral clustering based on this *fused* matrix (Fig. 1(d)). Our central idea was to iteratively update every matrix by diffusing information across subjects, making it more similar to others, until convergence [14]. To achieve this, for each subject-specific similarity matrix $\boldsymbol{A}^s$, we first computed a *full* kernel matrix $\boldsymbol{P}^s$ and a *sparse* kernel matrix $\boldsymbol{M}^s$ respectively as:

$$\boldsymbol{P}^s(i,j) = \begin{cases} \frac{\boldsymbol{A}^s(i,j)}{2\sum_{k\neq i}\boldsymbol{A}^s(i,k)}, & j \neq i \\ 1/2, & j = i \end{cases}, \text{ and } \boldsymbol{M}^s(i,j) = \begin{cases} \frac{\boldsymbol{A}^s(i,j)}{\sum_{k\in N_i}\boldsymbol{A}^s(i,k)}, & j\in N_i \\ 0, & \text{otherwise} \end{cases} \quad (1)$$

Herein, $\boldsymbol{P}^s$ encoded *full* similarity information among vertices and $\boldsymbol{M}^s$ captured reliable, high-similarity neighbors for each vertex [14]. N_i represented K nearest neighbors of vertex i. Given N subjects, $\boldsymbol{P}^s$ of each subject at iteration t was then updated as: $\boldsymbol{P}_t^s = \boldsymbol{M}^s \times \left(\frac{\sum_{k\neq s}\boldsymbol{P}_{t-1}^{(k)}}{N-1}\right) \times (\boldsymbol{M}^s)^T,\ s,k \in \{1,\ldots,N\}$. In this way, the isolated weak similarities disappeared, while the strong similarities were added to others. Meanwhile, the weak similarities supported by all matrices were retained, depending on their neighborhood connections across subjects. After T iterations, the *fused* matrix (average of all subjects' $\boldsymbol{P}_T^s$) was used for parcellation based on spectral clustering.

3 Results

We performed developmental trajectories based surface atlas parcellation using surface area and local gyrification, by utilizing a total of 202 MRI scans from 35 healthy infants. In all results, we set K as 30 experimentally. The *left* panel of Fig. 2 shows the parcellation results based on the trajectories of surface area with different numbers of clusters from 2 to 12, using the proposed method of *nonlinear fusion* of individuals' similarity matrices, in comparison to *simple averaging* of individuals' similarity matrices [6]. For direct comparison with parcellations based on the trajectories of cortical thickness [6] and genetic correlation of surface area [5], we set the maximum cluster number as 12 as in [5, 6]. As shown, the proposed method led to biologically much more meaningful parcellations. For example, at 2-cluster parcellation, the proposed method revealed an anterior-posterior division to partition the unimodal motor, somatosensory, visual, and auditory cortices from the high-order prefrontal, inferior temporal, and insula cortices. In contrast, the averaging-based method grouped high-order frontal pole area with unimodal cortices, thus leading to less meaningful results. Of note, the anterior-posterior division revealed by the proposed method was generally consistent with the genetic patterning of surface area in adults [5]. More importantly, the proposed method revealed a naturally hierarchical organization of developmental patterning of surface area, in line with the findings of hierarchical organization of genetic patterning of surface area [5]. This means that, when increasing the cluster numbers, a new region is created largely without changing existing boundaries of parcellation. For example, the boundaries between the prefrontal cortex and motor cortex (indicated by the blue arrows) and the boundaries between visual cortex and temporal cortex (indicated by the green arrows) were well-preserved from 4-cluster to 12-cluster parcellation using the proposed method, while the corresponding boundaries, by the averaging-based method, were quite unstable across different numbers of clusters. In addition, as highlighted by the gray arrows, the cluster of the auditory cortex was well-preserved from 4-cluster to 12-cluster parcellation by the proposed method, whereas this cluster disappeared from 8-cluster to 10-cluster parcellation, when using the averaging-based method [6]. Moreover, as indicated by the red arrows, the averaging-based method led to many isolated fragments in its parcellations. To further verify the parcellation, we performed seed-based analysis as in [5, 6]. Specifically, for each of the 26 uniformly distributed seeds on the atlas, its correlation with all other vertices, based on the population mean correlation maps, was shown by a respective color-coded small surface map. As shown in Fig. 3(a), seeds in the same cluster yielded largely the similar correlation patterns, while seeds across the boundaries of clusters (purple curves) led to quite different patterns. For example, the seed in the cluster of the auditory cortex had a unique correlation map, in comparison with the nearby seeds, confirming the rationality of our parcellation.

The *right* panel of Fig. 2 shows the surface atlas parcellations based on the developmental trajectories of *local gyrification* with different numbers of clusters. At 2-cluster parcellation, both methods identified a dorsal-ventral division to separate frontal and parietal cortices from temporal, insula, and visual cortices. However, with the number of clusters increasing, the proposed method revealed a more meaningful hierarchical organization of the developmental patterning of local gyrification. For example, the boundaries between prefrontal and insula cortices (green arrows), the boundaries between supramarginal gyrus and insula cortex (yellow arrows), and the boundaries between occipital and temporal cortices (blue arrows) were well-preserved from 4-cluster to 12-cluster parcellation by the proposed method, while the corresponding boundaries, by the averaging-based method, were quite variable across different numbers of clusters, showing unstableness of these clusters. As performed in verifying surface area based parcellation, we also performed seed-based analysis of the population mean correlation patterns of developmental trajectories of local gyrification, by using 26 uniformly distributed seeds on the atlas. As shown in Fig. 3(b), seeds in the same cluster yielded largely the similar correlation patterns, while seeds across the boundaries of clusters (purple curves) led to quite different patterns.

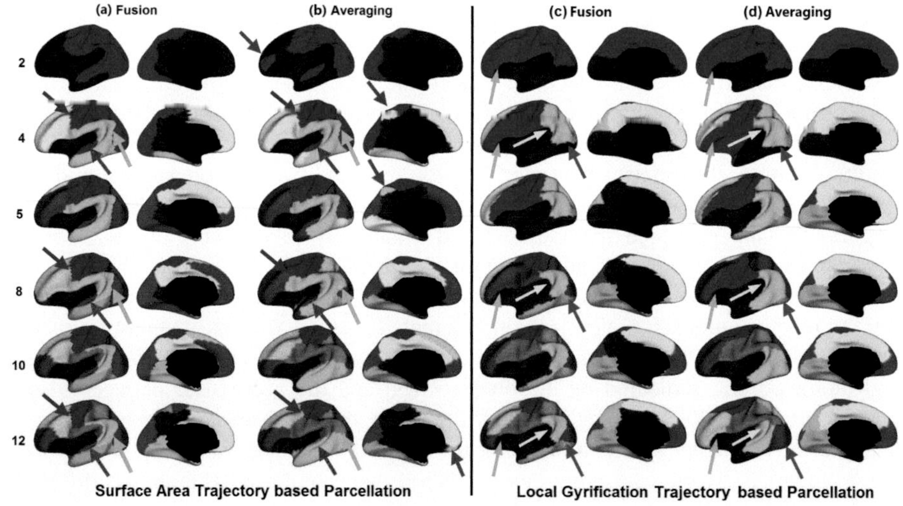

Fig. 2. Surface atlas parcellations based on the developmental trajectories of *surface area* (left panel) and *local gyrification* (right panel), respectively, by (a) and (c) fusion of individuals' similarity matrices, and (b) and (d) averaging of individuals' similarity matrices.

Fig. 4 shows a comparison of our parcellations with the parcellation based on genetic correlation of surface area of adults [5] and cortical thickness trajectories of infants [6]. In our 12-cluster parcellations based on developmental trajectories, all clusters largely corresponded to functional specializations, with their names provided in leftmost and rightmost columns. In general, surface area, local gyrification, and cortical thickness each exhibited distinct parcellation patterns based on its developmental trajectories, in line with the reports that each has distinct genetic underpinning, cellular mechanism, and developmental trajectories [7-9]. Interestingly, parcellations based on trajectories of surface area and local gyrification revealed several similar clusters, e.g., superior parietal (cluster 2), inferior parietal (cluster 3), and precuneus regions (cluster 6). In addition, parcellations based on trajectories of surface area and cortical thickness (Fig. 4(d)) [6] identified several similar clusters, e.g., perisylvian (cluster 4), visual (cluster 5), and medial temporal cortices (cluster 9). Moreover, several clusters in the parcellation based on trajectories of surface area and the genetic correlation of surface area (Fig. 4(c)) [5] appeared similar, e.g., visual (cluster 5), precuneus (cluster 6), and superior parietal cortices (cluster 2).

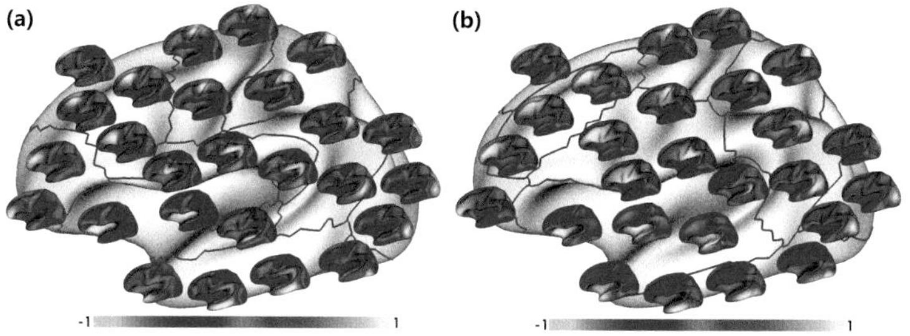

Fig. 3. Seed-based analysis of population mean correlation patterns of **(a)** *surface area* developmental trajectories and **(b)** *local gyrification* developmental trajectories from 35 infants, for verifying the parcellations in **Fig. 2**. For each of 26 seeds, its correlations with all other vertices are shown as a respective color-coded small surface map.

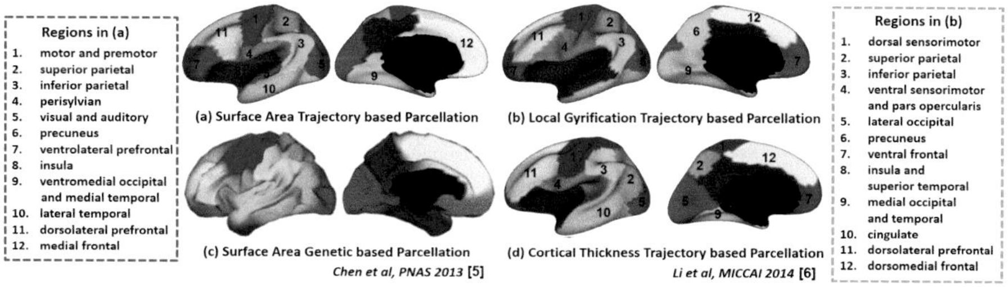

Fig. 4. Comparison with parcellation based on genetic correlation of surface area of adults [5] and parcellation based on cortical thickness trajectories of infants [6].

4 Conclusion

This paper has two major contributions. First, based on the work in [6], we propose a novel method to parcellate surface atlases, using cortical developmental trajectories, through *nonlinear fusion of* individuals' similarity matrices, which better capitalizes on both common and complementary information across subjects. Second, leveraging this new method, we derived the *first* infant cortical surface atlas parcellations based solely on dynamic developmental trajectories of surface area and local gyrification, respectively, revealing their distinct and biologically meaningful growth patterning. As there is no ground truth for developmental trajectories based parcellations, we validate our results by 1) using existing neuroscience knowledge, 2) performing seed-based analysis, and 3) comparing with the results using the existing method. In the future work, we will investigate the different numbers of clusters in parcellations and find the optimal cluster number, according to silhouette coefficient [5]. We will further comprehensively and quantitatively compare our parcellations with existing parcellations [4-6], and apply them to early brain development studies. As each cortical attribute defines a distinct parcellation, to study a specific attribute, its corresponding parcellation would better be adopted, as this encodes unique growth patterning.

References

1. Van Essen, D.C., Dierker, D.L.: Surface-based and probabilistic atlases of primate cerebral cortex. Neuron 56, 209–225 (2007)
2. Desikan, R.S., Segonne, F., Fischl, B., Quinn, B.T., Dickerson, B.C., Blacker, D., Buckner, R.L., Dale, A.M., Maguire, R.P., Hyman, B.T., Albert, M.S., Killiany, R.J.: An automated labeling system for subdividing the human cerebral cortex on MRI scans into gyral based regions of interest. Neuroimage 31, 968–980 (2006)
3. Zilles, K., Amunts, K.: TIMELINE Centenary of Brodmann's map - conception and fate. Nature Reviews Neuroscience 11, 139–145 (2010)
4. Yeo, B.T., Krienen, F.M., Sepulcre, J., Sabuncu, M.R., Lashkari, D., Hollinshead, M., Roffman, J.L., Smoller, J.W., Zollei, L., Polimeni, J.R., Fischl, B., Liu, H., Buckner, R.L.: The organization of the human cerebral cortex estimated by intrinsic functional connectivity. J. Neurophysiol. 106, 1125–1165 (2011)
5. Chen, C.H., Fiecas, M., Gutierrez, E.D., Panizzon, M.S., Eyler, L.T., Vuoksimaa, E., Thompson, W.K., Fennema-Notestine, C., Hagler, D.J., Jernigan Jr., T.L., Neale, M.C., Franz, C.E., Lyons, M.J., Fischl, B., Tsuang, M.T., Dale, A.M., Kremen, W.S.: Genetic topography of brain morphology. Proc. Natl. Acad. Sci. U. S. A. 110, 17089–17094 (2013)
6. Li, G., Wang, L., Shi, F., Lin, W., Shen, D.: Constructing 4D infant cortical surface atlases based on dynamic developmental trajectories of the cortex. Med. Image Comput. Comput. Assist. Interv. 17, 89–96 (2014)
7. Raznahan, A., Shaw, P., Lalonde, F., Stockman, M., Wallace, G.L., Greenstein, D., Clasen, L., Gogtay, N., Giedd, J.N.: How does your cortex grow? J. Neurosci. 31, 7174–7177 (2011)
8. Lyall, A.E., Shi, F., Geng, X., Woolson, S., Li, G., Wang, L., Hamer, R.M., Shen, D., Gilmore, J.H.: Dynamic Development of Regional Cortical Thickness and Surface Area in Early Childhood. Cereb Cortex (2014)
9. Li, G., Wang, L., Shi, F., Lyall, A.E., Lin, W., Gilmore, J.H., Shen, D.: Mapping longitudinal development of local cortical gyrification in infants from birth to 2 years of age. J. Neurosci. 34, 4228–4238 (2014)
10. Wang, L., Shi, F., Yap, P.T., Gilmore, J.H., Lin, W., Shen, D.: 4D multi-modality tissue segmentation of serial infant images. PLoS One 7, e44596 (2012)
11. Li, G., Nie, J., Wu, G., Wang, Y., Shen, D.: Consistent reconstruction of cortical surfaces from longitudinal brain MR images. Neuroimage 59, 3805–3820 (2012)
12. Yeo, B.T., Sabuncu, M.R., Vercauteren, T., Ayache, N., Fischl, B., Golland, P.: Spherical demons: fast diffeomorphic landmark-free surface registration. IEEE Trans. Med. Imaging 29, 650–668 (2010)
13. Ng, A.Y., Jordan, M.I., Weiss, Y.: On spectral clustering: Analysis and an algorithm. Adv. Neur. In. 14, 849–856 (2002)
14. Wang, B., Mezlini, A.M., Demir, F., Fiume, M., Tu, Z., Brudno, M., Haibe-Kains, B., Goldenberg, A.: Similarity network fusion for aggregating data types on a genomic scale. Nature Methods 11, 333–337 (2014)

Graph-Based Motion-Driven Segmentation of the Carotid Atherosclerotique Plaque in 2D Ultrasound Sequences

Aimilia Gastounioti[1,3,*], Aristeidis Sotiras[2], Konstantina S. Nikita[1], and Nikos Paragios[3]

[1] Biomedical Simulations and Imaging Laboratory, School of Electrical and Computer Engineering, National Technical University of Athens, Athens, Greece
gaimilia@biosim.ntua.gr, knikita@ece.ntua.gr
[2] Center for Biomedical Image Computing and Analytics, Department of Radiology, University of Pennsylvania, Philadelphia, USA
sotar22@gmail.com
[3] Center for Visual Computing, Department of Applied Mathematics, Ecole Centrale de Paris, Paris, France
nikos.paragios@ecp.fr

Abstract. Carotid plaque segmentation in ultrasound images is a crucial step for carotid atherosclerosis. However, image quality, important deformations and lack of texture are prohibiting factors towards manual or accurate carotid segmentation. We propose a novel fully automated methodology to identify the plaque region by exploiting kinematic dependencies between the atherosclerotic and the normal arterial wall. The proposed methodology exploits group-wise image registration towards recovering the deformation field, on which information theory criteria are used to determine dominant motion classes and a map reflecting kinematic dependencies, which is then segmented using Markov random fields. The algorithm was evaluated on 120 cases, for which manually-traced plaque contours by an experienced physician were available. Promising evaluation results showed the enhanced performance of the algorithm in automatically segmenting the plaque region, while future experiments on additional datasets are expected to further elucidate its potential.

Keywords: segmentation, carotid plaque, image registration, ultrasound.

1 Introduction

Carotid plaques are buildups of fatty substances, scar tissue and cholesterol deposits in the inner lining of the carotid artery and they are caused by a chronic degenerative arterial disease called atherosclerosis. The direct association of these arterial lesions with stroke events and the limitations of the current risk-stratification practice both underline the need for the development of computer-aided-diagnosis (CAD) systems for carotid plaques [1]. In particular, the development of effective CAD schemes, which are based on B-mode ultrasound (US) image analysis, is considered a grand challenge by the scientific

N. Navab et al. (Eds.): MICCAI 2015, Part III, LNCS 9351, pp. 551–559, 2015.
DOI: 10.1007/978-3-319-24574-4_66

community, due to the fact that this modality holds a prominent position in screening and follow-up exams of patients with carotid atherosclerosis. In this line of work, and given that manual tracing of regions of interest is always a time-consuming and strenuous task, automated plaque segmentation in B-mode US is a critical step towards user-independent measurements of novel biomarkers: (a) total plaque area [2], (b) plaque surface irregularities [3], (c) plaque deformations during the cardiac cycle [4], and (d) the underlying material composition of the plaque (texture descriptors) [1].

An attempt to provide a short overview of related studies [5]-[10] is presented in Table 1. It should be noted that there is quite limited work on the segmentation of the carotid plaque in 2D B-mode US of longitudinal sections of the carotid artery. Recent work explore either well known and well studied active-contours on the image features domain [5] or a conventional Bayesian formulation [7]. Full automatization is achieved only in [5]. It is also important to note that both approaches are applied separately to each frame of the sequence and they are based on local intensity values to segment the carotid plaque; the deformation field is used either to initialize the segmentation process in subsequent frames [5] or to ensure cohesion between segmentation results in different time points [7]. However, US is characterized by low image quality and texture features may vary significantly over different devices, image settings, and operators. Moreover, a frame-wise concept of segmenting the carotid plaque may limit the overall performance of the algorithm due to image artifacts in isolated frames, the view point of the sensor, the important displacements, and the variations of image intensities; it can also be more time-consuming than simultaneously using all frames (one-shot approach).

In this study, we aim to tackle aforementioned limitations and, motivated by recent findings suggesting that the kinematic activity of the carotid plaque differs from that of non-atherosclerotic arterial-wall segments [4], we introduce a novel fully automated one-shot segmentation approach, the core of which is the exploitation of motion as segmentation feature. The algorithm relies on group-wise image registration towards recovering the deformation field, on which information theory criteria are used to determine dominant motion classes and a map reflecting kinematic dependencies, which is then segmented using Markov random fields (MRFs). The designed algorithm is evaluated on 120 B-mode US video recordings of patients with carotid atherosclerosis.

Table 1. Previous work on developing computerized methodologies for segmenting the carotid plaque in B-mode ultrasound.

Study	Sample	Imaging modality	Fully Automatic
[5]	43	2D B-mode video - Longitudinal view	√
[6]	7	2D B-mode image - Transverse view	×
[7]	33	2D B-mode video - Longitudinal view	×
[8]	1	3D B-mode image - Transverse view	√
[9]	21	3D B-mode video - Transverse view	×
[10]	22	3D B-mode image – Longitudinal & Transverse view	×

2 The Proposed Methodology

The use of motion as segmentation feature involves three challenges; (i) the estimation of the deformation vectors, (ii) the identification of dominant kinematic hypotheses, and the (iii) segmentation of the image domain according to these hypotheses.

The proposed approach aims to explore motion differences as a feature vector towards carotid segmentation. Such an approach can either be addressed through a sequential approach, where either optical flow is estimated sequentially or all frames are mapped to a reference frame. The first approach is proned to accumulation of errors, which can be critical if motion vectors are used as segmentation features, while the latter can be quite sensitive in the presence of important displacements throughout the sequence while it introduces also a significant bias depending on the choice of the reference frame. Recent studies have shown that population (group-wise) registration methods perform in general more reliably compared to the ones exploiting the pair-wise assumption.

2.1 Group-Wise Image Registration

In this step, the deformation field is estimated by registering the entire image sequence through an one-shot optimization approach. Let us now consider without loss of generality a sequence of N frames where each frame is deformed according to a deformation model T_i. Inspired from the ideas presented in [11], we adopt a discrete optimization framework which aims to estimate all deformations at a single step. The central idea is to deform the grids simultaneously, such that meaningful correspondences between the N images are obtained and their mapping to the geometry (reference pose, R) creates a statistically compact variable. The described graphical model is expressed in the form of a MRF and the objective function in an abstract level can be expressed as follows:

$$\begin{aligned} E(T_i, R) = \alpha \sum_{i=1}^{N} \sum_{j=1}^{N} \iint_{\Omega} \rho(I_i(T_i), I_j(T_j)) d\omega + \\ \beta \sum_{i=1}^{N} \iint_{\Omega} \psi(T_i) d\omega + \gamma \iint_{\Omega} \eta(R, I_1(T_1), \cdots, I_N(T_N)) \end{aligned} \quad (1)$$

seeking to optimize an objective function which consists of three terms weighted by factors α, β, and γ; one that measures the similarity (ρ) between two images, a second term which incorporates a convex function, ψ, imposing smoothness at each deformation field and a third term which measures the similarity, η, of the images on the intersection of the deformed images to enforce pair-wise correspondences.

This is a coupled optimization problem that is discretized towards reducing complexity. Deformations are expressed through reduced complexity grids endowed with an interpolation strategy (free-form deformations), while reference image intensities are discretized as well. The optimization is, then, performed with the efficient linear programming method which is described in detail in [12]. The outcome of this inference process consists of N- deformation models mapped all to a common pose and reference frame where each pixel is associated with an $N \times 2$-dimensional feature vector (vertical and horizontal displacements towards the estimated reference space). Reasoning on this space requires estimation of the dominant hypotheses.

2.2 A Mutual-Information Map Reflecting Kinematic Dependencies

Let us denote the resultant of an $N \times 2$-dimensional feature vector as MTD (magnitude of total displacement). In this step, each pixel is associated with an MTD vector and the goal is to identify dominant motion classes and elucidate kinematic dependencies among pixels. We empirically found that the application of independent component analysis (ICA) on the MTD vector set mostly captured the motion of the plaque, with a number of 50 independent components sufficiently explaining variance in kinematic activity. Therefore, a subset of $K = 50$ independent MTD vectors (IVs) are first isolated using ICA.

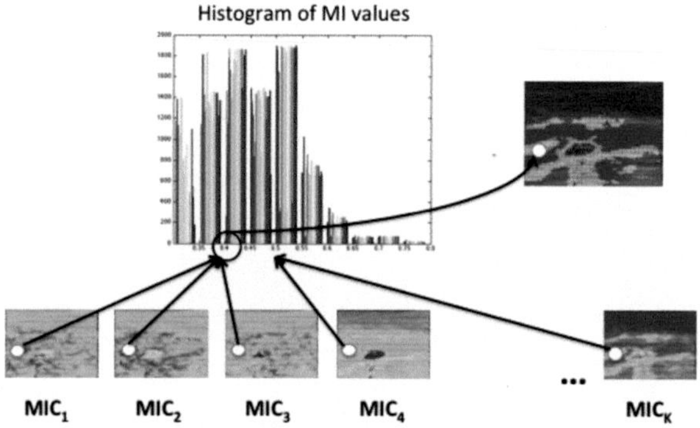

Fig. 1. Combining K mutual information color maps (MIC), each representing the mutual information (in [0: blue - 1: red]) between an independent vector and MTD vectors, to estimate a final mutual information value for each pixel.

Having isolated motion vectors that mainly describe plaque motion, the next step is to discriminate regions where the kinematic activity mostly depends on those vectors. To this end, each MTD vector is mapped to the IVs (ICA base) using the mutual information (MI), which was empirically found to perform better than simple projection to the ICA base, as follows. K colormaps, each representing the MI values of every MTD vector with the kth IV ($k \in [1, K]$), are produced and a final MI value is attributed to each pixel through majority voting. Specifically, based on the histogram of all K color maps, each pixel is associated with the center of the bin where the majority of the corresponding MI values belong (Fig. 1).

2.3 Graph-Based Segmentation of the Mutual-Information Map

At this stage, the final MI map is segmented by following again the concepts of graphical models and MRFs. A grid is superimposed onto the map, with each pixel corresponding to a node and the edge system is constructed by assuming an 8-neighbor connectivity for smoother segmentation results (Fig. 2), giving rise to a binary labeling problem (label 1: "plaque" and label 2: "non plaque").

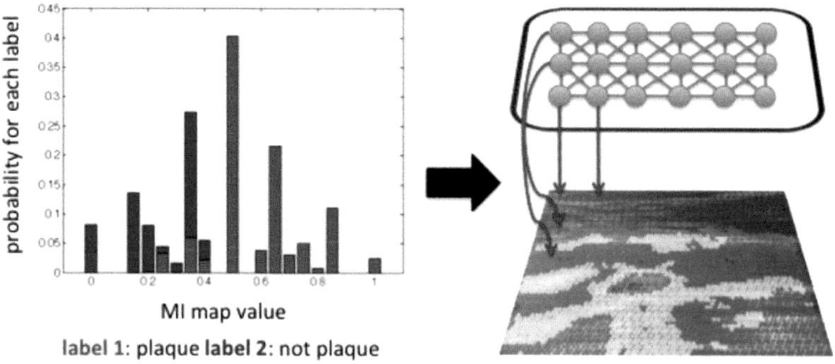

Fig. 2. (Right) Rough presentation of the underlying graph which is used in graph-based segmentation of the final color map; for simplicity reasons, only a subset of nodes and edges is displayed. The red edges represent the relationship between the grid nodes and the pixels of the color map, while the blue ones correspond to the pairwise potentials. The singleton potentials are given by the likelihood of a label given the MI map value (bar chart on the left).

The objective function to be optimized consists of two terms, one singleton representing the node-labeling costs ($\bar{\mathbf{g}}$) and one pair-wise standing for the costs to split neighboring nodes ($\bar{\mathbf{f}}$):

$$\varepsilon(\bar{\mathbf{g}}, \bar{\mathbf{f}}) = \min_{u} \sum_{p \in V} \bar{g}_p(u_p) + \lambda \sum_{(p,q) \in E} \bar{f}_{pq}(u_p, u_q) \quad (2)$$

where V and E denote, respectively, the vertices and edges of the graph. The labeling costs for each node are considered to be proportional to the likelihood of a label given the final MI map value for the corresponding pixel. These likelihood values are already learned in a training step (see also section 3). The pair-wise potentials are considered to be equal to 1 and 0 for neighboring pixels with different or the same labels, respectively, assuming equal weights for all connections. The optimization problem is solved again with a previously presented linear programming method [12].

3 Evaluation Process and Results

The study dataset consisted of 120 patients with established carotid atherosclerosis; the atherosclerotic lesions were mainly soft plaques causing mild or moderate lumen stenosis, which are more often clinically encountered and prone-to-rupture. For each subject, the carotid artery was scanned in the longitudinal direction and a B-mode US image sequence was recorded at a rate higher than 25 frames/s for at least one cardiac cycle. The algorithm was empirically parameterized with 32×32 grids and α, β and γ equal to 2, 1 and 18, respectively, for the group-wise image registration. Optimal graph-based segmentation of the final MI maps was achieved with weights equal to 1 for all connections.

The algorithm was evaluated on the dataset following leave-one-out cross validation, by repeating the following phases for each patient m (with $m \in [1, 120]$) considering that the mth patient was the testing case and the other patients formed the training set. In the training phase, the final MI maps for the training cases, together with the ground-truth plaque regions (as manually traced by an experienced vascular physician), were fed to Adaboost in order to learn the likelihood distributions of each label over different MI values. Then, the algorithm was applied to the testing case and the agreement between the segmentation result and the corresponding ground-truth plaques was measured in terms of the true negative (TNF) and the true positive (TPF) fractions, the Dice coefficient, the overlap index, and the mean contour distance (MCD). In all repetitions, the "plaque" label was associated with statistically higher MI values than the "non plaque" label (Wilcoxon rank-sum test, $p < 0.05$).

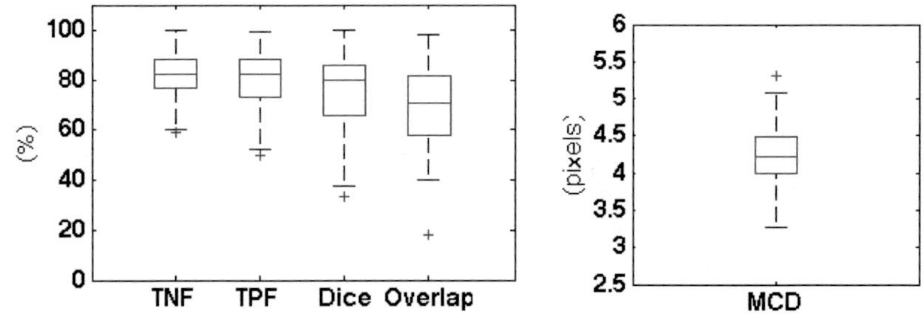

Fig. 3. Boxplots of the evaluation results for all patients.

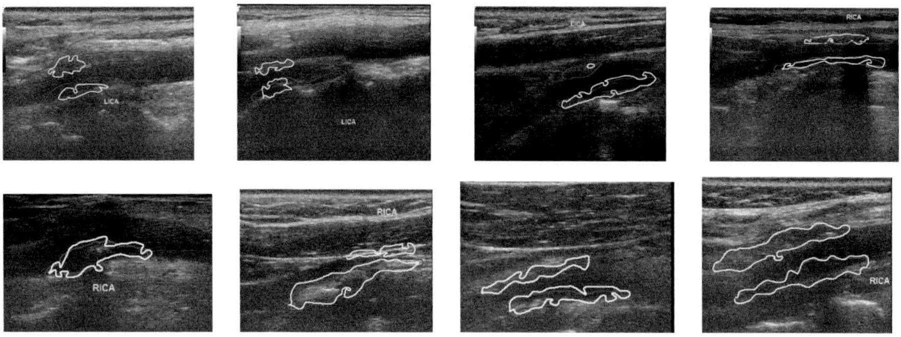

Fig. 4. Outlines of plaque regions as estimated by the proposed algorithm (yellow) and as manually traced by experienced vascular physicians (red) for cases of minimum (1st row, TNF=60-65%, TPF=61-64%, Dice=45-52%, Overlap=40-50%, MCD=4.5-5.0 pixels) and maximum (2nd row, TNF=82-87%, TPF=80-85%, Dice=79-81%, Overlap=75-80%, MCD=3.5-4.0 pixels) performance of the algorithm.

The evaluation results for all patients are summarized in the boxplots of Fig. 3. Fig. 4 illustrates examples of the segmentation results and the corresponding ground-truth boundaries. The evaluation results are in line with those presented in the limited number of related studies which are available in the literature [5,7]. Although straightforward comparisons are not possible due to different datasets, the promising performance of the proposed algorithm is further enhanced considering that (a) the algorithm achieved similar segmentation accuracy on a 3-times larger database (Table 1), (b) it uses motion, which is more reliable and more robust over different US image recordings than texture, as segmentation feature, and (c) it is an one-shot approach which, as explained in section 1, limits many drawbacks of US imaging. Moreover, it is important to note that plaque segmentation in US is a very challenging task, with low agreement even in manual delineation by expert operators [13].

4 Discussion

This study introduced a fully automated algorithm for graph-based motion-driven segmentation of the carotid plaque in 2D ultrasound image sequences. Future experiments, including datasets of different US scanners and scanner settings, as well as ground-truth plaque outlines by multiple experienced physicians, are expected to further elucidate the potential of the algorithm. In a future perspective, integration of visual and motion features within the segmentation framework is a natural extension of the proposed framework. In terms of methodological view point, integration of motion hypotheses generation along with segmentation can be done jointly if the task is considered as an unsupervised clustering problem where both assignments, number of clusters and cluster centers are unknown. Furthermore, the entire chain can be considered as a single optimization problem if the "segmentation" labels are integrated to the population registration framework a "singleton" likelihoods acting on the reconstructed reference image in the form of a higher order potential. This will allow - given a predefined set of motion hypotheses - to jointly register and segment all images at once and eventually will improve both segmentation and registration results since their solutions will mutually benefit from their association.

References

1. Golemati, S., Gastounioti, A., Nikita, K.S.: Toward novel noninvasive and low-cost markers for predicting strokes in asymptomatic carotid atherosclerosis: the role of ultrasound image analysis. IEEE Trans. Biomed. Eng. (Special issue on grand challenges in engineering life sciences and medicine) 60(3), 652–658 (2013)
2. Destrempes, F., Meunier, J., Giroux, M.F., Soulez, G., Cloutier, G.: Segmentation of plaques in sequences of ultrasonic b-mode images of carotid arteries based on motion estimation and a Bayesian model. IEEE Trans. Biomed. Eng. 58(8), 2202–2211 (2011)
3. Prabhakaran, S., Rundek, T., Ramas, R., Elkind, M.S., Paik, M.C., Boden-Albala, B., Sacco, R.L.: Carotid plaque surface irregularity predicts ischemic stroke: the northern Manhattan study. Stroke 37(11), 2696–2701 (2006)
4. Gastounioti, A., Golemati, S., Stoitsis, J.S., Nikita, K.S.: Adaptive block matching methods for carotid artery wall motion estimation from B-mode ultrasound: in silico evaluation & in vivo application. Phys. Med. Biol. 58, 8647–8661 (2013)
5. Loizou, C., Petroudi, S., Pantziaris, M., Nicolaides, A., Pattichis, C.: An integrated system for the segmentation of atherosclerotic carotid plaque ultrasound video. IEEE Trans. Ultrason. Ferroelectr. Freq. Control 61(1), 86–101 (2014)
6. Mao, F., Gill, J., Downey, D., Fenster, A.: Segmentation of carotid artery in ultrasound images: Method development and evaluation technique. Med. Phys. 27(8), 1961–1970 (2000)
7. Destrempes, F., Meunier, J., Giroux, M.F., Soulez, G., Cloutier, G.: Segmentation of plaques in sequences of ultrasonic b-mode images of carotid arteries based on motion estimation and a Bayesian model. IEEE Trans. Biomed. Eng. 58(8), 2202–2211 (2011)
8. Zahalka, A., Fenster, A.: An automated segmentation method for three-dimensional carotid ultrasound images. Phys. Med. Biol. 46(4), 1321–1342 (2001)
9. Ukwatta, E., Awad, J., Ward, A.D., Buchanan, D., Samarabandu, J., Parraga, G., Fenster, A.: Three-dimensional ultrasound of carotid atherosclerosis: semiautomated segmentation using a level set-based method. Med. Phys. 38(5), 2479–2493 (2011)
10. Buchanan, D., Gyacskov, I., Ukwatta, E., Lindenmaier, T., Fenster, A., Parraga, G.: Semi-automated segmentation of carotid artery total plaque volume from three dimensional ultrasound carotid imaging. In: Proc. SPIE, vol. 8317, pp. 83170I–83170I-7 (2012)

11. Sotiras, A., Komodakis, N., Glocker, B., Deux, J.-F., Paragios, N.: Graphical models and deformable diffeomorphic population registration using global and local metrics. In: Yang, G.-Z., Hawkes, D., Rueckert, D., Noble, A., Taylor, C. (eds.) MICCAI 2009, Part I. LNCS, vol. 5761, pp. 672–679. Springer, Heidelberg (2009)
12. Komodakis, N., Tziritas, G., Paragios, N.: Performance vs computational efficiency for optimizing single and dynamic mrfs: Setting the state of the art with primal-dual strategies. Comput. Vis. Imag. Und. 112(1), 14–29 (2008)
13. Polak, J.F., Pencina, M.J., OLeary, D.H., DAgostino, R.B.: Common-carotid artery intima-media thickness progression as a predictor of stroke in multi-ethnic study of atherosclerosis. Stroke 42(11), 3017–3021 (2011)

Cortical Surface-Based Construction of Individual Structural Network with Application to Early Brain Development Study

Yu Meng[1,2], Gang Li[2], Weili Lin[2], John H. Gilmore[3], and Dinggang Shen[2]

[1] Department of Computer Science, University of North Carolina at Chapel Hill, NC, USA
[2] Department of Radiology and BRIC, University of North Carolina at Chapel Hill, NC, USA
[3] Department of Psychiatry, University of North Carolina at Chapel Hill, NC, USA

Abstract. Analysis of anatomical covariance for cortex morphology in individual subjects plays an important role in the study of human brains. However, the approaches for constructing individual structural networks have not been well developed yet. Existing methods based on patch-wise image intensity similarity suffer from several major drawbacks, i.e., 1) *violation of cortical topological properties*, 2) *sensitivity to intensity heterogeneity*, and 3) *influence by patch size heterogeneity*. To overcome these limitations, this paper presents a novel cortical surface-based method for constructing individual structural networks. Specifically, our method first maps the cortical surfaces onto a standard spherical surface atlas and then uniformly samples vertices on the spherical surface as the nodes of the networks. The similarity between any two nodes is computed based on the biologically-meaningful cortical attributes (e.g., cortical thickness) in the spherical neighborhood of their sampled vertices. The connection between any two nodes is established only if the similarity is larger than a user-specified threshold. Through leveraging spherical cortical surface patches, our method generates biologically-meaningful individual networks that are comparable across ages and subjects. The proposed method has been applied to construct cortical-thickness networks for 73 healthy infants, with each infant having two MRI scans at 0 and 1 year of age. The constructed networks during the two ages were compared using various network metrics, such as degree, clustering coefficient, shortest path length, small world property, global efficiency, and local efficiency. Experimental results demonstrate that our method can effectively construct individual structural networks and reveal meaningful patterns in early brain development.

Keywords: Individual networks, infant, cortical thickness, development.

1 Introduction

In the last decade, analysis of functional and structural connectivity has received increasing attentions in human brain studies, as it opens up a new approach in understanding brain development, aging and disorders. Generally, functional connectivity is identified by exploring the correlation of regional fMRI or EEG/MEG

N. Navab et al. (Eds.): MICCAI 2015, Part III, LNCS 9351, pp. 560–568, 2015.
DOI: 10.1007/978-3-319-24574-4_67

signals [1], while structural connectivity is usually established by tracking the fibers in white matters (WM) using diffusion-weighted images (DWI). Recently, there has been rising interests in studying anatomical covariance in the cortical gray matter (GM) using MR images [1]. This can help identify direct and indirect correlations between cortical regions and help reveal genetic influence on brain morphology. In contrast to the conventional studies of functional and structural connectivity that examine the correlation of brain regions within an individual, most existing studies of anatomical covariance in GM explore the correlation among morphological measures across a population [1]. To better understand the human brain, studying individual anatomical covariance in GM is also considerably indispensable. However, the methods for constructing meaningful individual anatomical networks have not been well developed yet. Although several methods based on the patch-wise similarity of image intensity have been recently proposed and reported interesting results [2-4], they all suffer from several major limitations: 1) *violation of cortical topological properties*, 2) *sensitivity to intensity heterogeneity*, and 3) *influence by patch size heterogeneity*.

Violation of Cortical Topological Properties. In image-patch-based methods, each patch is considered as a node in the constructed network. However, anatomically-distinct and geodesically-distant cortical regions may be included in the same patch, causing the respective node and its connections to be less meaningful. For example, as shown in Fig. 1(a), two gyral regions (x and y) are partially included in the red patch, although they are geodesically far away from each other.

Sensitivity to Intensity Heterogeneity. Most existing methods compute the similarity between two patches based on their image intensity values. However, the intensity lacks clearly defined anatomical meanings, and the same intensity value may stand for different tissues in different MR scans, making it incomparable across subjects and longitudinal scans of the same subject. This problem is particularly pronounced in early brain development studies, where the intensity of MRI varies regionally considerably and changes temporally dynamically. For example, as shown in Fig. 1(b), the MR images of the same infant have completely different intensity levels at different ages. Thus, 'Similarity 0' and 'Similarity 1' are not comparable, though they measure the anatomical covariance in corresponding regions.

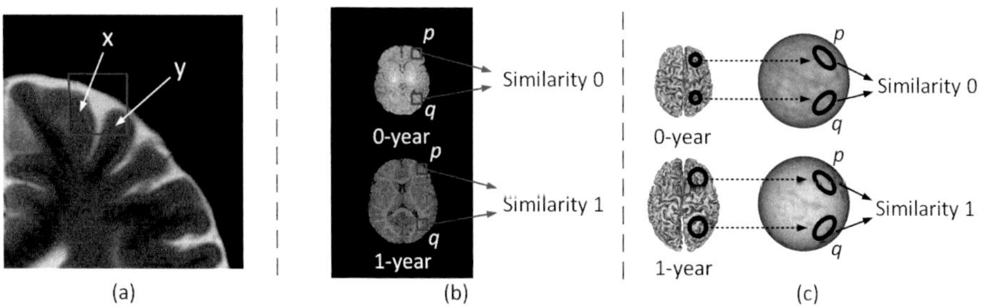

Fig. 1. Limitations of existing methods (a, b), and the advantages of the proposed method (c).

Influence by Patch Size Heterogeneity. Since the volumes of human brains are quite variable across subjects and ages, it is impossible to determine a unique size of image patch for each individual, while keeping the patches comparable across subjects. Even for the scans of the same subject at different ages, simply adjusting the patch size according to changes in brain volume still does not achieve comparable patches, as the brain develops nonlinearly and regionally heterogeneously.

To address the above limitations, this paper proposes a novel cortical surface-based method to construct individual structural networks. Specifically, in our method, the cortical surfaces are first mapped onto a standard spherical surface and aligned onto the spherical surface atlas. Then, patches on the aligned spherical surface are used to define the nodes in the individual network, as shown in Fig. 1(c). This guarantees that each surface patch strictly represents geodesically and anatomically meaningful cortical regions. Moreover, the similarity between two spherical patches is computed using cortical anatomical attributes with clear biological meanings, such as cortical thickness [5] and cortical folding. This similarity is fully comparable across subjects and also across ages for the same subject. Furthermore, since the patches are selected from aligned spherical surfaces, the size of the patch is independent from brain volume. As a result, each patch will always represent the anatomically corresponding cortical regions across different subjects and ages.

The proposed method has been applied to construct individual cortical-thickness networks for 73 healthy infants, with each infant having two MRI scans at 0 and 1 year of age. The constructed networks at the two ages were compared using various network metrics, such as degree, clustering coefficient, shortest path length, small world property, global efficiency, and local efficiency. The experimental results demonstrate that our method can effectively construct individual structural networks and reveal meaningful patterns in early brain development.

2 Methods

Subjects and Image Acquisition. MR images were acquired for 73 healthy infants (42 males and 31 females), using a Siemens head-only 3T scanner with a circular polarized head coil. For each subject, images were longitudinally collected at term birth (0-year-old) and 1 year of age (1-year-old). Both T1-weighted (resolution $=1\times1\times1$ mm^3) and T2-weighted (resolution$=1.25\times1.25\times1.95$ mm^3) MR images were collected.

Image Preprocessing. All MR images were processed by the following pipeline as in [6]. First, each T2-weighted image was linearly aligned onto the corresponding T1-weighted image, and then resampled to the resolution of $1\times1\times1$ mm^3. Second, skull, cerebellum and brain stem were removed automatically, and intensity inhomogeneity was corrected using N3 method [7]. Third, each image was rigidly aligned to the age-matched infant brain atlas [8]. Fourth, tissue segmentation was performed by using a longitudinally-guided coupled level-sets method [9]. Finally, non-cortical structures were filled, with each brain further separated into left and right hemispheres [10].

Cortical Surface Reconstruction and Registration. For each hemisphere of each image, topologically correct inner and outer cortical surfaces (represented by triangular meshes) were reconstructed using a deformable surface method [11]. Cortical thickness of each vertex was computed as the closest distance between the inner and outer cortical surfaces. To establish both inter-subject and left-right cortical correspondences, all cortical surfaces of the left hemisphere and mirror-flipped right hemisphere at the same age were mapped onto a spherical space and nonlinearly aligned to the age-matched unbiased surface atlases [11]. Longitudinal cortical correspondences were established by aligning the cortical surfaces at birth to the corresponding cortical surfaces at 1 year of age using Spherical Demons [12].

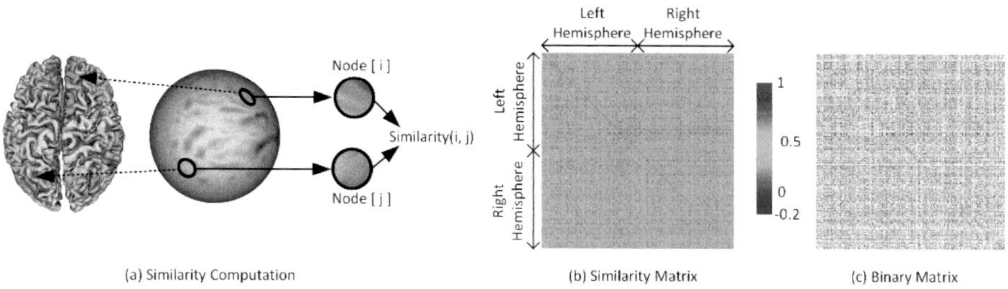

Fig. 2. Illustration of construction of individual structural network based on cortical surface.

Construction of Individual Networks. The individual network is constructed with the following three major steps: (1) defining the nodes of the network, (2) computing similarity matrix between nodes, and (3) binarizing the similarity matrix.

In Step (1), N vertices are uniformly sampled on the aligned spherical surfaces of two hemispheres. For each sampled vertex, its neighborhood is selected and defined as a node of the network, as shown in Fig. 2(a). The size of the neighborhood (also namely node area) is constrained by two factors. First, any position on the spherical surface must be covered by at least one node area. Second, the portion of overlapping among node areas is no more than a user-specified threshold $T_{overlap}$. We experimentally set N as 1284 and $T_{overlap}$ as 10% in our implementation.

In Step (2), as shown in Fig. 2(b), the similarity matrix is built by calculating the similarity between any two node areas. Specifically, in the area of each node i, a certain number of vertices are uniformly sampled. Then, a feature vector $\boldsymbol{v}_i \in \mathbb{R}^n$ is constructed using the cortical morphological attributes (e.g., cortical thickness in our implementation) at all sampled vertices, where n is the number of sampled vertices in the node area. To obtain the similarity of two areas of nodes i and j, Pearson's correlation coefficient r_{ij} is computed using their feature vectors $\boldsymbol{v}_i$ and $\boldsymbol{v}_j$ as: $r_{ij} = \frac{\sum_{k=1}^{n}(v_{ik}-\bar{v}_i)(v_{jk}-\bar{v}_j)}{\sqrt{\sum_{k=1}^{n}(v_{ik}-\bar{v}_i)^2}\sqrt{\sum_{k=1}^{n}(v_{jk}-\bar{v}_j)^2}}$. Since the similarity of two node areas is directionally sensitive, for any two nodes i and j, the Pearson's correlation coefficient r_{ij} is repetitively computed for every θ angle rotation of the spherical patches in its tangential plane. The maximum value is used as the similarity s_{ij} for these two nodes. This process can be formulated as: $s_{ij} = \max_m r_{ij}(m\theta)$. In our implementation, we set θ as $\pi/10$, which indicates that 10 different correlation coefficients are computed for each pair of nodes. We also tested using the smaller θ, but the results showed no significant changes.

In Step (3), the similarity matrix is binarized using a subject-specific threshold, which is determined automatically for each subject based on an expected level of statistical significance. Specifically, the matrix of Pearson's correlation coefficients is first transformed to a p-value matrix, and then the false discovery rate (FDR) technique is applied to the p-value matrix with an expected p-value τ [13]. A corrected p-value τ' is produced by FDR. Finally, each element in the p-value matrix is compared with τ'. If it is less than τ', the corresponding element in the similarity matrix is set as 1; otherwise, it is set as 0. The FDR process is necessary because it can effectively control the proportion of false positives for multiple comparisons under an expected level. Generally speaking, by using FDR technique, for any subject the chance of including false correlations in its network is limited to $100\tau\%$. We chose τ to be 0.022 since the average sparsity degree of the network for this value was 22~23%, which was similar to that of previous studies [3, 14, 15].

By using the above three steps, an individual network of cortical thickness can be established. Leveraging spherical cortical surface patches, our method generates biologically-meaningful individual networks, of which the node areas are comparable across ages and subjects. Note that, connections in the individual network may reflect the direct or indirect fiber connectivity in white matter or similar genetic influence between two regions [1] or intrinsic micro-structural connectivity in gray matter [16]. This method can also be used to construct individual networks using other cortical attributes, such as sulcal depth and cortex folding degree.

Network Metrics. The constructed individual cortical thickness network is an undirected and unweighted graph represented by a binary matrix. To measure these individual networks, we employ the following widely used metrics in graph theory, including: *node degree*, *clustering coefficient*, *shortest path length*, *small world property*, *global efficiency*, and *local efficiency*, as in [3, 17]. Specifically, in an undirected graph, *node degree* α_i is the number of edges of a node i. Assume the subnetwork G_i consists of all the direct neighbors of node i and their connections, the *clustering coefficient* c_i of the node i is defined as the number (N_{G_i}) of edges in G_i divided by the number of all possible connections, formulated as: $c_i = \frac{2N_{G_i}}{\alpha_i(\alpha_i - 1)}$. The *shortest path length* L_i of a node i is the average value over its shortest path lengths to all other nodes. Of note, in our network, the path length between two directly connected nodes is 1. The *small world property* of a network G is denoted as $\sigma = \gamma/\lambda$, where γ is defined as the sum of clustering coefficients for all nodes in G divided by the sum of clustering coefficients for all nodes in a random network G_{rand}, formulated as: $\gamma = \frac{\sum_{i \in G} c_i}{\sum_{i \in G_{rand}} c_i}$. And λ is defined as the sum of shortest path lengths for all nodes in G divided by the sum of shortest path lengths for all nodes in G_{rand}, formulated as: $\lambda = \frac{\sum_{i \in G} L_i}{\sum_{i \in G_{rand}} L_i}$. Of note, the random network G_{rand} is generated by reconnecting the nodes (changing the edges) in G, while preserving the node degrees [18]. A network is considered to own small world property if and only if the following two conditions are satisfied simultaneously: $\gamma > 1$ and $\lambda \approx 1$. The *global efficiency* of a network G is defined as the average of the inverse of all shortest path lengths, formulated as: $E_{global} = \frac{2}{N(N-1)} \sum_{i \neq j \in G} \frac{1}{d_{ij}}$. Herein, d_{ij} is the shortest path length between nodes i and j; and N is the number of nodes in G. The *local efficiency* of a node i, $E_g(G_i)$, is defined as the global efficiency of the local network G_i. Then the *local efficiency* of a network G is defined as the average of local efficiencies of all nodes, formulated as: $E_{local} = \frac{1}{N} \sum_{i \in G} E_g(G_i)$.

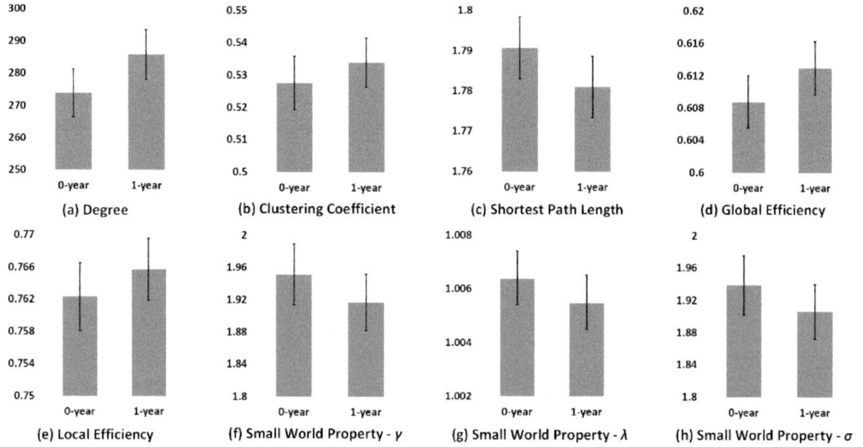

Fig. 3. Network metrics of 73 subjects at 0-year-old and 1-year-old, respectively.

3 Results

We constructed individual cortical thickness networks for 73 health infants at age 0 and age 1, and measured each individual network using the metrics introduced in Section 2. Fig. 3 reports the distributions of network measures of the whole population. As we can see, from 0 to 1 year of age, all the metrics change dramatically, indicating that our method is able to reveal network differences during early brain development. Specifically, the degree, clustering coefficient, global efficiency, and local efficiency of the cortical thickness network increase, while the shortest path length decreases in the first year. The increase of global and local efficiency is generally consistent with the results in early brain development study of population-based anatomical networks [19]. We also launched paired t-test for each metric to evaluate the difference between the networks at 0-year-old and 1-year-old. With all p-values being far less than 0.01, we can conclude that all those metrics derived from individual networks of cortical thickness are significantly different at the two time points.

We further investigated the small world property for the cortical thickness networks at age 0 and 1. Although the metric σ changes significantly during the first year as shown in Fig. 3, the cortical thickness network consistently has the small world property. Fig. 4 shows the comparison between constructed networks and their corresponding randomized networks for 10 randomly selected individuals. We can see that, at both age 0 (Fig. 4a) and age 1 (Fig. 4e), the clustering coefficient of constructed network for each individual is consistently larger than that of the randomized network, which has the same degree distribution with our constructed network. Moreover, the shortest path length of our constructed network for each individual is consistently approximately equivalent to that of the randomized network at both age 0 (Fig. 4c) and age 1 (Fig. 4g). The similar observation can also be seen from the average metrics for 73 subjects (Fig. 4b, d, f, and h). Therefore, for both ages, the metric γ is always larger than 1 and the metric λ is always approximately equal to 1, indicating that the small world property of the cortical thickness network constructed by our method is retained in the first year, which is consistent with results reported in early brain development study of population-based anatomical networks [19].

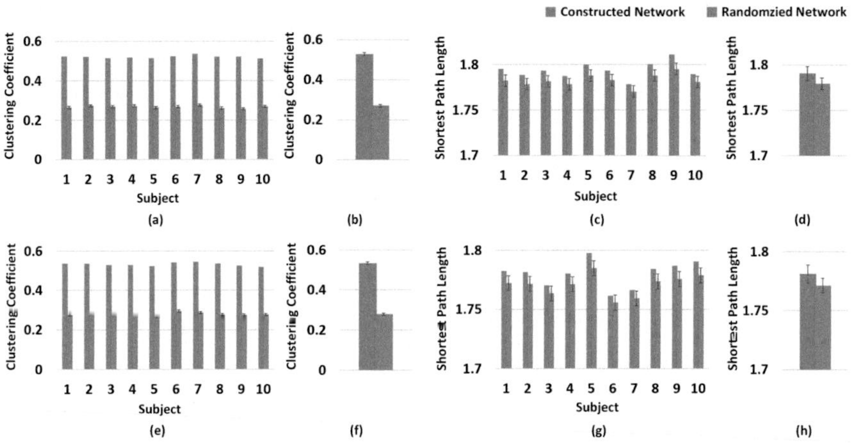

Fig. 4. Comparison of constructed networks and randomized networks for 10 randomly selected individuals (a, c, e, and g) and the whole population of 73 subjects (b, d, f, and h). The first row shows the metrics of 0-year-old networks, and the second row shows the metrics of 1-year-old networks.

4 Conclusion

This paper presents a novel method for cortical surface-based construction of individual structural networks. Compared to the existing intensity patch based methods [2-4], the proposed method has three major advantages. First, surface-based patch (node area) guarantees that each patch corresponds to anatomically meaningful and geodesically neighboring cortical regions, in contrast to an image patch that might contain geodesically-distant regions. Second, the cortical morphology-defined similarity ensures that this similarity is comparable across subjects and ages, in contrast to image intensity, which is quite variable across ages and subjects and has less meaningful anatomical meanings. Third, since patches are defined on the standard spherical surface atlas space, the patch size is independent of the brain volume, which makes both the cross-subject and longitudinal comparisons more meaningful. The proposed method has been applied to 73 healthy infants at age 0 and age 1, leading to meaningful discoveries of early brain development. In the future, we will construct individual networks using other cortical attributes, e.g., sulcal depth, cortical folding and cortical local gyrification [20], and further compare them with the structural networks derived from DTI and also the functional networks derived from fMRI.

References

1. Evans, A.C.: Networks of anatomical covariance. NeuroImage 80, 489–504 (2013)
2. Batalle, D., Munoz-Moreno, E., et al.: Normalization of similarity-based individual brain networks from gray matter MRI and its association with neurodevelopment in infants with intrauterine growth restriction. NeuroImage 83, 901–911 (2013)
3. Tijms, B.M., Series, P., et al.: Similarity-based extraction of individual networks from gray matter MRI scans. Cerebral Cortex 22, 1530–1541 (2012)
4. Kandel, B.M., Wang, D.J., Gee, J.C., Avants, B.B.: Single-subject structural networks with closed-form rotation invariant matching improve power in developmental studies of the cortex. In: Golland, P., Hata, N., Barillot, C., Hornegger, J., Howe, R. (eds.) MICCAI 2014, Part III. LNCS, vol. 8675, pp. 137–144. Springer, Heidelberg (2014)
5. Raj, A., Mueller, S.G., et al.: Network-level analysis of cortical thickness of the epileptic brain. NeuroImage 52, 1302–1313 (2010)
6. Meng, Y., Li, G., et al.: Spatial distribution and longitudinal development of deep cortical sulcal landmarks in infants. NeuroImage 100, 206–218 (2014)
7. Sled, J.G., Zijdenbos, A.P., et al.: A nonparametric method for automatic correction of intensity nonuniformity in MRI data. IEEE Transactions on Medical Imaging 17, 87–97 (1998)
8. Shi, F., Yap, P.T., et al.: Infant brain atlases from neonates to 1- and 2-year-olds. PloS One 6, e18746 (2011)
9. Wang, L., Shi, F., et al.: Longitudinally guided level sets for consistent tissue segmentation of neonates. Human Brain Mapping 34, 956–972 (2013)
10. Li, G., Nie, J., et al.: Mapping longitudinal hemispheric structural asymmetries of the human cerebral cortex from birth to 2 years of age. Cerebral Cortex 24, 1289–1300 (2014)
11. Li, G., Nie, J., et al.: Measuring the dynamic longitudinal cortex development in infants by reconstruction of temporally consistent cortical surfaces. NeuroImage 90, 266–279 (2014)
12. Yeo, B.T., Sabuncu, M.R., et al.: Spherical demons: fast diffeomorphic landmark-free surface registration. IEEE Transactions on Medical Imaging 29, 650–668 (2010)
13. Yekutieli, D., Benjamini, Y.: Resampling-based false discovery rate controlling multiple test procedures for correlated test statistics. J. Stat. Plan. Infer. 82, 171–196 (1999)
14. Zhu, W., Wen, W., et al.: Changing topological patterns in normal aging using large-scale structural networks. Neurobiology of Aging 33, 899–913 (2012)
15. Sanabria-Diaz, G., Melie-Garcia, L., et al.: Surface area and cortical thickness descriptors reveal different attributes of the structural human brain networks. NeuroImage 50, 1497–1510 (2010)
16. Ecker, C., Ronan, L., et al.: Intrinsic gray-matter connectivity of the brain in adults with autism spectrum disorder. PNAS 110, 13222–13227 (2013)
17. Nie, J., Li, G., et al.: Longitudinal development of cortical thickness, folding, and fiber density networks in the first 2 years of life. Human Brain Mapping 35, 3726–3737 (2014)

18. Maslov, S., Sneppen, K.: Specificity and stability in topology of protein networks. Science 296, 910–913 (2002)
19. Fan, Y., Shi, F., et al.: Brain anatomical networks in early human brain development. NeuroImage 54, 1862–1871 (2011)
20. Li, G., Wang, L., et al.: Mapping longitudinal development of local cortical gyrification in infants from birth to 2 years of age. The Journal of Neuroscience 34, 4228–4238 (2014)

Quantitative Image Analysis IV: Classification, Detection, Features, and Morphology

NEOCIVET: Extraction of Cortical Surface and Analysis of Neonatal Gyrification Using a Modified CIVET Pipeline

Hosung Kim[1], Claude Lepage[2], Alan C. Evans[2], A. James Barkovich[1], Duan Xu[1]

[1] Department of Radiology and Biomedical Imaging, University of California, San Francisco, San Francisco, CA

[2] McConnell Brain Imaging Center, Montreal Neurological Institute and Hospital, McGill University, Montreal, Quebec, Canada

hosung.kim@ucsf.edu

Abstract. Cerebral cortical gyration becomes dramatically more complex in the fetal brain during the 3rd trimester of gestation; the process proceeds in a similar fashion *ex utero* in children who are born prematurely. To quantify this morphological development , it is necessary to extract the interface between gray matter and white matter. We employed the well-established CIVET pipeline to extract this cortical surface, with point correspondence across subjects, using a surface-based spherical registration. We developed a variant of the pipeline, called NEOCIVET, that addresses the well-known problems of poor and temporally-varying gray/white contrast in neonatal MRI. NEOCIVET includes a tissue classification strategy that combines i) local and global contrast features, ii) neonatal template construction based on age-specific sub-groups, and iii) masking of non-interesting structures using label-fusion approaches. These techniques replaced modules that might be suboptimal for regional analysis of poor-contrast neonatal cortex. In the analysis of 43 preterm-born neonates, many with multiple scans (n=65; 28-40 wks PMA at scan), NEOCIVET identified increases in cortical folding over time in numerous cortical regions (mean curvature: +0.004/wk) while folding did not change in major sulci that are known to develop early (corrected $p<0.05$). Cortical folding increase was disrupted in the presence of severe types of perinatal WM injury. The proposed pipeline successfully mapped cortical structural development, supporting current models of cerebral morphogenesis.

Keywords: neonatal brain MRI, cortical folding, surface extraction, CIVET.

1 Introduction

Cerebral cortical gyration is one of the most striking morphological changes that occur in the fetal brain during the 3rd trimester of gestation; the process proceeds in a similar manner *ex utero* in children who are born prematurely. To quantify such early morphological development, it is necessary to extract cortical surface, especially the interface of the gray matter (GM) and white matter (WM). Only a few packages [1, 2] have been proposed to perform this task. To enable regional analysis, they co-register

N. Navab et al. (Eds.): MICCAI 2015, Part III, LNCS 9351, pp. 571–579, 2015.
DOI: 10.1007/978-3-319-24574-4_68

an individual lobar atlas to each subject's cortical surface. However, this approach lacks point-wise correspondence across subjects and, consequently, spatial sensitivity.

Pure surface-based packages such as the MNI's CIVET pipeline or FreeSurfer extract triangulated cortical surface [3, 4] and define point correspondence using surface-based spherical registration [5]. However, these packages have not been optimized for fetal/neonatal analyses. Different degrees of myelination, neuronal proliferation, and cell migration among various cortical and subcortical regions, which are distinctive features of developing brain, are manifested as regionally- and temporally-varying GM/WM contrast in structural MRI. This spatiotemporally dynamic tissue contrast challenges tissue classification techniques used in most pipelines since they are usually based on a tissue contrast histogram constructed from the whole brain across time.

Techniques that combine a feature of local intensity variations into the original classification scheme have recently been proposed. Among them, a level-set-based approach developed by Li et al. [6] displayed excellent segmentation performance in images with locally distorted intensity distribution. To enable the analysis of cortical morphology in neonates, we developed a variant of the CIVET pipeline, called NEOCIVET. This pipeline includes a number of new modifications and parameter tunings. In particular, we optimized Li's method for the cortical GM segmentation by including additional features. Also, we constructed age-specific surface templates to improve the surface registration performance across subjects.

2 Methods

NEOCIVET includes a series of image processing steps to achieve the goal of extracting the interface between GM and WM. Briefly we describe the flow of the pipeline as in Fig 1: **A**) MRI images underwent intensity non-uniformity correction using N3 [7]; **B**) These images were linearly registered to the NIH neonatal template that was averaged across 0-2 month-old babies (http://www.bic.mni.mcgill.ca/ServicesAtlases/NIHPD-obj2); **C**) We segmented the cerebrum and cerebellum using a patch-based brain extraction algorithm (BEaST) [8]; **D**) These masked brains were re-registered to the template to improve the intracranial fitting; **E**) MRI intensities were re-corrected using N3 and normalized within the brain mask; **F**) the GM and WM were classified within the mask using a level-set-based deformable model that uses global and local contrasts as well as a cortical thickness constraint. The intensity of CSF voxels neighboring the cortex or residing within the sulci resembled that of normal neonatal WM due to the partial volume effect. Thus, we corrected their classification in a post-processing step using their geometric characteristics: i.e., the CSF partial volumes located exterior to the GM were masked. We eroded WM voxels 5 times and applied iterative region-growing to the remaining WM voxels until they met a GM voxel; **G**) A nonlinear registration and label-fusion approach [9] was used to mask out uninteresting structures: deep GM, ventricles and the periventricular germinal zone (which looks like GM as neural cells extend into this area in neonates) and the cerebellum. While the cerebellum was removed, other masked structures were merged into the WM class; **H**) Segmentation of the corpus callosum in the mid-plane divided the WM into hemispheres. This separation allowed for analysis of hemispheric asymmetry in morphometry by co-registering the flipped right hemisphere to the left; **I**) we parameterized the WM boundary by evolving an ellipsoid, triangulated using an icosahedral model and a multi-resolution deformation scheme, as in the CIVET [3]; **J**) To improve point correspondence across subjects, a surface-based registration [5] was performed with respect to age-specific templates; **K**) The cortical morphology was characterized by measuring mean curvature; **L**) Finally, these measurements were further re-sampled to the surface template using the transformation obtained in the surface registration, in order to allow inter-subject comparison.

In the following sections, we describe the new modules included in NEOCIVET and how they address technical challenges in neonatal brain MRI. We also discuss the choice of parameters for optimal performance. Finally, using a large dataset of preterm-born neonates we investigate the ability of NEOCIVET to assess developmental trajectory and its clinical utility.

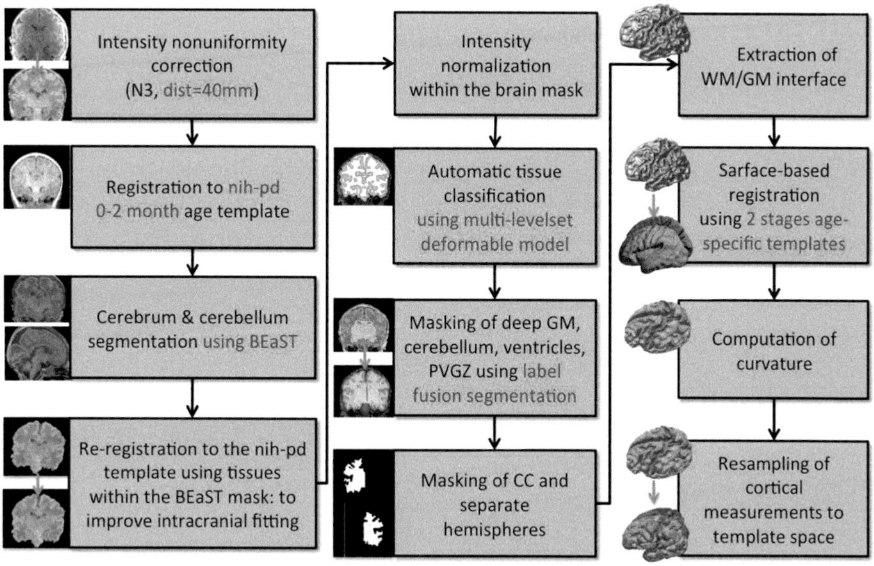

Fig. 1. Flowchart of NEOCIVET, a variant of CIVET used for neonatal brain analysis. New modules and parameters are in red. PVGZ: periventricular germinal zone.

2.1 Subjects and MRI Acquisition

Our initial dataset comprised 52 preterm newborns (mean postmenstrual age [PMA]= 28.7±1.8 wks; range 24.7-32.2 wks), admitted to UCSF Benioff Children's Hospital San Francisco between July 2011 and June 2014. All patients were scanned post-natally as soon as clinically stable, and 30 patients were re-scanned before discharge at late preterm age (34-38 wks corrected gestational age). Due to severe motion artifact, 9 baseline and 8 follow-up scans were excluded. The final database included 43 baseline (PMA=32.3±2.0 wks) and 22 follow-up scans (35.9±1.5 wks). 3T MRI scans were acquired using a specialized high-sensitivity neonatal head coil built within an MRI-compatible incubator. T1-weighted images were acquired using sagittal 3-dimensional inversion recovery spoiled gradient echo (TR = minimum; TE = minimum; FOV = 180°; NEX = 1.00; FA = 15°), yielding images with $0.7\text{x}0.7\text{x}1\text{mm}^3$ spatial resolution.

2.2 Classification of Brain Tissues

We expanded Li's deformable model [6] to constrain it for cortical GM segmentation. Let a given image be $I: \Omega_i \rightarrow \Re$. Ω_i (i=1, 2) is a region that defines foreground (i=1) or background (i=2). For a given 3D point $\mathbf{x} \in \Omega$ and intensity $I(\mathbf{x})$, Li's level-set formula is defined as:

$$\frac{\partial \phi}{\partial t} = -\delta_\epsilon(\phi)(\lambda_1 e_1 - \lambda_2 e_2) + v\delta_\epsilon(\phi)\nabla \cdot \left(\frac{\nabla\phi}{|\nabla\phi|}\right) + \mu\left(\nabla^2\phi - \nabla \cdot \frac{\nabla\phi}{|\nabla\phi|}\right) \quad (1)$$

where δ_ϵ is the smoothed Dirac delta function and e_1 and e_2 are terms combining global and local intensity fitting energy and are expanded as:

$$e_i(\mathbf{x}) = \int_{\Omega_i} K_\sigma(\mathbf{y} - \mathbf{x})|I(\mathbf{y}) - f_i(\mathbf{x})|^2 d\mathbf{y}, \ \ i = 1, 2 \quad (2)$$

K is 3D Gaussian kernel function that is centered at $\mathbf{x}$ and is scalable using σ ($\sigma > 0$). $f_1(\mathbf{x})$ and $f_2(\mathbf{x})$ are two values that approximate image intensities within Ω_1 and Ω_2. The term $\delta_\epsilon(\phi)(\lambda_1 e_1 - \lambda_2 e_2)$ in Eq (1) evolves the level-set to the regional boundary whereas the other terms maintain the regularity of the level-set. More details are found in the original publication [6].

To optimize GM/WM segmentation, we feed the algorithm an initial segmentation based on the EM algorithm performed on the whole brain (Fig. 2B). We also enhance the image $I(\mathbf{x})$ using non-local mean de-noising: $I'(\mathbf{x}) = NL(I(\mathbf{x}))$. Some cortical areas consistently appeared to be dark or thin in the MRI due to chemical shift misregistration. To address this, we introduced a cortical thickness constraint. The cortical thickness $T(\mathbf{x})$ is computed by the Laplacian transform within the GM mantle as in [10]. We invert this as:

$$T^{-1}(\mathbf{x}) = \frac{1}{T(\mathbf{x})} \text{ if } T(\mathbf{x}) > 0; \ \ T^{-1}(\mathbf{x}) = 0 \text{ if } T(\mathbf{x}) = 0 \quad (3)$$

A large T^{-1} describes voxel clusters of the "artificially" thin or missing cortex. Finally $I(\mathbf{x})$ in Eq. (2) is replaced with $I'(\mathbf{x}) + \lambda_{thick}\tilde{T}^{-1}(\mathbf{x})$,where $\tilde{T}^{-1}(\mathbf{x}) = K_{\sigma T}\ (T^{-1}(\mathbf{x}))$ is a smooth version of T^{-1} (Fig. 2C) and λ_{thick} is a weight constant. The thickness was re-computed every 40 iterations. An improved segmentation is illustrated in Fig. 2E.

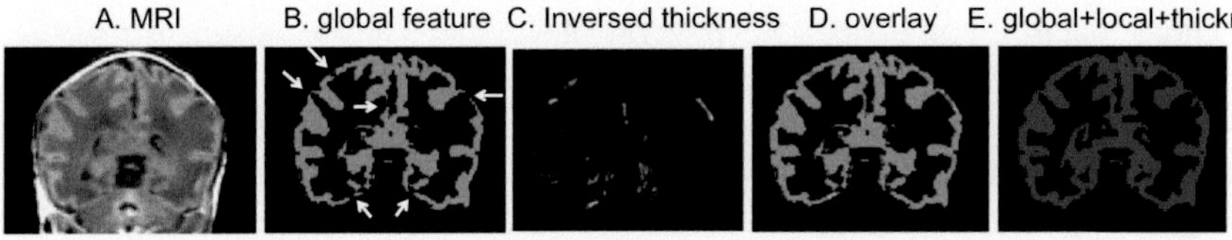

Fig. 2. Tissue classification. Initial segmentation using a global histogram shows missing GM voxels (arrows). Combining the inverted thickness constraint with local contrast term in the level-set formulation makes a marked recovery in GM segmentation and topology (red).

2.3 Surface Fitting

The WM/GM interface was extracted by deforming an ellipsoid triangulated using icosahedral sampling [4]. The initial surface was sampled with 320 triangles and deformed towards the boundary of the hemispheric WM. The surface was up-sampled to 81,920 triangles at the end of each deformation cycle.

2.4 Surface-Based Morphological Measurements

In most applications, CIVET is primarily used to measure cortical thickness between the inner and outer cortical surfaces. In contrast, NEOCIVET aims to characterize the cortical folding at the WM/GM interface (=inner surface) by computing mean curvature that captures concavity/convexity (Fig. 3).

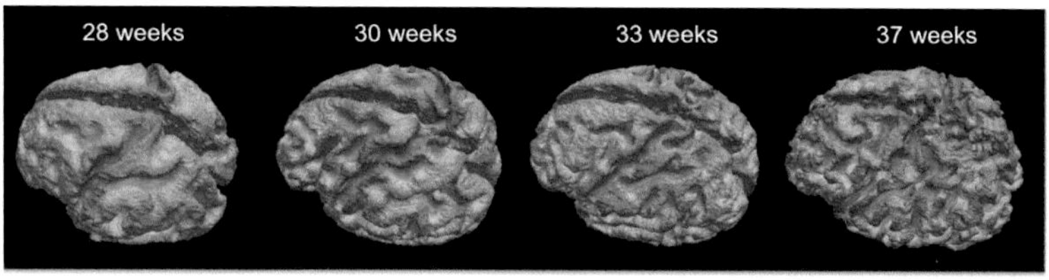

Fig. 3. Mean curvature as cortical folding measurement.

2.5 Construction of Age-Specific Surface Templates and Registration

As seen in Fig. 3, cortical folding changes dramatically during perinatal development. This emphasizes the importance of constructing templates that capture the precise cortical morphology at specific age ranges, so as to ensure the accuracy of registration. We therefore subdivided our dataset into four age ranges: 28-30 (n=12), 31-33 (n=15), 34-36 (n=19) and 37-40 (n=13) weeks PMA. For each group, we constructed a surface template using *SURFTRACC*, a surface registration algorithm included in CIVET [5] and an unbiased template construction framework [11]. In brief, *SURFTRACC* first transposes individual sulcal depth maps into icosahedral spheres. It then iteratively searches for local optimal vertex correspondence between an individual and a template sphere based on a matching of a given feature (in this case, depth potential function [12]). Mapping the deformed meshes back to the original cortical surface coordinates allows a registration of the individual to the template surface. Inclusion of a regularization step further preserves local surface topology. This procedure was integrated into a hierarchical framework that allows for registration from coarse to fine scale. An initial template was created by a simple averaging of vertices among the surfaces in each age group. Thereafter, an iterative alignment proceeds from low dimensional warping of all individuals to the initial template, and towards higher dimensional warping to a new template that is constructed from the previous warping cycle (similar to the process shown in Table). Left and "flipped-right" hemispheres from all subjects were pooled to avoid subject- and hemisphere-specific bias in the evolution and averaging. After construction, the youngest-age template was registered to the 2nd youngest and so on such that each template was registered to its closest older template, yielding a temporally continuous transformation. For inter-subject analyses, any given subject was first registered to the corresponding age template and then was ultimately transformed to the oldest template space (shown in Fig. 4-5) by concatenating the sequence of transformations between age-specific templates.

2.6 Other Technical Considerations and Parameter Selection

For optimal performance in our neonatal dataset, parameters in the NEOCIVET were empirically chosen. Also, some CIVET modules were updated with more recent publicly available techniques. Below, we describe these modifications in some detail so as to guide NEOCIVET users in their parameter selection with respect to MRI field strength, pulse sequence and spatial resolution:

a) For intensity inhomogeneity correction using N3, we found that a smoothing distance for RF wavelength as 40mm yielded best performance in brain masking and tissue classification, which also agreed with the result from a previous extensive analysis using 3T MRI data [13].

b) The FSL-BET-based brain masking and single atlas-based masking of deep GM and ventricles performed poorly for neonatal brains due to rapid changes in volume and intensity. We addressed this issue by introducing publicly available techniques that use patches of multiple templates or fuse multiple templates based on a similarity measure [8, 9]. The use of a minimum of 15-20 manually labeled atlases for various age ranges achieved excellent segmentation accuracy (Dice>0.87%).

c) Our data were scanned with an in-plane resolution of $0.7x0.7mm^2$ with 1mm thickness whereas the NIH neonatal template was sampled at $1mm^3$. Registration to this template caused image data loss. We thus up-sampled this template to $0.5x0.5x0.5mm^3$. However, this step did not necessarily improve registration, which was optimized ultimately using the age-specific surface templates described in 2.5.

d) Parameters in the level-set tissue segmentation were chosen empirically as: λ_1=1, λ_2=1, λ_{thick}=1, σ=3, σ_T=1, ϵ=1, μ=1, ν=12.5, time step=0.005, #iteration=400. On a single core of Intel^{TM} i7-3770K, 3.5GHz, the segmentation step and the whole pipeline process for a neonatal MRI took 10 minutes and 2.1 hours, respectively.

3 Application and Clinical Utility of NEOCIVET

Here, we investigated the ability of the pipeline to assess developmental trajectory and the impact of brain injury on cortical structural development.

3.1 Statistical Analyses

Statistical analysis was performed using SurfStat (http://www.math.mcgill.ca/keith/surfstat/). Mixed-effect linear models were used to address both inter-subject effects and within-subject changes between serial MRI scans by permitting multiple measurements per subject and thus increasing statistical power. We assessed developmental trajectory of cortical complexity by correlating the magnitudes of sulcal depth and curvature with postmenstrual age (PMA) at the time of scanning. Given that severe perinatal WM injury (WMI) often disrupts postnatal brain growth, we assessed the association between cortical complexity changes and the presence of WMI (a score of 2 or higher on the clinical grading system). To this end, we used a linear model that included WMI and PMA as independent variables and cortical measurements as the dependent variable set. We then analyzed an interaction term of WMI x PMA. Multiple comparisons were adjusted using false discovery rate [14].

3.2 Results

NEOCIVET identified significant increases in cortical folding in numerous cortical regions in relation to growth in preterm-born neonates (mean curvature: + 0.004/wk), whilst folding did not change in major sulci (Sylvian, central, parieto-occipital, and calcarine fissures) that are known to develop early (corrected p<0.05; Fig. 4) [15].

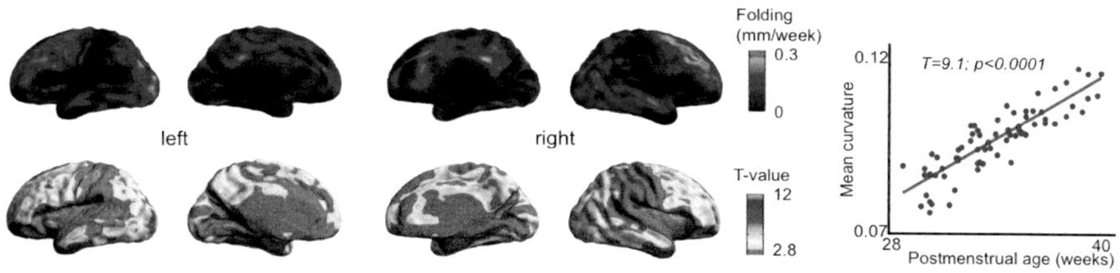

Fig. 4. Developmental trajectory of cortical folding. Left: Patterns show increased sulcal folding/week (top) and the significance map in T-value (p<0.05; bottom); Right: Plotted is mean curvature changes versus increase in PMA in the areas displaying significance.

In broad areas, including both early and late developing cortices, the cortical folding increase was disrupted in the presence of severe perinatal WMI (p<0.001; Fig. 5). The pattern of folding disruption was hemispherically symmetric. WMI is known to occur perinatally, mostly in the late second and the third trimester. The broad effect of WMI even on some of major sulcal areas may indicate disruption of late neuronal or astrocyte migration.

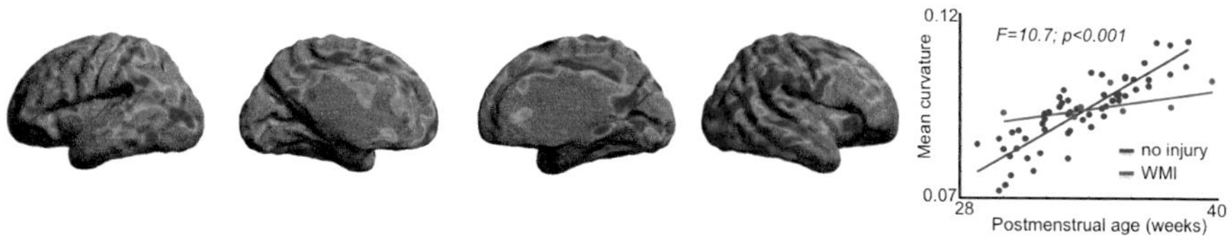

Fig. 5. Disrupted postnatal cortical folding in relation to severe WMI. Significant disruption is found in areas in blue (T>2.8; corrected p<0.05).

4 Discussion and Conclusion

We have proposed NEOCIVET, a variant of the CIVET pipeline that was designed to extract the cortical surface and measure relative morphometrics, for application to neonatal MRI. NEOCIVET successfully characterized the developmental trajectory of cortical folding by improving a series of processes in CIVET. NEOCIVET revealed cortical developmental disruption in the presence of perinatal WMI, demonstrating its potential to provide biomarkers of prematurity-related developmental outcome.

Volumetric registration can be biased by differences in anatomical maturation between preterm babies and the normal neonatal template. However, the volume registration in our analysis was only for coarse spatial normalization, specifically for brain size. The size normalization combined with use of a fixed number of vertices in surface modeling should minimize bias related to maturation that affects the parameters in segmentation and depth potential calculation for surface registration. Maturation-related anatomical variability was further addressed in the surface space where we measure actual cortical folding, using age-specific preterm brain templates.

The main weakness of the contemporary fetal/neonatal pipelines is using age-specific tissue probability maps to correct for local tissue intensity variations [16], which can bias the tissue segmentation in abnormal brains. Another weakness is the lack of point-wise correspondence between subjects, which challenges group-wise analysis of regional changes [1-2]. We overcame these weaknesses using a segmentation method with a local tissue contrast model without prior information as well as a surface registration technique that re-arranges mesh triangulation based on cortical folding similarity between subjects, thus optimizing point correspondence.

We note that the current set of templates is preliminary, as Lyttelton et al. [11] pointed out that a minimum of 30 subjects is required for a stable template construction. We are currently recruiting more preterm-born neonates and plan to re-create those templates with a sufficient sample size. We plan to include NEOCIVET in a future CIVET release that is open to the public through CBRAIN, a web-based platform for distributed processing and exchange of 3D/4D brain imaging data (http://mcin-cnim.ca/neuroimagingtechnologies/cbrain/).

References

1. Wright, R., Kyriakopoulou, V., Ledig, C., Rutherford, M.A., et al.: Automatic quantification of normal cortical folding patterns from fetal brain MRI. Neuroimage 91, 21–32 (2014)
2. Melbourne, A., Kendall, G.S., Cardoso, M.J., Gunny, R., et al.: Preterm birth affects the developmental synergy between cortical folding and cortical connectivity observed on multimodal MRI. Neuroimage 89, 23–34 (2014)
3. Kim, J.S., Singh, V., Lee, J.K., Lerch, J., et al.: Automated 3-D extraction and evaluation of the inner and outer cortical surfaces using a Laplacian map and partial volume effect classification. Neuroimage 27(1), 210–221 (2005)
4. MacDonald, D., Kabani, N., Avis, D., Evans, A.C.: Automated 3-D extraction of inner and outer surfaces of cerebral cortex from MRI. Neuroimage 12(3), 340–356 (2000)

5. Robbins, S., Evans, A.C., Collins, D.L., Whitesides, S.: Tuning and comparing spatial normalization methods. Med. Image Anal. 8(3), 311–323 (2004)
6. Li, C.M., Kao, C.Y., Gore, J.C., Ding, Z.H.: Minimization of region-scalable fitting energy for image segmentation. IEEE Transactions on Image Processing 17(10), 1940–1949 (2008)
7. Sled, J.G., Zijdenbos, A.P., Evans, A.C.: A nonparametric method for automatic correction of intensity nonuniformity in MRI data. IEEE Trans. Med. Imaging 17, 87–97 (1998)
8. Eskildsen, S.F., Coupe, P., Fonov, V., Manjon, J.V., et al.: BEaST: brain extraction based on nonlocal segmentation technique. Neuroimage 59(3), 2362–2373 (2012)
9. Wang, H.Z., Suh, J.W., Das, S.R., Pluta, J.B., et al.: Multi-Atlas Segmentation with Joint Label Fusion. IEEE Trans. on Pattern Analysis and Machine Intelligence 35(3), 611–623 (2013)
10. Jones, S.E., Buchbinder, B.R., Aharon, I.: Three-dimensional mapping of cortical thickness using Laplace's equation. Hum. Brain Mapp. 11(1), 12–32 (2000)
11. Lyttelton, O., Boucher, M., Robbins, S., Evans, A.: An unbiased iterative group registration template for cortical surface analysis. Neuroimage 34(4), 1535–1544 (2007)
12. Boucher, M., Whitesides, S., Evans, A.: Depth potential function for folding pattern representation, registration and analysis. Medical Image Analysis 13(2), 203–214 (2009)
13. Boyes, R.G., Gunter, J.L., Frost, C., Janke, A.L., et al.: Intensity non-uniformity correction using N3 on 3-T scanners with multichannel phased array coils. Neuroimage 39(4), 1752–1762 (2008)
14. Benjamini, Y., Hochberg, Y.: Controlling the false discovery rate: a practical and powerful approach to multiple testing. J. Royal Stat. Soc. 57(1), 289–300 (1995)
15. Kostovic, I., Vasung, L.: Insights from in vitro fetal magnetic resonance imaging of cerebral development. Semin. Perinatol. 33(4), 220–233 (2009)
16. Habas, P.A., Scott, J.A., Roosta, A., Rajagopalan, V., et al.: Early folding patterns and asymmetries of the normal human brain detected from in utero MRI. Cereb. Cortex 22(1), 13–25 (2012)

Learning-Based Shape Model Matching: Training Accurate Models with Minimal Manual Input

Claudia Lindner, Jessie Thomson, The arcOGEN Consortium, and Tim F. Cootes

Centre for Imaging Sciences, University of Manchester, U.K.

Abstract. Recent work has shown that statistical model-based methods lead to accurate and robust results when applied to the segmentation of bone shapes from radiographs. To achieve good performance, model-based matching systems require large numbers of annotations, which can be very time-consuming to obtain. Non-rigid registration can be applied to unlabelled images to obtain correspondences from which models can be built. However, such models are rarely as effective as those built from careful manual annotations, and the accuracy of the registration is hard to measure. In this paper, we show that small numbers of manually annotated points can be used to guide the registration, leading to significant improvements in performance of the resulting model matching system, and achieving results close to those of a model built from dense manual annotations. Placing such sparse points manually is much less time-consuming than a full dense annotation, allowing good models to be built for new bone shapes more quickly than before. We describe detailed experiments on varying the number of sparse points, and demonstrate that manually annotating fewer than 30% of the points is sufficient to create robust and accurate models for segmenting hip and knee bones in radiographs. The proposed method includes a very effective and novel way of estimating registration accuracy in the absence of ground truth.

Keywords: Random Forest regression-voting, bone segmentation, radiographs, statistical shape models, machine learning.

1 Introduction

There are many research questions which can be answered by analysing the large databases of tens of thousands of medical images which are now becoming available, both from large studies and from growing electronic archives of clinical data. A key first step in such analysis is often locating the outlines of the structures of interest. Recently, it has been shown that robust and accurate annotations can be automatically obtained using shape-based model matching algorithms [2,4,8,9]. Unfortunately, building such models requires accurate annotation of large numbers of points on several hundred images. This creates a significant bottleneck, hampering the ability to analyse large datasets efficiently.

This paper addresses the problem of building effective shape model matching systems from large sets of images with as little manual intervention as possible.

N. Navab et al. (Eds.): MICCAI 2015, Part III, LNCS 9351, pp. 580–587, 2015.
DOI: 10.1007/978-3-319-24574-4_69

We use a pragmatic, but effective, approach in which we use a *small number* of manually annotated points on each image to initialise a dense groupwise non-rigid registration (GNR) [10] to establish correspondences across the set of images, allowing us to propagate a dense annotation from one image to all the rest and then to use these to build a detailed model to be matched to new images.

One option to also consider for the generation of dense annotations is fully automatic GNR. However, while this can work well for some reasonably homogeneous datasets, problems often occur where images have been gathered from multiple sources. This tends to be the case in large epidemiological studies where images will have been collected retrospectively, from various centres and without consistent imaging protocols in place. Furthermore, even when the registration works well, models built from such automated correspondences are generally less effective than those built from careful manual annotations. This is because the registration is likely to smooth out details and fail to match to unusual variations. Fully automatic GNR often works well on examples close to the average but performs poorly on outliers. Many failures in the registration are one of two types, (a) gross failures where the registration has converged to the wrong place completely, or (b) localised failures where one part of the object has been poorly matched. Both types can be substantially mitigated if the user supplies a small number of manually annotated landmarks, integrating human expertise into the annotation procedure (see e. g. [6,11]).

Although registration techniques are widely used to establish correspondences and build shape models (particularly in 3D data) [1,3,5], we make a number of key contributions. We show on the challenging, but representative, datasets that we examine that *(i)* model matching systems built from GNR initialised only with the correct initial pose (from two manually annotated points) perform significantly worse than those built from dense manual annotations, particularly on the harder images; *(ii)* the robustness of the resulting model matching system improves monotonically with the number of additional manual points used for initialising the GNR; *(iii)* only small numbers of manually annotated points are required to achieve model matching results very similar to those of the best dense manual models; and *(iv)* we propose a novel method of estimating GNR accuracy in the absence of ground truth annotations.

Some of the most robust and accurate shape model matching results have been achieved using Random Forest regression-voting in the Constrained Local Model (RFRV-CLM) framework [7]. It was shown that RFRV-CLMs can successfully be applied as part of a fully automatic segmentation system to accurately and robustly segment bone shapes in 2D radiographs [8,9]. In this paper, we explore the effect of different annotation schemes on RFRV-CLM performance.

2 Methods

2.1 Groupwise Non-rigid Registration

The aim of GNR is to identify dense correspondences across images. We use a coarse-to-fine approach similar to that suggested in [3]. At each stage, the deformation field is represented by the location of the nodes of a triangulated mesh, and piece-wise affine interpolation is used to estimate the correspondence of any internal point. Early stages use coarse meshes with few points. Later stages use denser point sampling. Each stage involves two steps: 1) Build a GNR-model by warping the target images into the reference frame using the current points; and 2) Optimise the positions of the points on each image in turn to better match to the current GNR-model.

The process is usually initialised with an affine registration. However, if some manual annotations are available, they can be used to give a better start. In the following, we use a Thin Plate Spline to deform a reference mesh (defined on one image) to each of the other images, guided by the available manual sparse annotations. This gives a better initialisation for the GNR process. A dense annotation of a bone in one image, as in Fig. 1(a), is propagated to all other images using the deformated meshes from the GNR, and the resulting dense points are used to build an RFRV-CLM.

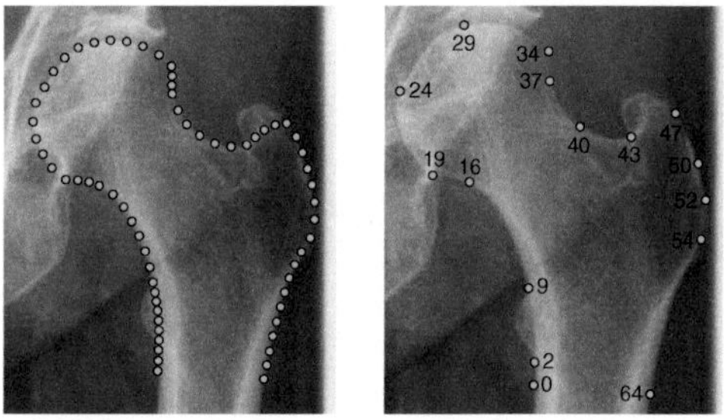

(a) (b)

Fig. 1. Points used for a model of the femur using 65 points: (a) manual ground truth, and (b) sparse subset points.

2.2 RF Regression-Voting in the CLM Framework

Recent work has shown that one of the most effective approaches to matching a statistical shape model to a new image is to train RFs to vote for the likely position of each model point and then to find the shape model parameters which optimise the total votes over all point positions. Full details are given in [7].

3 Experiments and Evaluation

We performed a set of experiments to analyse GNR accuracy and the performance of RFRV-CLMs built on annotations generated via GNR, as we vary the number of manually annotated points used to initialise the GNR. Extensive experiments were run on the segmentation of the proximal femur from pelvic radiographs by outlining its contour using a dense annotation of 65 points as shown in Fig. 1(a). We also provide results for a subset of experiments performed on the segmentation of the proximal tibia from knee radiographs using 37 points.

Datasets: The hip dataset comprised anteroposterior (AP) pelvic radiographs of 420 subjects suffering from unilateral hip osteoarthritis. All images were provided by the arcOGEN Consortium and were collected under relevant ethical approvals. The knee dataset comprised AP knee radiographs of 500 subjects from the Multicenter Osteoarthritis Study and the Osteoarthritis Initiative public use datasets.

For each test, we performed two-fold cross-validation experiments, averaging results from training on each half of the data and testing on the other half. All evaluations are based on manually annotated ground truth. The performance is summarised by the cumulative distribution function (CDF) for the the point-to-curve error (i. e. the shortest distance between each model point and the curve through the manual points, averaged over all points per image).

3.1 Guided Groupwise Non-rigid Registration and Refinement

On the hip dataset, we first investigate the effect of using increasing numbers of manual landmark points to initialise the GNR. We assume that between 2 and 16 points are available on each image. These are used to initialise the mesh used for the registration. The registration involves six stages, each refining the result of the previous stage. On completion of the GNR, the 65 points from one image are projected to all the others using the resulting deformation fields.[1]

We performed experiments for subsets of 2 (sparse2: 29,54), 4 (sparse4: sparse2 + 2,19), 6 (sparse6: sparse4 + 34,47), 8 (sparse8: sparse6 + 9,43), 10 (sparse10: sparse8 + 24,37), and 12 (sparse12: sparse10 + 0,64) 14 (sparse14: sparse12 + 16,50), and 16 (sparse16: sparse14 + 40,52) points. Fig. 1(b) shows the positions of all sparse points. The first two points (sparse2), 29 and 54, were chosen to define the location, size and orientation of the proximal femur. Subsequent pairs of points were chosen so as to sparsely capture the outline of the structure and the main areas of variation. This was assisted by identifying which regions were least well registered using the current set of points, qualitatively evaluating the "crispness" of the contours of the mean reference image (Fig. 2).

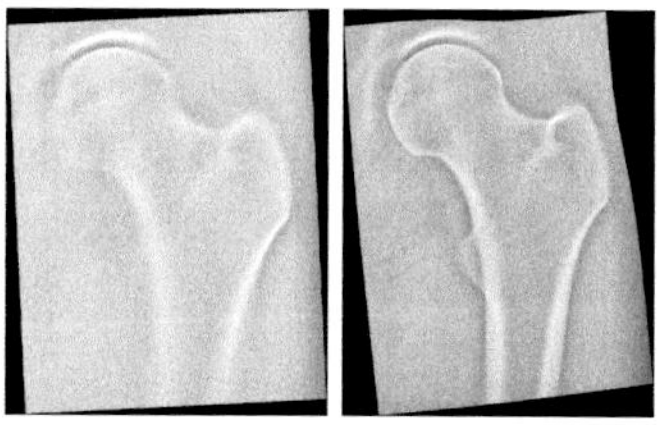

Fig. 2. Mean reference images after GNR for one of the two proximal femur cross-validation sets containing 210 images, for sparse2 and sparse12.

The quantitative GNR results in Fig. 3(a) show that with only two points for initialisation, GNR performs fairly poorly, with a median error of over 2mm and significant numbers of images with large errors. Thus, the 2-point GNR results are unlikely to be good enough for building an effective shape model matching system. As more points are added the performance gets better, particularly with the dramatic reduction in outliers. Gains beyond 12 points are marginal.

The results of the GNR and landmark propagation are a set of 65 points placed on every image. These can be used to train a two-stage RFRV-CLM; we

[1] In these experiments, all points were propagated from one of the training images. Better results are achievable when propagating the annotations from the reference image as this will be the best "match" to each of the images. This was not done here so as to have consistent points across the subset experiments (the reference image changes for each subset) and because for the smaller subsets the reference image was not good enough to reliably place points in all areas (e.g. sparse2 and the medial femoral head area, see Fig. 2).

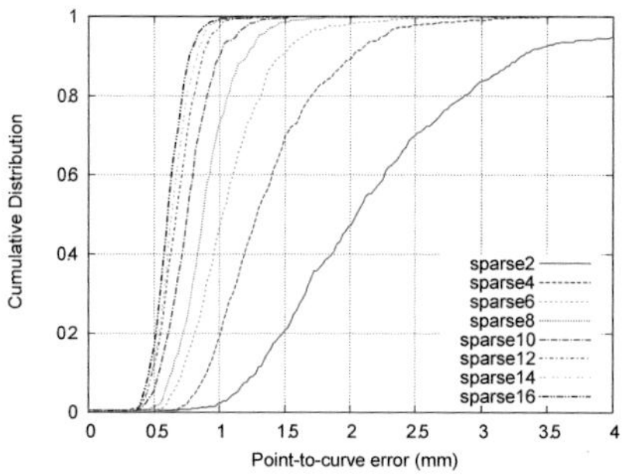

(a) Groupwise registration result (GNR)

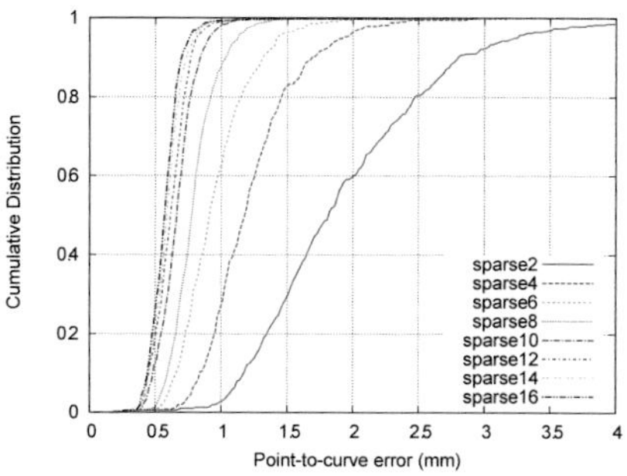

(b) GNR + RFRV-CLM

Fig. 3. Registration accuracy on the proximal femur training set compared to manual ground truth annotations: (a) without, and (b) with additional RFRV-CLM search.

used the same model parameters as those used in [8]. Fig. 3(b) shows the results of applying this RFRV-CLM to the *training set* itself, initialising the search with the sparse points used for GNR and comparing the search results with the ground truth labels. This demonstrates that, in every case, refining the points resulting from GNR using the RFRV-CLM actually leads to improvements in accuracy; though the improvement is largest for the cases with fewer landmarks for initialisation. Our experiments also showed that training another RFRV-CLM on these results led to no further improvement in accuracy (data not shown).

3.2 Estimation of GNR Accuracy in the Absence of Ground Truth

In the above, we trained on points which we know to be incorrect, because the registration is not accurate. In order to evaluate the performance of the registration, we also compared the above search results of the GNR-based RFRV-CLM with the dense points generated from the GNR stage.

Fig. 4(a) shows the quantitative evaluation of the performance of the registration by comparing the performance of the RFRV-CLM on the manual ground truth with its performance on the points generated by GNR (i. e. the points the RFRV-CLM was trained on), for sparse2 to sparse16 as above. Here the line gives the best fit to the 99%ile results (blue squares), demonstrating a strong correlation. This suggests that the performance of the GNR-based RFRV-CLM on the training set (when compared to the GNR results) can be used to estimate the overall accuracy of the registration for various subsets *in the absence of dense ground truth annotations*.

We obtain similar results when repeating the experiments on segmenting the proximal tibia in knee radiographs as shown in Fig. 4(b).

3.3 Performance of GNR-trained RFRV-CLM on New Images

To evaluate the segmentation performance of the RFRV-CLMs trained on the results of the GNR, we use them to search *unseen* test images. We incorporate the RFRV-CLMs built on the GNR results into a fully automatic shape model

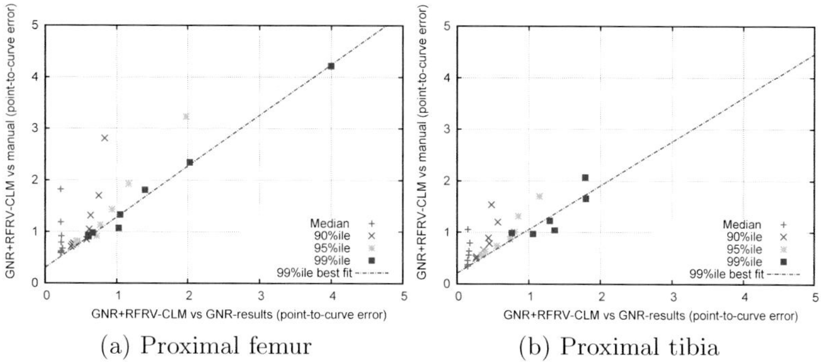

Fig. 4. Comparison of the GNR + RFRV-CLM search results vs manual ground truth with the GNR + RFRV-CLM search results vs the points generated by GNR (one marker per sparse subset per evaluated percentile). The strong correlation provides a means for the estimation of GNR accuracy in the absence of ground truth annotations.

matching system, which uses a Hough Forest to perform a global search of the whole image, followed by local refinement with the RFRV-CLM (similar to [8]).

Fig. 5(a) shows the results of running the hip system over the test images, using different training sets. The "ground truth" curve corresponds to the results of a model trained from the full set of 65 manually placed points. The results demonstrate that the fully automatic system works well, and that the results are strongly effected by the quality of the annotations on the training set. As more manual landmarks are added to initialise the GNR of the training set, the performance of the resulting model matching system improves, though adding more points beyond 12 leads to only very small further improvements. In terms of robustness, the RFRV-CLMs trained on the GNR annotations are similar to the models built on the manual ground truth annotations for subsets with at least 10 points, achieving sub-millimetre accuracy for at least 95% of all images. However, there remains a small (0.2mm) gap between the best median result from the GNR-based models and the dense manual model. This is partially explained by the choice of reference image used for propagating the dense points based on the GNR results. Annotating the mean reference image instead of one of the training images leads to a considerable improvement in performance (data not shown). For example, for sparse12 this achieves a point-to-curve error of within 1.1mm for 99% of all images and a median accuracy of less than 0.5mm, reducing the gap between medians to about 0.1mm. Though this does not quite reach the performance of the fully automatic system trained on the dense manual ground truth, the robustness of the two systems is comparable and the GNR-based models require significantly less manual input.

Fig. 5(b) gives the results of the fully automatic tibia segmentation system tested on *unseen* images. Building a fully automatic system based on just 10 manually annotated points achieved a point-to-curve-error of within 1.1mm for 99% of all images and a median accuracy of less than 0.5mm.

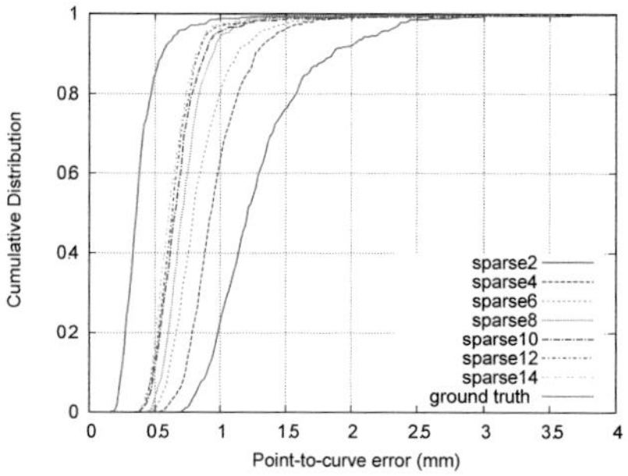

(a) Proximal femur

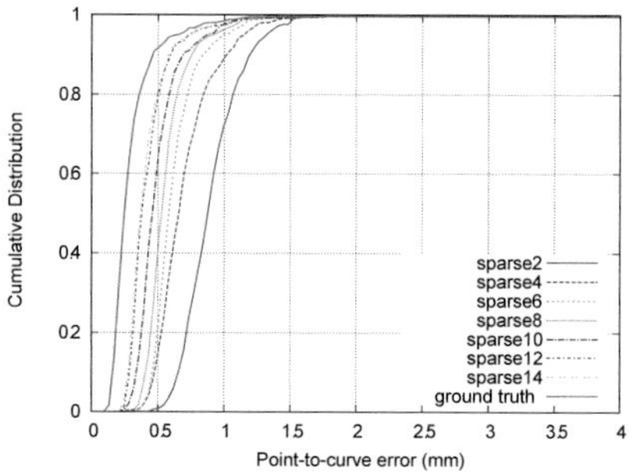

(b) Proximal tibia

Fig. 5. Search results of GNR-trained fully automatic RFRV-CLM model matching systems on unseen test images compared to manual ground truth annotations.

4 Discussion and Conclusions

We have shown that it is possible to use guided groupwise non-rigid registration to build segmentation models from large sets of images which are almost (but not quite) as effective as those built from careful dense manual annotations.

For segmenting the bone contours of the proximal femur, annotating 12 points on each image reduces the workload by over 80% but leads to a system whose median point-to-curve accuracy is only about 0.1mm worse than that of one built from dense 65-points manual annotations per image, and is almost as robust (both achieve over 98% of results with less than 1mm error). It should be noted that because the 12 points were chosen as well-defined landmarks, they are easier for a human to place than the intermediate points along a boundary – so in practice this will reduce the manual annotation time by even more than 80%. Applying the same approach to segmenting the contours of the proximal tibia shows that 10 points are sufficient to train a system that achieves a median accuracy of less than 0.5mm and that is as robust (99%ile $\leq$ 1.1mm) as one built from dense 37-points manual annotations, reducing the workload by over 70%.

Given a set of accurately annotated sparse points, this approach is equally applicable to the training of 3D models (e. g. using GNR methods as in [3]). Since the sparse points are used only to initialise the registration, small annotation errors in the sparse subsets are likely to be corrected for during the GNR process.

Fig. 4 shows a strong correlation between the ability of the RFRV-CLM to relocate the training points and the accuracy of those points compared to the ground truth. This holds the tantalising prospect of allowing an estimate of the accuracy of groupwise registration on new data in the absence of dense ground truth annotations. Furthermore, it provides an estimate of the improvement in accuracy by adding additional sparse points during GNR and hence is supportive in deciding on whether adding additional sparse points are likely to lead to significant improvements in overall accuracy.

For very large datasets (several hundreds to thousands of images) a cascaded approach might be followed to further minimise the manual input required: train a RFRV-CLM based on sparse annotations for a subset of all images and then use this to find the sparse annotations in all remaining images to initialise the GNR. Further work is needed to automate the selection of *suitable* sparse points to be used for the GNR initialisation, and to investigate the impact of a cascaded approach on performance. Overall this method will make it much easier to build effective models of different bone shapes from large datasets. This opens up opportunities to use bone shape analyses in more medical studies, allowing analysis of the change in shape across populations and of links between shape and disease.

Acknowledgments. arcOGEN is funded by Arthritis Research UK, J.T. by the Manchester Musculoskeletal Biomedical Research Unit (NIHR) and C.L. by the Engineering and Physical Sciences Research Council, UK (EP/M012611/1).

References

1. Baker, S., Matthews, I., Schneider, J.: Automatic construction of active appearance models as an image coding problem. IEEE TPAMI 26(10), 1380–1384 (2004)
2. Chen, C., Xie, W., Franke, J., Grutzner, P., Nolte, L.P., Zheng, G.: Automatic X-ray landmark detection and shape segmentation via data-driven joint estimation of image displacements. Medical Image Analysis 18(3), 487–499 (2014)
3. Cootes, T., Twining, C., Petrovic, V., Babalola, K., Taylor, C.: Computing accurate correspondences across groups of images. IEEE TPAMI 32(11), 1994–2005 (2010)
4. Donner, R., Menze, B.H., Bischof, H., Langs, G.: Fast anatomical structure localization using top-down image patch regression. In: Menze, B.H., Langs, G., Lu, L., Montillo, A., Tu, Z., Criminisi, A. (eds.) MCV 2012. LNCS, vol. 7766, pp. 133–141. Springer, Heidelberg (2013)
5. Frangi, A.F., Rueckert, D., Schnabel, J.A., Niessen, W.J.: Automatic 3D ASM construction via atlas-based landmarking and volumetric elastic registration. In: Insana, M.F., Leahy, R.M. (eds.) IPMI 2001. LNCS, vol. 2082, pp. 78–91. Springer, Heidelberg (2001)
6. Langs, G., Donner, R., Peloschek, P., Bischof, H.: Robust autonomous model learning from 2D and 3D data sets. In: Ayache, N., Ourselin, S., Maeder, A. (eds.) MICCAI 2007, Part I. LNCS, vol. 4791, pp. 968–976. Springer, Heidelberg (2007)
7. Lindner, C., Bromiley, P., Ionita, M., Cootes, T.: Robust and Accurate Shape Model Matching using Random Forest Regression-Voting. IEEE TPAMI 37(9), 1862–1874 (2015)
8. Lindner, C., Thiagarajah, S., Wilkinson, M., The arcOGEN Consortium, Wallis, G., Cootes, T.: Fully Automatic Segmentation of the Proximal Femur Using Random Forest Regression Voting. IEEE TMI 32(8), 1462–1472 (2013)
9. Lindner, C., Thiagarajah, S., Wilkinson, J.M., arcOGEN Consortium, Wallis, G.A., Cootes, T.F.: Accurate bone segmentation in 2D radiographs using fully automatic shape model matching based on regression-voting. In: Mori, K., Sakuma, I., Sato, Y., Barillot, C., Navab, N. (eds.) MICCAI 2013, Part II. LNCS, vol. 8150, pp. 181–189. Springer, Heidelberg (2013)
10. Sotiras, A., Davatzikos, C., Paragios, N.: Deformable Medical Image Registration: A Survey. IEEE TMI 32(7), 1153–1190 (2013)
11. Zhang, P., Adeshina, S.A., Cootes, T.F.: Automatic learning sparse correspondences for initialising groupwise registration. In: Jiang, T., Navab, N., Pluim, J.P.W., Viergever, M.A. (eds.) MICCAI 2010, Part II. LNCS, vol. 6362, pp. 635–642. Springer, Heidelberg (2010)

Scale and Curvature Invariant Ridge Detector for Tortuous and Fragmented Structures*

Roberto Annunziata[1],**, Ahmad Kheirkhah[2], Pedram Hamrah[2], and Emanuele Trucco[1]

[1] School of Computing, University of Dundee, Dundee, UK
r.annunziata@dundee.ac.uk
[2] Massachusetts Eye and Ear Infirmary, Harvard Medical School, Boston, USA

Abstract. Segmenting dendritic trees and corneal nerve fibres is challenging due to their uneven and irregular appearance in the respective image modalities. State-of-the-art approaches use hand-crafted features based on local assumptions that are often violated by tortuous and point-like structures, e.g., straight tubular shape. We propose a novel ridge detector, SCIRD, which is simultaneously rotation, scale and curvature invariant, and relaxes shape assumptions to achieve enhancement of target image structures. Experimental results on three datasets show that our approach outperforms state-of-the-art hand-crafted methods on tortuous and point-like structures, especially when captured at low resolution or limited signal-to-noise ratio and in the presence of other non-target structures.

1 Introduction

Segmenting automatically curvilinear structures such as blood vessels, dendritic arbors, or corneal nerve fibres has been the subject of much research as a fundamental pre-processing step, e.g. for lesion quantification and evaluation of therapy progress [1–9]. Most of the methods estimate a local *tubularity measure* (e.g. *vesselness* in [2,9]) based on hand-crafted features (henceforth, HCFs) modelling local geometrical properties of ideal tubular structures; enhancement filters are then built based on such models [2,3,5,9]. Recently, combining hand-crafted and learned filters, or using HCF in the learning process, has been shown to improve detection [7,8]. It is therefore important to identify HCF sets leading to high detection performance, to be used either separately or in combination with learning; this is the purpose of this paper. While HCF methods are typically fast, they are based on assumptions that might be violated in some cases. For instance, highly fragmented and tortuous structures violate two usual assumptions of most

* This research was supported by the EU Marie Curie ITN REVAMMAD, n° 316990. The authors are grateful to S. McKenna, J. Zhang (CVIP, Dundee) for valuable comments and to Amos Sironi (CVlab, EPFL) for providing the VC6 and BF2D datasets.

** Corresponding author.

N. Navab et al. (Eds.): MICCAI 2015, Part III, LNCS 9351, pp. 588–595, 2015.
DOI: 10.1007/978-3-319-24574-4_70

HCF models, i.e. continuous and locally straight tubular shapes. While discontinuity can be addressed by elongated kernels (e.g., Gabor [3]), no *hand-crafted* ridge detector for non-straight tubular shapes has been proposed so far. Here we present a novel hand-crafted ridge detector, *SCIRD (Scale and Curvature Invariant Ridge Detector)* which is simultaneously rotation, scale and curvature invariant, and removes the assumption of locally straight tubular structures by introducing a *curved-support Gaussian model* (Figure 1). Our tubularity measure is obtained by convolving the image with a filter bank of second-order directional derivatives of such curved-support Gaussians. To cope with irregular, point-like structures, we generate a subsets of directionally elongated kernels, similar to a Gabor filter bank [3]. Experimental results on three challenging datasets [7] show that our approach outperforms state-of-the-art HCF methods on tortuous structures.

2 Methods

Curved-Support Gaussian Models. Our HCF model is inspired by the curved-Gaussian models introduced by Lin and Dayan [10] who analyzed the correlation between currencies in time (exchange rate curvature analysis). Consider a multivariate zero-mean (n-D) Gaussian function with diagonal covariance matrix,

$$G(\boldsymbol{\varphi};\boldsymbol{\sigma}) = \frac{1}{\sqrt{(2\pi)^n \prod_{i=1}^{n} \sigma_i^2}}\, e^{-\sum_{i=1}^{n} \frac{\varphi_i^2}{2\sigma_i^2}} \quad (1)$$

where $\boldsymbol{\varphi} = (\varphi_1, \varphi_2, \ldots, \varphi_n)$ represents a point in the $\{\varphi\}$ coordinate system, and $\boldsymbol{\sigma} = (\sigma_1, \sigma_2, \ldots, \sigma_n)$ describes its amount of dispersion around the average (set to 0 without loss of generality). To bend the support of this Gaussian, we consider a volume-preserving non-linear transformation $\mathcal{T} : \mathbb{R}^n \mapsto \mathbb{R}^n$ with $\mathcal{T}(\boldsymbol{x}) = \boldsymbol{\varphi} = (\varphi_1, \varphi_2, \ldots, \varphi_n)$ of the form

$$\varphi_n = x_n + \sum_{i=1}^{n} k_{ni} m_{ni}(x_1, x_2, \ldots, x_{n-1}) \quad (2)$$

where k_{ni} are weights (see below) and the non-linear functions $m_{ni}(x_1, x_2, \ldots, x_{n-1})$ (and their inverses) have continuous partial derivatives [10]. Now, using the change of variable theorem, the non-linear transformation of the normalised $G(\boldsymbol{\varphi};\boldsymbol{\sigma})$ in the $\{\varphi\}$ coordinate system will be already normalised in the new $\{x\}$ coordinate system since the transformation considered is volume-preserving. In the 2-D case (i.e. $n = 2$), the application of the transformation $\mathcal{T}$ to $G(\boldsymbol{\varphi};\boldsymbol{\sigma})$ in Eq. (1) leads to the curved-support bivariate Gaussian function:

$$\mathrm{G}(x_1, x_2; \boldsymbol{\sigma}, \boldsymbol{k}) = \frac{1}{\sqrt{4\pi^2\sigma_1^2\sigma_2^2}}\, e^{-\frac{(x_1+k_{11})^2}{2\sigma_1^2} - \frac{[x_2+k_{20}m_{20}(x_1)+k_{21}m_{21}(x_1)+k_{22}m_{22}(x_1)]^2}{2\sigma_2^2}} . \quad (3)$$

If we now consider *quadratic* non-linear functions $m_{ni} = x_i^2$ for $0 < i < n$ and $m_{n0} = 1$, some of the parameters k_{ni} have the intuitive interpretation of

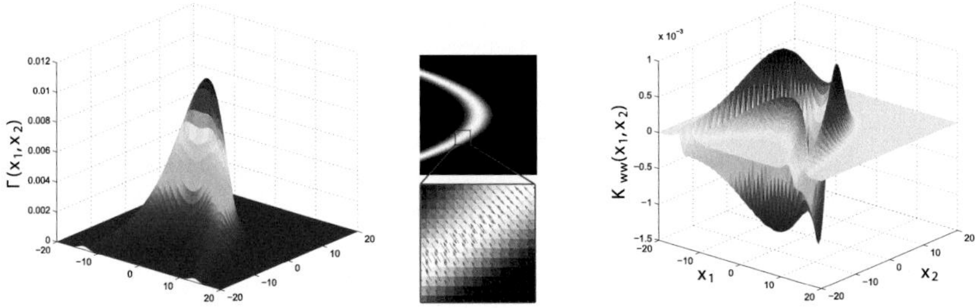

Fig. 1. An example of our "curved" shape model (left), its gradients map (centre) and the derived filter used to detect tortuous and point-like structures (right).

curvatures [10]. In fact, we observe that k_{11} controls the elongation *imbalance* of the shape (i.e. $k_{11} \neq 0$ makes one side tail longer than the other), k_{21} its curvature and k_{20} is simply a translation parameter. We are now in a position to define our shape model:

$$\Gamma(x_1, x_2; \boldsymbol{\sigma}, k) = \underbrace{\frac{1}{\sqrt{2\pi\sigma_1^2}} e^{-\frac{x_1^2}{2\sigma_1^2}}}_{\text{longitudinal}} \underbrace{\frac{1}{\sqrt{2\pi\sigma_2^2}} e^{-\frac{\left(x_2 + k x_1^2\right)^2}{2\sigma_2^2}}}_{\text{orthogonal}} . \tag{4}$$

where (x_1, x_2) is a point in the principal component coordinate system of the target structure [1], (σ_1, σ_2) control the elongation of the shape ("memory") and its width, respectively; in fact, the first term of $\Gamma(x_1, x_2; \boldsymbol{\sigma}, k)$ controls the longitudinal Gaussian profile of the model, while the second controls the cross-sectional Gaussian profile. We set $k_{11} = 0$ and $k_{20} = 0$. Importantly, we add a new parameter, k, to control the curvature of the Gaussian support (see Figure 1 - left).

Unsupervised SCIRD. Various detectors of tubular image structures compute the contrast between the regions inside and outside the tube or ridge [2,3,9]. We extend this idea to curved-support Gaussian models by computing the second-order directional derivative in the gradient direction at each pixel.

Let $I(x, y)$ represent the grey-level of a monochrome image at the location (x, y) in image coordinates. The grey-level at this location can be expressed using the first-order gauge coordinate system $(\boldsymbol{v}, \boldsymbol{w})$, where $\boldsymbol{w} = \frac{\nabla I(x,y)}{\|\nabla I(x,y)\|}$ and $\boldsymbol{v} = \boldsymbol{w}_{\perp}$. Our "curved tubularity" measure is

$$I_{ww}(x, y) = D_{\boldsymbol{w}}\left[D_{\boldsymbol{w}} I(x, y)\right] = D_{\boldsymbol{w}}\left[\boldsymbol{w}^T \nabla I(x, y)\right] \triangleq \boldsymbol{w}^T H_I \boldsymbol{w}, \tag{5}$$

where $D_{\boldsymbol{w}}$ is the directional derivative operator along $\boldsymbol{w}$.

$$H_I = \begin{bmatrix} I_{xx}(x, y) & I_{xy}(x, y) \\ I_{yx}(x, y) & I_{yy}(x, y) \end{bmatrix} \tag{6}$$

[1] Notice that this formulation requires a prior knowledge of the structure orientation. Later, we remove this constraint using multiple rotated kernels.

is the Hessian matrix, and $\nabla I(x, y) = [I_x(x, y), I_y(x, y)]^T$ is the gradient of $I(x, y)$. Substituting Eq. (6) in Eq. (5):

$$I_{ww} = \frac{(I_x I_{xx} + I_y I_{yx})I_x + (I_x I_{xy} + I_y I_{yy})I_y}{I_x^2 + I_y^2}. \quad (7)$$

where we have omitted arguments $(x, y; \boldsymbol{\sigma}, k)$ for compactness. However, computing these differential operators separately and then combining them is very expensive; hence we differentiate by convolving with derivatives of curved-support Gaussian, which simultaneously smooths noise [2]. This leads to an efficient tubularity enhancement filter:

$$I_{ww}(x, y; \boldsymbol{\sigma}, k) = I(x, y) * K_{ww}(x, y; \boldsymbol{\sigma}, k), \quad (8)$$

where K_{ww} represents our *tubularity* probe kernel (see example in Figure 1 - right):

$$K_{ww} = \frac{(\tilde{\Gamma}_x \Gamma_{xx} + \tilde{\Gamma}_y \Gamma_{yx})\tilde{\Gamma}_x + (\tilde{\Gamma}_x \Gamma_{xy} + \tilde{\Gamma}_y \Gamma_{yy})\tilde{\Gamma}_y}{\tilde{\Gamma}_x^2 + \tilde{\Gamma}_y^2}. \quad (9)$$

Here, $\tilde{\Gamma}$ is a curved-support Gaussian model (our model) with a constant (i.e. non-Gaussian) longitudinal profile, whose gradient direction is orthogonal to the centreline (Figure 1 - centre). To achieve scale and curvature invariance in the discrete domain, we create a filter bank from multiple kernels generated by making σ_2 and k span scale and curvature range for the specific application at hand. Rotation invariance is obtained augmenting our filter bank with kernel replicas rotated by angles $\theta \in [0, 2\pi)$, i.e., symbolically, $K_{ww}(x, y; \boldsymbol{\sigma}, k, \theta)$. Fragmented (point-like) structures are dealt with by tuning the "memory" parameter σ_1 (see Section 3 for how to tune σ_1). Figure 2(a) shows some of the kernels used in our experiments. Finally, SCIRD selects the maximum response over all kernels. Notice that since we are interested in ridge-like structures, we set $\text{SCIRD}(x, y) = 0$ for all (x, y) locations such that $\text{SCIRD}(x, y) < 0$ [2].

We observed that in some cases, e.g. *in vivo* confocal microscopy, non-linear contrast variations across the image can make interesting structures appear thin and poorly contrasted. In other cases, e.g. bright-field micrographs, such structures may not be interesting and therefore they should not be enhanced. To address this, we introduce a contrast normalization term and a parameter $\alpha \in \mathbb{R}$ that is positive in the former case (enhancement required) and negative in the latter, obtaining

$$\text{SCIRD}(x, y) = \frac{\max_{\boldsymbol{\sigma}, k, \theta} I_{ww}(x, y; \boldsymbol{\sigma}, k, \theta)}{1 + \alpha \, I^C(x, y)}, \quad (10)$$

where

$$I^C(x, y) = \frac{1}{(N+1)^2} \sum_{i=x-\frac{N}{2}}^{x+\frac{N}{2}} \sum_{j=y-\frac{N}{2}}^{y+\frac{N}{2}} \max_{\sigma_2} ||\nabla I(i, j; \sigma_2)|| \quad (11)$$

is a contrast measure based on multiscale gradient magnitude estimation averaged on a patch $(N+1) \times (N+1)$ around the pixel (x, y). Notice, N is not a free parameter, but the width (and height) of the largest filter in the SCIRD filter bank ($N = 8\sigma_{2max}$)[2]. Since SCIRD is designed to respond maximally at the centreline, it can be employed for both curvilinear structure segmentation *and* centreline detection. The former is achieved, e.g., by thresholding directly the *tubularity map* obtained from Eq. (10). The latter is achieved, e.g., by Canny-like non-maxima suppression.

Supervised SCIRD. Segmentation and centreline detection using unsupervised SCIRD can be improved by introducing a supervised classifier. Hence, we combine n feature maps ($I_{ww}^{(i)},\ i = 1, \ldots, n$) obtained using our filter bank with unsupervised SCIRD to form a feature vector $\boldsymbol{f}$:

$$\boldsymbol{f} = \left[\ \text{SCIRD}, I_{ww}^{(1)}, I_{ww}^{(2)}, \cdots, I_{ww}^{(n)}\ \right]^T. \tag{12}$$

We employ a Random Decision Forest [7,11] to classify each pixel. Thresholding directly the resulting probability map (which can be seen as a tubularity map) leads indeed to a more accurate and less noisy segmentation (see precision-recall curves in Section 3). Supervised centreline detection is obtained using Canny-like non-maxima suppression on the tubularity map. As local orientation for both supervised and unsupervised centreline detection we choose that of the kernel responding maximally.

3 Experiments and Results

Datasets. We validate SCIRD on 3 datasets including low and high resolution images of corneal nerve fibres and neurons, showing very diverse curvilinear structures as illustrated in Figure 2(b). **IVCM** [1] is a dataset of 100 384 $\times$ 384 confocal microscopy images of the corneal subbasal nerve plexus with different grades of tortuosity. Nerve centrelines were manually traced by a specialist as ground truth. Low resolution, non-uniform and poor contrast, tortuosity, and fibre fragmentation make this dataset particularly challenging. As usually done to evaluate methods extracting onepixel-wide curves [12], we introduce a tolerance factor ρ: a predicted centreline point is considered a true positive if it is at most ρ distant from a ground truth centreline point. In our experiments we set $\rho = 2$ pixel. Following the usual benchmarking procedure [7], we average performance measures over 10 random sub-sampling cross-validation runs, using 50 images for training and the rest for testing in each run. The resulting precision-recall curves are reported in Figure 4 (mean and standard deviation of the results from individual runs). The **BF2D** dataset [7] consists of two minimum intensity projections of bright-field micrographs that capture neurons, annotated by an expert. The images have a high resolution (1024 $\times$ 1792 and 768 $\times$ 1792) but a low signal-to-noise ratio because of irregularities in the staining process; the dendrites often appear as point-like (fragmented) structures easily mistaken for noise. As a consequence, the quality of the annotations themselves is

[2] Source code available at `http://staff.computing.dundee.ac.uk/rannunziata/`.

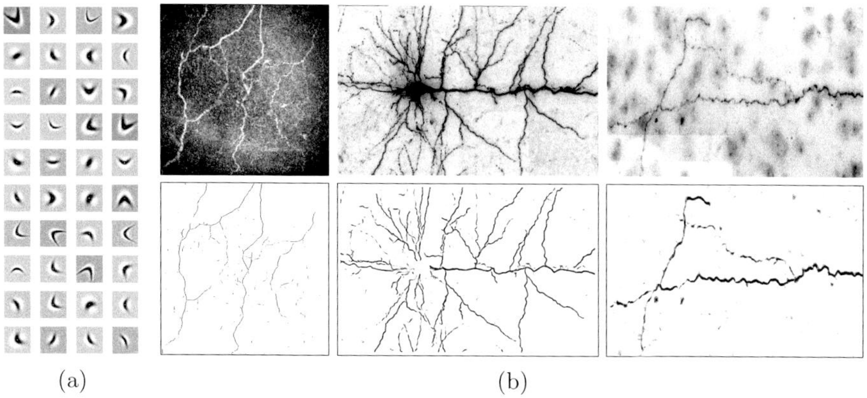

Fig. 2. (a) A subset of SCIRD filters used in our experiments. Notice, the model includes straight support too; (b) original images (top), supervised SCIRD *tubularity* maps (bottom) from IVCM (left), BF2D (centre), VC6 (right) testing sets.

limited [7]. We adopted the same set partition described in [7]. The **VC6** dataset was created by the authors in [7] from a set of publicly available 3D images showing dendritic and axonal subtrees from one neuron in the primary visual cortex. It consists of three images obtained computing minimum intensity projections of a subset of 3-D images, with numerous artifacts and poor contrast, hence challenging for automatic segmentation. We retained two images for training and the third one for testing, adopting the same set partition in [7].

Parameters Setting. SCIRD's key parameters are σ_1, σ_2 and k controlling the filter memory, width and curvature, respectively. The ranges of σ_1 over datasets were chosen considering the level of fragmentation. We set σ_2 values taking into account the maximum and minimum width of the target structures in each dataset as they depend on resolution; curvature values were set according to the level of tortuosity shown by the specific curvilinear structures. The contrast normalisation parameter α was set as discussed in Section 2. We set the range of θ and k for all the datasets: $\theta = \left\{\frac{\pi}{12}, \frac{\pi}{6}, \cdots, 2\pi\right\}$, and $k = \{0, 0.025, \cdots, 0.1\}$. We set other parameters separately, given the significant difference in resolution between datasets. For the IVCM, $\sigma_1 = \{2, 3, 4\}$, $\sigma_2 = \{2, 3\}$, $\alpha = 1$; for the BF2D dataset, $\sigma_1 = 5$, $\sigma_2 = \{2, 3, 4\}$, $\alpha = -0.075$; for the VC6, $\sigma_1 = 3$, $\sigma_2 = \{2, 3\}$, $\alpha = 0$. For the supervised SCIRD, we used the same range of θ and k, but we doubled the discretisation steps for computational efficiency. We trained Random Forests with the number of decision trees and maximum number of samples in each leaf set using the out-of-bag error. We randomly selected 50,000 pixels from the training set for each dataset. Parameters for SCIRD and baseline methods were tuned separately to achieve their best performance on each dataset to provide a fair comparison.

Results and Discussion. We compare SCIRD against 3 HCF ridge detectors: Frangi [2], based on Hessian matrix eigenvalue analysis, Gabor [3] and the recent Optimally Oriented Flux (OOF) [5], widely acknowledged as excellent tubular

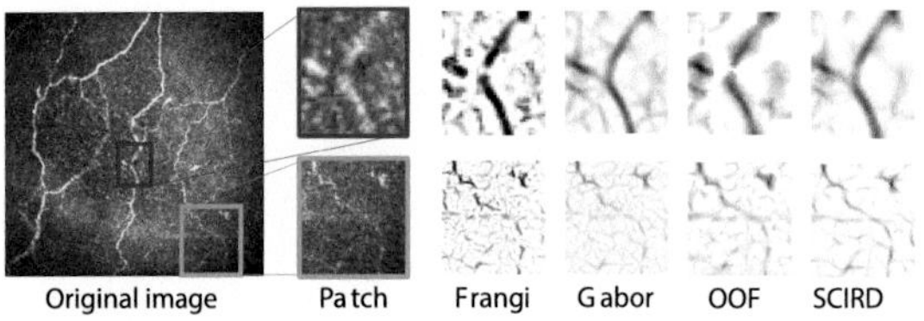

Fig. 3. Qualitative comparison: tubularity estimation results on IVCM. SCIRD (our approach) shows better connectivity and higher signal-to-noise ratio than others.

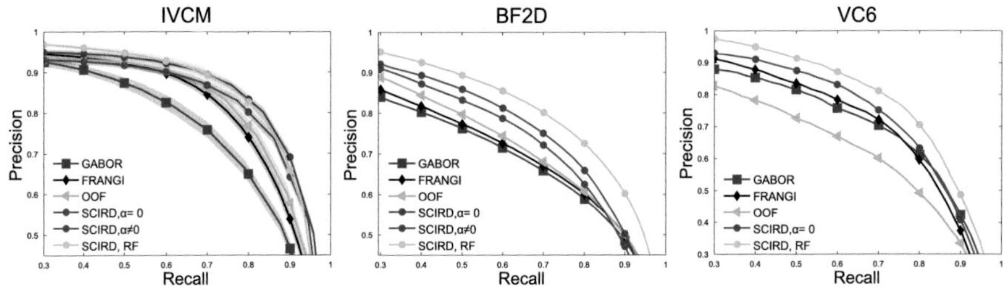

Fig. 4. Precision-recall curves for SCIRD and baselines on IVCM, BF2D and VC6 datasets. Curves are obtained applying different thresholds on the *tubularity* maps.

structure detectors. Qualitative (Figure 3) and quantitative (Figure 4) results show that SCIRD outperforms the other methods on all datasets. Specifically, SCIRD shows higher precision from medium to high recall values for the IVCM dataset, suggesting that our filters behave better than others at low resolution and low SNR when dealing with tortuous and fragmented structures. The low number of false positives when false negatives are low, implies that SCIRD selects target structures with higher confidence. Notice that contrast enhancement ("SCIRD $\alpha \neq 0$", $\alpha = 1$) boosts performance on this dataset achieving the level of performance obtained in the supervised setting ("SCIRD, RF"), at a lower computational cost. For the BF2D dataset, unsupervised SCIRD shows a significant improvement from low to high recall values, suggesting that fewer non-target structures are detected and targets are enhanced with higher accuracy (e.g. point-like structures are correctly reconnected, tortuous structure profiles are better preserved). Contrast reduction ("SCIRD $\alpha \neq 0$", $\alpha = -0.075$) proves helpful for these images. Supervised classification improves performance further. For the VC6 dataset, SCIRD shows better performance from low to medium recall values, indicating a better discrimination between curvilinear structures and artifacts, in addition to a more accurate profile segmentation for tortuous structures. Contrast enhancement did not help for this dataset, while supervised classification contributes significantly to improve results. The time to run SCIRD on Intel i7-4770 CPU @ 3.4 GHz and MATLAB code is 0.86s (IVCM), 0.62s (VC6) and 8.75s (BF2D). Since SCIRD is highly parallelizable the time to run can be reduced further.

4 Conclusion

We designed a novel HCF ridge detector based on curved-support Gaussians, which is simultaneously invariant to orientation, scale, and, unlike its peers, curvature invariant. Experimental results show that SCIRD outperforms current state-of-the-art HCF ridge detectors on 3 challenging datasets, two of which used in the recent literature for similar methods. Our future work will investigate the combination of SCIRD with learned filters (e.g. [13]) in order to capture or discard structures difficult to model (e.g. crossings and artifacts).

References

1. Annunziata, R., Kheirkhah, A., Aggarwal, S., Cavalcanti, B.M., Hamrah, P., Trucco, E.: Tortuosity classification of corneal nerves images using a multiple-scale-multiple-window approach. In: OMIA Workshop, MICCAI (2014)
2. Frangi, A.F., Niessen, W.J., Vincken, K.L., Viergever, M.A.: Multiscale vessel enhancement filtering. In: Wells, W.M., Colchester, A.C.F., Delp, S.L. (eds.) MICCAI 1998. LNCS, vol. 1496, p. 130. Springer, Heidelberg (1998)
3. Soares, J.V., Leandro, J.J., Cesar, R.M., Jelinek, H.F., Cree, M.J.: Retinal vessel segmentation using the 2-d gabor wavelet and supervised classification. IEEE TMI (2006)
4. Santamaría-Pang, A., Colbert, C.M., Saggau, P., Kakadiaris, I.A.: Automatic centerline extraction of irregular tubular structures using probability volumes from multiphoton imaging. In: Ayache, N., Ourselin, S., Maeder, A. (eds.) MICCAI 2007, Part II. LNCS, vol. 4792, pp. 486–494. Springer, Heidelberg (2007)
5. Law, M.W.K., Chung, A.C.S.: Three dimensional curvilinear structure detection using optimally oriented flux. In: Forsyth, D., Torr, P., Zisserman, A. (eds.) ECCV 2008, Part IV. LNCS, vol. 5305, pp. 368–382. Springer, Heidelberg (2008)
6. González, G., Aguet, F., Fleuret, F., Unser, M., Fua, P.: Steerable features for statistical 3D dendrite detection. In: Yang, G.-Z., Hawkes, D., Rueckert, D., Noble, A., Taylor, C. (eds.) MICCAI 2009, Part II. LNCS, vol. 5762, pp. 625–632. Springer, Heidelberg (2009)
7. Rigamonti, R., Lepetit, V.: Accurate and efficient linear structure segmentation by leveraging ad hoc features with learned filters. In: Ayache, N., Delingette, H., Golland, P., Mori, K. (eds.) MICCAI 2012, Part I. LNCS, vol. 7510, pp. 189–197. Springer, Heidelberg (2012)
8. Becker, C., Rigamonti, R., Lepetit, V., Fua, P.: Supervised feature learning for curvilinear structure segmentation. In: Mori, K., Sakuma, I., Sato, Y., Barillot, C., Navab, N. (eds.) MICCAI 2013, Part I. LNCS, vol. 8149, pp. 526–533. Springer, Heidelberg (2013)
9. Hannink, J., Duits, R., Bekkers, E.: Crossing-preserving multi-scale vesselness. In: Golland, P., Hata, N., Barillot, C., Hornegger, J., Howe, R. (eds.) MICCAI 2014, Part II. LNCS, vol. 8674, pp. 603–610. Springer, Heidelberg (2014)
10. Lin, J.K., Dayan, P.: Curved gaussian models with application to the modeling of foreign exchange rates. In: Computational Finance. MIT Press (1999)
11. Criminisi, A., Shotton, J.: Decision forests for computer vision and medical image analysis. Springer (2013)
12. Sironi, A., Lepetit, V., Fua, P.: Multiscale centerline detection by learning a scale-space distance transform. In: CVPR (2014)
13. Annunziata, R., Kheirkhah, A., Hamrah, P., Trucco, E.: Boosting hand-crafted features for curvilinear structures segmentation by learning context filters. In: Frangi, A. et al. (eds.) MICCAI 2015, Part III. LNCS, vol. 9351, pp. 596-603. Springer, Heidelberg (2015)

Boosting Hand-Crafted Features for Curvilinear Structure Segmentation by Learning Context Filters*

Roberto Annunziata[1,**], Ahmad Kheirkhah[2], Pedram Hamrah[2], and Emanuele Trucco[1]

[1] School of Computing, University of Dundee, Dundee, UK
r.annunziata@dundee.ac.uk
[2] Massachusetts Eye and Ear Infirmary, Harvard Medical School, Boston, USA

Abstract. Combining hand-crafted features and learned filters (i.e. feature boosting) for curvilinear structure segmentation has been proposed recently to capture key structure configurations while limiting the number of learned filters. Here, we present a novel combination method pairing hand-crafted appearance features with learned context filters. Unlike recent solutions based only on appearance filters, our method introduces *context information* in the filter learning process. Moreover, it reduces the potential redundancy of learned appearance filters that may be reconstructed using a combination of hand crafted filters. Finally, the use of k-means for filter learning makes it fast and easily adaptable to other datasets, even when large dictionary sizes (e.g. 200 filters) are needed to improve performance. Comprehensive experimental results using 3 challenging datasets show that our combination method outperforms recent state-of-the-art HCFs and a recent combination approach for both performance and computational time.

1 Introduction

Clinical research has shown that morphometric properties of curvilinear structures in the human body, e.g. blood vessels, are associated with a wide range of sub-clinical (e.g. atherosclerosis) and clinical cardiovascular diseases (e.g. diabetes, hypertension, stroke) [1]. Automated systems would allow cost-effective large screening programs aimed at early diagnosis.

To measure automatically morphometric properties such as tortuosity [2], these structures have to be segmented accurately. Many solutions have been proposed to cope with the multiple challenges involved, including low signal-to-noise ratio at small scales, confounding non-target structures, non-uniform illumination and complex configurations [3–11]. Most approaches are based on a local

* This research was supported by the EU Marie Curie ITN 316990 "REVAMMAD". The authors are grateful to Amos Sironi (CVlab, EPFL) for providing the VC6 and BF2D datasets and to Max Law (Western University) for the OOF code.

** Corresponding author.

N. Navab et al. (Eds.): MICCAI 2015, Part III, LNCS 9351, pp. 596–603, 2015.
DOI: 10.1007/978-3-319-24574-4_71

tubularity measure estimated via hand-crafted features (henceforth, HCFs) [3, 4, 6, 7, 10], or learned from training data [5, 9, 11]. Although HCFs can be fast, they may rely on assumptions violated in some cases (e.g. at bifurcations and crossing points). For this reason, Honnorat et al. [7] use a graphical model after HCF-based tubularity estimation to improve guide-wire tracking during cardiac angioplasty interventions. Other methods are based on fully learned architectures capturing key configurations on training data, but can be demanding computationally since they typically require more filters than efficient HCFs [3, 6]. Recently, Rigamonti et al. [8] proposed a novel, hybrid approach combining HCFs with learned appearance filters (i.e. feature boosting) to exploit the efficiency of fast HCFs while limiting the amount of learned filters. It employs sparse coding (henceforth, SC) to learn 9 appearance filters and combines them with state-of-the-art HCFs. Although this method outperforms state-of-the-art approaches such as [3, 6], our work is motivated by limitations including the amount of false positives far from target structures and modest success in segmenting fragmented or weakly connected structures such as corneal nerve fibres and neurons (Section 3). Integrating *context* information with *appearance* features has been recently found to address these shortcomings, albeit at an extra computational cost as multiple discriminative models are learned sequentially [12].

In this paper, we propose a novel combination approach in which efficient HCFs capturing the *appearance* are paired with learned *context* filters. Overall, our method has three key advantages over recently proposed methods (e.g. [8]): 1) it includes context information recently found to improve results over appearance-only frameworks [12] while still learning a *single* discriminative model; 2) it implicitly reduces or eliminate the redundancy of learned filters; 3) it is fast and easily adaptable to other datasets, even when large dictionary sizes (e.g. 200 filters) are needed to improve performance.

2 Proposed Approach

Unsupervised Filter Learning. k-means clustering has been successfully used for filter/dictionary learning, often competing with more complex state-of-the-art methods [13]. Although k-means is not designed to learn "distributed" representations, like sparse coding or independent component analysis, experiments suggest that k-means tends to discover sparse projections of the data [13] with sufficiently large numbers of training patches given the patch size and patch-level whitening to remove correlations between nearby pixels. Because of this and given the large amount of our training data (Section 3), we employ k-means clustering to learn filters instead of algorithms explicitly designed to obtain sparse representations like SC used in [8]. We use the k-means filter learning algorithm described in [13] which we summerize succinctly.

Our goal is to learn a dictionary $\mathbf{D} \in \mathbb{R}^{n \times k}$ of k vectors so that a data vector $\mathbf{x}^{(i)} \in \mathbb{R}^n, i = 1, \ldots, m$ can be mapped to a code vector that minimizes the reconstruction error. Before running the learning algorithm we normalize the brightness and contrast of each input data point (i.e. patch) $\mathbf{x}^{(i)}$. Then, we apply patch-level

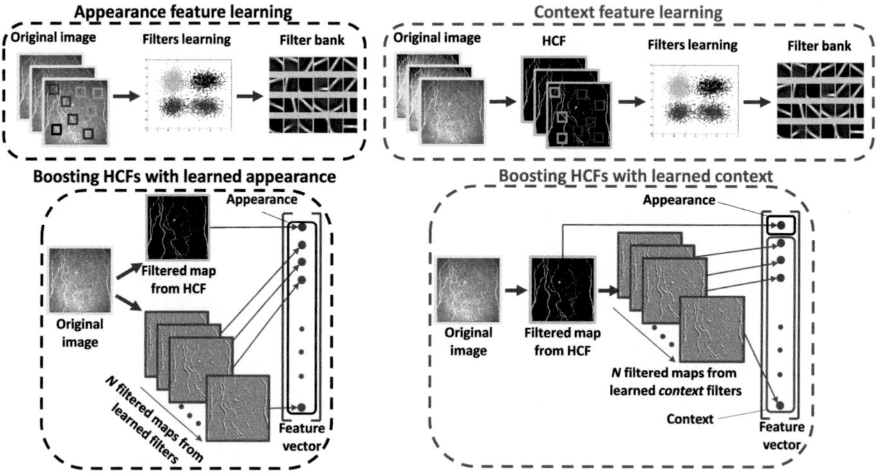

Fig. 1. Boosting HCFs with learned appearance and context filters. In the former, learned filters are applied to original image; HCF maps are used in the latter.

whitening through the ZCA transform so that $\mathbf{x}_{ZCA}^{(i)} = \mathbf{V}(\mathbf{\Sigma}+\epsilon_{ZCA}\mathbf{I})^{-1/2}\mathbf{V}^T\mathbf{x}^{(i)}$, where $\mathbf{V}$ and $\mathbf{\Sigma}$ are computed from the eigenvalue decomposition of the data points covariance $\mathbf{V}\mathbf{\Sigma}\mathbf{V}^T = \mathrm{cov}(\mathbf{X})$, and ϵ_{ZCA} is a small constant (Section 3) controlling the trade-off between whitening and noise amplification. After pre-processing the patches, we solve the optimization problem

$$\underset{\mathbf{D},\mathbf{c}}{\mathrm{argmin}} \sum_i \left\| \mathbf{D}\mathbf{c}^{(i)} - \mathbf{x}_{ZCA}^{(i)} \right\|_2^2 \tag{1}$$

subject to $||\mathbf{c}^{(i)}||_0 \leq 1, \forall i = 1, \ldots, m$ and $||\mathbf{d}^{(j)}||_2 = 1, \forall j = 1, \ldots, k$, where $\mathbf{c}^{(i)}$ is the code vector related to input $\mathbf{x}_{ZCA}^{(i)}$, and $\mathbf{d}^{(j)}$ is the j-th column of the dictionary $\mathbf{D}$.

Combining appearance filters learned through k-means (or SC) with HCFs leads to the combination approach proposed in [8] based on appearance-only features (see Figure 1 left).

Learning Context Filters. Hand-crafted and learned appearance features are designed to capture object-specific properties. In the case of curvilinear structures, they detect characteristics that make them *appear* as ridge-, vessel- or tube-like shapes. However, appearance features do not take into account specific inter-object relationships, *context* information that has been found recently to improve performance significantly in segmentation tasks over methods employing appearance features only. One well-known method including context information is auto-context [12], which learns multiple discriminative models sequentially. This imposes an extra computational cost over learning a single discriminative model, as in traditional methods based on features representing object pixels and a single classifier to infer their labels. While an extra computational cost may have little impact on training/testing time for applications involving small datasets or small images, it may become impractical with large volumes of images data. This is the case, for instance, with large screening programs based on images, e.g., diabetic retinopathy [1]. For this reason, our goal is to include context information in a learning method without increasing the computational cost with respect to the solution in [8]. This is achieved by learning a *single* discriminative model which takes as input both *appearance* (i.e. likelihood computed on the original image) and, unlike the method in [8], *context information* (i.e. relations between objects). To model appearance, we employ the fast Optimally Oriented Flux (OOF) feature [6], shown to outperform other HCFs on the datasets we use for our tests [8]. We include context information by learning context filters to be used in combination with the HCFs in a new hybrid model to segment curvilinear structures. Learning context filters has two clear advantages: 1) including high-level information in a hybrid framework; 2) high efficiency and adaptability since convolution with filter banks is very fast on standard computers. In addition, our proposed method has a key advantage over methods learning appearance filters (e.g. [8]): it implicitly eliminates, or reduces significantly, the redundancy of learned filters. In fact, learned appearance filters may be reconstructed through a combination (linear or non-linear) of the HCFs already used to model appearance, thus reducing the discrimination power of the feature set. Figure 1 shows the difference between the proposed approach (right) and the combination method proposed in [8] (left). Notice, while appearance filters are learned on the same layer where HCFs are applied (original image), context filters are learned on a *different* layer (i.e. after HCFs are applied).

Description Vector and Supervised Classification. Learned filters are applied to the input image to compute multiple feature maps efficiently using correlation:

$$\mathbf{L}^{(j)} = \mathbf{D}^{(j)} \circ \mathbf{I}_n, \tag{2}$$

where $\mathbf{D}^{(j)}$ is the j-th learned filter, $\mathbf{I}_n$ is the normalized input image (i.e., zero mean and unit standard deviation) and the $\circ$ symbol denotes correlation. We have also experimented with normalizations of the input image at patch level (including whitening), measuring the squared distance between the pre-processed patch and each filter; experiments (omitted given space limits) show that these normalizations, although important during the filter learning procedure, do not improve performance significantly and increase the computational cost. Thus, for each image location (u, v), we construct the following description vector:

$$[\underbrace{\mathbf{OOF}(u,v),}_{\textbf{appearance}} \ \underbrace{\mathbf{L}^{(1)}(u,v), \ldots, \mathbf{L}^{(N)}(u,v)}_{\textbf{context}} \ ]^T, \tag{3}$$

including appearance and learned context features ($N \leq 200$ in our experiments). We then apply a Random Decision Forest to classify each pixel. Centreline detection is obtained using Canny-like non-maxima suppression on the tubularity map. Local orientation is estimated using OOF.

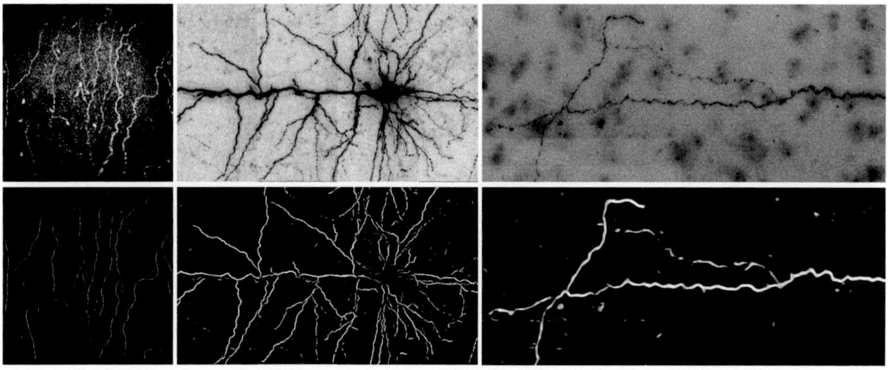

Fig. 2. Original images (top) and tubularity maps (bottom) obtained with our approach on IVCM (left), BF2D (centre), VC6 (right) datasets.

3 Experiments

Datasets. We validate our combination method using 3 datasets including low and high resolution images of corneal nerve fibres and neurons, showing very diverse images of curvilinear structures as shown in Figure 2.

IVCM [2] is a dataset of 100 384×384 confocal microscopy images capturing corneal nerve fibres with different grades of tortuosity, annotated by the clinical authors. Low resolution, non-uniform and poor contrast, tortuosity, and fibre fragmentation make this dataset particularly challenging. Following [11], we introduce a tolerance factor ρ for centreline detection: a predicted centreline point is considered a true positive if it is at most ρ pixels distant from a ground truth centreline point ($\rho = 2$ pixels [11]). Random sub-sampling is used to test performance on this dataset, using 50 images for training and the rest for testing in each cross-validation runs.

The **BF2D** dataset [8] consists of two minimum intensity projections of bright-field micrographs that capture neurons, annotated by an expert. The images have a high resolution (1024×1792 and 768×1792) but a low signal-to-noise ratio; the dendrites often appear as point-like structures easily mistaken for noise. We adopted the same dataset partition as in [8].

The **VC6** dataset [8] shows dendritic and axonal subtrees from one neuron in the primary visual cortex. It consists of three images obtained computing minimum intensity projections of 3D images, with numerous artifacts and poor contrast, hence challenging for automatic segmentation. We adopted the same dataset partition as in [8], selecting two images for training, and the third for testing. For all the datasets we averaged results over 10 random trials.

Experimental Setup. First, images are normalised to have zero mean and unit standard deviation. When HCFs are used as baselines, all parameters are tuned separately for each dataset to achieve best performance. To reduce the number of parameters to be optimised over datasets and test generalization, we fixed the OOF parameters range, the whitening parameter ϵ_{ZCA} and filters size in our filter banks to the same for *all* datasets. For OOF, we set $\sigma =$

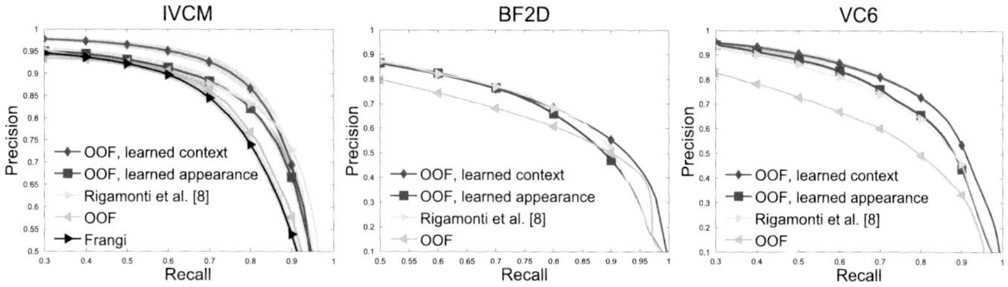

Fig. 3. Precision-recall curves for pixel-level classification. Shaded color bands represent 1 standard deviation of the results from individual runs.

$\{2, 3, 4\}$ (Eq. (8) [6]) and $R = \{2, 3, 4\}$ (Eq. (5) [14]). ϵ_{ZCA} was set to 0.001, considering the trade-off between noise amplification and filters sharpness [13]. Filters size was set to 11×11 pixels. Notice that the chosen patch size allows us to collect a sufficient number of patches to learn dictionaries, in agreement with the guidelines in [13][1]. We adopt filter banks of 100 filters (i.e., $N = 100$) for our method as good compromise between accuracy and speed. We used Random Decision Forests with 100 random trees to make predictions fast. We trained classifiers using the same number of positive and negative samples and priors estimated empirically. Experiments were run on a 8-core 64-bit architecture using MATLAB implementations.

We compare our method, combining appearance and context filters, with the one recently introduced in [8] based only on appearance. Therefore, we report results obtained with the original implementation of [8] using 9 appearance filters learned through SC ("*Rigamonti et al. [8]*" in Figure 3)[2]. We also report experiments using k-means to learn appearance filters ("*OOF, learned appearance*") and the same dictionary size we adopted to learn context filters.

Results and Discussion. As Figure 3 shows, our feature boosting method ("*OOF, learned context*") outperforms the baselines on all datasets, especially on IVCM and VC6. The variability of the datasets allows us to compare performance with very diverse data characteristics: with tortuous, fragmented structures and low signal-to-noise ratio (IVCM), our method shows a better precision for low recall values as it better segments fragmented structures; when structures have better contrast but point-like appearance (BF2D), our method shows higher precision at high recall values as it reduces the false positives due to point-like non-target structures and increases the connectivity; when dealing with complex non-target structures (e.g. blobs in VC6), our approach shows better performance from medium to high recall values, since it reduces the amount of false positives due to such structures.

Since our main goal is to compare learned context with learned appearance regardless of the learning algorithm used (k-means or SC), we evaluate the effect

[1] We selected 340,000 patches in the worst case represented by a single training image of the BF2D dataset. Notice that, in [13] 100,000 16×16 patches are considered sufficient.

[2] Original code at: `https://bitbucket.org/roberto_rigamonti/med_img_pc`.

Table 1. Effect of patch and dictionary size on the area under precision-recall curves (mean/standard deviation). Our method outperforms the baseline in all conditions.

IVCM	Patch size (pixels)			Number of learned filters (N)		
	11 × 11	15 × 15	21 × 21	10	100	200
OOF, learned context	0.8928/0.0056	0.9078/0.0043	0.9133/0.0052	0.8866/0.0033	0.8928/0.0056	0.8976/0.0037
OOF, learned appearance	0.8665/0.0114	0.8878/0.0059	0.8870/0.0102	0.8557/0.0069	0.8665/0.0114	0.8878/0.0039
	100 learned filters			**Patch size:** 11 × 11 **pixels**		

BF2D	Patch size (pixels)			Number of learned filters (N)		
	11 × 11	15 × 15	21 × 21	10	100	200
OOF, learned context	0.8057/0.0017	0.8010/0.0029	0.7948/0.0021	0.7966/0.0043	0.8057/0.0017	0.8054/0.0022
OOF, learned appearance	0.7881/0.0060	0.7888/0.0035	0.7908/0.0036	0.7857/0.0026	0.7881/0.0060	0.7824/0.0044
	100 learned filters			**Patch size:** 11 × 11 **pixels**		

VC6	Patch size (pixels)			Number of learned filters (N)		
	11 × 11	15 × 15	21 × 21	10	100	200
OOF, learned context	0.8272/0.0052	0.8295/0.0035	0.8069/0.0063	0.7911/0.0070	0.8272/0.0052	0.8368/0.0041
OOF, learned appearance	0.7905/0.0063	0.7904/0.0045	0.7809/0.0032	0.7460/0.0053	0.7905/0.0063	0.7905/0.0062
	100 learned filters			**Patch size:** 11 × 11 **pixels**		

of patch and dictionary size on the performance measured using Area Under Precision-Recall Curve (AUPRC) for both combination methods using k-means as learning method. As Table 1 shows, combining OOF with learned context (proposed here) outperforms the combination with learned appearance [8] in terms of AUPRC regardless of the chosen patch and dictionary size. Moreover, learning as little as 10 context filters gives the same or even better performance than learning 100 appearance filters, thus confirming that our approach reduces potential redundancy.

As expected, learning appearance filters using SC [8] improves performance over k-means (at a parity of dictionary size), but it is much slower: AUPRC are 0.8748 vs 0.8557 on IVCM, 0.77 vs 0.7460 on VC6, 0.7955 vs 0.7857 on BF2D; speed 25-30 mins vs a few seconds. However, learning 10 context filters with k-means yields better AUPRC than [8] (0.8866 vs 0.8748 on IVCM, 0.7911 vs 0.77 on VC6, 0.7966 vs 0.7955 on BF2D), although in [8] SC is used. Also, while learning with SC is time-consuming for filter banks larger than 100 (several days are reportedly needed to learn a filter bank of 121 filters), a few minutes are required to learn as many as 200 context filters with k-means, in case a larger dictionary is needed (e.g. for VC6). As a result, our method combining OOF with context filters learned using k-means outperforms significantly the method proposed in [8]: best AUPRC figures are 0.9078 vs 0.8748 on IVCM, 0.8368 vs 0.7700 on VC6, 0.8057 vs 0.7955 on BF2D.

4 Conclusion

Boosting hand-crafted features with learned filters has recently emerged as a successful technique to compensate for limits of HCFs and fully-learned approaches. We have proposed a novel combination method in which HCFs are paired with learned context filters to enhance pixel representation including inter-object relationships. Quantitative results suggest that our segmentation framework for curvilinear structures can be used for different image modalities and get top-rank performance running in a few minutes only. Our future work will investigate the combination of learned context filters with our recently proposed HCF,

SCIRD [15], and the design of new ones to exploit optimally the information obtained by the appearance model.

References

1. Ikram, M., Ong, Y., Cheung, C., Wong, T.: Retinal vascular caliber measurements: Clinical significance, current knowledge and future perspectives. Ophthalmologica (2013)
2. Annunziata, R., Kheirkhah, A., Aggarwal, S., Cavalcanti, B.M., Hamrah, P., Trucco, E.: Tortuosity classification of corneal nerves images using a multiple-scale-multiple-window approach. In: OMIA, MICCAI (2014)
3. Frangi, A.F., Niessen, W.J., Vincken, K.L., Viergever, M.A.: Multiscale vessel enhancement filtering. In: Wells, W.M., Colchester, A.C.F., Delp, S.L. (eds.) MICCAI 1998. LNCS, vol. 1496, pp. 130–137. Springer, Heidelberg (1998)
4. Soares, J.V., Leandro, J.J., Cesar, R.M., Jelinek, H.F., Cree, M.J.: Retinal vessel segmentation using the 2-d gabor wavelet and supervised classification. IEEE TMI (2006)
5. Santamaría-Pang, A., Colbert, C.M., Saggau, P., Kakadiaris, I.A.: Automatic centerline extraction of irregular tubular structures using probability volumes from multiphoton imaging. In: Ayache, N., Ourselin, S., Maeder, A. (eds.) MICCAI 2007, Part II. LNCS, vol. 4792, pp. 486–494. Springer, Heidelberg (2007)
6. Law, M.W.K., Chung, A.C.S.: Three dimensional curvilinear structure detection using optimally oriented flux. In: Forsyth, D., Torr, P., Zisserman, A. (eds.) ECCV 2008, Part IV. LNCS, vol. 5305, pp. 368–382. Springer, Heidelberg (2008)
7. Honnorat, N., Vaillant, R., Paragios, N.: Graph-based geometric-iconic guide-wire tracking. In: Fichtinger, G., Martel, A., Peters, T. (eds.) MICCAI 2011, Part I. LNCS, vol. 6891, pp. 9–16. Springer, Heidelberg (2011)
8. Rigamonti, R., Lepetit, V.: Accurate and efficient linear structure segmentation by leveraging ad hoc features with learned filters. In: Ayache, N., Delingette, H., Golland, P., Mori, K. (eds.) MICCAI 2012, Part I. LNCS, vol. 7510, pp. 189–197. Springer, Heidelberg (2012)
9. Becker, C., Rigamonti, R., Lepetit, V., Fua, P.: Supervised feature learning for curvilinear structure segmentation. In: Mori, K., Sakuma, I., Sato, Y., Barillot, C., Navab, N. (eds.) MICCAI 2013, Part I. LNCS, vol. 8149, pp. 526–533. Springer, Heidelberg (2013)
10. Hannink, J., Duits, R., Bekkers, E.: Crossing-preserving multi-scale vesselness. In: Golland, P., Hata, N., Barillot, C., Hornegger, J., Howe, R. (eds.) MICCAI 2014, Part II. LNCS, vol. 8674, pp. 603–610. Springer, Heidelberg (2014)
11. Sironi, A., Lepetit, V., Fua, P.: Multiscale centerline detection by learning a scale-space distance transform. In: CVPR (2014)
12. Tu, Z., Bai, X.: Auto-context and its application to high-level vision tasks and 3d brain image segmentation. IEEE TPAMI (2010)
13. Coates, A., Ng, A.Y.: Learning feature representations with k-means. In: Neural Networks: Tricks of the Trade (2012)
14. Law, M.W.K., Chung, A.C.S.: An oriented flux symmetry based active contour model for three dimensional vessel segmentation. In: Daniilidis, K., Maragos, P., Paragios, N. (eds.) ECCV 2010, Part III. LNCS, vol. 6313, pp. 720–734. Springer, Heidelberg (2010)
15. Annunziata, R., Kheirkhah, A., Hamrah, P., Trucco, E.: Scale and curvature invariant ridge detector for tortuous and fragmented structures. In: A. Frangi et al. (eds.) MICCAI 2015, Part III. LNCS vol. 9351, pp. 588–595. Springer, Heidelberg (2015)

Kernel-Based Analysis of Functional Brain Connectivity on Grassmann Manifold

Luca Dodero[1], Fabio Sambataro[2], Vittorio Murino[1,4] and Diego Sona[1,3]

[1] Pattern Analysis and Computer Vision, PAVIS, Istituto Italiano di Tecnologia, Genova, Italy
[2] pRED, NORD DTA, Hoffmann-La Roche, Ltd Basel, Switzerland
[3] NeuroInformatics Laboratory, Fondazione Bruno Kessler, Trento, Italy
[4] University of Verona, Department of Computer Science, Strada Le Grazie 15 Verona, Italy

Abstract. Functional Magnetic Resonance Imaging (fMRI) is widely adopted to measure brain activity, aiming at studying brain functions both in healthy and pathological subjects. Discrimination and identification of functional alterations in the connectivity, characterizing mental disorders, are getting increasing attention in neuroscience community.

We present a kernel-based method allowing to classify functional networks and characterizing those features that are significantly discriminative between two classes.

We used a manifold approach based on Grassmannian geometry and graph Laplacians, which permits to learn a set of sub-connectivities that can be used in combination with Support Vector Machine (SVM) to classify functional connectomes and for identifying neuroanatomically different connections.

We tested our approach on a real dataset of functional connectomes with subjects affected by Autism Spectrum Disorder (ASD), finding consistent results with the models of aberrant connections in ASD.

Keywords: Manifold, Grassmann, fMRI, Classification, Connectivity, Autism.

1 Introduction

Resting-state Functional Magnetic Resonance Imaging (rs-fMRI) is commonly used to study functional process at brain-scale. A common way to describe functional brain activity is through network representation, defining a set of nodes corresponding to brain areas, and a set of weighted links describing the amount of correlated functionality between regions time-series during rest or specific tasks. An important goal in functional connectivity studies is to discriminate healthy from pathological subjects affected with mental disorders like autism or schizophrenia and in the meantime determine which features (i.e. brain areas or connections) are significantly different.

To solve this problem, *Support Vector Machine* (SVM) [1] has been widely adopted to classify brain graphs, using the time-series correlation between brain

N. Navab et al. (Eds.): MICCAI 2015, Part III, LNCS 9351, pp. 604–611, 2015.
DOI: 10.1007/978-3-319-24574-4_72

regions as features [2, 3]. These features, however, lie on the Euclidean space, which does not reflect the real geometry of the data, making classification more difficult.

To cope with this issue, sparse connectivity learning based on the properties of semi-positive definite matrices has been proposed to define and classify sub-connectivity patterns [4].

Manifold approaches have been recently proposed for functional connectivity classification, in particular taking into account the properties of positive definite matrices, which form a Riemannian Manifold. In particular, transport on the manifold of covariance matrices has been successfully applied for longitudinal studies [5]. A regularized version of graph Laplacians has been recently adopted to classify both functional and structural connectomes on the Riemannian Manifold [6]. This approach, however, does not allow to delineate the discriminative connections in the graph populations.

Aiming at characterizing connections across groups, brain functional network extracted through Independent Component Analysis (ICA) [7], have been analyzed on Grassmann Manifold [8]. Although this approach reaches good classification performance, the analysis of functional networks is limited to the networks extracted by ICA (i.e. default mode network, visual, sensory motor, etc.).

In this work, we propose a classification algorithm able to classify functional connectomes through subspace learning. Indeed, using graph Laplacians and the corresponding eigenspaces, which underlie functional sub-connectivity patterns, in combination with the properties of Grassmann Manifold and spectral theory, we defined a positive definite kernel which can be directly used with SVM for classification.

We compared our approach with kernel-based methods on Riemannian Manifold and on Euclidean space using a public dataset of functional connectivity with patients affected by Autism Spectrum Disorder (ASD). Results showed that our analysis on Grassmann Manifold outperforms other approaches. We also proposed a strategy to reconstruct the connectivity described by the subspace learned through the classification step, allowing to find aberrant connectivities typically involved in ASD disease with results in line with the literature.

2 Functional Connectivity Classification on Manifold

Our method has two main goals, classification of functional connectomes between healthy and pathological subjects and subsequently identification of discriminative connections between classes.

Starting from a set of connectivity graphs $W_s \in \mathbb{R}^{n \times n}$, $s = 1...S$ with positive weights $w_{ij} \geq 0$, where n is the number of nodes in the graph and S is the total number of samples belonging to two different classes $y_s \in \{-1, 1\}$, we computed for each W_s the corresponding Normalized Graph Laplacian, defined as follow:

$$L_s = D_s^{-\frac{1}{2}}(D_s - W_s)D_s^{-\frac{1}{2}} \tag{1}$$

where $D_s = \text{diag}\left(\sum_j w_{ij}\right)$ is the degree matrix of W_s.

Taking into account the properties of Laplacians, we can decompose each L_s as follow:

$$L_s = B_s \Lambda_s B_s' \tag{2}$$

where $B_s = [b_s^1, ..., b_s^n]$ is the eigenspace and Λ_s is the diagonal matrix with corresponding eigenvalues. Since Laplacians are *semi-definte positive matrices*, λ_s are always positives $0 = \lambda_1 \leq ..... \leq \lambda_n$.

Functional connectivity is often better described in a lower dimensional space of the graph spectrum [9]. Hence, in order to analyze functional differences in mental disorders, we used the corresponding eigenspace of the graph Laplacians. An interesting property of the eigenspace is that each eigenvector b_s^i or a combination of k eigenvectors, which define a subspace of B, highlights a set of connectivity patterns of the whole graph (i.e. a sub-graph) [10].

Reordering the eigenvectors of each sample in ascending order, where the smallest hold the most connected components of the graph, it is possible to analyze functional brain networks on Grassmann Manifold, allowing to identify the smallest subspace able to classify functional graphs with the best performance.

2.1 Grassmann Manifold

Given a space $\mathbb{R}^n$, the set of linear subspaces of dimension k, $0 < k \leq n$ does not lie on the Euclidean space but on the Riemannian manifold known as Grassmann manifold defined as $\mathcal{G}(k, n)$. Each subspace is represented as an orthonormal matrix $X \in \mathbb{R}^{n \times k}$, where $X^T X = I$, whose columns span the corresponding k-dimensional subspace of $\mathbb{R}^n$, denoted as $span(X)$.

On the manifold, each subspace is mapped as a point and the distance between two points is defined as geodesic distance, which is the length of the shortest path in the manifold connecting the two points. Afterwards, the distance between points on the manifold or between the two subspaces $span(X)$ and $span(Y)$ can be computed through the principal angles, $0 \leq \theta_1 \leq \theta_2 \leq ... \leq \theta_k \leq \pi/2$ as follow:

$$\begin{aligned} \cos(\theta_i) = & \max_{u_i \in span(X)} \max_{v_i \in span(Y)} u_i^T v_i \\ & \text{s.t. } ||u_i||_2 = 1 \;\; ||v_i||_2 = 1 \\ & \qquad u_i^T u_j = 0 \;\; v_i^T v_j = 0 \end{aligned} \tag{3}$$

where the principal angle θ_1 is the smallest one between two subspaces.

Through the notion of principal angles, geodesic distance on the manifold can be easily computed as:

$$d_g(X, Y) = ||\Theta||_2, \qquad \Theta = \theta_1, ..., \theta_n \tag{4}$$

However, in order to use this distance for classification tasks, a kernel function has to be defined. Closely related to the principal angles, *projection metric* is an approximation of the geodesic distance widely adopted as alternative metric between subspaces on $\mathcal{G}$ [11]:

$$d_{proj} = ||X^T Y||_F^2 = \sum_i^k \cos^2(\theta_i) \tag{5}$$

where $\cos(\theta_i)$ can be computed through Singular Values Decomposition:

$$X^T Y = USV^T \tag{6}$$

where $S = \text{diag}(\cos\theta_1 ... \cos\theta_k)$, X and Y represent in our framework the subspace of Laplacians with fixed dimension k. Projection metric defines a positive definite kernel, known as Grassmannian kernel, denoted by $K(X,Y) = ||X'Y||_F^2$ that can be directly used in kernel-based classification algorithms like SVM.

In order to classify healthy and pathological subjects, with the minimal subset of connectivity patterns, we investigated all linear subspaces $B_s^k = [b_s^1, ..., b_s^k]$ varying their dimension from $k = 1, ..., n$. The aim was to identify through a classification step which subset of connectivity is more discriminative between healthy and pathological subjects.

Hence, we computed the projection metric (Eq. 5) to define the kernel matrix for each B_s^k and we adopted SVM classifier, using *lib-SVM* [1]. We used leave-one-out cross-validation for all the experiments, using as training set $S-1$ samples, where S is the total number of subjects and one subject as testing. We performed parameter tuning to reach the best classification accuracy.

2.2 Identification of Discriminative Functional Connections

Once evaluated the performance for each k, we identified the subspace of dimension k that gives the highest classification performance. Therefore, we approximated the original Laplacians only using the information embedded in the subspace described by the k connectivities, catching discriminative information through the outer product of the k eigenvectors as follows:

$$\tilde{L_s} = B_s^k {B_s^k}^T \tag{7}$$

We approximated each sample with the corresponding $\tilde{L_s}$ and on the new representation of functional brain connectivity, we performed two sample t-test analysis for each connections in the graph. The output of this procedure, after False Discovery Rate correction ($p < 0.05$), is a set of connectivity candidates that can be seen as the discriminative connections between healthy and pathological subjects.

3 Material

In our experiments, we tested our framework using functional connectivity dataset extracted from Autism Spectrum Disorder (ASD) connectome database released by UCLA [12], based on Power Atlas, describing the brain in terms of 264

Algorithm 1. Classification of Functional Connectivity on Grassmann Manifold

Data: Similarity matrix for each Subject: $W_s \in \mathbb{R}^{n \times n}$
Result: Identification of discriminative connections through subspace learning
Normalized Graph Laplacian $L_s = D_s^{-\frac{1}{2}} (D_s - W_s) D_s^{-\frac{1}{2}}$
Eigenvector Decomposition $[B_s, \Lambda_s] = \text{eig}(L_s)$
for $k = 1$ *to* n **do**
  $K(s,t) = ||B_s^{k^T} B_t^k||_F^2 \quad \forall s \neq t \in \{1, ..., S\}$
  Leave one out SVM: $P(k) = \text{SVM}(K)$
Connectivity Matrices Approximation: $\hat{k} = \underset{k}{\text{argmax}}\ P(k)$
$\tilde{L_s} = B_s^{\hat{k}} B_s^{\hat{k}^T}$
Connection-wise Two-sample t-test on $\tilde{L_s}$

regions (ROIs) [13]. ASD dataset contains two groups of rs-fMRI connectomes, with 37 healthy and 42 pathological subjects, respectively, built computing pair-wise Pearson correlation connectivity matrices (z-transformed). Further details of acquisition and pre-processing are explained in [14]. As commonly done with functional connectivity based on cross-correlation, we focused our attention only on positive correlations.

4 Results and Discussion

We applied our kernel-based approach using projection metric on Grassmann Manifold (**Grass-Kernel**) and we compared the results in term of classification accuracy with kernel-based method on Riemannian manifold using Log-Euclidean distance (**GK-LogE**) computed using regularized Laplacians as done in [6]. Finally, we also compared the method with baseline solutions directly using the vectorized connectivity matrices with Gaussian kernel SVM (**GK**) and linear kernel SVM (**LK**) in the Euclidean space.

Fig. 1 shows the trend of classification accuracy in autism functional dataset with varying k. We obtained two peaks, for $k = 11$ and $k = 24$. Overall, we obtained the best performance of accuracy using less than 5% of the whole information.

Tab. 1 shows the results of classification accuracy for each tested method. Our approach based on Grassmann-Kernel reaches the best performances, with an overall improvement of 4% wrt to LK baseline. We also computed sensitivity (patients correctly identified) as well as the specificity (percentage of controls correctly identified) reaching a sensitivity of 73.81% and specificity of 51.35%. Our classification algorithm produces a low number of false positive, being successful in patients identification, however it produces many false negatives.

These results highlight the importance of subspace learning. In fact, we outperforms kernel-based methods on Riemannian Manifold and in the Euclidean space, where the information of the whole network is used with less success.

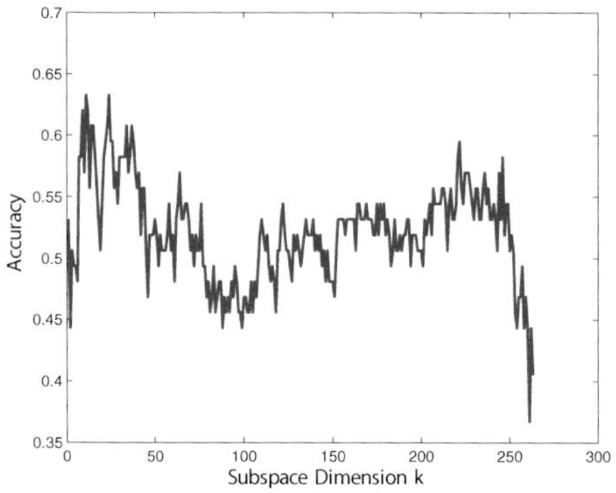

Fig. 1. Classification Accuracy varying the subspace dimension k

Even in our approach, considering the entire eigenspace (i.e. all the connectivity information) causes low accuracy (see Fig. 1).

Beyond the improved performance, the subspace learning framework proposed, allows a further investigation. The analysis on Grassmann Manifold permits to reconstruct the original connectivity graphs using low-rank approximation through Eq. 7. The eigenvalues are not used in the low-rank approximation as they were not used during classification. It is therefore possible to find discriminative connections that characterize a specific mental disorder, which are better represented in this low-rank approximation.

Fig. 2 shows qualitative results of significant connections. Red connections identify higher connectivity in healthy subjects while blue connections identify an higher connectivity strength in pathological subjects. We decided to use $k = 24$ in order not to loose the information belonging to the first k eigenvectors.

Our results showed widespread alterations of brain connectivity in individuals with autism within the motor system. In particular, the connectivity within precentral gyrus was decreased [16], whereas the connectivity of this region with striatal regions was increased [17]. Also, we found ectopic connectivity of precentral and striatal and occipital regions [18]. This results are consistent with a general model of aberrant connectivity in ASD. Furthermore, they suggest the importance of motor dysfunction which has been associated with difficulties in learning and performing gestures that are important for social and communicative behavior [16].

Table 1. Classification accuracy of all compared methods

	Manifold Laplacian		Euclidean Space	
	Grass-Kernel	GK-LogE	GK	LK
Accuracy	**63.29**%	60.76%	56%	59.49%

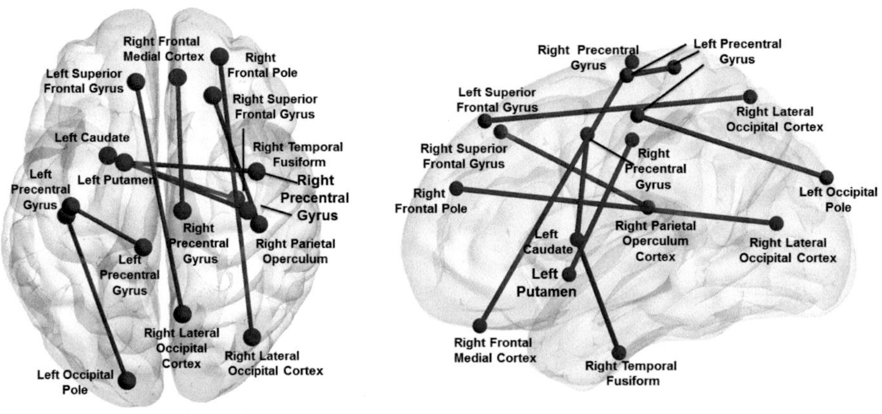

Fig. 2. Significant discriminative connections in ASD dataset using $k = 24$. **Left**: 2D Axial view. **Right**: 2D Sagittal view. Significant connections were visualized with the BrainNet Viewer [15]

5 Conclusion

In this work, we have presented a framework to classify connectivity graphs of healthy and pathological subjects, which helps to identify aberrant connections characterizing functional connectivity in Autism Spectrum Disorder. Managing the information of the eigenspace of graph Laplacians into Grassmann manifold classification framework, we are able to learn which subspace contains the most discriminative neuroanatomical information of functional connectivity across two classes.

Classification through subspace learning permits to approximate network connectivity, discarding those connectivity that can be seen as unnecessary for discrimination. In fact, thanks to this new representation, it is possible to perform a posterior analysis of connectivity patterns in the subspace, finding aberrations in the motor system of the human brain that were recently described in neuroscientific ASD studies [16, 17, 18].

References

1. Chang, C.-C., Lin, C.-J.: Libsvm: a library for support vector machines. ACM Transactions on Intelligent Systems and Technology (TIST) 2(3), 27 (2011)
2. Satterthwaite, T.D., Wolf, D.H., Ruparel, K., Erus, G., Elliott, M.A., Eickhoff, S.B., Gennatas, E.D., Jackson, C., Prabhakaran, K., Alex, Smith, o.: Heterogeneous impact of motion on fundamental patterns of developmental changes in functional connectivity during youth. Neuroimage 83, 45–57 (2013)
3. Craddock, R.C., Holtzheimer, P.E., Hu, X.P., Mayberg, H.S.: Disease state prediction from resting state functional connectivity. Magnetic Resonance in Medicine 62(6), 1619–1628 (2009)

4. Eavani, H., Satterthwaite, T.D., Filipovych, R., Gur, R.E., Gur, R.C., Davatzikos, C.: Identifying sparse connectivity patterns in the brain using resting-state fmri. NeuroImage 105, 286–299 (2015)
5. Ng, B., Dressler, M.: Transport on riemannian manifold for functional connectivity-based classification. In: Golland, P., Hata, N., Barillot, C., Hornegger, J., Howe, R. (eds.) Medical Image Computing and Computer-Assisted Intervention MICCAI 2014. LNCS, vol. 8674, pp. 405–412. Springer, Heidelberg (2014)
6. Dodero, L., Quang, M.H., Biagio, M.S., Murino, V., Sona, D.: Kernel-based classification for brain connectivity graphs on the riemannian manifold of positive definite matrices. In: IEEE International Symposium of Biomedical Imaging ISBI 2015 (2015)
7. Calhoun, V.D., Liu, J., Adalı, T.: A review of group ica for fmri data and ica for joint inference of imaging, genetic, and erp data. Neuroimage 45(1), 163 (2009)
8. Fan, Y., Liu, Y., Wu, H., Hao, Y., Liu, H., Liu, Z., Jiang, T.: Discriminant analysis of functional connectivity patterns on grassmann manifold. Neuroimage 56(4), 2058–2067 (2011)
9. Ghanbari, Y., Bloy, L., Shankar, V., Edgar, J.C., Roberts, T.L., Schultz, R., Verma, R.: Functionally driven brain networks using multi-layer graph clustering. In: Golland, P., Hata, N., Barillot, C., Hornegger, J., Howe, R. (eds.) Medical Image Computing and Computer-Assisted Intervention MICCAI 2014. LNCS, vol. 8675, pp. 113–120. Springer, Heidelberg (2014)
10. Dodero, L., Gozzi, A., Liska, A., Murino, V., Sona, D.: Group-wise functional community detection through joint laplacian diagonalization. In: Golland, P., Hata, N., Barillot, C., Hornegger, J., Howe, R. (eds.) Medical Image Computing and Computer-Assisted Intervention MICCAI 2014. LNCS, vol. 8674, pp. 708–715. Springer, Heidelberg (2014)
11. Hamm, J., Lee, D.D.: Grassmann discriminant analysis: a unifying view on subspace-based learning. In: Proceedings of the 25th International Conference on Machine Learning, pp. 376–383. ACM (2008)
12. Brown, J.A., Rudie, J.D., Bandrowski, A., Van Horn, J.D., Bookheimer, S.Y.: The ucla multimodal connectivity database: a web-based platform for brain connectivity matrix sharing and analysis. Frontiers in Neuroinformatics 6 (2012)
13. Power, J.D., Schlaggar, B.L., Petersen, S.E.: Studying brain organization via spontaneous fmri signal. Neuron 84(4), 681–696 (2014)
14. Rudie, J.D., Brown, J.A., Beck-Pancer, D., Hernandez, L.M., Dennis, E.L., Thompson, P.M., Bookheimer, S.Y., Dapretto, M.: Altered functional and structural brain network organization in autism. NeuroImage: Clinical (2012)
15. Xia, M., Wang, J., He, Y.: Brainnet viewer: a network visualization tool for human brain connectomics. PloS One 8(7), e68910 (2013)
16. Nebel, M.B., Eloyan, A., Barber, A.D., Mostofsky, S.H.: Precentral gyrus functional connectivity signatures of autism. Frontiers in Systems Neuroscience 8 (2014)
17. Di Martino, A., Kelly, C., Grzadzinski, R., Zuo, X.N., Mennes, M., Mairena, M.A., Lord, C., Castellanos, F.X., Milham, M.P.: Aberrant striatal functional connectivity in children with autism. Biological Psychiatry 69(9), 847–856 (2011)
18. Noonan, S.K., Haist, F., Müller, R.A.: Aberrant functional connectivity in autism: evidence from low-frequency bold signal fluctuations. Brain Research 1262, 48–63 (2009)

A Steering Engine: Learning 3-D Anatomy Orientation Using Regression Forests

Fitsum A. Reda, Yiqiang Zhan, and Xiang Sean Zhou

Syngo Innovation, Siemens Healthcare, Malvern 19355, PA, USA
{fitsum.reda,yiqiang.zhan,xiang.zhou}@siemens.com

Abstract. Anatomical structures have intrinsic orientations along one or more directions, e.g., the tangent directions at points along a vessel central-line, the normal direction of an inter-vertebral disc or the base-to-apex direction of the heart. Although auto-detection of anatomy *orientation* is critical to various clinical applications, it is much less explored compared to its peer, "auto-detection of anatomy *location*". In this paper, we propose a novel and generic algorithm, named as "steering engine", to detect anatomy orientation in a robust and efficient way. Our work is distinguished by three main contributions. (1) Regression-based colatitude angle predictor: we use regression forests to model the highly non-linear mapping between appearance features and anatomy colatitude. (2) Iterative colatitude prediction scheme: we propose an algorithm that iteratively queries colatitude until longitude ambiguity is eliminated. (3) Rotation-invariant integral image: we design a spherical coordinates-based integral image from which Haar-like features of any orientation can be calculated efficiently. We validate our method on three diverse applications (different imaging modalities and organ systems), i.e., vertebral column tracing in CT, aorta tracing in CT and spinal cord tracing in MRI. In all applications (tested on a total of 400 scans), our method achieves a success rate above 90%. Experimental results suggest our method is fast, robust and accurate.

1 Introduction

"Where is the anatomical structure?", "What is the orientation of the anatomical structure?"- these are two fundamental questions frequently asked during medical image interpretation. Here, "anatomy orientation" denotes one or more intrinsic directions of an anatomical structure. These directions can be defined by local landmarks or global organ shapes, and are consistent across population. Some examples of anatomy orientations (see Fig. 1) include the tangent directions at points along a vessel central-line, the normal direction of an intervertebral disc or the base-to-apex direction of the heart. The ability to automatically detect anatomy orientation will not only benefit various clinical use cases, e.g., automatic MR scan planning [6], but will also pave a way to other high-level medical image analysis tasks. For example, predicting a local vessel orientation is a fundamental task for tracing algorithms [1], [2].

N. Navab et al. (Eds.): MICCAI 2015, Part III, LNCS 9351, pp. 612–619, 2015.
DOI: 10.1007/978-3-319-24574-4_73

Early studies of anatomy orientation detection often exploit prior knowledge of specific anatomies. For example, template matching that relies on the Matched Filter Theorem or eigenanalysis of Hessian matrix has been widely used to determine local vessel orientation and perform tracing [1], [2]. These methods are dependent on strong priors of the anatomy under study, and do not generalize to other anatomies, such as the heart or the vertebral-column.

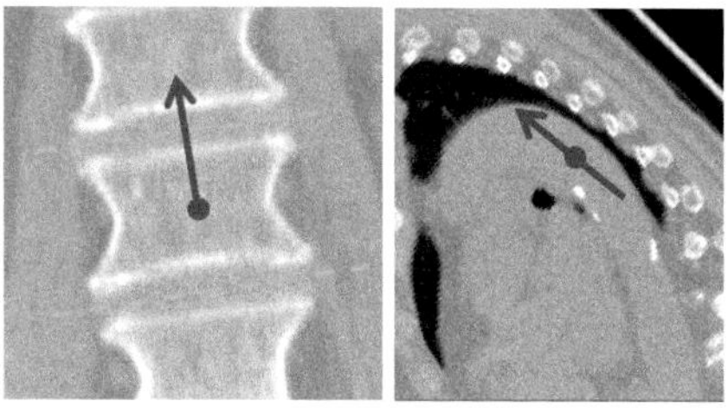

Fig. 1. Anatomy orientation (red arrow) of a vertebral column (left) and an aorta segment (right).

From another perspective, machine learning technologies have revolutionized the landscape of medical image analysis. In the areas of anatomy detection or segmentation, learning-based approaches have provided generic solution to different organs in different modalities [3]-[7]. However, learning technologies in detecting anatomy orientation remain under explored. One pioneer work is the marginal space learning (MSL) [8] which formulates the detection of anatomy orientation as a classification problem. This technique uses a classification model trained to detect a desired orientation. During testing, it uniformly samples the orientation space and performs an exhaustive test, which induces significant computational cost.

In contrast to classification, regression methods directly estimate the most probable hypothesis (anatomy orientation in our study) without exhaustively testing the hypothesis space. In fact, recent works have shown the power of regression-based approaches for medical image analysis, including landmark localization [4],[6], object detection [5],[7], and segmentation [3],[11]. Inspired by these works, we resort to regression paradigm and propose a method for efficient detection of anatomy orientation in a generic fashion (across modalities and organ systems), which is named as "steering engine". Our steering engine has three major novelties. (1) Regression-based colatitude angle predictor: we use regression forests to model the highly nonlinear mapping between appearance features and anatomy colatitude. (2) Iterative colatitude prediction scheme: we propose an algorithm that iteratively queries colatitude until longitude ambiguity is eliminated. (3) Rotation-invariant integral image: we design a spherical coordinates-based integral image from which Haar-like features of any orientation can be calculated very efficiently. With these three hallmarks, our method is able to detect anatomy orientations robustly and efficiently. In addition, thanks to the nature of machine learning techniques, our method is highly scalable to different organ systems and imaging modalities.

2 Methods

2.1 Problem Definition

Given a 3-D image patch $\wp$ (black cuboid in Fig 2a) containing an anatomy of interest (blue cuboid in Fig 2a), the goal of our steering engine is to determine the anatomy orientation $\hat{\boldsymbol{v}}$ using appearance features. In this paper, we assume the anatomy is roughly located at the center of the patch. In practice, this can be achieved by existing anatomy detection algorithms or manual operators. The anatomy orientation $\hat{\boldsymbol{v}}$ is parameterized as (α, β), where $\alpha \in [0°, 90°]$ is the colatitude, which is the complement of the latitude or the angle measured from the positive z-axis (North Pole), and $\beta \in [0°, 360°)$ is the longitude, which is the counter-clockwise angle in the xy-plane measured from the positive x-axis (see Fig. 2b). This work does not discuss the prediction of the ϕ degree-of-freedom, which describes the anatomy's spinning around its own axis (see Fig 2b). In fact, after $\hat{\boldsymbol{v}}$ is determined, prediction of ϕ is a 2D orientation detection problem, which can also be solved by our steering engine. We plot the 3D orientation space (α, β) in a 2-D polar system, with α as the radius and β as the angle measured from the polar axis. As shown in Fig 2c, each black dot denotes a hypothesis in the orientation space. Fig 2d shows the corresponding 3D orientation space, in which the red dot denotes the North Pole.

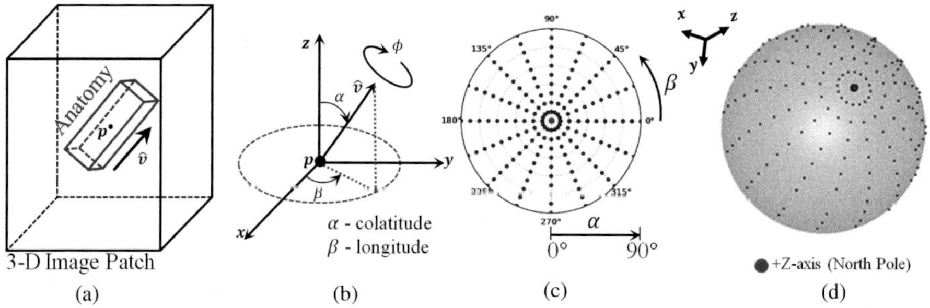

Fig. 2. Problem definition and orientation space.

2.2 Regression-Based Anatomy Colatitude Prediction

To achieve a generic solution, learning-based approaches are preferred. Recall one of the representative learning-based approaches, Marginal Space Learning (MSL) [8], in which orientation prediction is formulated as a classification problem as

$$(\alpha, \beta)_{\text{opt}} = \text{argmax}_{\alpha \in [0°, 90°], \beta \in [0°, 360°)}\, C(\wp_{\alpha,\beta}), \tag{1}$$

where $\wp_{\alpha,\beta}$ is the original patch $\wp$ rotated by (α, β), and $C(\cdot)$ is a pre-trained classifier that maps $\wp_{\alpha,\beta}$ to a score which indicates if the anatomy orientation within the patch is along the desired direction. As shown in Eq. 1, at run-time, each (α, β) hypothesis needs to be evaluated by $C(\cdot)$ and the hypothesis that maximizes the score is the predicted anatomy orientation. Assuming the orientation space is quantized into a 1° resolution, Eq. 1 needs to evaluate 32,400 (360×90) hypotheses, which induces high computational cost.

To achieve efficient orientation detection, we resort to regression paradigm. Mathematically, the orientation prediction is formulated as

$$(\alpha, \beta)_{\text{opt}} = \boldsymbol{R}(\wp). \tag{2}$$

At run-time, the pre-trained regressor $\boldsymbol{R}(\cdot)$ evaluates $\wp$ only *once* to estimate orientation. Compared to classification paradigm, which uses exhaustive test, the regression-based method has immense potential for run-time efficiency. The remaining challenge is how to learn the highly non-linear function that maps visual features of $\wp$ to anatomy orientation (α, β). In this study, we select random forests (RF) [10] as the regressor. Since RF comprises a set of non-linear decision trees with feature selection capability, it is able to model the highly non-linear mapping between visual features (observable variables) and anatomy orientation (latent variables). In addition, we simplify the regressand from the orientation vector (α, β) to the colatitude variable α. This strategy is designed for two reasons. First, a single-regressand mapping function is usually less complex to learn than a multi-regressand mapping function. Second, since the longitude β is a circular variable, the longitude statistics required by standard RF training cannot be calculated in a trivial way.

The colatitude predictor can then be described as

$$\alpha = \boldsymbol{RF}(\boldsymbol{\mathcal{F}}(\wp)), \tag{3}$$

where $\boldsymbol{RF}$ denotes a trained regression forest, and $\boldsymbol{\mathcal{F}}(\wp)$ denotes the visual features of $\wp$ [6], [12]. In this study, we use Haar-like features which comprise one or multiple cuboids (refer to [6] for more details). These features are automatically selected in the regression forest training stage. We train the regression forest as suggested in [10].

2.3 Iterative Colatitude Prediction and Patch Reorientation

Since Eq. 3 predicts only anatomy colatitude, it still cannot provide complete 3D anatomy orientation. To address this problem, we design an iterative algorithm exploiting a unique property of the 3D orientation space that all longitudes converge at the North Pole. In other words, as shown in Fig 2c, the smaller the colatitude the less the ambiguity of 3-D orientations with respect to different longitudes. For example, while orientations on the equator (colatitude = 90°) vary a lot with different longitudes, the orientation at the North Pole (colatitude = 0°) is not affected by longitude at all. Accordingly, our algorithm iteratively performs colatitude prediction and patch reorientation until the predicted colatitude from the reoriented patch is close to zero, i.e., until the orientation ambiguity from the unknown longitude is eliminated.

A schematic explanation of our algorithm is shown in Fig. 3. We denote a patch $\wp$ rotated by (α, β) as $\wp_{\alpha,\beta}$, and let $\wp_{\alpha_0,\beta_0}$ $(\alpha_0 = 0°, \beta_0 = 0°)$ is the original patch. The green dot in Fig 3a denotes the ground truth of the anatomy orientation in $\wp_{\alpha_0,\beta_0}$. Our algorithm first predicts the anatomy colatitude $\alpha_1 = \boldsymbol{RF}\left(\boldsymbol{\mathcal{F}}\left(\wp_{\alpha_0,\beta_0}\right)\right)$, which narrows down the orientation hypothesis to the yellow circle in Fig 3a. Due to possible prediction errors, the narrowed hypothesis may not include the ground truth (whose colatitude is $\hat{\alpha}_0$). To further reduce the size of the hypothesis space along the longitude, we sample M uniformly spread hypothesis along the longitude (blue points on the yellow circle in Fig. 3a). Intuitively, the "best" hypothesis (the dark-blue point in Fig 3a) should be the one that is closest to the ground truth (green point), i.e., the hypothesis with the minimum *relative* colatitude to the ground truth. Mathematically the optimal longitude β_1 is determined by,

$$\beta_{i+1} = \arg\min_{\{\beta_{ij}|j=1,\ldots,M\}} \boldsymbol{RF}\left(\boldsymbol{\mathcal{F}}\left(\wp_{\alpha_{i+1},\beta_{ij}}\right)\right). \tag{4}$$

Then, $\wp_{\alpha_0,\beta_0}$(Fig. 3b) is re-oriented to $\wp_{\alpha_1,\beta_1}$ (Fig. 3d), and its orientation space is re-centered at α_1, β_1 (dark-blue point in Fig. 3a moved to orientation space center in Fig. 3c). Comparing Fig. 3b and 3d, the colatitude $\hat{\alpha}_0$ in $\wp_{\alpha_0,\beta_0}$has decreased to $\hat{\alpha}_1$ in $\wp_{\alpha_1,\beta_1}$. Hence, the longitude ambiguity (yellow circles in Fig. 3a and 3c) has greatly reduced. The colatitude prediction and patch reorientation steps are then iterated until the colatitude is less than a small threshold.

Although Eq. 4 looks similar to the classification-based approach (Eq. 1), it essentially has much higher run-time efficiency due to two reasons. First, the colatitude predictor shrinks the full hypothesis space to a circle at each iteration (yellow band in Fig 3a). Second, along with the iterations, even the sizes of the shrunk hypothesis reduce dramatically (yellow circle shrinks from Fig. 3a to Fig. 3c).

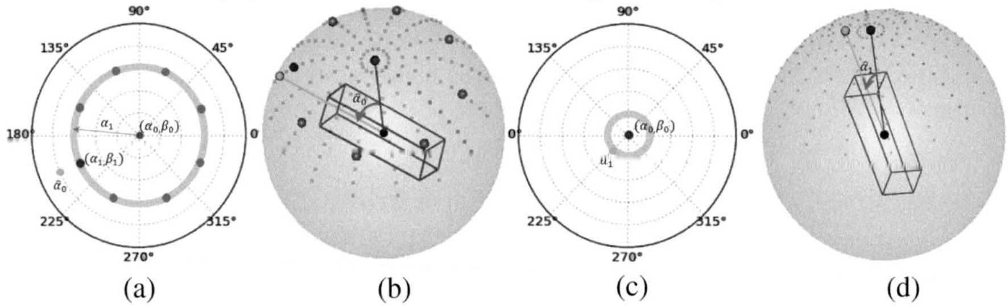

Fig. 3. Illustration of iterative colatitude prediction and patch reorientation.

2.4 Rotation-Invariant Integral Image for Fast Feature Calculation

The colatitude predictor uses Haar-like features, which can be efficiently computed using the integral image [9]. However, during the iterative colatitude prediction and patch re-orientation, the integral image needs to be recalculated, since it is not rotationally invariant. To speed-up this computationally expensive task, we propose a rotation-invariant integral image built on the spherical coordinate system. We illustrate our idea in 2D first. Given a 2-D image I (Fig. 4a), its integral image II (Fig. 4c) can be built on the polar-coordinate system as,

$$II(r,\theta) = \textstyle\sum_{r'<r,\theta'<\theta} I(r'\cos\theta', r'\sin\theta'). \tag{5}$$

$II(r,\theta)$ is equal to the sum of the intensities within the red sector in Fig 4a. The basic element of Haar-like features, i.e., the sum of the intensity within a circular trapezoid (Fig. 4b) (approximation of a rectangle), can be quickly calculated using four entries in the integral image as,

$$A = II(r_2, \theta_2) + II(r_1, \theta_1) - II(r_2, \theta_1) - II(r_1, \theta_2) \ . \tag{6}$$

To calculate the same Haar element on a rotated image (rotated by $\Delta\theta$), instead of re-computing the integral image, we only change the coordinates of the four entries in the integral image as:

$$A' = II(r_2, \theta_2 + \Delta\theta) + II(r_1, \theta_1 + \Delta\theta) - II(r_2, \theta_1 + \Delta\theta) - II(r, \theta_2 + \Delta\theta) \tag{7}$$

Eq. 6 and Eq. 7 show the "rotation-invariant" property of the polar coordinate system-based integral image. The same integral image can be reused to calculate Haar-like features at any orientation. The same idea can be extended to 3-D using the spherical coordinate system.

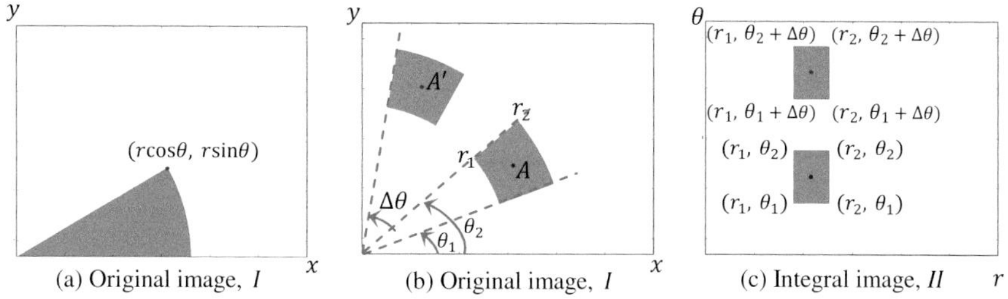

Fig. 4. Illustration of the rotation-invariant integral image in 2D.

3 Experimental Results

We evaluate our method on different anatomical structures, organ-systems and imaging modalities. The datasets have large variability due to different scanners (GE, Siemens and Philips), exposure time, field of view, or contrast level. Voxel resolutions range from 0.5 to 5 mm. To validate the generalization ability of our method, we use the same RF training parameters: number of trees (100), minimum sample size to split (20), maximum node size (10), number of features to examine per node (100).

Local Anatomy Orientation Detection: This experiment aims to evaluate the performance of our steering engine on local orientation detection on two anatomical structures, vertebrae and aorta segments (see Fig 1 for orientation definition). The input of the algorithm is a fixed-size volume of interest (VOI) containing the anatomical structure, which is roughly located at the center of the VOI. We compare the steering engine with (a) classification-based approach (as described in Eq. 1) and (b) Steering engine w/o RIII: steering engine without using the rotation-invariant integral image (RIII).

Table I shows the results on 280 vertebrae VOIs (the steering engine is trained from another 100 CTs). We achieved <4° average error, <8° error in ~95% VOIs with run-time speed of ~1.33 seconds (a single thread implementation on an Intel Xeon 2.3GHz CPU). The classification-based approach achieved inferior accuracy/robustness and is ~65 times slower. Without using RIII, the accuracy is similar but the speed is ~3 times slower. We conduct similar comparison on 220 aorta VOIs (trained by another 50 CTs). Despite the lack of contrast in 50% of the VOIs, our steering engine is still accurate, robust and fast. The comparisons across the detection methods show similar pattern as the vertebrae use case.

Table 1. Quantitative comparison of orientation detection methods

Vertebrae	Accuracy (°)	Robustness (%)				Speed (seconds)
		<1°	<2°	<4°	<8°	
Classification	4.13±2.01	0.00%	11.36%	49.54%	97.27%	86.13±13.81
Steering engine w/o RIII	3.75±1.88	**5.00%**	19.09%	80.90%	97.73%	4.47±1.09
Steering engine	**3.74±2.17**	4.54%	**22.72%**	**85.91%**	95.90%	**1.33±0.42**
Aorta	Accuracy (°)	Robustness (%)				Speed (seconds)
		<1°	<2°	<4°	<8°	
Classification	5.09±2.45	0.19%	9.26%	39.67%	83.01%	29.29±5.25
Steering engine w/o RIII	**4.86±2.45**	2.41%	9.92%	33.97%	**84.98%**	0.88±0.23
Steering engine	4.97±2.75	**4.42%**	**22.12%**	**39.82%**	83.18%	**0.32±0.14**

Anatomical Structure Tracing: We further evaluate the steering engine on more clinically relevant applications - tracing anatomical structures. Given a starting location, we (a) identify anatomy orientation using the steering engine, (b) step to a new location along the orientation, and (c) iterate (a) and (b) until a maximum number of steps or a stopping location is reached. We tested it on tracing (a) the aorta in 100 CTs (with varying level of contrast, and some with no contrast), (b) the vertebral column in 100 CTs, and (c) the spinal cord in 200 DIXON-sequence MRIs, and achieved a success rate (based on evaluation of experienced professionals) of 95%, 96% and 90%, respectively. Fig 5 shows representative example tracing results. Tracing was successful despite the large anatomical shape variation in a scoliosis subject (Fig 5a), and a kyphosis subject (Fig 5b), the lack of contrast in the CT (Fig 5d), the noisy reconstruction CT kernel (Fig 5c) and large shape and intensity variation surrounding the spinal cord (Fig 5e and 5f).

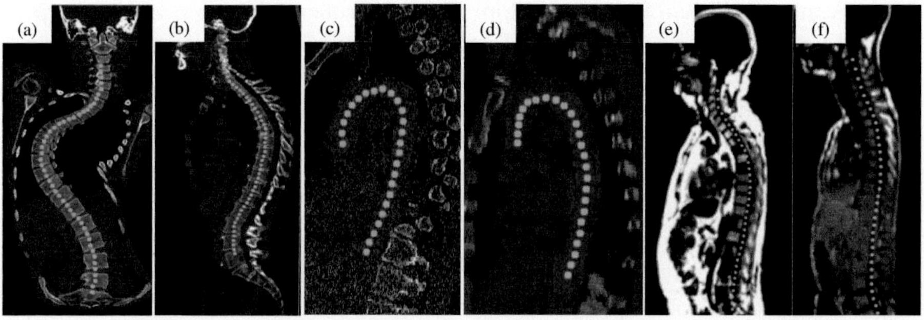

Fig. 5. Representative results of anatomy tracing in different use cases.

4 Conclusions

We presented a novel and generic steering engine to automatically detect anatomy orientation in a robust and efficient fashion. We employ regression forests to learn the highly non-linear relationship between anatomy visual features and anatomy colatitude. By exploiting a unique property of the 3D orientation space, we design an iterative algorithm to determine anatomy orientation by fully relying on colatitude prediction. In addition, we design a rotation-invariant integral image to efficiently calculate Haar-like features at any orientations. We tested our steering engine on both local anatomy orientation detection and anatomy tracing. In all three applications, including different imaging modalities (CT and MRI Dixon) and anatomies (vertebral column, spinal cord and aorta), experimental results show that our method is fast, robust and accurate.

References

1. Friman, O., Hindennach, M., Kühnel, C., Peitgen, H.: Multiple hypothesis template tracking of small 3D vessel structures. MedIA, 14(2010), 160–171 (2010)
2. Frangi, A.F., Niessen, W.J., Vincken, K.L., Viergever, M.A.: Multiscale vessel enhancement filtering. In: Wells, W.M., Colchester, A.C.F., Delp, S.L. (eds.) MICCAI 1998. LNCS, vol. 1496, pp. 130–137. Springer, Heidelberg (1998)
3. Lindner, C., Thiagarajah, S., Wilkinson, J.M., Consortium, T.A., Wallis, G.A., Cootes, T.F.: Fully Automatic Segmentation of the Proximal Femur Using Random Forest Regression Voting. IEEE Trans. Med. Imag. 32(8), 181–189 (2013)
4. Glocker, B., Feulner, J., Criminisi, A., Haynor, D.R., Konukoglu, E.: Automatic localization and identification of vertebrae in arbitrary field-of-view CT scans. In: Ayache, N., Delingette, H., Golland, P., Mori, K. (eds.) MICCAI 2012, Part III. LNCS, vol. 7512, pp. 590–598. Springer, Heidelberg (2012)
5. Yaqub, M., Kopuri, A., Rueda, S., Sullivan, P.B., McCormick, K., Noble, J.A.: A Constrained Regression Forests Solution to 3D Fetal Ultrasound Plane Localization for Longitudinal Analysis of Brain Growth and Maturation. In: Wu, G., Zhang, D., Zhou, L. (eds.) MLMI 2014. LNCS, vol. 8679, pp. 109–116. Springer, Heidelberg (2014)
6. Zhan, Y., Dewan, M., Harder, M., Krishnan, A., Zhou, X.S.: Robust automatic knee mr slice positioning through redundant and hierarchical anatomy detection. IEEE Trans. Med. Imag. 30(12), 2087–2100 (2011)
7. Criminisi, A., Robertson, D., Konukoglu, E., Shotton, J., Pathak, S., White, S., Siddiqui, K.: Regression Forests for Efficient Anatomy Detection and Localization in Computed Tomography Scans. MedIA 17(8), 1293–1303 (2013)
8. Zheng, Y., Barbu, A., Georgescu, B., Scheuering, M., Comaniciu, D.: Four-Chamber Heart Modeling and Automatic Segmentation for 3D Cardiac CT Volumes using Marginal Space Learning and Steerable Features. IEEE Trans. Med. Imag. 27(11), 1668–1681 (2008)
9. Viola, P., Jones, M.: Rapid object detection using a boosted cascade of simple features. In: Proc. IEEE CVPR, pp. 1-511 (2001)
10. Breiman, L.: Random forests. Machine Learning 45(1), 5–32 (2001)
11. Gao, Y., Shen, D.: Learning distance transform for boundary detection and deformable segmentation in ct prostate images. In: Proc. MLMI, pp. 93–100 (2014)
12. Skibbe, H., Reisert, M., Schmidt, T., Brox, T., Ronneberger, O., Burkhardt, H.: Fast Rotation Invariant 3D Feature Computation Utilizing Efficient Local Neighborhood Operators. IEEE PAMI 34(8), 1563–1575 (2012)

Automated Localization of Fetal Organs in MRI Using Random Forests with Steerable Features

Kevin Keraudren[1], Bernhard Kainz[1], Ozan Oktay[1], Vanessa Kyriakopoulou[2], Mary Rutherford[2], Joseph V. Hajnal[2], and Daniel Rueckert[1]

[1] Biomedical Image Analysis Group, Imperial College London
[2] Department Biomedical Engineering, King's College London

Abstract. Fetal MRI is an invaluable diagnostic tool complementary to ultrasound thanks to its high contrast and resolution. Motion artifacts and the arbitrary orientation of the fetus are two main challenges of fetal MRI. In this paper, we propose a method based on Random Forests with steerable features to automatically localize the heart, lungs and liver in fetal MRI. During training, all MR images are mapped into a standard coordinate system that is defined by landmarks on the fetal anatomy and normalized for fetal age. Image features are then extracted in this coordinate system. During testing, features are computed for different orientations with a search space constrained by previously detected landmarks. The method was tested on healthy fetuses as well as fetuses with intrauterine growth restriction (IUGR) from 20 to 38 weeks of gestation. The detection rate was above 90% for all organs of healthy fetuses in the absence of motion artifacts. In the presence of motion, the detection rate was 83% for the heart, 78% for the lungs and 67% for the liver. Growth restriction did not decrease the performance of the heart detection but had an impact on the detection of the lungs and liver. The proposed method can be used to initialize subsequent processing steps such as segmentation or motion correction, as well as automatically orient the 3D volume based on the fetal anatomy to facilitate clinical examination.

1 Introduction

Although the main focus of fetal Magnetic Resonance Imaging (MRI) is in imaging of the brain due to its crucial role in fetal development, there is a growing interest in using MRI to study other aspects of fetal growth, such as assessing the severity of intrauterine growth restriction (IUGR) [4]. In this paper, we present a method to automatically localize fetal organs in MRI (*heart*, *lungs* and *liver*), which can provide automated initialization for subsequent processing steps such as segmentation or motion correction [8].

The main challenge for the automated localization of fetal organs is the unpredictable orientation of the fetus. Two methodological approaches can be identified from the current literature on the localization of the fetal brain in MRI. The first approach seeks a detector invariant to the fetal orientation [6,9,7]. The second approach learns to detect fetuses in a known orientation and rotates the

N. Navab et al. (Eds.): MICCAI 2015, Part III, LNCS 9351, pp. 620–627, 2015.
DOI: 10.1007/978-3-319-24574-4_74

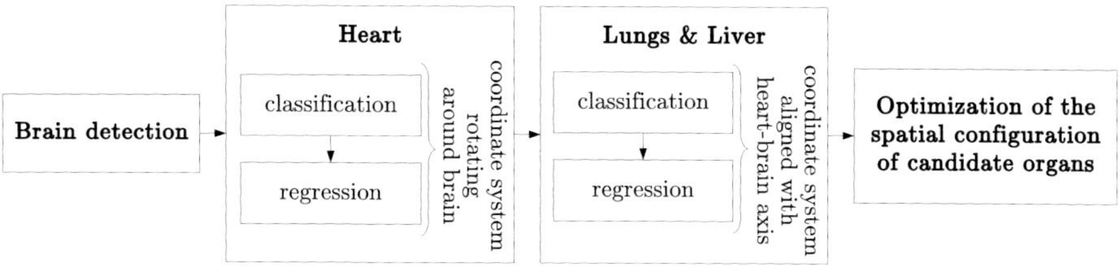

Fig. 1. Overview of the proposed pipeline for the automated localization of fetal organs in MRI.

test image [1]. We adopt this second approach in the present paper, but as illustrated by *steerable features* [12], it is more efficient to extract features in a rotating coordinate system than to rotate the whole 3D volume. We thus propose to extend the Random Forests (RF) framework for organ localization [10] with the extraction of features in a local coordinate system specific to the anatomy of the fetus.

A RF classifier [3] is an ensemble method for machine learning which averages the results of decision trees trained on random subsets of the training dataset, a process called *bagging*. Similarly, a RF regressor is an ensemble of regression trees. A RF classifier assigns a label to each voxel, resulting in a segmentation of the input image while a RF regressor assigns an offset vector to each voxel, allowing it to vote for the location of landmarks. Classification and regression forests can be combined so that only voxels assigned to a certain class can vote for the location of specific landmarks. This is of particular relevance when detecting landmarks within the fetus whose position has little correlation with surrounding maternal tissues. While [5] proposed to form trees that randomly alternate decision and regression nodes (*Hough Forest*), we chose to sequentially apply a classification and a regression forest. This enables us to benefit from generic RF implementations [11] while focusing on the key step of feature extraction.

At training time, image features are learnt in a coordinate system that is normalized for the age of the fetus and defined by the anatomy of the fetus (Fig. 2). At test time, assuming that the center of the brain is known, image features are extracted in a coordinate system rotating around the brain in order to find the heart. The lungs and liver are then localized using a coordinate system in which one axis is parallel to the heart-brain axis. An overview of our proposed pipeline is presented in Fig. 1. In the remainder of this paper, we will present our proposed method in Section 2 and evaluate it in Section 3 on two datasets of MRI scans. The first dataset, used for training and leave-one-out cross validation, consists of scans of 30 healthy and 25 IUGR subjects without significant motion artifacts. The second dataset (64 subjects) is used to evaluate the performance of the proposed method in the presence of motion artifacts.

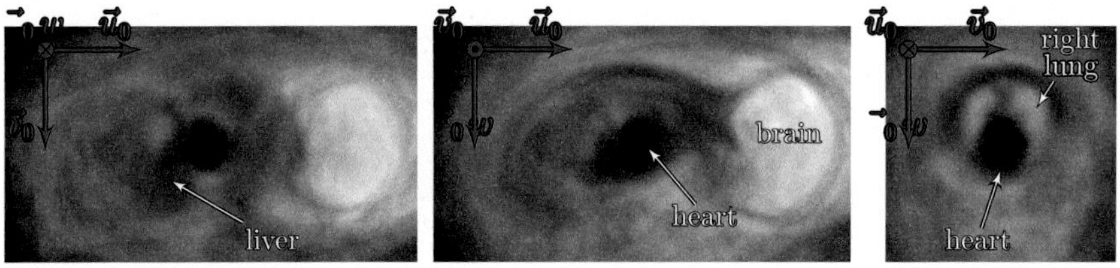

Coronal plane Sagittal plane Transverse plane

Fig. 2. Average image of 30 healthy fetuses after resizing (Section 2) and alignment defined by anatomical landmarks (Section 2). It highlights the characteristic intensity patterns in fetal MRI for the brain, heart, lungs and liver.

2 Method

Preprocessing: There is a large variability in the MR scans of fetuses due to fetal development. In particular, the length of the fetus increases by 50% between 23 weeks and term (40 weeks) [2]. We thus propose to normalize the size of all fetuses by resampling the images to an isotropic voxel size s_{ga} that is a function of the gestational age (GA), so that a fetus of 30 weeks is resampled to a voxel size s_{30}: $s_{ga} = \text{CRL}_{ga}/\text{CRL}_{30} \times s_{30}$, where CRL denotes the *crown-rump length* [2]. This differs from previously proposed methods which either ignored the GA [1,6,7] or only used it to define size constraints [9]. Moreover, fetal MRI is typically acquired as stacks of 2D images that freeze in-plane motion but form a 3D volume corrupted by fetal and maternal motion. The images are thus preprocessed using median filtering to attenuate motion artifacts.

Detecting Candidate Locations for the Heart: In theory, a detector could be trained on aligned images while at test time, it would be applied to all possible rotated versions of the 3D volume. However, in practice it would be too time consuming to explore an exhaustive set of rotations. In particular, the integral image that is used to extract intensity features would need to be computed for all tested rotations. Instead of rotating the image itself, we thus propose to rotate the sampling grid of the image features. This is done by defining a local orientation of the 3D volume for every voxel.

When training the classifier, all voxels are oriented using the anatomy of the fetus (Fig. 2 and Fig. 3a): $\vec{u}_0$ points from the heart to the brain, $\vec{v}_0$ from the left lung to the right lung and $\vec{w}_0$ from back to front ($\vec{w}_0 = \vec{u}_0 \times \vec{v}_0$). When applying the detector to a new image, in theory, all possible orientations $(\vec{u}, \vec{v}, \vec{w})$ should be explored. However, assuming that the location of the brain is already known [9], $\vec{u}$ can be defined as pointing from the current voxel x to the brain (Fig. 3b). In this case, only the orientation of the plane $\mathcal{P}_{x,\vec{u}}$ passing through x and orthogonal to $\vec{u}$ remains undefined. $(\vec{v}, \vec{w})$ are then randomly chosen so that they form an orthonormal basis of $\mathcal{P}_{x,\vec{u}}$. The rationale for this definition of $\vec{u}$ is that when x is positioned at the center of the heart, $\mathcal{P}_{x,\vec{u}}$ is the transverse plane of the fetal anatomy (Fig. 2). To address the sensitivity to the brain localization, a random offset is added to the estimated brain center with a 10mm range comparable to

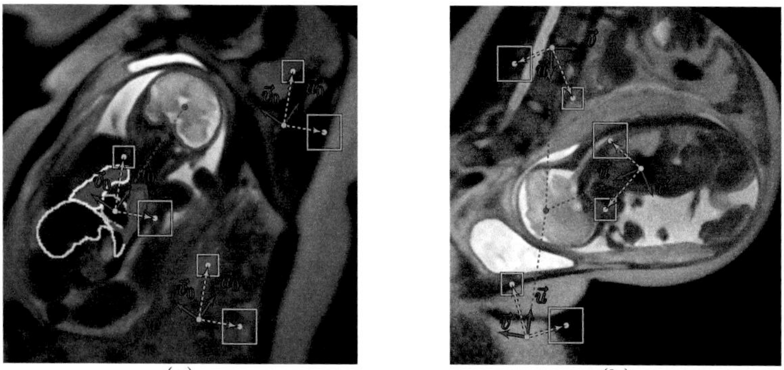

(a) (b)

Fig. 3. (a) When training the classifier, features (*light blue* squares) are extracted in the anatomical orientation of the fetus: $\vec{u}_0$ points from the heart (*green*) to the brain (*red*), and $\vec{v}_0$ points from the left lung (*blue*) to the right lung (*yellow*). The *pink* contour corresponds to the liver. (b) At testing time, features are extracted in a coordinate system rotating around the brain.

the prediction errors reported in [9]. Additionally, knowing the location of the brain, the search for the heart only needs to explore the image region contained between two spheres of radii R_1 and R_2 (Fig. 4) that are independent of the GA thanks to the size normalization.

The localization of the heart is performed in two stages: a classification forest is first applied to obtain for each voxel x a probability $p(x)$ of being inside the heart (Fig 5a). All voxels with $p(x) > 0.5$ are then passed on to a regression forest, which predicts for each of them the offset to the center of the heart. Using the predicted offsets, the probabilities are then accumulated in a voting process, and the voxels receiving the highest sum of probabilities are considered as candidate centers for the heart (Fig 5b). During classification, in order to increase the number of true positives, an initial random orientation of the plane $\mathcal{P}_{x,\vec{u}}$ is chosen and the detector is successively applied by rotating $(\vec{v}, \vec{w})$ with an angular step θ. The value of $(\vec{v}, \vec{w})$ maximizing the probability of the current voxel to be inside the heart is selected, and only this orientation of $\mathcal{P}_{x,\vec{u}}$ is passed on to the regression step.

Four types of features are used in the RFs: tests on image intensity, gradient magnitude, gradient orientation and distance from the current voxel to the brain. In order to be invariant to intensity shifts [10], image intensity or gradient magnitude features select two axis-aligned cube patches of random sizes at random offsets from the current voxel and compare their mean intensity. All features are extracted in the local orientation $(\vec{u}, \vec{v}, \vec{w})$. Similarly, during the voting process, the predicted offsets are computed with the same local orientation.

Detecting Candidate Locations for the Lungs and Liver: For each candidate location of the heart, candidate centers for the lungs and liver are detected. Similarly to the heart detection, a classification RF first classifies each voxel as either heart, left lung, right lung, liver or background. For each organ, a

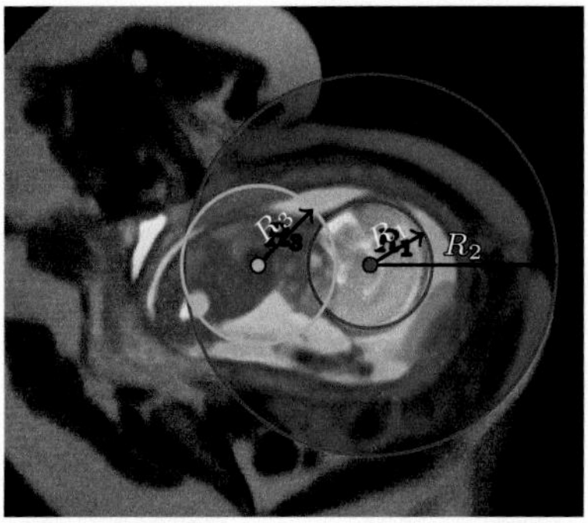

Fig. 4. Knowing the location of the brain, the search for the heart can be restricted to a narrow band within two spheres of radius R_1 and R_2 (*red*). Similarly, knowing the location of the heart, the search for the lungs and the liver can be restricted to a sphere of radius R_3 (*green*).

regression RF is then used to vote for the organ center. During training, the images are oriented according to the fetal anatomy (Fig. 2). During testing, both the location of the brain and heart are known and only the rotation around the heart-brain axis needs to be explored. For each voxel x, we can hence set $\vec{u} = \vec{u}_0$, and only the orientation of the plane $\mathcal{P}_{x,\vec{u}_0}$ remains unknown. $(\vec{v}, \vec{w})$ are thus randomly chosen to form an orthonormal basis of $\mathcal{P}_{x,\vec{u}_0}$.

In the set of features for the RFs, the distance from the current voxel to the brain, which was used in the detection of the heart, is now replaced by the distance to the heart. Additionally, the projection of the current voxel on the heart-brain axis is used in order to characterize whether the current voxel is below or above the heart relative to the brain. Similarly to the heart detection, the detector is run with an angular step θ. For each voxel, the value of θ maximizing the probability of being inside one of the organs of the fetus is selected.

Spatial Optimization of Candidate Organ Centers: The voting results from the regression RF are first smoothed with a Gaussian kernel. Local maxima are then extracted to form a set of candidates x_l for the center of each organ, $l \in L = \{$ heart, left lung, right lung, liver $\}$, along with their individual scores $p(x_l)$. Each combination of candidate centers is assigned a score (Eq. 1) based on the individual scores $p(x_l)$ and the spatial configuration of all organs:

$$\sum_{l \in L} \lambda p(x_l) + (1 - \lambda) e^{-\frac{1}{2}(x_l - \bar{x}_l)^\top \Sigma_l^{-1} (x_l - \bar{x}_l)} \tag{1}$$

where $\bar{x}_l$ is the mean position and Σ_l the covariance matrix for the organ l in the training dataset, computed in the anatomical coordinate system of the fetus. λ is a weight between individual scores and the spatial configuration of organs. Once the organ centers have been localized, the voting process can be reversed in order to obtain a rough segmentation (Fig. 5c).

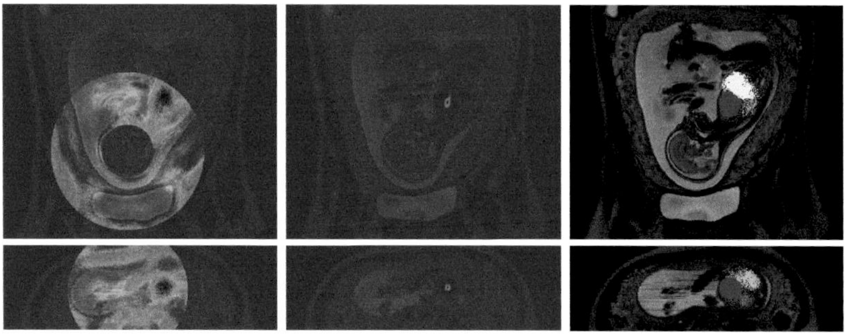

(a) (b) (c)

Fig. 5. (a) Probability of a voxel to be inside the heart. (b) Accumulated regression votes for the center of the heart. (c) After all organs have been located, the voting process can be reversed, resulting in a rough segmentation for each organ: heart (*blue*), left lung (*red*), right lung (*green*), liver (*yellow*).

3 Experiments

Datasets: Two datasets of 1.5T T2-weighted ssTSE images were used in this paper. The first dataset was used to train and validate the model in a leave-one-out cross validation, in the absence of motion artifacts. It consists of 55 scans covering the whole uterus for 30 healthy subjects and 25 IUGR subjects (scanning parameters: TR 1000ms, TE 98ms, 4mm slice thickness, 0.4mm slice gap). The second dataset is used to test the model in the presence of motion artifacts. There are 224 scans, from 64 healthy subjects, which do not all fully cover the fetal body (scanning parameters: TR 15000ms, TE 160ms, 2.5mm slice thickness, 1.5mm slice overlap). A ground truth segmentation for all fetal organs was provided by an expert for the first dataset. Due to the large number of images and the presence of motion artifacts, only the center of each organ has been manually annotated in the second dataset. The location of the brain is passed to the detector for the first dataset in order to evaluate the proposed method on its own while the method of [9] is used to localize the brain automatically in the second dataset, thus evaluating a fully automated localization of fetal organs. Both datasets cover the range of gestational ages from 20 to 38 weeks.

Results: The results are reported as detection rates in Table 1, where a detection is considered successful for the organ l if the predicted center is within the ellipsoid defined by $(x_l - y_l)^\top \Sigma_l^{-1}(x_l - y_l) < 1$ where y_l is the ground truth center. For the first dataset, Σ_l is the covariance matrix of the ground truth segmentation while for the second dataset, it is defined from training data as in Section 2. The distance error between the predicted centers and their ground truth are reported in Fig. 6. Although healthy and IUGR subjects were mixed in the training data, results are reported separately to assess the performance of the detector when fetuses are small for their gestational age. Training two detectors on each subset of the data did not improve the results. The higher detection

Table 1. Detection rates for each organs.

	Heart	Left lung	Right lung	Liver
1st dataset: healthy	90%	97%	97%	90%
1st dataset: IUGR	92%	60%	80%	76%
2nd dataset	83%	78%	83%	67%

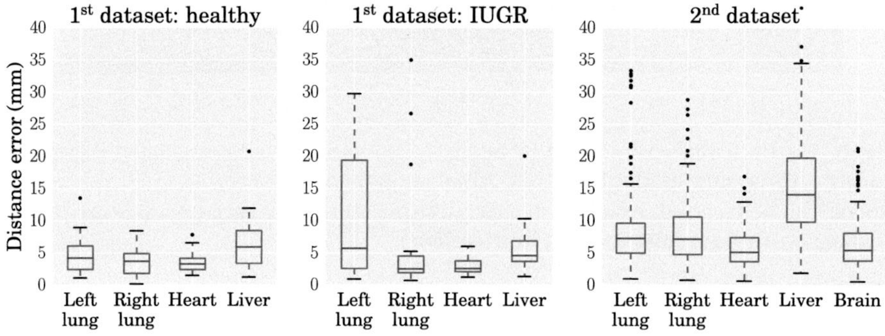

Fig. 6. Distance error between the predicted organ centers and their ground truth for the first dataset (30 healthy fetuses and 25 IUGR fetuses) and the second dataset (64 healthy fetuses).

rate for the lungs than for the heart for the healthy subjects of the first dataset (Table 1) is due to the detector overestimating the size of the heart (Fig 5c), which can be linked to the signal loss when imaging the fast beating heart. A decrease in performance can be observed for the detection of the lungs in IUGR fetuses, which can be associated with a reduction in lung volume reported in [4]. The asymmetry in the performance of the detector between the left and right lungs can be explained by the presence of the liver below the right lung, leading to a stronger geometric constraint in Eq. 1.

For the second dataset, the largest error for the detection of the brain detection using the method of [9] is 21mm, which is inside the brain and is sufficient for the proposed method to succeed. In 90% of cases, the detected heart center is within 10mm of the ground truth, which suggests that the proposed method could be used to provide an automated initialization for the motion correction of the chest [8]. Beside motion artifacts, the main difference between the first and second dataset is that the second dataset does not fully cover the fetal abdomen in all scans, which could explain its lower performance when detecting the liver. Training the detector takes 2h and testing takes 15min on a machine with 24 cores and 128 GB RAM. The parameters in the experiments were chosen as follows: $s_{30} = 1mm$, maximal patch size 30 pixels, maximal offset size 20 pixels, $\lambda = 0.5$, $\theta = 90°$.

4 Conclusion

We presented a pipeline which, in combination with automated brain detection, enables the automated localization of the lungs, heart and liver in fetal MRI. The localization results can be used to initialize a segmentation or motion correction, as well as to orient the 3D volume with respect to the fetal anatomy to facilitate clinical diagnosis. The key component to our method is to sample the image features in a local coordinate system in order to cope with the unknown orientation of the fetus. During training, this coordinate system is defined by the fetal anatomy while at test time, it is randomly oriented, within constraints set by already detected organs. In future work, the possibility to merge the classification and regression steps into a Hough Forest [5] will be investigated.

References

1. Anquez, J., Angelini, E., Bloch, I.: Automatic Segmentation of Head Structures on Fetal MRI. In: ISBI, pp. 109–112. IEEE (2009)
2. Archie, J.G., Collins, J.S., Lebel, R.R.: Quantitative Standards for Fetal and Neonatal Autopsy. American Journal of Clinical Pathology 126(2), 256–265 (2006)
3. Breiman, L.: Random Forests. Machine Learning 45(1), 5–32 (2001)
4. Damodaram, M., Story, L., Eixarch, E., Patkee, P., Patel, A., Kumar, S., Rutherford, M.: Foetal Volumetry using Magnetic Resonance Imaging in Intrauterine Growth Restriction. Early Human Development (2012)
5. Gall, J., Lempitsky, V.: Class-specific Hough Forests for Object Detection. In: CVPR, pp. 1022–1029. IEEE (2009)
6. Ison, M., Donner, R., Dittrich, E., Kasprian, G., Prayer, D., Langs, G.: Fully Automated Brain Extraction and Orientation in Raw Fetal MRI. In: Workshop on Paediatric and Perinatal Imaging, MICCAI, pp. 17–24. Springer (2012)
7. Kainz, B., Keraudren, K., Kyriakopoulou, V., Rutherford, M., Hajnal, J.V., Rueckert, D.: Fast Fully Automatic Brain Detection in Fetal MRI using Dense Rotation Invariant Image Descriptors. In: ISBI, pp. 1230–1233. IEEE (2014)
8. Kainz, B., Malamateniou, C., Murgasova, M., Keraudren, K., Rutherford, M., Hajnal, J., Rueckert, D.: Motion Corrected 3D Reconstruction of the Fetal Thorax from Prenatal MRI. In: Golland, P., Hata, N., Barillot, C., Hornegger, J., Howe, R. (eds.) MICCAI 2014, Part II. LNCS, vol. 8674, pp. 284–291. Springer, Heidelberg (2014)
9. Keraudren, K., Kyriakopoulou, V., Rutherford, M., Hajnal, J.V., Rueckert, D.: Localisation of the Brain in Fetal MRI Using Bundled SIFT Features. In: Mori, K., Sakuma, I., Sato, Y., Barillot, C., Navab, N. (eds.) MICCAI 2013, Part I. LNCS, vol. 8149, pp. 582–589. Springer, Heidelberg (2013)
10. Pauly, O., Glocker, B., Criminisi, A., Mateus, D., Möller, A., Nekolla, S., Navab, N.: Fast Multiple Organ Detection and Localization in Whole-Body MR Dixon Sequences. In: Fichtinger, G., Martel, A., Peters, T. (eds.) MICCAI 2011, Part III. LNCS, vol. 6893, pp. 239–247. Springer, Heidelberg (2011)
11. Pedregosa, F., et al.: Scikit-learn: Machine Learning in Python. Journal of Machine Learning Research 12, 2825–2830 (2011)
12. Zheng, Y., Barbu, A., Georgescu, B., Scheuering, M., Comaniciu, D.: Fast Automatic Heart Chamber Segmentation from 3D CT Data using Marginal Space Learning and Steerable Features. In: ICCV, pp. 1–8. IEEE (2007)

A Statistical Model for Smooth Shapes in Kendall Shape Space*

Akshay V. Gaikwad, Saurabh J. Shigwan, and Suyash P. Awate

Computer Science and Engineering Department,
Indian Institute of Technology (IIT) Bombay
suyash@cse.iitb.ac.in

Abstract. This paper proposes a novel framework for learning a statistical shape model from image data, automatically without manual annotations. The framework proposes a *generative model* for image data of individuals within a group, relying on a model of group shape variability. The framework represents shape as an equivalence class of pointsets and models group shape variability in Kendall shape space. The proposed model captures a novel shape-covariance structure that incorporates *shape smoothness*, relying on Markov regularization. Moreover, the framework employs a novel model for data likelihood, which lends itself to an inference algorithm of low complexity. The framework infers the model via a novel expectation maximization algorithm that *samples* smooth shapes in the Riemannian space. Furthermore, the inference algorithm normalizes the data (via similarity transforms) by optimal *alignment* to (sampled) individual shapes. Results on simulated and clinical data show that the proposed framework learns better-fitting compact statistical models as compared to the state of the art.

Keywords: Statistical shape model, Kendall shape space, geodesic distance, Markov model, shape sampling, shape alignment, image data normalization.

1 Introduction and Related Work

The typical notion of object shape [4,13] is an equivalence class of object boundaries / silhouettes, where the equivalence relation is given by a similarity transformation. These geometric invariance properties make shape space non-Euclidean. Following Kendall [8], representing shapes via pointsets with known correspondences, we model (i) preshape space as a subset of Euclidean space, i.e., an intersection of the unit hypersphere (for scale invariance) with a hyperplane through the origin (for translation invariance) and (ii) shape space with an additional rotational-invariance structure. While typical pointset-based shape models ignore this structure, the proposed method adapts shape modeling and inference to this Riemannian structure.

Unlike typical pointset-based shape models, the proposed model incorporates prior information that real-world objects have *smooth* boundaries. Such information is useful during (i) model learning: as regularization to counter the noise in image data (even errors in manual landmark placement) to produce more compact models; and (ii) model

* Thanks to the Royal Academy of Engineering 1314RECI076 and IIT Bombay 14IRCCSG010.

N. Navab et al. (Eds.): MICCAI 2015, Part III, LNCS 9351, pp. 628–635, 2015.
DOI: 10.1007/978-3-319-24574-4_75

application (e.g., segmentation with shape priors): to more effectively regularize the learned covariance, having several near-zero eigenvalues, to enforce smoother shapes.

Many early methods for statistical shape analysis rely on manually defined landmarks on image data [3] or templates [11]. Later methods optimize point positions relying on model covariance or information-theoretic criteria [2,4], but do *not* propose generative models. Medial representations [13] lead to sophisticated Riemannian statistical shape modeling approaches [6], but are limited to non-branching objects.

Some advanced approaches capture shape variability through nonlinear diffeomorphic warps of object boundaries [1,5,7,14]. Unlike our approach, such approaches entail joint statistical analysis in the very large dimensional Riemannian spaces of nonlinear diffeomorphisms coupled with the aligned boundaries. Some such approaches [5] enforce shape smoothness via current distance [14], which is a metric, but is computationally expensive as compared to the shape dissimilarity in our approach. Others [1] models object boundaries as missing data by treating deformations as hidden variables, somewhat analogous to our approach in Kendall shape space.

We propose a novel generative statistical model that relies on Kendall shape space and pointset-based shape representation. It introduces a novel prior on shape smoothness. It treats each individual shape pointset as a random variable, thereby modeling its distribution that can lead to more robust inference via expectation maximization (EM). The proposed EM relies on a novel algorithm for sampling smooth shapes.

2 Methods

We present a shape model in Kendall shape space including a Markov prior for shape smoothness, a computationally-efficient likelihood model for the observed image data given individual shapes, and EM inference involving sampling smooth shapes.

2.1 Statistical Shape Model Using Riemannian Distances and Smoothness Priors

We model each shape as an equivalence class of pointsets, where equivalence is defined via translation, rotation, and isotropic scaling. During model learning, given the correspondences between points in the mean shape and points in each individual shape, we infer point locations within each shape. The known correspondences allow us to order the points in each pointset and thereby represent each pointset as a vector.

Consider I individuals labeled $i = 1, \cdots, I$ with 3-dimensional anatomical shapes represented using pointsets of cardinality N. Let the *hidden* random vector Z_i model the shape for individual i, where an instance $z_i \in \mathbb{R}^D, D = 3N$. Let the *parameters* $\{\mu, C, \beta\}$ model the probability density function (PDF) of individual *shape pointsets*, i.e., $P(Z_i|\mu, C, \beta)$, where $\mu \in \mathbb{R}^D$ represents the group *mean*, $C \in \mathbb{R}^{D \times D}$ represents the unregularized group *covariance*, and $\beta \in \mathbb{R}^+$ represents the *smoothness* of the spatial variation of point locations in each shape. Without loss of generality, we constrain the mean shape μ and the individual shapes z_i to (i) have the centroid at the coordinate-space origin and (ii) be of unit norm. Thus, μ and $\{z_i\}_{i=1}^I$ lie in preshape space.

We propose to model a PDF on preshape space to capture the covariance structures of population shape variability and shape smoothness, by relying on the (i) approximate Normal law [10] that models a Gaussian PDF in the hypersphere's tangent space at mean μ and (ii) Markov-based Gibbs energy that penalizes deviation of each point's location from its neighbors' locations. We extend this PDF to shape space, enforcing rotation invariance. The Normal law relies on the logarithmic map $\text{Log}_\mu(\cdot)$ and the exponential map $\text{Exp}_\mu(\cdot)$. Let $z_{in} \in \mathbb{R}^3$ be the n-th point in the shape pointset for the i-th individual. The Markov model relies on a neighborhood system $\mathcal{N} := \{\mathcal{N}_n\}_{n=1}^N$, where $\mathcal{N}_n$ gives the set of neighbors of the n-th point. We enforce the same $\mathcal{N}$ for all pointsets. We propose to model shape variability, for all individuals i, via $P(z_i|\mu, C, \beta) :=$

$$\frac{1}{\eta(\mu, C, \beta)} \exp\left(-\frac{1}{2}(\text{Log}_\mu(z_i))^T C^{-1} \text{Log}_\mu(z_i) - \frac{\beta}{2} \sum_n \sum_{m \in \mathcal{N}_n} \|z_{in} - z_{im}\|_2^2\right), \quad (1)$$

where $\eta(\mu, c, \beta)$ is the normalization constant.

2.2 Efficient Model of Likelihood of Image Data Given Object Shape

Let random vector X_i model the observed image data for individual i. We propose a novel generative model for the observed individual data $\{x_i\}_{i=1}^I$ given individual shapes $\{z_i\}_{i=1}^I$. This paper considers the data to represent the object boundary by the set of pixels on the zero crossing of a level set fitted to the 0.5-valued isosurface of the fuzzy segmentation. Each *data pointset* x_i can have a different number of points M_i.

The proposed model relies on a novel dissimilarity measure $\delta(x_i, z_i)$ between two pointsets x_i and z_i of different cardinality, where the pointset z_i represents shape (in shape space). We design this dissimilarity measure by measuring the dissimilarity between pointsets, modulo translation t, rotation R, and scale s, as follows:

$$\delta(x_i, z_i) := \min_{s,R,t} \left(\sum_{n=1}^{N} \min_m \|x_{im}^{sRt} - z_{in}\|_2^2 + \sum_{m=1}^{M} \min_n \|x_{im}^{sRt} - z_{in}\|_2^2\right), \quad (2)$$

where data pointset x_i comprises M points $\{x_{im}\}_{m=1}^M$, shape pointset z_i comprises N points $\{z_{in}\}_{n=1}^N$, $s \in \mathbb{R}$ represents isotropic scaling, $R \in \mathbb{R}^{D \times D}$ represents rotation as an orthogonal matrix with determinant 1, $t \in \mathbb{R}^D$ represents translation, and $x_m^{sRt} := sRx_m + t$ is the location of the similarity-transformed point x_m.

The dissimilarity $\delta(\cdot, \cdot)$ is non-negative and symmetric. Ensuring pointsets x_i and z_i to be devoid of coincident points, which is straightforward, $\delta(x_i, z_i) = 0$ if and only if $x_i = z_i$. Thus, except the triangular inequality, $\delta(\cdot, \cdot)$ satisfies all metric properties. Moreover, unlike methods [5,15] using current distance having quadratic complexity in either pointset cardinality, $\delta(x_i, z_i)$ can be well approximated efficiently using algorithms of complexity close to $O(M + N)$ instead of $O(MN)$, by maintaining a list of nearest inter-pointset neighbors and updating it intermittently (see Section 2.3).

Thus, we model $P(x_i|z_i) := \exp(-\delta(x_i, z_i))/\gamma$, with normalization constant γ.

2.3 Parameter Inference Using Expectation Maximization

We fit the model to the data $\bar{\mathbf{x}} := \{x_i\}_{i=1}^I$ by computing the maximum-likelihood estimate (MLE) for the parameters. In this paper, β is a user-defined parameter. Denoting $\theta := \{\mu, C\}$, we solve for the MLE $\arg\max_\theta P(\bar{\mathbf{x}}|\theta)$, treating the shape pointsets $\bar{\mathbf{z}} := \{z_i\}_{i=1}^I$ as hidden / latent variables, via iterative EM optimization.

At iteration t, given parameter estimates $\theta^t := \{\mu^t, C^t\}$, the *E step* defines

$$Q(\theta;\theta^t) := E_{P(\bar{\mathbf{Z}}|\bar{\mathbf{x}},\theta^t)}[\log P(\bar{\mathbf{x}},\bar{\mathbf{Z}}|\theta)], \text{ where } P(\bar{\mathbf{x}},\bar{\mathbf{z}}|\theta) = \prod_{i=1}^{I} P(x_i|z_i)P(z_i|\theta). \quad (3)$$

The expectation is difficult to evaluate analytically and, hence, we approximate it using Monte-Carlo simulation of shape pointsets $\bar{\mathbf{z}}$ (see Section 2.4) as follows:

$$Q(\theta;\theta^t) \approx \widehat{Q}(\theta;\theta^t) := \frac{1}{S}\sum_{s=1}^{S} \log P(\bar{\mathbf{x}},\bar{\mathbf{z}}^s|\theta), \text{ where } \bar{\mathbf{z}}^s \sim P(\bar{\mathbf{Z}}|\bar{\mathbf{x}},\theta^t). \quad (4)$$

The *M step* obtains parameter updates $\theta^{t+1} := \arg\max_\theta \widehat{Q}(\theta;\theta^t)$. Given data $\bar{\mathbf{x}}$ and the sample individual shapes $\{\bar{\mathbf{z}}^s\}_{s=1}^S$, we alternatingly optimize the shape-distribution parameters μ, C and the internal parameters $\{s_i, R_i, t_i\}_{i=1}^I$, until convergence.

Update Mean μ: Given C and $\{\bar{\mathbf{z}}^s\}_{s=1}^S$, the optimal shape mean estimate $\widehat{\mu}$ is:

$$\arg\min_\mu \sum_{s=1}^{S}\sum_{i=1}^{I} (\text{Log}_\mu(z_i^s))^T C^{-1} \text{Log}_\mu(z_i^s). \quad (5)$$

The gradient of the objective function is the vector $C^{-1}\sum_s\sum_i \text{Log}_\mu(z_i^s)$ in the tangent space at μ. At a local minimum, the gradient magnitude must be zero. For all real-world data with finite variance, the null space of C^{-1} contains only the zero vector. So, the gradient magnitude can be zero only when $\sum_s\sum_i \text{Log}_\mu(z_i^s)$ is zero. We iteratively seek μ satisfying the aforementioned condition, via projected gradient descent (projection via C) where the iterative update, with a step size $\tau \in (0,1)$, is: $\widehat{\mu} \leftarrow \text{Exp}_{\widehat{\mu}}((\tau/SI)\sum_{s=1}^S\sum_{i=1}^I \text{Log}_{\widehat{\mu}}(z_i^s))$. We set $\tau = 0.5$ and find that a few iterations suffice for convergence.

Update Covariance C: We observe that the Markov regularization term enforcing shape smoothness, i.e., $\sum_n\sum_{m\in\mathcal{N}_n} 0.5\beta \parallel z_{in} - z_{im} \parallel_2^2$, is a quadratic function of z_i and can be rewritten as $0.5 z_i^T \Omega z_i$ where Ω is a sparse precision matrix that has (i) all diagonal elements $= 2\beta$, (ii) off-diagonal elements in row n and column $m \neq n$ as $(-\beta)$ when points n and m are neighbors, and (iii) all other off-diagonal elements $= 0$.

Given shape mean μ and shape-smoothness parameter β, the optimal covariance is

$$\arg\min_C \sum_{s=1}^{S}\sum_{i=1}^{I} \frac{1}{2}(\text{Log}_\mu(z_i^s))^T C^{-1}\text{Log}_\mu(z_i^s) + \frac{1}{2}(z_i^s)^T \Omega z_i^s + \log\eta(\mu,C,\beta). \quad (6)$$

The normalization constant $\eta(\mu,C,\beta)$ is difficult to evaluate analytically (even for the Normal law [10] alone). Nevertheless, we propose a novel scheme to achieve a good approximation for practical utility that is evident from the results in this paper. We assume that the distribution of shapes $P(Z_i|\theta)$ has sufficiently low variance such that the Gaussian PDF on $\text{Log}_\mu(z_i)$, in the tangent space at μ, can be approximated by a Gaussian PDF on $z_i - \mu$ in the tangent space. That is, we approximate locations z_i to the tangent-space locations $\breve{z}_i := \mu + \text{Log}_\mu(z_i)$. This observation allows us to treat $P(Z_i|\theta,\beta)$

as a product of two Gaussian PDFs in $\mathbb{R}^D$, i.e., (i) a Gaussian PDF $P(Z_i|\theta)$ with mean μ and covariance C restricted to the tangent space at μ, capturing the population shape variability, and (ii) a Gaussian PDF $P(Z_i|\beta)$ enforcing shape smoothness via a Markov-based Gibbs energy, with mean 0 and covariance Ω^{-1}. We know that the product of two Gaussian PDFs is also a Gaussian PDF where the normalization constant is easy to compute. In our case, the product Gaussian $P(Z_i|\theta)P(Z_i|\beta) \approx P(Z_i|\theta,\beta)$ has mean μ and covariance $C_{\text{reg}} = (C^{-1} + \Omega)^{-1}$ that is restricted to the tangent space at μ, which makes the normalization constant $\eta(\mu, C, \beta) \approx (2\pi)^{D/2}|C_{\text{reg}}|^{1/2}$. Thus, the optimal covariance $\widehat{C}_{\text{reg}}$ is the sample covariance of $\breve{z}_i^s$ in the tangent space: $\widehat{C}_{\text{reg}} = (1/(IS)) \sum_{s=1}^{S} \sum_{i=1}^{I} \text{Log}_\mu(z_i^s)\text{Log}_\mu(z_i^s)^T$. The optimal covariance $\widehat{C} = (\widehat{C}_{\text{reg}}^{-1} - \Omega)^{-1}$.

Update Similarity Transforms: Given sample shapes $\{\overline{\mathbf{z}}^s\}_{s=1}^S$, we optimize the similarity transforms modeled by $\{s_i, R_i, t_i\}_{i=1}^I$ independently for each individual i via

$$\arg\min_{s_i,R_i,t_i} \sum_{s=1}^{S} \left(\sum_{n=1}^{N} \min_m \| x_{im}^{s_i R_i t_i} - z_{in} \|_2^2 + \sum_{m=1}^{M} \min_n \| x_{im}^{s_i R_i t_i} - z_{in} \|_2^2 \right) \quad (7)$$

that optimally aligns the data pointset x_i to the set of sampled shape pointsets $\{z_i^s\}_{s=1}^S$. We optimize $\{s_i, R_i, t_i\}_{i=1}^I$ using gradient descent that relies on an efficient gradient computations. The objective function depends on mappings between each point in one pointset and the closest point in the other pointset (say, $\phi(\cdot)$ and $\psi(\cdot)$, detailed next). While the data pointset x_i has a large number of points densely distributed along the object boundary, the shape pointset z_i^s has far fewer points distributed sparsely along the object boundary (sufficient to model object shape). Assuming the parameter updates to be sufficiently small, (i) for most points x_{im} in the data pointset, the nearest point $z_{i\phi(m)}^s$ in the shape pointset before and after the update is unchanged and (ii) for most points z_{in}^s in the shape pointset, the displacement vector to the nearest point $x_{i\psi(n)}$ in the data pointset before and after the update is unchanged. This leads to a good approximation of the gradient of the objective function. For parameter t_i, the gradient is

$$\sum_{s=1}^{S} \left(\sum_{n=1}^{N} 2(x_{i\psi(n)}^{s_i R_i t_i} - z_{in}^s)^T \frac{\partial x_{i\psi(n)}^{s_i R_i t_i}}{\partial t_i} + \sum_{m=1}^{M} 2(x_{im}^{s_i R_i t_i} - z_{i\phi(m)}^s)^T \frac{\partial x_{im}^{s_i R_i t_i}}{\partial t_i} \right), \quad (8)$$

where $\partial x_{ij}^{s_i R_i t_i} / \partial t_i = \mathbb{I}$, the identity matrix. Similarly, for parameter s_i, $\partial x_{ij}^{s_i R_i t_i} / \partial s_i = R_i x_{ij}$. Equating each gradient to zero gives closed-form updates for s_i and t_i. To update the rotation matrix R_i, we perform projected gradient descent on the manifold on rotation matrices, with the gradient in ambient space as

$$\sum_{s=1}^{S} \left(\sum_{n=1}^{N} 2 s_i x_{i\psi(n)} (x_{i\psi(n)}^{s_i R_i t_i} - z_{in}^s)^T + \sum_{m=1}^{M} 2 s_i x_{im} (x_{im}^{s_i R_i t_i} - z_{i\phi(m)}^s)^T \right). \quad (9)$$

2.4 Sampling Smooth Shapes in Kendall Shape Space

The E step in Section 2.3 relies on Monte-Carlo approximation to the expectation by sampling, for all individuals i, shape pointsets $\{z_i^s\}_{s=1}^S$ from the posterior PDF

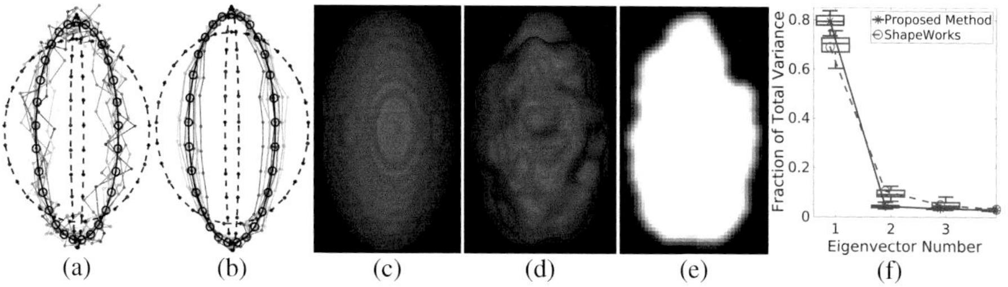

Fig. 1. Smooth-Shape Sampling using HMC. HMC-sampled shapes (colored), **(a)** without shape smoothness ($\beta = 0$) and **(b)** with shape smoothness ($\beta > 0$), from a distribution (on 2D ellipses, for easy viewing); solid black ellipse $\equiv$ mean pointset (point locations $\equiv$ small circles) and the principal mode of variation $\equiv$ dotted black ellipses. **Results on** 40 **Simulated Ellipsoids. (c)** Uncorrupted segmentation. **(d)** Corrupted segmentation with **(e)** a 2D slice of its distance transform (thresholded beyond $[-2, 2]$ mm for viewing). **(f)** Box plot showing fraction of total variance modeled by eigenvectors of estimated shape covariance.

$P(Z_i|\theta^t, \beta, x_i)$ that is proportional to $P(x_i|Z_i)P(Z_i|\theta^t, \beta)$. We sample using a novel adaptation of Hamiltonian Monte Carlo (HMC) [9] to the Riemannian space.

Following the analysis in Section 2.3 (used for updating C), which models the prior $P(Z_i|\theta^t, \beta)$ as a flat Gaussian on the tangent space of the hypersphere at μ^t, we consider the (i) likelihood $P(x_i|Z_i)$ as a non-flat PDF in $\mathbb{R}^D$ and (ii) posterior $P(Z_i|\theta^t, \beta, x_i)$ as a flat PDF on the tangent space at μ^t. Thus, we sample shapes z_i^s by (i) first sampling tangent vectors t^s in the tangent space at μ from the posterior PDF that is restricted to the tangent space and (ii) then producing shape samples $\{z_i^s\}_{s=1}^S$ by taking the exponential map $\text{Exp}_\mu(t^s)$. HMC sampling requires the gradient of $\log P(Z_i|\theta^t, \beta, x_i)$ with respect to Z_i, upto an additive constant. Because we represent the flat posterior PDF (of dimensionality $< D$) in the ambient D-dimensional space, a naive gradient computation can result in a gradient with a component orthogonal to the tangent space of shape space. Hence, within HMC, we replace the naive gradient by a (i) projected gradient onto the tangent space of preshape space followed by (ii) a rotational alignment with the shape mean μ. Figures 1(a)–(b) clearly shows that enforcing shape smoothness ($\beta > 0$) enables modeling realistic shape variations leading to realistic shape samples.

3 Results

We compare the proposed method with ShapeWorks [2,12] that optimizes point locations within shape pointsets, but restricts the points to the object-boundary isosurface in the (fuzzy) segmentation and neither enforces shape smoothness nor realigns data. Both methods use (i) $N = 64$ points in the shape model and (ii) similarity-transform-aligned distance transforms of the object boundaries as input. We initialize shape mean μ, and the neighborhood system $\mathcal{N}$, using the vertices and edges of a triangular mesh fitted to the object surface in one of the input images. After getting optimal θ^* via EM, we solve for optimal (i) individual pointsets z_i^* as $\arg\max_{z_i} P(z_i|x_i, \theta^*, \beta)$ and (ii) aligned data pointsets $x_i^{s_i^*, R_i^*, t_i^*}$ to aid evaluation (described next).

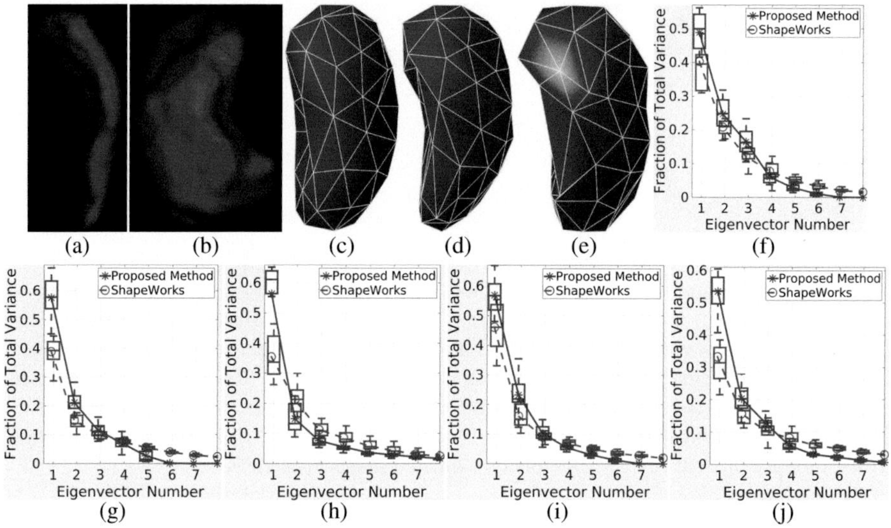

Fig. 2. Results on 186 **Clinical Brain MR Images.** A segmentation for **(a)** caudate, **(b)** thalamus. **(c)–(e)** Sampled thalamic shapes. Fraction of total variance modeled by eigenvectors of estimated shape covariance for **(f)** caudate, **(g)** globus pallidus, **(h)** hippocampus, **(i)** putamen, **(j)** thalamus.

Validation on Simulated Data: We generate 40 images of ellipsoids (Figure 1(c)) by introducing 1 major mode of variation, keeping 2 of the ellipsoid axis lengths to be fixed (40 mm) and varying the third (between 40–80 mm). The proposed method with $\beta = 0$ (without enforcing shape smoothness) and ShapeWorks were both able to learn this variation correctly, producing only 1 non-zero eigenvalue for the learned covariance matrix (in our case, C_{reg}). The optimal point locations z_{in}^*, within shape pointsets, were virtually exactly on the object boundary seen in the input images. We then *corrupt* the segmentation data with random perturbations to each object boundary (Figures 1(d)–(e)), get optimal shape-model parameter estimates θ^*, and repeat 20 times. With the corrupted data, the proposed method correctly detects a single mode of variation (Figure 1(f)). We set $\beta = 2$ to be sufficiently small to ensure that, within the optimal shape pointsets, point locations z_{in}^* were still within about 1 mm of the *uncorrupted* object boundary (mean 0.9 mm, standard deviation 0.2 mm). ShapeWorks incorrectly detected ≥ 2 modes of variation (Figure 1(f)), which is a less compact statistical model.

ShapeWorks restricts the shape pointset to lie on the segmented object boundary, asssuming it to be devoid of errors from, e.g., random noise or inhomogeneity. ShapeWorks may treat coarse- or fine-scale random spatial perturbations in object boundary's segmentation as part of the true signal, leading to inflated covariance. We prevent this by allowing a small deviation of the shape pointset from segmented object boundary.

Evaluation on Clinical Data: We used 186 T1-weighted magnetic resonance (MR) brain images (voxel size 1 mm^3 isotropic) with expert segmentations for the caudate, globus pallidus, hippocampus, putamen, and thalamus (Figures 2(a)–(e)) provided by the National Alliance for Medical Image Computing (`www.na-mic.org`).

The proposed method used $\beta = 2$ for all structures except the hippocampus where we set $\beta = 0.2$ (weaker smoothness enforced) because of the more complex hippocampal shape. We set β to be sufficiently small to ensure that distances between (i) points z^*_{in} in each optimal shape pointset and (ii) the closest point $x^{s^*_i, R^*_i, t^*_i}_{i\phi(n)}$ in the realigned data pointset were about the same as the distances in case of $\beta = 0$. To evaluate the robustness of the proposed method, we bootstrap sample 40 brains from the 186 brains, estimate the shape model, and repeat 20 times. Compared to ShapeWorks, the proposed method is able to learn more compact models (Figures 2(f)–(j)) by capturing a larger fraction of the total variance in fewer eigenvectors / dimensions.

Conclusions. The results show that the proposed method produces more compact shape models consistently for several anatomical structures, using novel contributions in the form of (i) Riemannian statistical shape modeling, (ii) Markov regularity for shape smoothness, (iii) optimal realignment of data during model learning, and (iv) a generative model that effectively deals with corrupted data via EM inference. We also propose a novel method for sampling smooth shapes in Kendall shape space. The proposed generic regularized shape model can be used for other applications.

References

1. Allassonniere, S., Kuhn, E., Trouve, A.: Construction of Bayesian deformable models via a stochastic approximation algorithm: A convergence study. Bernoulli 16(3), 641–678 (2010)
2. Cates, J., Fletcher, P.T., Styner, M., Shenton, M., Whitaker, R.: Shape modeling and analysis with entropy-based particle systems. In: Info. Proc. Med. Imag., pp. 333–345 (2007)
3. Cootes, T., Taylor, C., Cooper, D., Graham, J.: Active shape models - their training and application. Comp. Vis. Image Understanding 61(1), 38–59 (1995)
4. Davies, R., Twining, C., Taylor, C.: Statistical Models of Shape: Optimisation and Evaluation. Springer (2008)
5. Durrleman, S., Pennec, X., Trouve, A., Ayache, N.: Statistical models of sets of curves and surfaces based on currents. Med. Imag. Anal. 13(5), 793–808 (2009)
6. Fletcher, T., Lu, C., Pizer, S., Joshi, S.: Principal geodesic analysis for the study of nonlinear statistics of shape. IEEE Trans. Med. Imag. 23(8), 995–1005 (2004)
7. Glasbey, C.A., Mardia, K.V.: A penalized likelihood approach to image warping. J. Royal Statistical Society, Series B 63(3), 465–514 (2001)
8. Kendall, D.: A survey of the statistical theory of shape. Statist. Sci. 4(2), 87–99 (1989)
9. Neal, R.: MCMC using Hamiltonian dynamics. In: Handbook of Markov Chain Monte Carlo, pp. 113–162. Chapman and Hall, CRC Press (2010)
10. Pennec, X.: Intrinsic statistics on Riemannian manifolds: Basic tools for geometric measurements. J. Mathematical Imaging and Vision 25(1), 127–154 (2006)
11. Rangarajan, A., Coughlan, J., Yuille, A.: A Bayesian network framework for relational shape matching. In: Int. Conf. Comp. Vis., pp. 671–678 (2003)
12. SCI Institute: ShapeWorks: An open-source tool for constructing compact statistical point-based models of ensembles of similar shapes that does not rely on specific surface parameterization (2013), http://www.sci.utah.edu/software/shapeworks.html
13. Siddiqi, K., Pizer, S.: Medial Representations: Mathematics, Algorithms and Applications. Springer, Heidelberg (2008)
14. Vaillant, M., Glaunes, J.: Surface matching via currents. In: Info. Proc. Med. Imag., pp. 381–392 (2005)
15. Yu, Y., Fletcher, P., Awate, S.: Hierarchical Bayesian modeling, estimation, and sampling for multigroup shape analysis. In: Med. Image Comput. Comp. Assist. Interv., pp. 9–16 (2014)

A Cross Saliency Approach to Asymmetry-Based Tumor Detection

Miri Erihov, Sharon Alpert, Pavel Kisilev, and Sharbell Hashoul

IBM Research - Haifa, University of Haifa Campus, Haifa, 3498825, Israel

Abstract. Identifying regions that break the symmetry within an organ or between paired organs is widely used to detect tumors on various modalities. Algorithms for detecting these regions often align the images and compare the corresponding regions using some set of features. This makes them prone to misalignment errors and inaccuracies in the estimation of the symmetry axis. Moreover, they are susceptible to errors induced by both inter and intra image correlations. We use recent advances in image saliency and extend them to handle pairs of images, by introducing an algorithm for image cross-saliency. Our cross-saliency approach is able to estimate regions that differ both in organ and paired organs symmetry without using image alignment, and can handle large errors in symmetry axis estimation. Since our approach is based on internal patch distribution it returns only statistically informative regions and can be applied as is to various modalities. We demonstrate the application of our approach on brain MRI and breast mammogram.

1 Introduction

Identifying regions that break the inherent symmetry of the human anatomy is widely used to detect abnormalities and tumors in MRIs', CTs' and mammograms. These regions are computed by either comparing paired organs (e.g. breast), or within an organ, by dividing it along some symmetry axis (e.g. brain mid-sagittal plain). Regardless of the modality, automatic detection relies on accurate image alignment and symmetry axis estimation [4,2]. Both are able to achieve good performance on relatively similar images, meaning that abnormalities are nearly absent. Nevertheless, the existence of a tumor inherently violates the symmetry assumption making the images in question far less similar. In these cases, robust image alignment and symmetry axis estimation can be highly challenging unless the tumor location is known before hand.

Our approach attempts to solve this chicken and egg problem. It does so by formulating the problem as an image cross saliency problem. Our approach is motivated by recent advances in image saliency [7] that eliminate internal patch correlations. We extend this notion by also eliminating cross patch correlations between the two organ parts. By measuring only cross and internal patch statistics, image alignment is not needed and errors in symmetry axis estimation are simply translated to variations in patch statistics. Since the number of patches is large, small variations have only minor effect on salient regions.

N. Navab et al. (Eds.): MICCAI 2015, Part III, LNCS 9351, pp. 636–643, 2015.
DOI: 10.1007/978-3-319-24574-4_76

Much of the work and the literature on this topic is modality and organ specific. In a brain MRI [11], a non-rigid 3D registration was used after reflecting around the mid-sagittal plane and then an L_1 distance was applied to compare the two halves. The tumor detection survey [4], points out several asymmetry-based algorithms. The most prominent studies use symmetry constraint levels sets [6] and Bhattacharya coefficient [10] to model the differences between the images. Breast mammogram is another field in which such symmetry is important. The survey [2], points out that the vast majority of algorithms, first align the left and right breasts followed by extraction of the glandular tissue. Then various features like tumor appearance [5] are used to detect significant changes. In addition to brain MRI and breast mammogram, asymmetry detection is also used in prostate MRI [8] and breast MRI [1]. Where the later work, suggested using non localized features to avoid using 3D registration. However, exact tumor localization cannot be obtained using this approach.

2 Cross Saliency

The guiding principle of our approach is that a salient object consists of pixels whose local neighborhood (region or patch) is distinctive both internally and across its symmetric pair. We do that by constructing a saliency function that integrates two measures: cross pattern distinctness and cross image patch flow. Cross pattern distinctness assigns a score to each pixel based on a rectangular region (patch) around it. The guiding principle is that a pixel is salient if the pattern of the patch around it cannot be explained well by other image patches. The second measure patch flow is based on an assumption commonly used in natural images that the flow field between two similar images is smooth [3]. Basically, this assumption asserts that adjacent patches in one image, corresponds to adjacent patches in the other image. The guiding principle is that a patch is not likely to be salient if it behaves well under this assumption. The combination of both measures is important to handle the complex nature of images. This is best illustrated in Fig. 2 (bottom) where different cues mark different parts of the edema as salient. The combined measure marks the entire edema as salient. Next, we explain in details how each measure is computed.

2.1 Cross Patch Distinctness

Patch distinctness (PD) is determined by considering the internal statistics of the patches in the image. Again, the guiding principle is that a pixel is salient if the patch surrounding it cannot be explained well by other image patches. The common solution to measure patch distinctness is based on comparing each image patch to all other image patches using some L_p-distance. This solution overlooks the correlation between pixels and requires numerous patch-to-patch distance calculations. To circumvent that, Margolin et al. [7] suggested computing the L_1-distance between each patch to the average patch along the principal components (PC) of all $n \times n$ patches in the image. Therefore, for a given patch $p_{x,y}$ centered at (x, y) the distinctness measure is computed by:

$$PD(p_{x,y}) = \sum_{k=1}^{n} |p_{x,y} w_k^T| \tag{1}$$

where $p_{x,y}$ is a vectorized patch and w_k^T is the k'th principal component of the distribution of all $n \times n$ patches in the image.

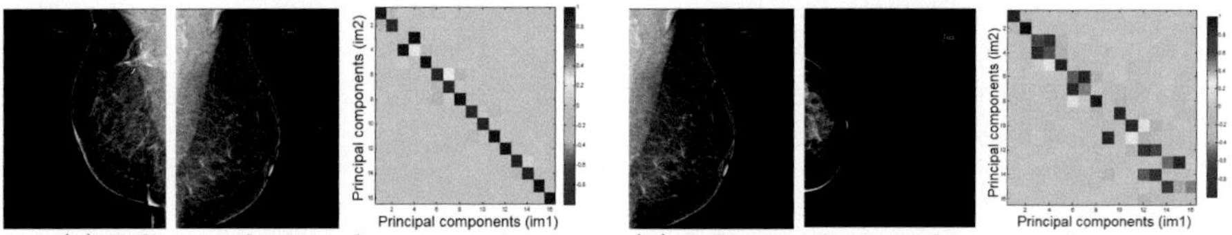

(a) PC's similarity of same patient (b) PC's similarity of two random patient

Fig. 1. Cosine similarity between the principal components (sorted according to variance) of left and right mammograms (a) same patient (b) different patients. Note in (a) the switch in location between the 3rd and 4th principal components.

We extend the patch distinctness shown above by considering cross correlations between images as well as internal image correlations. We achieve that, by computing the patch distinctness measure only on a subset of informative principal components. Our observation is that we are dealing with images of paired organs or an organ divided along some symmetry axis. It is reasonable to assume that their respective patch distributions would have some degree of similarity. This can be seen by analyzing their respective principal components, which would have similar directions but the relative amount of variance each principal component represents would be different. This is illustrated in Fig. 1 where pairs of left & right mammograms from the same patient (a) and two random patients (b) are shown. For each pair the distance matrix shows the cosine of the angle between the principal components of each image sorted according to relative variance. The matrix in (a) is nearly diagonal implying nearly identical directions of the principal components. However, in (a) we can see that the third principal component of the first image and the fourth principal component of the second image switch places. This indicates that this principal component is more informative to that image since it captures more variance.

To model correlations across images, we derive a cross patch distinctness measure (CPD) by extending the PD measure (eq. 1) using an additional gating variable C. This variable controls the influence of each PC based on cross-correlations between the images. Therefore, the CPD measure is defined as:

$$CPD(p_{x,y}) = \sum_{j=1} c_j |p_{x,y} w_k^T| \quad c_j \in C, C \in \{0,1\}^n \tag{2}$$

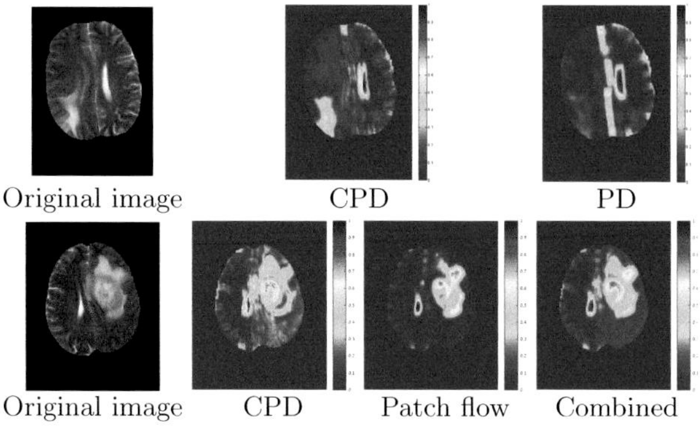

Fig. 2. Top: Comparison of CPD and PD measure: Our CPD measure (middle), gives high scores for the brain edema seen on the right parietal side of the brain, while the PD measure (right) assigns low scores similar to a regular tissue. **Bottom: Contribution of the CPD and Patch flow** the CPD marked most of the necrotic core and part of the edema while the Patch flow completed the other part of the edema.

Fig. 2 shows the difference between the PD and our suggested CPD.

The subset of principal components for the CPD (eq. 2) is computed separately for each image. Having the PC' for each image, we first establish a correspondence between the PC's of the two image by pairing then according angular similarity. Then, we estimate gating vectors (one for each image) $C_{1,2}$ by maximizing the following expression:

$$C_1 = \arg\max \sum_j c_j(v_j^1 - v_j^2) - \lambda \|C_1\|_1, \quad c_j \in \{0,1\} \tag{3}$$

$$C_2 = \arg\max \sum_j c_j(v_j^2 - v_j^1) - \lambda \|C_2\|_1, \quad c_j \in \{0,1\} \tag{4}$$

where v_j^1, v_j^2 is the relative variance captured by the j'th PC in each image.

2.2 Patch Flow

Patch flow measures, how well a patch fits the smooth motion field assumption between two similar images. It is important to stress that unlike rigid or non rigid registration patch flow allows each patch to move independently from other patches. We measure the flow field by applying a fast, randomized, correspondence algorithm called PatchMatch [3]. This algorithm uses the smooth motion field assumption to compute a dense flow field for each pixel by considering an $n \times n$ patch around it. Initially, for each pixel location (x, y) it assigns a random displacement vector T that marks the location of its corresponding patch in the other image. Then, the quality of the displacement T is measured by computing the L_2 distance between the corresponding patches:

$$D(p_{x,y}, p_{x+T_x,y+T_y}) = \sum_{i=x-n/2}^{i=x+n/2} \sum_{j=y-n/2}^{j=y+n/2} \|I_1(i,j) - I_2(i+T_x, j+T_y)\|_2 \tag{5}$$

where $I_{1,2}$ represents the corresponding images intensity values. The algorithm attempts to improve the displacement for each location by testing new hypotheses generated from the displacement vectors of neighboring patches in the same image. The algorithm progresses by iterating between the random and propagation steps, where the best estimate according to the L_2 distance is kept. Usually, the algorithm requires 4 to 5 iterations to converge to a fairly good approximation of the flow field under the smooth motion field assumption. The algorithm is applied to find for each patch (in both images) its corresponding nearest neighbor in the other image. Then, we measure how well a patch fits the smooth motion field assumption by its nearest neighbor error (NNE):

$$NNE(p_{x,y}) = \min_{T} D(p_{x,y}, p_{x+T_x,y+T_y}). \tag{6}$$

2.3 Combining the Measures

We seek patches that are salient in and across the input images. Therefore, we compute the CPD and NNE with various patch sizes and down sampling rates (scales). Then, we compute the cross saliency score (CS) by averaging across all scales:

$$CS(x,y) = \frac{1}{2l} \sum_{s=1}^{l} CPD(p_{x,y}) + NNE(p_{x,y}) \tag{7}$$

where the CPD and NNE measures are pre-normalized to the range of $[0 \ldots 1]$. To avoid uninformative scales, we discard scales in which the difference in variance is negligible, or if the distribution of NNEs is nearly Gaussian (using skewness).

3 Experiments

In this section we apply our approach to both paired organs and in-organ symmetry, in two different modalities. Initially, we apply it to the brain MRI and test the correlation between the most salient region and high-grade gliomas. Then, we apply the same algorithm and evaluate its contribution to tumor detection in breast mammograms. Lastly, we provide empirical evaluation of our approach preforms under perturbations in symmetry axis. In our experiments we set λ to select three principal components in the CPD measure ($\lambda \approx 0.05$).

3.1 Unsupervised Tumor Detection on BRATS2014

The BRATS2014 training set contains 20 skull-stripped multi-modal MR images ($T_1, T_{1contrast}, T_2, Flair$) high-grade gliomas. It is desirable, that a saliency algorithm would produce results highly correlated with the gliomas. Another challenge is that the saliency algorithm should account for the multi-modal nature of the data. We apply our algorithm as in sec. 2 with mid-saggital line detection [12]. For each slice, we computed the cross saliency by considering $3 \times 3 \times 4$ cubes in two scale (original, down-sample by 2). The third dimension represents the four MRI channels (stacked). To find the most salient volume, we segment the cross saliency map of each slice into a set of salient regions using Mean-shift clustering algorithm. Then, we match regions that have similar cluster centroid and shape between consecutive slices. This forms a chain of regions that are consistent between slices. To select the most salient 3D region in the volume, we seek in each slice the region that has the maximum saliency score in its centroid. Then, the chain with the highest number of maximum saliency regions is considered as the salient volume.

We evaluate the correlation between the most salient volume and the ground truth using the Dice score on the complete tumor. Fig. 3 shows the results obtained by our unsupervised approach. As far as we are know, there aren't any unsupervised approaches applied on the BRATS challenge. For reference only we show the results shown in [13] as it is the only study that provides Dice score for each case. Our average Dice score was 0.753 ± 0.039 which is comparable to the Zikic et al. RF approach [13] that had average score of 0.763 ± 0.027.

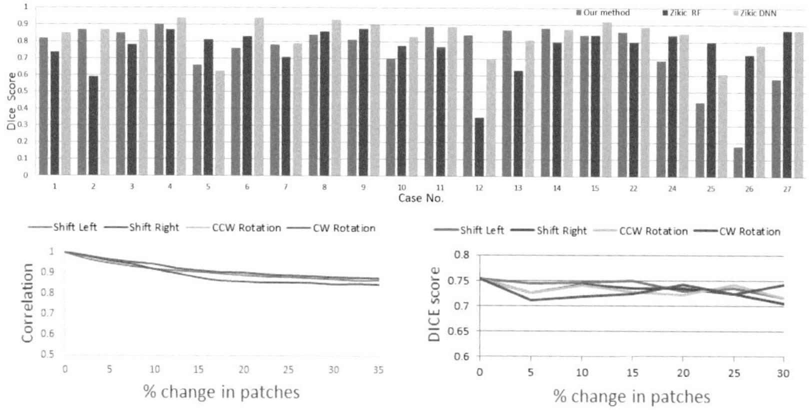

Fig. 3. (Top) dice score of the tumor detection in BRATS2014 our approach (blue) vs. results obtained by [13]. (Bottom) variations under perturbation of the mid-sagittal line - (left) Correlation with correctly estimated mid-sagittal line (right) changes in the Dice score (top) as a function of the perturbation in the mid-sagittal line.

3.2 Tumor Detection in Breast Mammogram

Tumor detection in breast mammogram is one case where symmetry is estimated between paired organs (left and right breasts). We tested three features variants for detecting tumors. The first uses spatial features [9]. The features include: patch intensity histogram, mean intensity, standard deviation of intensities and relative position to the nipple (in polar coordinates). The second algorithm, uses the same spatial features and an earth movers distance (EMD) flow vector between two corresponding regions in a pair of aligned mammograms. The alignment process was done using Thin-Plate spline (TPS) as shown in [2]. The third algorithm, uses spatial features and the CPD (eq. 2) and NNE (eq. 6) measures computed on 9×9 patches in four down-sampling factors (2,4,8,16).

Our evaluation data contains FFD mammograms of 40 different patients; we had left and right MLO scans for each patient. The images were annotated by a radiologist by delineating the boundaries of each tumor. Out of the 40 patients 38 had a single tumor and the other had bilateral tumors. This amounts to a total of 42 tumors with long axis length between 4 to 83mm.

For each of the three features variants we trained a Random Forest classifier in a leave-one-out manner and tested its accuracy in a pixel wise manner. Table 1 summarizes the performance of the three classifier. We can see that our approach has added 16% to the sensitivity compared with the spatial features and 6% compered to the TPS+EMD. However, the TPS+EMD had a drop in specificity of 10% while our approach retained its high specificity. As for the AUC, our approach showed an increase of 5% compared to all the other approaches.

Table 1. Accuracy of the three classifiers applied to mammogram tumor detection.

Measure	spatial features	spatial features+cross saliency	spatial features+TPS+EMD
AUC	0.88	**0.93**	0.88
Sensitivity	0.72 ± 0.05	**0.88** ± 0.03	0.82 ± 0.002
Specificity	0.82 ± 0.013	**0.82** ± 0.018	0.73 ± 0.008

3.3 Stability under Variation in Mid-Sagittal Plane Estimation

We preformed two tests to measure performance under symmetry axis errors. The first, we changed the mid-sagittal used in sec. 3.1 and measured the changes in the Dice score. Since this test uses automatic estimation of the mid-sagittal line errors are not unlikely. Therefore, in the second test we randomly selected 60 slices (3 from each case) where we validated that the mid-sagittal line is estimated correctly. Then we introduced changes the mid-sagittal line and measured the correlation in the cross saliency score with the unchanged estimation. In all cases we simulated errors in the mid-sagittal line by shifting the line from 1 to 15 pixels in each direction or rotating it between 1 to 15 degrees (both CW and CCW). Each single shift or rotation moves around 2.5% of the patches from one side to the other. Fig. 3 (bottom-right) summarizes the average Dice scores for each perturbation. We can see that most of average scores fall well within the standard error range of the unmodified score (0.753 ± 0.039). Indicating that most of the changes do not introduced significant changes to the overall detection. This is supported by the second experiment Fig. 3 (bottom-left) showing high correlation ≥ 0.95 for a patch change of up to 7.5% and a correlation ≥ 0.90 for a patch change of up to 22.5%. Indicating that even large changes in the symmetry axis have a relatively small effect on the cross correlation maps.

4 Conclusion

We have proposed an unsupervised cross saliency algorithm for both paired organs and in-organ symmetry. Our approach attempts to solve the inherent difficulty when tumors are present, by eliminating image alignment and reduce the effect of errors in symmetry axis estimation. We have demonstrated the advantages of our method in tumor detection in both mammogram and MRI.

References

1. Alterson, R., Plewes, D.B.: Exploring symmetries in breast mri scan. In: Ellis, R.E., Peters, T.M. (eds.) MICCAI 2003. LNCS, vol. 2879, pp. 754–761. Springer, Heidelberg (2003)
2. Bandyopadhyay, S.K.: Breast asymmetry-tutorial review. Breast (2010)
3. Barnes, C., Shechtman, E., Finkelstein, A., Goldman, D.B.: Patchmatch: A randomized correspondence algorithm for structural image editing. In: SIGGRAPH (2009)
4. Bauer, S., Wiest, R., Nolte, L.P., Reyes, M.: A survey of mri-based medical image analysis for brain tumor studies. Physics in Medicine and Biology (2013)
5. Good, W.F., Wang, X.H., Maitz, G.S.: Feature-based differences between mammograms. In: Medical Imaging 2003 (2003)
6. Khotanlou, H., Colliot, O., Atif, J., Bloch, I.: 3d brain tumor segmentation in mri using fuzzy classification, symmetry analysis and spatially constrained deformable models. Fuzzy Sets and Systems (2009)
7. Margolin, R., Tal, A., Zelnik-Manor, L.: What makes a patch distinct? In: CVPR (2013)
8. Qiu, W., Yuan, J., Ukwatta, E., Sun, Y., Rajchl, M., Fenster, A.: Fast globally optimal segmentation of 3d prostate mri with axial symmetry prior. In: Mori, K., Sakuma, I., Sato, Y., Barillot, C., Navab, N. (eds.) MICCAI 2013, Part II. LNCS, vol. 8150, pp. 198–205. Springer, Heidelberg (2013)
9. Rangayyan, R.M., Ayres, F.J., Desautels, J.L.: A review of computer-aided diagnosis of breast cancer: Toward the detection of subtle signs. JFI (2007)
10. Saha, B.N., Ray, N., Greiner, R., Murtha, A., Zhang, H.: Quick detection of brain tumors and edemas: A bounding box method using symmetry. Comput. Med. Imag. Grap (2012)
11. Zhao, L., Wu, W., Corso, J.J.: Semi-automatic brain tumor segmentation by constrained mrfs using structural trajectories. In: Mori, K., Sakuma, I., Sato, Y., Barillot, C., Navab, N. (eds.) MICCAI 2013, Part III. LNCS, vol. 8151, pp. 567–575. Springer, Heidelberg (2013)
12. Zhao, L., Ruotsalainen, U., Hirvonen, J., Hietala, J., Tohka, J.: Automatic cerebral and cerebellar hemisphere segmentation in 3d mri: adaptive disconnection algorithm. Medical Image Analysis (2010)
13. Zikic, D., Ioannou, Y., Brown, M., Criminisi, A.: Segmentation of brain tumor tissues with convolutional neural networks (2014)

Grey Matter Sublayer Thickness Estimation in the Mouse Cerebellum

Da Ma[1], Manuel J. Cardoso[1], Maria A. Zuluaga[1], Marc Modat[1], Nick Powell[1], Frances Wiseman[3], Victor Tybulewicz[4], Elizabeth Fisher[3], Mark F. Lythgoe[2], and Sébastien Ourselin[1]

[1] Translational Imaging Group, CMIC, University College London, UK
[2] Centre for Advanced Biomedical Imaging , University College London, UK
[3] Institute of Neurology, University College London, UK,
[4] Crick Institute, UK

Abstract. The cerebellar grey matter morphology is an important feature to study neurodegenerative diseases such as Alzheimer's disease or Down's syndrome. Its volume or thickness is commonly used as a surrogate imaging biomarker for such diseases. Most studies about grey matter thickness estimation focused on the cortex, and little attention has been drawn on the morphology of the cerebellum. Using *ex vivo* high-resolution MRI, it is now possible to visualise the different cell layers in the mouse cerebellum. In this work, we introduce a framework to extract the Purkinje layer within the grey matter, enabling the estimation of the thickness of the cerebellar grey matter, the granular layer and molecular layer from gadolinium-enhanced *ex vivo* mouse brain MRI. Application to mouse model of Down's syndrome found reduced cortical and layer thicknesses in the transchromosomic group.

1 Introduction

Grey matter thickness measurements have been widely used for quantitative analysis of neurodegenerative diseases. Studies have been limited to the cerebrum, even though this type of diseases also affect the cerebellum. Clinical studies have shown that diseases such as Down's Syndrome correlate with morphological changes in the cerebellar grey matter [1]. Although cerebellar grey matter thickness measurements could provide more insights about neurodegenerative diseases and phenotype identification, these are currently limited by the resolution of clinical MRI and the highly convoluted nature of the human brain.

Thanks to the high resolution of preclinical MRI scanners and to the anatomical similarities between human and mouse brains, the latter represents a promising model to further understand how the cerebellum is affected by the progression of neurodegenerative diseases. To date most of the quantitative analysis on mice cerebellum has focused on volumetric analysis and, to the best of our knowledge, no previous studies have addressed the problem of estimating the cerebellar cortical thickness.

N. Navab et al. (Eds.): MICCAI 2015, Part III, LNCS 9351, pp. 644–651, 2015.
DOI: 10.1007/978-3-319-24574-4_77

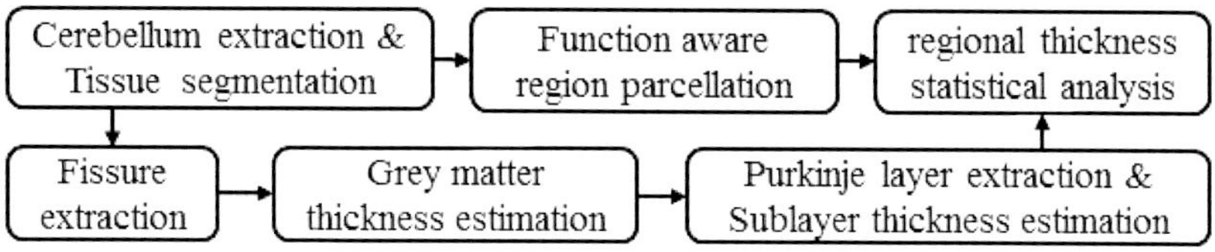

Fig. 1. Schematic diagram of the proposed framework.

In this work, we propose to not only estimate the thickness of the mouse cerebellar grey matter, but also extract and measure the thickness of two anatomical cerebellar layers (*i.e.* the granular, and the molecular layer) from high resolution MRI. The presented framework explores and extends the Laplace equation based cortical thickness estimation method to multiple layers. These layers are defined through surface segmentation and, when not visible, extrapolated using the Laplace equation.

2 Methods

In this section we introduce the proposed framework for cerebellum sublayer thickness estimation. The overall pipeline is presented in Fig. 1. The first steps of the framework include the extraction of the cerebellum, the white matter (WM) and grey matter (GM) tissue segmentation, the fissure extraction and the parcellation of the cerebellum based on the functional characteristics of the tissues. The later steps include the extraction of the Purkinje layer, which enables the estimation of sublayer thickness.

2.1 Cerebellum Extraction and Tissue Segmentation

Based on a T2-weighted MR image, the cerebellum is extracted using a multi-atlas segmentation propagation framework [2]. In order to obtain an accurate thickness estimation, one needs first to obtain an accurate segmentation of the WM and GM tissues. Ashburner & Friston based their approach on a Gaussian mixture model of tissue classes, and segmented the tissues within an expectation-maximisation framework [3]. This framework gains in robustness by using a priori spatial information in the form of tissue probabilistic maps. Since there are currently no publicly available tissue probability maps for mouse cerebellum, we use a semi-automatic approach to first generate tissue probability maps, and then segment the tissues.

The intensity distribution in the cerebellar area for all MR images in the study is standardised using landmark-based piecewise linear intensity scaling introduced by Nyúl *et al.* [4] with 11 histogram landmarks. Using an iterative groupwise scheme, we then create an average image. A symmetric block-matching approach [5] is used for the global registration steps and an symmetric scheme based on a cubic B-Spline parametrisation of a stationary velocity field [6] is employed for the local registration stages.

Using a Gaussian mixture model of tissue classes, we first segment the group average image into 4 tissues without using anatomical priors. The segmentation of the group image is then manually corrected in order to generate an anatomically correct segmentation, e.g. disconnect misclassified Purkinje layer voxels from the white matter class. Note that this step only needs to be done once, as the groupwise tissue segmentation can be used to segment new subjects.

Using the backward transformations obtained during the groupwise registration step, the segmented tissues are propagated back to the initial input images. As proposed by Chakravarty *et al.* [7], all input images and their newly generated tissue segmentations are then considered as a template database for a multi-atlas segmentation propagation scheme. Using a leave-one-out framework, for each image, a spatial anatomical prior is generated by first propagating all the tissue segmentations from every other images to the target dataset, followed by a fusion step [2]. Each image is then segmented using a Gaussian mixture model of tissue classes combined with the image specific probability maps.

2.2 Fissure Extraction

The morphology of mouse cerebellum consists of folia lobes separated by fissures. Most of these thin fissures are subject to partial volume effect, resulting in incorrect tissue segmentations. In order to appropriately extract the fissures, even when highly corrupted by PV, a distance-based skeletonisation technique [8] is used here. A geodesic distance transform $D(x)$ is obtained by solving the Eikonal equation $F(x)|\nabla D(x)| = 1$ from the white/grey matter boundary. Here, $D(x)$ is the geodesic distance and $F(x)$ is the speed function, in the computational domain Ω, defined as $F = I * \mathcal{G}_\sigma$, with I being the image and $\mathcal{G}_\sigma$ being a Gaussian kernel with $\sigma = 1.5$ voxels. The fissures are then extracted by first finding the local maxima of $D(x)$ only along the direction of $\nabla D(x)$, followed by a recursive geodesic erosion in order to ensure single voxel thick fissure segmentations.

2.3 Grey Matter Thickness Estimation

As proposed by Jones *et al.* [9], cortical thickness is estimated here by modelling the anatomical laminar layers as Laplacian field level-set analogues. The Laplace equation is solved using the Jacobi method. We first reconstruct the pial surface by combining the extracted fissures with the outer boundary of cerebellum mask. The thickness of each voxel is defined as the length of the streamlines perpendicularly passing through the isosurface of the Laplacian field. The streamlines are integrated along the direction of the normalised vector field $\hat{V}$, and are calculated using the Eulerian PDE method proposed by Yezzi and Prince [10]. At each voxel, the length of the streamlines along the direction $\hat{V}$, when measured from the pial surface is denoted by D_{Pial}, and when measured from the WM is denoted D_{WM}. The thickness at each voxel x can thus be estimated by adding $D_{WM}(x)$ and $D_{\text{Pial}}(x)$, i.e. $T_{GM}(x) = D_{WM}(x) + D_{\text{Pial}}(x)$.

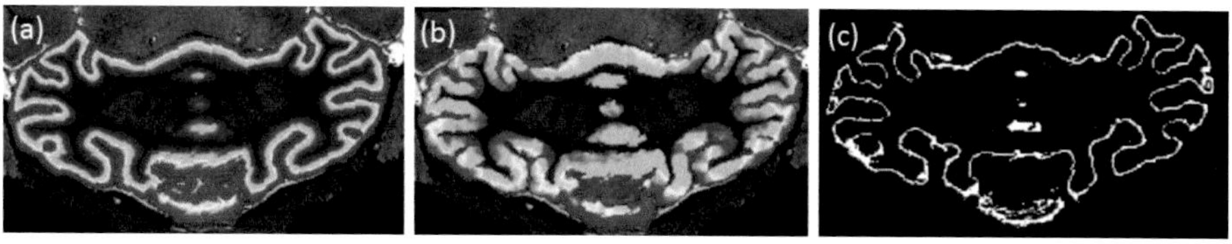

Fig. 2. (a) White matter distance ratio map R_{WM}. (b) Gaussian smoothed map for the ratio map of Purkinje layer R_{P_S}. (c) Map of λ.

2.4 Purkinje Layer Extraction and Sublayer Thickness Estimation

In this step, we extract the narrow layer that sits in the middle of the grey matter - the Purkinje layer. This will allow us to obtain the thickness of the other two grey matter sublayers - the molecular layer and the granular layer. Segmentation is obtained by exploiting both the intensity information and the laminar nature of the Purkinje layer.

The Purkinje layer is an anatomical surface. Thus, a modified Frangi vesselness filter [11] is used here to find and enhance planar structures *P(s)* (instead of tubular ones) within the GM region at fixed scale $s = 0.04$:

$$P(s) = \begin{cases} 0 & \text{if } \lambda_2 > 0 \text{ or } \lambda_3 > 0 \\ exp(-\frac{R_A^2}{2\alpha^2})exp(-\frac{R_B^2}{2\beta^2})(1 - exp(-\frac{S^2}{2c^2})) & \end{cases}, \quad (1)$$

where α,β and c are thresholds, $R_A = \frac{|\lambda_2|}{|\lambda_3|}$, $R_B = \frac{|\lambda_1|}{\sqrt{|\lambda_2\lambda_3|}}$, and λ_k are the k-*th* smallest eigenvalue decomposition ($|\lambda_1| \leqslant |\lambda_2| \leqslant |\lambda_3|$).

Areas with significant filter response are used as an initial estimates of the Purkinje layer M_{P^0}. Voxels touching the white matter or the sulcal region are removed through conditional morphological erosion.

The above method does not capture the Purkinje in its entirety, mostly due to problems with local intensity contrast, partial volume effect, image noise, and adjacency to the grey matter boundary. Thus, the initial estimate of the Purkinje layer is used to extrapolate the remaining locations. In order to enhance the Purkinje layer segmentation, we first define the white matter thickness ratio as $R_{WM} = D_{WM}/T_{GM}$ (see Fig 2(a)), and the Purkinje layer distance ratio $R_P = R_{WM} * M_{P^0}$ at each grey matter voxel.

A multi-level Gaussian smoothing is applied on R_P to all voxel $x \in R_{WM} \cap x \notin M_{P^0}$. 10 Gaussian smoothing levels with exponentially decreasing variances between 15 and 1 voxels were used in this work. This multi level Gaussian smoothly propagates and averages the value of R_P to neighbouring regions, providing an estimate of R_P for voxels outside M_{P^0}. The smoothed version of R_P is here denoted R_{P_S} (Fig 2(b)). If the the Gaussian smoothed map R_{P_S} is equal to R_{WM} at location x, then the voxel x should be part of the Purkinje layer. We thus define the $\lambda = |R_{P_S} - R_{WM}|$ as a measurement of distance between the two maps (see Fig 2(c)).

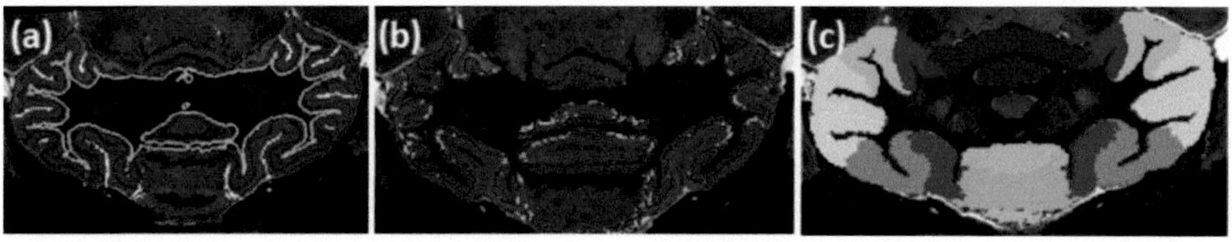

Fig. 3. (a) Results of preprocessing steps. Red: cerebellum extraction; Green: White matter extraction; Yellow: Fissure extraction. (b) Purkinje layer extraction. Red: initial extraction; Green: final extraction. (c) Parcellated grey matter function regions.

In order to robustly find locations where $\lambda \approx 0$, we find local minima of λ only along the direction of the vector field $\hat{V}$. The recovered local minima λ_{min} are then added to the initial Purkinje layer mask, i.e. the final segmentation of the Purkinje layer is given by $M_{P^F} = M_{P^0} \cup \lambda_{min}$.

Lastly, all relevant thicknesses, including whole grey matter thicknesses T_{GM}, granular layer thicknesses T_{Gran}, and molecular layer thickness T_{Mol} are measured at the Purkinje layer location M_{P^F}. The granular layer thickness is here defined as the distance from the WM, given by $T(x)_{Gran} = D_{WM}(x)\ \forall x \in M_{P^F}$, the molecular layer thickness is defined as the distance from the pial layer, given by $T(x)_{Mol} = D_{Pial}(x)\ \forall x \in M_{P^F}$, and the total GM thickness at the Purkinje layer voxels, denoted by $T_{GM_{P^F}}$, is given by $T_{GM_{P^F}}(x) = T_{GM}(x) \forall x \in M_{P^F}$.

2.5 Grey Matter Function Aware Region Parcellation

Similarly to studies on human cortical thickness [12], we measure the average thickness (T_{GM}, T_{Gran} and T_{Mol}) in regions of interest. The grey matter subregions are parcellated automatically using the high resolution mouse cerebellum atlas database published by Ullmann *et al.* [13]. This atlas divides the cerebellum into multiple regions based on their neuronal function. As previously, we use the approach by Chakravarty *et al.* [7] to obtain image specific parcellations based on a leave-on-out segmentation propagation scheme.

3 Experimental Data and Validation

The proposed method has been assessed on a data set which includes 28 gadolinium-enhanced *ex vivo* T2 MRI scan of mouse brains: 14 wildtype and 14 transchromosomic that model Down's syndrome [14]. All theses images have been processed as previously described. Fig. 3(a) shows an example of an extracted cerebellar grey matter. Fig. 3(b) shows the initial and final Purkinje layer extraction. Fig. 3(c) shows the parcellated cerebellar structures.

We compare the full grey matter thickness as well as the sublayer thicknesses between the wild type and the transchromosomic groups for each parcellated region. To regress out the effect of the gross brain size, we also normalised the thickness to the total intracranial volume (TIV). The results are presented in Fig. 4. We corrected for multiple comparisons with a false discovery rate set to

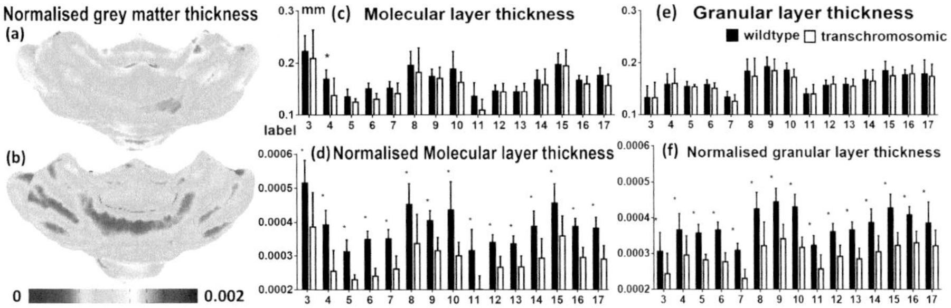

Fig. 4. Normalised grey matter thickness map of (a) wildtype group, and (b)transgenic group, as well as the thicknesses of parcellated regions of (c,d) molecular layer, (e,f) granular layer before and after normalisation with TIV. *: Significant difference between the wildtype and the transchromosomic group.

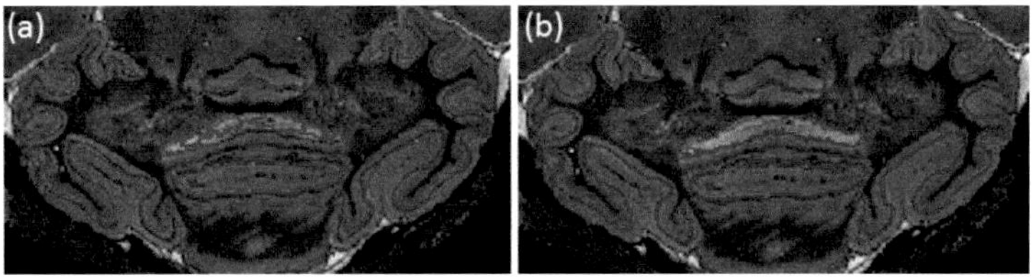

Fig. 5. Comparison between the (a) central surface and (b) the Purkinje layer.

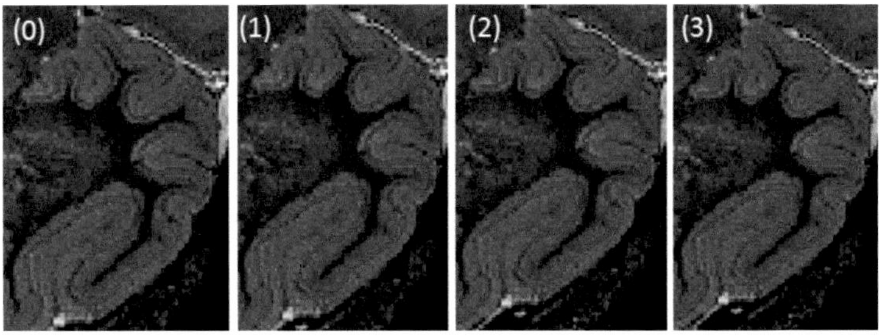

Fig. 6. Iterative multi-kernel Gaussian smoothness gradually recover the Purkinje layer (0) Initial extracted Purkinje layer. (1-3) Recovered Purkinje layer after each iteration.

$q = 0.1$. Both the granular and molecular layer of the transchromosomic group are thinner over all the subregions when compared with the wild type group. Significant differences were found in a subregion of the molecular layer. After normalising with TIV, the difference becomes significant over all subregions for both sublayers. Our results agree with previous findings by Baxter *et al.*, in which measurements from histological slides also showed thickness reduction of granular layer and molecular layer in mouse model of Down's syndrome[15].

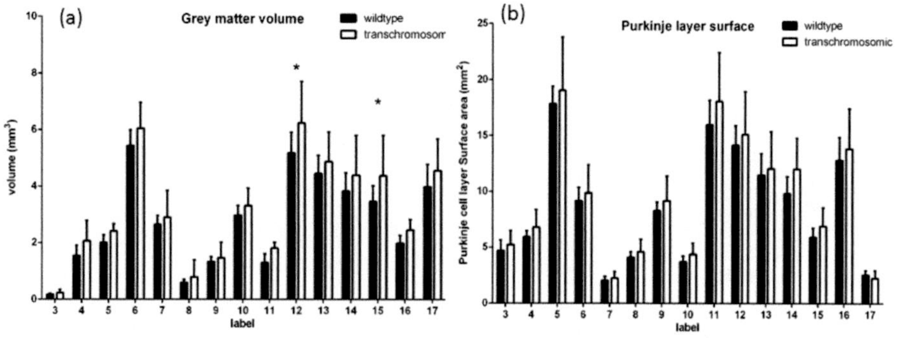

Fig. 7. (a) Volume of the parcellated grey matter subregions. (b) Surface area of Purkinje layer.

4 Conclusion and Discussion

We presented a framework for mouse cerebellar grey matter sublayer thickness estimation. Sublayer measurements were enabled by a 2-step extraction of the Purkinje layer. The framework has been evaluated on *ex vivo* MRI data of a mouse model of Down's syndrome, where data suggests a reduction in regional average thickness in mice that model Down's Syndrome.

Within most current studies, the grey matter thickness estimation is commonly projected onto the central surface in order to perform quantitative statistical analyses [8]. However, this model is limited by the spatial variability in sublayer thickness within the grey matter (see in Fig. 5). The information of the Purkinje layer location could provide robust information consistently across subjects, when performing groupwise analyses. Fig 5 shows the difference between the central surface and the Purkinje layer.

The fissure (sulcal) extraction is an important preprocessing step for cerebellar (cortical) thickness estimation. Previous studies have been using tissue membership functions to guide the skeletisation when extracting deep sulcal lines [8]. While the proposed method can greatly improve the Purkinje layer segmentation accuracy (see Fig 6), due to complex intensity patterns and the presence of inter-layer contrast in the mouse cerebellum, an accurate tissue/Purkinje segmentation remains challenging. Future work will explore a joint model for the segmentation of the cerebellar tissues and Purkinje layer.

To understand why the grey matter of the transchromosomic mouse is overall thinner, we also measured the volume of each parcellated grey matter region and the surface area of the Purkinje layer. The obtained results are shown in Fig. 7. The larger volume and longer surface area of the Purkinje layer in the mice that model Down's Syndrome suggests that the morphology of the cerebellar grey matter of the transcromosomic mice could be more convoluted than the one of the wild type mice. Further investigation is necessary to confirm these findings.

References

1. Aylward, E.H., Habbak, R., Warren, A.C., Pulsifer, M.B., Barta, P.E., Jerram, M., Pearlson, G.D.: Cerebellar volume in adults with down syndrome. Archives of Neurology 54(2), 209–212 (1997)
2. Ma, D., Cardoso, M.J., Modat, M., Powell, N., Wells, J., Holmes, H., Wiseman, F., Tybulewicz, V., Fisher, E., Lythgoe, M.F., et al.: Automatic structural parcellation of mouse brain MRI using multi-atlas label fusion. PLoS One 9(1) (2014)
3. Ashburner, J., Friston, K.J.: Voxel-based morphometry the methods. Neuroimage 11(6), 805–821 (2000)
4. Nyúl, L.G., Udupa, J.K., Zhang, X.: New variants of a method of mri scale standardization. IEEE Transactions on Medical Imaging 19(2), 143–150 (2000)
5. Modat, M., Cash, D.M., Daga, P., Winston, G.P., Duncan, J.S., Ourselin, S.: Global image registration using a symmetric block-matching approach. Journal of Medical Imaging 1(2), 024003 (2014)
6. Modat, M., Daga, P., Cardoso, M., Ourselin, S., Ridgway, G., Ashburner, J.: Parametric non-rigid registration using a stationary velocity field. In: 2012 IEEE Workshop on Mathematical Methods in Biomedical Image Analysis (MMBIA), pp. 145–150 (2012)
7. Chakravarty, M.M., Steadman, P., Eede, M.C., Calcott, R.D., Gu, V., Shaw, P., Raznahan, A., Collins, D.L., Lerch, J.P.: Performing label-fusion-based segmentation using multiple automatically generated templates. Human Brain Mapping 34(10), 2635–2654 (2013)
8. Han, X., Pham, D.L., Tosun, D., Rettmann, M.E., Xu, C., Prince, J.L.: Cruise: cortical reconstruction using implicit surface evolution. NeuroImage 23(3), 997–1012 (2004)
9. Jones, S.E., Buchbinder, B.R., Aharon, I.: Three-dimensional mapping of cortical thickness using laplace's equation. Human Brain Mapping 11(1), 12–32 (2000)
10. Yezzi, A.J., Prince, J.L.: An Eulerian PDE Approach for computing tissue thickness. IEEE Transactions on Medical Imaging 22(10), 1332–1339 (2003)
11. Frangi, A.F., Niessen, W.J., Vincken, K.L., Viergever, M.A.: Multiscale vessel enhancement filtering. In: Wells, W.M., Colchester, A.C.F., Delp, S.L. (eds.) MICCAI 1998. LNCS, vol. 1496, pp. 130–137. Springer, Heidelberg (1998)
12. Grand'Maison, M., Zehntner, S.P., Ho, M.K., Hébert, F., Wood, A., Carbonell, F., Zijdenbos, A.P., Hamel, E., Bedell, B.J.: Early cortical thickness changes predict β-amyloid deposition in a mouse model of Alzheimer's disease. Neurobiology of Disease 54, 59–67 (2013)
13. Ullmann, J.F., Keller, M.D., Watson, C., Janke, A.L., Kurniawan, N.D., Yang, Z., Richards, K., Paxinos, G., Egan, G.F., Petrou, S., et al.: Segmentation of the c57bl/6j mouse cerebellum in magnetic resonance images. Neuroimage 62(3), 1408–1414 (2012)
14. O'Doherty, A., Ruf, S., Mulligan, C., Hildreth, V., Errington, M.L., Cooke, S., Sesay, A., Modino, S., Vanes, L., Hernandez, D., Linehan, J.M., Sharpe, P.T., Brandner, S., Bliss, T.V.P., Henderson, D.J., Nizetic, D., Tybulewicz, V.L.J., Fisher, E.M.C.: An aneuploid mouse strain carrying human chromosome 21 with down syndrome phenotypes. Science 309(5743), 2033–2037 (2005)
15. Baxter, L.L., Moran, T.H., Richtsmeier, J.T., Troncoso, J., Reeves, R.H.: Discovery and genetic localization of Down syndrome cerebellar phenotypes using the Ts65Dn mouse. Human Molecular Genetics 9(2), 195–202 (2000)

Unregistered Multiview Mammogram Analysis with Pre-trained Deep Learning Models*

Gustavo Carneiro[1], Jacinto Nascimento[2], and Andrew P. Bradley[3]

[1] ACVT, University of Adelaide, Australia
[2] ISR, Instituto Superior Tecnico, Portugal
[3] University of Queensland, Australia

Abstract. We show two important findings on the use of deep convolutional neural networks (CNN) in medical image analysis. First, we show that CNN models that are pre-trained using computer vision databases (e.g., Imagenet) are useful in medical image applications, despite the significant differences in image appearance. Second, we show that multiview classification is possible without the pre-registration of the input images. Rather, we use the high-level features produced by the CNNs trained in each view separately. Focusing on the classification of mammograms using craniocaudal (CC) and mediolateral oblique (MLO) views and their respective mass and micro-calcification segmentations of the same breast, we initially train a separate CNN model for each view and each segmentation map using an Imagenet pre-trained model. Then, using the features learned from each segmentation map and unregistered views, we train a final CNN classifier that estimates the patient's risk of developing breast cancer using the Breast Imaging-Reporting and Data System (BI-RADS) score. We test our methodology in two publicly available datasets (InBreast and DDSM), containing hundreds of cases, and show that it produces a volume under ROC surface of over 0.9 and an area under ROC curve (for a 2-class problem - benign and malignant) of over 0.9. In general, our approach shows state-of-the-art classification results and demonstrates a new comprehensive way of addressing this challenging classification problem.

Keywords: Deep learning, Mammogram, Multiview classification.

1 Introduction

Deep learning models are producing quite competitive results in computer vision and machine learning [1], but the application of such large capacity models in medical image analysis is complicated by the fact that they need large training sets that are rarely available in our field. This issue is circumvented in computer vision and machine learning with the use of publicly available pre-trained deep learning models, which are estimated with large annotated databases [2]

* This work was partially supported by the Australian Research Council's Discovery Projects funding scheme (project DP140102794). Prof. Bradley is the recipient of an Australian Research Council Future Fellowship(FT110100623).

N. Navab et al. (Eds.): MICCAI 2015, Part III, LNCS 9351, pp. 652–660, 2015.
DOI: 10.1007/978-3-319-24574-4_78

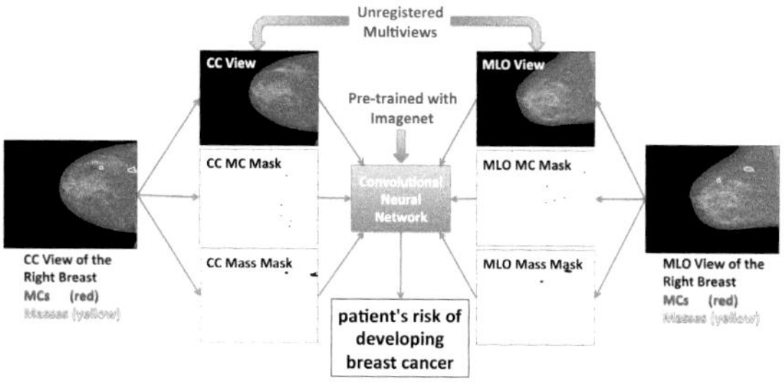

Fig. 1. Model proposed in this paper using unregistered CC/MLO views and MC/Mass segmentations of the same breast, where the classification of the patient's risk of developing breast cancer uses a CNN pre-trained with Imagenet [2].

and re-trained (or fine-tuned) for other problems that contain smaller annotated training sets. This fine-tuning process has been shown to improve the generalization of the model, compared to a model that is trained with randomly initialized weights using only the small datasets [1]. However, such pre-trained models are not available for medical image applications, so an interesting question is if models pre-trained in other (non-medical) datasets are useful in medical imaging applications. Another important potential advantage provided by deep learning methods is the automatic estimation of useful features that provide a high-level representation of the input data, which is robust to image transformations [3]. A pertinent question with regards to this point is if such features can be used in multiview classification without the need to pre-register the input views.

Literature Review: Deep learning has become one of the most exciting topics in computer vision and machine learning [4]. The main advantage brought by deep learning models, and in particular by deep convolutional neural networks (CNN) [3], is the high-level features produced by the top layers of the model that are shown to improve classification results, compared to previous results produced by hand-built features [4]. Moreover, these high-level features have also been shown to be robust to image transformations [5]. Nevertheless, the training process for CNNs requires large amounts of annotated samples (usually, in the order of 100Ks) to avoid overfitting to the training data given the large model capacity. This issue has been handled with transfer learning, which re-trains (in a process called fine-tuning) publicly available models (pre-trained with large datasets) using smaller datasets [1]. However, it is still not possible to utilize this approach in medical image analysis given the lack of large publicly available training sets or pre-trained models.

In spite of the issues above, we have seen the successful use of deep learning in medical imaging. Recently, Cireşan et al. [6] and Roth et al. [7] set up their training procedures in order to robustly estimate CNN model parameters, and in both cases (mitosis and lymph node detection, respectively), their results suparssed the current state of the art by a large margin. Another way of handling the issues above is with unsupervised training of deep autoencoders that are fine-tuned to specific classification problems [8,9,10,11]. Other interesting approaches using autoencoders for processing multiview data have been proposed [12,13], but they require pre-registered input data. However, to date we have not seen the use of pre-trained CNN models in medical imaging, and we have not seen the analysis of unregistered input images in multiview applications with CNN models.

The literature concerning the classification of the patient's risk of developing breast cancer using mammograms is quite vast, and cannot be fully covered here, so we focus on the most relevant works for our paper. In a recent survey, Giger et al. [14] describe recent methodologies for breast image classification, but these methods focus only on binary classification of microcalcification (MC) and mass like lesions. This is different from the more comprehensive approach taken here, where we aim at classifying a whole breast exam. The state-of-the-art binary classification of masses and MCs into benign/malignant [15,16] produces an area under the receiver operating characteristic (ROC) curve between $[0.9, 0.95]$, but these results cannot be used as baseline because they usually use databases and annotations that are not publicly available. More similar to our approach, the multimodal analysis that takes lesions imaged from several modalities (e.g., mammograms and sonograms) have been shown to improve the average performance of radiologists [17]. We believe that the new approach here proposed based on the combination of multiview analysis with MC and mass detection has the potential to improve the overall breast exam classification in terms of sensitivity and specificity.

Contributions: We show two results in this paper (see Fig. 1). First, we show that CNN models pre-trained with a typical computer vision database [2] can be used to boost classification results in medical image analysis problems. Second, we show that the high-level features produced by such CNN models allow the classification of unregistered multiview data. We propose a methodology that takes unregistered CC/MLO mammograms and MC/Mass segmentations and produce a classification based on Breast Imaging-Reporting and Data System (BI-RADS) score. Using two publicly available databases [18,19], containing a total of 287 patients and 1090 images, we show the benefits of these two contributions and also show that we demonstrate improved classification performance for this problem. Finally, given our use of publicly available datasets only, these results can be used as baseline for future proposals.

2 Methodology

Assume we have a dataset $\mathcal{D} = \{(\mathbf{x}^{(p,b)}, \mathbf{c}^{(p,b)}, \mathbf{m}^{(p,b)}, \mathbf{y}^{(p,b)})\}_{p,b}$, where $\mathbf{x} = \{\mathbf{x}_{\text{CC}}, \mathbf{x}_{\text{MLO}}\}$ denotes the two views (CC and MLO) available (with $\mathbf{x}_{\text{CC}}, \mathbf{x}_{\text{MLO}} : \Omega \rightarrow \mathbb{R}$ and Ω denoting the image lattice), $\mathbf{c} = \{\mathbf{c}_{\text{CC}}, \mathbf{c}_{\text{MLO}}\}$ is the MC segmentation in each view with $\mathbf{c}_{\text{CC}}, \mathbf{c}_{\text{MLO}} : \Omega \rightarrow \{0, 1\}$, $\mathbf{m} = \{\mathbf{m}_{\text{CC}}, \mathbf{m}_{\text{MLO}}\}$ represents

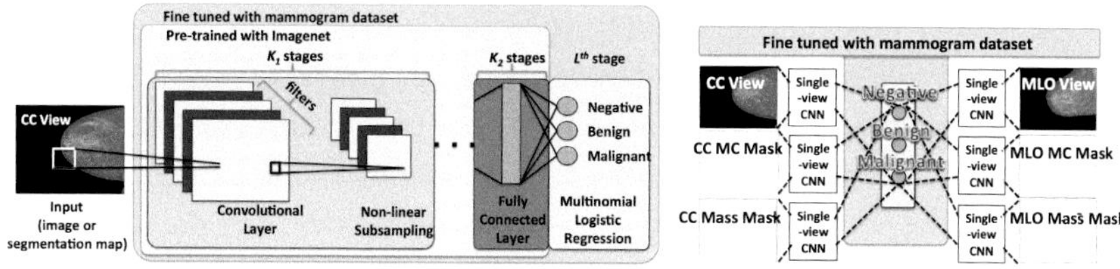

a) Single view CNN model b) Multiview CNN model

Fig. 2. Visualization of the single view (a) and multiview (b) CNN models with K_1 stages of convolutional and non-linear sub-sampling layers, K_2 stages of fully connected layers and one final layer of the multinomial logistic regressor.

the mass segmentation in each view with $\mathbf{m}_{\mathrm{CC}}, \mathbf{m}_{\mathrm{MLO}} : \Omega \rightarrow \{0, 1\}$, $\mathbf{y} \in \mathcal{Y} = \{0, 1\}^C$ denotes the BI-RADS classification with C classes, $p \in \{1, ..., P\}$ indexes the patients, and $b \in \{\text{left}, \text{right}\}$ indexes the patient's left and right breasts (each patient's breast is denoted as a case because they can be labeled different BI-RADS scores). The BI-RADS classification has 6 classes (1: negative, 2: benign finding(s), 3: probably benign, 4: suspicious abnormality, 5: highly suggestive of malignancy, 6: proven malignancy), but given the small amount of training data in some of these classes in the publicly available datasets (Fig. 3), we divide these original classes into three categories: negative or $\mathbf{y} = [1, 0, 0]^\top$ (BI-RADS=1), benign or $\mathbf{y} = [0, 1, 0]^\top$ (BI-RADS $\in \{2, 3\}$) and malignant or $\mathbf{y} = [0, 0, 1]^\top$ (BI-RADS $\in \{4, 5, 6\}$). We also have a dataset of non-medical image data for pre-training the CNN, $\widetilde{\mathcal{D}} = \{(\widetilde{\mathbf{x}}^{(n)}, \widetilde{\mathbf{y}}^{(n)})\}_n$, with $\widetilde{\mathbf{x}} : \Omega \rightarrow \mathbb{R}$ and $\widetilde{\mathbf{y}} \in \widetilde{\mathcal{Y}} = \{0, 1\}^{\widetilde{C}}$ (i.e., the set of $\widetilde{C}$ classes present in dataset $\widetilde{\mathcal{D}}$).

Convolutional Neural Network: A CNN model consists of a network with multiple processing stages, each comprising two layers (the convolutional layer, where the filters are applied to the image, and the non-linear subsampling layer, which reduces the input image size), followed by several fully connected layers and a multinomial logistic regression layer [4] (Fig. 2(a)). The convolution layers compute the output at location j from input at i using the filter $\mathbf{W}_k$ and bias b_k (at k^{th} stage) using $\mathbf{x}_k(j) = \sigma(\sum_{i \in \Omega(j)} \mathbf{x}_{k-1}(i) * \mathbf{W}_k(i, j) + b_k(j))$, where $\sigma(.)$ is a non-linear function [4] (e.g., logistic or rectification linear unit), $*$ represents the convolution operator, and $\Omega(j)$ is the input region addresses; while the non-linear subsampling layers are defined by $\mathbf{x}_k(j) = \downarrow(\mathbf{x}_{k-1}(j))$, where $\downarrow(.)$ denotes a subsampling function that pools (using the mean or max functions) the values from the region $\Omega(j)$ of the input data. The fully connected layers consist of the convolution equation above using a separate filter for each output location, using the whole input from the previous layer, and the multinomial logistic regression layer computes the probability of the ith class using the features $\mathbf{x}_L$ from the Lth layer with the softmax function $\mathbf{y}(i) = \frac{e^{\mathbf{x}_L(i)}}{\sum_j e^{\mathbf{x}_L(j)}}$. Inference consists of the application of this process in a feedforward manner, and training is carried out with stochastic gradient descent to minimize the cross entropy loss [4] over the training set (via back propagation).

The process of pre-training a CNN, represented by the model $\widetilde{\mathbf{y}}^* = f(\widetilde{\mathbf{x}};\widetilde{\theta})$ (with $\widetilde{\theta} = [\widetilde{\theta}_{cn}, \widetilde{\theta}_{fc}, \widetilde{\theta}_{mn}]$), is defined as training K_1 stages of convolutional and non-linear subsampling layers (represented by the parameters $\widetilde{\theta}_{cn}$), then K_2 fully connected layers (parameters $\widetilde{\theta}_{fc}$) and one multinomial logistic regression layer $\widetilde{\theta}_{mn}$ by minimizing the cross-entropy loss function [4] over the dataset $\widetilde{\mathcal{D}}$. This pre-trained model can be used by taking the first $K_1 + K_2$ layers to initialize the training of a new model [1], in a process called fine-tuning (Fig. 2(a)). Yosinski et al. [1] notice that using a large number of pre-trained layers and fine tuning the CNN is the key to achieve the best classification results in transfer learning problems. Following this result, we take the parameters $\widetilde{\theta}_{cn}, \widetilde{\theta}_{fc}$ and add a new multinomial logistic regression layer θ_{mn} (with random initial values), and fine tune the CNN model by minimizing the cross-entropy loss function using $\mathcal{D}$. This fine tuning process will produce six models per case: 1) MLO image $\mathbf{y} = f(\mathbf{x}_{\text{MLO}};\theta_{\text{MLO,im}})$, 2) CC image $\mathbf{y} = f(\mathbf{x}_{\text{CC}};\theta_{\text{CC,im}})$, 3) MLO MC map $\mathbf{y} = f(\mathbf{c}_{\text{MLO}};\theta_{\text{MLO,mc}})$, 4) CC MC map $\mathbf{y} = f(\mathbf{c}_{\text{CC}};\theta_{\text{CC,mc}})$, 5) MLO mass map $\mathbf{y} = f(\mathbf{m}_{\text{MLO}};\theta_{\text{MLO,ma}})$ and 6) CC mass map $\mathbf{y} = f(\mathbf{m}_{\text{CC}};\theta_{\text{CC,ma}})$. The final multiview training (Fig. 2(b)) takes the features from the last fully connected layer (i.e., $L-1^{th}$ layer, labeled as $\mathbf{x}_{\text{MLO},L-1}$ for the first model above, and similarly for the remaining ones) from the six models, and train a single multinomial logistic regression layer using those inputs (Fig. 2(b)), resulting in $\mathbf{y} = f(\mathbf{x}_{\text{MLO},L-1}, \mathbf{x}_{\text{CC},L-1}, \mathbf{c}_{\text{MLO},L-1}, \mathbf{c}_{\text{CC},L-1}, \mathbf{m}_{\text{MLO},L-1}, \mathbf{m}_{\text{MLO},L-1}; \theta_{mn})$, where θ_{mn} is randomly initialized in this multiview training.

3 Materials and Methods

We use the publicly available InBreast [18] and DDSM [19] mammogram datasets. InBreast [18] has 115 patients (410 images), and it does not have any division in terms of training and testing sets, so we run a 5-fold cross validation experiment, where we randomly divide the original set into 90 patients for training and validation and 25 for testing. DDSM [19] has 172 patients (680 images), obtained by joining the original MC and mass datasets proposed, but removing all cases that appear in the training set of mass and testing set of MC and vice versa. With DDSM, we run an experiment with the proposed 86 patients for training and 86 for testing. The distribution of patients in terms of BI-RADS for both datasets is depicted in Fig. 3. We use the MC and mass maps provided with these datasets, and if no mass or MC map is available for a particular case, we use a blank image of all zeros instead.

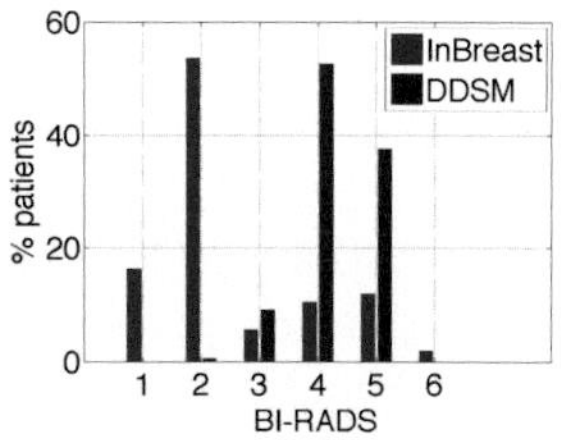

Fig. 3. Distribution of BI-RADS cases in InBreast (blue) and DDSM (red).

We use the publicly available CNN-F model from [20], consisting of a CNN that takes a 264×264 input image with four stages of convolution and non-linear sub-sampling layers, two stages of fully connected layers and a final multinomial logistic regression stage. Specifically, CNN-F has stage 1 with 64 11×11 filters and a max-pooling that sub-samples the input by 2, stage 2 with 256 5×5 filters and a max-pooling that sub-samples the input by 2, stages 3-5 with 256 3×3 filters (each) with no sub-sampling, stage 6-7 with 4096 nodes (each), and stage 8 containing the softmax layer. This model is pre-trained with Imagenet [2] (1K visual classes, 1.2M training, 50K validation and 100K test images), then we replace stage 8 with a new softmax layer containing only three classes (negative, benign and malignant) and fine tune for the CC and MLO views and the MC and mass segmentation maps (Fig. 2(a)). Finally, we take the features from stage 7 for the six models and train stage 8 of the multiview model (Fig. 2(b)). The use of the proposed pre-training can be seen as a regularization approach, which can be compared to other forms of regularization, such as data augmentation [4], obtained by artificially augmenting the training set with random geometric transformations applied to each original sample that generates new artificial training samples. Hence, we also run an experiment that uses the same CNN-F structure with no pre-training (i.e., with random weight initialization using an unbiased Gaussian with standard deviation 0.001) and runs the training with data augmentation by adding 10 or 20 new samples per training image. Each new training sample is built by cropping the original image using randomly defined top-left and bottom-right corners (within a range of $[1, 10]$ pixels from the original corners). For completeness, we also apply this data augmentation to the pre-trained CNN-F model. Finally, the learning rate $= 0.001$, and momentum $=$ 0.9. With this experimental design, we can then compare the pre-training and data augmentation regularizations.

The input CC and MLO views are pre-processed with local contrast normalization, then Otsu's segmentation [21] to remove most of the background. This pre-processing steps is found to improve the final results (Fig. 5 shows some samples of these pre-processed images). The classification accuracy is measured using volume under ROC surface (VUS) for a 3-class problem [22], and the area under ROC curve (AUC) for the benign/malignant classification of cases that have at least one finding (MC or mass).

4 Results

Figure 4 shows the VUS for the test sets of InBreast (average and standard deviation of 5-fold cross validation and the two breasts) and DDSM (average and standard deviation of the two breasts). We show the results for the six inputs per case (two views and four maps) and the result of the multiview model, and we also display the improvement achieved with the Imagenet pre-trained model compared to the randomly initialized model. Figure 5 shows four typical results of the pre-trained model (without data augmentation) on InBreast test cases. The classification of the cases into benign or malignant (where each case has at least an MC or a mass) produces an AUC of $0.91(\pm 0.05)$ on InBreast and $0.97(\pm 0.03)$ on DDSM using the pre-trained model with no data augmentation, where the same general trends can be observed compared to Fig. 4. Finally, the

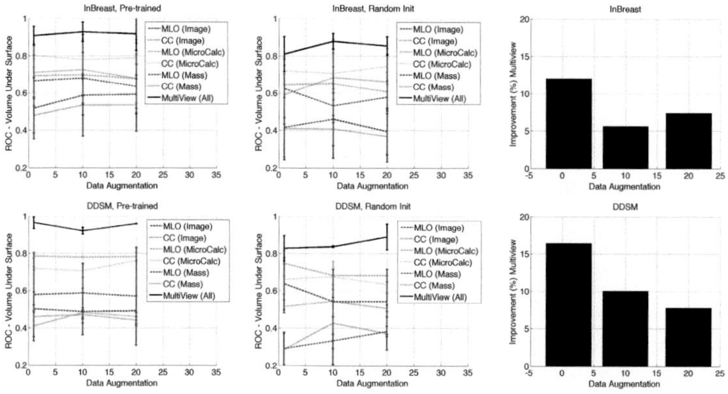

Fig. 4. VUS in terms of data augmentation on InBreast (top) DDSM (bottom). 1st column shows the results with the Imagenet pre-trained model, 2nd shows the randomly initialized models, and the third displays the average improvement in the results with pre-trained models, compared to the randomly initialized models.

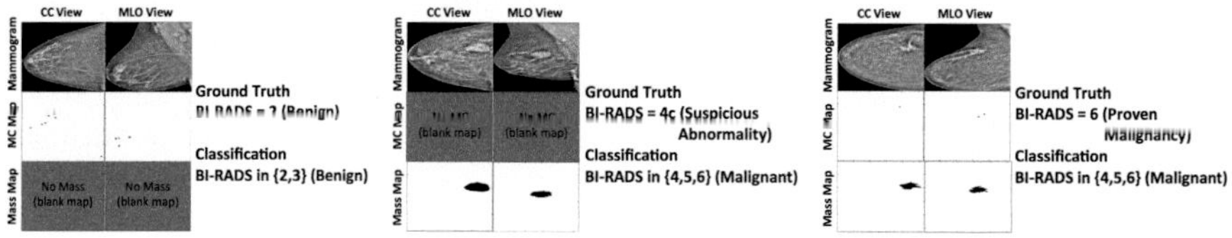

Fig. 5. InBreast test case results using Imagenet pre-trained model with no data augmentation (the ground truth and the automatic classifications are shown).

training time for all six models and the final multiview model (with no data augmentation) is one hour. With 10 additional training samples, the training time is four hours and with 20 additional training samples, the training time increases to 7.5 hours. These training times are obtained on InBreast, measured using Matconvnet training [20] on a 2.3GHz Intel Core i7 with 8GB, and graphics card NVIDIA GeForce GT 650M 1024 MB.

5 Discussion and Conclusion

The results show a clear improvement of multiview compared to single views, demonstrating that the high-level features of the individual CNN models provide a robust representation of the input images, which do not need to be registered. This is particularly important in mammograms, where registration is challenging due to non-rigid deformations. The poor performance of some single view classifications is due to: 1) including some MC view cases with BI-RADS > 1 that do not have annotation, which makes its classification difficult (similarly for some mass view cases); and 2) the classification using mammogram only is challenging because of the lack of sufficient detail in the image. We also notice that the pre-trained multiview model provides better classification results compared to the randomly initialized model, with improvements of 5% to 16%, where the largest differences happen with the no data augmentation test. This is expected given that this is the condition where the random initialized model is more likely to overfit the training data. These results are difficult to compare to previously published results in the field (see Sec. 1) given that: 1) most of the previously published results are computed with datasets that are not publicly available, and 2) these other results focus mostly on the specific classification of masses or MCs instead of the full breast exam. Nevertheless, looking exclusively at the AUC results, our methodology can be considered to be comparable (on InBreast) or superior (on DDSM) to the current state of the art, which present AUC between $[0.9, 0.95]$ for MCs and mass classification [15,16]. However, we want to emphasize that our results can be used as baseline in the field given that we only use public data and models, and consequently be fairly compared to other works, resolving one of the issues identified by Giger et al. [14]. We believe that our work opens two research fronts that can be applied to other medical image analysis applications, which are the use of pre-trained models from non-medical imaging datasets and the comprehensive analysis of unregistered multiview data.

References

1. Yosinski, J., Clune, J., Bengio, Y., Lipson, H.: How transferable are features in deep neural networks? In: Advances in Neural Information Processing Systems, pp. 3320–3328 (2014)
2. Russakovsky, O., Deng, J., Su, H., Krause, J., Satheesh, S., Ma, S., Huang, Z., Karpathy, A., Khosla, A., Bernstein, M., Berg, A.C., Fei-Fei, L.: ImageNet Large Scale Visual Recognition Challenge (2014)
3. Bengio, Y.: Learning deep architectures for ai. Foundations and trends® in Machine Learning 2(1), 1–127 (2009)
4. Krizhevsky, A., Sutskever, I., Hinton, G.E.: Imagenet classification with deep convolutional neural networks. In: NIPS, vol. 1, p. 4 (2012)
5. Zou, W., Zhu, S., Yu, K., Ng, A.Y.: Deep learning of invariant features via simulated fixations in video. In: Advances in Neural Information Processing Systems, pp. 3212–3220 (2012)
6. Cireşan, D.C., Giusti, A., Gambardella, L.M., Schmidhuber, J.: Mitosis detection in breast cancer histology images with deep neural networks. In: Mori, K., Sakuma, I., Sato, Y., Barillot, C., Navab, N. (eds.) MICCAI 2013, Part II. LNCS, vol. 8150, pp. 411–418. Springer, Heidelberg (2013)
7. Roth, H.R., Lu, L., Seff, A., Cherry, K.M., Hoffman, J., Wang, S., Liu, J., Turkbey, E., Summers, R.M.: A new 2.5 d representation for lymph node detection using random sets of deep convolutional neural network observations. In: Golland, P., Hata, N., Barillot, C., Hornegger, J., Howe, R. (eds.) MICCAI 2014, Part I. LNCS, vol. 8673, pp. 520–527. Springer, Heidelberg (2014)
8. Fakoor, R., Ladhak, F., Nazi, A., Huber, M.: Using deep learning to enhance cancer diagnosis and classification. In: Proceedings of the ICML Workshop on the Role of Machine Learning in Transforming Healthcare (WHEALTH), Atlanta, GA (2013)

9. Carneiro, G., Nascimento, J.C.: Combining multiple dynamic models and deep learning architectures for tracking the left ventricle endocardium in ultrasound data. IEEE Transactions on Pattern Analysis and Machine Intelligence 35(11), 2592–2607 (2013)
10. Cruz-Roa, A.A., Arevalo Ovalle, J.E., Madabhushi, A., González Osorio, F.A.: A deep learning architecture for image representation, visual interpretability and automated basal-cell carcinoma cancer detection. In: Mori, K., Sakuma, I., Sato, Y., Barillot, C., Navab, N. (eds.) MICCAI 2013, Part II. LNCS, vol. 8150, pp. 403–410. Springer, Heidelberg (2013)
11. Li, R., Zhang, W., Suk, H.-I., Wang, L., Li, J., Shen, D., Ji, S.: Deep learning based imaging data completion for improved brain disease diagnosis. In: Golland, P., Hata, N., Barillot, C., Hornegger, J., Howe, R. (eds.) MICCAI 2014, Part III. LNCS, vol. 8675, pp. 305–312. Springer, Heidelberg (2014)
12. Brosch, T., Yoo, Y., Li, D.K.B., Traboulsee, A., Tam, R.: Modeling the variability in brain morphology and lesion distribution in multiple sclerosis by deep learning. In: Golland, P., Hata, N., Barillot, C., Hornegger, J., Howe, R. (eds.) MICCAI 2014, Part II. LNCS, vol. 8674, pp. 462–469. Springer, Heidelberg (2014)
13. Guo, Y., Wu, G., Commander, L.A., Szary, S., Jewells, V., Lin, W., Shen, D.: Segmenting hippocampus from infant brains by sparse patch matching with deep-learned features. In: Golland, P., Hata, N., Barillot, C., Hornegger, J., Howe, R. (eds.) MICCAI 2014, Part II. LNCS, vol. 8674, pp. 308–315. Springer, Heidelberg (2014)
14. Giger, M.L., Karssemeijer, N., Schnabel, J.A.: Breast image analysis for risk assessment, detection, diagnosis, and treatment of cancer. Annual Review of Biomedical Engineering 15, 327–357 (2013)
15. Cheng, H., Shi, X., Min, R., Hu, L., Cai, X., Du, H.: Approaches for automated detection and classification of masses in mammograms. Pattern Recognition 39(4), 646–668 (2006)
16. Wei, L., Yang, Y., Nishikawa, R.M., Jiang, Y.: A study on several machine-learning methods for classification of malignant and benign clustered microcalcifications. IEEE Transactions on Medical Imaging 24(3), 371–380 (2005)
17. Horsch, K., Giger, M.L., Vyborny, C.J., Lan, L., Mendelson, E.B., Hendrick, R.E.: Classification of breast lesions with multimodality computer-aided diagnosis: Observer study results on an independent clinical data set. Radiology 240(2), 357–368 (2006)
18. Moreira, I.C., Amaral, I., Domingues, I., Cardoso, A., Cardoso, M.J., Cardoso, J.S.: Inbreast: toward a full-field digital mammographic database. Academic Radiology 19(2), 236–248 (2012)
19. Heath, M., Bowyer, K., Kopans, D., Moore, R., Kegelmeyer, P.: The digital database for screening mammography. In: Proceedings of the 5th International Workshop on Digital Mammography, pp. 212–218 (2000)
20. Chatfield, K., Simonyan, K., Vedaldi, A., Zisserman, A.: Return of the devil in the details: Delving deep into convolutional nets. arXiv preprint arXiv:1405.3531 (2014)
21. Otsu, N.: A threshold selection method from gray-level histograms. Automatica 11(285-296), 23–27 (1975)
22. Landgrebe, T.C., Duin, R.P.: Efficient multiclass roc approximation by decomposition via confusion matrix perturbation analysis. IEEE Transactions on Pattern Analysis and Machine Intelligence 30(5), 810–822 (2008)

Automatic Craniomaxillofacial Landmark Digitization via Segmentation-Guided Partially-Joint Regression Forest Model

Jun Zhang[1], Yaozong Gao[1,2], Li Wang[1], Zhen Tang[3], James J. Xia[3,4], and Dinggang Shen[1]

[1] Department of Radiology and BRIC, UNC at Chapel Hill, NC, USA
[2] Department of Computer Science, UNC at Chapel Hill, NC, USA
[3] Houston Methodist Hospital, Houston, TX, USA
[4] Weill Medical College, Cornell University, New York, USA

Abstract. Craniomaxillofacial (CMF) deformities involve congenital and acquired deformities of the head and face. Landmark digitization is a critical step in quantifying CMF deformities. In current clinical practice, CMF landmarks have to be manually digitized on 3D models, which is time-consuming. To date, there is no clinically acceptable method that allows automatic landmark digitization, due to morphological variations among different patients and artifacts of cone-beam computed tomography (CBCT) images. To address these challenges, we propose a segmentation-guided partially-joint regression forest model that can automatically digitizes CMF landmarks. In this model, a regression voting strategy is first adopted to localize landmarks by aggregating evidences from context locations, thus potentially relieving the problem caused by image artifacts near the landmark. Second, segmentation is also utilized to resolve inconsistent landmark appearances that are caused by morphological variations among different patients, especially on the teeth. Third, a partially-joint model is proposed to separately localize landmarks based on coherence of landmark positions to improve digitization reliability. The experimental results show that the accuracy of automatically digitized landmarks using our approach is clinically acceptable.

1 Introduction

Craniomaxillofacial (CMF) deformities involve congenital and acquired deformities of the head and face [10]. In diagnosis and treatment planning, computed tomography (CT) scans (including multi-slice (MS) and cone-beam (CB) CT) are typically processed using the following procedures: segmentation, reconstruction of 3D models, placing anatomical landmarks on the 3D models (called landmark digitization), and quantitative measurements based on the landmarks (called cephalometry). Compared with MSCT, CBCT has short scanning time, reduced radiation dose, low cost, and the potential for in-office imaging, which is increasingly being used to scan CMF patients.

N. Navab et al. (Eds.): MICCAI 2015, Part III, LNCS 9351, pp. 661–668, 2015.
DOI: 10.1007/978-3-319-24574-4_79

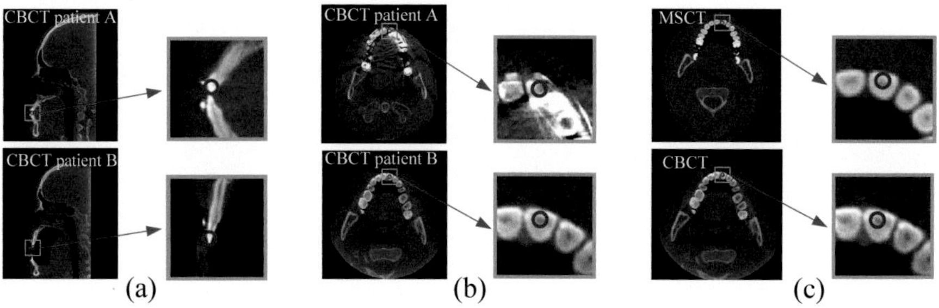

Fig. 1. Various morphological appearances. (a) Inconsistent patch appearances of the same tooth landmark. (b) Inconsistent patch appearances caused by metal effects. (c) Similar patch appearances in both MSCT and CBCT images.

Accurate landmark digitization is a critical step to quantitatively assess the CMF anatomy. In current practice, all anatomical CMF landmarks are manually digitized on 3D models, which is time-consuming. To date, there is no effective method that allows automatic landmark digitization in clinical use, because of two major challenges. 1) Morphological variations among different patients. For example, local morphological appearance of the same landmark could be significantly different across different patients, as shown in Fig. 1 (a) for a tooth landmark. 2) Artifacts of CBCT images from amalgam dental fillings and orthodontic wires, bands and braces. For example, the top image of Fig. 1 (b) shows artifacts from orthodontic braces, while the bottom image does not have such artifacts. In this example, the metal brace caused artifacts and made the local patch appearances, near the teeth landmarks, inconsistent.

So far, there are a few reports on automatic CMF landmark digitization from CBCT images. Cheng *et al.* adopted random forest, combined with constrained search space, to detect dent-landmarks [1]. Keustermans *et al.* used sparse shape and appearance models to localize cephalometric landmarks [5]. Shahidi *et al.* used a registration-based method to detect craniofacial landmarks [9]. However, the performances of these methods are tempered due to the fact that they did not consider the problems in morphological variations and imaging artifacts.

In this paper, we present a Segmentation-guided Partially-joint Regression Forest (S-PRF) model for landmark digitization from CBCT. First, a regression voting strategy is adopted to localize each landmark by aggregating evidences from context locations, thus potentially relieving the problem caused by image artifacts near the landmark. Second, segmentation is also utilized to reduce inconsistent landmark appearances caused by morphological variations among different patients, especially on teeth landmarks. Third, a partially-joint model is further proposed to separately localize landmarks, based on the coherence of landmark positions, to improve digitization reliability. In addition, we also enhance performance by including MSCT scans into the training dataset, since MSCT shares many similar local patch appearances with CBCT as shown in Fig. 1 (c), which allows for potential improvement in digitization performance.

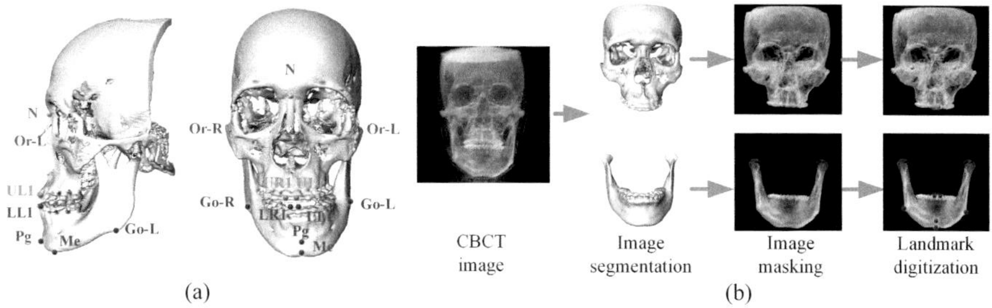

Fig. 2. Segmentation-guided landmark digitization. (a) CMF landmarks shown on segmentation. (b) Flow chart of segmentation-guided landmark digitization.

2 Automatic CMF Landmark Digitization

In our method, we use segmentation to guide landmark digitization. Specifically, our method consists of three steps: 1) using an automatic segmentation method to separate mandible from maxilla, thus obtaining two segmentation masks; 2) utilizing the obtained 3D segmented maxilla and mandible to mask the maxilla and mandible in CBCT images; 3) detecting landmarks on mandible and maxilla separately by using our partially-joint random forest model on the respective masked images. Fig. 2 (a) shows the CMF landmarks and Fig. 2 (b) shows the flowchart of proposed framework.

2.1 Traditional Regression Forest Model for Landmark Digitization

Regression forest based methods have demonstrated their superiority in anatomy detection for different organs and structures [2, 12, 6, 3, 4]. Specifically, in the training stage, the regression forest can be used to learn a non-linear mapping between a voxel's local appearance and its 3D displacement to the target landmark. Generally, Haar-like features are used to describe a voxel's local appearance. However, in this application, the Haar-like features could be easily affected by the local inhomogeneity caused by artifacts. In this paper, we compute multi-scale statistical features based on oriented energies [11], which are invariant to local inhomogeneity, and can potentially relieve the effects of artifacts. Instead of using N-ray coding [11] for vector quantization, we adopt the bag-of-words strategy to achieve relatively low feature dimension. Moreover, since multi-scale representation captures both coarse and fine structural information, which can help describe local appearance more effectively.

In the testing stage, the learned regression forest can be used to estimate a 3D displacement from every voxel in the image to the potential landmark position, based on local appearance features extracted from the neighborhood of this voxel. Using the estimated 3D displacement, each voxel can cast one vote to the potential landmark position. By aggregating all votes from all voxels, a voting map can be obtained, from which the landmark position can be easily identified as the location with the maximum vote.

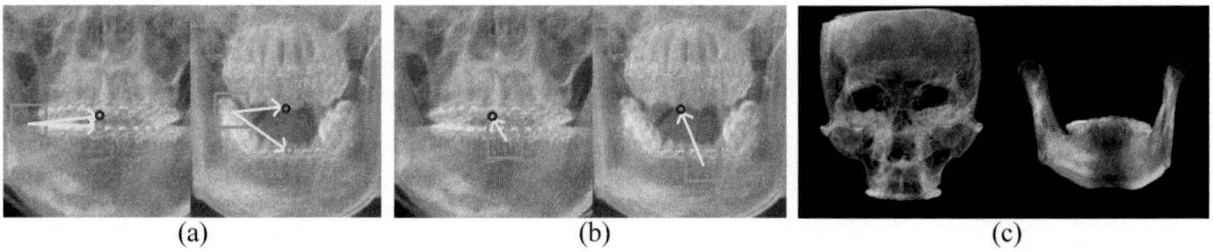

Fig. 3. Displacement and voting map. (a-b) Two cases of incoherent displacements happened near teeth landmarks. (c) A typical voting map overlaid with 3D rendering skull.

2.2 Segmentation-Guided Partially-Joint Regression Forest (S-PRF) Model

Despite its popularity, the traditional regression-forest-based methods still suffer from two limitations: 1) all landmarks are often jointly localized without considering the incoherence of landmark positions. Among the CMF landmarks, the landmark positions, respectively, from different anatomical regions, could change dramatically because of morphological differences across patients. 2) All image voxels are equally treated in the regression voting stage. Thus, the voting map may be negatively influenced by the voxels that are uninformative to the target landmark position. To address these two limitations, we propose two respective strategies: partially-joint regression forest model, and segmentation-guided landmark digitization, with both detailed below.

Partially-Joint Regression Forest Model: A fully-joint model predicts the displacements of a voxel to multiple landmarks. The fully-joint model assumes that similar local appearances correspond to coherent multiple displacements. However, this assumption is invalid in this application. For example, Fig. 3 (a) shows two CBCT images, where the displacements to a lower tooth and a upper tooth are not coherent. Since regression forest predicts the displacement based solely on the input appearance features, the ambiguous displacements associated with voxels of same appearances could mislead the training procedure, which could eventually lower the accuracy of landmark digitization.

To address this issue, we exploit the coherence of landmark positions. Specifically, we propose a partially-joint regression forest model by dividing all CMF landmarks into several groups. To form groups, landmarks are clustered, based on a dissimilarity matrix, where each entry is the variance of pair-wise landmark distances across subjects. Fig. 2 (a) shows the partition result where the landmarks with the same color belong to the same group. Then, we learn several fully-joint models, one for each group of landmarks. Using this approach, the ambiguous displacement problem can be largely avoided.

Segmentation-Guided Strategy: As stated above, one limitation of traditional regression-forest-based methods is the failure to consider the voting confidence of each voxel and equally treating their votes. Since different voxels have different voting confidences, it is necessary to associate voting weight for each voxel. Here, we consider two types of uninformative voxels.

The first type of uninformative voxels is faraway voxels. For those voxels, an intuitive way is to assign large voting weights only for the voxels near the landmark, while small voting weights are assigned for those faraway voxels, as they are not informative to precise landmark location. Specifically, we use $w = e^{-\frac{\|\tilde{\mathbf{d}}\|}{\alpha}}$ to define the voting weight of a voxel, where $\tilde{\mathbf{d}}$ is the estimated 3D displacement from this voxel to the target landmark, and α is a scaling coefficient.

The second type of uninformative voxels is voxels misleading prediction. In our application, voxels in mandible often have consistent 3D displacements to the lower teeth landmarks, but may have ambiguous 3D displacements to the upper teeth landmarks. For example, Fig. 3 (b) shows that the teeth of one patient closely bite, while the other does not. This causes the votes from voxels in the lower teeth region to be unreliable for localizing the upper teeth landmarks.

To address this issue, we use image segmentation as guidance to remove those uninformative voxels. As shown in Fig. 2 (b), the original CBCT image is segmented into mandible and maxilla using an automatic segmentation method [8]. Specifically, the deformable registration method was first used to warp all atlases to the current testing image. Then, a sparse representation based label propagation strategy was employed to estimate a patient-specific atlas from all aligned atlases. Finally, the patient-specific atlas was integrated into a Bayesian framework for accurate segmentation. By using the segmented mandible and maxilla as masks, we can separate mandible from maxilla in the original CBCT image. Therefore, landmarks on mandible and maxilla can now be separately digitized using our partially-joint model on the respectively masked CBCT images. By using segmentation as guidance, those uninformative voxels can be removed for localizing the landmark. Fig. 3 (c) shows a voting map of digitizing one patient's CMF landmarks.

3 Experiments, Results and Discussion

3.1 Data Description and Parameter Setup

Fifteen sets of CBCTs (in 0.4 mm of isotropic voxel) of patients with nonsyndromic dentofacial deformity were used (IRB# IRB0413-0045). In addition, 30 sets of MSCTs ($0.488 \times 0.488 \times 1.25mm^3$) were used as a part of training dataset. In this experiment, 11 commonly used anatomical landmarks were used to test our automatic digitization algorithm. They were manually digitized by two experienced CMF surgeons, serving as ground-truth landmarks (Fig. 2 (a)).

The parameters in our approach were defined as follows. The local patch sizes were set as $7.5mm$,$15mm$ and $30mm$ isotropically. The number of trees was set at 10 and the tree depth was set at 20. In the regression voting, the scaling coefficient α for the weight was set at 20.

3.2 Experimental Results

We conducted a two-fold cross validation for 15 patient's CBCTs to evaluate the performance of our S-PRF model. Note that 30 MSCTs were added into the

Table 1. Digitization errors of two-fold cross validation.

Landmark	Go-R	Go-L	Me	Pg	LR1	LL1	N	Or-R	Or-L	UR1	UL1
CBCT (mm)	1.66	1.41	1.35	1.37	1.48	1.62	1.63	1.22	1.25	1.20	1.38
MSCT (mm)	1.70	1.52	1.14	1.23	1.30	1.41	1.71	1.41	1.63	1.14	1.19

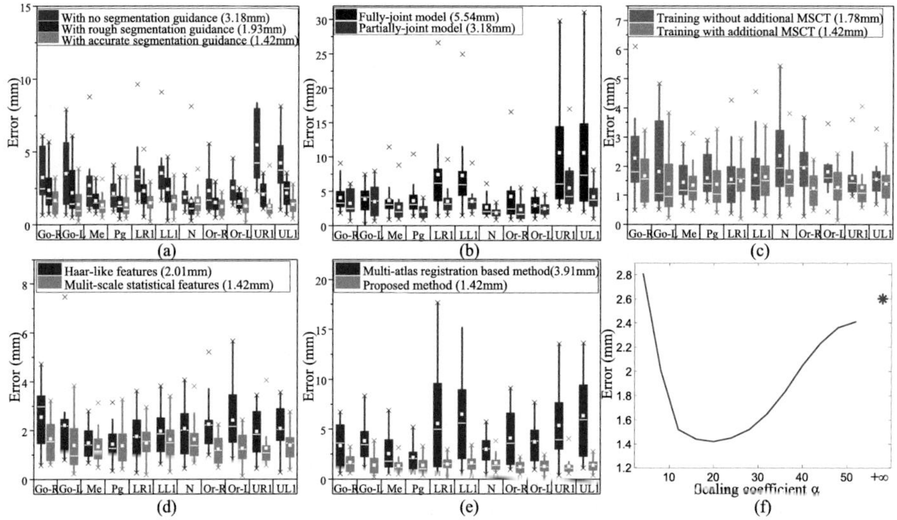

Fig. 4. Quantitative comparisons. The results of same color across different subfigures are the same, and the number inside the parenthesis is the mean error for all the landmarks and patients. (a) Digitization errors with different segmentation accuracies. (b) Digitization errors of using partially-joint model and fully-joint model. (c) Digitization errors with and without MSCT for training. (d) Digitization errors of using Haar-like features and multi-scale statistical features. (e) Digitization errors of using registration-based landmark digitization. (f) Digitization errors of using different scaling coefficients.

training dataset in each cross validation, to enlarge the sample size of training data. Table 1 shows the mean errors of the landmarks automatically detected using our approach, in comparison to the ground truth. All the errors are less than $2mm$, which is clinically acceptable [7]. Moreover, two-fold cross validation was also performed for 30 MSCT data as shown in Table 1. We also completed a group of additional two-fold cross validations to evaluate the effects of each strategy used in our approach. They are described below in details.

Effect on the Segmentation-Guided Strategy: We first compared the performance of our method among three situations: 1) using rough segmentation, 2) using accurate segmentation, and 3) using no segmentation as guidance. Here, a rough segmentation was obtained by simple majority voting with aligned multiple atlases (which offers the average Dice ratio of 0.78). An accurate segmentation was obtained by using the patch-based sparse representation segmentation method [8] (which offers the average Dice ratio of 0.89). The results in Fig. 4 (a) show that the landmark digitization performance is significantly improved even using rough segmentation, due to significant reduction of morphological variations by separating the mandible from the maxilla.

Effect on the Use of Partially-Joint Versus Fully-Joint Models: In order to evaluate the effect of morphological variations to the joint estimation of landmarks, we further completed an experiment to compare the performance of landmark digitization using either a partially-joint model or a fully-joint model, both without using segmentation as guidance. In the fully-joint model, all the landmarks are jointly estimated. The partially-joint model is the same as our proposed approach (except using segmentation as guidance), to separately estimate the landmarks from different groups. As shown in Fig. 4 (b), the partially-joint model achieves better performance than the fully-joint model. These results further support our observation that positional relationships among all the landmarks are not stable, due to morphological variations.

Effect on Adding Additional MSCT Images into the Training Dataset: We compared performance by using or removing the additional 30 MSCTs from the training dataset. Although CBCT and MSCT are different modalities, they have very similar morphology as shown in Fig. 1 (c). The results in Fig. 4 (c) show that the performance of automatic landmark digitization can be significantly improved by using additional MSCTs to help training.

Effect on Features: We also compared Haar-like features and multi-scale statistical features in our framework. The results in Fig. 4 (d) show that our framework, with multi-scale statistical features, achieves better digitization accuracy compare to that of Haar-like features. This can explain the effectiveness of our features in CBCT landmark digitalization.

Comparison with Registration-Based Landmark Detection: We implemented a multi-atlas landmark digitization approach, where the landmark was localized by averaging the corresponding positions in the aligned atlases. The result is shown in Fig. 4 (e). Due to registration error, the detection error obtained by simple multi-atlas-based method is relatively large.

Effect on the Use of Scaling Coefficient: Fig. 4 (f) shows the effect of using different scaling coefficients α. The digitization performance is significantly improved by using proper scaling coefficient.

4 Conclusion

We proposed a new S-PRF model to automatically digitize CMF landmarks. Our model has addressed the challenges of both inter-patient morphological variations and imaging artifacts. Specifically, by using regression based voting, our model can potentially resolve the issue of imaging artifacts near the landmark. Also, by using image segmentation as guidance, our model can address the issue of inconsistent landmark appearances, especially for teeth. Finally, by using a partially-joint model, the digitization reliability can be further improved through the best utilization of coherence in landmark positions. The experimental results show that the accuracy of our automatically digitized landmarks is clinically acceptable.

References

[1] Cheng, E., Chen, J., Yang, J., Deng, H., Wu, Y., Megalooikonomou, V., Gable, B., Ling, H.: Automatic dent-landmark detection in 3-d cbct dental volumes. In: 2011 Annual International Conference of the IEEE Engineering in Medicine and Biology Society, EMBC, pp. 6204–6207 (2011)
[2] Cootes, T.F., Ionita, M.C., Lindner, C., Sauer, P.: Robust and accurate shape model fitting using random forest regression voting. In: Fitzgibbon, A., Lazebnik, S., Perona, P., Sato, Y., Schmid, C. (eds.) ECCV 2012, Part VII. LNCS, vol. 7578, pp. 278–291. Springer, Heidelberg (2012)
[3] Criminisi, A., Robertson, D., Konukoglu, E., Shotton, J., Pathak, S., White, S., Siddiqui, K.: Regression forests for efficient anatomy detection and localization in computed tomography scans. Medical Image Analysis 17(8), 1293–1303 (2013)
[4] Gao, Y., Shen, D.: Context-aware anatomical landmark detection: Application to deformable model initialization in prostate ct images. In: Wu, G., Zhang, D., Zhou, L. (eds.) MLMI 2014. LNCS, vol. 8679, pp. 165–173. Springer, Heidelberg (2014)
[5] Keustermans, J., Smeets, D., Vandermeulen, D., Suetens, P.: Automated cephalometric landmark localization using sparse shape and appearance models. In: Suzuki, K., Wang, F., Shen, D., Yan, P. (eds.) MLMI 2011. LNCS, vol. 7009, pp. 249–256. Springer, Heidelberg (2011)
[6] Lindner, C., Thiagarajah, S., Wilkinson, J.M., Consortium, T., Wallis, G., Cootes, T.: Fully automatic segmentation of the proximal femur using random forest regression voting. IEEE Transactions on Medical Imaging 32(8), 1462–1472 (2013)
[7] Lou, L., Lagravere, M.O., Compton, S., Major, P.W., Flores-Mir, C.: Accuracy of measurements and reliability of landmark identification with computed tomography (ct) techniques in the maxillofacial area: a systematic review. Oral Surgery, Oral Medicine, Oral Pathology, Oral Radiology, and Endodontology 104(3), 402–411 (2007)
[8] Wang, L., Chen, K.C., Gao, Y., Shi, F., Liao, S., Li, G., Shen, S.G., Yan, J., Lee, P.K., Chow, B., et al.: Automated bone segmentation from dental cbct images using patch-based sparse representation and convex optimization. Medical Physics 41(4), 043503 (2014)
[9] Shahidi, S., Bahrampour, E., Soltanimehr, E., Zamani, A., Oshagh, M., Moattari, M., Mehdizadeh, A.: The accuracy of a designed software for automated localization of craniofacial landmarks on cbct images. BMC Medical Imaging 14(1), 32 (2014)
[10] Xia, J.J., Gateno, J., Teichgraeber, J.F.: A new clinical protocol to evaluate cranio-maxillofacial deformity and to plan surgical correction. Journal of Oral and Maxillofacial Surgery: Official Journal of the American Association of Oral and Maxillofacial Surgeons 67(10), 2093 (2009)
[11] Zhang, J., Liang, J., Zhao, H.: Local energy pattern for texture classification using self-adaptive quantization thresholds. IEEE Transactions on Image Processing 22(1), 31–42 (2013)
[12] Zhang, S., Zhan, Y., Dewan, M., Huang, J., Metaxas, D.N., Zhou, X.S.: Towards robust and effective shape modeling: Sparse shape composition. Medical Image Analysis 16(1), 265–277 (2012)

Automatic Feature Learning for Glaucoma Detection Based on Deep Learning

Xiangyu Chen[1], Yanwu Xu[1], Shuicheng Yan[2], Damon Wing Kee Wong[1], Tien Yin Wong[3], and Jiang Liu[1]

[1] Institute for Infocomm Research, Agency for Science, Technology and Research, Singapore
[2] Department of Electrical and Computer Engineering, National University of Singapore
[3] Department of Ophthalmology, National University of Singapore

Abstract. Glaucoma is a chronic and irreversible eye disease in which the optic nerve is progressively damaged, leading to deterioration in vision and quality of life. In this paper, we present an Automatic feature Learning for glAucoma Detection based on Deep LearnINg (ALADDIN), with deep convolutional neural network (CNN) for feature learning. Different from the traditional convolutional layer that uses linear filters followed by a non-linear activation function to scan the input, the adopted network embeds micro neural networks (multilayer perceptron) with more complex structures to abstract the data within the receptive field. Moreover, a contextualizing deep learning structure is proposed in order to obtain a hierarchical representation of fundus images to discriminate between glaucoma and non-glaucoma pattern, where the network takes the outputs from other CNN as the context information to boost the performance. Extensive experiments are performed on the *ORIGA* and *SCES* datasets. The results show area under curve (AUC) of the receiver operating characteristic curve in glaucoma detection at 0.838 and 0.898 in the two databases, much better than state-of-the-art algorithms. The method could be used for glaucoma diagnosis.

1 Introduction

Glaucoma is a chronic eye disease that leads to vision loss, in which the optic nerve is progressively damaged. It is one of the common causes of blindness, and is predicted to affect around 80 million people by 2020 [8]. Glaucoma is characterized by the progressive degeneration of optic nerve fibres, which leads to structural changes of the optic nerve head, the nerve fibre layer and a simultaneous functional failure of the visual field. As the symptoms only occur when the disease is quite advanced, glaucoma is called the silent thief of sight. Although glaucoma cannot be cured, its progression can be slowed down by treatment. Therefore, timely diagnosis of this disease is important.

Glaucoma diagnosis is typically based on the medical history, intra-ocular pressure and visual field loss tests together with a manual assessment of the Optic

N. Navab et al. (Eds.): MICCAI 2015, Part III, LNCS 9351, pp. 669–677, 2015.
DOI: 10.1007/978-3-319-24574-4_80

Disc (OD) through ophthalmoscopy. OD or optic nerve head is the location where ganglion cell axons exit the eye to form the optic nerve, through which visual information of the photo-receptors is transmitted to the brain. In 2D images, the OD can be divided into two distinct zones; namely, a central bright zone called the optic cup (in short, cup) and a peripheral region called the neuroretinal rim. The loss in optic nerve fibres leads to a change in the structural appearance of the OD, namely, the enlargement of cup region (thinning of neuroretinal rim) called cupping. Since one of the important indicators is the enlargement of the cup with respect to OD, various parameters are considered and estimated to detect the glaucoma, such as the vertical cup to disc ratio (CDR) [9], disc diameter [10], ISNT rule [11], and peripapillary atrophy (PPA) [12]. Since all these measurements focus on the study of OD and most of them only reflect one aspect of the glaucoma disease, effectively capturing the hierarchical deep features of OD to boost the glaucoma detection is our main interest in this paper.

Unlike natural scene images, where typical analysis tasks are related to object detection of regions that has an obvious visual appearance (e.g. texture, shape or color), glaucoma fundus images reveal a complex mixture of visual hidden patterns. These patterns could be only observed by the training and expertise of the examiner. Deep learning (DL) architectures are formed by the composition of multiple linear and non-linear transformations of the data, with the goal of yielding more abstract and ultimately more useful representations [13]. Convolutional neural networks (CNNs) are deep learning architectures, are recently been employed successfully for image segmentation and classification tasks [14,13,15]. DL architectures are an evolution of multilayer neural networks (NN), involving different design and training strategies to make them competitive. These strategies include spatial invariance, hierarchical feature learning and scalability [13][17].

In this paper, we develop a novel deep learning architecture to capture the discriminative features that better characterize the important hidden patterns related to glaucoma. The adopted DL structure consists of convolutional layers which use multilayer perceptrons to convolve the input. This kind of layers could model the local patches better [4]. Unlike conventional CNN, we develop a contextualizing training strategy, which is employed to learn deep hidden features of glaucoma. In the proposed deep CNN, the context takes the responsibility of dynamically adjusting the model learning of CNN, which exploit to effectively boost glaucoma detection by taking the outputs from one CNN as the context of the other one. In addition, to reduce the overfitting problem, we adopt response-normalization layers and overlapping-pooling layers . In order to further boost the performance, dropout and data augmentation strategies are also adopted in the proposed DL architecture.

2 Method

2.1 Feature Learning Based on Deep Convolutional Neural Network

The overview of our proposed automatic feature learning for glaucoma detection is shown in Fig.1, the net of CNN contains 6 layers: five multilayer perceptron

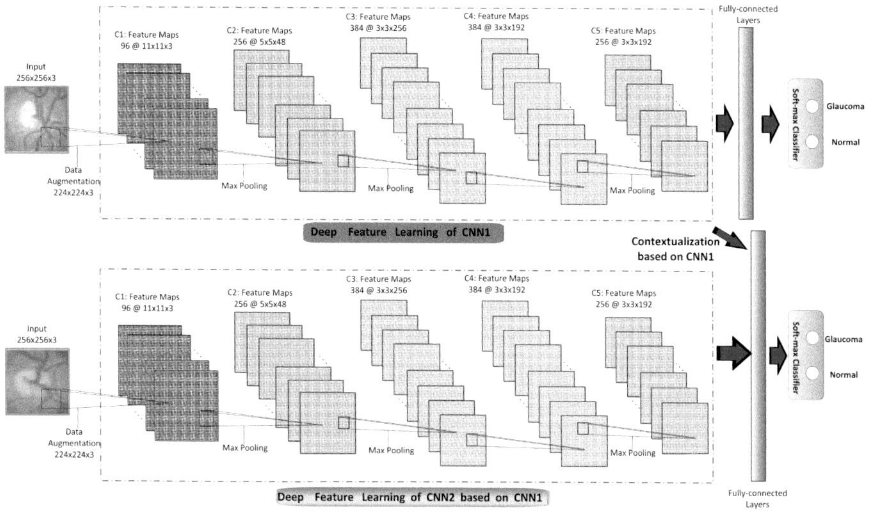

Fig. 1. System overview of our proposed automatic feature learning for glaucoma detection. The net of CNN contains 6 layers: five multilayer perceptron convolutional layers and one fully-connected layer. Data Augmentation is done by extracting random 224×224 patches from the input images. $256 \times 256 \times 3$ denotes the dimension of input image. $96@11 \times 11 \times 3$ denote 96 kernels of size $11 \times 11 \times 3$.

convolutional layers [4] and one fully-connected layer. Response-normalization layers and overlapping layers are also employed in our proposed learning architecture as in [14].

Convolutional Layers. Convolutional layers are used to learn small feature detectors based on patches randomly sampled from a large image. A feature in the image at some location can be calculated by convolving the feature detector and the image at that location. We denote $\mathbf{L}^{(n-1)}$ and $\mathbf{L}^{(n)}$ as the input and output for the n-th layer of CNN. Let $\mathbf{L}^{(0)}$ be the 2D input image patch and $\mathbf{L}^{(N)}$ be the output of the last layer N. Let $M_I^{(n)} \times M_I^{(n)}$ and $M_O^{(n)} \times M_O^{(n)}$ be the size of the input and the output map, respectively, for layer n. Denote $P_I^{(n)}$ and $P_O^{(n)}$ as the number of input and output maps respectively for the n-th layer. Since the input to n-th layer is the output of $(n-1)$-th layer, $P_I^{(n)} = P_O^{(n-1)}$ and $M_I^{(n)} = M_O^{(n-1)}$. Let $\mathbf{L}_j^{(n)}$ be the j-th output-feature-map of n th layer. As the input-feature-maps of the n th layer are actually the output-feature-maps of the $(n-1)$-th layer, $\mathbf{L}_i^{(n-1)}$ is the i-th input-feature-map of layer n. Finally, we could get the output of a convolutional layer:

$$\mathbf{L}_j^{(n)} = f(\Sigma_i \mathbf{L}_i^{(n-1)} * \mathbf{w}_{ij}^{(n)} + b_j^{(n)} \mathbf{1}_{M_O^{(n)}}), \quad (1)$$

where $\mathbf{w}_{ij}^{(n)}$ is the kernel linking i-th input map to j-th output map, $*$ denotes the convolution, $0 \leq i \leq P_I^{(n-1)}, 0 \leq j \leq P_O^{(n-1)}$, and $b_j^{(n)}$ is the bias element for j-th output-feature-map of n-th layer.

Multilayer Perceptron Convolution Layers. The convolution filter in traditional CNN is a generalized linear model (GLM) for the underlying data patch, and it is observed that the level of abstraction is low with GLM [4]. In this section, we replace the GLM with a more potent nonlinear function approximator, which is able to enhance the abstraction ability of the local model. Given no priors about the distributions of the latent concepts, it is desirable to use a universal function approximator for feature extraction of the local patches, as it is capable of approximating more abstract representations of the latent concepts. Radial basis network and multilayer perceptron are two well known universal function approximators.

There two reasons for employing multilayer perceptron in the proposed DL architecture: First, multilayer perceptron is compatible with the structure of convolutional neural networks, which is trained using back-propagation; Second, multilayer perceptron can be a deep model itself, which is consistent with the spirit of feature re-use. This type of layer is denoted as mlpconv in this paper, in which MLP replaces the GLM to convolve over the input. Here, Rectified linear unit is used as the activation function in the multilayer perceptron. Then, the calculation performed by mlpconv layer is shown as follows:

$$f_{i,j,k_1}^1 = \max(w_{k_1}^1 x_{i,j} + b_{k_1}, 0), \tag{2}$$

$$f_{i,j,k_1}^n = \max(w_{k_n}^n f_{i,j}^{n-1} + b_{k_n}, 0), \tag{3}$$

where n is the number of layers in the multilayer perceptron. (i, j) is the pixel index in the feature map, x_{ij} stands for the input patch centered at location (i, j), and k is used to index the channels of the feature map.

Contextualizing Training Strategy. Different from the traditional CNNs, training neural network independently, we adopt a contextualizing training for our proposed DL architecture, where the whole deep CNN is called Contextualized Convolutional Neural Network (C-CNN). For CNN training, we takes the outputs from one learned CNN as the context input of its own fully-connected layer. The context takes the responsibility of adjusting the model learning of CNN, and thus the contextualized convolutional neural network is achieved. Fig.1 gives an illustration of the algorithmic pipeline. As shown in Fig.1, CNN2 is trained by above mentioned C-CNN strategy, which takes the output of convolutional layers of CNN1 as a contextualized input for its own fully-connected layer. The C-CNN comprises the five multilayer perceptron convolution layers of CNN1 and whole network of CNN2. Then the prediction result of glaucoma is from the soft-max classifier of CNN2.

2.2 Glaucoma Classification

Disc Segmentation. Since optic disc is the main area for glaucoma diagnosis, disc images are the input images of our proposed C-CNN. To segment the optic disc from a retinal fundus image, we employ the method of Template Matching as adopted in [19]. The adopted disc segmentation method is based on peripapillary atrophy elimination, where the elimination is done through edge filtering, constraint elliptical Hough transform and peripapillary atrophy detection. Then each segmented disc image is down-sampled to a fixed resolution of 256×256. Finally, the mean value over all the pixels in the disc image is subtracted from each pixel to remove the influence of illumination variation among images.

Dropout and Data Augmentation. To reduce overfitting on image data, we employ data augmentation to artificially enlarge the dataset using label-preserving transformations, and dropout for model combination. Dropout consists of setting to zero the output of each hidden neuron with probability 0.5 [16]. If the neurons in CNN are dropped out, they do not contribute to the forward pass and do not participate in back propagation. During testing, we use all the neurons but multiply their outputs by 0.5. We use dropout in the fully-connected layer in our proposed deep learning architecture.

Data augmentation consists of generating image translations and horizontal reflections [14]. At training time, we perform the data augmentation by extracting random 224×224 patches including their horizontal reflections from the 256×256 images, and training our network on these extracted patches. The size of our training dataset will be increased by a factor of 2048. If we do not adopt this scheme, our network will suffer from substantial overfitting. At test time, the CNN makes a prediction by extracting five 224×224 patches including the four corner patches and the center patch, as well as their horizontal reflections, and averaging the predictions made by the network soft-max layer on these ten patches. We refer to this test strategy as multi-view test (MVT).

Automatic Classification by Softmax Regression. A softmax regression is a generalization of a logistic regression classifier, which considers as input the condensed feature maps of the pooling layer. For the binary classification setting, the classifier is trained by minimizing the following cost function:

$$J(\Omega) = 1/k[\sum_{i=1}^{k} y_i \log h_\Omega(v_i) + (1 + y_i) \log(1 - h_\Omega(v_i))], \tag{4}$$

where $(v_1, y_1), ..., (v_k, y_k)$ is the training set containing k images, and $h_\Omega(v_i) = 1/(1 + \exp(-\Omega^T v_i))$. For the i-th image, $v_i \in \Re^q$ is the image representation obtained from the output of the pooling layer and $y_i \in \{0, 1\}$ is class label. Ω is a weight vector of $q \times z$ (z is the pool dimension).

3 Experiments

To evaluate the glaucoma diagnosis performance of our proposed C-CNN method, we perform experiments on two glaucoma fundus image datasets ORIGA[5] and

Table 1. The AUCs of different CNN architectures on the ORIGA and SCES datasets. $ORIGA^m$ means that all results in this row are obtained based on various CNN structures without multi-view test strategy on ORIGA. $ORIGA^d$ means that all results in this row are obtained based on various CNN structures without dropout on ORIGA.

Methods	CNN	3 CNN	5 CNN	7 CNN	C-CNN	3 C-CNN	5 C-CNN	7 C-CNN
ORIGA	82.4 %	82.4 %	82.6%	82.5%	82.9%	83.0%	**83.8%**	83.7%
SCES	86.9 %	87.0%	87.7%	87.6%	88.6%	88.9%	**89.8%**	89.8%
$ORIGA^m$	82.0 %	82.0 %	82.3%	82.1%	82.6%	82.6%	**83.2%**	83.2%
$SCES^m$	86.4 %	86.5%	87.2%	87.1%	88.0%	88.1%	**89.0%**	89.0%
$ORIGA^d$	81.6 %	81.7 %	82.0%	82.0%	82.3%	82.4%	**83.0%**	82.9%
$SCES^d$	86.0 %	86.1%	86.7%	86.6%	87.5%	87.5%	**88.4%**	88.3%

SCES[6]. We compare our algorithm to state-of-the-art reconstruction-based [7], pixel [1], sliding window [2] and superpixel [3][18] based methods. In addition, we compare our system against the current clinical standard for glaucoma detection using intra-ocular pressure (IOP) and to CDR values from expert graders. To validate the effectiveness of our proposed C-CNN architecture, we also perform extensive experiments for glaucoma prediction utilizing different types of CNN architectures and testing strategies.

3.1 Evaluation Criteria

In this work, we utilize the area under the curve (AUC) of receiver operation characteristic curve (ROC) to evaluate the performance of glaucoma diagnosis. The ROC is plotted as a curve which shows the tradeoff between sensitivity TPR (true positive rate) and specificity TNR (true negative rate), defined as

$$TPR = \frac{TP}{TP + FN}, \; TNR = \frac{TN}{TN + FP}, \tag{5}$$

where TP and TN are the number of true positives and true negatives, respectively, and FP and FN are the number of false positives and false negatives, respectively.

3.2 Experimental Setup

We adopt the same settings of the experiments for glaucoma diagnosis in [7] in this work to facilitate comparisons. The ORIGA dataset with clinical glaucoma diagnoses, is comprised of 168 glaucoma and 482 normal fundus images. The SCES dataset contains 1676 fundus images, and 46 images are glaucoma cases.

3.3 Comparison of Different Types of CNN Architectures

We systematically compare our proposed C-CNN with different types of CNN architectures and testing strategies as listed in Table 1. Amongst them,

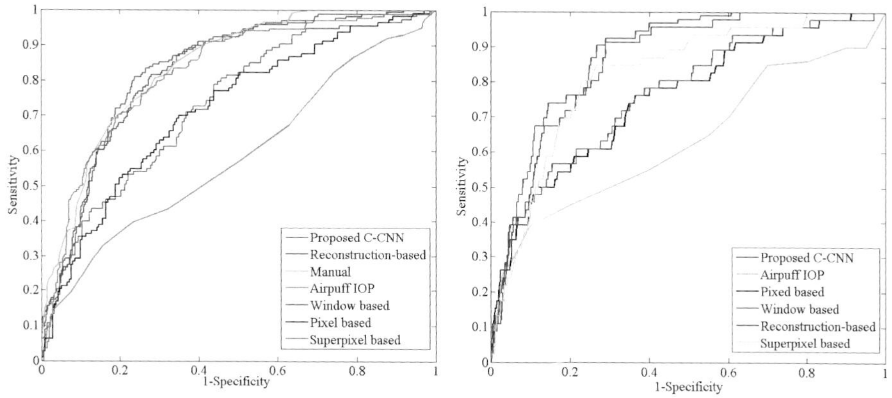

Fig. 2. Glaucoma diagnosis performance on *ORIGA* dataset (left) and *SCES* dataset (right).

- *CNN* means that the final prediction is just from one CNN.
- *3 CNN* means that the final prediction of glaucoma is obtained by averaging three similar CNNs.
- *C-CNN* means the net has 2 CNNs (the five multilayer perceptron convolution layers of CNN1 and whole network of CNN2) as shown in Fig. 1. The prediction result is from CNN2.
- *5 C-CNN* means that we have 5 CNNs and they have the concatenated structure as shown in Fig. 1.
- *7 C-CNN* means that we have 7 CNNs and they have the similar concatenated structure as shown in Fig. 1.

From the quantitative results from Table 1, we are able to observe that: 1) the method of *5 C-CNN* outperforms all the competing methods on *ORIGA* and *SCES* datasets, 2) under six different setting ($ORIGA$, $ORIGA^m$, $ORIGA^d$, $SCES$, $SCES^m$, $SCES^d$), *5 C-CNN* has the best performance. In this work, we use the *5 C-CNN* strategy to validate the glaucoma diagnosis.

3.4 Glaucoma Diagnosis

To validate the effectiveness of our method C-CNN on glaucoma diagnosis accuracy, we compare the predictions of C-CNN (here we use the 5 C-CNN) to state-of-the-art algorithms. In addition, we compare to the current standard of care for glaucoma detection using IOP, as well as CDR grading results from an expert grader. For *ORIGA* dataset, we adopt the same setting of [7]. The training set contains a random selection of 99 images from the whole 650 images, and the remaining 551 images are used for testing. For *SCES* dataset, we use the 650 images from *ORIGA* for training, and the whole 1676 images of *SCES* are the test data.

As shown in Fig. 2, the proposed C-CNN method outperforms previous automatic methods and IOP on *ORIGA* and *SCES* datasets. The AUC values of our method on *ORIGA* and *SCES* are 0.838 and 0.898, respectively. For the state-of-the-art reconstruction-based method, the AUC values are 0.823 and 0.860. On *SCES* dataset, our proposed algorithm has better boost performance than that of *ORIGA*. The reason is that the size of training set on *ORIGA* is only 99.

4 Conclusion

In this paper, we present an automatic feature learning scheme for glaucoma detection based on deep convolutional neural network, which is able to capture the discriminative features that better characterize the hidden patterns related to glaucoma. The adopted DL structure consists of convolutional layers which use multilayer perceptrons to convolve the input. Moreover, we develop a contextualizing training strategy, which is employed to learn deep features of glaucoma. In the proposed deep CNN, the context takes the responsibility of dynamically adjusting the model learning of CNN, which exploit to effectively boost glaucoma detection by taking the outputs from one CNN as the context of the other one. In future work, we plan to extend our study of deep leaning architecture based on C-CNN to multiple ocular diseases detection.

References

1. Wong, D.W.K., Lim, J.H., Tan, N.M., Zhang, Z., Lu, S., Li, H., Teo, M., Chan, K., Wong, T.Y.: Intelligent Fusion of Cup-to-Disc Ratio Determination Methods for Glaucoma Detection in ARGALI. In: Int. Conf. Engin. In: Med. and Biol. Soc., pp. 5777–5780 (2009)
2. Xu, Y., Xu, D., Lin, S., Liu, J., Cheng, J., Cheung, C.Y., Aung, T., Wong, T.Y.: Sliding Window and Regression based Cup Detection in Digital Fundus Images for Glaucoma Diagnosis. In: Fichtinger, G., Martel, A., Peters, T. (eds.) MICCAI 2011, Part III. LNCS, vol. 6893, pp. 1–8. Springer, Heidelberg (2011)
3. Xu, Y., Liu, J., Lin, S., Xu, D., Cheung, C.Y., Aung, T., Wong, T.Y.: Efficient Optic Cup Detection from Intra-image Learning with Retinal Structure Priors. In: Ayache, N., Delingette, H., Golland, P., Mori, K. (eds.) MICCAI 2012, Part I. LNCS, vol. 7510, pp. 58–65. Springer, Heidelberg (2012)
4. Lin, M., Chen, Q., Yan, S.: Network In Network. In: International Conference on Learning Representations 2014 (2014)
5. Zhang, Z., Yin, F., Liu, J., Wong, D.W.K., Tan, N.M., Lee, B.H., Cheng, J., Wong, T.Y.: Origa-Light: An Online Retinal Fundus Image Database for Glaucoma Analysis and Research. In: IEEE Int. Conf. Engin. in Med. and Biol. Soc., pp. 3065–3068 (2010)
6. Sng, C.C., Foo, L.L., Cheng, C.Y., Allen, J.C., He, M., Krishnaswamy, G., Nongpiur, M.E., Friedman, D.S., Wong, T.Y., Aung, T.: Determinants of Anterior Chamber Depth: the Singapore Chinese Eye Study. Opthalmology 119(6), 1143–1150 (2012)
7. Xu, Y., Lin, S., Wong, T.Y., Liu, J., Xu, D.: Efficient Reconstruction-Based Optic Cup Localization for Glaucoma Screening. In: Mori, K., Sakuma, I., Sato, Y., Barillot, C., Navab, N. (eds.) MICCAI 2013, Part III. LNCS, vol. 8151, pp. 445–452. Springer, Heidelberg (2013)

8. Quigley, H.A., Broman, A.T.: The number of people with glaucoma worldwide in 2010 and 2020. In: Ophthalmol 2006 (2006)
9. Damms, T., Dannheim, F.: Sensitivity and specificity of optic disc parameters in chronic glaucoma. In: Invest. Ophth. Vis. Sci. (1993)
10. Michael, D., Hancox, O.D.: Optic disc size, an important consideration in the glaucoma evaluation. In: Clinical Eye and Vision Care 1999 (1999)
11. Harizman, N., Oliveira, C., Chiang, A., Tello, C., Marmor, M., Ritch, R., Liebmann, J.M.: The isnt rule and differentiation of normal from glaucomatous eyes. In: Arch Ophthalmol 2006 (2006)
12. Jonas, J.B., Fernandez, M.C., Naumann, G.O.: Glaucomatous parapapillary atrophy occurrence and correlations. In: Arch Ophthalmol (1992)
13. Bengio, Y., et al.: Representation learning: A review and new perspectives. In: Arxiv 2012 (2012)
14. Krizhevsky, A., Sutskever, I., Hinton, G.E.: Imagenet classification with deep convolutional neural networks. In: Neural Information Processing Systems, NIPS (2012)
15. Le, Q.V., et al.: Building high-level features using large scale unsupervised learning. In: International Conference on Machine Learning, ICML (2011)
16. Hinton, G.E., Srivastava, N., Krizhevsky, A., Sutskever, I., Salakhutdinov, R.R.: Improving neural networks by preventing co-adaptation of feature detectors. In: Arxiv 2012 (2012)
17. Tu, Z.: Auto-context and its application to high-level vision tasks. In: Computer Vision and Pattern Recognition, CVPR (2008)
18. Xu, Y., Duan, L., Lin, S., Chen, X., Wong, D.W.K., Wong, T.Y., Liu, J.: Optic Cup Segmentation for Glaucoma Detection Using Low-Rank Superpixel Representation. In: Golland, P., Hata, N., Barillot, C., Hornegger, J., Howe, R. (eds.) MICCAI 2014, Part I. LNCS, vol. 8673, pp. 788–795. Springer, Heidelberg (2014)
19. Cheng, J., Liu, J., Wong, D.W.K., Yin, F., Cheung, C.Y., Baskaran, M., Aung, T., Wong, T.Y.: Automatic Optic Disc Segmentation with Peripapillary Atrophy Elimination. In: IEEE Int. Conf. Engin. in Med. and Biol. Soc., pp. 6224–6227 (2011)

Fast Automatic Vertebrae Detection and Localization in Pathological CT Scans - A Deep Learning Approach

Amin Suzani[1], Alexander Seitel[1], Yuan Liu[1], Sidney Fels[1], and Robert N. Rohling[1,2], and Purang Abolmaesumi[1]

[1] Department of Electrical and Computer Engineering
[2] Department of Mechanical Engineering, University of British Columbia, Vancouver, Canada

Abstract. Automatic detection and localization of vertebrae in medical images are highly sought after techniques for computer-aided diagnosis systems of the spine. However, the presence of spine pathologies and surgical implants, and limited field-of-view of the spine anatomy in these images, make the development of these techniques challenging. This paper presents an automatic method for detection and localization of vertebrae in volumetric computed tomography (CT) scans. The method makes no assumptions about which section of the vertebral column is visible in the image. An efficient approach based on deep feed-forward neural networks is used to predict the location of each vertebra using its contextual information in the image. The method is evaluated on a public data set of 224 arbitrary-field-of-view CT scans of pathological cases and compared to two state-of-the-art methods. Our method can perform vertebrae detection at a rate of 96% with an overall run time of less than 3 seconds. Its fast and comparably accurate detection makes it appealing for clinical diagnosis and therapy applications.

Keywords: Vertebrae localization, vertebrae detection, deep neural networks.

1 Introduction

Automatic vertebrae detection and localization in spinal imaging is a crucial component for image-guided diagnosis, surgical planning, and follow-up assessment of spine disorders such as disc/vertebra degeneration, vertebral fractures, scoliosis, and spinal stenosis. It can also be used for automatic mining of archived clinical data (PACS systems in particular). Furthermore, it can be a pre-processing step for approaches in spine segmentation, multi-modal registration, and statistical shape analysis.

The challenges associated with building an automated system for robust detection and localization of vertebrae in the spine images arise from: 1) restrictions in field-of-view; 2) repetitive nature of the spinal column; 3) high inter-subject variability in spine curvature and shape due to spine disorders and pathologies; and 4) image artifacts caused by metal implants.

N. Navab et al. (Eds.): MICCAI 2015, Part III, LNCS 9351, pp. 678–686, 2015.
DOI: 10.1007/978-3-319-24574-4_81

Several methods have been proposed in the literature for automatic vertebrae detection and localization in Computed Tomography (CT) [8,9,11,16,10] and Magnetic Resonance Imaging (MRI) volumes [10,15,14,1]. Several studies either concentrate on a specific region of the spine, or make assumptions about the visible part of the vertebral column in the image. A few recent studies claim handling arbitrary-field-of-view scans in a fully-automatic system [8,9,11,16]. The methods proposed in [8] and [16] rely on a generative model of shape and/or appearance of vertebrae. As a result, these methods may be challenged with pathological subjects, especially when metal implants produce artifacts in the image. The most promising method reported [9], uses classification forests to probabilistically classify each voxel of the image as being part of a particular vertebra. Based on predicted probabilities, the centroid of these points are obtained using the mean-shift algorithm. Although excellent results are obtained on a challenging data set, this method requires an additional post-processing step for removing false positives. This step adds to the computation time. In fact, this approach [9], which is the fastest method reported to-date, has a computation time of about a minute. Slow computation time can limit the application of automatic methods for image-guided tasks in clinics. A method with a faster computation time, on the order of seconds, has the potential to be used during guided interventions and may broaden the scope of such automatic analysis techniques.

In this work, we aim to find a faster solution to the problem of vertebra localization in general clinical CT scans by using deep neural networks [2]. No assumptions are made about which and how many vertebrae are visible in the images. The computation of image features is adopted from [8,9]. To allow for low computation times, our method does not require computationally expensive post-processing steps. We evaluate our method on a publicly-available data set, and compare it against the methods proposed by Glocker et al. [8,9] that use the same data set.

2 Methods

The vertebrae localization problem is parametrized as a multi-variate non-linear regression. Similar to [8,9] intensity-based features are extracted from voxels in the image. The features represent the short-range contextual information of the reference voxel. The targets of the regression are the relative distances between the center of each vertebral body and the reference voxel. In other words, the vector from the reference voxel to the center of the vertebral body is considered as one target in the regression.

The number of observations in our regression problem is equal to the number of selected voxels from the image. Since the images of our CT data set are labeled with 26 landmarks (26 vertebral bodies), the target of our regression includes 26 three-dimensional vectors for each observation. Therefore, the vertebrae localization problem is parametrized as a multi-variate regression with 500 features and $26 \times 3 = 78$ targets.

For a test image, we first extract intensity-based features from all the voxels. We then use a deep neural network to predict the relative distance vector of

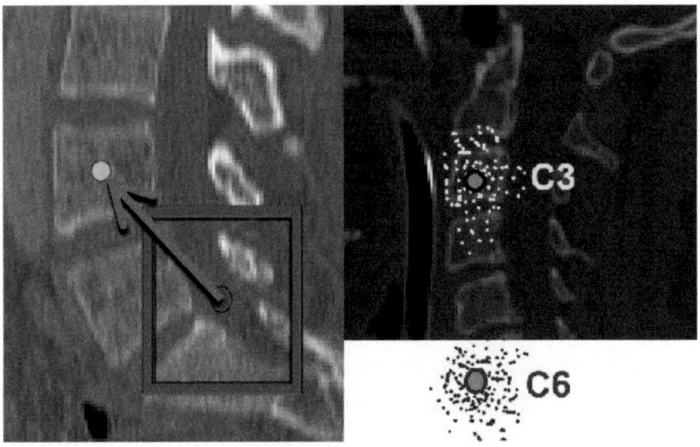

Fig. 1. Left: The vertebrae localization problem is parametrized as a regression problem. The targets of the regression are the vectors from the reference voxel to the center of each vertebral body (The orange arrow). The reference voxel is described by 500 intensity-based features which are extracted from the area around it. The green point is considered as the vote of the red voxel for a specific vertebra. Right: Location of each vertebra is estimated by getting the centroid of the votes of the voxels. This centroid may or may not be located inside the field of view of the image. In this case, C3 is considered as a true positive, and C6 is considered as a true negative.

each vertebral body with respect to the reference voxel. Knowing the location of the reference voxel and the relative distance vector to the center of a specific vertebral body, we can compute the predicted absolute location of the vertebral body on the test image. This absolute location is considered the vote of that voxel for the location of a vertebral body. Note that these votes might be either inside or outside of the field-of-view of the image. Each voxel in the image votes for the location of each vertebral body, so for each specific vertebral body, we compute the centroid of these votes to obtain a single prediction for the location of the vertebral body.

2.1 Point Selection

In our method, each vertebra is localized by aggregating the votes of the points in the image. However, in most of the images there are certain regions, like those in the background, that do not help with the prediction of vertebrae. Disregarding these points increases the accuracy and decreases the computational time. To this end, we use the Canny edge detector [5] and disregard points that are not close to the extracted edges.

2.2 Feature Extraction

The value of each feature is the mean intensity over a three-dimensional cuboid displaced with respect to the reference voxel position. The cuboid dimensions and the displacement of each feature are chosen randomly. For the reference voxel p, the feature vector $v(p) = (v_1, ..., v_j, ..., v_m)$ is computed as follows:

$$v_j = \frac{1}{|F_{p;j}|} \sum_{q \in F_{p;j}} I(q), \tag{1}$$

where $I(q)$ is the image intensity at position q in the image, and $q \in F_{p;j}$ are the image voxels within the cuboid. $F_{p;j}$ denotes the feature cuboid j displaced in respect to voxel p. Similar features are used in [8,7,6] for object detection and localization. Extracting mean intensity over cuboidal regions can be computed very quickly by using an integral image (introduced in [18]). These features are then used to train a regressor for vertebra localization.

2.3 Deep Neural Network

In recent years, state-of-the-art results have been produced by applying deep learning to various tasks in computer vision [12,17]. In this work, a deep feed-forward neural network with six layers is used for solving the multi-variate non-linear regression problem. The parameters of the network were set as an input layer holding 500 neurons, and four hidden layers with 200, 300, 200, and 150 neurons, followed by 78 neurons in the output layer. The intensity-based features of each selected voxel are given as the input to the network. The network output is the estimated relative distances of the voxel to the center of each vertebral body. These relative distances are then converted to absolute voxel positions in the image. We use a rectifier function, $g_{hidden}(x) = max(0, x)$, to activate the hidden layers, and a linear function, $g_{output}(x) = x$, to activate the output layer. The deep neural network is trained by using layerwise pre-training [3] and then, by fine-tuning the connection weights using conventional backpropagation. Layerwise pre-training involves breaking down the deep network into several shallow networks and training each of them greedily. Stochastic gradient descent (SGD) is used for minimizing the cost function in both pre-training and fine-tuning steps.

2.4 Centroid Estimation

In our approach, we used an adaptive kernel density estimation method [4] to obtain a fast and reliable density function for the voxel votes for each vertebral body. The global maximum of this density function is considered as the predicted location of the centroid of the vertebral body in the image. The main advantage of using this method as opposed to e.g. the popular Gaussian kernel density estimation is its lower sensitivity to outliers and its fast, automatic data-driven bandwidth selection that does not make any assumptions about normality of the input data [4,13].

2.5 Refinement

The predicted vertebra locations are refined by estimating the centroid of only the votes which are close to the predicted location. For each visible vertebra (according to the prediction of the previous step) in the image, the points around itself and its adjacent vertebrae (if present) are aggregated using kernel density estimation. The previously-localized points are then replaced by the points that are obtained from this step.

3 Experiments and Results

The performance of our method is evaluated on a publicly-available data set[1] consisting of 224 spine-focused CT scans of patients with varying types of pathologies. The pathologies include fractures, high-grade scoliosis, and kyphosis. Many cases are post-operative scans where severe image artifacts are caused by surgical implants. Various sections of the spine are visible in different images. The field-of-view is mostly limited to 5-15 vertebrae while the whole spine is visible in only a few cases.

In this work, *detection* records whether or not the input image contains a specific vertebra while *localization* determines the center of a specific vertebra in the image. After estimating the centroid of the votes of the voxels, our system may conclude that a specific vertebra is outside of the field-of-view of the image. If expert annotation confirms that the vertebra is not visible in the image, we consider it as a true negative (TN). Otherwise, if the image contains the vertebra, it will be a false negative (FN). Similarly, if our system concludes that the vertebra is in the field-of-view of the image and the expert annotations confirm, it is considered as a true positive (TP). Otherwise, it will be a false positive (FP). Based on these parameters, the detection rates are evaluated in terms of accuracy, precision, sensitivity, and specificity. Localization error is defined as the Euclidean distance between the estimated centroid of a vertebral body and its expert annotation. The mean and standard deviation of these localization errors are reported for each region and also for the whole vertebral column. Two-fold cross-validation is performed on two non-overlapping sets of volumetric CT scans with 112 images each. The results on data from fold 1 were obtained after training the deep neural network on fold 2, and vice versa. The folds are selected exactly as in [9] to enable comparing the results. All deep network parameters were set the same for this two-fold cross-validation. This approach also mitigates the risk of overfitting, as the training and testing are performed on two independent data sets.

Our final detection and localization results are presented in Table 1. Figure 2 illustrates exemplary localization results. The results show the capability of our method for detecting the vertebrae present in the image.

We compared our results to [8] and [9] and evaluated their methods on the same data set with a two-fold cross validation with exactly the same fold separation. The results of this comparison is summarized in Table 2.

[1] `http://spineweb.digitalimaginggroup.ca/`

Table 1. Detection rates and localization error for different regions of the vertebral column.

	Accuracy	Precision	Sensitivity	Specificity	Mean error	Std
All	96.0%	94.4%	97.2%	95.0%	18.2 mm	11.4 mm
Cervical	96.0%	91.2%	97.8%	95.0%	17.1 mm	8.7 mm
Thoracic	95.1%	93.9%	95.9%	94.5%	17.2 mm	11.8 mm
Lumbar	98.1%	97.5%	99.4%	96.1%	20.3 mm	12.2 mm

Table 2. Comparison of the detection rates and the mean localization error of our method with prior works. The same training and test sets are used in evaluations of all three methods.

	Accuracy	Precision	Sensitivity	Specificity	Mean error	Std
Ours	**96.0%**	**94.4%**	**97.2%**	**95.0%**	18.2 mm	11.4 mm
CF [9]	93.9%	93.7%	92.9%	94.7%	**12.4 mm**	11.2 mm
RF+HMM [8]	-	-	-	-	20.9 mm	20.0 mm

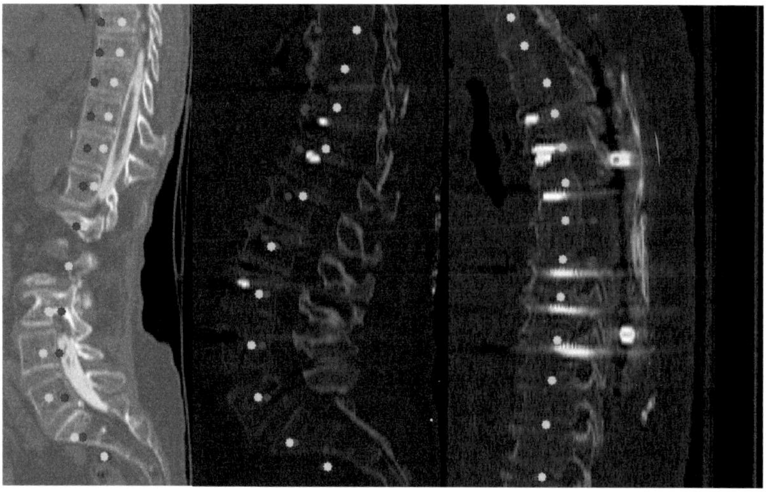

Fig. 2. Visual representation of the refinement step are shown on the mid-sagittal plane of three example images. The localization points before refinement are shown in red while the points after refinement by local centroid estimation are shown in cyan. Refined points have a better representation of the spine curvatures.

For evaluating the influence of Kernel Density Estimation (KDE) for centroid estimation, we repeated the experiments and used the mean and median of the points instead of the maximum of the density function. Using the median of the points instead of KDE reduced the overall accuracy from 96% to 93%, while using the mean of the points reduced it further to 88%.

4 Discussion

We proposed an approach for automatic and simultaneous detection and localization of vertebrae in three-dimensional CT scans using deep neural networks.

We evaluated our algorithm on a large publicly-available data set and compared it against two state-of-the-art methods. We achieved a localization accuracy of 96% which is comparable to results achieved by these methods. Detection and localization of all visible vertebrae can be performed in less then 3 seconds per CT volume which is significantly faster than reported for the methods of comparison that run in the order of minutes.

The key differences between the proposed method and the approaches introduced by Glocker et al. [8,9] are in the choice of the estimator (deep neural networks vs. random forests) and the method used for estimating the vertebra centroid (KDE vs. mean shift clustering). The deep learning approach allowed us to achieve comparably high localization accuracies while reducing the amount of post-processing needed. The influence of KDE in this matter can be regarded relatively low, as even a simple centroid estimation method using the median instead of the maximum of the density function achieves only slightly worse localization accuracies (93% using median vs. 96% using KDE) that are still in the range of the ones reported in [9]. While our results with deep neural networks are highly promising, deep neural networks has a very large number of parameters that need to be optimized preferably on very large data sets. We mitigate this issue in this work by using the greedy layerwise pre-training algorithm [3], which helps with tuning the network parameters layer-by-layer within a much smaller search space.

In [8], a voting framework based on regression forests is used to obtain a rough localization, and then a graphical model based on a hidden Markov model is used for refinement. The results of their method on this public data set is provided in [9]. They have reported lower localization errors on a data set of non-pathological cases. However, the performance of their method degrades significantly in this public pathological data set. A possible reason is that the graphical model cannot accommodate high variations in pathological cases and consequently fails to refine the predictions in this data set. Using a deep learning technique, we can eliminate the need for model-refinement which has relatively high computational cost and did not prove to be robust in pathological cases. The method presented in [9] uses a method based on classification forests that does not require any model-based refinements. While their approach has a lower mean error, our method shows higher accuracy, precision, sensitivity, and specificity. The computational cost of their method is adversely affected by adding extra steps such as a semi-automatic framework to provide dense annotations for the training data, mean shift clustering, and a post-processing step for removing false positives. The algorithms presented in [8] and [9] take about 2 minutes and 1 minute per image, respectively, on a desktop machine. In [8] a joint shape and appearance model in several scales is used to refine the predictions. In [9] centroid density estimates based on vertebra appearance are combined with a shape support term to remove false positives. Our method does not require any post-processing step and runs in less than 3 seconds on a desktop machine.

Combining the advantages of a deep neural network for regression and KDE for final centroid estimation allows us to efficiently detect and localize vertebrae in CT volumes with high accuracy. The low computational cost of our approach makes it appealing for clinical diagnosis and therapy applications.

Acknowledgement. This work is funded in part by the Natural Sciences and Engineering Research Council of Canada (NSERC), and the Canadian Institutes of Health Research (CIHR).

References

1. Alomari, R., Corso, J., Chaudhary, V.: Labeling of lumbar discs using both pixel- and object-level features with a two-level probabilistic model. IEEE Transactions on Medical Imaging 30(1), 1–10 (2011)
2. Bengio, Y.: Learning deep architectures for AI. Foundations and Trends® in Machine Learning 2(1), 1–127 (2009)
3. Bengio, Y., Lamblin, P., Popovici, D., Larochelle, H.: Greedy layer-wise training of deep networks. Advances in Neural Information Processing Systems 19, 153–168 (2007)
4. Botev, Z., Grotowski, J., Kroese, D., et al.: Kernel density estimation via diffusion. The Annals of Statistics 38(5), 2916–2957 (2010)
5. Canny, J.: A computational approach to edge detection. IEEE Transactions on Pattern Analysis and Machine Intelligence (6), 679–698 (1986)
6. Criminisi, A., Robertson, D., Pauly, O., Glocker, B., Konukoglu, E., Shotton, J., Mateus, D., Möller, A., Nekolla, S., Navab, N.: Anatomy detection and localization in 3D medical images. In: Decision Forests for Computer Vision and Medical Image Analysis, pp. 193–209. Springer, Heidelberg (2013)
7. Criminisi, A., Shotton, J., Bucciarelli, S.: Decision forests with long-range spatial context for organ localization in CT volumes. In: Proc MICCAI Workshop on Probabilistic Models for Medical Image Analysis, pp. 69–80 (2009)
8. Glocker, B., Feulner, J., Criminisi, A., Haynor, D.R., Konukoglu, E.: Automatic localization and identification of vertebrae in arbitrary field-of-view CT scans. In: Ayache, N., Delingette, H., Golland, P., Mori, K. (eds.) MICCAI 2012, Part III. LNCS, vol. 7512, pp. 590–598. Springer, Heidelberg (2012)
9. Glocker, B., Zikic, D., Konukoglu, E., Haynor, D.R., Criminisi, A.: Vertebrae localization in pathological spine CT via dense classification from sparse annotations. In: Mori, K., Sakuma, I., Sato, Y., Barillot, C., Navab, N. (eds.) MICCAI 2013, Part II. LNCS, vol. 8150, pp. 262–270. Springer, Heidelberg (2013)
10. Kelm, B., Wels, M., Zhou, S., Seifert, S., Suehling, M., Zheng, Y., Comaniciu, D.: Spine detection in CT and MR using iterated marginal space learning. Medical Image Analysis 17(8), 1283–1292 (2013)
11. Klinder, T., Ostermann, J., Ehm, M., Franz, A., Kneser, R., Lorenz, C.: Automated model-based vertebra detection, identification, and segmentation in CT images. Medical Image Analysis 13(3), 471–482 (2009)
12. Krizhevsky, A., Sutskever, I., Hinton, G.: Imagenet classification with deep convolutional neural networks. In: Advances in Neural Information Processing Systems, pp. 1097–1105 (2012)
13. Lim, P., Bagci, U., Bai, L.: Introducing Willmore flow into level set segmentation of spinal vertebrae. IEEE Transactions on Biomedical Engineering 60(1), 115–122 (2013)

14. Oktay, A., Akgul, Y.: Simultaneous localization of lumbar vertebrae and intervertebral discs with SVM-based MRF. IEEE Transactions on Biomedical Engineering 60(9), 2375–2383 (2013)
15. Peng, Z., Zhong, J., Wee, W., Lee, J.: Automated vertebra detection and segmentation from the whole spine MR images. In: 27th Annual International Conference of the Engineering in Medicine and Biology Society, IEEE-EMBS 2005, pp. 2527–2530. IEEE (2006)
16. Rasoulian, A., Rohling, R., Abolmaesumi, P.: Automatic labeling and segmentation of vertebrae in CT images. In: SPIE Medical Imaging, pp. 903623–903623. International Society for Optics and Photonics (2014)
17. Szegedy, C., Toshev, A., Erhan, D.: Deep neural networks for object detection. In: Advances in Neural Information Processing Systems, pp. 2553–2561 (2013)
18. Viola, P., Jones, M.: Robust real-time face detection. International Journal of Computer Vision 57(2), 137–154 (2004)

Guided Random Forests for Identification of Key Fetal Anatomy and Image Categorization in Ultrasound Scans

Mohammad Yaqub[1], Brenda Kelly[2], A.T. Papageorghiou[2], and J. Alison Noble[1]

[1] Institute of Biomedical Engineering, Engineering Science, University of Oxford
[2] Nuffield Department of Obstetrics & Gynaecology University of Oxford

Abstract. In this paper, we propose a novel machine learning based method to categorize unlabeled fetal ultrasound images. The proposed method guides the learning of a Random Forests classifier to extract features from regions inside the images where meaningful structures exist. The new method utilizes a translation and orientation invariant feature which captures the appearance of a region at multiple spatial resolutions. Evaluated on a large real world clinical dataset (~30K images from a hospital database), our method showed very promising categorization accuracy ($accuracy_{top1}$ is 75% while $accuracy_{top2}$ is 91%).

Keywords: Random Forests, Ultrasound, Image Categorization, Classification, Normalized Cross Correlation.

1 Introduction

Image categorization is a well-known open-research problem in computer vision for which many solutions have been proposed [1-3]. In medical image applications, image categorization is relatively under-investigated but nevertheless important. The volume of digital images acquired in the healthcare sector for screening, diagnosis or therapy is very large and increasing steadily.

Ultrasound based fetal anomaly screening is usually performed at 18 to 22 weeks of gestation. Several images of fetal structures are acquired following a standardized protocol. This screening scan aims to determine whether the fetus is developing normally by assessing several ultrasound images of different fetal structures. The number of different structures that are imaged and acquired in a complete scan varies, for example, the UK NHS Fetal Anomaly Screening Programme (FASP) recommends 21 views to be assessed and at least 9 images to be stored. The number of individual women undergoing a scan is often of the order of several thousands per department per annum. Most clinical departments save these scans to an archive system without any labeling of these images. This means it is not possible to recall images of body parts conveniently for later review or measurement nor to compare scans of the same fetus over time, or conduct automatic measurement post-acquisition.

Manual categorization is of course theoretically possible. However, it is expensive as it requires a good level of expertise alongside being tedious and time consuming. In this paper, we propose a method to automatically categorize fetal ultrasound images from anomaly scans. The new method is built on a machine learning classifier (Random

N. Navab et al. (Eds.): MICCAI 2015, Part III, LNCS 9351, pp. 687–694, 2015.
DOI: 10.1007/978-3-319-24574-4_82

Forests RF) in which we propose novel ideas to guide the classifier to focus on regions of interest (ROI). Although there are a number of methods which have been proposed to address different medical image categorization problems [4-6], very little research has been done in fetal ultrasound image categorization [4, 7, 8]. This may in part be explained because fetal ultrasound image categorization has unique challenges - the quality and appearance of the images vary for a number of reasons including variation of fetal position, sonographer experience, and maternal factors all affect the appearance of images. In addition, one fetal ultrasound image can contain one or more fetal and non-fetal structures. This implies that general classification methods applied to a whole image to output single-class fail to achieve this task robustly. Here we instead propose to restrict classification to candidate regions of interest.

The most closely related work to ours is [4] in which the authors proposed a machine learning method based on Probabilistic Boosting Tree (PBT) to automatically detect and measure anatomical structures in fetal ultrasound images. The method learns a PBT from coarse to fine resolution using Haar features to output object location. In our work, we also use a family of Haar features but ours are generalizable and allow capturing not only local but global appearance. In addition, the ultimate goal of [4] was to perform measurements on the detected object. Our goal is the more general goal of categorizing images by their content. Moreover, we evaluate our method on a much larger dataset (30K vs 5K). Finally, we base our solution on a RF classifier which has proven to outperform many state-of-the-art learners including boosting methods [9].

2 Guided Random Forests

In general, the proposed method first extracts novel features from 2D fetal ultrasound images to build a RF classifier which learns the anatomy within any image. The classifier learns eight classes which represent seven anatomical views 1) head in the trans-ventricular plane (Head TV), 2) head in the trans-cerebellar plane (Head TC), 3) 4-chamber view of the heart (cardio), 4) face (a coronal view of the lips), 5) abdomen (at the level where the abdominal circumference is measured), 6) femur (for the measurement of femur length), 7) spine and 8) a category called "Others" which may contain many other fetal structures e.g., limbs, kidneys, cord insertion, etc.

Learning is guided because the proposed features are extracted from regions where structures of interest exist. This helps avoid misleading anatomy within these images. We propose a method to build the features computed on these regions in a translation, orientation, and scaling invariant fashion that is key to make our proposed learning algorithm robust.

2.1 Localizing Object of Interests

The main objective in this method is to automatically localize a single object of interest. The proposed RF method samples features from within discriminative regions instead of looking blindly everywhere across the images. As noted earlier, this is important in ultrasound where there can be distracting regions of similar appearance. To achieve this we have built several multi-resolution and multi-orientation geometric templates which capture the geometric appearance of the main structures we are interested in classifying.

To find the best match between an image *I* and a template *T*, we compute the normalized cross-correlation between *I* and *T* in the Fourier domain. The parameters for the image region which produces the maximum correlation with the template are recorded. These 9 parameters are $\{corr, s, d, \underline{C}, \underline{P_1}, \underline{P_2}\}$ such that *corr* is the template correlation value (response), *s* is the relative size of the matched region with respect to the original image size, *d* is the Euclidean distance measured between the center of the region $\underline{C} = \{cx, cy\}$ and the center of the image, $\underline{P_1} = \{x_1, y_1\}$ is the location of the top left corner of the matched region within the image, and $\underline{P_2} = \{x_2, y_2\}$ is the location of the bottom right corner.

We utilize established clinical knowledge of fetal anatomy in the templates to ensure that their physical size correspond to the size of fetal structures. For instance, biparietal diameter (the minor axis of the fetal skull) of the fetal skull ranges from 40mm to 55mm [10]. Fig. 1 shows an example from each template type. Fig. 2 illustrates the matched regions of best-matched templates on three ultrasound images (see supplementary videos for further examples). We use *green* for skull, *blue* for spine, *red* for face, *magenta* for abdomen and *yellow* for femur. The width of the border of the box indicates the strength of the template response (*corr*).

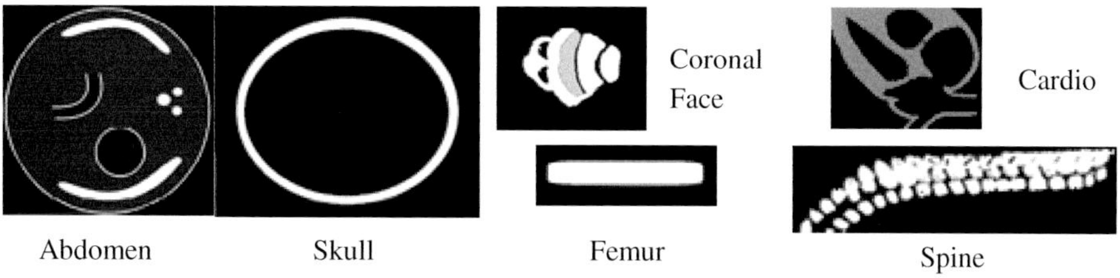

Fig. 1. Examples of a representative set of fetal structure templates.

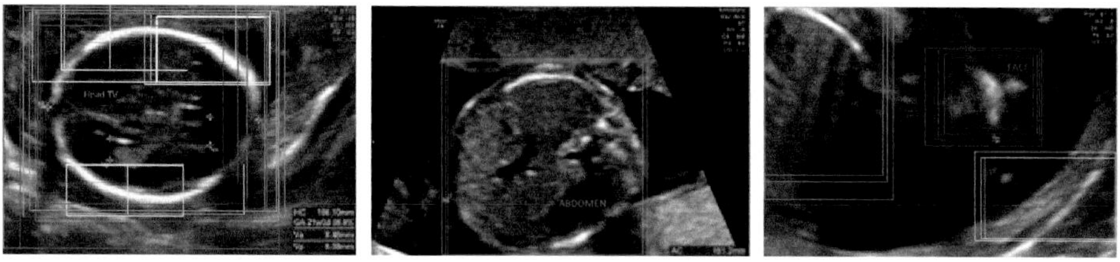

(a) Head TV (b) Abdomen (c) Face

Fig. 2. Template responses on three images (regions with high responses are only shown here for convenience). The template response is depicted as a colored rectangle (see text for color definition).

2.2 Feature Sets for the Learning Algorithm

Our machine learning solution utilizes two feature sets. The first feature set represents template metadata (*corr*, *s*, *d*) as defined in Section 2.1. These values are highly discriminative since *corr* provides an indication of how probable it is that a region contains a structure of interest, *s* indicates how large a region is within an image e.g., fetal face occupies a small region within an image while a skull is typically larger, and d is the Euclidian distance between a region and the center of the image i.e., in sonography the structure of interest typically appears in the middle of the image; therefore, if an image contains two anatomical structures, this feature will lean to classify the image according to the structure that appears closer to center of the image. The number of features in this feature set is small (77×3=231; here 77 is the number of templates) but highly discriminative between some structures e.g., head TV vs spine. However, this set is not rich enough alone for good discrimination. For instance, the skull template will not distinguish between head TV and head TC and the femur and spine templates look similar and can provide similar responses.

The second feature set captures the appearance of a region R by splitting the region into a number of rows r and columns c such that r and c are randomly selected by the learning algorithm. This random splitting allows multiresolution distinction between regions (scaling invariance). In other words, if r and c are small, global appearance of the region is captured while if r and c are as large as the number of rows and columns in the region then fine detail appearance is learned. Fig. 3 (a) shows a candidate region which is split into 12 blocks. In general, the mean intensity is computed inside each block $k : [1, (r{\times}c)]$. To compute the relative appearance between blocks within a region, a square feature matrix A (as in Fig. 3 (b)) of $(r{\times}c)$ rows and columns is computed as follows

$$\forall \begin{bmatrix} i = 1:(r \times c) \\ j - 1:(r \times c) \end{bmatrix}, \quad A_{k_i,k_j} = \begin{cases} Mean(block_{k_i}) & \mid i = j \\ Mean(block_{k_i}) - Mean\left(block_{k_j}\right) & \mid i \neq j \end{cases}, \quad (1)$$

As in [11], a feature value is then computed as

$$f = log_e\,(det(A)) \quad : \quad det\ is\ the\ determinant\ of\ a\ matrix \quad (2)$$

Because the location of a region is not fixed within the image, the computed feature over a region is translation invariant. In addition, because the matrix A represents the variance between a given block and the rest irrespective of block position within a region, this feature type robustly learns region appearance at different orientations.

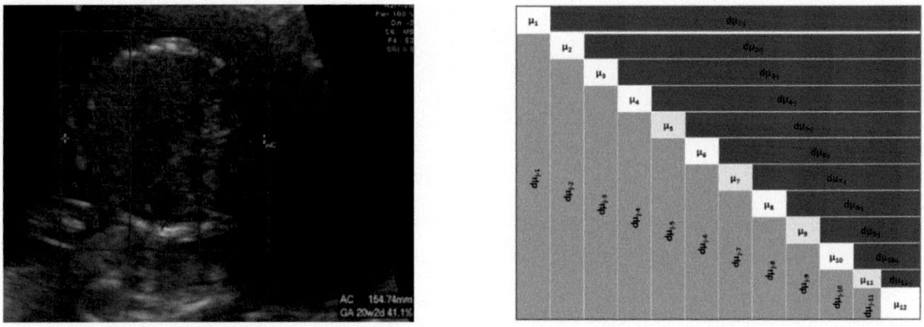

(a) splitting the region into random number of blocks

(b) Feature matrix A (12×12 in this example). *Green area* is mean(block$_i$) – mean(block$_j$) while *red* is the negative of it.

Fig. 3. An example region of 4×3 blocks on a fetal abdominal image and the feature matrix A.

2.3 Training and Testing

Before training and testing, all images are resized to the same pixel spacing to simplify correspondence between appearance features. We have developed a classifier based on RF which learns a fetal image category from a set of fetal ultrasound anomaly images. Training is performed on a set of images $\mathcal{I}=\{I_1, ..I_N\}$ such that N is the total number of images and their class labels $\mathcal{L}=\{L_1, ..L_N\}$ such that the ith training example is parameterized by $\{I_i, \{f_1, f_2, \ldots f_F\}, L_i\}$ where f is a feature from the feature pool of size F. The classifier learns the best combination of the features described in Section 2.2 to build a set of trees. Each tree node is created out of the best feature/threshold from a set of randomly sampled features from the feature pool. Once the best feature and threshold are found for a tree node, the list of training examples branch left and right and the training proceeds recursively on each subtree. A leaf node is created if the maximum tree depth is reached or if the number of training examples of a node is small. The set of training images reaching a leaf is used to create a distribution which can be used to classify unseen images during testing.

3 Experiments

3.1 Dataset

29858 2D fetal ultrasound images from 2256 routine anomaly scans undertaken in the 12 months of 2013 between 18 weeks + 0 days to 22 weeks + 6 days were used from a hospital database. These scans were acquired by 22 different sonographers so there is large (but typical) variation in image quality, machine settings, and zoom aspects. All images were manually categorized by 14 qualified sonographers. No attempt was made to reject or remove any scans from the dataset as we intended to evaluate our method on a real-world dataset. This means the reported results show potential performance in real world deployment. The dataset contained fetal head (TV and TC), abdomen, femur, spine, face, cardio, and several other categories as specified in the standard screening protocol in the hospital. Scans were acquired on a GE Voluson E8 machines (GE Healthcare, Milwaukee USA). All images were anonymized before analysis, and their use underwent institutional board approval.

3.2 Evaluation Protocol and Metrics

The accuracy of the template matching was visually assessed, see supplementary material. We investigated the effect of the new proposed features by comparing the guided RF with a traditional RF using standard generalized Haar wavelets used in many medical image applications including [11-16]. These features compute the difference of mean intensity of two random blocks. The whole image was considered when sampling features and the center of the image used as a reference point for those features. In addition, we investigated the categories that found confusing to gain further understanding of the algorithm performance.

We have performed 10-fold cross validation and we have selected RF parameters experimentally. These were then fixed in all reported experiments. Maximum tree depths of 18 and 30 trees were trained. RF produces probabilities during testing. An image is correctly classified (defined by the true positives *TP*), if its class has the maximum probability among all other class probabilities. We report the accuracy of a method as ($acc = TP / N$). However, due to the complexity of fetal images and the occurrence of multiple structures in many images, we also report $acc_{top2} = TP_{top2} / N$ (as used in many machine learning imaging papers e.g., [17, 18]). An image is considered in TP_{top2} if its class is within the top 2 probabilities of the algorithm. Finally, all experiments were implemented in Matlab and all RF methods were trained and tested in a parallel manner to achieve fast implementation. Given an unseen image, Guided RF categorizes it in approximately 0.32sec on a high end workstation with 20 processor units.

4 Results

Fig. 2 shows visual results of localization of objects of interest where boxes are drawn around the matched regions for the different templates. Only the best-matched templates are shown. Each color represents a different template type as described in Section 2.1 and the width of the box border signifies the strength of the template response. Further typical results can be found in the supplementary material. The overall accuracy of the traditional RF method was 65% while Guided RF achieved 75% accuracy. A detailed comparison on the different classes is shown in Fig. 4 (a). Fig. 4 (b) shows the $accuracy_{top2}$ result for both the traditional RF and the Guided RF. Guided RF increased to 91% accuracy when considering the top 2 probabilities from RF output while traditional RF increased to 79% accuracy. Finally, Fig. 5 shows the category confusion plot which presents the different categories in descending order with respect to how often images get classified in. Note that the most common error is for one of the eight classes to be mis-classified as "Others" as opposed to being confused with another named fetal class.

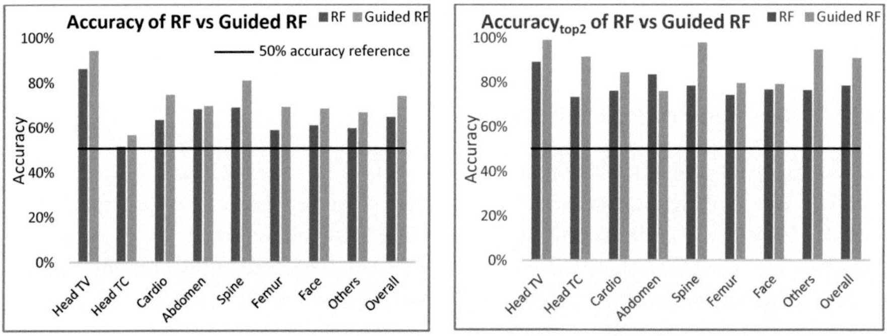

(a) Accuracy of both RFs on the top probability (b) Accuracy of both RFs on the top 2 probabilities

Fig. 4. Accuracy of the proposed method on the different image categories.

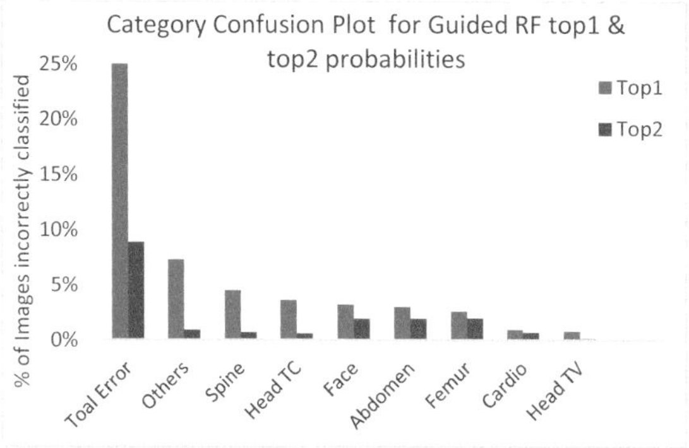

Fig. 5. Category Confusion Plot. From the 8 categories, this figure shows the misleading categories in descending order for the top1 categorization. Confusing categorizes is also shown for Top2. For instance, when a "Head TV" gets categorized as "Others" then the "Others" gets one more confusing case.

5 Discussion and Future Work

We have presented a new machine learning solution based on RF to categorize fetal ultrasound images. We showed how the RF classifier can be guided to provide good classification via guided sampling of features from ROIs. We first presented a method to detect ROIs using template matching to allow the classifier to learn from these regions and ignore misleading regions. We also presented a new feature type which captures a region within an image such that this feature is translation and orientation invariant. This type of feature proved to be important in our application because the position and orientation of fetal structures depends on the location of the fetus in the womb which is highly variable, see Fig. 4.

Because of the complexity of the "Others" group and the existence of many images in this group which look similar to the other 7 groups (e.g., cord insertion images are very similar to abdominal images), many images gets sorted as "Others". This can be seen in Fig. 5. Also, note that the "Spine" group may also be confusing as its appearance is similar to different structures, e.g., femur and diaphragm which is in the "Others" group. A multiclass solution which accommodates context of other labels may solve this problem and will be investigated in future work. Finally, while we have considered 2D ultrasound, the method is generalizable and could be extended to 3D ultrasound and other imaging modalities.

References

[1] Murray, R.F.: Classification images: A review. Journal of Vision 11 (2011)
[2] Bosch, A., Muñoz, X., Martí, R.: Review: Which is the best way to organize/classify images by content? Image Vision Computing 25, 778–791 (2007)
[3] Lu, D., Weng, Q.: A survey of image classification methods and techniques for improving classification performance. Int. J. Remote Sens. 28, 823–870 (2007)
[4] Carneiro, G., Georgescu, B., Good, S., Comaniciu, D.: Detection and Measurement of Fetal Anatomies from Ultrasound Images using a Constrained Probabilistic Boosting Tree. IEEE Transactions on Medical Imaging 27, 1342–1355 (2008)

[5] Prasad, B.G., Krishna, A.N.: Classification of Medical Images Using Data Mining Techniques. In: Das, V.V., Stephen, J. (eds.) CNC 2012. LNICST, vol. 108, pp. 54–59. Springer, Heidelberg (2012)
[6] Greenspan, H., Pinhas, A.T.: Medical Image Categorization and Retrieval for PACS Using the GMM-KL Framework. IEEE Transactions on Information Technology in Biomedicine 11, 190–202 (2007)
[7] Maraci, M., Napolitano, R., Papageorghiou, A., Noble, J.A.: Object Classification in an Ultrasound Video Using LP-SIFT Features. In: Menze, B., Langs, G., Montillo, A., Kelm, M., Müller, H., Zhang, S., et al. (eds.) Medical Computer Vision: Algorithms for Big Data (2014)
[8] Ni, D., Yang, X., Chen, X., Chin, C.-T., Chen, S., Heng, P.A., et al.: Standard Plane Localization in Ultrasound by Radial Component Model and Selective Search. Ultrasound in Medicine & Biology 40, 2728–2742 (2014)
[9] Fernández-Delgado, M., Cernadas, E., Barro, S., Amorim, D.: Do we Need Hundreds of Classifiers to Solve Real World Classification Problems? Journal of Machine Learning Research 15, 3133–3181 (2014)
[10] Papageorghiou, A.T., Ohuma, E.O., Altman, D.G., Todros, T., Ismail, L.C., Lambert, A., et al.: International standards for fetal growth based on serial ultrasound measurements: the Fetal Growth Longitudinal Study of the INTERGROWTH-21st Project. The Lancet 384, 869–879
[11] Criminisi, A., Shotton, J., Robinson, D., Konukoglu, E.: Regression Forests for Efficient Anatomy Detection and Localization in CT Studies. In: Presented at the MICCAI Workshop in Medical Computer Vision: Recognition Techniques and Applications in Medical Imaging, Beijing, China (2010)
[12] Chykeyuk, K., Yaqub, M., Noble, J.A.: Novel Context Rich LoCo and GloCo Features with Local and Global Shape Constraints for Segmentation of 3D Echocardiograms with Random Forests. In: Menze, B.H., Langs, G., Lu, L., Montillo, A., Tu, Z., Criminisi, A. (eds.) MCV 2012. LNCS, vol. 7766, pp. 59–69. Springer, Heidelberg (2013)
[13] Konukoglu, E., Glocker, B., Zikic, D., Criminisi, A.: Neighbourhood Approximation Forests. In: Ayache, N., Delingette, H., Golland, P., Mori, K. (eds.) MICCAI 2012, Part III. LNCS, vol. 7512, pp. 75–82. Springer, Heidelberg (2012)
[14] Pauly, O., Glocker, B., Criminisi, A., Mateus, D., Möller, A.M., Nekolla, S., Navab, N.: Fast Multiple Organs Detection and Localization in Whole-Body MR Dixon Sequences. In: Fichtinger, G., Martel, A., Peters, T. (eds.) MICCAI 2011, Part III. LNCS, vol. 6893, pp. 239–247. Springer, Heidelberg (2011)
[15] Yaqub, M., Javaid, M.K., Cooper, C., Noble, J.A.: Investigation of the Role of Feature Selection and Weighted Voting in Random Forests for 3-D Volumetric Segmentation. IEEE Transactions on Medical Imaging 33, 258–271 (2014)
[16] Yaqub, M., Kopuri, A., Rueda, S., Sullivan, P.B., McCormick, K., Noble, J.A.: A Constrained Regression Forests Solution to 3D Fetal Ultrasound Plane Localization for Longitudinal Analysis of Brain Growth and Maturation. In: Wu, G., Zhang, D., Zhou, L. (eds.) MLMI 2014. LNCS, vol. 8679, pp. 109–116. Springer, Heidelberg (2014)
[17] Alex, K., Sutskever, I., Geoffrey, E.H.: ImageNet Classification with Deep Convolutional Neural Networks. Advances in Neural Information Processing Systems, 1097–1105 (2012)
[18] Russakovsky, O., Deng, J., Su, H., Krause, J., Satheesh, S., Ma, S., et al.: ImageNet Large Scale Visual Recognition Challenge. Computer Vision and Pattern Recognition, arXiv:1409.0575 (2014)

Dempster-Shafer Theory Based Feature Selection with Sparse Constraint for Outcome Prediction in Cancer Therapy

Chunfeng Lian[1,2], Su Ruan[2], Thierry Denœux[1], Hua Li[4], and Pierre Vera[2,3]

[1] Sorbonne Universités, Université de Technologie de Compiègne, CNRS, UMR 7253 Heudiasyc, 60205 Compiègne, France
[2] Université de Rouen, QuantIF - EA 4108 LITIS, 76000 Rouen, France
[3] Centre Henri-Becquerel, Department of Nuclear Medicine, 76038 Rouen, France
[4] Washington University School of Medicine, Department of Radiation Oncology, Saint Louis, 63110 MO, USA

Abstract. As a pivotal task in cancer therapy, outcome prediction is the foundation for tailoring and adapting a treatment planning. In this paper, we propose to use image features extracted from PET and clinical characteristics. Considering that both information sources are imprecise or noisy, a novel prediction model based on Dempster-Shafer theory is developed. Firstly, a specific loss function with sparse regularization is designed for learning an adaptive dissimilarity metric between feature vectors of labeled patients. Through minimizing this loss function, a linear low-dimensional transformation of the input features is then achieved; meanwhile, thanks to the sparse penalty, the influence of imprecise input features can also be reduced via feature selection. Finally, the learnt dissimilarity metric is used with the Evidential K-Nearest-Neighbor (EK-NN) classifier to predict the outcome. We evaluated the proposed method on two clinical data sets concerning to lung and esophageal tumors, showing good performance.

Keywords: Outcome Prediction, PET, Feature Selection, Sparse Constraint, Dempster-Shafer Theory.

1 Introduction

Accurately predicting the treatment outcome prior to or even during cancer therapy is of great clinical value. It facilitates the adaptation of a treatment planning for individual patient. Medical imaging plays a fundamental role in assessing the response of a treatment, as it can monitor and follow up the evolution of tumor lesions non-invasively [8]. Up to now, the metabolic uptake information provided by fluoro-2-deoxy-D-glucose (FDG) positron emission tomography (PET) has been proven to be predictable for pathologic response of a treatment in several cancers, e.g., lung tumor [6,11] and esophageal tumor [15]. Abounding image features can be extracted from FDG-PET, such as standardized uptake values (SUVs), like SUV_{max}, SUV_{peak} and SUV_{mean}, that describe metabolic uptake

N. Navab et al. (Eds.): MICCAI 2015, Part III, LNCS 9351, pp. 695–702, 2015.
DOI: 10.1007/978-3-319-24574-4_83

in a region of interest, total lesion glycolysis (TLG) and metabolic tumor volume (MTV) [15]. In addition, some complementary analysis of PET images, e.g., image texture analysis [16], can also provide supplementary evidence for outcome evaluation. The quantification of these features before and during cancer therapy has been claimed to be predictable for treatment response [8]. Nevertheless, their further application is still hampered by some practical difficulties. First, compared to a relatively large amount of interesting features from the point of view of clinicians, we often have just a small sample of observations in clinical study. As a consequence, the predictive power of traditional statistical machine learning algorithms, e.g., K-nearest neighbor (K-NN) classifier, break down as the dimensionality of feature space increases. Secondly, due to system noise and limited resolution of PET imaging, the effect of small tumor volumes [1], as well as partly subjective quantification of clinical characteristics, some of these (texture, intensity and clinical) features are imprecise.

Dimensionality reduction is a feasible solution to the issues discussed above. However, traditional methods, including feature transformation methods, e.g., kernel principal component analysis (K-PCA) [13] and neighbourhood components analysis (NCA) [7], and feature selection, e.g., univariate and multivariate selection [12,17], are not designed to work for imperfect data tainted with uncertainty. As a powerful framework for representing and reasoning with uncertainty and imprecise information, Dempster-Shafer theory (DST) [14] has been increasingly applied in statistical pattern recognition [5,10] and information fusion for cancer therapy [2,9]. These facts motivated us to design a new DST-based prediction method for imprecise input features and small observation samples.

In this paper, we firstly develop a specific loss function with sparse penalty to learn an adaptive low-rank distance metric for representing dissimilarity between different patients' feature vectors. A linear low-dimensional transformation of input features is then achieved through minimizing this loss function. Simultaneously, using the $\ell_{2,1}$-norm regularization of learnt dissimilarity metric in the loss function, feature selection is also realized to reduce the influence of imprecise features. At last, we apply the learnt dissimilarity metric in the evidential K-nearest-neighbor (EK-NN) classifier [4] to predict the treatment outcome.

The rest of this paper is organized as follows. The fundamental background on DST is reviewed in Section 2. The proposed method is then introduced in Section 3, after which some experimental results are presented in Section 4. Finally, Section 5 concludes this paper.

2 Backgrounds on Dempster-Shafer Theory

DST is also known as evidence theory or theory of belief functions. As a generalization of both probability theory and set-membership approach, it acts as a framework for reasoning under uncertainty based on the modeling of evidence [14].

Specifically speaking, we assume ω be a variable taking values in a finite domain $\Omega = \{\omega_1, \cdots, \omega_c\}$, called the *frame of discernment*. An item of evidence regarding the actual value of ω can be represented by a *mass function* m from 2^{Ω} to [0,1], such that $\sum_{A\subseteq\Omega} m(A) = 1$. Each number $m(A)$ denotes a *degree of belief* attached to the hypothesis that "$\omega \in A$". Function m is said to be *normalized* if $m(\emptyset) = 0$, which is assumed in this paper.

Corresponding to a normalized mass function m, the *belief* and *plausibility function* for all $A \subseteq \Omega$ are further defined as:

$$Bel(A) = \sum_{B\subseteq A} m(B); \quad Pl(A) = \sum_{B\cap A\neq\emptyset} m(B). \tag{1}$$

Quantity $Bel(A)$ represents the degree to which the evidence *supports* A, while $Pl(A)$ represents the degree to which the evidence is *not contradictory* to A.

Different items of evidence can be aggregated to elaborate beliefs in DST. Let m_1 and m_2 be two mass functions derived from independent items of evidence. They can be combined via *Dempster's rule* to generate a refined mass function:

$$(m_1 \oplus m_2)(A) = \frac{1}{1-Q} \sum_{B\cap C=A} m_1(B)m_2(C) \tag{2}$$

for all $A \in 2^{\Omega} \setminus \emptyset$, where $Q = \sum_{B\cap C=\emptyset} m_1(B)m_2(C)$ measures the *degree of conflict* between these two pieces of evidence.

3 Method

Assume we have a collection of n labeled patients $\{(X_i, Y_i)|i = 1, \cdots, n\}$, in which $X_i = [x_1, \cdots, x_v]^T$ is the ith observation with v input features, and Y_i is the corresponding label taking values in a frame of discernment $\Omega = \{\omega_1, \cdots, \omega_c\}$.

Firstly, we need to learn a dissimilarity metric $d(X_i, X_j)$ on this training data set, so as to maximize the prediction performance of the EK-NN classifier on future testing patient. Alternatively, we regard this problem as learning a transformation matrix $A \in \mathbf{R}^{h\times v}$, from which the distance $d(X_i, X_j)$ is defined as

$$d(X_i, X_j) = (AX_i - AX_j)^T(AX_i - AX_j) = (X_i - X_j)^T A^T A(X_i - X_j). \tag{3}$$

Matrix A is further restricted to be of low-rank h (i.e., $h \ll v$), such that a low-dimensional linear transformation of the input feature space can be learnt, making the EK-NN classifier more efficient.

In the DST framework, if X_i is a query instance, then other labeled points in the training data set can be viewed as partial knowledge regarding X_i's prediction label. More precisely, each point X_j ($\neq i$) with $Y_j = \omega_q$ is a piece of evidence that increases the belief that X_i also belongs to ω_q. However, this piece of evidence is not 100% certainty. It is inversely proportional to the dissimilarity between X_i and X_j, and can be quantified as a mass function

$$\begin{cases} m_{ij}(\omega_q) & = \exp\left(-d(X_i, X_j)\right) \\ m_{ij}(\Omega) & = 1 - \exp\left(-d(X_i, X_j)\right) \end{cases}, \tag{4}$$

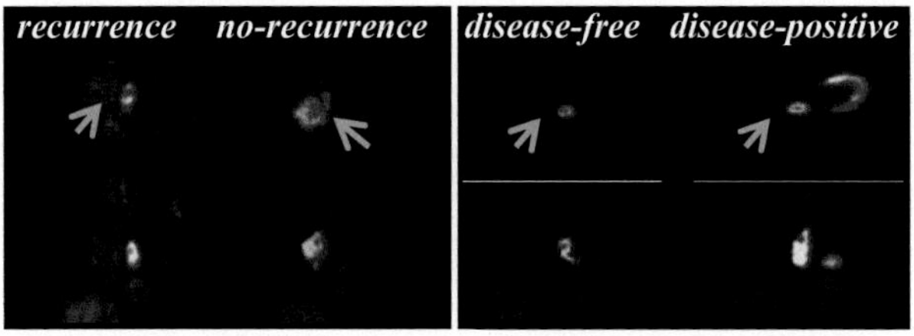

(a) Lung Tumors (b) Esophageal Tumors

Fig. 1. Examples of tumor uptakes on FDG-PET imaging from different views; (a) recurrence and no-recurrence instances before treatment of lung tumor; (b) disease-free and disease-positive instances before treatment of esophageal tumor.

where dissimilarity $d(X_i, X_j)$ is measured via Eq. (3). This mass function can be expressed by saying that, based on (X_j, Y_j), the belief can only partly be committed to ω_q, while the complementary of it is uncertainty, and can only be assigned to the whole frame Ω.

After modeling the evidence from all training samples (except X_i) using Eq. (4), they are further allocated into different groups Γ_q $(q = 1, \ldots, c)$ according to corresponding class labels. Then, after combination using Dempster's rule (Eq. (2)), the mass function for each group Γ_q is represented as

$$\begin{cases} m_i^{\Gamma_q}(\{\omega_q\}) & = 1 - \prod_{j \in \Gamma_q} \left[1 - \exp\left\{-(X_i - X_j)^T A^T A (X_i - X_j)\right\}\right] \\ m_i^{\Gamma_q}(\Omega) & = \prod_{j \in \Gamma_q} \left[1 - \exp\left\{-(X_i - X_j)^T A^T A (X_i - X_j)\right\}\right] \end{cases}. \tag{5}$$

The mass of belief $m_i^{\Gamma_q}(\Omega)$ for group Γ_q reflects the imprecision about the hypothesis that $Y_i = \omega_q$. If any hypothesis is true, the corresponding mass function should be more precise. For instance, *if the actual value of* Y_i *is* ω_q*, this imprecision should then close to zero, i.e.,* $m_i^{\Gamma_q}(\Omega) \approx 0$*; in contrast, imprecision pertaining to other hypotheses should close to one, i.e.,* $m_i^{\Gamma_r}(\Omega) \approx 1$*, for* $\forall r \neq q$. Based on this idea, we propose to represent the prediction loss for training sample (X_i, Y_i) as

$$loss_i = \sum_{q=1}^{c} t_{i,q} \cdot \left(1 - m_i^{\Gamma_q}(\omega_q) \cdot \prod_{r \neq q}^{c} m_i^{\Gamma_r}(\Omega)\right)^2, \tag{6}$$

where $t_{i,q}$ is the qth element of a binary vector $t_i = \{t_{i,1}, \ldots, t_{i,c}\}$, with $t_{i,q} = 1$ if and only if $Y_i = \omega_q$.

As a result, for all training samples, the average loss function with respect of the transformation matrix A can be expressed as

$$l(A) = \frac{1}{n} \sum_{i=1}^{n} loss_i + \lambda ||A||_{2,1}, \tag{7}$$

where $loss_i$ is calculated using Eq. (6). The $\ell_{2,1}$-norm sparse regularization, i.e., $||A||_{2,1} = \sum_{i=1}^{v}(\sum_{j=1}^{h} A_{i,j}^2)^{1/2}$, is added to select features in order to limit the influence of imprecise input features during the linear transformation. Scalar λ is a hyper-parameter that controls the influence of the regularization term.

As a differentiable function regarding matrix A, Eq. (7) is then minimized using a quasi-Newton method [3]. After that, we apply the learnt matrix A in Eq. (3), and use the EK-NN classifier to predict the treatment outcome of future testing patients.

Table 1. Comparing prediction accuracy (ave±std, in %) of different methods. ELT-FS* and ELT* denote, respectively, the proposed method with/without the $\ell_{2,1}$-norm sparse regularization.

Method	**Lung Tumor Data**		**Esophageal Tumor Data**	
	training	testing	training	testing
EK-NN	69.50±4.46	60.00±50.00	63.73±2.14	61.11±49.44
SVM	100.00±0.00	76.00±43.60	100.00±0.00	63.89±48.71
T-test	99.67±1.15	72.00±45.83	75.56±2.10	66.67±47.81
IG	86.50±3.86	68.00±47.61	88.57±2.37	75.00±43.92
SFS	95.67±2.24	84.00±37.42	85.63±1.60	52.78±50.56
SFFS	64.33±3.62	72.00±45.83	59.68±6.79	80.56±40.14
PCA	88.33±1.70	80.00±40.82	59.60±5.81	55.56±50.40
LDA	100.00±0.00	52.00±50.99	100.00±0.00	55.56±50.40
NCA	99.50±1.83	80.00±40.82	94.21±3.24	69.44±46.72
K-PCA	81.33±4.36	80.00±40.82	71.19±5.89	72.22±45.43
ELT*	95.83±3.80	**88.00±33.17**	88.02±4.03	63.89±48.71
ELT-FS*	100.00±0.00	**88.00±33.17**	97.46±1.64	**83.33±37.80**

4 Experimental Results

We compared the proposed method (called evidential low-dimensional transformation with feature selection, i.e., ELT-FS) with several feature transformation methods, namely PCA, linear discriminant analysis (LDA), NCA and K-PCA; and several feature selection methods, namely T-test, Information Gain (IG), Sequential Forward Selection (SFS) and Sequential Floating Forward Selection (SFFS) [12]. We used two real patient data sets:

1) Lung Tumor Data: Twenty-five patients with stage II-III non-small cell lung cancer treated with curative intent chemo-radiotherapy were considered. Totally 52 SUV-based (SUV_{max}, SUV_{mean}, SUV_{peak}, MTV and TLG) and texture-based (gray level size zone matrices (GLSZM) [16]) features were extracted from longitudinal PET images before and during the treatment. The extraction of GLSZM-based features consists of two main steps: firstly, homogenous areas were identified within the tumor, and then a matrix linking the size of each of these homogeneous areas to its intensity was constructed; after that, features characterizing regional heterogeneity were then calculated from this matrix, such as parameters that quantify the presence of a high-intensity large-area

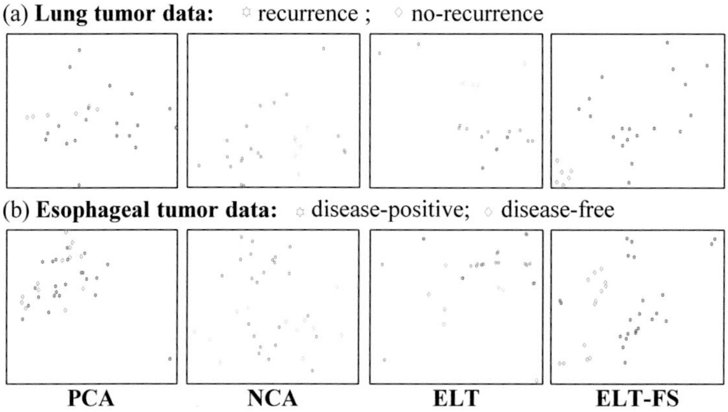

Fig. 2. Two-dimensional transformation results of PCA, NCA, our ELT (without feature selection, i.e., $\lambda = 0$) and ELT-FS.

emphasis or a low-intensity small-area emphasis. The definition of recurrence for patients at one year after the treatment was primarily clinical with biopsy and FDG-PET/CT. Local or distant *recurrence* was diagnosed on nineteen patients, while *no recurrence* was reported on the remaining six patients (example images can be seen in Fig. 1(a)).

2) Esophageal Tumor Data: Thirty-six patients with esophageal squamous cell carcinomas treated with chemo-radiotherapy were studied. Totally 29 SUV-based (SUV_{max}, SUV_{mean}, SUV_{peak}, MTV and TLG), GLSZM-based and patients' clinical features (gender, tumour stage and location, WHO performance status, dysphagia grade and weight loss from baseline) were extracted based on the baseline PET images. The disease-free evaluations include a clinical examination with PET/CT and biopsies. Finally, thirteen patients were labeled *disease-free* when neither loco regional nor distant tumor recurrence is detected, while the remaining twenty-three patients were diagnosed as *disease-positive* (as shown in Fig. 1(b)).

The leave-one-out cross-validation (LOOCV) procedure was used for evaluation. For been compared methods (except NCA, since it was designed specifically for the K-NN classifers), after learning a low-dimensional subspace, the SVM (Gaussian kernel with $\sigma = 1$ was empirically chosen) classifier was used to predict class labels of both training instances and the left testing instance; while the EK-NN classifier (K was empirically set as 3) was used with NCA and the proposed method. Hyper-parameter λ for ELT-FS was determined by a rough grid search strategy. The dimension of output subspace was chosen between two to five according to the minimum average testing error. Finally, the average training and testing accuracy for all methods are summarized in Table 1, in which results obtained by the SVM and EK-NN in the input space, and by our method without feature selection (namely with $\lambda = 0$) are also presented for comparison. It can be observed that the proposed method, especially ELT-FS, leads to higher testing performance than other methods. Although LDA results in larger training accuracy than our method, the worst testing performance is obtained too. It maybe because the studied data sets were too small, therefore the covariance matrix obtained by LDA has been badly scaled. It is also worth noting that ELT and ELT-FS have the same testing performance on the lung tumor data, while ELT-FS performs much better on the esophageal tumor data than ELT. This result maybe can be explained from two different aspects: firstly, the lung tumor data is easier to be separated than the esophageal tumor data, hence the difference became small; on the other hand, it perhaps also demonstrates that the sparse term can play a real role to improve the prediction under complex situation, such as on the esophageal tumor data.

Furthermore, we visualized the dimension reduction in 2D achieved using PCA, NCA, ELT and ELT-FS methods, as shown in Fig. 2. It can be seen that different classes in both data sets are better separated by our methods than using other methods. The best separation is achieved using our method with feature selection (ELT-FS).

5 Conclusion

In this study, a novel approach based on DST has been proposed to predict the outcome of a cancer treatment using PET image features and clinical characteristics. A specific loss function has been designed to tackle uncertainty and imprecision, so as to learn an adaptive dissimilarity metric for the EK-NN classifier. Through minimizing this loss function to obtain a low-rank transformation matrix A, we have realized a low-dimensional linear transformation of input features. Simultaneously, thanks to the $\ell_{2,1}$-norm regularization of A, a feature selection procedure has been implemented to reduce the influence of imprecise input features during prediction. Experimental results obtained on two clinical data sets show that the proposed method performs well as compared to some other methods. In the future, we will further evaluate it on more and larger data sets with different types of tumors, and study the influence of the regularization hyper-parameter λ. Moreover, to further improve the prediction accuracy, we will attempt to include more features that extracted from other complementary sources of information, such as CT, FLT-PET, FMISO-PET images, etc.

Acknowledgements. This work was partly supported by China Scholarship Council.

References

1. Brooks, F.J., Grigsby, P.W.: The effect of small tumor volumes on studies of intratumoral heterogeneity of tracer uptake. Journal of Nuclear Medicine 55(1), 37–42 (2014)
2. Chandana, S., Leung, H., Trpkov, K.: Staging of prostate cancer using automatic feature selection, sampling and Dempster-Shafer fusion. Cancer Informatics 7, 57 (2009)

3. Dennis, Jr., J.E., Schnabel, R.B.: Numerical methods for unconstrained optimization and nonlinear equations, vol. 16. SIAM (1996)
4. Denœux, T.: A K-nearest neighbor classification rule based on Dempster-Shafer theory. IEEE Transactions on Systems, Man and Cybernetics 25(5), 804–813 (1995)
5. Denœux, T.: Maximum likelihood estimation from uncertain data in the belief function framework. IEEE Transactions on Knowledge and Data Engineering 25(1), 119–130 (2013)
6. Erasmus, J.J., McAdams, H., Patz, J. E.F., Goodman, P.C., Coleman, R.E.: Thoracic FDG PET: state of the art. Radiographics 18(1), 5–20 (1998)
7. Goldberger, J., Roweis, S., Hinton, G., Salakhutdinov, R.: Neighbourhood components analysis. In: Advances in Neural Information Processing Systems, pp. 513–520 (2005)
8. Lambin, P., van Stiphout, R.G., Starmans, M.H., Rios-Velazquez, E., Nalbantov, G., Aerts, H.J., Roelofs, E., van Elmpt, W., Boutros, P.C., Pierluigi, Granone, O.: Predicting outcomes in radiation oncology—multifactorial decision support systems. Nature Reviews Clinical Oncology 10(1), 27–40 (2013)
9. Lelandais, B., Ruan, S., Denœux, T., Vera, P., Gardin, I.: Fusion of multi-tracer PET images for dose painting. Medical Image Analysis 18(7), 1247–1259 (2014)
10. Lian, C., Ruan, S., Denœux, T.: An evidential classifier based on feature selection and two-step classification strategy. Pattern Recognition 48(7), 2318–2327 (2015)
11. Mi, H., Petitjean, C., Dubray, B., Vera, P., Ruan, S.: Prediction of lung tumor evolution during radiotherapy in individual patients with PET. IEEE Transactions on Medical Imaging 33(4), 995–1003 (2014)
12. Pudil, P., Novovičová, J., Kittler, J.: Floating search methods in feature selection. Pattern Recognition Letters 15(11), 1119–1125 (1994)
13. Schölkopf, B., Smola, A., Müller, K.R.: Kernel principal component analysis. In: Gerstner, W., Hasler, M., Germond, A., Nicoud, J.-D. (eds.) ICANN 1997. LNCS, vol. 1327, pp. 583–588. Springer, Heidelberg (1997)
14. Shafer, G.: A mathematical theory of evidence, vol. 1. Princeton University Press, Princeton (1976)
15. Tan, S., Kligerman, S., Chen, W., Lu, M., Kim, G., Feigenberg, S., D'Souza, W.D., Suntharalingam, M., Lu, W.: Spatial-temporal [18 F]FDG-PET features for predicting pathologic response of esophageal cancer to neoadjuvant chemoradiation therapy. International Journal of Radiation Oncology* Biology* Physics 85(5), 1375–1382 (2013)
16. Tixier, F., Hatt, M., Le Rest, C.C., Pogam, A.L., Corcos, L., Visvikis, D.: Reproducibility of tumor uptake heterogeneity characterization through textural feature analysis in 18F-FDG PET. Journal of Nuclear Medicine 53(5), 693–700 (2012)
17. Zhang, N., Ruan, S., Lebonvallet, S., Liao, Q., Zhu, Y.: Kernel feature selection to fuse multi-spectral MRI images for brain tumor segmentation. Computer Vision and Image Understanding 115(2), 256–269 (2011)

Disjunctive Normal Shape and Appearance Priors with Applications to Image Segmentation

Fitsum Mesadi[1], Mujdat Cetin[2], and Tolga Tasdizen[1,2]

[1] Electrical and Computer Engineering Department, University of Utah, USA
[2] Faculty of Engineering and Natural Sciences, Sabanci University, Turkey

Abstract. The use of appearance and shape priors in image segmentation is known to improve accuracy; however, existing techniques have several drawbacks. Active shape and appearance models require landmark points and assume unimodal shape and appearance distributions. Level set based shape priors are limited to global shape similarity. In this paper, we present a novel shape and appearance priors for image segmentation based on an implicit parametric shape representation called disjunctive normal shape model (DNSM). DNSM is formed by disjunction of conjunctions of half-spaces defined by discriminants. We learn shape and appearance statistics at varying spatial scales using nonparametric density estimation. Our method can generate a rich set of shape variations by locally combining training shapes. Additionally, by studying the intensity and texture statistics around each discriminant of our shape model, we construct a local appearance probability map. Experiments carried out on both medical and natural image datasets show the potential of the proposed method.

1 Introduction

The use of prior information about shape and appearance is critical in many biomedical image segmentation problems. These include scenarios where the object of interest is poorly differentiated from surrounding structures in terms of its intensity, the object and the background have complex, variable appearances and where a significant amount of noise is present. Active shape models (ASM) and its extension active appearance models (AAM) [1] are powerful techniques for segmentation using priors. However, the explicit shape representation used in these models has some drawbacks. Annotating landmark points with correct correspondences across all example shapes can be difficult and time consuming. The extensions of the technique to handle topological changes and segment multiply-connected objects are not straightforward. Moreover, ASM and AAM use linear analysis tools such as principal component analysis (PCA), which limits the domain of applicability of these techniques to unimodal densities. To overcome the limitations of ASMs, level set based shape priors were proposed [2,3]. Because of their implicit nature, level set methods can easily handle topological changes. However, due to their non-parametric nature the use of shape priors in level-set segmentation framework has limited capability. For example, during segmentation using level set based shape priors, the candidate shapes are forced to move

N. Navab et al. (Eds.): MICCAI 2015, Part III, LNCS 9351, pp. 703–710, 2015.
DOI: 10.1007/978-3-319-24574-4_84

towards the globally similar training shapes without any consideration for any local shape similarity [2,3]. In addition, the region based shape similarity metrics used in shape prior computations do not always correspond to the true shape similarity observed by humans [2, 3]. Finally, appearance statistics in level sets framework is usually limited to a simple use of global histograms [4], and its extension to full appearance models is not straightforward.

We use an implicit and parametric shape model called Disjunctive Normal Shape Models (DNSM) [5], which were previously used for interactive segmentation, to construct novel shape and appearance priors. DNSM's parametric nature allows the use of a powerful local prior statistics, while its implicit nature removes the need to use landmark points. The major contributions of this paper include new global and semi-local shape priors for segmentation using DNSM (Section 3), and a new local appearance model for image segmentation that includes both texture and intensity (Section 4). We describe the overall segmentation algorithm that uses the proposed priors in Section 5. Section 6 uses ISBI 2013 prostate central gland segmentation and MICCAI 2012 prostate segmentation datasets, and reports state-of-the-art results on both challenges.

2 Disjunctive Normal Shape Model

DNSMs approximate the characteristic function of a shape as a union of convex polytopes which themselves are represented as intersections of half-spaces. Consider the characteristic function of a D-dimensional shape $f : \mathbf{R}^D \rightarrow B$ where $B = \{0, 1\}$. Let $\Omega^+ = \{\mathbf{x} \in \mathbf{R}^D : f(\mathbf{x}) = 1\}$ represent the foreground region. Ω^+ can be approximated as the union of N convex polytopes $\Omega^+ \approx \bigcup_{i=1}^N P_i$. The ith polytope is defined as the intersection $P_i = \bigcap_{j=1}^M H_{ij}$ of M half-spaces. The half-spaces are defined as $H_{ij} = \{\mathbf{x} \in \mathbf{R}^D : h_{ij}(\mathbf{x})\}$, where $h_{ij}(\mathbf{x}) = 1$ if $\sum_{k=1}^n w_{ijk} x_k \geq 0$, and $h_{ij}(\mathbf{x}) = 0$ otherwise. Therefore, Ω^+ is approximated by $\bigcup_{i=1}^N \bigcap_{j=1}^M H_{ij}$ and equivalently $f(\mathbf{x})$ is approximated by the disjunctive normal form $\bigvee_{i=1}^N \bigwedge_{j=1}^M h_{ij}(\mathbf{x})$ [6]. Converting the disjunctive normal form to a differentiable shape representation requires the following steps. First, De Morgan's rules are used to replace the disjunction with negations and conjunctions which yields $f(\mathbf{x}) \approx \bigvee_{i=1}^N \bigwedge_{j=1}^M h_{ij}(\mathbf{x}) = \neg \bigwedge_{i=1}^N \neg \bigwedge_{j=1}^M h_{ij}(\mathbf{x})$. Since conjunctions of binary functions are equivalent to their product and negation is equivalent to subtraction from 1, $f(\mathbf{x})$ can also be approximated as $1 - \prod_{i=1}^N (1 - \prod_{j=1}^M h_{ij}(\mathbf{x}))$. The final step for obtaining a differentiable representation is to relax the discriminants h_{ij} to sigmoid functions (Σ_{ij}), which gives

$$f(\mathbf{x}) = 1 - \prod_{i=1}^{N} \left(1 - \prod_{j=1}^{M} \frac{1}{e^{\sum_{k=1}^{D+1} w_{ijk} x_k}} \right), \tag{1}$$

where $\mathbf{x} = \{x, y, 1\}$ for 2-dimensional (2D) shapes and $\mathbf{x} = \{x, y, z, 1\}$ for 3-dimensional (3D) shapes. The only free parameters are w_{ijk} which determine the orientation and location of the sigmoid functions(discriminants) that define the half-spaces. The level set $f(x) = 0.5$ is taken to represent the interface between the foreground ($f(\mathbf{x}) > 0.5$) and background ($f(\mathbf{x}) < 0.5$) regions. DNSMs can be used for segmentation by minimizing edge-based and region-based energy terms when no training data are available [5]. The contributions of this paper are the construction of shape and appearance priors for the DNSM from training data and their use in segmentation.

3 DNSM Shape Priors

In this section, we describe how a DNSM shape prior can be constructed from a set of training shapes and used in the segmentation of new images. The set of parameters $\mathbf{W} = \{w_{ijk}\}$ of the DNSM are used to represent shapes; therefore, shape statistics will be constructed in this parameter space. In order to obtain pure shape statistics it is important to first remove the effects of pose variations (scale, rotation, and translation) in the training samples using image registration [7]. Then, the DNSM can be fit to the registered training shapes by choosing the weights that minimize the energy

$$E(\mathbf{W}^t) = \int_{\mathbf{x}\in\Omega} (f(\mathbf{x}) - q_t(\mathbf{x}))^2 d\mathbf{x} + \eta \sum_i \sum_{r\neq i} \int_{\mathbf{x}\in\Omega} g_i(\mathbf{x}) g_r(\mathbf{x}) d\mathbf{x} \qquad (2)$$

where $g_i(\mathbf{x}) = \prod_{j=1}^{M} \frac{1}{e^{\sum_{k=1}^{D+1} w_{ijk} x_k}}$ represents the individual polytopes of $f(x)$, $q_t(\mathbf{x})$ is the ground truth (1 for object and 0 for background) of the tth training sample and η is a constant. The first term fits the model to the training shape, while the second term minimizes the overlap between the different polytopes. An η value of 0.1 is experimentally found to be sufficient to avoid the overlapping of the polytopes. We have found that a common initialization for all training shapes together with the second term is sufficient to keep the correspondence between the discriminants and polytopes across the training shapes. Figure 1(d-f) shows the correspondence achieved between the polytopes across the shapes in (a-c).This is an advantage over ASMs which can require manually placed landmark points to ensure correspondence. Another reason for minimizing the overlap between polytopes will be further discussed in Section 4. We minimize (2) using gradient descent to obtain $\mathbf{W}^t$.

One of the major limitations of level set based shape priors is that the similarity between the candidate and training shapes are computed only globally [2,3]. Since no local shape similarity is considered, these approaches can not generate shape variations by locally combining training shapes. For instance, in Fig. 1, let shapes (a) and (b) be the training samples, and we want to segment the shape in (c). Since shape (c) is not in the training set, segmentation using global shape prior can only move the candidate shape towards the globally similar training sample. However, if shape similarities are considered locally at smaller spatial scales, then the hand positions of shape (c) are similar to shape (a), and the leg positions are similar to shape (b). Therefore, evaluating the similarity between shapes at semi-local scale, as will be defined in the next paragraph, helps to segment shape (c) in our example, by combining training shapes (a and b) at locations that are locally more similar to the candidate shape.

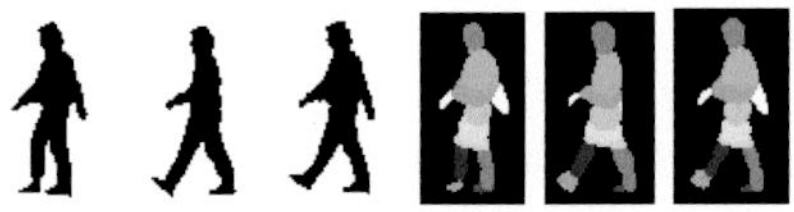

(a) (b) (c) (d) (e) (f)

Fig. 1. (a)-(c) are shapes from walking silhouettes dataset [3]. (d)-(f) show the non-overlapping polytopes(N=15) for shapes in (a)-(c) respectively, using DNSM. Each color corresponds to 1 polytope.

Let a given shape be represented by N polytopes and M discriminants per polytope using DNSM. Let us also assume that semi-local regions are represented by a single polytope (see Fig. 1(d-f)). We make this assumption for explanation purposes. It can be relaxed so that the semi-local region can be of any size. We will study the shape priors of each polytope independently by decoupling the entire shape in to N semi-local regions (polytopes). We can write the probability density function of the candidate's i^{th} polytope shape, represented by the weight $\mathbf{W_i}$, given the discriminant parameters of the training shapes for the corresponding polytope $\mathbf{W_i}^t$ as

$$p(\mathbf{W_i}) = \frac{1}{T}\sum_{t=1}^{T}\mathcal{K}(d(\mathbf{W_i}, \mathbf{W_i}^t), \sigma_i) \tag{3}$$

where T is the total number of training shapes, $\mathcal{K}$ is a Gaussian kernel of standard deviation σ_i, $d(\mathbf{W_i}, \mathbf{W_i}^t)$ is the ith polytope shape similarity distance between the candidate shape and t^{th} training sample. We define the distance between two polytopes as

$$d(\mathbf{W_i}, \mathbf{W_i}^\mathbf{t}) = \sum_{j=1}^{M}\sum_{k=1}^{D+1}\left(\left|\frac{\mathbf{W_{ijk}}}{\mathbf{W_{ikA}}} - \frac{\mathbf{W^t_{ijk}}}{\mathbf{W^t_{ikA}}}\right|\right) \tag{4}$$

where $\mathbf{W_{ijk}}$ is k^{th} weight of the jth discriminant of the ith polytope, and $\mathbf{W_{ikA}}$ is the average of the kth weight across all discriminants in i^{th} polytope. This normalization is necessary because the bias weights are typically much larger than the other weights. The shape energy for the ith polytope is defined as the negative logarithm of (3). During segmentation, the update to the discriminant weights, w_{ijk} of the ith polytope, is obtained by minimizing the polytope shape energy using gradient descent

$$\frac{\partial E_{\text{Shape},i}}{\partial w_{ijk}} = \frac{1}{p(\mathbf{W_i})n{\sigma_i}^2}\sum_{t=1}^{T}\mathcal{K}(d(\mathbf{W_i}, \mathbf{W_i}^\mathbf{t}), \sigma_i)(w_{ijk} - {w_{ijk}}^t). \tag{5}$$

Equation (5) shows that at local maxima, the candidate polytope shape is a weighted average of the corresponding polytope training shapes, where the weight depends on the similarity between the polytope of the candidate shape and that of the given training sample. Therefore, in the semi-local region represented by a given polytope, the shape prior term forces that part of the segmented image to move towards the semi-locally closest plausible shapes. The global shape prior used in level set based techniques [2,3] can be seen as a special case, where all polytopes are used together in (3). To use the global prior in our model, we let (4) be the distance between full parameter vectors $d(\mathbf{W}, \mathbf{W}^t)$.

4 DNSM Appearance Priors

Histograms of the global appearances of the object and background are commonly used in image segmentation. However, medical objects usually have spatially varying intensity distributions. In this section, we construct a local appearance prior using DNSM. The first step in appearance training is representing the training shapes with DNSM using (2). Then, each pixel in the region of interest is assigned to its closest discriminant plane using point-to-plane distance. In order to have a proper local appearance prior, the different polytopes should cover non overlapping regions, which is achieved by the second term in (2), as can also be seen from Fig. 1(d-f). During training, two separate histograms are built for each discriminant: one for the foreground pixels and the other for background pixels. That is, for a shape represented by $M \times N$ DNSM, there will be $2 \times M \times N$ different intensity histograms. In addition to intensity, eight features (energy, entropy, correlation, difference moment, inertia, cluster shade, cluster prominence, and Haralick's correlation) that summarize the texture of a given image are obtained using grey-level co-occurrence matrix texture measurements [8].

During segmentation, our goal is to compute the probability that the current pixel, with intensity I and texture vector T, belongs to the foreground region, based on the local appearance statistics obtained during the training. For each pixel, we first find its nearest discriminant ij, and then use the appearance statistics of that particular discriminant to compute the probability that the pixel belongs to the foreground

$$S(x) = \frac{H_{ij_{\text{Objct}}}(I)}{H_{ij_{\text{Objct}}}(I) + H_{ij_{\text{Backgrd}}}(I)} + \beta \frac{H_{ij_{\text{Objct}}}(T)}{H_{ij_{\text{Objct}}}(T) + H_{ij_{\text{Backgrd}}}(T)} \tag{6}$$

where H_{ij} refer to the normalized intensity and texture histograms for foreground and background regions for discriminant ij. β is a constant value between 0 and 1, and it controls how much the texture term contributes to the appearance prior. See Fig. 2(b) for an example of appearance probability map obtained from both intensity and texture for central gland. The energy from appearance term, $E_{Appr}(\mathbf{W})$, for the segmentation is then given as

$$E_{\text{Appr}}(\mathbf{W}) = \int_{\mathbf{x} \in \Omega} (S(\mathbf{x}) - f(\mathbf{x}))^2 d\mathbf{x} \tag{7}$$

where $f(\mathbf{x})$ is the level set value given as in (1), and $S(\mathbf{x})$ is given in (6). During segmentation, the update to the discriminant weights, w_{ijk} from the appearance prior is obtained by minimizing (7) using gradient descent, which is given as

$$\frac{\partial E_{\text{Appr}}}{\partial w_{ijk}} = -2\left(S(\mathbf{x}) - f(\mathbf{x})\right) \prod_{r \neq i} \left(1 - g_r(\mathbf{x})\right) g_i(\mathbf{x}) \left(1 - \Sigma_{ij}(\mathbf{x})\right) \mathbf{x}_k \tag{8}$$

5 Segmentation Algorithm

The segmentation is achieved by minimizing the weighted average of the shape and appearance prior energy terms. By applying gradient descent on the combined energy, the update to the discriminants w_{ijk} is then given as

$$w_{ijk} \leftarrow w_{ijk} - \alpha \frac{\partial E_{\text{Shape}}}{\partial w_{ijk}} - \gamma \frac{\partial E_{\text{Appr}}}{\partial w_{ijk}} \tag{9}$$

where $\frac{\partial E_{\text{Shape}}}{\partial w_{ijk}}$ and $\frac{\partial E_{\text{Appr}}}{\partial w_{ijk}}$ are as given in (5) and (8) respectively. α and γ are constants that determine the level of contributions from the shape and appearance priors. The steps involved in the segmentation algorithm can be summarized as follows:

1. Preprocessing: Intensity normalizations by histogram matching(for MRI).
2. Pose Estimation: The image of the appearance term (7), see Fig. 2(b), is used to find the approximate pose (location and size) of the object. This step improves segmentation accuracy, while also decreasing the number of iterations required to reach the final result.
3. Gradient Descent: Starting from the initial pose obtained in step 2 above, one gradient descent iteration involves: a) update the weights using the appearance prior term (8); b) register the current shape to the aligned training shapes [7]; c) update the weights using the shape prior term (5); d) register the current shape to its original pose. Note that registration of the current shape to the training shapes and back to its original pose are required for computation of the shape and appearance priors, respectively.

6 Experiments

Prostate Central Gland Segmentation: We use the NCI-ISBI 2013 Challenge - Automated Segmentation of Prostate Structures [9] MRI dataset to evaluate the effect of our shape priors. Automated segmentation of the central gland in MRI is challenging due to its variability in size, shape, location, and its similarity in appearance with the surrounding structures. Figure 2 shows one slice of the original MR image, the local appearance probability map, and the segmentation results with and without shape priors. Local appearance prior is used in the experiments of this section. Table 1 compares our segmentation algorithm using global and semi-local shape priors, with the top performing results from the NCI-ISBI challenge. Our algorithm shows a larger improvement over the 1st ranked result, compared to the improvement of the 1st rank over the 2nd rank [9] result, on both mean distance and DICE measurements. The table also shows that the semi-local shape prior outperforms the global shape prior.

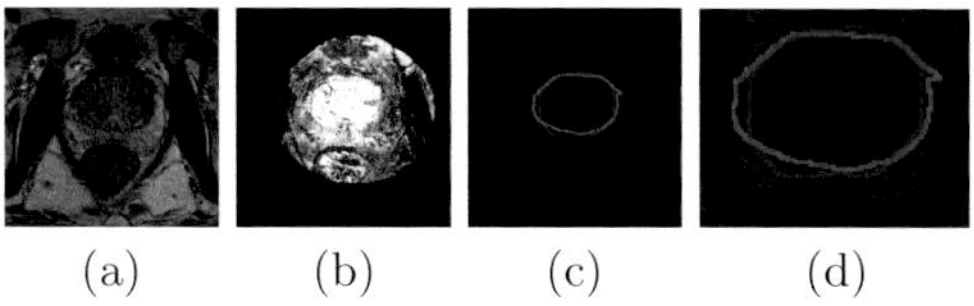

Fig. 2. Central gland segmentation: a) MRI section; b) Local appearance probability map (the brightness corresponds to the probability of the point to be a central gland); c) Segmentation results with and without shape prior in blue and red respectively; green is the ground truth. d) Result in (c) overlaid on the MRI and zoomed in.

Table 1. Central gland segmentation quantitative results

Method	Mean DICE	Mean distance
DNSM: Local Appearance + No Shape Prior	75.2	2.13
DNSM: Local Appearance + Global Shape	82.7	1.32
DNSM: Local Appearance + Semi-Local Shape	**83.8**	**1.28**
Atlas: Rusu et al. [9]	82.1	1.58
Interactive: RUNMC [9]	80.8	1.83

Full Prostate Segmentation: We use the MICCAI PROMISE2012 challenge dataset to compare the local and global appearance priors. The semi-local shape prior is used here since it was shown to provide better accuracy in the previous experiment. Since the prostate has two distinct regions, the central gland and the peripheral region, a single global histogram is suboptimal. Learning local appearance at different parts of the prostate during training improves accuracy, as shown in Table 2. Our approach performs comparably to or better than the best results from the challenge participants. Figure 3 shows sample segmentation result for one slice using local and global appearance priors.

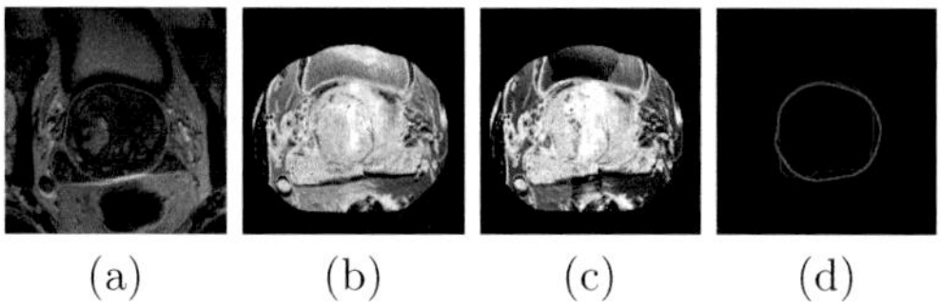

Fig. 3. Prostate segmentation: a) MRI section; b) Section of global appearance probability map; c) Local appearance probability map. d) Segmentation results with local and global appearance priors in blue and red respectively; green is the ground truth.

Table 2. Prostate segmentation quantitative results

Method	Mean DICE
DNSM: Semi-Local Shape + Global Appearance	84.1
DNSM: Semi-Local Shape + Local Appearance	**88.6**
DNSM: No Shape + Local Appearance	79.5
AAM: Vincent et al. [10]	88.0
Interactive: Malmberg et al. [10]	85.8

7 Conclusion

In this paper we presented shape and appearance priors based image segmentation using DNSM shape representation. Because of the implicit parametric nature of DNSM, we are able to learn the shape priors at semi-local and global scales. From the experiments we have seen that semi-local shape priors give better segmentation results. DNSMs also allow us to model appearance locally or globally. Our experimental results show that learning appearance statistics at small local neighborhoods give better results. Finally, our method is able to outperform state-of-the-art techniques in central gland and full prostate segmentations. Possible extensions of our work include, coupled segmentation of multiple objects and the joint modeling of shape and appearance.

Acknowledgments. This work is supported by NSF IIS-1149299, NIH 1R01-GM098151-01, TUBITAK-113E603 and TUBITAK-2221.

References

1. Cootes, T.F., Edwards, G.J., Taylor, C.J.: Active appearance models. IEEE Transactions on Pattern Analysis and Machine Intelligence, 484–498 (1998)
2. Kim, J., Cetin, M., Willsky, A.S.: Nonparametric shape priors for active contour-based image segmentation. Signal Processing 87(12), 3021–3044 (2007)
3. Cremers, D., Osher, S.J., Soatto, S.: Kernel density estimation and intrinsic alignment for shape priors in level set segmentation. International Journal of Computer Vision 69(3), 335–351 (2006)
4. Toth, R., et al.: Integrating an adaptive region-based appearance model with a landmark-free statistical shape model: application to prostate mri segmentation. In: SPIE Medical Imaging, vol. 7962. SPIE (2011)
5. Ramesh, M., Mesadi, F., Cetin, M., Tasdizen, T.: Disjunctive normal shape model. In: ISBI, IEEE International Symposium on Biomedical Imaging (2015)
6. Hazewinkel, M.: Encyclopaedia of Mathematics: An Updated and Annotated Translation of the Soviet Mathematical Encyclopaedia. Encyclopaedia of Mathematics, vol. 1. Springer (1997)
7. Zitova, B., Flusser, J.: Image registration methods: a survey. Image and Vision Computing 21(11), 977–1000 (2003)
8. Haralick, R.M.: Statistical and structural approaches to texture. Proceedings of the IEEE 67(5), 786–804 (1979)
9. NCI-ISBI Challenge. Automated segmentation of prostate structures (2013)
10. MICCAI Grand Challenge. Prostate mr image segmentation (2012)

Positive Delta Detection for Alpha Shape Segmentation of 3D Ultrasound Images of Pathologic Kidneys

Juan J. Cerrolaza[1], Christopher Meyer[1], James Jago[2], Craig Peters[1], and Marius George Linguraru[1,3]

[1] Sheikh Zayed Institute for Pediatric Surgical Innovation, Children´s National Health System, Washington DC, USA
{JCerrola,MLingura}@cnmc.org
[2] Philips Healthcare, Bothell, WA, USA
[3] School of Medicine and Health Sciences, George Washington Univ., Washington, DC, USA

Abstract. Ultrasound is the mainstay of imaging for pediatric hydronephrosis, which appears as the dilation of the renal collecting system. However, its potential as diagnostic tool is limited by the subjective visual interpretation of radiologists. As a result, the severity of hydronephrosis in children is evaluated by invasive and ionizing diuretic renograms. In this paper, we present the first complete framework for the segmentation and quantification of renal structures in 3D ultrasound images, a difficult and barely studied challenge. In particular, we propose a new active contour-based formulation for the segmentation of the renal collecting system, which mimics the propagation of fluid inside the kidney. For this purpose, we introduce a new positive delta detector for ultrasound images that allows to identify the fat of the renal sinus surrounding the dilated collecting system, creating an alpha shape-based patient-specific positional map. Finally, we incorporate a Gabor-based semi-automatic segmentation of the kidney to create the first complete ultrasound-based framework for the quantification of hydronephrosis. The promising results obtained over a dataset of 13 pathological cases (dissimilarity of 2.8 percentage points on the computation of the volumetric hydronephrosis index) demonstrate the potential utility of the new framework for the non-invasive and non-ionizing assessment of hydronephrosis severity among the pediatric population.

Keywords: Collecting system, 3D ultrasound, segmentation, monogenic signal, alpha shapes, kidney, hydronephrosis.

1 Introduction

Thanks to its non-invasive and non-irradiating properties, ultrasound (US) allows quick, safe, and relatively inexpensive evaluation of the kidney and the urinary tract in children. Hydronephrosis (HN), the dilation of the renal collecting system (CS) inside the kidney with distortion of the renal parenchyma caused by the obstruction of the urinary track (see Fig. 1(a)), is one of the most common abnormal finding in these studies, affecting 2-2.5% of children [1] in a wide spectrum of severity. Thus, an early

N. Navab et al. (Eds.): MICCAI 2015, Part III, LNCS 9351, pp. 711–718, 2015.
DOI: 10.1007/978-3-319-24574-4_85

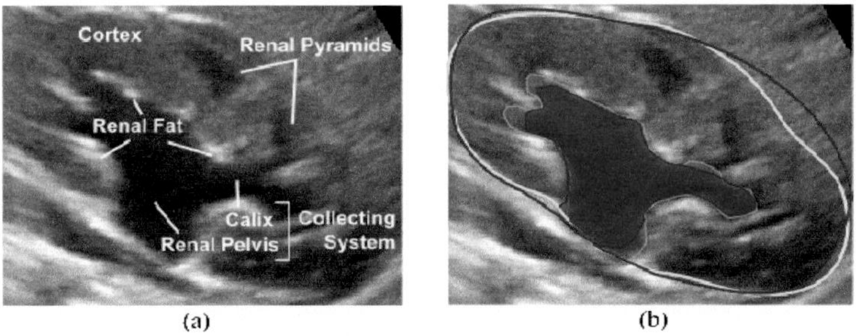

Fig. 1. Renal segmentation in US. (a) US longitudinal view of a hydronephrotic kidney and identification of relevant anatomical structures. (b) Ground truth (GT) and resulting segmentation (RS) for the kidney (GT: yellow; RS: red) and the collecting system (GT: green; RS: blue).

diagnosis is very important in order to identify those cases with severe obstruction of the urinary tract that require immediate surgical intervention. Based on the simple visual inspection of structural abnormalities, the Society for Fetal Urology (SFU) presented a 5-level grading system for classifying and standardizing the severity of HN [2], although its potential as diagnostic tool is limited by the subjective visual interpretation of radiologists. In the assessment of hydronephrosis, it is the effect on kidney function that is of most clincial importance. That assessment has typically been made using radionuclide imaging techniques (i.e., invasive procedures that include exposure to ionizing radiation) to measure relative kidney function and drainage. Though US can only represent the physical structure of the kidney, yet with robust analysis of kidney shape parameters, it has been shown that shape can define clinically relevant functional thresholds to simplify clinical evaluation and reduce the need for invasive imaging. Recently, some works [3,4] have demonstrated the potential value of automated US imaging processing for the quantitative, reproducible, and standardized assessment of HN, with the hydronephrosis index (HI) being one of the most popular methods [3]. HI is computed as $1 - V_{CS}/V_K$, where V_{CS} and V_K represent the volume of the CS and the entire kidney, respectively. In this context, the accurate parameterization and segmentation of the kidney anatomy becomes essential to guarantee an optimal performance and robustness.

Although the quality of US images has increased considerably in recent years, they still suffer from low signal-to-noise ratio, signal attenuation and dropout, and missing boundaries, making the evaluation of organs challenging. Despite the increasing interest in developing new segmentation methods for sonographic images [5] in other application areas like echocardiography, or transrectal ultrasound, there is a dearth of literature discussing the computerized analysis of renal structures. Recently, Cerrolaza et al. [7] proposed a new kidney segmentation framework combining statistical shape models and Gabor-based appearance model tailored to the particularities of the imaging physics of 3DUS. Mendoza et al.[6] presented one of the first approaches to segment both, the kidney and its CS from 2DUS images. However, the segmentation and thus the computation of HI can be significantly affected by the selection of the 2D US slice. To our knowledge, the 3D segmentation of CS remains an unsolved problem. Despite the fact that CS can be partially identified thanks to its hypoechoic nature in hydronephrotic renal US, its segmentation is particularly challenging due to undefined shape, blurred boundaries, heterogeneous structures of different shapes and intensities inside the kidney (i.e., the renal pyramids in very young children), which can confuse even the experienced eye (see Fig. 1(a)).

In this paper, we present, to the best of our knowledge, the first segmentation and quantification method of the CS in 3DUS. In Section 2.1 we introduce a new positive delta detector for ultrasound images derived from the monogenic signal formulation [9]. This delta detector allows to identify echogenic bands in US images, such as the fat of the renal sinus that surrounds the dilated collecting system. Based on this information, Section 2.2 presents an alpha shape-based patient-specific positional map that controls the evolution of the segmentation process. Section 2.3 presents an original active contour-based formulation, which allows to replicate the evolution of HN in the CS. Finally, the Gabor-based segmentation method for the kidney [7] is incorporated in Section 2.4 to create the complete segmentation framework for renal structures in 3DUS. The segmentation algorithm is tested in Section 3.

2 Methods

2.1 Local Phase-Based 3D Positive Delta Detection

Local phase-based boundary detection methods in US images have been exploited in previous work in the context of echocardiography images [12], showing promising results thanks to reduced sensitivity to speckle and intensity invariance. Given the complex-valued representation of a signal (i.e., the 1D analytic signal based on the Hilbert transform), the local amplitude includes intensity information, whereas the local phase contains local structural information (i.e., location and orientation of image features, such as transitions or discontinuities).

The monogenic signal [9] is a n-dimensional generalization of the 1D analytic representation by means of the Riesz transform. In the context of 3D image processing, the monogenic signal, $\boldsymbol{I}_M$, is defined as the 4D vector $\boldsymbol{I}_M = (\boldsymbol{I}, \boldsymbol{I}_R)$, where $\boldsymbol{I}: \Omega \rightarrow \mathbb{R}^+$ represents the 3D gray level image in the image domain $\Omega \in \mathbb{R}^3$, and $\boldsymbol{I}_R = \left(\boldsymbol{I}_{Rx}, \boldsymbol{I}_{Ry}, \boldsymbol{I}_{Rz}\right) = \left(\boldsymbol{I} * \boldsymbol{h}_x, \boldsymbol{I} * \boldsymbol{h}_y, \boldsymbol{I} * \boldsymbol{h}_z\right)$ represents the three Riesz filtered components. The spatial representation of the earlier filters is defied by $\boldsymbol{h}_k = -k / \left(2\pi(x^2+y^2+z^2)^{3/2}\right)$, where $k = x, y,$ or z. In practice, the original signal $\boldsymbol{I}$ should be first filtered by an isotropic bandpass filter such as a log-Gabor filter $\boldsymbol{g}_{LG,\omega}$, with central frequency ω. Therefore, the monogenic signal can be represented in a polar form by the scalar-valued even component, $even_\omega = \boldsymbol{g}_{LG,\omega} * \boldsymbol{I}$, and odd component, $odd_\omega = (\sum_{k=x,y,z}(\boldsymbol{g}_{LG,\omega} * \boldsymbol{I}_{Rk})^2)^{1/2}$. Using this representation of the monogenic signal, the local phase [13] can be defined as $\Phi_\omega = \mathrm{atan}\,(even_\omega / odd_\omega)$, with $\mathrm{atan}\,(.)$ being the inverse tangent in radians. Typically, the properties of the local phase are used to detect step edges in images identifying those points whose absolute value of the local phase is 0 (positive edges), or π (negative edges) [13]. However, local phase properties can also be exploited to detect symmetrical image features such as positive (ridge) or negative (valleys) deltas, identified with points whose local phase is $+\pi/2$, or $-\pi/2$, respectively. In particular,

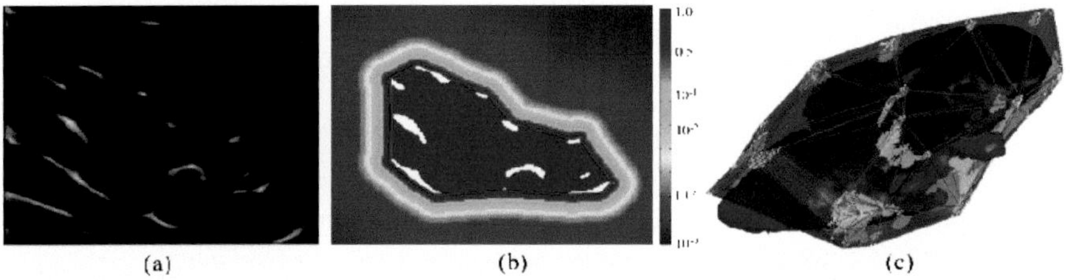

Fig. 2. Renal patient specific positional map. (a) Example of 3D positive delta detection for the US image shown in Fig. 1(a). (b) Alpha shape (red contour) and resulting positional map from the fat points inside the segmented kidney shown in Fig. 1(a). (c) 3D alpha shape (red) surrounding the collecting system (blue). The detected fat points are shown in yellow.

we are interested in relatively thin echogenic regions (i.e., ridges) inside the kidney, corresponding to fat tissue, originally located in the renal sinus and displaced towards the interior of the kidney due to the dilation of the CS in hydronephrotic cases. These bands of fat surround the dilated CS and constitute a key visual clue for the radiologist to differentiate the CS from other hypoechoic structures like the renal pyramids (see Fig. 1(a)). Inspired by the phase congruency theory proposed by Kovesi [13], we propose a multi-scale positive delta detector (PDD) identifying those regions where the local phase is $+\pi/2$, i.e., points where $|even_\omega| \gg |odd_\omega|$ and $sign(even_\omega \cdot odd_\omega) > 0$. Since positive deltas, like step edges, are scale-dependent features, the multiple-scales PDD is defined as

$$\mathrm{PDD} = \sum_\omega \frac{\lfloor ||even_\omega| - |odd_\omega| - T_\omega \rfloor \cdot sign(even_\omega \cdot odd_\omega) \rfloor}{\sqrt{{odd_\omega}^2 + {even_\omega}^2 + \varepsilon}}, \quad (1)$$

where the $\lfloor \cdot \rfloor$ operator zeros the negative values, ε is a small positive constant to prevent division by zero, and T_ω is a scale specific noise threshold defined as $T_\omega = \exp\left(mean[\log(({odd_\omega}^2 + {even_\omega}^2)^{1/2})]\right)$. In particular, PDD $\in [0,1]$, taking values close to 1 near bright bands (i.e., positive delta features), and close to zero otherwise (see Fig. 2(a)).

2.2 Patient Specific Positional Maps via Alpha Shapes

Having identified the fat areas inside the kidney, the goal is to create an anatomically-justified stopping criteria for the active contour formulation that prevents the leak of the contour outside the region delimited by the fat tissue. However, most of the existing surface reconstruction techniques from point sets (i.e., fat points located via PDD) assume a densely-sampled point cloud, which is not the case in most of hydronephrotic kidneys, where the scattered distribution of the inner thin fat results in an unstructured set of dispersed points. Here, we describe this region as the 3D alpha shape [14],S_α, defined by the fat points identified by PDD (see Fig.2(c)). Alpha shapes are a generalization of the concept of convex hull that allow to recover the shape of non-convex and even non-connected sets of points in 3D. In our case, alpha shapes provide an elegant and efficient solution to the problem of estimating the intuitive notion of the shape defined by the fat regions. In particular, the level of detail of the polyhedron is controlled by the single configuration parameter, $\alpha \in \mathbb{R}^+$, with S_∞ being equivalent to the convex hull defined by the points. Thus, the new stopping function can be defined as $\mathrm{SF}(\mathbf{x}) = 1/(1 + \lfloor D_{S_\alpha}(\mathbf{x}) \rfloor)^\tau$, where $\mathbf{x} \in \Omega$ defines a point in the image domain, $D_{S_\alpha}(\mathbf{x})$ is the signed distance to S_α, taking negative or positive values inside and outside S_α, respectively, and $\tau \in [1, +\infty)$ is a control variable (see Fig. 2(b) and (c)). Note that the computation of SF(.) can be performed offline for the entire image domain, Ω, since it does not depend on the evolution of the contour. This new stopping function is integrated in the active contour evolution equation in the next section.

2.3 Active Contours Formulation

To address the segmentation of the CS, we employ an active contour approach [8]. In particular, we propose a new energy functional that combines contour and intensity-based terms, incorporating the patient-specific positional map described above as additional stopping criteria.

Suppose $\boldsymbol{I}: \Omega \to \mathbb{R}^+$ represents a 3D gray level image in the image domain $\Omega \in \mathbb{R}^3$, and $\boldsymbol{U}: (t, \Omega) \to \mathbb{R}$ is an implicit representation of the surface $\boldsymbol{S}$, which coincides with the set of points $\boldsymbol{U}(t, .) = 0$. Following the geodesic active contours formulation proposed by Caselles et al. [8], the evolution of $\boldsymbol{U}$ is defined by $/\boldsymbol{\partial t} = g(\boldsymbol{I})|\nabla \boldsymbol{U}|(\kappa + c) + \nabla g(\boldsymbol{I}) \cdot \nabla \boldsymbol{U}$, where $\kappa = div(\nabla \boldsymbol{U}/|\nabla \boldsymbol{U}|)$ is the curvature term computed on the level set of $\boldsymbol{U}$, $c \in \mathbb{R}^+$ is a constant velocity term, and $g(\boldsymbol{I})$ is an inverse edge indicator function of the image $\boldsymbol{I}$. The constant expanding force represented by c prevents the contour to get stuck at local minimum when dealing with noisy and low contrast data in US images. Additionally, the constant expanding force represented by c can be interpreted as the expansive dilation force that pushes the dilation of CS inside the kidney. The directionality of the expansion process of the CS (i.e. the dilation of the CS is not uniform in space; see Fig. 1(a)) is controlled by the patient specific positional map described in Section 2.2. Typically, $g(\boldsymbol{I})$ is defined as $g(\boldsymbol{I}) = 1/(1 + |\nabla(G_\sigma * \boldsymbol{I})|)$, with G_σ representing a Gaussian kernel with standard deviation σ. However, this typical intensity-based method of boundary detection generally performs poorly in US due to the aforementioned drawbacks. As alternative, we use the feature asymmetry detector (FA) [13] (i.e., a local phase-based step function detector) whose satisfactory performance as edge detector in US images was emphasized by previous works [10,12]. Thus, the inverse edge indicator function can be defined as $(\boldsymbol{I}) = 1 - FA^\gamma$, with $\gamma \in [0,1]$.

The terms described above are all expansive forces controlled by the external image dependent stopping function, $g(\boldsymbol{I})$, whose main goal is to stop the evolving surface when it arrives to the object boundaries. However, it turns inefficient when segmenting objects with weak or missing boundaries. Here we combine the above gradient-based active contour model with the minimal variance formulation proposed by Chan and Vese [11], whose more general formulation defines the evolution of the contour as $\partial \boldsymbol{U}/t = (\lambda_{out}(\boldsymbol{I} - \mu_{out})^2 - \lambda_{in}(\boldsymbol{I} - \mu_{in})^2)|\nabla \boldsymbol{U}|$, where μ_{out}, and μ_{in} are the mean intensities in the exterior and the interior of the surface $\boldsymbol{S}$, respectively; λ_{out}

and λ_{in} are two control parameters generally defined as $\lambda_{out} = \lambda_{in} = 1$. With this formulation, the segmentation turns into an optimization process that looks for the best separating contour in $\boldsymbol{I}$, and the optimal expected values μ_{out} and μ_{in}. Given the hypoechoic nature of the CS in US images (i.e., $\mu_{in} \approx 0$), the second term of the above equation prevents the evolution of the contour into brighter areas, whereas the first term acts as expansive force toward dark areas (i.e., toward the CS). Finally, incorporating the alpha shape-based patient-specific positional map as additionally stopping function, the final evolution equation of the active contour is defined as

$$\frac{\partial U}{\partial t} = \mathrm{SF}(\boldsymbol{I})\left(\beta\left((\kappa + c)g(\boldsymbol{I})|\nabla \boldsymbol{U}| + \nabla \mathrm{g}(\boldsymbol{I}) \cdot \nabla \boldsymbol{U}\right) + (1-\beta)\left((\lambda_o(\boldsymbol{I} - \mu_o)^2 - \lambda_i(\boldsymbol{I} - \mu_i)^2)|\nabla \boldsymbol{U}|\right)\right), \quad (2)$$

where $\beta \in \mathbb{R}^{+}$ is a constant that balances the contour- and the intensity-based terms.

2.4 Complete Segmentation Framework of Renal Structures in 3DUS

The kidney (including CS) Gabor-based segmentation method recently proposed by Cerrolaza et al. [7] is now integrated with the CS segmentation approach described above, creating a complete framework for the segmentation and quantification of hydronephrosis in 3DUS. The semi-automatic algorithm proposed in [7] requires minimal user intervention, selecting two point clicks to roughly define the major axis of the kidney. Within the segmented kidney, the segmentation of CS is automatically initialized by selecting the darkest $3 \times 3 \times 3$ region within S_α. Using the initial segmentation of the kidney to filter those spurious adipose points outside the renal tissue, an estimation of S_α is obtained and the CS is segmented. Finally, the volumetric HI is automatically computed as explained in Section 1.

3 Results and Discussion

To validate the new framework for the analysis of renal structures, we used a set of 13 3DUS image of pathologic pediatric right kidneys diagnosed with hydronephrosis of varying severity. Image data were acquired from a Philips iU22 system with X6-1 xMATRIX Array transducer. The average image size was $484 \times 404 \times 256$ voxels, with a resolution range from 0.15 mm to 0.82 mm. For each image, the kidney and CS were delineated manually by an expert radiologist to provide the ground truth. The method was evaluated using the leave-one-out cross-validation. The statistical shape model used in the kidney segmentation method was refined using an additional set of 11 healthy kidney cases. The same configuration parameters described in [9] were used during the experiments. The rest of the configuration parameters were determined empirically using an iterated grid search approach. In particular, the selected values were: $c = 1$, $\lambda_{out} = \lambda_{in} = 1$, $\beta = 0.3$, $\alpha = 60$, and $\tau = 9$. For the local phase-based feature detection, we use a bank of log-Gabor filters with central frequencies $\omega = 0.04, 0.05$ and 0.06. Two point clicks were manually defined to initialize the segmentation of the kidney, while the CS was initialized automatically, as described in Section 2.4 A valid initialization seed (i.e., a $3 \times 3 \times 3$ region inside the CS) was automatically detected in 11 cases; in the other two images, the location of the seed was corrected manually. No significant difference was observed for different initializations, provided that the seed is located inside the CS.

Table 1 shows the segmentation error of both the kidney and CS. Although the method proposed here is the first segmentation framework for the CS in 3DUS, the performance of this new approach is compared with our 3D version of the graph cut-based method described by Mendoza et al. [8], originally conceived for 2DUS. It can be observed how the new framework provides not only better average results, but also lower standard deviation for the two accuracy metrics considered: Dice's coefficient (DC), and symmetric point-to-surface distance (SPSD). This improvement was statistically significant (p-value < 0.05 for both metrics), as assessed by means of a Wilcoxon paired signed non-parametric test. In particular, the new method provides an average DC of 0.75 ± 0.08, similar to the inter-user accuracy reported by [6], 0.76 ± 0.18 (p-value > 0.2 using a two-sample t-test between the mean values).

Table 1. Segmentation accuracy evaluation of the kidney and the CS segmentation using the new tailored active contour-based approach (CS-TAC), and the graph cut-based method proposed in [6] (CS-GC). The table present the average error and standard deviation for the Dice's coefficient (DC), and the symmetric point-to-surface distance (SPSD).

	Kidney		CS-TAC		CS-GC	
	MEAN	STD	MEAN	STD	MEAN	STD
DC	0.80	0.06	0.75	0.08	0.62	0.19
SPSD(mm)	2.30	0.80	0.98	0.27	1.35	1.20

Finally, the potential utility of the new segmentation framework for the assessment of pediatric hydronephrosis was evaluated computing the volumetric HI for all the cases (computed as percentage). The average error provided by the full semi-automatic framework detailed in Section 2.3 was 2.8 ± 3.30 percentage points. Compared to the subjective and commonly used SFU grading system, 3DHI provides a quantitative measurement for hydronephrosis severity, allowing objective longitudinal monitoring of the patient by US. The ability to objectively assess kidneys with hydronephrosis without using invasive imaging with ionizing radiation would be of great clinical value. This would permit establishment of thresholds where less complex imaging would be safe and effective for ongoing monitoring and assessment.

A Matlab® implementation of the framework was tested on a 64-bit 2.8 GHz processor, with an average execution time of 321 s (kidney: 96 s and CS: 225 s), which represents a considerable improvement over the several hours it takes for the unreproducible manual delineation by an operator.

4 Conclusions

In this paper, we present the first complete framework for the segmentation and quantification of renal structures in 3DUS. Thanks to the new positive delta detector introduced here, bands of fat inside the kidney are successfully identified, allowing us to define positional maps of the dilated collecting system via alpha shapes-based volume reconstruction. This patient-specific information is integrated into a hybrid contour-based formulation for the segmentation of the collecting system, combining contour- and intensity-based propagation terms. Finally, a Gabor-based semi-automatic segmentation of the kidney is incorporated to create the first complete ultrasound-based framework for the quantification of hydronephrosis. The promising results obtained in the segmentation and the estimation of the volumetric hydronephrosis index demonstrate the potential utility of the new proposed framework for the assessment of hydronephrosis among the pediatric population using non-invasive non-ionizing US images. In particular, the system provides objective and accurate information of the renal parenchymal status, which allows for better informed clinical decision making.

References

1. Peters, C., Chevalier, R.: Congenital Urinary Obstruction: Pathophysiology and Clinical Evaluation. In: Wein, A., Kavoussi, L., Novick, A., Partin, A., Peters, C. (eds.) Campbell-Walsh Textbook of Urology, vol. 4, pp. 3028–3047. Elsevier, Inc, Philadelphia
2. Fernbach, S.K., et al.: Ultrasound Grading of Hydronephrosis: Introduction to the System Used by the Society for Fetal Urology. Pediatric Radiology 23(6), 478–480
3. Shapiro, S., et al.: Hydronephrosis Index: A New Method to Track Patients with Hydronephrosis Quantitatively. Urology 72(3), 536–538 (2008)
4. Cerrolaza, J.J., et al.: Ultrasound Based Computer-Aided-Diagnosis of Kidneys for Pediatric Hydronephrosis. SPIE Medical Imaging, paper 9035 102 (2014)
5. Noble, J.A., et al.: Ultrasound image segmentation: a survey. IEEE Trans. on Med. Imag. 25(8), 987–1009 (2006)
6. Mendoza, C.S., et al.: Automatic Analysis of Pediatric Renal Ultrasound Using Shape, Anatomical and Image Acquisition Priors. In: Mori, K., Sakuma, I., Sato, Y., Barillot, C., Navab, N. (eds.) MICCAI 2013, Part I. LNCS, vol. 8151, pp. 259–266. Springer, Heidelberg (2013)
7. Cerrolaza, J.J., et al.: Segmentation of Kidney in 3D-Ultrasound Images Using Gabor-based Appearance Models. In: IEEE Int. Symp. on Biom. Imag., 633–636 (2014)
8. Caselles, V., et al.: Geodesic Active Contours. Int. Journal of Comp. Vis. 22(1), 61–79 (1997)
9. Felsberg, M., Sommer, G.: The Monogenic Signal. IEEE Trans. on Sig. Proc. 49(12), 3136–3144 (2001)
10. Belaid, A., et al.: Phase-Based Level Set Segmentation of Ultrasound Images. IEEE. Trans. on Inf. Tech. in Biomed. 15(1), 138–147 (2011)
11. Chan, T.F., Vese, L.A.: Active Contours Without Edges. IEEE Trans. Image Proc. 10(2), 266–277 (2001)
12. Rajpoot, K., et al.: Local-Pase Based 3D Boundary Detection Using Monogenic Signal and its Application to Real-Time 3-D Echocardiography Images. IEEE ISBI (2009)
13. Kovesi, P.: Image Features from Phase Congruency. J. Comput. Vis. Res. 1(3), 1–26 (1999)
14. Edelsbrunner, H., et al.: On the Shape of a Set of Points in the Plane. IEEE Trans. Inf. Theory 29(4), 551–559 (1983)

Non-local Atlas-guided Multi-channel Forest Learning for Human Brain Labeling

Guangkai Ma[1,2], Yaozong Gao[2,3], Guorong Wu[2], Ligang Wu[1], and Dinggang Shen[2]

[1] Space Control and Inertial Technology Research Center, Harbin Institute of Technology, Harbin, China
[2] Department of Radiology and BRIC, UNC at Chapel Hill, NC, USA
[3] Department of Computer Science, UNC at Chapel Hill, NC, USA

Abstract. Labeling MR brain images into anatomically meaningful regions is important in many quantitative brain researches. In many existing label fusion methods, appearance information is widely used. Meanwhile, recent progress in computer vision suggests that the context feature is very useful in identifying an object from a complex scene. In light of this, we propose a novel learning-based label fusion method by using both low-level appearance features (computed from the target image) and high-level context features (computed from warped atlases or tentative labeling maps of the target image). In particular, we employ a multi-channel random forest to learn the nonlinear relationship between these hybrid features and the target labels (i.e., corresponding to certain anatomical structures). Moreover, to accommodate the high inter-subject variations, we further extend our learning-based label fusion to a multi-atlas scenario, i.e., we train a random forest for each atlas and then obtain the final labeling result according to the consensus of all atlases. We have comprehensively evaluated our method on both LONI-LBPA40 and IXI datasets, and achieved the highest labeling accuracy, compared to the state-of-the-art methods in the literature.

1 Introduction

Automatic labeling of MR brain images has become a hot topic in the field of medical image analysis, since quantitative brain image analysis often relies on the reliable labeling of brain images. However, due to the high complexity of brain structures, it is still a challenging task for automatic brain labeling.

Recently multi-atlas based labeling methods have achieved a great success. In these methods, a set of already-labeled MR images, namely atlases, are used to guide the labeling of new target images [3, 9]. For example, Coupé et al. [6] proposed a non-local patch-based label fusion technique by using patch-based similarity as weight to propagate the neighboring labels from the aligned atlases to the target image, for potentially overcoming errors from registration. Instead of pair-wisely estimating the patch-based similarity, Wu et al. [7] adopted sparse representation to jointly estimate all patch-based similarities between a to-be-labeled target voxel and its neighboring voxels in all the atlases. However, the

N. Navab et al. (Eds.): MICCAI 2015, Part III, LNCS 9351, pp. 719–726, 2015.
DOI: 10.1007/978-3-319-24574-4_86

traditional multi-atlas based labeling techniques are still limited: the definition of patch-based similarity is often handcrafted based on the predefined features, which might not be effective for labeling all types of brain structures.

On the other hand, learning-based methods have also attracted much attention recently. In these methods, a strong classifier is typically trained for each label/ROI, based on the local appearance features. For example, Zikic et al. [2] proposed atlas forest, which encodes an atlas by learning a classification forest on it. The final labeling of a target image is achieved by averaging the labeling results from all the selected atlas forests. Tu et al. [5] adopted the probabilistic boosting tree (PBT) for labeling. To further boost the performance, an auto-context model (ACM) was also proposed to iteratively refine the labeling results. The learning-based methods often determine a target voxel's label solely based on the local image appearance, without getting clear assistance from the spatial information of labels encoded in the atlases. Accordingly, their labeling accuracy could be limited, since patches with similar local appearance could appear in different parts of the brain.

In this paper, we propose a novel atlas-guided multi-channel forest learning method for labeling multiple ROIs (Regions of Interest). Here, multi-channel means multiple representations of a target image, which include features extracted from not only the target (intensity) image but also the label maps of all aligned atlases. Instead of labeling each target voxel with only its local image appearance from the target image, we also utilize label information from the aligned atlas. To further refine the labeling result, Haar-based multi-class contexture model (HMCCM) is also proposed to iteratively construct a sequence of classification forests by updating the context features. The final labeling result is the average over all labeling results from all atlas-specific forests. Validated on both LONI-LBPA40 and IXI datasets, our proposed method consistently outperforms both traditional multi-atlas based methods and learning-based methods.

The rest of the paper is organized as follows. Section 2 describes the proposed labeling method and its application to single-ROI and multi-ROI labeling. Experiments are performed and analyzed in Section 3. Finally, discussion and conclusion are given in the last section.

2 Method

In this section, we will first present notations used in our paper. Then, we will explain the learning procedure of our atlas-guided multi-channel forest, followed by application of the learned forests to single-ROI and multi-ROI labeling. Finally, we present HMCCM to iteratively refine the labeling results.

Notations. An atlas library $\mathbf{A}$ consists of multiple atlases $\{A_i = (I_i, L_i)|i = 1, \ldots, N\}$, where I_i and L_i are the intensity image and the label image/map of the i-th atlas, and N is the total number of atlases in the library $\mathbf{A}$. Set $T = \{T_j = (H_j, B_j)|j = 1, \ldots, M\}$ represents the training set, where H_j and B_j are the intensity image and the label image/map of the j-th training sample, and M is the total number of training samples. $A_i^j = \{I_i^j, L_i^j\}, i = 1, \ldots, N, j =$

$1, \ldots, M$ denotes the intensity (I_i^j) and label (L_i^j) images of the i-th atlas after mapping to the j-th training image. Each brain ROI is assigned with a ROI/label s, $s = 1, \ldots, S$, where S is the total number of ROIs.

2.1 Atlas-guided Multi-channel Forest Learning

To increase the flexibility of our learning procedure, we will train one multi-channel random forest $F_{i,s}$ for each atlas i and each ROI s. In this way, when a new atlas is added into $\mathbf{A}$, only the new multi-channel forest needs to be trained with the new atlas, while all previously trained forests can be reused.

To label the s-th ROI, we will learn a multi-channel forest $F_{i,s}$ with each atlas, i.e., the i-th atlas. To obtain more accurate label information from atlas, registration and patch selection are performed. First, during the $F_{i,s}$ learning, we non-rigidly register the i-th atlas image I_i onto each training target image H_j, to obtain the warped atlas image I_i^j and label map L_i^j. For each sample voxel x in H_j, we first extract its appearance features from a local patch of H_j, centered at x. To reduce the registration error and further get more accurate label from the atlas, according to the similarity between local intensity patches of training image and warped atlas image, we search a nearest voxel $c_1(x)$ (with largest similarity) of x from the warped atlas image I_i^j. For efficiency, the overall intensity difference within the patch is used as the similarity measurement [6]. Then, we extract label features from the local patch of $c_1(x)$ in the aligned atlas label image L_i^j. Finally, both appearance features and label features are combined to jointly characterize the appearance and spatial label context information of each sample voxel, and use it for inferring label. Afterwards, the positive and negative samples are taken inside and outside of the s-th ROI from every training image for multi-channel forest learning, as detailed below. The flowchart shown in Fig. 1 gives an illustration for learning one multi-channel forest.

Sampling Strategy: The positive and negative samples used to train multi-channel forest for the s-th ROI are randomly sampled inside and outside the s-th ROI, respectively. Intuitively, voxels around the ROI boundary are more difficult to be correctly classified than other voxels. Therefore, more samples are drawn around the ROI boundary, as shown in the right bottom of Fig. 1, and also the numbers of positive and negative samples are kept the same.

Feature Extraction: To train multi-channel forests for the i-th atlas, as mentioned above, every training image $H_j, j = 1, \ldots, M$, will be associated with its respective aligned i-th atlas $A_i^j = \{I_i^j, L_i^j\}$. More specifically, there are $S + 1$ different channels of features extracted for: **1 channel** of local appearance features extracted from the training image (e.g., H_j), and S **channels** of local label context features extracted from the aligned i-th atlas label map (e.g., L_i^j) with respect to each of S ROIs.

Local Appearance Features. The local image appearance features extracted from a given (training) target image include: 1) patch intensities 2) outputs from the first-order difference filters (FODs), second-order difference filters (SODs),

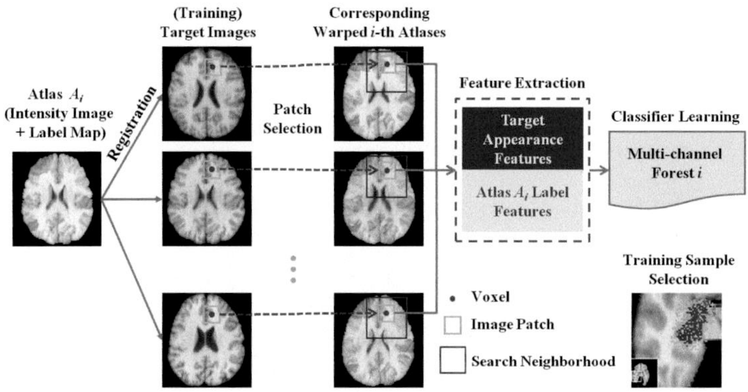

Fig. 1. The flowchart of our method for learning one multi-channel forest with the i-th atlas. An example for sample selection during the training stage is also given in the right-bottom corner, where blue points denote samples belonging to the ROI while green points denote samples belonging to the background. Note here that more samples are drawn around the ROI boundaries.

3D Hyperplan filters, 3D Sobel filters, Laplacian filters and range difference filters, and 3) the random 3D Haar-like features computed from a neighborhood. In addition, by randomly selecting different parameter values of features, the appearance features can capture rich texture information of the target image.

Local Label Context Features. To extract the label context features for each ROI, we first convert the multi-ROI atlas label map into S binary label maps, $L^j_{i,s}$, where $L^j_{i,s}$ corresponds to ROI s, with only voxels in ROI s having label 1 (positive) while all other voxels having label 0 (negative). Then, from each binary label map $L^j_{i,s}$, we uniformly and sparsely select 343 voxels within a $11 \times 11 \times 11$ neighborhood. Finally, a total of $125 \times S$ voxels are sampled, and their label values are served as local label context features.

2.2 Single-ROI and Multi-ROI Labeling

Single-ROI Labeling: To label a single ROI in a new target image, all atlases are first non-rigidly registered onto the target image. To effectively correct for inaccurate registration, we adopt the non-local strategy in the testing stage. Specifically, for a target voxel x to be labeled, we first perform a local patch search in the aligned atlas image (e.g. I^j_i) to select the top K atlas patches with similar appearance to the target patch centered at x. Here, the centers of the selected atlas patches are indexed as $c_k(x), k = 1, \ldots, K$. **1)** For each voxel $c_k(x)$, its label context features can be extracted from the binary label maps $\{L^j_{i,s}, s = 1, \ldots, S\}$. Then, these S channels of label context features and also one channel of appearance features computed from the target image can be combined as a feature representation of x. **2)** Afterwards, we apply the learned $F_{i,s}$ to estimate the label probability of x. **3)** We obtain K label probabilities

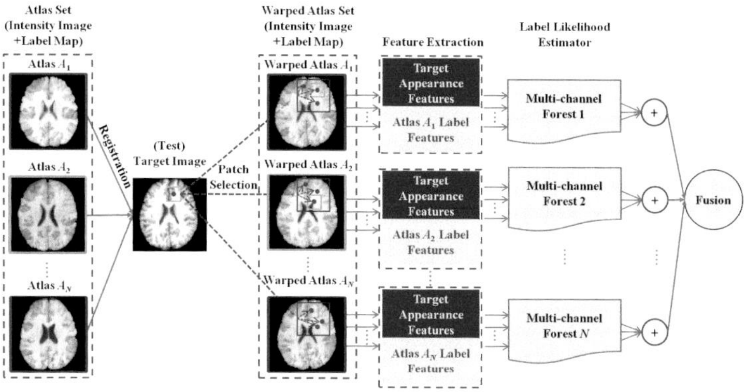

Fig. 2. A diagram for single-ROI labeling with our proposed atlas-guided multi-channel forest learning.

for K selected atlas patches, and then simply average them to obtain a final label for x. Note that, using the above step, each aligned atlas can use its own learned multi-channel forest for labeling the target image independently. Then, the labeling results from all N atlases can be further averaged to obtain the final labeling result for the target image. To increase the efficiency of voxel-wise labeling for the target image, we apply our method only to the voxels that receive votes from the warped atlas label maps. Fig. 2 gives an illustration of our single-ROI labeling method.

Multi-ROI Labeling: The extension from single-ROI labeling to multi-ROI labeling is straightforward. For each target voxel to be labeled, we first use labels of the corresponding voxels in the aligned atlases to find a set of candidate labels for this voxel. Then, we apply only the ROI classifiers responsible to those candidate labels for estimating the label probabilities of the target voxel, while all other ROI classifiers are excluded, and their corresponding label probabilities are simply set to zero. For all the ROIs, we can obtain S single-ROI labeling maps. To fuse these single-ROI labeling maps into one multi-ROI labeling map, the label of each target voxel is simply assigned by the one with the maximum probability across all different single-ROI label maps.

2.3 Haar-Based Multi-Class Contexture Model (HMCCM)

After applying our trained atlas-specific multi-channel forest to the target image, we can obtain a label probability map, which contains more relevant label context information (than the aligned atlas label map) for the target image. We, thus, further update the label context information from the newly obtained (tentative) label probability map, to learn a next multi-channel forest for refinement of labeling. By iterating this procedure, a sequence of classifiers (random forests) can be learned to iteratively improve the labeling result of the target image. In the following paragraphs, we detail the training and testing stages of HMCCM for the case of multi-ROI labeling.

Training: In the initial layer, for each atlas (e.g., the i-th atlas), we first train a set of atlas-specific multi-channel forests $\{F_{i,s}^1, s = 1, \ldots, S\}$. Then, by applying the trained $\{F_{i,s}\}$ to each training image, a set of initial label probability maps $P^1 = \{P_s^1\}$ can be obtained. In the second layer, we can extract the context information from the set of P^1, instead of binary label maps of the aligned atlas. Specifically, for each target voxel x in the target image, Haar-like features are extracted in the local patch centered at x from each P_s^1, for characterizing the multi-scale label context features. (Note that, in this study, for obtaining large-scale label context information, we adopt a large local patch). Then, we combine these updated label context features with the appearance features to re-train a next set of atlas-specific multi-channel forests $\{F_{i,s}^2\}$, which can be again used to estimate a next set of new label probability maps $P^2 = \{P_s^2\}$ for each training image. In the each of the following layers, the label context features are updated from the set of label probability maps computed in the previous layer, and then these updated features are combined with the appearance features of the target image to train a next set of atlas-specific multi-channel forests (corresponding to each ROI). Finally, after training totally O layers, we can obtain O subsequent sets of atlas-specific multi-channel forests, $\{F_{i,s}^o\}, o = 1, \ldots, O$.

Testing: For a new test H^t, each voxel is layer-wisely tested by the trained classifiers $\{F_{i,s}^o\}, o = 1, \ldots, O$. Specifically, for each atlas (e.g., the i-th atlas), we use the first layer of $\{F_{i,s}^1\}$ to obtain the initial label probability maps $P^{t,1} = \{P_s^{t,1}\}$ for H^t. In the following layer, we update the Haar-like features from the label probability maps of the previous layer as the context features. Then, these updated context features are combined with the appearance features of the test image and further input to the set of trained atlas-specific multi-channel forests of the current layer for obtaining a refined set of label probability maps of the test image. This procedure is iterated until reaching the last layer, thus, obtaining the final label probability maps for the test image (with the i-th atlas). The labeling results from all N atlases will be averaged to produce the final labeling.

3 Experimental Results

In this section, we apply our proposed method to the LONI-LPBA40 dataset [1] and IXI dataset (https://www.brain-development.org) for evaluating its performance in ROI labeling. We compared the proposed multiple atlas-guided multi-channel forest (MAMCF) and MAMCF+HCCM with two popular learning-based methods, i.e., standard random forests (SRF) [4] and auto-context model (ACM) [5]. Also, for comparison with multi-atlas based labeling methods, we apply majority voting (MV) and the conventional patch-based methods by non-local patch based labeling propagation (Nonlocal PBL) [6] and the recently proposed sparse patch-based labeling propagation (Sparse PBL) [6, 7]. To align each atlas image with the target image, affine registration is first performed by FLIRT. Then, diffeomorphic Demons is further performed for deformable registration. To quantitatively evaluate the labeling accuracy, we use the Dice Similarity Coefficient (DSC) to measure the overlap degree between automatic labeling and

Table 1. The mean and standard deviation of DSC (%) by MV, Non-local PBL, Sparse PBL, SRF, SRF+HMCCM and our method on LONI_LPBA40 and IXI datasets, respectively

Method	LONI-LPBA40	IXI
MV	78.55 ± 4.33	76.64 ± 4.56
Non-local PBL	78.58 ± 4.32	75.85 ± 4.70
Sparse PBL	80.21 ± 4.32	77.40 ± 4.52
SRF	72.48 ± 4.36	72.09 ± 4.98
SRF+ACM	73.83 ± 4.47	74.53 ± 4.49
MAMCF	81.89 ± 4.25	79.08 ± 4.41
MAMCF+HMCCM	82.56 ± 4.22	79.78 ± 4.34

manual labeling of each ROI. In the experiments, we use leave-one-out cross-validation to evaluate the performance of our method. For each test image, all other images are split into two equal parts: one used for training, and another used as an atlas images.

Parameters: For texture features (FODs, SODs etc.), parameter setting of each filter can be referred to [8]. For appearance patch size (11x11x11) and label patch size (11x11x11), we determine them by five-fold across validation on the training data. In first stage of our method, we extract total 2367 appearance features and 1331 label features for each ROI. In second stage of our method, we extract additional 500 haar-like features for each ROI from label probability maps. In the training stage, we train 20 trees for each multi-channel forest. The maximum tree depth is set to 20, and the minimum number of samples in the tree leaf node is set to 4.

LONI-LPBA40 Dataset: The dataset consists of 40 T1-weighted MRI brain images from 40 healthy volunteers, each with 54 manually labeled ROIs (excluding cerebrum and brainstem). Most of these ROIs are within the cortex. The second column of Table 1 shows the mean and standard deviation of DSC on 54 ROIs by the compared methods. Over the all 54 ROIs, the average DSCs achieved by MV, Nonlocal PBL, and Sparse PBL, SRF and SRF+ACM are $78.55\% \pm 4.33\%$, $78.58\% \pm 4.32\%$, $80.21\% \pm 4.32\%$, $72.48\% \pm 4.36\%$ and $73.83\% \pm 4.47\%$ respectively, which are lower than MAMCF ($81.89\% \pm 4.25\%$) and MAMCF+HMCCM ($82.56\% \pm 4.22\%$). In terms of average performance over all the ROIs, compared with other methods, MAMCF and MAMCF+HMCCM obtain statistically significant improvements ($p < 0.0001$) by the paired Student's t-test.

IXI Dataset: We use 30 images in the IXI dataset, which contains manual annotations of 80 structures (excluding cerebrum and brainstem). The third column of Table 1 shows the mean and standard deviation of DSC on all 80 ROIs. It can be observed that MAMCF+HMCCM ($79.78\% \pm 4.34\%$) methods are ranked top, followed by MAMCF (79.08%±4.41%), Sparse PBL (77.4%±4.52%), MV (76.64% ± 4.56%), Non-local PBL (75.85% ± 4.7%), SRF+ACM (74.53% ± 4.49%) and SRF (72.09% ± 4.98%). In terms of average performance over all the ROIs, compared with other methods, MAMCF and MAMCF+HMCCM obtain statistically significant improvements ($p < 0.0001$).

4 Conclusion

In this paper, we propose a novel atlas-guided multi-channel forest learning to effectively combine the advantages of both multi-atlas based labeling methods and learning-based labeling methods. Instead of labeling a target voxel based only on its own local image appearance, we also utilize label context information from the aligned atlas. A non-linear multi-channel forest is learned for automatically fusing all information. Furthermore, the Haar-based multi-class contexture model (HMCCM) is also proposed to enhance the structural and label context information of the target image. Specifically, we use Haar-like features to iteratively extract multi-scale label context information from the tentatively-estimated multi-ROI label probability maps of the target image. Our method shows more accurate labeling results than both the existing multi-atlas based labeling methods and learning-based labeling methods, on both LONI-LBPA40 and IXI datasets.

References

[1] Shattuck, D.W., Mirza, M., Adisetiyo, V., Hojatkashani, C., Salamon, G., Narr, K.L., Poldrack, R.A., Bilder, R.M., Toga, A.W.: Construction of a 3D probabilistic atlas of human cortical structures. Neuroimage 39(3), 1064–1080 (2007)
[2] Zikic, D., Glocker, B., Criminisi, A.: Atlas encoding by randomized forests for efficient label propagation. In: Mori, K., Sakuma, I., Sato, Y., Barillot, C., Navab, N. (eds.) MICCAI 2013, Part III. LNCS, vol. 8151, pp. 66–73. Springer, Heidelberg (2013)
[3] Wang, H., Sub, J.W., Das, S.R., Pluta, J.B., Craige, C., Yushkevich, P.A.: Multi-atlas segmentation with joint label fusion. IEEE Trans. Pattern Analysis and Machine Intelligence 35(3), 611–623 (2013)
[4] Breiman, L.: Random forests. Machine Learning 45(1), 5–32 (2001)
[5] Tu, Z., Bai, X.: Auto-context and its application to high-level vision tasks and 3d brain image segmentation. IEEE Trans. Pattern Analysis and Machine Intelligence 32(10), 1744–1757 (2010)
[6] Coupé, P., Manjón, J.V., Fonov, V., Pruessner, J., Robles, M., Collins, D.L.: Patch-based segmentation using expert priors: Application to hippocampus and ventricle segmentation. NeuroImage 54(2), 940–954 (2011)
[7] Wu, G., Wang, Q., Zhang, D., Shen, D.: Robust patch-based multi-atlas labeling by joint sparsity regularization. In: MICCAI Workshop STMI (2012)
[8] Hao, Y., Wang, T., Zhang, X., Duan, Y., Yu, C., Jiang, T., Fan, Y.: Local label learning (LLL) for subcortical structure segmentation: application to hippocampus segmentation. Human Brain Mapping 35(6), 2674–2697 (2014)
[9] Gao, Y., Liao, S., Shen, D.: Prostate segmentation by sparse representation based classification. Medical Physics 39(10), 6372–6387 (2012)

Model Criticism for Regression on the Grassmannian

Yi Hong[1], Roland Kwitt[3], and Marc Niethammer[1,2]

[1]University of North Carolina (UNC) at Chapel Hill, NC, US
[2]Biomedical Research Imaging Center, UNC-Chapel Hill, NC, US
[3]Department of Computer Science, University of Salzburg, Austria

Abstract. Reliable estimation of model parameters from data requires a suitable model. In this work, we investigate and extend a recent *model criticism* approach to evaluate regression models on the Grassmann manifold. Model criticism allows us to check if a model fits and if the underlying model assumptions are justified by the observed data. This is a critical step to check model validity which is often neglected in practice. Using synthetic data we demonstrate that the proposed model criticism approach can indeed reject models that are improper for observed data and that the approach can guide the model selection process. We study two real applications: degeneration of corpus callosum shapes during aging and developmental shape changes in the rat calvarium. Our experimental results suggest that the three tested regression models on the Grassmannian (equivalent to linear, time-warped, and cubic-spline regression in $\mathbb{R}^n$, respectively) can all capture changes of the corpus callosum, but only the cubic-spline model is appropriate for shape changes of the rat calvarium. While our approach is developed for the Grassmannian, the principles are applicable to smooth manifolds in general.

1 Introduction

In Euclidean space, regression models, e.g., linear least squares, are commonly used to estimate the relationship between variables. Recently, they have been successfully extended to manifolds, e.g., the manifold of diffeomorphisms [9], general Riemannian manifolds [2], and in particular the Grassmannian [6]. These models capture changes of data objects (e.g., images, or shapes) with respect to an associated descriptive variable, such as age. To measure the goodness-of-fit of these regression models, one usually computes the sum of squared errors (SSE), R^2 [2], or the mean squared error (MSE) using cross-validation.

While these measures assess fitting quality, they do not directly check if the underlying model assumptions hold. *Model criticism* does exactly that: it checks if a model's assumptions (including the noise model) are consistent with the observed data. It thereby provides valuable additional information beyond the classical measures for model fit. Recently, statistical model criticism [8] using a kernel-based two-sample test [3] has been proposed and its utility to evaluate regression models in Euclidean space was demonstrated.

N. Navab et al. (Eds.): MICCAI 2015, Part III, LNCS 9351, pp. 727–734, 2015.
DOI: 10.1007/978-3-319-24574-4_87

In this paper, we take this approach one step further and use the fact that the strategy of [8] depends on a suitable kernel function for the data and can thus be extended to manifolds given such a kernel function. Given a population of data samples on the Grassmannian, we (1) perform regression, then (2) generate samples from the regression model and (3) assess whether the observed data could have been generated by the fitted model. We demonstrate the approach by criticizing three different regression models on the Grassmannian [7] using both synthetic and real data. We argue that model criticism is complementary to traditional measures of model fit, but has the advantage of directly assessing the suitability of a statistical model and its fit for given observed data.

Contributions. We propose an extension of model criticism to regression models on the Grassmannian. In particular, we extend the approach of [8] by (1) providing a strategy to generate Gaussian-distributed samples with a specific variance on this manifold, and (2) incorporating existing kernels into the two-sample testing strategy used for model criticism. We then apply the approach to check the validity of different regression models. Our experimental results are based on both synthetic and real data, including corpus callosum and rat calvarium shapes, providing insight into the appropriateness of the regression models beyond the customary use of the R^2 statistic.

2 Model Criticism for Regression in Euclidean Space

The objective of model criticism for regression is to test for discrepancies between observed data and a model estimated from the data [8]. We assume the data observations are independently and identically distributed (i.i.d.) and that we can draw i.i.d. samples from the model respecting the noise assumptions; then, the key ingredient of model criticism is to measure whether these two samples are drawn from the same underlying distribution. To perform this *two-sample test*, a "kernelized" variant of the maximum mean discrepancy (MMD) [3] has been proposed as one choice of the test-statistic.

Review of Kernel-Based Two-Sample Testing [3]. Assume we have i.i.d. samples $X = \{x_i\}_{i=1}^m$ and $Y = \{y_i\}_{i=1}^n$, drawn randomly from distributions p, q, defined on a domain $\mathcal{X}$. The goal of two-sample testing is to assess if $p = q$. One choice of a test-statistic is the MMD, defined as

$$\mathrm{MMD}[\mathcal{F}, p, q] = \sup_{f \in \mathcal{F}} (\mathbb{E}_{x\sim p}[f(x)] - \mathbb{E}_{y\sim q}[f(y)]) \ , \tag{1}$$

where $\mathcal{F}$ is a suitable class of functions $f : \mathcal{X} \to \mathbb{R}$. To uniquely measure whether $p = q$, Gretton et al. [3] let $\mathcal{F}$ be the unit ball in a reproducing kernel Hilbert space (RKHS) $\mathcal{H}$, i.e., $\mathcal{F} = \{f \in \mathcal{H} : \|f\|_\mathcal{H} \le 1\}$, with associated reproducing kernel $k : \mathcal{X} \times \mathcal{X} \to \mathbb{R}$. The kernel can be written as $k(x, y) = \langle \phi(x), \phi(y) \rangle_\mathcal{H}$, where $\langle \cdot, \cdot \rangle_\mathcal{H}$ is the inner product in $\mathcal{H}$ and $\phi : \mathcal{X} \to \mathcal{H}$ denotes the feature map.

According to [3], Eq. (1) can then be expressed as the RKHS distance between the mean embeddings $\mu[p]$ and $\mu[q]$ of the distributions p and q, in particular

$\mu[p] := \mathbb{E}_{x\sim p}[\phi(x)]$. Since the mean embedding satisfies $\mathbb{E}_{x\sim p}[f(x)] = \langle \mu[p], f\rangle_{\mathcal{H}}$, Eq. (1) can be written as

$$\mathrm{MMD}[\mathcal{F}, p, q] = \sup_{\|f\|_{\mathcal{H}}\leq 1} \langle \mu[p] - \mu[q], f\rangle = \|\mu[p] - \mu[q]\|_{\mathcal{H}} \tag{2}$$

with the empirical estimate (using the kernel function k)

$$\widehat{\mathrm{MMD}}[\mathcal{F}, X, Y] = \left[\frac{1}{m^2}\sum_{i,j=1}^{m} k(x_i, x_j) - \frac{2}{mn}\sum_{i,j=1}^{m,n} k(x_i, y_j) + \frac{1}{n^2}\sum_{i,j=1}^{n} k(y_i, y_j)\right]^{\frac{1}{2}}. \tag{3}$$

In the following, we omit $\mathcal{F}$ and let $\widehat{\mathrm{MMD}}(X, Y)$ denote the computation of the MMD statistic on two samples X and Y using a suitable kernel function k.

Model Criticism Using Two-Sample Testing. Assume we have data observations $\{Y_i^{obs}\}_{i=1}^N$, drawn from some distribution p, conditioned on an associated independent value t_i. A regression model M is estimated from the tuples $\{(t_i, Y_i^{obs})\}_{i=1}^N$. If the regression model is based on a Gaussian noise assumption[1], we can generate i.i.d. samples from the model; let this distribution be denoted by q and a sample by $\{Y_i^{est} = M(t_i) + n_i\}_{i=1}^N$, where $n_i \sim N(0, \sigma^2)$ and σ is the standard deviation of the residuals. Criticizing the model M now means to perform a two-sample test between $\{(t_i, Y_i^{obs})\}_{i=1}^N$ and $\{(t_i, Y_i^{est})\}_{i=1}^N$ under the null-hypothesis $H_0 : p = q$. This is done by computing the test-statistic between data observations and samples drawn from the regression model, i.e., $T^* = \widehat{\mathrm{MMD}}(\{(t_i, Y_i^{obs})\}_{i=1}^N, \{(t_i, Y_i^{est})\}_{i=1}^N)$. Then, to obtain the distribution of T under H_0, we repeatedly draw (from q) N i.i.d. samples to form two populations, $\{(t_i, Y_i^a)\}_{i=1}^N$ and $\{(t_i, Y_i^b)\}_{i=1}^N$. For each such draw j, we compute $T_j = \widehat{\mathrm{MMD}}(\{(t_i, Y_i^a)\}_{i=1}^N, \{(t_i, Y_i^b)\}_{i=1}^N)$ and thereby obtain the empirical distribution of T under H_0. Note that in case of observations in $\mathbb{R}^n$, computing the MMD statistic for model criticism is straightforward, since we can simply add t_i as an additional dimension to our data, i.e., we obtain observations in $\mathbb{R}^{n+1}$. The well-known RBF kernel can then be used to compute Eq. (3). We will see that this needs to be handled differently on manifolds.

Finally, we count the number of times that the bootstrapped statistics under H_0 are larger than the test statistic T^*, which results in a p-value estimate. Because T^* will be affected by the added random noise, we can also sample it a large number of times, resulting in a distribution of T^* and associated p-values.

3 Model Criticism for Regression on the Grassmannian

We now extend the model criticism approach of the previous section to the Grassmann manifold. The test objects are regression models on the Grassmannian, i.e., generalizations of classical regression in Euclidean space which minimize the sum of squared (geodesic) distances to the regression curves. Noise in these models is assumed to be Gaussian. To generalize the model criticism idea, one

[1] Other noise models can also be used as long as one can sample from them.

key ingredient is to draw random samples on the Grassmannian at each point on the regression curves. The other key ingredient is a suitable kernel k for Eq. (3) and a strategy to include the independent value into the kernel.

Drawing Random Samples on the Grassmannian. Similar to the Euclidean case, we assume we have N data observations on the Grassmannian $\mathcal{G}(r,s)$[2] with associated independent values, i.e., $\{(t_i, \mathbf{Y}_i^{obs})\}_{i=1}^N$. Using a regression model M estimated from this data, we can compute the corresponding data points on the regressed curve for each t_i as $\bar{\mathbf{Y}}_i^{est} = M(t_i)$. To draw sample points at each t_i under a Gaussian noise model, we adhere to the following strategy (although, other approaches such as the one outlined in [11] are possible). First, we compute the empirical standard deviation of the residuals as

$$\sigma = \sqrt{\frac{\sum_{i=1}^N d^2(\mathbf{Y}_i^{obs}, \bar{\mathbf{Y}}_i^{est})}{N-1}} \ , \tag{4}$$

where $d(\cdot,\cdot)$ denotes the geodesic distance on $\mathcal{G}(r,s)$. For each estimated data point $\bar{\mathbf{Y}}_i^{est}$, we then generate a tangent vector $\dot{\mathbf{Y}}_i^{est}$ as the projection of an $s \times r$ random matrix $\mathbf{Z}_i = [z_{uv}]$, $z_{uv} \sim \mathcal{N}(0, \hat{\sigma}^2)$ onto the tangent space at $\bar{\mathbf{Y}}_i^{est}$; this is done via $\dot{\mathbf{Y}}_i^{est} = (\mathbf{I}_s - \bar{\mathbf{Y}}_i^{est}(\bar{\mathbf{Y}}_i^{est})^\top)\mathbf{Z}_i$ where $\mathbf{I}_s$ is the $s \times s$ identity matrix. The random point $\mathbf{Y}_i^{est}$ (at t_i), is eventually computed via the Riemannian exponontial map as

$$\mathbf{Y}_i^{est} = \mathrm{Exp}(\bar{\mathbf{Y}}_i^{est}, \dot{\mathbf{Y}}_i^{est}) \ . \tag{5}$$

We note that the standard deviation $\hat{\sigma}$ of the samples in $\mathbf{Z}_i$ is proportional to the standard deviation σ as computed by Eq. (4). In fact, it can be shown[3] that the resulting geodesic distance between $\bar{\mathbf{Y}}_i^{est}$ and $\mathbf{Y}_i^{est}$ has standard deviation $\hat{\sigma}\sqrt{rs}$. Consequently, we set $\hat{\sigma} = \sigma/\sqrt{rs}$ when creating the $\mathbf{Z}_i$.

Kernels for Model Criticism on the Grassmannian. The next step is to adjust the kernel-based two-sample test of [3] for model criticism on the $\mathcal{G}(r,s)$ by selecting a suitable kernel. In [5], several positive definite (and universal) kernels on $\mathcal{G}(r,s)$ have been proposed, e.g., RBF, Laplace and Binomial kernels. These kernels are constructed by using the Binet-Cauchy kernel k_{bc} [10] and the projection kernel k_p [4]. We selected the kernel $k_{l,p}(\mathbf{X},\mathbf{Y}) = \exp\left(-\beta\sqrt{r - \|\mathbf{X}^\top\mathbf{Y}\|_F^2}\right), \beta > 0$ from [5] for our experiments[4]. However, for model criticism as proposed in [8] to be used on regression models, we need to be able to compute the MMD test for $(t_i, \mathbf{Y}_i)$ (i.e., including the information about the independent variable). While this is simple in the Euclidean case (cf.

---

[2] The Grassmannian $\mathcal{G}(r,s)$ is the manifold of r-dimensional subspaces of $\mathbb{R}^s$. A point on $\mathcal{G}(r,s)$ is identified by an $s \times r$ matrix $\mathbf{Y}$ with $\mathbf{Y}^\top\mathbf{Y} = \mathbf{I}_r$.

[3] Say we have samples $\mathbf{Y}_1, \ldots, \mathbf{Y}_n$ with Fréchet mean $\bar{\mathbf{Y}}$. The Fréchet variance is defined as $\sigma^2 = \min_{\mathbf{Y}\in\mathcal{G}(r,s)} {}^1\!/_n \sum_{i=1}^n d^2(\mathbf{Y}, \mathbf{Y}_i)$; this can equivalently be written as $\sigma^2 = \frac{1}{n}\sum_{i=1}^n \mathrm{tr}(\dot{\mathbf{Y}}_i^\top\dot{\mathbf{Y}}_i)$ with $\dot{\mathbf{Y}}_i = \mathrm{Exp}^{-1}(\bar{\mathbf{Y}}, \mathbf{Y}_i)$. Expanding the trace yields $\sigma^2 = \sum_{j=1}^s\sum_{k=1}^r [{}^1\!/_n \sum_{i=1}^n y_{i,j,k}^2]$ where the term in brackets is $\hat{\sigma}^2$ since $y_{i,j,k}$ is i.i.d. as $\mathcal{N}(0,\hat{\sigma}^2)$. We finally obtain $\sigma^2 = rs\hat{\sigma}^2$.

[4] Here, r denotes the subspace dimension in $\mathcal{G}(r,s)$, as defined before.

Section 2), the situation on manifolds is more complicated since we cannot simply add t_i to our observations. Our strategy is to use an RBF kernel for the t_i, i.e., $k_{rbf}(t, t') = \exp(-(t-t')^2/(2\gamma^2))$ and then leverage the closure properties of positive definite kernels, which allow multiplication of positive definite kernels. This yields our *combined kernel* as

$$k((t_i, \mathbf{X}), (t_j, \mathbf{Y})) = \exp\left(-\frac{(t_i - t_j)^2}{2\gamma^2}\right) \cdot \exp\left(-\beta\sqrt{r - \|\mathbf{X}^\top \mathbf{Y}\|_F^2}\right) . \quad (6)$$

In all the experiments, we set both β and γ to 1 for simplicity.

Model Criticism on the Grassmannian. The computational steps for model criticism on the Grassmannian are listed below:

(1) Compute the points $\{\bar{\mathbf{Y}}_i^{est} = M(t_i)\}_{i=1}^N$ for each data observation $\mathbf{Y}_i^{obs}$ on $\mathcal{G}(r, s)$ from the estimated regression model M.
(2) Estimate the standard deviation of residuals, σ, using Eq. (4).
(3) Generate noisy samples, $\mathbf{Y}_i^{est}$ at each t_i using Eq. (5) and $\hat{\sigma}^2 = \sigma^2/(rs)$.
(4) Compute $T^* = \widehat{\text{MMD}}(\{(t_i, \mathbf{Y}_i^{est})\}_{i=1}^N, \{(t_i, \mathbf{Y}_i^{obs})\}_{i=1}^N)$ using Eqs. (3) & (6).
(5) Repeat (3) and (4) many times to obtain a population of T^*.
(6) Generate two groups of samples using (3), $\{(t_i, \mathbf{Y}_i^a)\}_{i=1}^N$, and $\{(t_i, \mathbf{Y}_i^b)\}_{i=1}^N$, and compute $T = \widehat{\text{MMD}}(\{(t_i, \mathbf{Y}_i^a)\}_{i=1}^N, \{(t_i, \mathbf{Y}_i^b)\}_{i=1}^N)$.
(7) Repeat (6) many times to obtain a distribution of T under H_0.
(8) Compute a p-value for each T^* in (5) with respect to the distribution of T from (7), resulting in a population of p-values. This allows to reject the null-hypothesis that the observed data distribution is the same as the sampled data distribution of the model at a chosen significance level α (e.g., 0.05).

4 Experimental Results

We criticize three different regression models on the Grassmannian [7]: Std-GGR, TW-GGR, and CS-GGR, which are generalizations of linear least squares, time-warped, and cubic-spline regression, respectively. These three models are estimated by energy minimization from an optimal-control point of view.

Synthetic Data. For easy visualization, we synthesize data on the Grassmannian $\mathcal{G}(1, 2)$, i.e., the space of lines through the origin in $\mathbb{R}^2$. Each point uniquely corresponds to an angle in $[-\pi/2, \pi/2]$ with respect to the horizontal axis.

(1) Different Data Distributions. The first experiment is to perform model criticism on *one* regression model, but for different data distributions. To generate this data, we select two points on $\mathcal{G}(1, 2)$ to define a geodesic curve, and then uniformly sample 51 points along this geodesic from one point at time 0 to the other point at time 1. Using the strategy described in Section 3, Gaussian noise with $\sigma = 0.05$ is then added to the sampled points along the geodesic, resulting in the 1st group (Group 1) of synthetic data. The 2nd group (Group 2) of synthetic data is simulated by concatenating two different geodesics. Again, 51 points are uniformly sampled along the curve and Gaussian noise is added. The left column in Fig. 1(a) shows the two synthetic data sets using their corresponding angles.

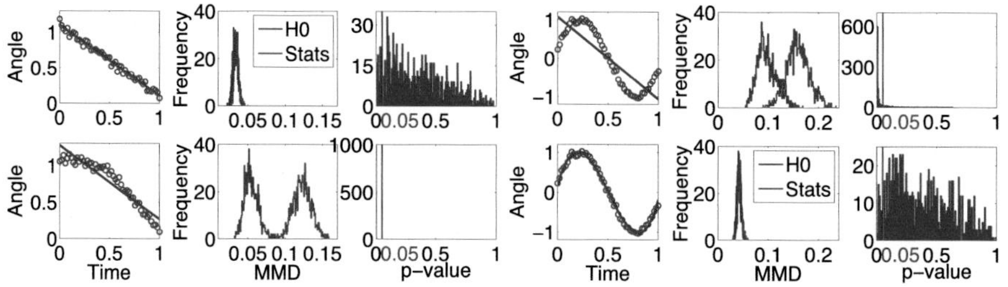

(a) Different data distributions (b) Different regression models

Fig. 1. Model criticism for synthetic data on the Grassmannian. (a) Different data distributions are fitted by one regression model (Std-GGR); (b) One data distribution is fitted by different regression models (*top*: Std-GGR, *bottom*: CS-GGR).

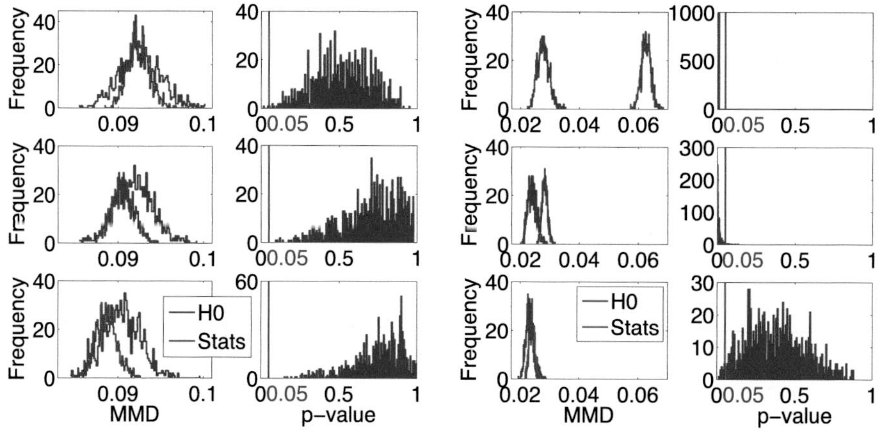

(a) Corpus callosum (b) Rat calvarium

Fig. 2. Model criticism for real data. From *top* to *bottom*: the regression model corresponds to Std-GGR, TW-GGR, and CS-GGR respectively.

Both groups are fitted using a standard geodesic regression model (Std-GGR); the qualitative and quantitative results of model criticism are reported in Fig. 1(a) and Table 1, respectively. Among 1000 trials, H_0 is rejected in only 8.1% of all cases for Group 1 (generated from one geodesic), but H_0 is always rejected for Group 2 (i.e., generated from two geodesics). As expected, Std-GGR is not an appropriate model to capture the distribution of the data belonging to multiple geodesics. Model criticism correctly identifies this, while the R^2 values are hard to interpret with respect to model suitability.

(2) Different Regression Models. The second experiment is to generate one data distribution, but to estimate different regression models. We first generate a section of a sine curve with x-axis as time and y-axis as the angle. Each angle θ corresponds to a point on the Grassmannian, i.e., $[\cos\theta; \sin\theta] \in \mathcal{G}(1,2)$. In this way, we can generate polynomial data on $\mathcal{G}(1,2)$ with associated time $t \in [0,1]$.

Table 1. Comparison of R^2 measure and model criticism for synthetic data.

	Different data distributions		**Different regression models**	
	Group 1	Group 2	Std-GGR	CS-GGR
R^2	0.99	0.89	0.73	0.99
%(p-values < 0.05)	8.1%	100%	88.0%	4.5%

Table 2. Comparison of R^2 measure and model criticism for real data.

	Corpus callosum			**Rat calvarium**		
	Std-GGR	TW-GGR	CS-GGR	Std-GGR	TW-GGR	CS-GGR
R^2	0.12	0.15	0.21	0.61	0.79	0.81
%(p-values < 0.05)	0.2%	0%	0%	100%	98.0%	1.3%

A visualization of the generated data with added Gaussian noise ($\sigma = 0.05$) is shown in the left column of Fig. 1(b). The data points are fitted by a standard geodesic regression model (Std-GGR) and its cubic spline variant (CS-GGR), respectively. The results of model criticism are shown in Fig. 1(b) and Table 1; in 88.0% of 1000 trials, H_0 is rejected for the Std-GGR model, while we only reject H_0 in 4.5% of all trials for CS-GGR. As designed, CS-GGR has better performance than Std-GGR and can appropriately capture the distribution of the generated data, as confirmed by model criticism.

Real Data. Two real applications, shape changes of the corpus callosum during aging and landmark changes of the rat calvarium with age, are used to evaluate model criticism for three regression models on the Grassmannian.

(1) Corpus Callosum Shapes. The population of corpus callosum shapes is collected from 32 subjects with ages varying from 19 to 90 years. Each shape is represented by 64 2D boundary landmarks. We represent each shape matrix as a point on the Grassmannian using an affine-invariant shape representation [1]. As shown in Fig. 2(a) and Table 2, although the R^2 values of the three regression models are relatively low, our model criticism results with 1000 trials suggest that all three models may be appropriate for the observed data.

(2) Rat Calvarium Landmarks. We use 18 individuals with 8 time points from the Vilmann rat data[5]. The time points range from 7 to 150 days. Each shape is represented by a set of 8 landmarks. We project each landmark-based rat calvarium shape onto the Grassmannian, using the same strategy as for the corpus callosum shapes. From the model criticism results shown in Fig. 2(b) and Table 2 we can see that the equivalent linear (Std-GGR) and time-warped (TW-GGR) models cannot faithfully capture the distribution of the rat calvarium landmarks. However, the cubic-spline model is not rejected by model criticism and therefore appears to be the best among the three models. This result is consistent with the R^2 values, and also provides more information about the

[5] Available online: `http://life.bio.sunysb.edu/morph/data/datasets.html`

regression models. As we can see, the R^2 values of TW-GGR and CS-GGR are very close, but the model criticism suggests CS-GGR is the one that should be chosen for regression on this dataset.

5 Discussion

We proposed an approach to *criticize* regression models on the Grassmannian. This approach provides complementary information to the existing measure(s) for checking the goodness-of-fit for regression models, such as the customary R^2 statistic. While we developed the approach for the Grassmannian, the general principle can be extended to other smooth manifolds, as long as one knows how to add the modeled noise into samples and a positive definite kernel is available for the underlying manifold. Two important ingredients of model criticism are the estimation of the parameters of the noise model on the manifold (in our case Gaussian noise and therefore we estimate the standard deviation) and the selection of the kernel. Exploring, in detail, the influence of the estimator and the kernel and its parameters is left as future work.

Acknowledgments. This work was supported by NSF grants EECS-1148870 and EECS-0925875.

References

1. Begelfor, E., Werman, W.: Affine invariance revisited. In: CVPR (2006)
2. Fletcher, P.T.: Geodesic regression and the theory of least squares on Riemannian manifolds. Int. J. Comput. Vision 105(2), 171–185 (2013)
3. Gretton, A., Borgwardt, K.M., Rasch, M.J., Schölkopf, B., Smola, A.: A kernel two-sample test. J. Mach. Learn. Res. 13, 723–773 (2012)
4. Hamm, J., Lee, D.D.: Grassmann discriminant analysis: a unifying view on subspace-based learning. In: ICML (2008)
5. Harandi, M.T., Salzmann, M., Jayasumana, S., Hartley, R., Li, H.: Expanding the family of Grassmannian kernels: An embedding perspective. In: Fleet, D., Pajdla, T., Schiele, B., Tuytelaars, T. (eds.) ECCV 2014, Part VII. LNCS, vol. 8695, pp. 408–423. Springer, Heidelberg (2014)
6. Hong, Y., Kwitt, R., Singh, N., Davis, B., Vasconcelos, N., Niethammer, M.: Geodesic regression on the Grassmannian. In: Fleet, D., Pajdla, T., Schiele, B., Tuytelaars, T. (eds.) ECCV 2014, Part II. LNCS, vol. 8690, pp. 632–646. Springer, Heidelberg (2014)
7. Hong, Y., Singh, N., Kwitt, R., Vasconcelos, N., Niethammer, M.: Parametric regression on the Grassmannian. `http://arxiv.org/abs/1505.03832`
8. Lloyd, J.R., Ghahramani, Z.: Statistical model criticism using kernel two sample tests (Preprint). `http://mlg.eng.cam.ac.uk/Lloyd/papers/`
9. Niethammer, M., Huang, Y., Vialard, F.X.: Geodesic regression for image time-series. In: Fichtinger, G., Martel, A., Peters, T. (eds.) MICCAI, vol. 6892, pp. 655–662. Springer, Heidelberg (2011)
10. Wolf, L., Shashua, A.: Learning over sets using kernel principal angles. J. Mach. Learn. Res. 4, 913–931 (2003)
11. Zhang, M., Fletcher, P.T.: Probabilistic principal geodesic analysis. In: NIPS, pp. 1178–1186 (2013)

Structural Edge Detection for Cardiovascular Modeling

Jameson Merkow[1], Zhuowen Tu[2], David Kriegman[3], and Alison Marsden[4]

[1] Electrical and Computer Engineering
[2] Cognitive Science
[3] Computer Science and Engineering
[4] Mechanical and Aerospace Engineering
University of California, San Diego

Abstract. Computational simulations provide detailed hemodynamics and physiological data that can assist in clinical decision-making. However, accurate cardiovascular simulations require complete 3D models constructed from image data. Though edge localization is a key aspect in pinpointing vessel walls in many segmentation tools, the edge detection algorithms widely utilized by the medical imaging community have remained static. In this paper, we propose a novel approach to medical image edge detection by adopting the powerful structured forest detector and extending its application to the medical imaging domain. First, we specify an effective set of medical imaging driven features. Second, we directly incorporate an adaptive prior to create a robust three-dimensional edge classifier. Last, we boost our accuracy through an intelligent sampling scheme that only samples areas of importance to edge fidelity. Through experimentation, we demonstrate that the proposed method outperforms widely used edge detectors and probabilistic boosting tree edge classifiers and is robust to error in *a prori* information.

1 Introduction

Building on advances in medical imaging technology, cardiovascular blood flow simulation has emerged as a non-invasive and low risk method to provide detailed hemodynamic data and predictive capabilities that imaging alone cannot [4]. A necessary precursor to these simulations is accurate construction of patient-specific 3D models via segmentation of medical image data. Currently available tools to aid model construction include ITK-SNAP (`http://www.itksnap.org`) for general medical image segmentation and SimVascular (`http://www.simvascular.org`) and vmtk (`http://www.vmtk.org`) which use specialized segmentation techniques for blood flow simulation. These packages implement automated segmentation tools, most of which rely heavily on region growers, active-contours and snakes. These methods can be effective for cardiovascular segmentation, however they often require finely-tuned algorithm parameters, hence manual segmentation is commonly used in practice. Model creation remains one of the main bottle-necks in widespread simulation

N. Navab et al. (Eds.): MICCAI 2015, Part III, LNCS 9351, pp. 735–742, 2015.
DOI: 10.1007/978-3-319-24574-4_88

of patient specific cardiovascular systems. Increased efficiency of the model construction process will enable simulations in larger cohorts of patients, increasing the clinical impact of simulation tools. Machine learning techniques produce robust results without manual interaction, which make them a powerful tool for model construction. There has been extensive research into learned edge detection in natural images but edge detection has not received the same attention in medical imaging.

In this paper, a machine learning based edge detection technique is proposed by leveraging diverse domain specific expert annotations in structured prediction labels and builds upon the structured forest classifier [1]. We contribute a novel combination of domain specific features, introduce *a priori* information, and devise an intelligent sampling scheme to correctly classify edges while using a minimum number of training samples.

2 Background and Relevant Work

Active contours are one of the most widely used strategies for segmentation in medical imaging. Active contours propagate segmentation labels using opposing internal and external forces. Internal forces update the contour via appearance criterion while external forces modulate the contour shape with geometric constraints. This technique enforces contour smoothness making it attractive for vascular segmentation for CFD. However, active contours run into difficulty under varying image conditions and often require finely tuned parameters to prevent segmentations from leaking into background pixels.

Alternative strategies use learning based methods and avoid parameter tuning by utilizing expert annotations to build statistical appearance and shape models. Zheng et. al employed probabilistic boosting trees (PBTs) with pixel transformations, gradient data, and atlas features to quickly generate vesselness labels in 46 cardiovascular CT volumes [8]. Schneider et al. used steerable features with hough decision forest voting to perform joint vessel and centerline segmentation [6].

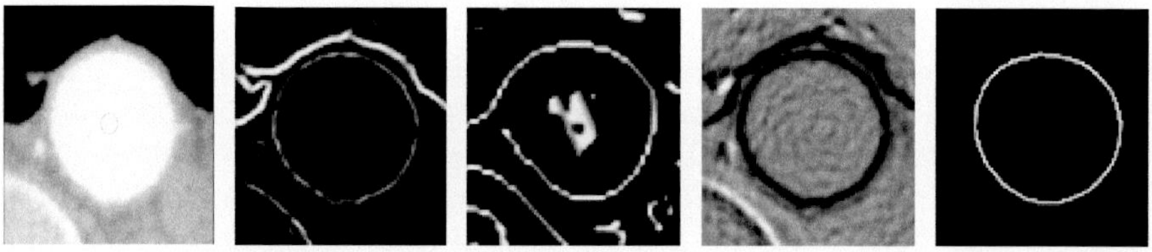

Fig. 1. Cross sectional appearance feature examples, from left to right: lumen intensity, gradient magnitude, Canny edge map, distance-gradient projection and ground truth.

Recent research shows that contextual information boosts learned classifier performance. Auto context models (ACM) learn important shape contexts and discriminative features with an iterative approach to segmentation. ACMs have been successful in a range of medical imaging tasks including brain segmentation, and segmentation of prostates [7,2]. However, ACM is best suited to regional label maps, making it sub-optimal for contour detection where ground truth is often a single voxel in thickness.

Despite an abundance of research into learned edge detection in natural images, edge detection in medical imaging has remained static. Ren and Bo calculated learned sparse coding features and SVM to localize image contours, successfully combined powerful oriented gradient features and dictionary learning to capture edge characteristics [5]. In [3], the authors used discrete sets of clustered local contour features, dubbed *sketch tokens*, to perform various segmentation tasks. Dollár and Zitnick used a clustering algorithm to train a structured forest edge detector [1].

Inspired by the success of contour detection in natural images, we propose a novel edge detection method specific to cardiovascular imaging. We build upon recent work on structured forests by extending the classifier to work in medical imaging. We define a novel set of domain specific features, incorporate *a priori* information into classification, and employing a specialized sampling scheme.

3 Methods

In this section, we describe the methodology used to train our classifier for edge detection. Our goal is to generate a forest of decision trees that produce high scores at edge aligned voxels, and low scores elsewhere. First, we begin by collecting randomized samples of lumen patches and edge ground truth from a training set of image volumes. Second, we compute feature channels from the input patches and find a discretization of the output space. Last, input features and edge ground truths are used to train a decision tree. This process is repeated N times to generate a forest of N trees.

3.1 Sampling Methodology

At each sample location a $16 \times 16 \times 16$ voxel patch and an $8 \times 8 \times 8$ edge ground truth patch are collected. Due to computational constraints of collecting 3D samples, fewer training samples could be collected so a specialized sampling scheme was devised. First, all positive samples were taken from vessel wall aligned overlapping patches to produce more precise edge responses. Second, negative samples were collected from two zones. We collected a majority of negative samples in the region just outside the vessel wall. However, to properly interpret *a priori* information, approximately 30% of the negative samples were taken from any negative region. These zones were determined based on the vessel wall location supplied by ground truth annotation. Figure 2 depicts 2D cross section diagram of our sampling method, we denote the positive sampling zone in blue, the vessel wall adjacent negative sample area in yellow (zone 1) and the general negative sampling region (zone 2) in red.

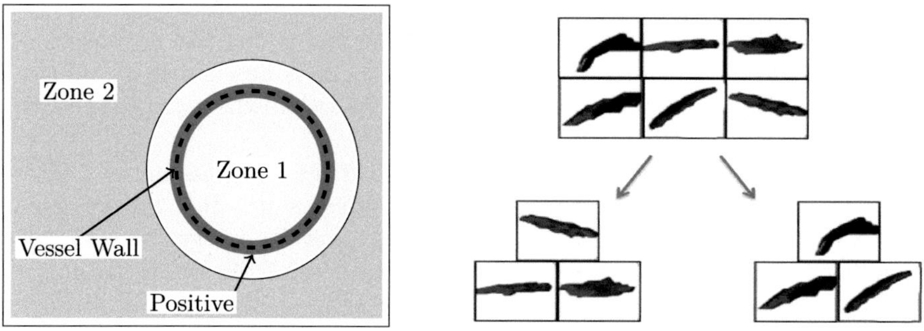

Fig. 2. (right) Sample zones depicted as a 2D cross section. (left) Example of structured labels grouped into discrete sets.

3.2 Topographical and Image Features

For each sample, a set of appearance and atlas-based feature channels are computed. We selected three appearance features: lumen intensity, gradient magnitude and Canny edge response, each of which are available at full and $\frac{1}{2}$ resolutions. In addition to appearance features, we incorporated *a prior* information by including a distance map from user-generated centerlines as an additional feature channel. Centerlines were created *a priori* during model construction by generating interpolated curves from user-supplied control points placed in vessel lumen. Typically, 15-30 control points are placed and approximately 300 points are generated through interpolation. This feature injects atlas information into the classifier but it is treated as any other feature channel. Next, we combined appearance and *a priori* features into a composite feature by projecting the image gradient onto the gradient of the distance map. This provides a strong response when the image gradient aligns with the normal direction of the path. Last, difference features were calculated by heavily blurring each feature channel then computing the piecewise paired differences of five voxel sub-patches.

3.3 Edge Detection

Classifier Training. Our approach employs a collection of de-correlated decision trees that classify input patches $\mathbf{x} \in X$ with a structured label map $\mathbf{y} \in Y$. Decision trees are trained by calculating information gain of the ith element across all j input vectors, $\mathbf{x}_j \in X, \mathbf{x}_j = (x_1, x_2, x_3, ..., x_i)_j$, for unique labels in $y_j \in \mathbf{Y}$. For binary classification, y_j has two possible values, $y_j = \{0, 1\}$, in multi-class systems y_j has k possible values, $y_j = \{1, 2, 3, ..., k\}$. When training decision trees with label patches, every permutation of the label patch could be considered a distinct class; this leads to an enormous number of potential classes of y_j. For example, a binary 8×8 label map, would result in $\binom{8\times8}{2} = 2016$ distinct classes, and this complexity increases exponentially with 3D patches, a $8 \times 8 \times 8$ label patch results in $\binom{8\times8\times8}{2} = 130,816$ classes. With a label space of this complexity, information gain is ill defined, and training a decision tree is ill posed. However, Dollár and Zitnick observed that contour labels have structure and can be mapped to a discrete label space. By mapping similar elements in $\mathbf{y} \in Y$ to the same discrete labels $c \in C, C = \{1, ..., k\}$, *approximate* information gain can be calculated across C, and normal training procedures can be used to train decision trees [1].

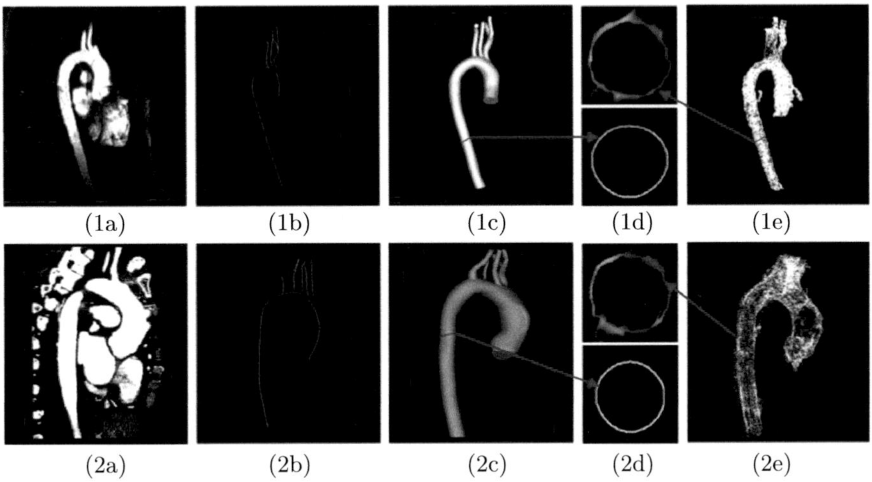

Fig. 3. Illustration of edge detection results. Columns from left to right: (a) Image data, (b) center line paths, (c) 3D ground truth, (d) vessel cross section (top: our result, bottom ground truth), (e) our result. Row 1 depicts an MR result, row 2 depicts a CT result.

To find a discrete label set C and an accompanying mapping $Y \rightarrow C$, similarity between individual labels $\mathbf{y} \in Y$ must be measured. Similarity between labels presents computational challenge since comparing two label patches results in $\binom{8 \cdot 8 \cdot 8}{2} = 130,816$ difference pairs. To avoid this complexity, we map Y to an intermediate space, Z, where similarity can be calculated efficiently. Intermediate label space Z is found by down-sampling Y to m samples then computing Principal Component Analysis (PCA) and keeping only the λ strongest components. This results in a parameterized mapping $\Pi_\phi : Y \rightarrow Z$ where $\phi = \{m, \lambda\}$. Using similarity calculated in Z, mapping $Y \rightarrow C$ becomes a straight forward calculation. Figure 2 shows of a mapping of labels into discrete sets. During training, decision trees are de-correlated by randomizing sample locations, randomly disregarding 50% of the features, and selecting a random down-sampled set when mapping $\Pi_\phi : Y \rightarrow Z$.

Classification. Since each tree classifies an entire neighborhood, we performed edge classification for patches centered at odd rows, odd columns, and odd aisles. Every voxel location receives multiple votes from each tree, $t_i \in T$ where

$T = (t_1, t_2, t_3, ...t_N)$. With $8\times8\times8$ label patches, each voxel receives $\approx 8^3 \cdot ||T||/8$ votes, in our experiments we set $||T|| = 8$. Votes were de-correlated by aggregating results from alternating trees at each location.

4 Experimentation and Results

We evaluated our method on a data set consisting of 21 MRI and 17 CT volumes for a total 38 volumes that include part or both of the thoracic and abdominal regions. 30 of the volumes in our dataset were provided to us from the vascular model repository (`http://www.vascularmodel.com`) the remaining eight were collected from local collaborators. Image volumes vary in resolution from $512 \times 512 \times 512$ to $512 \times 512 \times 64$. All volumes were captured from individual patients for clinically indicated purposes then expertly annotated with ground truth and verified by a cardiologist. Ground truth annotations include all visible arterial vessels except pulmonary and coronary arteries and each volume was annotated specifically for CFD simulation. For experimentation, our data set was divided into sets for training and testing. Our classifiers were trained on 29 randomly selected volumes, and the remaining 9 were used for testing, both sets include approximately 50% MRI and CT images.

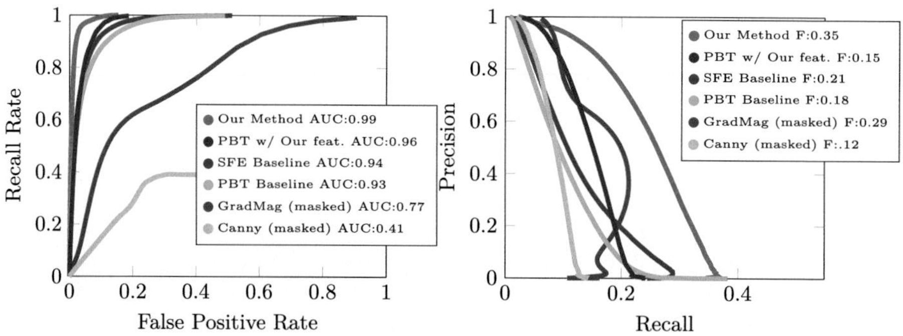

Fig. 4. Classifier performance comparison of our method, PBT edge detectors and commonly used edge detectors. (Left) Receiver operating curve. (Right): Precision vs Recall performance.

For experimentation, we trained our classifiers using a combination of C++ and Matlab implementations. Appearance feature extraction and manipulation was performed using the Insight Toolkit (ITK) (`http://www.itk.org`), and classifiers were trained using Piotr Dollár's Matlab toolbox (`http://vision.ucsd.edu/~pdollar/toolbox/doc`).

We performed two sets of experiments to examine different aspects of our algorithm. In our first set of experiments, we compared our method against a baseline structured forests model and two PBT forests models, one trained using our feature and sampling methodologies and another trained with baseline features and sampling. In our baseline models, positive samples included patches where any edge voxel is present and negative samples were collected from any negative region without restriction. We selected baseline features that closely mirror features used in natural images, these are: lumen intensity, gradient magnitude and oriented gradients. Oriented gradients were computed by projecting $\nabla F(x,y,z) = (\frac{df}{dx}, \frac{df}{dy}, \frac{df}{dz})$ onto the surface of an approximated unit sphere. In addition, we collected results of commonly used edge detection methods, gradient magnitude and Canny edge response. In our second set of experiments, we exam-

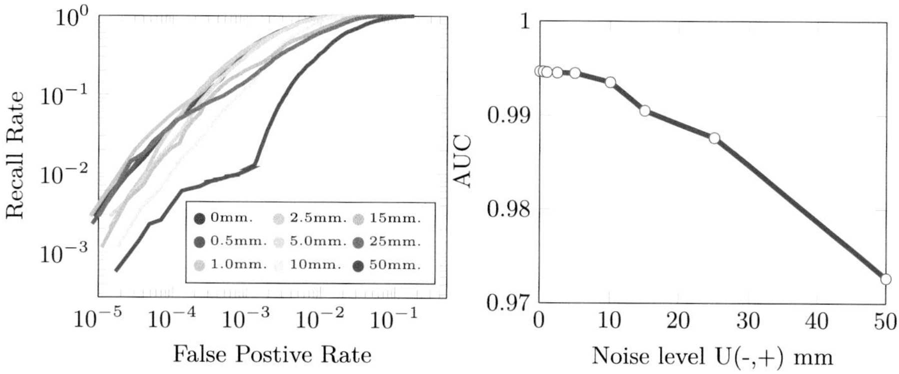

Fig. 5. Classifier performance after introducing centerline error through uniform additive noise on control points. (Left) Receiver operating curves. (Right) Classifier AUC at uniform noise levels.

ined our method's robustness to error in user-generated centerline annotations. For each test volume, the centerline control points were varied by additive uniform noise, centerlines were re-interpolated, and new edge maps were computed. This process was performed at increasing noise levels from $U(-.5\text{mm}, .5\text{mm})$ to $U(-50\text{mm}, 50\text{mm})$.

Performance statistics, in all experiments, were calculated by comparing edge responses against ground truth annotations. Hit, fall out and positive predictive voxel rates were calculated by tallying counts for each image and combining them to obtain rates for the entire test set. For our method, PBT and gradient magnitude, performance curves were generated by thresholding edge responses at different values. Canny performance curves were generated by sampling different combinations of input parameters. For each performance curve, area-under-the-curve (AUC) and top F-Measure scores were recorded and are included in our results. To fairly compare conventional methods against learned edge classifiers, only voxels within a 15 voxel radius of ground truth vessel walls were considered in performance calculations for Canny response and gradient magnitude.

Quantitative results for the first set of experiments are displayed in Figure 4. This figure shows that our method out-performs similarly trained PBT classifiers and out-performs commonly used edge detectors by a wide margin. We see both increased accuracy and improved precision when utilizing structured output labels and domain specific features. Figure 4 also indicates that our features and sampling methodology boost accuracy for other learned edge detectors. Figure 3 shows qualitative examples of classifier's results. Results of the second experiment appear in Figure 5. These curves suggest that our method is very robust to inaccurate annotation. We see only small a small drop in performance for noise levels up to $U(-5\text{mm}, 5\text{mm})$, and our method continues to achieve reasonable performance even with high noise introduced to the centerline.

5 Conclusion

In this work, we propose a novel method for edge classification in medical imaging. We contribute a novel set of domain specific features that effectively capture edge contours across modalities. In addition, we incorporate an atlas prior to edge classification to increase accuracy and precision. We show obtaining top accuracy and edge localization with a reduced number of sample is possible by constraining sampling regions to areas of interest. Our experiments indicate that our method out performs other edge detectors and is robust error in *a priori* information. Given that many medical imaging techniques are built upon edge fields we feel that this approach has significant potential in a variety of applications.

References

1. Dollár, P., Zitnick, C.L.: Structured forests for fast edge detection. In: ICCV, pp. 1841–1848. IEEE (2013)
2. Li, W., Liao, S., Feng, Q., Chen, W., Shen, D.: Learning image context for segmentation of the prostate in ct-guided radiotherapy. Physics in Medicine and Biology 57(5), 1283 (2012)
3. Lim, J.J., Zitnick, C.L., Dollar, P.: Sketch Tokens: A Learned Mid-level Representation for Contour and Object Detection. In: CVPR, pp. 3158–3165. IEEE (2013)
4. Marsden, A.L.: Optimization in cardiovascular modeling. Annual Review of Fluid Mechanics 46, 519–546 (2014)
5. Ren, X., Bo, L.: Discriminatively trained sparse code gradients for contour detection. In: NIPS (2012)
6. Schneider, M., Hirsch, S., Weber, B., Székely, G., Menze, B.H.: Joint 3-D vessel segmentation and centerline extraction using oblique Hough forests with steerable filters. Med. Image Analysis 19(1), 220–249 (2015)
7. Tu, Z., Bai, X.: Auto-context and its application to high-level vision tasks and 3d brain image segmentation. PAMI 32(10), 1744–1757 (2010)
8. Zheng, Y., Loziczonek, M., Georgescu, B., Zhou, S.K., Vega-Higuera, F., Comaniciu, D.: Machine learning based vesselness measurement for coronary artery segmentation in cardiac ct volumes. In: SPIE Medical Imaging, pp. 79621K–79621K. International Society for Optics and Photonics (2011)

Sample Size Estimation for Outlier Detection

Timothy Gebhard[1], Inga Koerte[1,2], and Sylvain Bouix[1]

[1] Psychiatry Neuroimaging Laboratory, Brigham and Women's Hospital, Harvard Medical School
[2] Department of Child and Adolescent Psychiatry, Psychosomatic, and Psychotherapy, Ludwig-Maximilians-Universität München

Abstract. The study of brain disorders which display spatially heterogeneous patterns of abnormalities has led to a number of techniques aimed at providing subject specific abnormality (SSA) maps. One popular method to identify SSAs is to calculate, for a set of regions, the z-score between a feature in a test subject and the distribution of this feature in a normative atlas, and identify regions exceeding a threshold. While sample size estimation and power calculations are well understood in group comparisons, describing the confidence interval of a z-score threshold or estimating sample size for a desired threshold uncertainty in SSA analyses have not been thoroughly considered. In this paper, we propose a method to quantify the impact of the size and distribution properties of the control data on the uncertainty of the z-score threshold. The main idea is that a z-score threshold confidence interval can be approximated by using Gaussian Error Propagation of the uncertainties associated with the sample mean and standard deviation. In addition, we provide a method to estimate the sample size of the control data required for a z-score threshold and associated desired width of confidence interval. We provide both parametric and resampling methods to estimate these confidence intervals and apply our techniques to establish confidence of SSA maps of diffusion data in subjects with traumatic brain injury.

Keywords: Confidence interval, outlier rejection, sample size estimation, diffusion MRI, TBI.

1 Introduction

In the last 15 years, diffusion-tensor imaging (DTI) has become an increasingly popular tool in neuroimaging and has been used to study a number of disorders including schizophrenia (see [3] for a review), mild traumatic brain injury (mTBI) (see [6] for a review) and many others. Most neuroimaging analyses utilize a group-comparison approach which aims at detecting spatially consistent patterns of brain alterations in a group of patients when compared to healthy controls (HC). However, the underlying assumptions behind this are not necessarily true. For example, the effects of mTBI significantly depend on the circumstances of the injury, and it is unlikely that all mTBI patients would show a

N. Navab et al. (Eds.): MICCAI 2015, Part III, LNCS 9351, pp. 743–750, 2015.
DOI: 10.1007/978-3-319-24574-4_89

common pattern of brain matter alterations, especially at the acute stage of the injury. It has therefore been acknowledged by the medical imaging community that there is a need for the detection of subject-specific abnormalities (SSA) [1,4].

A popular approach to identifying SSAs is to calculate a reference distribution (an atlas) from a group of HC, and then compare a single subject's data against this distribution [7], effectively turning the detection of SSAs into a problem of outlier detection. In the "pothole" method, as presented in [8], a white matter skeleton is extracted from DTI data for both a group of patients and HC. Fractional Anisotropy (FA) values for this skeleton are then z-transformed voxel-wise, using mean and standard deviation as calculated from only the HC cohort. Each voxel is then classified as either "normal" or "abnormal" by applying a z-score threshold of 2. This corresponds to the FA values of abnormal voxels being in at least the 95th percentile. Usually this is also combined with a threshold on the number of contiguous abnormal voxels to reduce the number of false positives. Multiple comparison corrections can also be included, e.g. through Bonferroni correction.

An improvement on this approach was presented in [1] by using a "leave-one-out" approach which accounts for the potential bias that may arise if one z-transforms the data of an individual using statistical moments that were calculated from a sample which included the subject that is being transformed. Therefore in this method, all HC are z-transformed using a mean and standard deviation that was calculated from all *other* HC, while patients are still transformed using the parameters from all HC. Other approaches to detecting SSAs include one versus many t-tests, the use of binomial distributions and machine learning algorithms (see [4] and references therein).

However, most of these methods do not pay enough attention to the impact of sample size and distribution properties. For example, it can be shown that the distribution of the z-transformed FA values will generally not be the same for patients and HC and that equivalent z-score thresholds are not necessarily applicable to HC and patients (especially for small sample sizes) [4].

In this paper, we turn our attention to the impact of sample size of subjects used to estimate the reference distribution. In particular, we investigate the uncertainty associated with the z-threshold used for the outlier classification. We present a method to approximate a confidence interval (CI) for the z-threshold using Gaussian error propagation (GEP) of the uncertainties associated with the estimation of the mean and standard deviation. In addition, we provide a technique to estimate the minimum sample size necessary for a given desired z-threshold uncertainty. We show how parametric and non-parametric techniques can be used to estimate the z-score CI, and apply these techniques to establish confidence in SSA maps of diffusion data in subjects with mTBI.

2 Methods

To detect outliers in a data set, one commonly makes use of the z-score:

$$z = \frac{v - \mu}{\sigma} \tag{1}$$

with μ denoting the arithmetic mean and σ the standard deviation of the population. Data points with an absolute z-score $|z|$ exceeding a threshold z_0 are classified as outliers. In most cases, one sets $z_0 = 1.96$ as it corresponds to a 5% probability for the measurement to belong to the distribution. Unfortunately, the values of μ and σ are rarely truly known. Instead, they are estimated from a sample and have an associated uncertainty, which is usually represented by a *confidence interval* at a particular $1 - \alpha$ confidence level (α is often set to 0.05). While confidence intervals for μ and σ are well understood, their impact on the z_0 threshold is not well known. Our first aim is therefore to find a confidence interval for z_0 based on the uncertainties of μ and σ and a given fixed $v = v_0$.

2.1 A Confidence Interval for z_0

We assume that the parameter uncertainties follow a normal distribution so that we can use Gaussian error propagation to estimate the uncertainty associated with z_0. Given $y = y(x_1, \cdots, x_n)$, whose variables $x_1, \cdots, x_n$ have uncertainties $u_1, \cdots, u_2$, then the uncertainty of y is given as:

$$u_y = \sqrt{\sum_{i=1}^{n} \left(\frac{\partial y}{\partial x_i} \cdot u_i \right)^2 + \sum_{i=1}^{n-1} \sum_{k=i+1}^{n} \frac{\partial y}{\partial x_i} \frac{\partial y}{\partial x_k} \cdot \mathrm{Cov}(x_i, x_k)} \tag{2}$$

In the special case of eq. (1), we assume μ, σ to be independent so that $\mathrm{Cov}(\mu, \sigma) = 0$. Evaluating eq. (2), for $z_0(\mu, \sigma)$ yields:

$$u_{z_0} = \frac{1}{\sigma} \sqrt{u_\mu^2 + \frac{(v_0 - \mu)^2}{\sigma^2} u_\sigma^2} = \frac{1}{\sigma} \sqrt{u_\mu^2 + z_0^2 u_\sigma^2} \tag{3}$$

We now estimate u_μ and u_σ through their confidence intervals. The mean of a normal distribution is itself normally distributed [5], therefore its confidence interval $I_{\alpha,\mu}$ is expected to be symmetric around μ and u_μ can be defined as its half-width: $u_\mu = \frac{1}{2} \cdot \|I_{\alpha,\mu}\|$. The variance, however, follows an asymmetric scaled χ^2-distribution [5], hence the confidence interval of σ is not symmetric around σ so left and right uncertainties need to be introduced. Let $I_{\alpha,\sigma} = [A, B]$ be a confidence interval for σ for the confidence level $1 - \alpha$. We then define: $u_{\sigma,\mathrm{l}} = \sigma - A$ and $u_{\sigma,\mathrm{r}} = B - \sigma$. From eq. (3), it then follows that the confidence interval for z_0 is given as:

$$I_{\alpha,z_0} = \left[z_0 - \frac{1}{\sigma} \sqrt{u_\mu^2 + z_0^2 u_{\sigma,\mathrm{l}}^2} \, , \; z_0 + \frac{1}{\sigma} \sqrt{u_\mu^2 + z_0^2 u_{\sigma,\mathrm{r}}^2} \right] \tag{4}$$

We now turn to the estimation of I_μ and I_σ and propose a parametric and resampling approach to estimate these confidence intervals.

Parametric Approach: If we assume the data to be normally distributed, the confidence interval of the mean and standard deviation are known [5] and u_μ, $u_{\sigma,\mathrm{l}}$, $u_{\sigma,\mathrm{r}}$ can be computed directly from these intervals. For the mean we have:

$$u_\mu = t_{(1-\frac{\alpha}{2};n-1)} \frac{s}{\sqrt{n}} \tag{5}$$

where s^2 is the unbiased estimator of the sample variance and $t_{(1-\alpha/2;n-1)}$ is the $(1-\frac{\alpha}{2})$-quantile of a t-distribution with $n-1$ degrees of freedom. For the standard deviation we have:

$$u_{\sigma,\mathrm{l}} = \sigma - s\sqrt{\frac{n-1}{\chi^2_{(1-\frac{\alpha}{2};n-1)}}} \qquad u_{\sigma,\mathrm{r}} = s\sqrt{\frac{n-1}{\chi^2_{(\frac{\alpha}{2};n-1)}}} - \sigma \tag{6}$$

where $\chi^2_{(1-\alpha/2;n-1)}$ is the $(1-\frac{\alpha}{2})$-quantile of a χ^2-distribution with $n-1$ degrees of freedom, and s is the unbiased estimator of the sample standard deviation.

Resampling Approach: If we want to stay clear of strong assumptions on the sample distribution, we propose to use bootstrapping to estimate I_μ and I_σ. Given a sample S we draw repeatedly (e.g. N=1000) a sample S' from S with the same size (sampling with replacement). For each S', we then calculate $p(S')$ and look at the distribution. The $(\frac{\alpha}{2} \cdot 100)$-th and $((1-\frac{\alpha}{2}) \cdot 100)$-th percentile span the bootstrap confidence interval for $p(S)$ for the confidence level $1-\alpha$.

2.2 Estimating Sample Sizes

In real experiments, one will be interested in knowing the minimum sample size so that the distance between the desired z_0 and the upper bound $z_0{}'$ of its 95% confidence interval is no bigger than a given threshold ε. This problem is equivalent to solving the following equation for n if one uses the parametric estimates for the uncertainties of μ and σ:

$$\varepsilon = z_0{}' - z_0 = \sqrt{\frac{1}{n} t^2_{(1-\frac{\alpha}{2};n-1)} + z_0^2 \left(1 - \sqrt{\frac{n-1}{\chi^2_{(\frac{\alpha}{2};n-1)}}}\right)^2} \tag{7}$$

While there is no closed form solution for n, eq. (7) is monotonically decreasing and a sequential evaluation using increasing n quickly leads to the minimum sample size necessary to achieve ε.

3 Experiments

All experiments were performed on an Apple MacBook Pro running Mac OS X 10.9, and were programmed in Python 2.7.8. Additional libraries that were used are NumPy 1.9.1 and SciPy 0.15.1. Plots were created using Matplotlib 1.4.2.

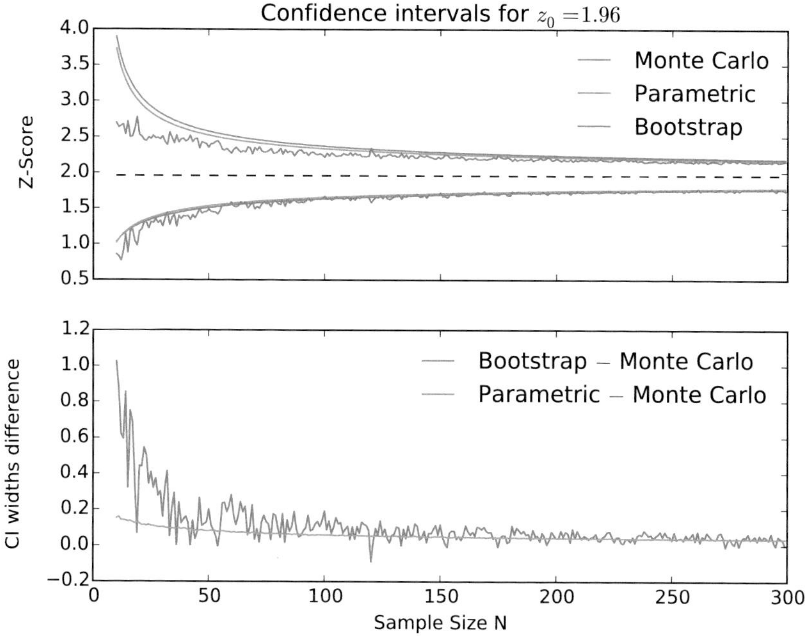

Fig. 1. Top: CI for $z_0 = 1.96$ for increasing sample size as predicted by eq. (4) using a parametric model and a bootstrap estimate vs. the Monte Carlo estimate. **Bottom:** Difference between the interval widths, i.e. $||\text{CI}_{\text{Parametric}}|| - ||\text{CI}_{\text{Monte Carlo}}||$ and $||\text{CI}_{\text{Bootstrap}}|| - ||\text{CI}_{\text{Monte Carlo}}||$.

3.1 Plausibility Test: Our Formula vs. Monte Carlo Estimate

The aim of this experiment was to verify whether the computation of the CI through eq. (4) accurately match CI estimated through Monte Carlo simulation. We design the following procedure to perform this test:

1. Choose a significance level α and a value for z_0. For this experiment, $\alpha = 5\%$ and $z_0 = 1.96$ were used. We also chose to set a seed for the random number generator to receive reproducible results.
2. From a normal distribution (we used $\mu = 0$, $\sigma = 1$ for this experiment) draw a sample S_N of size N. Calculate the sample mean $\mu^*_{S_N}$ and the sample standard deviation $\sigma^*_{S_N}$.
3. Calculate the $(1 - \alpha)$ confidence intervals for $\mu^*_{S_N}$ and $\sigma^*_{S_N}$, both parametrically and via bootstrapping (using 1000 samples that are drawn from S_N with replacement).
4. From these confidence intervals, randomly draw numbers $\mu^i_{S_N}$ and $\sigma^i_{S_N}$ n times. Calculate $z^i_{0,S_N} = \frac{(\mu^i_{S_N} + z_0 \cdot \sigma^i_{S_N}) - \mu^*_{S_N}}{\sigma^*_{S_N}}$. Repeat this step (we used 10^5 iterations).

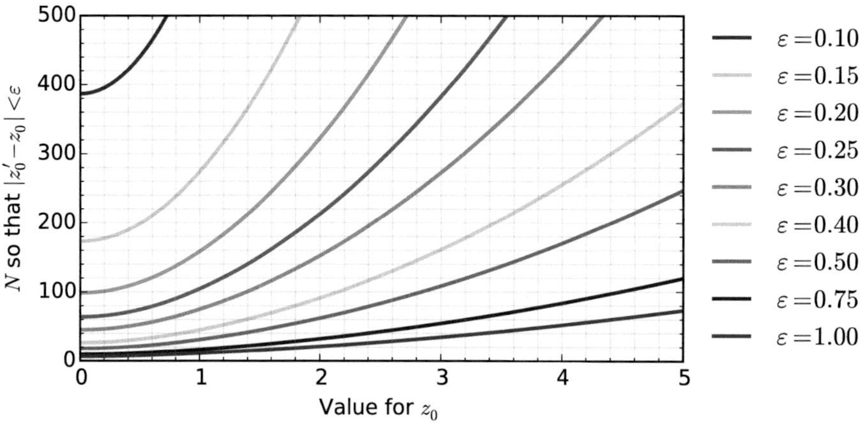

Fig. 2. Minimum sample sizes so that the difference between z_0 and the upper boundary of its confidence interval is equal to ε.

5. Cut off the top and bottom $(\frac{\alpha}{2} \cdot 100)$-th percentile of the distribution of z_0^i generated through the Monte Carlo process to estimate the $1-\alpha$ CI of z_{0,S_N}.
6. Do this for $N = \{10, 11, \cdots, 299, 300\}$, and plot the Monte Carlo estimate and the prediction from eq. (4) (using both the parametric and the bootstrap method).

Our results are given in fig. 1. As one can see the CI calculated via eq. (4) closely match those estimated via our Monte Carlo procedure. We repeated this test for a range of $z_0 \in [0, 5]$ and found a similar trend for all values tested.

3.2 Sample Size Estimation for Given ε

In this experiment, we calculated, for different values of ε and z_o, the minimum sample size that is necessary so that $|z_0' - z_0| < \varepsilon$.

1. Choose a value for the threshold ε, and the significance level $\alpha = 0.05$.
2. For every $z_0 = \{0.0, 0.05, \cdots, 4.95, 5.00\}$, numerically solve eq. (7) for n.
3. Plot the found values for n over z_0.

The results are presented in fig. 2 for different ε. One can observe that the sample size needs to be relatively large (by medical imaging standards) even for relaxed ε. For example at $z_0 = 2$, $\varepsilon = 0.4$ the sample size needed is close to 100 samples and $\varepsilon = 0.25$ requires over 200 samples.

3.3 Application to Real Data

As a last experiment, we applied our method to a real data set of subjects with mTBI. The data consisted of average FA values in 145 regions of interests (ROIs) extracted using Freesurfer [2] in 45 healthy controls and 11 patients with

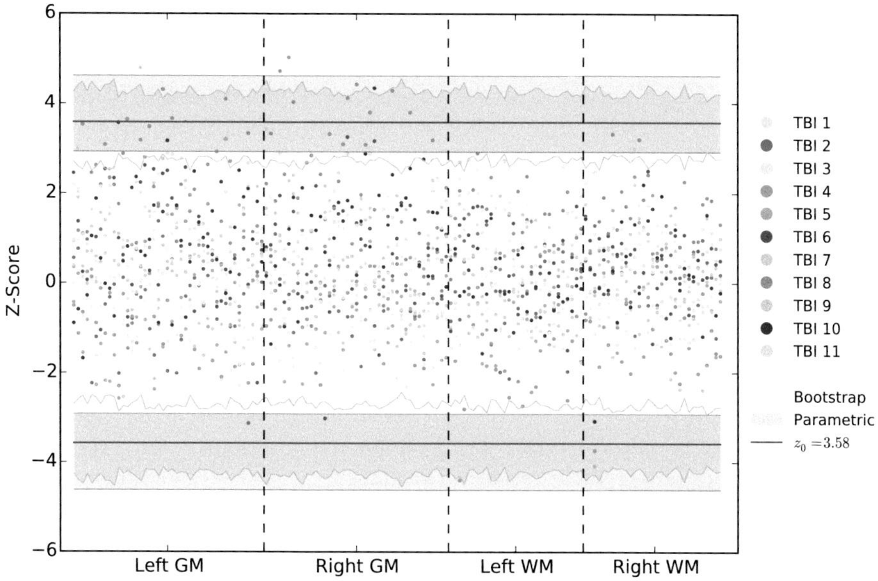

Fig. 3. The x-axis represent individual ROIs (145 in total), for each ROI the z-score of the 11 mTBI subjects are displayed on the y-axis. The red line represents a z-score threshold of $z_0 = 3.58$. The blue bar represents our parametric estimate for the CI, while the green bar is the bootstrap estimate of the CI.

mTBI. In [1], a simple threshold of $z_0 = 3.58$ (the Bonferroni corrected threshold equivalent to $z_0 = 1.96$) was used to classify data points as outliers, and thus identify SSAs. We estimated the $z_0 = 3.58$ CIs for each ROI in our sample using both the parametric and bootstrap approach. As can be seen from eq. (7), the parametric estimate for the z_0-confidence interval only depends on the sample size, hence the resulting confidence interval is the same for all ROIs. For the bootstrap estimate we drew 10^5 samples from the HC (with replacement) which had the same size as the original HC sample (i.e. 45 subjects). For all these samples, we calculated the mean μ and standard deviation σ. We sorted the values for μ and σ and cut off the top and bottom 2.5^{th}-percentile, giving us the bootstrap estimate for the 95%-confidence interval for both the mean and the standard deviation. This gave us estimates for the uncertainties of μ and σ, which we used to evaluate eq. (4). We reproduced part of figure 2 of [1], with the addition of the parametric and bootstrap CIs. The result is presented in fig. 3. One can observe that the bootstrap and parametric CIs overall agree although, the bootstrap estimates are tighter and more symmetric than the parametric intervals. Most importantly, the figure show that at this $z_0 = 3.58$ level only a few measurements lie outside the outer edge of the CIs for this sample size.

4 Conclusion

In this paper we have investigated the confidence interval of a z-score threshold for the purpose of outlier detection. Parametric and bootstrap approaches were presented to estimate this confidence interval. In addition, we presented a method to estimate the minimum sample size necessary to achieve a confidence interval at a particular z_0 threshold. Our results show that our method is in agreement with confidence intervals generated through Monte Carlo simulations. We further provided illustration of sample sizes needed for various z_0 thresholds and tolerance ε, which emphasized that relatively large sample sizes of a reference population are needed for outlier detection. Finally, we applied our technique on real data and further demonstrated the impact of sample size on the confidence of detecting outliers. Our results strongly suggest that uncertainties associated with detecting subject specific abnormalities are significant enough that they should be taken into account when designing an experiment or at least acknowledged when reporting results.

Acknowledgement. This work was supported by the German Academic Exchange Service, the Else Kroner-Fresenius Stiftung, Germany, a VA Merit Award and NIH grant R01-MH082918 and DoD grant W81XWH-08-2-0159.

References

1. Bouix, S., Pasternak, O., Rathi, Y., Pelavin, P.E., Zafonte, R., Shenton, M.E.: Increased gray matter diffusion anisotropy in patients with persistent post-concussive symptoms following mild traumatic brain injury. PLoS One 8(6), e66205 (2013)
2. Fischl, B., Salat, D.H., Busa, E., Albert, M., Dieterich, M., Haselgrove, C., van der Kouwe, A., Killiany, R., Kennedy, D., Klaveness, S., Montillo, A., Makris, N., Rosen, B., Dale, A.M.: Whole brain segmentation: automated labeling of neuroanatomical structures in the human brain. Neuron 33(3), 341–355 (2002)
3. Kubicki, M., McCarley, R., Westin, C.-F., Park, H.-J., Maier, S., Kikinis, R., Jolesz, F.A., Shenton, M.E.: A review of diffusion tensor imaging studies in schizophrenia. Journal of Psychiatric Research 41(12), 15–30 (2007)
4. Mayer, A.R., Bedrick, E.J., Ling, J.M., Toulouse, T., Dodd, A.: Methods for identifying subject-specific abnormalities in neuroimaging data. Human Brain Mapping 35(11), 5457–5470 (2014)
5. Riffenburgh, R.H.: Statistics in Medicine, 3rd edn. Elsevier Science (2012)
6. Shenton, M., Hamoda, H., Schneiderman, J., Bouix, S., Pasternak, O., Rathi, Y., Vu, M.-A., Purohit, M., Helmer, K., Koerte, I., Lin, A., Westin, C.-F., Kikinis, R., Kubicki, M., Stern, R., Zafonte, R.: A review of magnetic resonance imaging and diffusion tensor imaging findings in mild traumatic brain injury. Brain Imaging and Behavior 6(2), 137–192 (2012)
7. Viviani, R., Beschoner, P., Jaeckle, T., Hipp, P., Kassubek, J., Schmitz, B.: The bootstrap and cross-validation in neuroimaging applications: Estimation of the distribution of extrema of random fields for single volume tests, with an application to ADC maps. Human Brain Mapping 28(10), 1075–1088 (2007)
8. White, T., Schmidt, M., Karatekin, C.: White matter 'potholes' in early-onset schizophrenia: A new approach to evaluate white matter microstructure using diffusion tensor imaging. Psychiatry Research: Neuroimaging 174(2), 110–115 (2009)

Multi-scale Heat Kernel Based Volumetric Morphology Signature

Gang Wang[1,2] and Yalin Wang[2,⋆]

[1] Ludong University, School of Information and Electrical Engineering, Yantai, 264025 China
[2] Arizona State University, School of Computing, Informatics, and Decision Systems Engineering, Tempe, AZ, 878809 USA

Abstract. Here we introduce a novel multi-scale heat kernel based regional shape statistical approach that may improve statistical power on the structural analysis. The mechanism of this analysis is driven by the graph spectrum and the heat kernel theory, to capture the volumetric geometry information in the constructed tetrahedral mesh. In order to capture profound volumetric changes, we first use the volumetric Laplace-Beltrami operator to determine the point pair correspondence between two boundary surfaces by computing the streamline in the tetrahedral mesh. Secondly, we propose a multi-scale volumetric morphology signature to describe the transition probability by random walk between the point pairs, which reflects the inherent geometric characteristics. Thirdly, a point distribution model is applied to reduce the dimensionality of the volumetric morphology signatures and generate the internal structure features. The multi-scale and physics based internal structure features may bring stronger statistical power than other traditional methods for volumetric morphology analysis. To validate our method, we apply support vector machine to classify synthetic data and brain MR images. In our experiments, the proposed work outperformed FreeSurfer thickness features in Alzheimer's disease patient and normal control subject classification analysis.

Keywords: Heat kernel, Volumetric Laplace-Beltrami operator, Point distribution model, Support vector machine.

1 Introduction

In Alzheimer's disease (AD) research, several MRI-based measures of atrophy, including cortical thickness, hippocampal atrophy or ventricular enlargement, are closely correlated with changes in cognitive performance, supporting their validity as biomarkers of early AD identification. As we know, the MRI imaging

⋆ This work was partially supported by the joint special fund of Shandong province Natural Science Fundation (ZR2013FL008), National Natural Science Foundation of China (61471185), National Health Institutes (R21AG043760,U54EB020403) and National Science Foundation (DMS-1413417,IIS-1421165).

N. Navab et al. (Eds.): MICCAI 2015, Part III, LNCS 9351, pp. 751–759, 2015.
DOI: 10.1007/978-3-319-24574-4_90

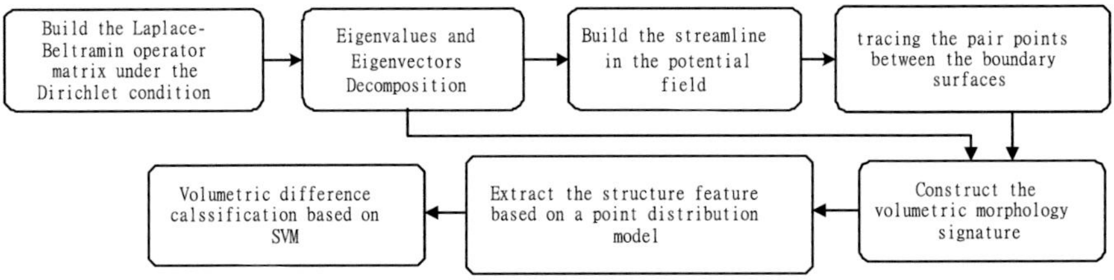

Fig. 1. Pipeline of the volumetric morphology signature computation.

measurement of medial temporal atrophy is not sufficiently accurate on its own to serve as an absolute diagnostic criterion for the clinical diagnosis of AD at the mild cognitive impairment (MCI) stage. A key research question is how to select the features which have a high discriminatory power. For example, the cortical thickness was the popular feature which has been used to capture the difference between different clinical groups. Currently, there are two different computational paradigms on brain cortical thickness, with methods generally classified as either surface or voxel based [1,2]. However, all measured distances are unitary distances between boundary points and they are unitary values that suggest only global trends and cannot capture topological variations (e.g. the regional information along the connecting curves is not considered). To address these difficulties, we introduce diffusion geometry methods to compute multi-scale intrinsic volumetric morphology signatures. Because the 2D shape analysis cannot offer the internal volumetric structure information within the solid volume such as brain grey matter. Based on some recent work [3,4] which studied volumetric heat kernel and the volumetric Laplace-Beltrami operator [5], here we propose a multi-scale heat kernel statistic to describe the transition probability by random walk between white-grey matter and CSF-grey matter boundary point pairs. With the tetrahedral mesh representation, our work may achieve sub-voxel numerical accuracy. They provide quantitative measures of brain changes which are important for evaluating disease burden, progression and response to interventions.

In our work, a new set morphological descriptors is used to represent the volumetric structure information, which depends on heat transmission time and is somewhat influenced by the topological properties on the heat transmission path. Following that, a point distribution model (PDM) is applied to reduce the feature dimensionality to make classification feasible. With the support vector machine (SVM), we extract the most discriminative features that expose the brain abnormal changes. We also test the effectiveness of our framework in classification experiments.

A major innovation here is that our formulations make it possible for profoundly analyzing the internal structural information. The multi-scale and physics based geometric features may offer more statistical power on the topological change analysis in grey matter morphology as preclinical AD biomarkers.

2 Methods

Fig. 1 shows the pipeline of the volumetric morphology signature system.

2.1 Theoretical Background

The heat kernel diffusion on differentiable manifold M with Riemannian metric is governed by the heat equation:

$$\triangle_M f(x,t) = \frac{\partial f(x,t)}{\partial t} \tag{1}$$

where $f(x,t)$ is the heat distribution of the volume at the given time. Given an initial heat distribution $F : M \to \mathcal{R}$, let $H_t(F)$ denotes the heat distribution at time t, and $\lim_{t\to 0} H_t(F) = F$. $H(t)$ is called the *heat operator*. Both $\triangle_M$ and H_t share the same eigenfunctions, and if λ_i is an eigenvalue of $\triangle_M$, then $e^{-\lambda_i t}$ is an eigenvalue of H_t corresponding to the same eigenfunction.

For any compact Riemannian manifold, there exists a function $l_t(x,y) : \mathbb{R}^+ \times M \times M \to \mathbb{R}$, satisfying the formula

$$H_t F(x) = \int_M l_t(x,y) F(y) dy \tag{2}$$

where dy is the volume form at $y \in M$. The minimum function $l_t(x,y)$ that satisfies Eq. 2 is called the *heat kernel* [6], and can be considered as the amount of heat that is transferred from x to y in time t given a unit heat source at x. In other words, $l_t(x,\cdot) = H_t(\delta_x)$ where δ_x is the Direc delta function at $x : \delta_x(z) = 0$ for any $z \neq x$ and $\int_M \delta_x(z) = 1$.

According to the theory of the spectral analysis, for compact M, the heat kernel has the following eigen-decomposition heat diffusion distance:

$$l_t(x,y) = \sum_{i=0}^{\infty} e^{-\lambda_i t} \phi_i(x) \phi_i(y) \tag{3}$$

where λ_i and ϕ_i are the ith eigenvalue and eigenfunction of the Laplace-Beltrami operator, respectively. The heat kernel $l_t(x,y)$ can be interpreted as the transition density function of the Brownian motion on the manifold.

2.2 Discrete Multi-scale Volumetric Morphology Signature

On volumetric structure represented by a tetrahedral mesh, we can estimate the boundary point pairs (x and y) based on the heat propogation, e.g. [5]. Then we can compute the eigenfunctions and eigenvalues of L_p and then estimate the heat diffusion distance $l_t(x,y)$ by evaluating Eqn. 3. We define the evaluation of $l_t(x,y)$ between surface point pairs, x and y, with varying time t, as the *volumetric morphology signature (VMS)*. To establish measurements on the unified template for statistical analysis, the weighted spherical harmonic representation [7] is applied to build surface correspondence between the different surfaces.

In order to reveal the internal structure features in a way that best explains the variance in the *VMS*, we apply a point distribution model(PDM) [8] to extract the most informative features. Given a group of N tetrahedral meshes, we apply the eigenanalysis of the covariance matrix Σ of the *VMS* as follows:

$$\begin{aligned} \Sigma &= \frac{1}{N-1}\sum_{i=1}^{N}(\mathbf{T}_i - \overline{\mathbf{T}})(\mathbf{T}_i - \overline{\mathbf{T}})^T \\ \Sigma P &= DP \end{aligned} \tag{4}$$

where $\mathbf{T}_i$ is the *VMS* of the ith tetrahedral mesh and $\overline{\mathbf{T}}$ is the mean *VMS* of N objects. The columns of P hold eigenvectors, and the diagonal matrix D holds eigenvalues of Σ. The eigenvectors in P can be ordered according to respective eigenvalues, which are proportional to the variance explained by each eigenvector. The first few eigenvectors (with greatest eigenvalues) often explain most of variance in the *VMS* data. Now any volumetric morphology signature $\mathbf{T}_i$ can be obtained using

$$\mathbf{T}_i = \overline{\mathbf{T}} + Pv_i \tag{5}$$

where v_i is a vector containing the principal components which are called the *internal structure features*. It can be used to represent the principal internal structure information of the individual tetrahedral mesh in a new basis of the deformation models.

2.3 Internal Structure Feature Selection

Generally speaking, the additional features are theoretically helpful to improve the classifier performance. However, in practice, each additional feature adds a parameter to the classifier model which needs to be estimated, and mis-estimations that result from the less informative features can actually degrade performance. This is a form of overfitting. So there is a need to order the features from more information to less information. This tactics can improve the classification accuracy. We adopt a t-test on each feature and obtain a p-value associated with the statistical group difference. Thus, a lower p-value implies a more significant feature. In the following experiments, we will test the classification accuracies according to two different feature orderings.

3 Experimental Results

3.1 Synthetic Data Results

We conduct classification experimental studies on a synthetic data set. Fig. 2 shows two classes of 12 synthetic volumetric geometrical structures each, Class 1 shows the cylinders with a sphere hole and Class 2 shows the cylinders with a bump-sphere hole. First we compute the streamlines between the outer cylinder surface and the inner spherical surface and establish the measurements on the unified template [5]. Then the VMS can be obtained with Eqn. 3. Fig. 3(a) shows a volumetric tetrahedral mesh. The point pairs between the outer cylinder surface and the inner spherical surface is shown in (b). The VMS of this tetrahedral mesh is shown in (c), where the horizontal axis is $log(t)$ and the vertical axis is the VMS value. Apply Eqn. 4 and Eqn. 5, we obtain the first 23 internal

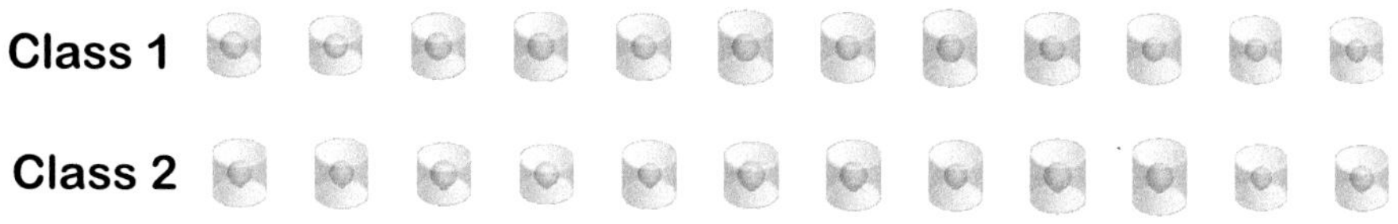

Fig. 2. Two classes of synthetic volumetric geometrical structures.

structure features of every object. Then the features have been scaled to $[-1, +1]$ before the classification. The main advantage of scaling is to avoid attributes in greater numeric ranges dominating those in smaller numeric ranges. In (d), we validate the classification performance of the two different feature orderings using the leave-one-out cross-validation method based on the SVM classifier. One is the standard ordering according to the order of the eigenvalue of the covariance matrix Σ generated from the training data , which indicates the variance amount of every feature from large to small. The other is the p-value ordering of the features from the training data. From the results, we can see that the internal structure features based on VMS have the high discriminative power. The mean accuracy of p-value ordering is 93.7% and the mean accuracy of standard ordering is 84.8%. And the two orderings can achieve the best accuracy 100% with fewer features. Moreover, the main computation is the eigenanalysis of the covariance matrix. By using the Gram matrix for eigenanalysis,the computational time for PDM can be improved to $O(n_s^2 * n_l)$ time. n_s is the number of shapes and n_l is the resolution.

In addition, we illustrate the importance of the feature selection in the projection space. The direction vectors of the classification hyperplane from the training data can be calculated as $proj\_value = x_\delta^T * w$, where $x_\delta = x - \bar{x}$ indicates the heat diffusion distance difference between the individual and the average. $proj\_value$ is the projected value and w is the direction vectors of the classification hyperplane. Fig. 4 shows the classification results in the projection space, with the horizontal coordinate representing the projection data, and with the vertical coordinate used for the posterior probability of belonging to the particular class. (a) and (b) represent the training data distributions with the first ith feature number (i.e., 6 and 23) according to the p-value respectively. The symbol $\diamondsuit$ and $\divideontimes$ indicate the two classes. From the results we can see that the phenomenon of the data piling has become apparent with the increasing of the feature number.(c) and (d) are the test classification results based on the first 6 and 23 features respectively. And the symbol $\diamondsuit$ and $\divideontimes$ with red mark indicate the misclassification results. From the results in Fig. 4, when all the features are used in training data, is associated with low in-sample error rate and high out-of-sample error rate.

3.2 Application to Alzheimer's Disease

To validate whether VMS can improve the statistical power on brain MRI analysis, we apply it to study the volumetric differences associated with AD

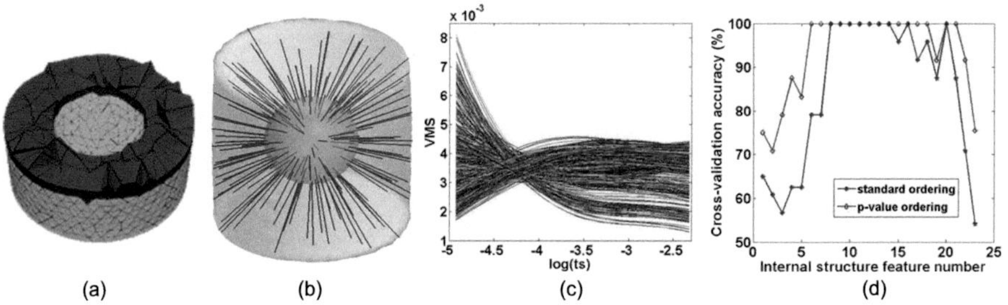

Fig. 3. Illustration of streamlines, VMS and classification accuracies on the synthetic cylinder with inner spherical hole.

and Control groups on the Alzheimer's Disease Neuroimaging Initiative (ADNI) dataset [9]. We used the baseline T1-weighted images from 81 subjects consisting of 41 healthy controls (CTL) and 40 patients of Alzheimer's (AD). We apply FreeSurfer software [10] for skull stripping, tissue segmentation and surface reconstruction. Given the white matter and pial surfaces, the tetrahedral meshes are generated by an adaptively sized tetrahedral mesh modeling method [11]. After the boundary point pairs are estimated, we resample all the brain surface to a common template which contains 40962 sample points. This allows us to compare the VMS measurements across different cortical surfaces. Next we apply the point distribution model (PDM) to the VMS to obtain v_i which contains 80 internal structure features for every individual grey matter tetrahedral mesh. After the scaling process, all the features are scaled to the interval $[-1, 1]$. We apply a t-test on each feature and obtain a p-value associated with the test statistic. The results are shown in Fig. 5 (a). The second feature corresponds to $p = 2.29 \times 10^{-9}$, the third and fourth features correspond to $p = 1.34 \times 10^{-6}$ and $p = 1.51 \times 10^{-6}$ respectively, and for all the other features are above 1×10^{-3}. Based on the SVM classifier, we investigate the leave-one-out cross-validation accuracies using the first i features from the two different ordering of the features. The results are shown in Fig. 5 (b). From the results, we can see that the best accuracy (97.5%)can be achieved using few (e.g.,34) features based on the p-value ordering, while on the standard ordering, a good accuracy (88.9%) can be achieved using 42 features. Moreover, the mean cross-validation accuracy based on the p-value ordering is higher about (5%) than the standard ordering. From the Eqn. 5, the specific eigenvector has the weights to create the specific feature. Therefore, the most informative feature should correspond to the specific eigenvector with the most significant contribution for the group differences. We compute the L_2 norm of the specific eigenvector to obtain these weights according to the template surface. The weights from the first four eigenvectors are shown on the mean outer surface in Fig. 5. From (c) to (f), they are the computed weights from the first eigenvector to the fourth eigenvector. Large weights correspond to locations with the most discrimination power. The weights are later color coded on the surface template point with the group difference p-map by different principal components. The values increase as the color goes from blue

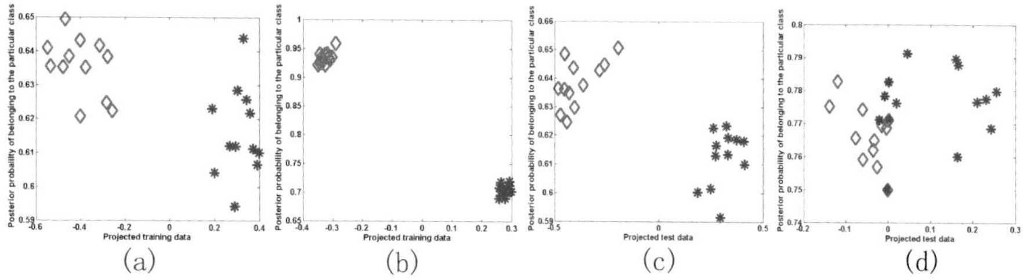

Fig. 4. The training and test data classification results with the different feature number in the projection space .

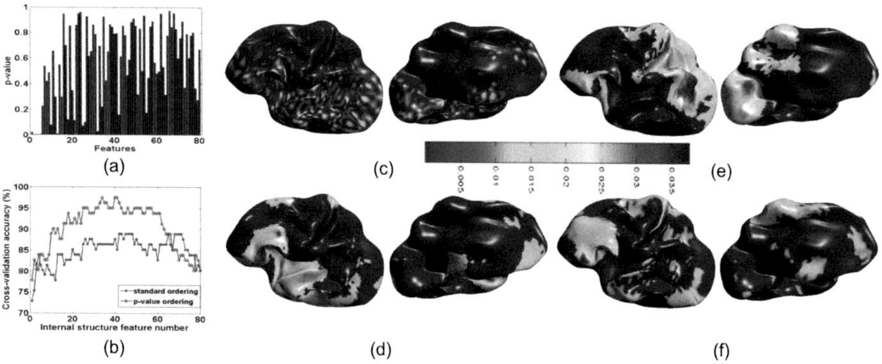

Fig. 5. Illustration of the SVM classification accuracy and the contrubutions from the four eigenvectors color coded on the mean outersurface of AD and Control subjects.

to yellow and to red. Because the second principal component has the smallest p-value, a significant difference exists in the medial temporal lobe region represented in Fig. 5 (d), supporting the fact that the medial temporal atrophy is the hallmark of AD disease.

3.3 Comparison with Freesurfer Thickness Feature

In this section, we compare the classification performance about the VMS and the thickness based on the Freesurfer method [10]. Here we apply the receiver operating characteristic (ROC) analysis to compare the discriminative power of the two analysis framework, which is created by plotting the true positive rate against the false positive rate at various threshold settings. After obtaining the thickness values on the unified template, we apply the PDM to the thickness to obtain v_i as the thickness feature. Through varying the threshold value which can determine the SVM classifier boundary, we can obtain the true positive rate, false positive rate and draw a ROC curve. The ROC curve is shown in Fig. 6 and

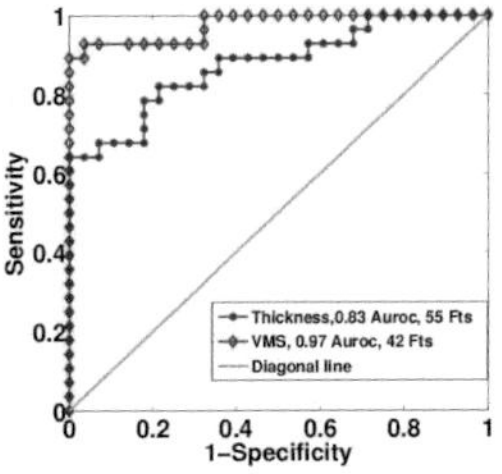

Fig. 6. ROC analysis for comparison using VMS and thickness features.

the legend shows the two data set, the area under the ROC curve (AUROC) and the number of features used. Here we choose 42 VMS features and 55 cortical thickness features computed by Freesurfer to achieve the maximum AUROC according to the p-value feature selection scheme. And a completely random guess would give a diagonal line from the left bottom to the top right corners. The points above the diagonal represent good classification results (better than random), points below the line represent poor results (worse than random). From the result, we can see that the features of the VMS have the higher discriminative power than the cortical thickness.

A key reason for better classification is that VMS can not only compute geodesic distance between the point pairs, but it also compare the immediate neighboring volume changes along the geodesics. It may provide new insights to grey matter morphology study.

4 Conclusions and Future Work

Based on heat kernel analysis, we propose a novel multi-scale volumetric morphology signature. This has many applications in brain imaging research. Whether or not our new method provides a more relevant shape analysis power than those afforded by other criteria (folding, surface curvature, cortical thickness) requires careful validation for each application. Because different geometric properties produce different models, we plan to compare them in future for detecting subtle differences in brain structure for preclinical AD research.

References

1. Jones, S.E., Buchbinder, B.R., Aharon, I.: Three-dimensional mapping of cortical thickness using Laplace's equation. Hum. Brain Mapp. 11(1), 12–32 (2000)
2. Fischl, B., Dale, A.M.: Measuring the thickness of the human cerebral cortex from magnetic resonance images. Proc. Natl. Acad. Sci. U.S.A. 97(20), 11050–11055 (2000)
3. Raviv, D., Bronstein, M.M., Bronstein, A.M., Kimmel, R.: Volumetric heat kernel signatures. In: Proc. Intl. Workshop on 3D Object Retrieval (3DOR), pp. 39–44. ACM Multimedia (2010)
4. Castellani, U., Mirtuono, P., Murino, V., Bellani, M., Rambaldelli, G., Tansella, M., Brambilla, P.: A new shape diffusion descriptor for brain classification. In: Fichtinger, G., Martel, A., Peters, T. (eds.) MICCAI 2011, Part II. LNCS, vol. 6892, pp. 426–433. Springer, Heidelberg (2011)
5. Wang, G., Zhang, X., Su, Q., Shi, J., Caselli, R.J., Wang, Y.: A novel cortical thickness estimation method based on volumetric Laplace-Beltrami operator and heat kernel. Med. Image Anal. 22(1), 1–20 (2015)

6. Coifman, R.R., Lafon, S., Lee, A.B., Maggioni, M., Nadler, B., Warner, F., Zucker, S.W.: Geometric diffusions as a tool for harmonic analysis and structure definition of data: multiscale methods. Proc. Natl. Acad. Sci. U.S.A. 102(21), 7432–7437 (2005)
7. Chung, M.K., Dalton, K.M., Shen, L., Evans, A.C., Davidson, R.J.: Weighted Fourier representation and its application to quantifying the amount of gray matter. IEEE Transactions on Medical Imaging 26, 566–581 (2007)
8. Shen, L., Ford, J., Makedon, F., Saykin, A.: A surface-based approach for classification of 3D neuroanatomic structures. Intelligent Data Analysis 8, 519–542 (2004)
9. Mueller, S.G., Weiner, M.W., Thal, L.J., Petersen, R.C., Jack, C., Jagust, W., Trojanowski, J.Q., Toga, A.W., Beckett, L.: The Alzheimer's disease neuroimaging initiative. Neuroimaging Clin. N. Am. 15(4), 869–877 (2005)
10. Fischl, B., Sereno, M.I., Dale, A.M.: Cortical surface-based analysis. II: Inflation, flattening, and a surface-based coordinate system. Neuroimage 9(2), 195–207 (1999)
11. Lederman, C., Joshi, A., Dinov, I., Vese, L., Toga, A., Van Horn, J.D.: The generation of tetrahedral mesh models for neuroanatomical MRI. Neuroimage 55(1), 153–164 (2011)

Structural Brain Mapping

Muhammad Razib[1], Zhong-Lin Lu[2], and Wei Zeng[1]

[1] Florida International University, Miami, Florida 33199, USA
[2] The Ohio State University, Columbus, Ohio 43210, USA

Abstract. Brain mapping plays an important role in neuroscience and medical imaging fields, which flattens the convoluted brain cortical surface and exposes the hidden geometry details onto a canonical domain. Existing methods such as conformal mappings didn't consider the anatomical atlas network structure, and the anatomical landmarks, e.g., gyri curves, appear highly curvy on the canonical domains. Using such maps, it is difficult to recognize the connecting pattern and compare the atlases. In this work, we present a novel brain mapping method to efficiently visualize the convoluted and partially invisible cortical surface through a well-structured view, called the *structural brain mapping*. In computation, the brain atlas network ("node" - the junction of anatomical cortical regions, "edge" - the connecting curve between cortical regions) is first mapped to a planar straight line graph based on Tutte graph embedding, where all the edges are crossing-free and all the faces are convex polygons; the brain surface is then mapped to the convex shape domain based on harmonic map with linear constraints. Experiments on two brain MRI databases, including 250 scans with automatic atlases processed by FreeSurfer and 40 scans with manual atlases from LPBA40, demonstrate the efficiency and efficacy of the algorithm and the practicability for visualizing and comparing brain cortical anatomical structures.

1 Introduction

Brain mapping was introduced to map the genus zero 3D brain cortical surface (usually brain hemisphere) onto a unit sphere or a planar canonical domain (e.g., a unit disk, a rectangle domain), so that the convoluted and invisible cortical folds are flattened and the geometric details are fully exposed onto the canonical domain. A plausible category of methods is conformal mapping, which preserves angles (local shapes) and therefore is highly desired for brain morphometry study in neuroscience and medical imaging fields. It has been well studied in recent works using spherical harmonic mapping [1], Ricci curvature flow [2] and other methods [3]. Another commonly used category of methods is area-preserving brain mapping [4,5], computed based on optimal mass transportation theory.

Brain anatomical landmarks including gyri and sulci curves are used to help shape registration and analysis applications. One method [2] is to slice the brain surface open along these curves, and map the new surface to a unit disk with circular holes or a hyperbolic polygon; the curves are mapped to circular holes or hyperbolic lines for generating intrinsic shape signatures. The other method [6]

N. Navab et al. (Eds.): MICCAI 2015, Part III, LNCS 9351, pp. 760–767, 2015.
DOI: 10.1007/978-3-319-24574-4_91

is to map the whole brain surface with interior curve straightening constraints based on holomorphic 1-form method, without changing surface topology; the interior curves are mapped to canonically-shaped segments, e.g., straight lines in a rectangle or circular arcs in a unit disk. Brain anatomical connectivity between cortical regions (atlas) is also one significant anatomical feature. To date, none of the existing methods integrate the anatomical atlas structure into the mapping, and makes the atlas well-shaped in the mapping.

Brain networks, the so-called brain graphs [7], have been intensively studied in neuroscience field. Bullmore et al. [7] gave thorough reviews and methodological guide on both structural and functional brain network analysis. In this work, we focus on brain structural network on cortical surface, i.e., cortical network. It has been used to discover the relation of its disorganization to diseases such as Alzheimer's disease [8]. One important task within this is brain network visualization and comparison. To date, it still needs a lot of efforts to explore a more perceptively straightforward and visually plausible graph drawing.

In summary, the motivation of this work is to provide a well-structured convex shape view for convoluted atlas structure, which is more accessible for reading than pure surface mapping (e.g. conformal) views with curvy landmarks and more efficient for anatomical visualization and comparison.

Brain Net. The cortical network studied in this work is *different* from the definition of structural "brain graph" in [7], where the node denotes the cortical region, the edge denotes the connectivity between two cortical regions, and it is completely a topological graph. In this work, we define the node as the junction of anatomical cortical regions and the edge as the common curvy boundary of two neighboring cortical regions. This anatomical graph (see Fig. 1 (b)) is embedded on the 3D genus zero cortical surface, has physically positioned nodes and *crossing-free curvy edges*, and therefore is planar in theory [9]. For simplicity and differentiation, we call it "brain net". In terms of topology, it is the "dual graph" of the brain graph in [7]. We have verified this in our experiments. In this work, brain net is used to drive a canonical surface mapping (the regions and the whole domain are convex). We call this technique *brain-net mapper*.

Approach. This work presents a novel method for brain cortical anatomical structure mapping. It employs the special properties of the anatomical brain net: 1) planar and 2) 3-connected (after testing and minor filtering). The computational strategy is to employ the planar graph embedding as guidance for *structural* brain surface mapping using constrained harmonic map. In detail, first, the 3-connected planar brain net graph is embedded onto the Euclidean plane without crossing graph edges and every face is convex based on Tutte embedding theorem [10]; then, using the obtained convex target domain with convex subdivision as constraints, a harmonic map of the brain surface is computed. The mapping is unique and diffeomorphic, which can be proved by generalizing Radó theorem [11]. The algorithm solves sparse linear systems, therefore is efficient and robust to topology and geometry noises. The resulting mapping exposes invisible topological connectivity and also details cortical surface geometry.

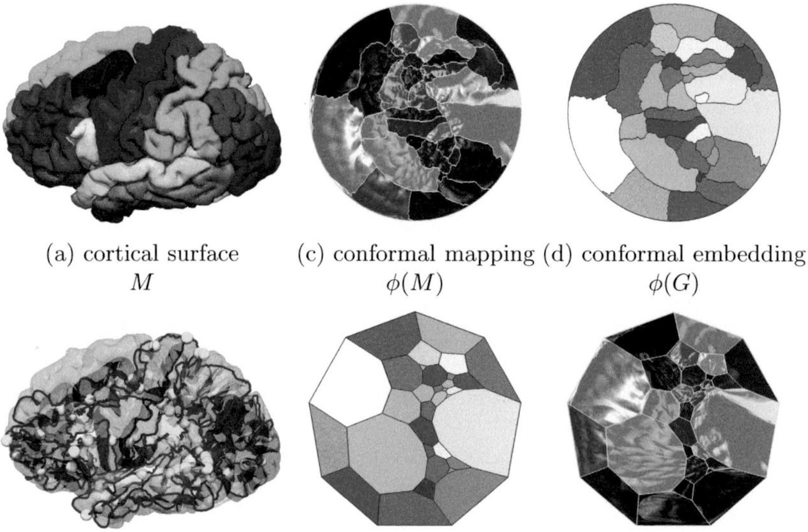

(a) cortical surface M (c) conformal mapping $\phi(M)$ (d) conformal embedding $\phi(G)$

(b) cortical net G (e) Tutte embedding $\eta(G)$ (f) structural mapping $h(M, G)$

Fig. 1. Brain net embeddings for brain A_1 (left hemisphere).

Figure 1 gives an example where regions are denoted in different colors (a). The brain net G (b) is mapped to a planar polygonal mesh (e), where each face is convex and assigned with the corresponding region's color. The planar representation (f) is the final map guided by (e), with *visually plausible structure*, i.e., planar straight lines and convex faces with interior surface harmonically flattened (stretches minimized). It illustrates the cortical anatomical structure (a). We call this mapping *structural brain mapping.* In contrast, conformal map (c) generates the planar graph embedding but with curvy graph edges (d).

To our best knowledge, this is the *first* work to present a structural view of brain cortical surface associated with anatomical atlas by making all anatomical regions in convex polygonal shapes and minimizing stretches. Experiments were performed on 250 brains with automatic parcellations and 40 brains with manual atlas labels to verify the 3-connected property of brain nets (anatomical connectivity) and test the efficiency and efficacy of our algorithm for brain cortical anatomical atlas visualization and further cortical structure comparison.

2 Theoretic Background

This section briefly introduces the theoretic background. For details, we refer readers to [9] for graph embedding and [11] for harmonic mappings.

Graph Embedding. In graph theory, a graph G is k-connected if it requires at least k vertices to be removed to disconnect the graph, i.e., the vertex degree of the graph $deg(G) \geq k$. A planar graph is a graph that can be embedded in the plane, i.e., it can be drawn on the plane in such a way that its edges intersect only at their endpoints. Such a drawing is called the planar embedding of a graph, which maps the nodes to points on a plane and the edges to straight lines or curves on that plane without crossings.

A 3-connected planar graph has special property that it has planar crossing-free straight line embedding. Tutte (1963) [10] gave a computational solution, the classical *Tutte embedding*, where the outer face is prescribed to a convex polygon and each interior vertex is at the average (barycenter) of its neighboring positions. Tutte's spring theorem [10] guarantees that the resulting planar embedding is unique and always crossing-free, and specially, every face is convex.

Harmonic Map. Suppose a metric surface $(S, \mathbf{g})$ is a topology disk, a genus zero surface with a single boundary. By Riemann mapping theorem, S can be conformally mapped onto the complex plane, $\mathbb{D} = \{z \in \mathbb{C} | |z| < 1\}$, $\phi : S \rightarrow \mathbb{D}$, which implies $\mathbf{g} = e^{2\lambda(z)} dz d\bar{z}$, where λ is the conformal factor.

Let $f : (\mathbb{D}, |dz|^2) \rightarrow (\mathbb{D}, |dw|^2)$ be a Lipschitz map between two disks, $z = x+iy$ and $w = u + iv$ are complex parameters. The *harmonic energy* of the map is defined as $E(f) = \int_{\mathbb{D}} (|w_z|^2 + |w_{\bar{z}}|^2) dxdy$. A critical point of the harmonic energy is called a *harmonic map*, which satisfies the Laplace equation $w_{z\bar{z}} = 0$. In general, harmonic mapping is unnecessarily diffeomorphic. Radó theorem [11] states that if the restriction on the boundary is a homeomorphism, then the map from a topological disk to a convex domain is a diffeomorphism and unique.

3 Computational Algorithms

The computation steps include: 1) compute graph embedding; and 2) compute harmonic map using graph embedding constraints (see Algorithm 1).

The brain cortical surface is represented as a triangular mesh of genus zero with a single boundary (the black region is cut off), denoted as $M = (V, E, F)$, where V, E, F represent vertex, edge and face sets, respectively. Similarly, the brain net is denoted as a graph $G = (V_G, E_G, F_G)$ (3-connected and planar, embedded on M) (see Fig. 1(b)). Thus, we use (M, G) as the input.

Step 1: Isomorphic Graph Embedding. The first step is to compute a straight line convex graph embedding of G, $\eta : G \rightarrow \hat{G}$ by Tutte embedding [10]. We first place the graph nodes on boundary ∂M onto the unit circle uniformly, and then compute the mapping positions $\eta(v_i)$ for interior nodes v_i as the barycenters of the mapping positions of neighboring nodes v_j, $\{\eta(\hat{v}_i) = \Sigma_{(v_i,v_j) \in E_G} \lambda_{ij} \eta(\hat{v}_j)\}$. We use $\lambda_{ij} = 1/deg(v_i)$, where $deg(v_i)$ denotes the degree of node v_i in G. Solving the sparse linear system, we obtain the Tutte embedding result $\hat{G}$, which defines a convex planar domain Ω (see Fig. 1(e)).

Step 2: Constrained Harmonic Mapping. The second step is to compute a surface mapping $h : (M, G) \rightarrow (\Omega, \hat{G})$ to restrict graph G to the planar Tutte embedding result $\hat{G}$ by a constrained harmonic map (see Fig. 1(f)). We map the whole surface M onto the convex planar domain Ω by minimizing the discrete harmonic energy under graph constraints, formulated as $\min\{E(\phi(v_i)) = \Sigma_{[v_i,v_j] \in E} w_{ij} (\phi(v_i) -$

Algorithm 1. Graph Embedding for Surface Mapping

Input: A triangular mesh with decorative graph (M, G)
Output: A planar triangular mesh with straight line decorative graph $(\Omega, \hat{G})$
1: Compute Tutte embedding $\eta : G \to \hat{G}$
2: Compute harmonic map $\phi : (M, G) \to (\Omega, \hat{G})$ with constraints $\phi(G) = \hat{G}$

$\phi(v_j))^2, \forall v_i \in V\}$, s.t., $\phi(l_k) = \hat{l}_k, \forall l_k \in G, \hat{l}_k = \eta(l_k)$, i.e., l_k is the curvy edge of graph G, and $\hat{l}_k$ is the corresponding edge on the planar graph embedding $\hat{G}$. The solution to the harmonic energy minimization problem is equivalent to solving the linear system $\Delta\phi = 0$ (Δ is the Laplacian operator), descreterized as the linear equations $\{\Sigma_{[v_i,v_j]\in E} w_{ij}(\phi(v_i) - \phi(v_j)) = 0, \forall v_i \in V\}$.

We only specify the target positions for the two end vertices of l_k. Other interior vertices on l_k are constrained to $\hat{l}_k$ through a linear combination of two neighbors on $\hat{l}_k$. The linear constraints between coordinates x, y on straight line $\hat{l}_k$ can be plugged into the above system. We employ the mean value coordinates to guarantee the edge weight w_{ij} to be positive. Then in our construction, for each vertex there is a convex combination of neighbors. According to Tutte's spring theorem [10], Radó theorem [11] and generalized Tutte embedding [12], the solution achieves a unique and diffeomorphic surface mapping.

4 Experiments

The proposed algorithms were validated on two databases with different atlas types: 1) the own captured 250 brain MRI scans, we use FreeSurfer to automatically extract triangular cortical surfaces and anatomical atlas (see Figs. 1, 2(a)); and 2) the public 40 brains with manual atlas labels provided by LPBA40 [13] (see Fig. 2(b-c)), we use BrainSuite to correlate the triangular cortical surface with manual labels. All the brains come from human volunteers.

Brain Net Extraction. We extract the brain nets from cortical surface using anatomical region id or color assigned. To employ Tutte embedding, we then test the 3-connected property of all the brain nets using two conditions: (a) every node has ≥ 3 neighboring regions; (b) every region has ≥ 3 boundary nodes. If both are satisfied, then the brain net is 3-connected, a "good" one.

Our tests show that all brain nets satisfy condition (a). All the "bad" regions detected contain 2 nodes, i.e., 2 boundary edges, which contradicts (b). There may be (i) 1, (ii) 2, or (iii) 3 bad regions. Table 1 gives the number of brains for each above case. We use (lh, rh) to denote the percentage of left and right hemisphere brain nets satisfying both (a-b): FreeSurfer $(22.8\%, 100\%)$, LPBA40 $(12.5\%, 82.5\%)$, both $(21.4\%, 97.6\%)$. The tests give that most exception cases are with $1 \sim 2$ "bad" regions, for which we only map one boundary edge to straight line and ignore the other in next structural brain mapping procedure. If the region is totally interior, we randomly select one; if it is adjacent to the brain surface boundary, then we select the boundary one, as shown in Fig. 2(b-c).

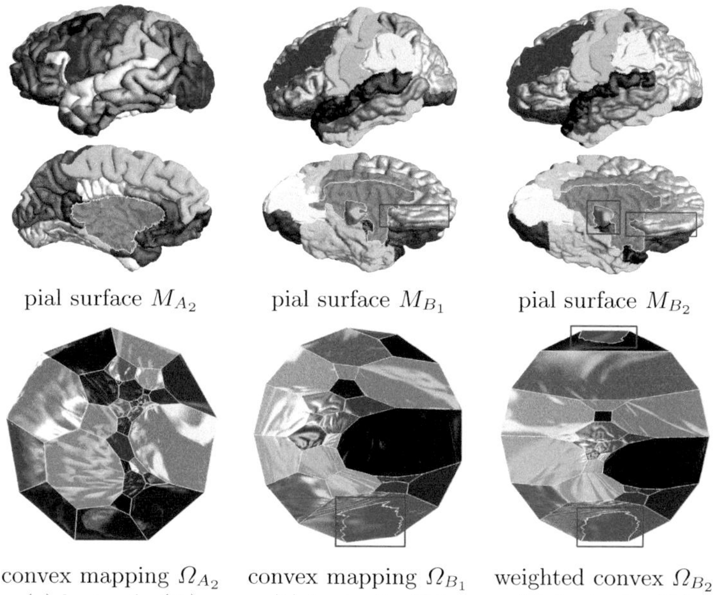

(a) brain A_2 (lh) (b) brain B_1 (lh) (c) brain B_2 (lh)

Fig. 2. Structural brain mappings driven by graph embedding.

Table 1. Statistics on brain nets, meshes and time. lh (rh) - left (right) hemisphere.

Data	FreeSurfer (lh)	FreeSurfer (rh)	LPBA40 (lh)	LPBA40 (rh)
#region,#node	33~35, 62~70	33~35, 41~52	24~28, 64~72	20~22, 39~55
#triangle,time	277k, 20 secs	279k, 20 secs	131k, 10 secs	131k, 10 secs
#good (a-b)	57	250	5	33
#bad (i/ii/iii)	193/0/0	0/0/0	24/10/1	7/0/0

Structural Brain Mapping. The algorithms were tested on a desktop with 3.7GHz CPU and 16GB RAM. The whole pipeline is automatic, stable and robust for all the tests. Table 1 gives the averaged running time. Figures 1-2 show various results, by which it is visually straightforward to figure out local topology (adjacency of regions) and tell whether two atlases are isomorphic (or topologically same); in contrast, it is hard to do so in a 3D view. Note that the polygonal shape is solely determined by the combinatorial structure of the brain net. Brains with consistent atlases are mapped to the same convex shape (see brains A_1, A_2), which fosters direct comparison. Brains B_1, B_2 from LPBA40 are with different brain nets, especially around the exception regions. Even though the unselected edges of the bad regions appear irregular, the mapping results are visually acceptable and functionally enough for discovering local and global structures and other visualization applications, such brain atlas comparison.

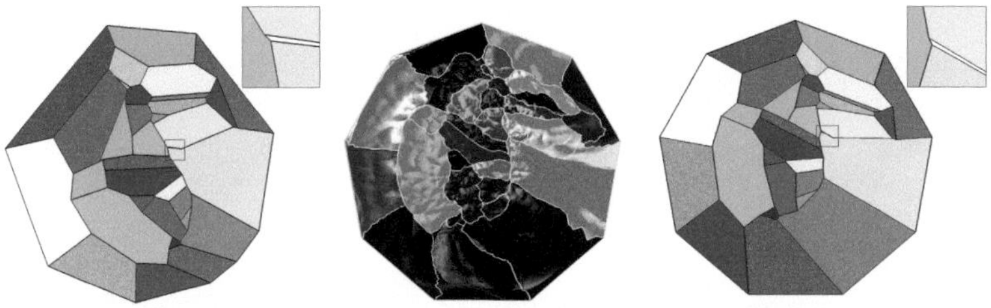

(a) straight line drawing of Fig. 1(c) (b) convex harmonic mapping of Fig. 1(a) (c) straight line drawing of (b)

Fig. 3. Straight line graph drawings induced by conformal and harmonic mappings.

5 Discussion

This work focuses to present a novel brain mapping framework based on Tutte embedding and harmonic map with convex planar graph constraint. For better understanding the method and its potentials, we have the discussions as follows.

Convex Shape Mapping: The cortical surface can be directly mapped to canonical domains such as conformal map to a disk [2] (Fig. 1(c)) and harmonic map to a convex domain [1] (Fig. 3(b)). Each map can define a planar straight line graph embedding (Fig. 3(a,c)) by simply connecting the nodes on the planar domain, but it may generate concave and skinny faces and cannot guarantee "crossing-free" and further the diffeomorphic brain mapping. Our method can solve these, and the diffeomorphism property has been verified in all the tests. If the graph is not 3-connected, we use valid subgraph for guiding the mapping. The unselected part is ignored and won't affect the diffeomorphism.

Topology and Geometric Meanings: This work studies "graph on surface" and its influence to surface mapping. The convex map preserves the topology of the graph on the canonical domain and minimizes the constrained harmonic energy (preserving angles as much as possible under constraints), therefore is more accessible and perceptually easy to capture global and local structures.

Advantages: In theory, the method is rigorous, based on the classical Tutte graph embedding for 3-connected planar graphs (Tutte's spring theorem [10]), and the harmonic map with linear convex constraints with uniqueness and diffeomorphism guarantee (Radó theorem [11], generalized Tutte embedding [12]). *In practice,* all the algorithms solve sparse linear systems and are easy to implement, practical and efficient, and robust to geometry or topology noises. The framework is general for surfaces decorated with graphs.

Extensions: This method is able to reflect more original geometry by introducing weighted graph embeddings, and can be extended to handle high genus cases by using advanced graph embeddings.

Potentials for Brain Mapping and Other Biomedical Research: The structural brain mapping can help understand anatomical structures and monitor anatomy progression, and has potential for brain cortical registration with atlas constraints.

This anatomy-aware framework is general for other convoluted natural shapes decorated with feature graphs (e.g., colons), and can be applied for their anatomy visualization, comparison, registration and morphometry analysis.

6 Conclusion

This work presents a brain cortical surface mapping method considering cortical anatomical structure, such that the complex convoluted brain cortical surface can be visualized in a well-structured view, i.e., a convex domain with convex subdivision. The algorithms based on Tutte embedding and harmonic map are efficient and practical, and are extensible for other applications where 3-connected feature graphs are associated. We will further employ weighted graph embeddings to reflect the original geometry in the mapping, and explore the potentials for solving brain surface registration and analysis problem in future works.

Acknowledgments. Wei Zeng is supported by NSF CCF-1544267.

References

1. Gu, X., Wang, Y., Chan, T., Thompson, P., Yau, S.T.: Genus zero surface conformal mapping and its application to brain surface mapping. IEEE Transactions on Medical Imaging 23(7) (2004)
2. Wang, Y., Shi, J., Yin, X., Gu, X., Chan, T.F., Yau, S.T., Toga, A.W., Thompson, P.M.: Brain surface conformal parameterization with the Ricci flow. IEEE Transactions on Medical Imaging 31(2), 251–264 (2012)
3. Haker, S., Angenent, S., Tannenbaum, A., Kikinis, R., Sapiro, G., Halle, M.: Conformal surface parameterization for texture mapping. IEEE Transactions on Visualization and Computer Graphics 6, 181–189 (2000)
4. Su, Z., Zeng, W., Shi, R.: Y. Wang, J.S., Gu, X.: Area preserving brain mapping. In: IEEE Conf. on Computer Vision and Pattern Recognition, CVPR 2013 (2013)
5. Haker, S., Zhu, L., Tannenbaum, A., Angenent, S.: Optimal mass transport for registration and warping. Int. J. of Computer Vision 60(3), 225–240 (2004)
6. Zeng, W., Yang, Y.-J.: Surface matching and registration by landmark curve-driven canonical quasiconformal mapping. In: Fleet, D., Pajdla, T., Schiele, B., Tuytelaars, T. (eds.) ECCV 2014, Part I. LNCS, vol. 8689, pp. 710–724. Springer, Heidelberg (2014)
7. Bullmore, E., Bassett, D.: Brain graphs: graphical models of the human brain connectome. Annu. Rev. Clin. Psychol. 7, 113–140 (2011)
8. He, Y., Chen, Z., Evans, A.: Structural insights into aberrant topological patterns of large-scale cortical networks in Alzheimer's disease. J. Neurosci. 28(18), 4756–4766 (2008)
9. Lando, S.K., Zvonkin, A.K.: Graphs on Surfaces and their Applications. Encyclopaedia of Mathematical Sciences, vol. 141. Springer (2004)
10. Tutte, W.T.: How to draw a graph. In: Proc. Lond. Math. Soc., pp. 743–767 (1963)
11. Schoen, R., Yau, S.T.: Lectures on Harmonic Maps. International Press (1997)
12. Floater, M.S.: One-to-one piecewise linear mappings over triangulations. Mathematics of Computation 72(242), 685–696 (2003)
13. Shattuck, D., Mirza, M., Adisetiyo, V., Hojatkashani, C., Salamon, G., Narr, K., Poldrack, R., Bilder, R., Toga, A.: Construction of a 3d probabilistic atlas of human cortical structures. NeuroImage, doi:10.1016/j.neuroimage.2007.09.031

Author Index